The Oxford Handbook of Infant, Child, and Adolescent Sleep and Behavior

OXFORD LIBRARY OF PSYCHOLOGY

Editor in Chief PETER E. NATHAN

The Oxford Handbook of Infant, Child, and Adolescent Sleep and Behavior

Edited by

Amy R. Wolfson

Hawley E. Montgomery-Downs

OXFORD
UNIVERSITY PRESS

OXFORD
UNIVERSITY PRESS

Oxford University Press is a department of the University of Oxford.
It furthers the University's objective of excellence in research, scholarship,
and education by publishing worldwide.

Oxford New York
Auckland Cape Town Dar es Salaam Hong Kong Karachi
Kuala Lumpur Madrid Melbourne Mexico City Nairobi
New Delhi Shanghai Taipei Toronto

With offices in
Argentina Austria Brazil Chile Czech Republic France Greece
Guatemala Hungary Italy Japan Poland Portugal Singapore
South Korea Switzerland Thailand Turkey Ukraine Vietnam

Published in the United States of America by
Oxford University Press
198 Madison Avenue, New York, NY 10016

Library of Congress Cataloging-in-Publication Data
The Oxford handbook of infant, child, and adolescent sleep and behavior / edited by
Amy R. Wolfson, Hawley Montgomery-Downs.
pages cm.—(Oxford library of psychology)
Includes bibliographical references.
ISBN 978–0–19–987363–0
1. Sleep disorders in children—Handbooks, manuals, etc. 2. Sleep disorders in adolescence—Handbooks, manuals, etc.
3. Children—Sleep—Handbooks, manuals, etc. I. Wolfson, Amy R. II. Montgomery–Downs, Hawley.
III. Title: Handbook of infant, child, and adolescent sleep and behavior.
RJ506.S55O947 2013
618.92′8498—dc23
2013003516

9 7 8 6 5 4 3 2 1
Printed in the United States of America
on acid-free paper

SHORT CONTENTS

OXFORD LIBRARY OF PSYCHOLOGY

The *Oxford Library of Psychology*, a landmark series of handbooks, is published by Oxford University Press, one of the world's oldest and most highly respected publishers, with a tradition of publishing significant books in psychology. The ambitious goal of the *Oxford Library of Psychology* is nothing less than to span a vibrant, wide-ranging field and, in so doing, to fill a clear market need.

Encompassing a comprehensive set of handbooks, organized hierarchically, the *Library* incorporates volumes at different levels, each designed to meet a distinct need. At one level are a set of handbooks designed broadly to survey the major subfields of psychology; at another are numerous handbooks that cover important current focal research and scholarly areas of psychology in depth and detail. Planned as a reflection of the dynamism of psychology, the *Library* will grow and expand as psychology itself develops, thereby highlighting significant new research that will impact on the field. Adding to its accessibility and ease of use, the *Library* will be published in print and, later on, electronically.

The *Library* surveys psychology's principal subfields with a set of handbooks that capture the current status and future prospects of those major subdisciplines. This initial set includes handbooks of social and personality psychology, clinical psychology, counseling psychology, school psychology, educational psychology, industrial and organizational psychology, cognitive psychology, cognitive neuroscience, methods and measurements, history, neuropsychology, personality assessment, developmental psychology, and more. Each handbook undertakes to review one of psychology's major subdisciplines with breadth, comprehensiveness, and exemplary scholarship. In addition to these broadly-conceived volumes, the *Library* also includes a large number of handbooks designed to explore in depth more specialized areas of scholarship and research, such as stress, health and coping, anxiety and related disorders, cognitive development, or child and adolescent assessment. In contrast to the broad coverage of the subfield handbooks, each of these latter volumes focuses on an especially productive, more highly focused line of scholarship and research. Whether at the broadest or most specific level, however, all of the *Library* handbooks offer synthetic coverage that reviews and evaluates the relevant past and present research and anticipates research in the future. Each handbook in the *Library* includes introductory and concluding chapters written by its editor to provide a roadmap to the handbook's table of contents and to offer informed anticipations of significant future developments in that field.

An undertaking of this scope calls for handbook editors and chapter authors who are established scholars in the areas about which they write. Many of the nation's and world's most productive and best-respected psychologists have agreed to edit *Library* handbooks or write authoritative chapters in their areas of expertise.

For whom has the *Oxford Library of Psychology* been written? Because of its breadth, depth, and accessibility, the *Library* serves a diverse audience, including graduate students in psychology and their faculty mentors, scholars, researchers, and practitioners in psychology and related fields. Each will find in the *Library* the information they seek on the subfield or focal area of psychology in which they work or are interested.

Befitting its commitment to accessibility, each handbook includes a comprehensive index, as well as extensive references to help guide research. And because the *Library* was designed from its inception as an online as well as a print resource, its structure and contents will be readily and rationally searchable online. Further, once the *Library* is released online, the handbooks will be regularly and thoroughly updated.

In summary, the *Oxford Library of Psychology* will grow organically to provide a thoroughly informed perspective on the field of psychology, one that reflects both psychology's dynamism and its increasing interdisciplinarity. Once published electronically, the *Library* is also destined to become a uniquely valuable interactive tool, with extended search and browsing capabilities. As you begin to consult this handbook, we sincerely hope you will share our enthusiasm for the more than 500-year tradition of Oxford University Press for excellence, innovation, and quality, as exemplified by the *Oxford Library of Psychology.*

Peter E. Nathan
Editor-in-Chief
Oxford Library of Psychology

ABOUT THE EDITORS

Amy R. Wolfson

Dr. Wolfson is the Associate Dean for Faculty and a Professor Psychology at the College of the Holy Cross in Worcester, Massachusetts. She completed her Bachelors' degree at Harvard University and her Doctorate in Clinical Psychology from Washington University, St. Louis. In addition, she was a Post-Doctoral researcher at Stanford University and spent two sabbaticals at the Chronobiology and Sleep Research Laboratory, E. P. Bradley Hospital, Warren Alpert Medical School of Brown University. Amy Wolfson's research focuses on developmental and psychosocial changes in sleep-wake patterns in children and adolescents. In addition to her numerous research articles and book chapters, she is the author of *The Woman's Book of Sleep*, published in 2001 and she recently completed the *Young Adolescent Sleep-Smart Pacesetter* study of urban, middle school students' sleep patterns, sleep hygiene, and daytime functioning funded by NIH-National Institute of Child Health and Human Development.

Hawley E. Montgomery-Downs

Dr. Montgomery-Downs is an Associate Professor of Psychology in the Behavioral Neuroscience program at West Virginia University. She studies the developmental psychobiology of pediatric sleep disordered breathing and postpartum sleep disturbance. She has published over 30 papers and her work has been supported by the United States National Institutes of Health.

CONTRIBUTORS

Candice A. Alfano
Department of Psychology
University of Houston
Houston, TX

Erica R. Appleman
Department of Psychology
Boston University
Boston, MA

Kristen H. Archbold
Department of Biobehavioral Health Systems
Department of Pediatrics
College of Medicine
College of Nursing
University of Arizona
Tucson, AZ

Rhoda Au
Department of Neurology
Framingham Heart Study
Boston University School of Medicine
Boston, MA

R. Robert Auger
Mayo Center for Sleep Medicine
Department of Psychiatry & Psychology
Mayo Clinic College of Medicine
Rochester, MN

Kristin T. Avis
Department of Pediatrics, Pulmonary Division
University of Alabama at Birmingham
Children's of Alabama Pediatric Sleep Disorders Center
Birmingham, AL

Erika Bagley
Human Development and Family Studies
Auburn University
Auburn, AL

John E. Bates
Department of Psychological and Brain Sciences
Indiana University
Bloomington, IN

Sarah N. Biggs
The Ritchie Centre
Monash Institute of Medical Research
Monash University
Melbourne, Australia

Neville M. Blampied
Department of Psychology
University of Canterbury
Christchurch, New Zealand

Richard R. Bootzin
Department of Psychology
University of Arizona
Tucson, AZ

Joseph A. Buckhalt
College of Education
Auburn University
Auburn, AL

Melissa M. Burnham
Human Development and Family Studies
University of Nevada, Reno
Reno, NV

Patrina HY Caldwell
The Children's Hospital at Westmead and Discipline of Paediatrics and Child Health
University of Sydney
Sydney, Australia

Mary A. Carskadon
Alpert Medical School
Brown University
E.P. Bradley Hospital
Providence, RI

Jamie Cassoff
Attention, Behavior and Sleep Lab
Douglas Mental Health University Institute
Department of Psychology
McGill University
Montreal, Quebec, Canada

Greg Clarke
Kaiser Permanente Center for Health Research
Portland, OR

Evelyn Constantin
Department of Pediatrics
McGill University
Montreal Children's Hospital
McGill University Health Centre
Montreal, Quebec, Canada

Penny Corkum
Department of Psychology and Neuroscience
Dalhousie University
Department of Pediatrics
IWK Health Centre
Colchester East Hants ADHD Clinic
CEHHA
Halifax, Nova Scotia, Canada

J. Aimée Coulombe
CIHR Better Nights Better Days Pediatric Sleep Team
Department of Psychology
Dalhousie University
Halifax, Nova Scotia, Canada

Jennifer C. Cousins
Department of Psychology
University of Pittsburgh
Pittsburgh, PA

Valerie McLaughlin Crabtree
Department of Psychology
St. Jude Children's Research Hospital
Memphis, TN

Stephanie J. Crowley
Biological Rhythms Research Laboratory
Department of Behavioral Sciences
Rush University Medical Center
Chicago, IL

Mona El-Sheikh
Human Development and Family Studies
Auburn University
Auburn, AL

Robin S. Everhart
Department of Psychology
Virginia Commonwealth University
Richmond, VA

Heather L. Gamble
Department of Psychology
St. Jude Children's Research Hospital
Memphis, TN

Michael Gradisar
School of Psychology
Flinders University
Adelaide, Australia

Reut Gruber
Attention, Behavior and Sleep Lab
Douglas Mental Health University Institute
Department of Psychiatry
McGill University
Montreal, Quebec, Canada

Lauren Hale
Program in Public Health
Department of Preventive Medicine
School of Medicine
Stony Brook University
Stony Brook, NY

Sara Harkness
Department of Human Development and Family Studies
University of Connecticut
Storrs, CT

Chantelle N. Hart
Department of Psychiatry and Human Behavior
Alpert Medical School
Brown University
Weight Control & Diabetes Research Center
The Miriam Hospital
Providence, RI

Allison G. Harvey
Department of Psychology
University of California, Berkeley
Berkeley, CA

Nicola Hawley
Department of Psychiatry and Human Behavior
Alpert Medical School
Brown University
Weight Control & Diabetes Research Center
The Miriam Hospital
Providence, RI

Shelley Hershner
Department of Neurology
University of Michigan
Ann Arbor, MI

Rosemary S.C. Horne
The Ritchie Centre
Monash Institute of Medical Research
Monash University
Melbourne, Australia

Anna Ivanenko
Feinberg School of Medicine
Northwestern University
Division of Child and Adolescent Psychiatry
Ann and Robert H. Lurie Children's Hospital of Chicago
Chicago, IL

Elissa Jelalian
Department of Psychiatry and Human Behavior
Alpert Medical School
Brown University
Weight Control & Diabetes Research Center
The Miriam Hospital
Providence, RI

Monica R. Kelly
Department of Psychology
University of Arizona
Tucson, AZ

John Declan Kennedy
Department of Respiratory and Sleep Medicine
Women's and Children's Hospital
Adelaide, Australia

Daphne Koinis Mitchell
Bradley/Hasbro Children's Research Center
Department of Psychiatry and Human Behavior
Brown Medical School
Providence, RI

Elizabeth Kuhl
Department of Psychiatry and Human Behavior
Alpert Medical School of Brown University
Weight Control & Diabetes Research Center
The Miriam Hospital
Providence, RI

Kymberly Larson
Meier Clinics
Wheaton, IL

Kenneth L. Lichstein
Department of Psychology
University of Alabama
Tuscaloosa, AL

Kurt Lushington
School of Psychology, Social Work, and Social Policy
University of South Australia
Adelaide, Australia

James Martin
Department of Respiratory and Sleep Medicine
Women's and Children's Hospital
Adelaide, Australia

Lisa J. Meltzer
Department of Pediatrics
National Jewish Health
Denver, CO

Sonia Michaelsen
Attention, Behavior and Sleep Lab
Douglas Mental Health University Institute
Verdun, Quebec, Canada

Jodi A. Mindell
Children's Hospital of Philadelphia
Saint Joseph's University
Philadelphia, PA
Providence, RI

Dennis L. Molfese
Department of Psychology
University of Nebraska—Lincoln
Lincoln, NE
Victoria J. Molfese
Department of Child, Youth, and Family Studies
University of Nebraska—Lincoln
Lincoln, NE
Hawley Montgomery-Downs
Department of Psychology
West Virginia University
Morgantown, WV
Melisa Moore
Children's Hospital of Philadelphia
Philadelphia, PA
Louise M. O'Brien
Sleep Disorders Center
Department of Oral & Maxillofacial Surgery
Department of Neurology
University of Michigan
Ann Arbor, MI
Tonya M. Palermo
Seattle Children's Research Institute
Department of Anesthesiology and Pain Medicine
University of Washington
Seattle, WA
Yvonne Pamula
Department of Respiratory and Sleep Medicine
Women's and Children's Hospital
Adelaide, Australia
Victoria Parente
Graduate Program in Public Health
School of Medicine
Stony Brook University
Stony Brook, NY
Gwendolyn K. Phillips
Graduate Program in Public Health
School of Medicine
Stony Brook University
Stony Brook, NY
Amanda M. Rach
Department of Psychology
University of Memphis
Memphis, TN
Amanda L. Richdale
Olga Tennison Autism Research Centre
La Trobe University
Melbourne, Australia
Brandy M. Roane
Department of Internal Medicine
UNT Health Science Center
Fort Worth, TX
Kathleen Moritz Rudasill
Department of Educational Psychology
University of Nebraska—Lincoln
Lincoln, NE
Stephen H. Sheldon
Feinberg School of Medicine
Northwestern University
Director, Sleep Medicine Center
Ann and Robert H. Lurie Children's Hospital of Chicago
Chicago, IL
Michelle A. Short
Centre for Sleep Research
University of South Australia
Adelaide, Australia
James C. Spilsbury
Center for Clinical Investigation
Case Western Reserve School of Medicine
Cleveland, OH
Karen Spruyt
Section of Pediatric Sleep Medicine
Department of Pediatrics
Comer Children's Hospital
Pritzker School of Medicine
The University of Chicago
Chicago, IL
Angela D. Staples
Department of Psychology
University of Virginia
Charlottesville, VA
Karina Stavitsky
VA Boston Healthcare System
Boston, MA
Sally Stevens
Southwest Institute of Research on Women
University of Arizona
Tucson, AZ

Robyn Stremler
Lawrence S. Bloomberg Faculty of Nursing
University of Toronto
The Hospital for Sick Children (SickKids)
Toronto, Ontario, Canada

Charles M. Super
Department of Human Development and Family Studies
University of Connecticut
Storrs, CT

Leila Tarokh
Alpert Medical School of Brown University
Institute of Pharmacology and Toxicology
University of Zurich
Zurich, Switzerland

Daniel J. Taylor
Department of Psychology
University of North Texas
Denton, TX

Pamela V. Thacher
Department of Psychology
St. Lawrence University
Canton, NY

S. Justin Thomas
Department of Psychology
University of Alabama
Tuscaloosa, AL

Colleen M. Walsh
Division of Sleep Medicine
University of Pennsylvania School of Medicine
Philadelphia, PA

Karen Waters
The Children's Hospital at Westmead and
Discipline of Paediatrics and Child Health
University of Sydney
Sydney, Australia

Amy R. Wolfson
Department of Psychology
College of Holy Cross
Worcester, MA

Lissy Zaremba
Rainbow Babies and Children's Hospital
University Hospitals-Case Medical Center
Cleveland, OH

CONTENTS

CHAPTER

1

Introduction to *The Oxford Handbook of Infant, Child, and Adolescent Sleep and Behavior*

Amy R. Wolfson

Abstract

This introductory chapter outlines the history and the theoretical basis for studying child and adolescent sleep and development. Furthermore, this chapter celebrates the progress the field has made in the last few decades, and makes the case for the crucial role sleep plays in child development. The chapter describes the organization of the handbook, outlining the many foundation and topical areas of sleep and child development covered in the text.

Key Words: child, adolescent, sleep, behavior, development, psychology

Welcome to *The Oxford Handbook of Infant, Child, and Adolescent Sleep and Behavior* that has the honor of being a part of the Oxford Library of Psychology. Recognition of the significance of sleep in the cognitive and behavioral development and emotional well being of infants, children, and adolescents is relatively recent. Over the last three decades, there has been an explosion in research focused on developmental changes in sleep and circadian rhythms from birth through adolescence. Further study has led to the characterization and assessment of sleep disorders unique to different developmental stages. Links between sleep problems and overall health, as well as emotional and behavioral disorders including depression, attention deficithyperactivity disorder (ADHD), neurodevelopmental disorders, and post-traumatic stress disorder, are now more established in children and adolescents.

Ahead of psychologists in the field, graduate programs, and psychology's professional associations, the editors of the Oxford Library of Psychology recognized the importance of including a volume on infant, child, and adolescent sleep and behavior in their Psychology Handbook series. My co-editor and I were thrilled to be a part of this significant and historic venture. As a child clinical psychologist, I was deeply committed to inviting experimental, clinical, school, and developmental psychologists as well as other behavioral clinicians and social and behavioral science researchers to author and coauthor chapters for what would become *The Oxford Handbook of Infant, Child, and Adolescent Sleep and Behavior*. Psychologists play a crucial role in developing and contributing to what is known as pediatric and adolescent sleep medicine; however, psychology, as a discipline, has only gradually recognized the importance of sleep in child development and developmental psychopathology research and in clinical, counseling, and school psychology undergraduate and graduate education. It is our hope that this first psychology handbook on child and adolescent sleep will inform child and adolescent clinical psychology practice, raise the importance of including child and adolescent sleep as a part of graduate programs in psychology and related fields, and provide future questions and directions for research in psychology and in the behavioral sciences.

As a child clinical psychologist, I have devoted my research program to studying sleep and daytime functioning in infants, children, and adolescents, as well as pregnant and postpartum women, since my graduate school days in the 1980s. At that time, few psychology graduate programs or individual faculty offered graduate-level courses on sleep or circadian rhythms. Psychologists, however, were beginning to lead a movement toward cognitive-behavioral approaches to treating insomnia. For example, while I was a graduate student in clinical psychology at Washington University in St. Louis (1982–1987), two faculty members, Patricia Lacks and Amy Bertelson, studied sleep in adults. Patricia Lacks developed stimulus control techniques for treating insomnia and wrote one of the first books on the treatment of insomnia, *Behavioral Treatment for Persistent Insomnia* (1987), and Amy Bertelson taught an exciting and popular undergraduate course on sleep. In contrast, scholarship on the development of sleep patterns over the course of infancy, childhood, and adolescence or on understanding and treating children's sleep problems was far less common. Observing my mentors' passion for helping adults improve their sleep and daytime lives, I was determined to study and understand how psychologists could contribute to improving children's sleep. As a graduate student, I began my ongoing, nearly 30-year inquiry into understanding how children's nighttime behaviors and sleep experiences influence not only their own daytime functioning, but also the lives of their parents and families.

Focused on the impact of healthy lifestyles as an approach to preventing mental health and behavioral difficulties in children, I started reading some of the mid-1980s publications, written by parents as well as pediatricians, on infant sleep. In particular, I focused on two parenting books: pediatrician Richard Ferber's *Solve Your Child's Sleep Problems* (2006) and parents' Joanne Cuthbertson and Susanna Schevill's *Helping Your Child Sleep Through the Night* (1985). Utilizing behavioral and social learning theories of behavior change and Cuthbertson and Schevill's insights on self-soothing and infants' developing ability to *sleep through the night*, I developed a preventive-intervention program that gave parents sleep knowledge and strategies along with a sense of self-competence to handle their infant's sleep during the first year. The empirical findings from this preventive approach were published (see Chapters 37 and 39 for summaries) in the *Journal of Consulting and Clinical Psychology* (Wolfson, Lacks, & Futterman, 1992), launching early attention to parenting and young children's sleep in the psychology literature. It took some time, however, before the child psychology discipline recognized that there were developmental changes in sleep and clear clinical and behavioral consequences for inadequate and poor quality sleep on developing youth. For example, when I presented my doctoral research on the effects of parent training on infants' sleep patterns at the 1988 Association for the Advancement of Behavior Therapy's (AABT) annual meeting, Jodi Mindell (coauthor of Chapter 37) and I gave the only presentations focused on behavioral approaches for improving children's sleep and at the 1995 biannual meeting of the Society for Research on Child Development (SRCD) only 0.3% of the peer-reviewed posters and presentations were related to children's sleep. In fact, in a shared van ride to that 1995 Seattle meeting of SRCD, a school psychologist asked me *if sleep was developmental?* With that story in mind, it was particularly meaningful to publish "Sleep Schedules and Daytime Functioning in Adolescents" in *Child Development* (Wolfson & Carskadon, 1998) with my coauthor and mentor, Mary Carskadon (coauthor of Chapter 8). Sleep, in striking contrast, is considered a focal area for the 2013 biannual meeting of the SRCD. The publication of this handbook underscores how far the behavioral and developmental sciences have come in recent years in the study, treatment, and public awareness of sleep and behavior in children and adolescents.

Over the last three decades, psychologists, pediatricians, and other health care providers have established an increasingly distinct understanding of children and adolescents' sleep demands, circadian timing, underlying bioregulatory processes, and environmental constraints. At the beginning of this handbook, in Chapters 2 and 3, respectively, Stephen Sheldon provides an overview of the history of child and adolescent sleep medicine and Tonya Palermo offers insights and historical background regarding psychology's historical contributions to infant, child, and adolescent sleep research. Studies have documented the clear consequences of insufficient and inconsistent sleep over the course of development, such as early behavioral and cognitive problems, poor academic performance, substance abuse, and emotion regulation difficulties. This critical area of child development and health research has begun to inspire public policy discussions and debates in areas such as school start times, regulation of preschool napping, and adolescent drivers' education laws and programs. Likewise, much of this research has practice implications and applications not only for infants, children, and adolescents with sleep disorders, but also for those who have no demonstrable sleep disorders. In other words, school pressures and schedules, family socioeconomic status, and a range of environmental constraints and challenges compromise the sleep of increasingly greater numbers of infants, children, adolescents, and emerging adults. Furthermore, children and adolescents who present with academic and behavior problems may in fact have primary sleep difficulties. The basic research and clinical presentations that are discussed in this handbook have clear implications for the overall health, development, emotional well being, and academic performance of children and adolescents.

The scientific study of sleep is a still a relatively young discipline, but tremendous gains in knowledge have been achieved over the last two decades, including advancing our understanding of sleep's role in memory consolidation and learning processes, associations between sleep deprivation and obesity, and the sleep and the circadian systems' regulatory influence on immune functions (Besedovsky, Born, & Lange, 2012; Knutson, Zhao, Mattingly, Galli, & Cizza, 2012; Walker & Stickgold, 2006). Although the preponderance of research on sleep has been conducted in adult populations, a significant body of knowledge and current research now focuses on the sleep patterns, disruptions, and disorders in infants, children, and adolescents.

This handbook offers a unique and important contribution to the field of child and adolescent sleep patterns, difficulties, and disorders. It provides behavioral and developmental approaches to understanding sleep and circadian timing development, assessment of sleep patterns and problems, etiology of sleep disorders, and preventive/intervention approaches in working with children, adolescents, and their families. We have brought together psychologists and other behavioral and developmental clinicians and developmental scientists to discuss developmental changes in sleep and circadian rhythms; the factors that influence, mediate, and moderate sleep patterns and problems over infancy, childhood, and adolescence; and the assessment and behavioral treatment of infant, child, and adolescent sleep problems and disorders. The authors are from a range of countries and include psychologists, pediatricians, psychiatrists, nurses, child life specialists, and other health care providers and researchers with expertise on infant, child, and adolescent sleep.

Research on children's sleep can be organized into seven areas, which are reflected here. The first section focuses on *Sleep and Development,* since one of the most significant factors affecting sleep is age or developmental stage. Following the two historical chapters mentioned earlier, Angela Staples and Jack Bates articulate what it means to consider sleep from a developmental perspective, so that developmental psychologists and other researchers might consider the role of sleep and circadian rhythms in development, and to remind sleep researchers how sleep changes from infancy through adolescence. Sleep and circadian rhythms change over the course of development from infancy into the emerging adult years, as highlighted and documented in the chapters by Kurt Lushington, Yvonne Pamula, Alfred James Martin, John Declan Kennedy and by Mary Carskadon and Leila Tarokh in Chapters 5, 6 and 8, respectively. An infant's sleep plays a particularly significant role in the lives of new parents, and Robyn Stremler's Chapter 7 examines the impact of infants' sleep and behavior on parents including marital satisfaction, coping strategies, postpartum depression, and the parents' own sleep-wake patterns. Although this section does not include a separate chapter on elementary school children's sleep, school-age children's sleep is discussed throughout the book with particular emphasis in Chapters 10, 11, 15, 21, 22, 27, and 34. Toward the end of Mary Carskadon and Leila Tarokh's chapter, they discuss an understudied developmental stage: emerging adulthood. Historically, sleep researchers, similar to researchers in other behavioral sciences, have invited college-age students to participate in studies and then generalized to wider adult populations. However, the American Psychological Association considers youth ages 10–18 as adolescents and emerging adults ages 19–29. Psychologist Jeffrey Arnett argues that emerging adulthood, or the "winding road from the late teens through the twenties," is a distinct and normative developmental or life stage (Arnett, 2004). Recent studies point out that first-year college students exhibit weeknight bed and rise times that are over an hour later than high school–age adolescents, as well as significantly later bed and rise times than older third and fourth-year college students (i.e., Lund, Reider, Whiting, & Prichard, 2010). Similarly, Roennberg, Kuehnle, Pramstaller, and colleagues found that after age 20, sleep midpoint times became increasingly earlier again; in other words, sleep schedules seem to become increasingly delayed over the course of adolescence, yet this pattern seems to change by the third or fourth year of college—which generally corresponds to about ages 20–22 (Roennberg, Kuehnle, Pramstaller, et al., 2004). As I emphasize in my 2010 *Journal of Adolescent Health* editorial, these remarkable cross-sectional findings suggest a developmental change; however, more research is needed to better understand and inform developmental science researchers, educators, and health care providers regarding the longitudinal trajectory of sleep and circadian timing over the late adolescence / emerging adulthood years (Wolfson, 2010).

Likewise, with each developmental period a myriad of different factors influence an infant's, child's, or adolescent's sleep patterns and, likewise, the sleep environment (i.e., college dorm room vs. family sleep environment), context, and other factors such as culture and socioeconomic status, interact with developmental changes in sleep. I was quite disturbed to learn that a 12-year-old in my National Institute of Child Health and Human Development (NICHD)–funded study of urban middle schoolers was sleeping in his neighbor's apartment until about midnight on school nights until his mother got home to awaken and escort him back to their apartment building for the remainder of the night—not an easy way to obtain the sufficient and consistent sleep needed for a developing adolescent. The second section of the book focuses on the *Complexity of Issues and Factors Influencing Sleep*. Here, authors Charles Super and Sara Harkness, Lauren Hale, Michael Gradisar and Michelle Short, Melissa Burnham, Lisa Meltzer, and James Spilsbury discuss and critique the newest research on the social, cultural, and economic determinants of children's sleep, with focus on the consequences of chronic illness and violent environments, and the rapidly changing role of technology that is interfering with childrens' and adolescents' ability to sustain healthy sleep-wake patterns. For example, in the National Sleep Foundation's 2011 Sleep in America Poll about in one in ten of 13–18-year-olds (9%) acknowledge that they are awakened after they go to bed every night or almost every night by a phone call, text message, or email, and nearly one in five of 13–29-year-olds note that this happens at least a few nights per week (NSF, 2011). In other words, adolescents' and emerging adults' lifestyle choices are creating a sleep disorder-like phenomenon with smart phones.

Parts three and four reflect the substantial literature on disordered sleep and sleep problems that manifest over the course of infancy, childhood, and adolescence. Section Three, *Assessment of Sleep and Sleep Problems*, articulates the range of clinical and research-based approaches for assessing and estimating sleep and circadian rhythms in infant, child, and adolescent populations. Authors Neville Blampied, Rosemary Horne and Sarah Biggs, Stephanie Crowley, Karen Spruyt, Valerie Crabtree, Amanda Rach, and Heather Gamble; Lissy Zaremba, and Joseph Buckhalt cover behavioral analysis, use of actigraphy and diaries or logs for estimating sleep patterns, and self-report measures, as well as school psychologists' roles and clinical lab protocols. Although the field has progressed in recent years, validation of retrospective self- and parent report sleep measures, prospective sleep-wake diaries, and actigraphy are still needed. It remains difficult to study children's sleep longitudinally, since few measures have been validated across developmental stages. Moreover, although actigraphy (in corroboration with sleep diaries) is a more objective means to estimate sleep in child and adult populations, researchers and clinicians need to establish unambiguous guidelines and standards for the scoring and reporting of actigraphy findings. Pending such standards, psychologists, other behavioral scientists, and health care providers need to be conscientious when using actigraphy and clearly report scoring rules and variables. As my colleagues and I have discussed extensively, scoring rules should be established a priori, with a research or consultation group available to evaluate ambiguous nights (Acebo & LeBourgeois, 2006; Acebo, Sadeh, Seifer, et al., 1999; Meltzer, Montgomery-Downs, Insana, et al., 2012; Wolfson, Carskadon, Acebo et al., 2003).

In Part Four, *Sleep Challenges, Problems, and Disorders*, authors Brandy Roane and Daniel Taylor, Robert Auger and Stephanie Crowley, Anna Ivanenko and Kymberly Larson, Kristen Archbold, and Patrina Caldwell and Karen Waters discuss some of the common sleep problems that children, adolescents, and their families confront including insomnia, delayed sleep phase disorder, nightmares and parasomnias, sleep apnea, and nocturnal enuresis. Many such sleep problems receive the attention of pediatricians and increasingly more psychologists, and there are also numerous books available for parents and professionals (e.g., Ferber, 2006; Ivanenko, 2008; Mindell, 2005; Owens & Mindell, 2003/2010). Many problems of sleep in young children are resolved before school attendance, but these difficulties sometimes come to the attention of child clinical and school psychologists. Sleep disorders with substantial prevalence in adulthood, such as obstructive sleep apnea, insomnia, and restless legs syndrome are also prevalent in children. This section reviews the diagnostic and treatment outcome literature and provides suggestions for behavioral interventions that can be implemented by psychologists and other clinicians.

Part Five focuses on the *Consequences of Insufficient Sleep,* with chapters by Erika Bagley and Mona El-Sheikh; Victoria Molfese, Kathleen Moritz Rudasill and Dennis Molfese; Louise O'Brien; Chantelle Hart, Nicola Hawley, Elizabeth Kuhl and Elissa Jelalian; and Shelley Hershner. These chapters discuss the preponderance of evidence that insufficient sleep, inconsistent sleep-wake schedules, sleep problems, and poor sleep hygiene habits are associated with health and behavior problems including internalizing and externalizing behaviors, emotion dysregulation, hyperactivity, inattention, school adjustment, and ineffective cognitive skills in children and adolescents. Shelly Hershner emphasizes that inadequate and erratic sleep in adolescents and emerging adults can have substantial consequences—that is, "sleepy driver" and "fall asleep at the wheel" driving accidents. Some locations have regulated when young drivers can be on the road and include education materials on sleep and the consequences of sleep deprivation in drivers education programs (e.g., *Curriculum Scope and Sequence Modules for Driver Education in Virginia,* 2001; *Driver Education Program,* Massachusetts Department of Transportation, 2010). In many ways, this section is only the tip of the iceberg, as, in addition to the areas covered by these authors, research has demonstrated that insufficient, inconsistent, and disordered sleep has negative consequences for cognitive development, substance use and abuse, work-related accidents, immune system functioning, and a range of other health, behavioral, and cognitive factors.

Sleep Difficulties Associated with Developmental and Behavioral Risks are examined in Part Six. Authors Daphne Koinis Mitchell and Robin Everhart; Amanda Richdale, Penny Corkum and J. Aimee Coulombe; Alison Harvey, Candice Alfano, and Greg Clarke; and Richard Bootzin, Jennifer Cousins, Monica Kelly, and Sally Stevens examine children, adolescents, and emerging adults with asthma and allergies, developmental disabilities, attention deficit hyperactivity disorder, affective disorders, and struggles with substance abuse. A prevalence of comorbid sleep problems is not uncommon for children and adolescents with behavioral and emotional disorders (e.g., Quine, 2001; Redline, Tishler, Schluchter, et al., 1999; Snell, Adam, & Duncan, 2007; Stores & Wiggs, 2001; Wolfson & Armitage, 2009). Of course, psychologists regularly work with children with these difficulties, but they may be less familiar with the associated sleep problems and behavioral consequences. In some situations, intervening and treating the sleep problems might mitigate the presenting and often challenging behavioral difficulties.

The Oxford Handbook of Infant, Child, and Adolescent Sleep and Behavior concludes with, perhaps, the most important area, Part Seven: *Prevention and Intervention.* These final five chapters (authors Melissa Moore and Jodi Mindell; Rhoda Au, Erica Appleman and Karina Stavitsky; Reut Gruber, Evelyn Constantin, Jamie Cassoff, and Sonia Michaelson; Pamela Thatcher; and S. Justin Thomas, Kristin Avis, and Kenneth Lichstein) focus on interventions and preventive approaches for families with young children; systemic countermeasures such as delaying school start times; prevention strategies and social learning-based programs for elementary, middle, and high school students; and approaches for working with college students and emerging adults struggling with disordered sleep. For example, my research team's Young Adolescent Sleep-Smart Pacesetter Program (funded by the National Institute of Child Health and Human Development) is evaluating the efficacy of a social learning–based, preventive intervention program designed to help early adolescents develop healthy sleep hygiene practices including decreasing caffeine use, obtaining adequate sleep, and maintaining consistent sleep schedules. Preliminary results suggest that the school-based *Sleep-Smart* program improved early adolescents' sleep patterns, hygiene practices, and sleep competence (Johnson, Harkins, Marco, Ludden, & Wolfson, 2012). Sleep-Smart participants also evidenced fewer health and behavioral difficulties and better grades following the program, whereas their comparison peers' behaviors remained the same during 7th grade.

The authors of this handbook have committed their academic and/or clinical careers to understanding the development of sleep patterns and the potential hurdles that prevent infants, children, and adolescents—along with their families—from obtaining sufficient and regular sleep. I am certain that they would agree with me and my coeditor, Hawley Montgomery-Downs, that high-quality, sound, and restorative sleep can improve our daily experiences, competence, and overall physical and emotional health. It is our hope that the research, guidance, and future directions discussed in each of the chapters in the *The Oxford Handbook of Infant, Child, and Adolescent Sleep and Behavior* will help psychologists and other behavioral scientists to understand and continue to study sleep and circadian rhythms in the context of psychological development and children's health, and in the prevention and treatment of sleep and behavioral disorders. As I recall, at about age 9, my son exclaimed one night: "Just because you study sleep, doesn't mean that I have to have a bedtime!" In looking back, I think he really meant to say: "Duh . . . you do not have to be a psychologist to know that a 9-year-old like me needs to get a good night's sleep!"

References

Acebo, C., Sadeh, A., Seifer, R., Tzischinsky, O., Wolfson, A., et al. (1999). Estimating sleep patterns with activity monitoring in children and adolescents: How many nights are necessary for reliable measures? *Sleep, 22*(1), 95–103.

Acebo, C, & LeBourgeois, M.K. (2006). Actigraphy. *Respiratory Care Clinics, 12*, 23–30.

Arnett, J. J. (2004). *Emerging adulthood: The winding road from the late teens through the twenties.* New York: Oxford University Press.

Besedovsky, L., Born, J., & Lange, T. (2012). Blockade of mineralocorticoid receptors enhances naïve T-helper cell counts during early sleep in humans. *Brain Behavior Immununology, 26*(7), 1116–1121.

Cuthbertson, J. & Schevill, S. (1985/2002). *Helping your child sleep through the night.* New York: Double Day/Broadway Books, Randome House.

Ferber, R. (1985/2006). *Solve your child's sleep problems.* New York: Simon and Schuster.

Ivanenko, A. (2008). *Sleep and psychiatric disorders in children and adolescents.* New York: Informa Healthcare USA, Inc.

Johnson, M., Harkins, E., Marco, C., Ludden, A., & Wolfson, A. (June 2012). *Effects of the Sleep-Smart Program on Early Adolescents' Perceived Health, Emotional Well-Being, and Caffeine Use.* Presented at the annual meeting of the Associated Professional Sleep Societies (Sleep 2012), Boston, MA.

Knutson, K.L., Zhao, X., Mattingly, M., Galli, G., & Cizza, G. (2012). Predictors of sleep-disordered breathing in obese adults who are chronic short sleepers. *Sleep Medicine, 13*(5), 484–489.

Lacks, Patricica. (1987). *Behavioral Treatment for Persistent Insomnia.* New York: Pergamon Books.

Lund, H.G., Reider, B.D., Whiting, A.B., & Prichard, J.R. (2010). Sleep patterns and predictors of disturbed sleep in a large population of college students. *Journal of Adolescent Health, 46(*2), 124–132.

Massachusetts Registry of Motor Vehicles (2010). *Driver Education Program.* Massachusetts Department of Transportation.

Meltzer, L. J., Montgomery-Downs, H. E., Insana, S. P., Walsh, C. M. (2012). Use of actigraphy for assessment in pediatric sleep research. *Sleep Medicine Reviews, 16*, 463–475.

Mindell, J.A. (2005). *Sleeping through the night: How infants, toddlers and their parents can get a good night's sleep.* New York: HarperCollins Publishers Inc.

National Sleep Foundation (2011). *Sleep in America Polls: Technology Use and Sleep.*

Owens J. A. & Mindell, J.A. (2003/2010). *A clinical guide to pediatric sleep: Diagnosis and management of sleep problems.* Philadephia, PA: Lippincott, Williams, and Wilkins.

Quine, L. (2001). Sleep problems in primary school children: comparison between mainstream and special school children. *Child: Care, Health and Development, 3*, 201–221.

Redline, S., Tishler, P.V., Schluchter, M., et al. (1999). Risk factors for sleep-disordered breathing in children: Associations with obesity, race, and respiratory problems. *American Journal of Respiratory Critical Care Medicine, 159*, 1527–1532.

Roennberg T, Kuehnle T, Pramstaller P, et al. (2004). A marker for the end of adolescence. *Current Biology, 14*:R1038–R1039.

Snell, E.K., Adam, E.K., & Duncan, G. (2007). Sleep and the Body Mass Index and overweight status of children and adolescents. *Child Development, 78*(1), 309–323.

Stores, G.S. & Wiggs, L. (2001). *Sleep disturbance in children and adolescents with disorders of development: Its significance and management.* London: MacKeith Press.

Virginia Department of Education (2001). *Curriculum Scope and Sequence Modules for Driver Education in Virginia.* Virginia Department of Motor Vehicles.

Walker, M.P., & Stickgold, R. (2006). Sleep, memory and plasticity. *Annual Review of Psychology, 10*, 139–166.

Wolfson, A., Lacks, P., & Futterman, A. (1992). The effects of parent training on infant sleeping patterns, parents' stress and perceived competence. *Journal of Consulting and Clinical Psychology, 60*(1), 41–48.

Wolfson, A. R., & Carskadon, M. A. (1998). Sleep schedules and daytime functioning in adolescents. *Child Development, 69*(4), 875–887.

Wolfson, A.R., Carskadon, M.A., Acebo, C., Seifer, R., Fallone, G., Labyak, S.E., & Martin, J. L. (2003). Evidence for the validity of a sleep habits survey for adolescents. *Sleep, 26*(2), 213–216.

Wolfson, A.R. & Armitage, R. (2009). Sleep and its relationship to adolescent depression. In: Nolen-Hoeksema, S. & Hilt, L.M. (Eds.) *Handbook of depression in adolescents.* New York: Routledge.

Wolfson, A.R. (2010). Adolescents and Emerging Adults' Sleep Patterns: New Developments. *Journal of Adolescent Health* (invited editorial), *46*, 97–99.

PART 1

Sleep and Development

CHAPTER

2 Overview of the History of Child and Adolescent Sleep Medicine

Stephen H. Sheldon

Abstract

Development of pediatric and adolescent sleep medicine parallels the development of pediatric health care in the United States. Historical development of health care for children, as well as development of sleep medicine as a necessary and important medical discipline for adults, provides insight into the current position of pediatric and adolescent sleep medicine and future directions for clinical practice and research. An understanding of the evolution of sleep medicine into a clinical and research discipline will create important perspective. Juxtaposition of disciplines will sensitize the reader to the need for state-of-the-art evaluation of sleep and its pathologies seen in infants, children, and adolescents.

Key Words: pediatric sleep medicine, adolescent sleep medicine, childhood and adolescent sleep disorders, history of pediatric sleep medicine

Introduction

The development of pediatric and adolescent sleep medicine parallels the development of pediatric health care in the United States. Historical development of health care for children, as well as development of sleep medicine for adults as a necessary and important medical discipline, provides insight into the current position of pediatric and adolescent sleep medicine and future directions for clinical practice and research.

Development of Pediatrics as a Unique Discipline

Prior to the beginning of the twentieth century, health care for children and adolescents was virtually nonexistent. Health care for children was provided by the family. Mortality rates for infants were high. More than one-third of infants died before their fifth birthday (Holt, 1943). Despite this high incidence of infant mortality, little was done and few took particular notice. Health care for children by the medical profession was provided using adult criteria, definition of disease/disorder, and therapeutic techniques (Cone, 1979). Medical practitioners who limited their practice to children were few and considered "baby feeders." At the turn of the century it has been estimated that there were not more than fifty medical practitioners in the United States who were particularly interested in the health care of children, and less than a dozen limited their practice exclusively to children (Smith, 1951). Locations for clinical evaluation specifically designed for children were nonexistent (Cone, 1979). Being considered property of their parents, children were and typically remain neither a political nor economic force. Diseases were widespread. Prevention was the underlying principle. Approaches to treatment of illness during childhood included tea, barley water, and protein milk. Floating hospitals and country sanatoria were occasionally utilized for treatment of childhood illness, since sun, fresh air, and isolation were managements of choice. But, for the most part, care of children remained in the home (Powers, 1939). Evaluation of childhood disease/disorders was based primarily on clinical signs and symptoms. Even congenital malformations were thought by many child health care practitioners to be due to maternal influences (Cone, 1979). Treatment was principally based on either adult medical interventions or was purely empiric. Climate therapy was common. Exposure to sunlight was prescribed for various illnesses including but not limited to tuberculosis, cutaneous abnormalities, anemia, and rickets. Some treatments were effective, but most were relatively ineffective. For example, treatment of pneumonia often included administration of digitalis, camphor, strychnia, and alcohol.

Child health care practitioners were thrust into the forefront of preventive medicine with the discovery and development of pasteurization of milk and immunizations for a variety of diseases. Antibiotics and the development of corticosteroids were instrumental in decreasing high childhood mortality rates existing during the first half of the twentieth century.

Subsequently, there had been rapid progress in pediatric medicine and surgery. Practice of pediatric medicine has turned from principally treatment of infectious diseases to comprehensive preventive programs, school health, community pediatrics, developmental pediatrics, and comprehensive adolescent medicine. Extensive morbidities have been identified, resulting in extensive efforts in behavioral disorders, family violence, child maltreatment, drug misuse, learning problems, school health, and developmental disabilities. Priorities have shifted, and identification of many pediatric disorders requires a multidisciplinary and interdisciplinary approach to diagnosis and management.

Development of Sleep Medicine as a Unique Discipline

Although there has been a fascination with sleep since antiquity, the scientific investigation of sleep and its disorders can be traced back to 1930 when Berger first described spontaneous EEG activity in the brains of sleeping subjects (Berger, 1930); differentiation of sleep into specific and distinct states by Harvey, Loomis, and Hobart in 1937 (Harvey, Loomis, & Hobart, 1937); and the first description of rapid eye movement (REM) sleep by Aserensky and Kleitman at the University of Chicago in 1953 (Aserensky & Kleitman, 1953). In 1955, Aserinsky and Kleitman observed sleeping infants and described a "rest–activity" cycle during sleep. These periods were characterized by quiet periods, where there were no body or eye movements, and active periods of body movements and rapid eye movements under closed lids (Aserensky & Kleitman, 1955). Two years later, Dement and Kleitman reported the cycling of REM sleep and non-rapid eye movement (NREM) sleep throughout the sleep period, proposed a classification system of NREM sleep into four distinct stages, and hypothesized the association of eye movements in REM sleep with dream mentation (Dement & Kleitman, 1957a, 1957b).

It had become clear that these discoveries ushered in the realization that it was not enough to evaluate health and disease during only waking hours but throughout the 24-hour continuum. A new era of medical and scientific research emerged focusing on physiological, pharmacological, pathophysiological, and even anatomical that are different during sleep than during the waking state (Orem & Barnes, 1980). Sleep research provided the groundwork and basis for the realization that clinical evaluation and management of patients might differ during sleep when compared to wake, resulting in the emergence of clinical sleep medicine (Carskadon & Roth, 1989).

At first, clinical sleep medicine evolved from patient self-referrals. Most sleep complaints were related to problem insomnia. However, it became clear that the common belief that the majority of etiologies of insomnia were purely psychiatric in origin was false (Carskadon & Roth, 1989). Obstructive sleep apnea had been identified in Europe, but there had been little notice of the condition in the United States. In 1970, Lugaresi and colleagues published remarkable success of tracheostomy in the treatment of obstructive sleep apnea (Lugaresi, Coccagna, Mantovani, & Brignani, 1970). Nonetheless, similar evaluation and management of obstructive sleep apnea was not yet accepted. In 1972, Guilleminault demonstrated remarkable results in managing uncontrollable hypertension in a $10^{1/2}$-year-old boy with tracheostomy (Dement, 1994). *It is stunning that the demonstration of the first successful treatment of sequelae of obstructive sleep apnea in the United States was in a child.*

Physiological evaluation of sleep had also progressed with adaptation of polygraphy, used in monitoring EEG, to evaluate other physiological variables during sleep. Termed *polysomnography,* its use by Holland (Holland, Dement, & Raynal, 1974) changed the face of clinical assessment of sleep in adult patients. Now there were methods for both basic evaluation by history and physical examination, as well as physiological assessment of sleep-related complaints in a clinical laboratory setting.

By the end of the 1970s, clinical sleep disorders medicine became an accepted area of medical inquiry, although practice of sleep disorders medicine was still couched in other disciplines of pulmonology, psychiatry, neurology, and internal medicine. In 1968, the *Manual of Standardized Terminology, Techniques, and Scoring System for Sleep Stages of Human Subjects* was published (Rechtschaffen & Kales, 1968). This was a significant step forward in standardizing sleep stage scoring in adults and eliminating unreliability and inconsistencies in laboratory evaluation of sleep, both between laboratories and within laboratories. It was clear at that time that this standardization was not appropriate for identification of stages of sleep and evaluation of sleep in newborns, infants, and children. Anatomical and physiological variables differed markedly from those of the adult. Similar standardization of sleep stage identification was a daunting task due to the rapid and constantly changing biology of the maturing and developing child. Therefore, the newborn infant became a starting point for a similar process that was started by Drs. Rechtschaffen and Kales in 1968. Drs. Thomas Anders, Robert Emde, and Arthur Parmelee were pioneers in bringing the science of sleep in infants and children to child health care practitioners. Because of their seminal work related to sleep in infants and children, Drs. Anders, Emde, and Parmelee co-chaired an ad hoc committee to provide similar standards, and the result was the publication in 1971 of *A Manual for Standardized Techniques and Criteria for Scoring of States of Sleep and Wakefulness in Newborn Infants* (Anders, Emde, & Parmelee, 1971). Strikingly, since publication of this manual, 42 years later there has been no similar effort for infants older than 2 months of age and children older than the beginning of puberty. Many problems precluded this task. Standardization in the pediatric age group is a formidable endeavor. First, there are rapid and dynamic changes that occur during the first two decades of life. The nervous system is constantly changing, structurally and functionally, during this period of life. Attempting to define cross-sectional criteria for evaluation of children both within same-age subjects and between subjects is extraordinarily difficult because of normal internal and external variability. Normal ranges can be extensive. Limitations include number of evaluations required for appropriate power. External reliability and validity can also be quite difficult to establish. Several longitudinal points are often required for appropriate comparison of polysomnographic variables. This has been suggested to be termed *developmental polysomnography* (Sheldon, 1996). This would then take into account normal progression of maturation, rather than evaluating a single polygraphic study at a single point in time. Because of these immense difficulties, little evidence-based standardized information has been available to provide accurate and reproducible normative data, despite evidence that sleep and its normal structure and maturation has far-reaching implications for growth, development, and learning (Karni, Tanne, Rubenstein, Askenasy, & Sagi, 1994; Wilson & McNaughton, 1994).

Identification of effective noninvasive treatments for many sleep-related disorders developed (for example, treatment of obstructive sleep apnea in adults with nasal CPAP), resulting in rapid development of therapeutic protocols and widespread use. The combination of high prevalence of obstructive sleep apnea in the adult population, management of the obstructive sleep-disordered breathing with nasal continuous positive airway pressure (CPAP), a relatively innocuous procedure, and effective management of sequelae led to the rapid expansion of sleep medicine into a unique medical discipline. Sleep disorders medicine has become an accepted and distinct specialty within the medical community.

Beginning in 1978, the American Board of Sleep Medicine (ABSM) provided an examination in clinical polysomnography to assure quality of practitioners practicing sleep disorders medicine and interpreting polysomnograms. The first examination certified 21 candidates. During the next 28 years, the ABSM certified more than 3400 individuals (Quan, Berry, Buyssee, Collop, Grigg-Damberger, Harding et al., 2008). This examination was not specialty-specific and was taken by internists, psychiatrists, psychologists, neurologists, family practitioners, and pediatricians. Successful applicants became diplomats of the ABSM. Indeed, sleep disorders medicine as a new and unique discipline became the focus of more clinical practitioners.

Pediatric and adolescent sleep medicine has become an outgrowth of this sleep disorders medicine practice. Inspiration has come from several directions: scientific and clinical interest in sudden infant death syndrome (SIDS); identification of obstructive sleep apnea and other sleep-related breathing disorders occurring with significant prevalence in the pediatric population; identification of the importance of sleep in the origin of daytime behavioral difficulties; and the influence of sleep disorders and insufficient sleep on children's daytime performance and learning.

In the early 1980s the practice of pediatrics was a highly respected medical discipline. One of the principal textbooks utilized by most students and practitioners of health care for children was entitled *Nelson's Textbook of Pediatrics* (Behrman, 1992). Nevertheless, the 14th edition of this text published in 1992 had a total of only *eleven paragraphs* uniquely devoted to sleep disorders in children.

Between 1978 and 1987, several seminal works were published. Publication of three books for parents, entitled *Solve Your Child's Sleep Problems* (Ferber, 1985), *Helping Your Child Sleep Through the Night* (Cuthbertson & Schevill, 1985), and *Healthy Sleep Habits, Happy Child* (Weissbluth, 1987), focused on different techniques parents might employ to affect their child's sleep. Interestingly, these books tended to employ different approaches, creating considerable controversy in the child health care community and parental confusion. A compilation of scientific articles was published in 1978 and was entitled *Sleep and Its Disorders in Children,* edited by Dr. Christian Guilleminault (Guilleminault, 1987). This book gathered groundbreaking scientific papers on normative data providing a basis for future direction in the scientific study of sleep and sleep-wake cycles during infancy, childhood, and adolescence.

More changes occur in anatomy, physiology, and sleep—wake patterns during the first 15 years of life than over the next four decades. Nonetheless, while the work in this volume attests to the high-quality empirical work conducted, comparatively little information has been published regarding this transformation. Prevalence and impact of dysfunctional sleep on the developing child requires large population-based studies. It is imperative to determine how sleep and its organization develop in infancy and early childhood, since disruption of normal progression of development during these vastly important stages in human maturation may have lifelong consequences.

Clinical pediatric sleep medicine has had to rely on nosology developed for adults (Thorpy, 1990). Adaptations have been attempted (Sheldon, Spire, & Levy, 1992), but it is clearly apparent that adapting adult criteria to infants and children can lead to many false starts and wrong turns. Most sleep-related problems in children might carry similar nomenclature, but children and adolescents are clearly different. It would be inappropriate, improper, and incongruous to apply adult sleep medicine anatomical, physiological, and pathological criteria to children.

Yet, the general pediatric community has been very slow to grasp the significance of the entirety of pediatric sleep disorders. Child health care practitioners have been resistant to absorb the importance of sleep physiology and sleep structure to human development and behavior. However, over the past 5 to 10 years, pediatric pulmonologists, otolaryngologists, neurologists, psychiatrists, and psychologists have increasingly recognized the importance of sleep and its disorders and have incorporated this large portion of the child's life into clinical and academic endeavors, with particular focus on sleep-related breathing abnormalities. With an apparent "epidemic" of obstructive sleep apnea in the pediatric population, this again seems to be an outgrowth of adult sleep medicine. To this end, child health care professionals began in 2005 to meet to discuss priorities for research, patient care, policy, and education. This first conference was sponsored by Brown University, Alpert Medical School, and was attended by more than 100 participants. There has been continued and ongoing excitement about this meeting, along with continued and rapid growth. In 2010, the first international conference was held in Rome, Italy, with more than 400 attendees. These conferences are now are now held biannually in alternate years.

In 2002, the American Academy of Sleep Medicine (AASM) applied to the Accreditation Council on Graduate Medical Education (ACGME) for establishment of sleep medicine training programs under the auspices of the ACGME as part of a comprehensive plan, along with the American Board of Medical Specialists, to accept sleep medicine as an independent medical specialty. In 2003 this was approved, and a consensus plan was developed for establishment of a new multidisciplinary specialty examination in sleep medicine to be jointly offered by the American Board of Internal Medicine, American Board of Psychiatry and Neurology, American Board of Pediatrics, American Board of Family Medicine, and the American Board of Otolaryngology, Head and Neck Surgery (Quan et al., 2008). The first examination was administered in 2007. Considerations and disorders unique to childhood comprised 2% of the first examination. Although pediatrics is a required portion of a sleep medicine fellowship curriculum, it is unclear how much pediatric medicine and sleep disorders in children is afforded to internists, otolaryngologists, psychiatrists, and neurologists studying general sleep medicine in these programs. It is also unclear whether training in developmental medicine and children's health care can be translated into practice of sleep medicine without a comprehensive underpinning of pediatric medicine.

Success in incorporating pediatric sleep medicine objectives into undergraduate, graduate, and postgraduate training curricula will depend upon outcome and cost-effectiveness. Integrating disciplines (including but not limited to medicine and psychology) is crucial in development of successful and effective sleep medicine services for children. Interdisciplinary and multidisciplinary approaches to diagnosis and management of sleep-related disorders in infancy, childhood, and adolescence requires this model. Many questions remain. First, can the provision of comprehensive sleep medicine services to children by pediatricians specializing and devoting full time to the practice of pediatric sleep medicine have a significant impact on comorbid medical illnesses such as sickle cell anemia, cystic fibrosis, neuromuscular disorders, craniofacial malformations, or congenital/acquired cardiovascular disease? Second, what effect does early disruption of sleep and/or sleep–wake cycling have on learning, memory, and cognitive development? Finally, can understanding sleep and its disorders in childhood contribute to a better understanding of behavioral disorders, problems of attention, and learning disabilities? The work described in this book illustrates the exciting, ongoing work that is being done. The authors of these chapters also highlight the most important future directions in each of their areas. The mystery of establishing and integrating neural networks required for early brain development and later executive functioning may be locked within the sleeping brain.

As was true of the development of pediatrics as a unique medical discipline, further appreciation of the development of sleep and its structure, as well as the effects of disruption of its normal maturation, might lead to improved diagnosis, treatment, and prevention of a wide variety of disorders unique to both children and adults. It is evident that the present is only the beginning of the understanding of pediatric sleep and pediatric sleep medicine.

Summary

Pediatric and adolescent sleep medicine has followed a similar path in its maturation to the development of pediatrics as a recognized and unique medical discipline. There has been a very significant increase in evidence-based knowledge regarding sleep and its disorders in infants, children, and adolescents over the past decade. Nonetheless, what is known now about the importance of sleep in normal human development and sleep in health and disease is likely only the "tip of the iceberg." The future of pediatric and Adolescent Sleep Medicine is truly before us. Many questions remain:

1. How important is the basic rest–activity cycle during gestation in growth and maturation of the central nervous system, neuronal migration, and neural network development?
2. What impact does disruption of normal sleep and/or its continuity during the first few years of life have on future human development and performance?
3. What effect does sleep deprivation during adolescence have on health and well-being as an adult? How might this contribute to chronic illness affecting these individuals as adults?

References

Anders, T., Emde, R., & Parmelee, A. H., eds. (1971). *A Manual of Standardized Terminology, Techniques and Criteria for Scoring of States of Sleep and Wakefulness in Newborn Infants.* UCLA Brain Information Service, NINDS Neurological Information Network, Los Angeles.

Aserensky, E., & Kleitman, N. (1953). Regularly recurring periods of eye motility, and concomitant phenomena, during sleep. *Science, 118*, 273–274.

Aserensky, E, & Kleitman, N. (1955). A motility cycle in sleeping infants as manifested by ocular and gross bodily activity. *Journal of Applied Physiology, 8*, 11–18.

Behrman, R. E., ed. (1992). *Nelson's Textbook of Pediatrics*, 14th Edition. Philadelphia: WB Saunders.

Berger, H. (1930). Uber das Elekoenkeephalogramm des Menchen. *Journal fur Psychologie und Neurologie, 40*, 160–179.

Carskadon, M. A., & Roth, T. (1989). Normal sleep and its variations. In M. Kryger, T. Roth, & W. C. Dement(Eds.), *Principles and Practice of Sleep Medicine* (pp. 3–15). Philadelphia: WB Saunders.

Cone, T. E. Jr. (1979). *History of American Pediatrics* (pp. 99–130). Boston: Little Brown.

Cuthbertson, J., & Schevill, S., *Helping Your Child Sleep Through the Night* (p. 237). New York: Doubleday, 1985.

Dement, W. C., & Kleitman, N. (1957a). Cyclic variations in EEG during sleep and their relation to eye movements, body motility, and dreaming. *Electroencephalography and Clinical Neurophysiolology, 9*, 673–690.

Dement, W. C., & Kleitman, N. (1957b). The relation of eye movements during sleep to dream activity: an objective method for the study of dreaming. *Journal of Experimental Psychology, 53*, 339–346.

Dement, W. C. (1994). History of sleep physiology and medicine. In Kryger, M., Roth, T., & Dement, W. C., eds. (1994). *Principles and Practice of Sleep Medicine*, 2nd Edition (pp. 3–15). Philadelphia: WB Saunders.

Ferber, R. (1985). *Solve Your Child's Sleep Problems.* New York: Simon & Schuster.

Freeman, R. G. (1916). Fresh air in pediatric practice. *Transactions of the American Pediatric Society, 28,* 7.
Guilleminault, C. (1987). *Sleep and Its Disorders in Children.* New York: Raven Press.
Harvey, E. N., Loomis, A. L., & Hobart, G. A. (1937). Cerebral states during sleep as studied by human brain potentials. *Science, 85,* 443–444.
Holland, V., Dement, W., & Raynal, D. (1974). *Polysomnography: responding to a need for improved communication.* Presentation to the Annual Meeting of the Sleep Research Society, Jackson Hole, Wyoming.
Holt, L. E. (1943). Infant mortality ancient and modern. An historical sketch. *Arch Pediatr, 30,* 885.
Karni, A., Tanne, D., Rubenstein, B. S., Askenasy, J. J. M., & Sagi, D. (1994). Dependence on REM sleep of overnight improvement of a perceptual skill. *Science, 265,* 679–682.
Lugaresi, E., Coccagna, G., Mantovani, M., & Brignani, F. (1970). Effects de la tracheotomie dans les hypersomnies avec respiration periodique. *Revue Neurologique, 123,* 267–268.
Orem, J., & Barnes, C. D. (1980). *Physiology in Sleep.* New York: Academic Press.
Powers, G. F. (1939). Developments in pediatrics in the past quarter century. *Yale Journal of Biology and Medicine, 12,* 1.
Quan, S. F., Berry, R. B., Buyssee, D., Collop, N. A., Grigg-Damberger, M., Harding, S. M., et al. (2008). Development and results of the first ABMS subspecialty certification examination in sleep medicine. *Journal of Clinical Sleep Medicine, 4,* 505–508.
Rechtschaffen, A., & Kales, A. (1968). *A Manual of Standardized Terminology, Techniques and Scoring System for Sleep Stages of Human Subjects.* Los Angles: BIS/BRI, UCLA.
Sheldon, S. H., Spire, J. P., & Levy, H. B. (1992). *Pediatric Sleep Medicine* (pp. 185–240). Philadelphia: WB Saunders.
Sheldon, S. H. (1996). *Evaluating Sleep in Infants and Children* (p. 276). New York: Lippincott-Raven.
Smith, R. M. (1951). Medicine as a science: pediatrics. *New England Journal of Medicine, 244,* 176.
Thorpy, M., chairman, Diagnostic Classification Steering Committee. (1990). *International Classification of Sleep Disorders: Diagnostic and Coding Manual.* Rochester, MN: American Sleep Disorders Association.
Weissbluth, M. (1987). *Healthy Sleep Habits, Happy Child* (p. 492). New York: Ballantine Books.
Wilson, M. A., & McNaughton, B. L. (1994). Reactivation of hippocampal ensemble memories during sleep. *Science, 265,* 676–679.

CHAPTER

3

A Brief History of Child and Adolescent Sleep Research: Key Contributions in Psychology

Tonya M. Palermo

Abstract

The scientific understanding of sleep in infants, children, and adolescents has expanded significantly over the past few decades. Within psychology, key discoveries have been made in several important areas including (1) the understanding of prevalence and impact of childhood sleep problems and disorders; (2) the development and evaluation of behavioral treatments for childhood sleep problems; (3) the development of conceptual models of children's sleep and sleep dysfunction; (4) the measurement of sleep patterns, behaviors, and disorders in children; and (5) the identification of sleep-related concerns in pediatric medical, neurodevelopmental, and psychiatric populations. Sleep is now recognized as a cross-cutting issue in child and pediatric psychology. Expanding opportunities within psychology for involvement in pediatric sleep research and sleep clinical training are part of this evolving history. A research agenda building from these key discoveries will move the field of pediatric sleep medicine forward over the next several decades.

Key Words: history, psychology, pediatric, sleep research

Introduction

Within the field of psychology, important contributions have been made to the scientific understanding of sleep in infants, children, and adolescents. Over the past three decades, scholarly work in psychology has expanded the evidence base of pediatric sleep medicine, led to practice changes in treatment of childhood sleep problems, produced policy changes (e.g., school start times), and led to increased emphasis on training in behavioral sleep medicine (e.g., certification in Behavioral Sleep Medicine, postdoctoral training). This has all been accomplished in a relatively short time, as the focus on infants, children, and adolescents within sleep research is recent.

The aim of this chapter is to highlight key areas of research contribution in psychology to the understanding of children's sleep. Specifically, five areas of key discoveries in child sleep research are reviewed, including: *(1)* prevalence and impact of sleep problems and disorders; *(2)* evaluation of behavioral treatments for pediatric sleep problems; *(3)* conceptual models of children's sleep and sleep dysfunction; *(4)* measurement of sleep behaviors, sleep patterns, and sleep disorders in children; and *(5)* sleep in special populations of children with medical, neurodevelopmental, and psychiatric conditions. Each of these areas is considered from a historical perspective in this chapter, highlighting key findings that moved the field forward. This chapter is not intended to provide a comprehensive historical overview of sleep research in psychology; rather, it is meant to draw attention to key discoveries and provide examples to demonstrate the progression of research.

Prevalence and Impact of Sleep Problems and Disorders

Three decades ago, relatively little was known about normative patterns and variation in children's sleep, and most advice about proper sleep patterns was based on personal observation and opinion. Thus, an important focus of psychology research aimed to describe infant, child, and adolescent sleep patterns and to identify the frequency of problematic sleep patterns and behaviors in childhood in order to establish scientific data on this topic. A number of cross-sectional survey studies emerged to fill in this gap in knowledge. Developmental changes in patterns of sleep including average bedtimes, wake times, and sleep duration of children across the pediatric age span were described (e.g., Anders & Keener, 1985; Carskadon, 1990; Levy, Gray-Donald, Leech, Zvagulis, & Pless,1986; Sadeh, Lavie, Scher, Tirosh, & Epstein, 1991). Moreover, studies were conducted to identify parental concerns about problematic child sleep behaviors (e.g., Blader, Koplewicz, Abikoff, & Foley, 1997; Johnson, 1991; Richman, 1981). Screening measures for sleep disorders were developed in community samples, identifying the prevalence of a range of behaviorally based and physiologically based sleep disorders to understand potential treatment needs. Progress was made in the investigation of behaviorally based sleep disorders; for example, prevalence data emerged showing that 12% to 16% of adolescents have clinically significant insomnia (Morrison, McGee, & Stanton, 1992; Ohayon, Caulet, & Lemoine, 1998; Roberts, Lee, Hemandez, & Solari, 2004). Researchers also recognized the importance of studying the course of sleep problems longitudinally, finding, for example, that a significant portion of children who experience sleep disturbances at earlier ages continue to do so over time (e.g., Kataria, Swanson, & Trevathan, 1987; Pollock, 1992) and that sleep disturbances may be chronic or persistent (e.g., Roberts, Roberts, & Duong, 2008). Together, data on the prevalence and course of sleep behaviors and sleep disorders were compelling in demonstrating that childhood sleep problems were an important pediatric health problem worthy of study.

Beyond prevalence and epidemiology, the impact of sleep problems became an important research topic in psychology. There was interest in understanding how sleep problems may affect children and families in a variety of domains. In infants and young children, researchers asked questions about the impact of the child's problematic sleep on adult caregivers in regard to their own sleep, mood and affect, and parenting stress (e.g., Hiscock & Wake, 2002). It was recognized that the child's sleep could impact the entire family. This followed from similar theoretical movements in the fields of pediatric and child psychology, where family systems theories were developing in the conceptualization of child illness (e.g., Kazak, 1989). The study of childhood sleep in the context of the family has continued to date; in particular, research has focused on the complexity for sleep in the family when a child has a chronic illness or developmental disorder (Meltzer & Montgomery-Downs, 2011).

Efforts were also directed toward describing the functional impact of disrupted sleep on children. Research in psychology showed clearly that children were affected by sleep loss and sleep disruption in a multitude of domains. For example, key findings emerged demonstrating that children and adolescents who experience excessive daytime sleepiness due to insufficient or interrupted sleep are at greater risk for mood disturbances, behavioral disruption, impaired cognitive functioning, reduced academic performance, attentional difficulties, and increased school absences (e.g., Fallone, Owens, & Deane, 2002; Gozal, 1998; Wolfson & Carskadon, 1998). Poor sleep was also linked with socioemotional problems, particularly symptoms of anxiety and depression, behavior problems, and substance abuse in youth (Johnson & Breslau, 2001; Smedje, Broman, & Hetta, 2001).

In child neuropsychology research, these functional indicators were further explored. Comprehensive studies were undertaken to examine neurocognitive function and sleep in children, finding that disturbed sleep is associated with problems with cognitive functioning, learning, and attention (Sadeh, Gruber, & Raviv, 2002, 2003). Neurocognitive function was studied in children with known sleep disorders such as sleep disordered breathing (SDB), as well as in children who are otherwise healthy. These data extended the study of consequences that had been defined in the adult literature related to SDB where neurocognitive deficits, which may be a consequence of sleep fragmentation or hypoxemia, had been reported. For example, investigations within neuropsychology of children with SDB showed similar deficits (as in adults) in neurocognitive performance, behavioral impairments, and reduced school performance (e.g., Blunden, Lushington, & Kennedy, 2001; Gozal, 1998; Lewin, Rosen, England, & Dahl, 2002; Owens, Spirito, McGuinn, & Nobile, 2000). Further research attempted to describe whether these deficits may be completely or partially reversible with treatment of SDB (Gozal, 1998; Lewin et al., 2002; Owens, Spirito, McGuinn et al., 2000). Major research discoveries have continued over the last decade providing new data on the consequences of SDB on children. This continues to be an important topic of study. For example, several recent investigations have examined whether behavioral and neurocognitive functions of children with obstructive sleep apnea syndrome (OSAS) improve after adenotonsillectomy (e.g., Landau et al., 2012; Redline et al., 2011). Findings to date suggest that the impact of OSAS on behavioral and cognitive functions begins in early childhood.

Contemporary research in neuropsychology is focusing on sleep restriction and neurocognitive function in otherwise healthy children (e.g., Beebe, Difrancesco, Tlustos, McNally, & Holland, 2009), using brain imaging methods. This innovative work continues to increase understanding of the broad impact of sleep disruption on children. Part Five of this book provides a contemporary focus on consequences of insufficient sleep.

In addition to neurocognitive effects, elegant work has emerged on the impact of OSAS on children's health care use (Tarasiuk et al., 2007). In this study, findings demonstrated that children with OSAS have higher health care use starting from the first year of life, and the majority of the health service use was due to higher occurrence of respiratory tract morbidity (Tarasiuk et al., 2007). Further research is needed to demonstrate the potential health economic impact of other sleep disturbances in infants, children, and adolescents.

Research discoveries in psychology in the area of prevalence and impact of childhood sleep problems have also been translated into public policy changes. One of the best exemplars of this is the topic of sleep in adolescents. In the 1980s, extending descriptive research on sleep to adolescents, Carskadon conducted pioneering studies that contributed knowledge of normal sleep-related changes in adolescence, identifying the optimal sleep needs of adolescents and serving to highlight the significant deficit in sleep obtained by most youth (Carskadon et al., 1980; see Carskadon and Tarokh, Chapter 8). This line of research on sleep regulation in adolescents has now spanned several decades and has led to increased understanding of sleep problems and impact on behavior in adolescents (e.g., Carskadon, Acebo, & Jenni, 2004; Carskadon, Wolfson, Acebo, Tzischinsky, & Seifer, 1998). These findings fueled a tremendous interest in the study of sleep in adolescents as well as advocacy efforts, particularly around school start times and consideration of how changes in policy may help to prevent sleep problems (see Au, Appleman, and Stavitsky, Chapter 38).

An influential study was published in 1998 by Wolfson, Carskadon, and colleagues specifically on the relationship between inadequate sleep quantity and quality and adolescent school performance. Using high school records of academic performance, this study clearly linked inadequate sleep to problems with attendance and reduced academic performance (Wolfson & Carskadon, 1998). This work became critical in a national debate about school start times. Over the subsequent years, a number of school districts have responded to these research findings regarding the prevalence of inadequate sleep among high school students with a policy change of delaying school start times (e.g., from starting at 7:30 a.m. to starting at 8:30 a.m.) to allow adolescents to sleep longer in the morning. Many school districts continue to debate the issue, and psychology research is active in extending these data to the study of sleep in middle school students (Wolfson, Spaulding, Dandrow, & Baroni, 2007).

The conclusions from this body of work in psychology are that sleep problems are common across the pediatric age span and, importantly, that they are also associated with major sources of child and family functional impact, highlighting the significance of directing efforts toward prevention and treatment of sleep problems in children.

Evaluating Behavioral Treatments for Sleep Problems in Children

In the 1980s and 1990s, pediatric sleep medicine was emerging as a legitimate clinical specialty. Psychologists began consulting with and collaborating alongside sleep medicine physicians to provide behavioral treatment to children with a range of sleep disorders. A number of books for health professionals on children's sleep emerged during this time (e.g., Ferber & Kryger, 1995; Guilleminault, 1987), focused broadly on describing sleep disorders in children and adolescents. Moreover, key books about children's sleep were published during this time specifically for a parent audience (e.g., Cuthbertson & Schevill, 1985; Ferber, 1986; Mindell, 1997; Weissbluth, 1987). Importantly, behavioral treatment strategies were introduced in these books, such as the application of behavioral techniques to treat bedtime resistance in young children. Clearly moving the field forward, many of the treatment and intervention strategies presented in these early professional and lay books continue to be used today.

Given that the most frequent childhood sleep problems involve bedtime resistance and night wakings in infants and young children (Meltzer & Mindell, 2006), the thrust of the treatment research in psychology has been in this area. Published reports of behavioral treatments for pediatric sleep problems emerged in the 1980s and 1990s with mostly case series and small treatment studies (e.g., France & Hudson, 1990; Rapoff, Christophersen, & Rapoff, 1982). Important review articles were written by psychologists describing treatment of sleep disorders in children (e.g., Mindell, 1993) and summarizing priorities for research. For example, Mindell (1993) highlighted a number of methodological problems in studies on sleep disorders in children including the large number of case studies and uncontrolled trials, the lack of long-term follow-up, subjectivity of the outcome data on sleep, and large gaps in research. Since Mindell's review was published, it has been exciting to see research in psychology address many of these research gaps and limitations, due to the concerted efforts to study sleep interventions in controlled trials in children and to improve on the measurement of sleep and related outcomes.

A solid body of literature now exists supporting the use of evidence-based behavioral management strategies to treat bedtime problems and night wakings in infants, toddlers, and preschoolers. An influential program of research on behavioral interventions is the work conducted by Mindell and colleagues, including randomized controlled trials of behavioral interventions for bedtime settling and night waking problems, as well as systematic reviews synthesizing this treatment literature (Mindell, 1999; Mindell, Kuhn, Lewin, Meltzer, & Sadeh, 2006). A recent systematic review was used in practice parameters developed by the American Academy of Sleep Medicine (AASM) presenting recommendations for the use of behavioral treatments for bedtime problems and night wakings in young children (Morgenthaler et al., 2006) based on this scientific evidence. Several specific behavioral treatments had enough evidence to be considered "standards" for treatment of bedtime problems and night wakings. These specific treatments include unmodified extinction, extinction with parental presence (see Blampied, Chapter 15), and preventive parent education. These were all rated as individually effective therapies in the treatment of bedtime problems and night wakings, producing reliable and significant clinical improvement in children's sleep.

Treatment directed toward the sleep problems of older children and adolescents has been relatively slow to develop in contrast to the tremendous surge of treatment research conducted over the past two decades in younger children. However, there are recent examples within psychology of research focused on the development and evaluation of interventions with older children and adolescents with insomnia (Bootzin & Stevens, 2005; Paine & Gradisar, 2011) and delayed sleep phase (Gradisar et al., 2011), and this is an area ripe for future investigation. Part Seven of this book highlights contemporary work on prevention and intervention of childhood sleep problems.

Conceptual Models of Sleep and Sleep Dysfunction

Within psychology, a number of conceptual models of childhood sleep and sleep dysfunction have been put forth over the years. Many of these models are intended to establish links between child and family risk of perpetuating factors for sleep problems, and consequences of sleep dysfunction, with the intent of identifying areas to intervene. Similar to conceptual models proposed in the child psychology literature more broadly (e.g., biopsychosocial models) to describe factors that influence children's adjustment to medical conditions, most models of childhood sleep are integrated in developmental models of sleep within the larger context of the child's biology, psychological factors, and social systems.

For example, one of the early models proposed by Sadeh and Anders (1993) was a transactional model of infant sleep which identified multiple etiological sources for infant sleep problems from a systems perspective. This model linked etiology to methods of assessment of sleep disturbances and application of specific intervention methods for the specific system involved. Similarly, in understanding adolescent sleep, Carskadon (2011) has described the convergence of biologic, psychological, and sociocultural influences on sleep. Other models have expanded understanding of family and culture to incorporate that children's sleep is shaped and interpreted by cultural values and beliefs (e.g, Boergers & Koinis-Mitchell, 2010).

Within childhood sleep research, conceptual models provide useful organizing frameworks helping to shape and focus research efforts in psychology. One example of how a conceptual model influenced subsequent research in psychology is in the area of children's pain and sleep. In 1999, Lewin and Dahl published a theoretical paper describing a model to explain the links between the regulation of sleep and pediatric pain. The primary tenet of the framework is that there are bidirectional effects between pain and sleep. Pain can directly affect sleep by prolonging sleep onset and interfering with the depth and continuity of sleep states, and the psychological and physiological sequelae of insufficient sleep (e.g., worry, negative thoughts, and decrements in behavioral control) may have deleterious effects on pain management. After the publication of this model, descriptions of sleep in children and adolescents with chronic pain became a topic of growing interest in psychology and pediatrics (e.g., Bruni, Russo, Violani, & Guidetti, 2004; Bruusgaard, Smedbraten, & Natvig, 2000; Haim et al., 2004; Palermo & Kiska, 2005). Researchers began to examine both directions of the pain–sleep relationship and focused attention on describing the impact of sleep disturbances on children's functional outcomes and health-related quality of life (LaPlant, Adams, Haftel, & Chervin, 2007).

Conceptual and theoretical models of childhood sleep are a major contribution within psychology, guiding subsequent research efforts. The continued focus on sleep within the child's broader systems of influence will remain a critical guide to further intervention development. Current research priorities on factors influencing sleep are described in Part Two of this book.

Measurement of Sleep Behaviors, Sleep Patterns, and Sleep Disorders

Because sleep is a multidimensional construct, measurement approaches have also been multimodal. In psychology, many contributions have been made over the past few decades to the measurement of sleep patterns, behaviors, and disorders in children. Research to describe patterns of children's sleep has encompassed both self-report of sleep and the measurement of activity patterns to derive sleep times using actigraphy (see Horne and Biggs, Chapter 16). For example, in the 1980s and 1990s, in validating actigraphy in child populations, the important work of Acebo, Sadeh, and colleagues (e.g., Carskadon, Acebo, Richardson, Tate, & Seifer, 1997; Sadeh & Acebo, 2002; Sadeh, Hauri, Kripke, & Lavie, 1995; Sadeh et al., 1991) supported this measurement technique as a viable option in child sleep research. Early publications focused on actigraphy procedures, scoring, and validity, guiding the approach to the use of actigraphy in child sleep research. Actigraphy validation and scoring in children remains an important contemporary area of scientific inquiry (e.g., Meltzer, Montgomery-Downs, Insana, & Walsh, 2012).

During the last 20 years, the number of pediatric subjective sleep measures (see Spruyt, Chapter 18) used in psychology research has increased significantly. Many specific measures have been developed to provide developmentally appropriate assessment of sleep across the entire pediatric age span from infancy to adolescence. There are now many available well-validated subjective measures to describe sleep habits, sleep quality, sleep beliefs, daytime sleepiness, and sleep disorders in children and adolescents; for example, see review by Lewandowski et al. (2011). Many of these instruments were developed with the contributions of psychologists.

One of the most widely used multidimensional measures of children's sleep is the *Children's Sleep Habits Questionnaire* (Owens, Spirito, & McGuinn, 2000). The publication of this measure was important in child sleep research, as it provided a tool to screen broad pediatric populations for sleep dysfunction and sleep disorders. It was widely available and quickly translated into many languages. More recent research on sleep measures has also involved validating subjective questionnaires against other forms of sleep assessment. For example, validation studies for both the *Brief Infant Sleep Questionnaire* (Sadeh, 2004) and the *Sleep Habits Survey* have demonstrated associations with actigraphy (Wolfson et al., 2003). Similarly, the sleep-related breathing disorder subscale of both the *Pediatric Sleep Questionnaire* (Chervin, Hedger, Dillon, & Pituch, 2000) and the *Sleep Disturbance Scale for Children* (Ferreira et al., 2009) have been validated with polysomnography. Important progress in measurement has greatly expanded available options in the study of children's sleep.

Accurate assessment of sleep disturbance and associated behaviors has practical applications in research and clinical care. As one example, the Ped-IMMPACT consensus group, charged with developing recommendations for relevant outcome domains in clinical trials for pediatric pain management, identified sleep as a core outcome domain (McGrath et al., 2008) in therapeutic trials for youth with chronic pain, recommending several validated subjective measures of sleep for outcome assessment.

Sleep in Special Populations: Children with Medical, Neurodevelopmental, and Psychiatric Conditions

The study of sleep in special populations of children with medical, neurodevelopmental, and psychiatric conditions emerged in the 1980s and 1990s as an important clinical topic in psychological or behavioral treatment of individuals with sleep problems and comorbidities. Published applications of behavioral strategies (e.g., positive routines, graduated extinction, and scheduled wakings; see Blampied, Chapter 15) to treat sleep problems in special pediatric populations are a significant part of this early history (e.g., Bramble, 1996, 1997; Durand, Gerner-Dott, & Mapstone, 1996; Milan, Mitchell, Berger, & Pierson, 1981). Because children with special health needs represent a large number of visits to child and pediatric psychologists, the treatment of sleep problems represented an important clinical challenge. For example, the majority of adolescents presenting for treatment of insomnia in a sleep clinic have been found to have a diagnosis of a psychiatric disorder, often a mood disorder (Ivanenko, Barnes, Crabtree, & Gozal, 2004; see Harvey, Alfano, and Clarke, Chapter 35).

Case series of behavioral interventions (e.g., positive routines, faded bedtimes, response cost) demonstrated that interventions used in physically healthy populations could be modified to successfully treat bedtime resistance in children with neurodevelopmental disorders (see Richdale Chapter 33,). For example, Piazza conducted a series of intervention studies in the 1990s with children with developmental disabilities (Piazza & Fisher, 1991a, 1991b; Piazza, Fisher, & Moser, 1991; Piazza, Fisher, & Sherer, 1997); finding improvements from behavioral interventions in children's sleep behaviors. Later that decade, Durand (1997) published a book appropriate to both health professionals and parents on treatment of childhood sleep problems, with particular emphasis on children with neurodevelopmental disorders. This collection of treatment studies on children with special needs propelled a much broader research focus on sleep in children with autism (see Richdale, Chapter 33, this volume), attention deficit disorder (see Corkum and Coulombe, Chapter 34), and other developmental and psychiatric conditions. Part Six of this handbook is devoted to sleep difficulties associated with developmental and behavioral risks and showcases the significant ongoing work being done in this area.

The clinical observations made by psychologists spurred additional research on the prevalence and impact of sleep disturbances in children with developmental disorders, chronic medical conditions (see Meltzer and Walsh, Chapter 13), and psychiatric conditions. A robust body of literature developed over the past decade demonstrated that the presence of chronic medical or developmental conditions in children is associated with increased prevalence of sleep problems (e.g., Hysing, Sivertsen, Stormark, Elgen, & Lundervold, 2009; Long, Krishnamurthy, & Palermo, 2008; Sivertsen, Posserud, Gillberg, Lundervold, & Hysing, 2012). Multiple factors including both acute and chronic pain, underlying disease processes, concurrent medications, the impact of hospitalization, and comorbid psychiatric conditions such as depression and anxiety have been identified as important to consider in assessing the bidirectional relationship of sleep problems and acute and chronic illness in children (Lewandowski, Ward, & Palermo, 2011). In recognition of the emerging focus on these populations within psychology, two special issues were published in the *Journal of Pediatric Psychology* in 2008 (Owens & Palermo, 2008; Palermo & Owens, 2008) on the topics of sleep in children with medical conditions and neurodevelopmental disorders. Current priorities in this area are dedicated to developing and evaluating behavioral interventions for special populations of children with sleep problems (e.g., Vriend, Corkum, Moon, & Smith, 2011).

My own interest in sleep was sparked by a desire to treat sleep problems in child medical populations. As a pediatric psychologist engaged in clinical services and research related to children with chronic pain, I had observed that sleep was an important issue interwoven with children's experiences with chronic pain and in their daily functioning. However, I stumbled upon sleep medicine in my early career in the late 1990s as a junior faculty member at Rainbow Babies and Children's Hospital, where I was asked to provide behavioral services within a children's sleep program. At that time, I was unaware of the emerging literature underlying the connection between sleep and health outcomes. I found the provision of behavioral sleep services to children and families to be highly satisfying and was drawn to merging sleep with my research interest in chronic pain. The theoretical model proposed by Lewin and Dahl (1999) was extremely influential in how I approached the study of pain and sleep in children. Thus, my work included description of sleep characteristics, patterns, and behaviors in youth with chronic pain (e.g., Long et al., 2008; Palermo & Kiska, 2005; Palermo, Toliver-Sokol, Fonareva, & Koh, 2007), and the bidirectional relationship between sleep, pain, and functional outcomes (e.g., Lewandowski, Palermo, De la Motte, & Fu, 2010; Palermo, Fonareva, & Janosy, 2008; Palermo, Wilson, Lewandowski, Toliver-Sokol, & Murray, 2011). My current research aims to develop and evaluate behavioral interventions for insomnia in youth with chronic pain. In my own career, I have straddled the fields of pediatric psychology, pain management, and sleep medicine; at the nexus is exactly where my passion lies.

Conclusion

Sleep is now recognized as a cross-cutting issue in child and pediatric psychology, one that inextricably connects health, mental health, and infant, child, and adolescent development. As such, investigators with diverse backgrounds may work toward addressing similar research questions. Conclusions from the last few decades of research on childhood sleep in psychology are that sleep problems are not only common across the pediatric age span in healthy as well as medical and psychiatric populations, but that they are also associated with significant child and family functional impact. Research findings have reinforced the importance of directing efforts toward prevention and treatment of sleep problems across the pediatric age span.

From the work in psychology, a solid body of literature now exists supporting the use of behavioral interventions to treat bedtime problems and night wakings in infants, toddlers, and preschoolers. Conceptual and theoretical models have guided subsequent research efforts in these areas, and are an important contribution within psychology. Strides have been made in the measurement of multiple domains of sleep, sleep behavior, and sleep disorders in children, and valid methods are available for outcome assessment in sleep intervention research.

Future Directions

Many topics in pediatric sleep research remain to be addressed within psychology. Based on the five areas of key research contribution covered in this chapter, the following questions, if solved, would provide important future direction for the field.

- What factors predict success of behavioral treatment for specific infants, children, adolescents, and families?
- Which sleep disturbances in childhood are associated with elevated health care utilization and costs?
- What behavioral treatments are effective for managing the sleep problems of older children and adolescents?
- How do we best measure insomnia symptoms in children and adolescents?
- Are existing sleep measures valid in culturally and racially diverse pediatric populations?
- Which interventions are effective for sleep problems in special populations of children with acute and chronic medical conditions and mental health and psychiatric disturbances?

References

Anders, T. F., & Keener, M. (1985). Developmental course of nighttime sleep-wake patterns in full-term and premature infants during the first year of life. I. *Sleep, 8*(3), 173–192.

Beebe, D. W., Difrancesco, M. W., Tlustos, S. J., McNally, K. A., & Holland, S. K. (2009). Preliminary fMRI findings in experimentally sleep-restricted adolescents engaged in a working memory task. *Behavioral and Brain Functions, 5*, 9.

Blader, J. C., Koplewicz, H. S., Abikoff, H., & Foley, C. (1997). Sleep problems of elementary school children. A community survey. *Archives of Pediatrics & Adolescent Medicine, 151*(5), 473–480.

Blunden, S., Lushington, K., & Kennedy, D. (2001). Cognitive and behavioural performance in children with sleep-related obstructive breathing disorders. *Sleep Medicine Reviews, 5*(6), 447–461.

Boergers, J., & Koinis-Mitchell, D. (2010). Sleep and culture in children with medical conditions. *Journal of Pediatric Psychology, 35*(9), 915–926.

Bootzin, R. R., & Stevens, S. J. (2005). Adolescents, substance abuse, and the treatment of insomnia and daytime sleepiness. *Clinical Psychology Review, 25*(5), 629–644.

Bramble, D. (1996). Consumer opinion concerning the treatment of a common sleep problem. *Child: Care, Health, and Development, 22*(6), 355–366.

Bramble, D. (1997). Rapid-acting treatment for a common sleep problem. *Developmental Medicine & Child Neurology, 39*(8), 543–547.

Bruni, O., Russo, P. M., Violani, C., & Guidetti, V. (2004). Sleep and migraine: an actigraphic study. *Cephalalgia, 24*(2), 134–139.

Bruusgaard, D., Smedbraten, B. K., & Natvig, B. (2000). Bodily pain, sleep problems and mental distress in schoolchildren. *Acta Paediatrica, 89*(5), 597–600.

Carskadon, M. A., Harvey, K., Duke, P., Anders, T. F., Litt, I. F., & Dement, W. C. (1980). Pubertal changes in daytime sleepiness. *Sleep, 2*(4), 453–460.

Carskadon, M. A. (1990). Patterns of sleep and sleepiness in adolescents. *Pediatrician, 17*(1), 5–12.

Carskadon, M. A., Acebo, C., Richardson, G. S., Tate, B. A., & Seifer, R. (1997). An approach to studying circadian rhythms of adolescent humans. *Journal of Biological Rhythms, 12*(3), 278–289.

Carskadon, M. A., Wolfson, A. R., Acebo, C., Tzischinsky, O., & Seifer, R. (1998). Adolescent sleep patterns, circadian timing, and sleepiness at a transition to early school days. *Sleep, 21*(8), 871–881.

Carskadon, M. A., Acebo, C., & Jenni, O. G. (2004). Regulation of adolescent sleep: implications for behavior. *Annals of the New York Academy of Sciences, 1021*, 276–291. Carskadon, M. A. (2011). Sleep in adolescents: the perfect storm. *Pediatric Clinics of North America, 58*(3), 637–647. Chervin, R. D., Hedger, K., Dillon, J. E., & Pituch, K. J. (2000). Pediatric sleep questionnaire (PSQ): Validity and reliability of scales for sleep-disordered breathing, snoring, sleepiness, and behavioral problems. *Sleep Medicine, 1*(1), 21–32.

Cuthbertson, J., & Schevill, S. (1985). *Helping Your Child Sleep Through the Night.* Garden City, *New York:* Doubleday.

Durand, P., Gerner-Dott, E., & Mapstone, E. (1996). Treatment of sleep disorders in children with developmental disabilities *Journal of the Association for Persons with Severe Handicaps, 21*(3), 114–122.

Durand, V. M. (1997). *Sleep Better! A Guide to Improving Sleep for Children with Special Needs* (1st Edition). Baltimore: Paul H. Brookes.

Fallone, G., Owens, J. A., & Deane, J. (2002). Sleepiness in children and adolescents: Clinical implications. *Sleep Medicine Reviews, 6*(4), 287–306.

Ferber, R. (1986). *Solve Your Child's Sleep Problems.* New York: Fireside.

Ferber, R., & Kryger, M. (Eds.). (1995). *Principles and Practice of Sleep Medicine in the Child.* Philadelphia: Saunders.

Ferreira, V. R., Carvalho, L. B., Ruotolo, F., de Morais, J. F., Prado, L. B., & Prado, G. F. (2009). Sleep disturbance scale for children: translation, cultural adaptation, and validation. *Sleep Medicine, 10*(4), 457–463.

France, K. G., & Hudson, S. M. (1990). Behavior management of infant sleep disturbance. *Journal of Applied Behavioral Analysis, 23*(1), 91–98.

Gozal, D. (1998). Sleep-disordered breathing and school performance in children. *Pediatrics, 102*(3 Pt 1), 616–620.

Gradisar, M., Dohnt, H., Gardner, G., Paine, S., Starkey, K., Menne, A., et al. (2011). A randomized controlled trial of cognitive-behavior therapy plus bright light therapy for adolescent delayed sleep phase disorder. *Sleep, 34*(12), 1671–1680.

Guilleminault, C. (Ed.). (1987). *Sleep and its Disorders in Children. New York*: Raven Press.

Haim, A., Pillar, G., Pecht, A., Lerner, A., Tov, N., Jaffe, M., & Hardoff, D. (2004). Sleep patterns in children and adolescents with functional recurrent abdominal pain: Objective versus subjective assessment. *Acta Paediatrica, 93*(5), 677–680.

Hiscock, H., & Wake, M. (2002). Randomised controlled trial of behavioural infant sleep intervention to improve infant sleep and maternal mood. *British Medical Journal, 324*(7345), 1062–1065.

Hysing, M., Sivertsen, B., Stormark, K. M., Elgen, I., & Lundervold, A. J. (2009). Sleep in children with chronic illness, and the relation to emotional and behavioral problems—a population-based study. *Journal of Pediatric Psychology, 34*(6), 665–670.

Ivanenko, A., Barnes, M. E., Crabtree, V. M., & Gozal, D. (2004). Psychiatric symptoms in children with insomnia referred to a pediatric sleep medicine center. *Sleep Medicine, 5*(3), 253–259.

Johnson, C. M. (1991). Infant and toddler sleep: A telephone survey of parents in one community. *Journal of Devopmental & Behavioral Pediatrics, 12*(2), 108–114.

Johnson, E. O., & Breslau, N. (2001). Sleep problems and substance use in adolescence. *Drug and Alcohol Dependence, 64*(1), 1–7.

Kataria, S., Swanson, M. S., & Trevathan, G. E. (1987). Persistence of sleep disturbances in preschool children. *Journal of Pediatrics, 110*(4), 642–646.

Kazak, A. E. (1989). Families of chronically ill children: A systems and social-ecological model of adaptation and challenge. *Journal of Consulting and Clinical Psychology, 57*(1), 25–30.

Landau, Y. E., Bar-Yishay, O., Greenberg-Dotan, S., Goldbart, A. D., Tarasiuk, A., & Tal, A. (2012). Impaired behavioral and neurocognitive function in preschool children with obstructive sleep apnea. *Pediatric Pulmonology, 47*(2), 180–188.

LaPlant, M. M., Adams, B. S., Haftel, H. M., & Chervin, R. D. (2007). Insomnia and quality of life in children referred for limb pain. *Journal of Rheumatology, 34*(12), 2486–2490.

Levy, D., Gray-Donald, K., Leech, J., Zvagulis, I., & Pless, I. B. (1986). Sleep patterns and problems in adolescents. *Journal of Adolescent Health Care, 7*(6), 386–389.

Lewandowski, A. S., Palermo, T. M., De la Motte, S., & Fu, R. (2010). Temporal daily associations between pain and sleep in adolescents with chronic pain versus healthy adolescents. Pain, *151*, 220–225.

Lewandowski, A. S., Toliver-Sokol, M., & Palermo, T. M. (2011). Evidence-based review of subjective pediatric sleep measures. *Journal of Pediatric Psychology, 36*(7), 780–793.

Lewandowski, A. S., Ward, T. M., & Palermo, T. M. (2011). Sleep problems in children and adolescents with common medical conditions. *Pediatric Clinics of North America, 58*(3), 699–713.

Lewin, D. S., & Dahl, R. E. (1999). Importance of sleep in the management of pediatric pain. *Journal of Developmental & Behavioral Pediatrics, 20*(4), 244–252.

Lewin, D. S., Rosen, R. C., England, S. J., & Dahl, R. E. (2002). Preliminary evidence of behavioral and cognitive sequelae of obstructive sleep apnea in children. *Sleep Medicine, 3*(1), 5–13.

Long, A. C., Krishnamurthy, V., & Palermo, T. M. (2008). Sleep disturbances in school-age children with chronic pain. *Journal of Pediatric Psychology, 33*(3), 258–268.

McGrath, P. J., Walco, G. A., Turk, D. C., Dworkin, R. H., Brown, M. T., Davidson, K., et al. (2008). Core outcome domains and measures for pediatric acute and chronic/recurrent pain clinical trials: PedIMMPACT recommendations. *Journal of Pain, 9*(9), 771–783.

Meltzer, L. J., & Mindell, J. A. (2006). Sleep and sleep disorders in children and adolescents. *Psychiatric Clinics of North America, 29*(4), 1059–1076; abstract x.

Meltzer, L. J., & Montgomery-Downs, H. E. (2011). Sleep in the family. *Pediatric Clinics of North America, 58*(3), 765–774.

Meltzer, L. J., Montgomery-Downs, H. E., Insana, S. P., & Walsh, C. M. (2012). Use of actigraphy for assessment in pediatric sleep research. *Sleep Medicine Reviews, 16*(5), 463–475.

Milan, M. A., Mitchell, Z. P., Berger, M. I., Pierson, D. F. (1981). Positive routines: A rapid alternative to extinction for elimination of bedtime tantrum behavior. *Child Behavior Therapy, 3*, 13–25.

Mindell, J. (1997). *Sleeping Through the Night: How Infants, Toddlers, and Their Parents Can Get a Good Night's Sleep.* New York: Collins.

Mindell, J. A. (1993). Sleep disorders in children. *Health Psychology, 12*(2), 151–162.

Mindell, J. A. (1999). Empirically supported treatments in pediatric psychology: Bedtime refusal and night wakings in young children. *Journal of Pediatric Psychology, 24*(6), 465–481.

Mindell, J. A., Kuhn, B., Lewin, D. S., Meltzer, L. J., & Sadeh, A. (2006). Behavioral treatment of bedtime problems and night wakings in infants and young children. *Sleep, 29*(10), 1263–1276.

Morgenthaler, T. I., Owens, J., Alessi, C., Boehlecke, B., Brown, T. M., Coleman, J., Jr.,et al. (2006). Practice parameters for behavioral treatment of bedtime problems and night wakings in infants and young children. *Sleep, 29*(10), 1277–1281.

Morrison, D. N., McGee, R., & Stanton, W. R. (1992). Sleep problems in adolescence. *Journal of the American Academy of Child and Adolescent Psychiatry, 31*(1), 94–99.

Ohayon, M. M., Caulet, M., & Lemoine, P. (1998). Comorbidity of mental and insomnia disorders in the general population. *Comprehensive Psychiatry, 39*(4), 185–197.

Owens, J., & Palermo, T. (2008). Introduction to the special issue: Sleep in children with neurodevelopmental and psychiatric disorders. *Journal of Pediatric Psychology, 33*(4), 335–338.

Owens, J. A., Spirito, A., & McGuinn, M. (2000). The Children's Sleep Habits Questionnaire (CSHQ): Psychometric properties of a survey instrument for school-aged children. *Sleep, 23*(8), 1043–1051.

Owens, J. A., Spirito, A., McGuinn, M., & Nobile, C. (2000). Sleep habits and sleep disturbance in elementary school-aged children. *Journal of Developmental & Behavioral Pediatrics, 21*(1), 27–36.

Paine, S., & Gradisar, M. (2011). A randomised controlled trial of cognitive-behaviour therapy for behavioural insomnia of childhood in school-aged children. *Behaviour Research and Therapy, 49*(6–7), 379–388.

Palermo, T. M., & Kiska, R. (2005). Subjective sleep disturbances in adolescents with chronic pain: Relationship to daily functioning and quality of life. *Journal of Pain, 6*(3), 201–207.

Palermo, T. M., Toliver-Sokol, M., Fonareva, I., & Koh, J. L. (2007). Objective and subjective assessment of sleep in adolescents with chronic pain compared to healthy adolescents. *Clinical Journal of Pain, 23*(9), 812–820.

Palermo, T. M., Fonareva, I., & Janosy, N. R. (2008). Sleep quality and efficiency in adolescents with chronic pain: Relationship with activity limitations and health-related quality of life. *Behavioral Sleep Medicine, 6*(4), 234–250.

Palermo, T. M., & Owens, J. (2008). Introduction to the special issue: Sleep in pediatric medical populations. *Journal of Pediatric Psychology, 33*(3), 227–231.

Palermo, T. M., Wilson, A. C., Lewandowski, A. S., Toliver-Sokol, M., & Murray, C. B. (2011). Behavioral and psychosocial factors associated with insomnia in adolescents with chronic pain. *Pain, 152*(1), 89–94.

Piazza, C. C., & Fisher, W. (1991a). A faded bedtime with response cost protocol for treatment of multiple sleep problems in children. *Journal of Applied Behavioral Analysis, 24*(1), 129–140.

Piazza, C. C., & Fisher, W. W. (1991b). Bedtime fading in the treatment of pediatric insomnia. *Journal of Behavior Therapy and Experimental Psychiatry, 22*(1), 53–56.

Piazza, C. C., Fisher, W., & Moser, H. (1991). Behavioral treatment of sleep dysfunction in patients with the Rett syndrome. *Brain and Development, 13*(4), 232–237.

Piazza, C. C., Fisher, W. W., & Sherer, M. (1997). Treatment of multiple sleep problems in children with developmental disabilities: Faded bedtime with response cost versus bedtime scheduling. *Developmental Medicine & Child Neurology, 39*(6), 414–418.

Pollock, J. I. (1992). Predictors and long-term associations of reported sleeping difficulties in infancy. *Journal of Reproductive and Infant Psychology, 10*(3), 151–168.

Rapoff, M. A., Christophersen, E. R., & Rapoff, K. E. (1982). The management of common childhood bedtime problems by pediatric nurse practitioners. *Journal of Pediatric Psychology, 7*(2), 179–196.

Redline, S., Amin, R., Beebe, D., Chervin, R. D., Garetz, S. L., Giordani, B., et al. (2011). The Childhood Adenotonsillectomy Trial (CHAT): Rationale, design, and challenges of a randomized controlled trial evaluating a standard surgical procedure in a pediatric population. *Sleep, 34*(11), 1509–1517.

Richman, N. (1981). A community survey of characteristics of one- to two- year-olds with sleep disruptions. *Journal of the American Academy of Child Psychiatry, 20*(2), 281–291.

Roberts, R. E., Lee, E. S., Hemandez, M., & Solari, A. C. (2004). Symptoms of insomnia among adolescents in the lower Rio Grande Valley of Texas. *Sleep, 27*(4), 751–760.

Roberts, R. E., Roberts, C. R., & Duong, H. T. (2008). Chronic insomnia and its negative consequences for health and functioning of adolescents: A 12-month prospective study. *Journal of Adolescent Health, 42*(3), 294–302.

Sadeh, A., Lavie, P., Scher, A., Tirosh, E., & Epstein, R. (1991). Actigraphic home-monitoring sleep-disturbed and control infants and young children: A new method for pediatric assessment of sleep-wake patterns. *Pediatrics, 87*(4), 494–499.

Sadeh, A. & Anders, T. F. (1993). Infant sleep problems: Origins, assessment, interventions. *Infant Mental Health Journal, 14*(1), 17–34.

Sadeh, A., Hauri, P. J., Kripke, D. F., & Lavie, P. (1995). The role of actigraphy in the evaluation of sleep disorders. *Sleep, 18*(4), 288–302.

Sadeh, A., & Acebo, C. (2002). The role of actigraphy in sleep medicine. *Sleep Medicine Reviews, 6*(2), 113–124.

Sadeh, A., Gruber, R., & Raviv, A. (2002). Sleep, neurobehavioral functioning, and behavior problems in school-age children. *Child Development, 73*(2), 405–417.

Sadeh, A., Gruber, R., & Raviv, A. (2003). The effects of sleep restriction and extension on school-age children: What a difference an hour makes. *Child Development, 74*(2), 444–455.

Sadeh, A. (2004). A brief screening questionnaire for infant sleep problems: Validation and findings for an Internet sample. *Pediatrics, 113*(6), e570–e577.

Sivertsen, B., Posserud, M. B., Gillberg, C., Lundervold, A. J., & Hysing, M. (2012). Sleep problems in children with autism spectrum problems: A longitudinal population-based study. *Autism, 16*(2), 139–150.

Smedje, H., Broman, J. E., & Hetta, J. (2001). Associations between disturbed sleep and behavioural difficulties in 635 children aged six to eight years: A study based on parents' perceptions. *European Child & Adolescent Psychiatry, 10*(1), 1–9.

Tarasiuk, A., Greenberg-Dotan, S., Simon-Tuval, T., Freidman, B., Goldbart, A. D., Tal, A., & Reuveni, H. (2007). Elevated morbidity and health care use in children with obstructive sleep apnea syndrome. *American Journal of Respiratory and Critical Care Medicine, 175*, 55–61.

Vriend, J. L., Corkum, P. V., Moon, E. C., & Smith, I. M. (2011). Behavioral interventions for sleep problems in children with autism spectrum disorders: Current findings and future directions. *Journal of Pediatric Psychology, 36*(9), 1017–1029.

Weissbluth, M. (1987). *Healthy Sleep Habits, Happy Child.* New York: Random House.

Wolfson, A. R., & Carskadon, M. A. (1998). Sleep schedules and daytime functioning in adolescents. *Child Development, 69*(4), 875–887.

Wolfson, A. R., Carskadon, M. A., Acebo, C., Seifer, R., Fallone, G., Labyak, S. E., & Martin, J. L. (2003). Evidence for the validity of a sleep habits survey for adolescents. *Sleep, 26*(2), 213–216.

Wolfson, A. R., Spaulding, N. L., Dandrow, C., & Baroni, E. M. (2007). Middle school start times: The importance of a good night's sleep for young adolescents. *Behavioral Sleep Medicine, 5*(3), 194–209.

CHAPTER 4

Developmental Science in the Study of Sleep

Angela D. Staples *and* John E. Bates

Abstract

Developmental research has typically focused on daytime behaviors. However, the burgeoning interest in the role of sleep in the development of cognitive, social, emotional, academic, and health outcomes (Beebe, 2006; Beebe & Gozal, 2002; Carskadon, Acebo, & Jenni, 2004; Ednick et al., 2009; 2009; El-Sheikh, 2011; Ohayon, Carskadon, Guilleminault, & Vitiello, 2004; Sadeh, Raviv, & Gruber, 2000) calls for a consideration of sleep as a developmental process that co-occurs, co-regulates, and is causally linked with other developmental processes. This chapter discusses what it means to consider sleep from a developmental perspective. We hope this chapter will be useful for both developmental researchers who want to consider sleep as a variable of interest and for sleep researchers who want to take a more developmental approach to understanding sleep as a behavior that undergoes dramatic change from infancy through adolescence. The chapter is organized around three questions. First, what does it mean to have a developmental perspective? Second, how does one approach the study of sleep from a developmental perspective? Finally, how do we incorporate the study of sleep into the study of other areas of development?

Key Words: developmental science, sleep, developmental systems

Introduction

> "Sleep, in its ubiquity, seeming nonsociality, apparent universality, and presumed biologically driven uniformity, has been overlooked [by anthropology] as a background variable" (Worthman & Melby, 2002, p. 69).

Although sleep is universal and certainly biologically driven to some extent, research on sleep and sleep-related behaviors has begun to define the ways in which sleep is social, is influenced by forces other than biology, and varies between people as well as across the lifespan. This chapter discusses what it means to consider sleep from a developmental perspective. We hope this chapter will be useful for both developmental researchers who want to consider sleep as a variable of interest and for sleep researchers who want to take a more developmental approach to understanding sleep. The chapter is organized around three questions. First, what does it mean to have a developmental perspective? Second, how does one approach the study of sleep from a developmental perspective? Finally, how do we incorporate the study of sleep into the study of other areas of development?

Developmental Perspective

> "Major concerns of the developmental orientation are understanding when and how behavioral changes occur and the potential in development for optimal adaptations" (Cairns, Costello, & Elder, 2001, p. 228).

The central question that separates developmental research from other areas of research is the quest to understand how both change and continuity occur. Broadly speaking, developmental science is concerned with understanding the process of human development over the course of the lifespan. How is it that an infant transitions from crawling to walking? How do infants' vowel and vowel consonant sounds play a role in the development of language? How do children develop skills for regulating their attention, emotion, and behavior? How do adolescents form their identities? It is not enough to merely list a sequence of milestones, for example to say that 6-month-olds do not walk and 12-month-olds walk. Developmental science strives to understand and quantify the conditions that promote or hinder qualitative and quantitative shifts in development across the lifespan. In other words, it seeks to understand *process* in both change and continuity.

Developmental science, like other areas of science, has become increasingly multidisciplinary in its approach to understanding the process of development. Today, researchers from the areas of developmental psychology, pediatrics, clinical and educational psychology, psychiatry, biology, neuroscience, sociology, and epidemiology work together on a wide variety of research topics. The broad, multidisciplinary field of developmental psychopathology (Cicchetti, 2006), which seeks to integrate multiple levels of organization from biology to social systems, as well as to consider both typical and atypical development, is a dominant example of how developmental science has been growing. Along with the increased emphasis on interdisciplinary research, theories of development are evolving to link changes that occur on time scales from the millisecond (e.g., neuronal activity), hourly (e.g., cellular activity), daily (e.g., cortisol fluctuation), yearly (e.g., mastering addition or calculus), or lifespan (e.g., identity, interpersonal relationships) with other facets of life such as family stress, health problems, school settings, and neighborhood quality.

To impose some structure on the vast diversity of developmental phenomena, we turn to the systems theories of Ford and Lerner (1992), Bronfenbrenner and Morris (2006), Fogel (1993), and Thelen and Smith (1994) among others. Each of these theorists provides a slightly different emphasis on how to approach development from a systems perspective. For example, Ford and Lerner emphasize the lifespan perspective and use systems terminology to target qualitative changes in development (Keller, 2005). In contrast, the systems approaches advocated by Thelen and Smith (1994) and colleagues (see Adolph & Robinson, 2008; Simmering & Spencer, 2008; Spencer, Perone, & Buss, 2011) as well as van Geert and colleagues (Steenbeek, 2007; van Geert, 2011) emphasize rigorous mathematical quantification of change processes that are biologically plausible. Adding to the complexity, Bronfenbrenner urges consideration of the nested, interconnected systems in which development occurs through the framework of studying process, person, context, and time (Bronfenbrenner & Morris, 2006). Together, these systems perspectives challenge developmental researchers to consider continuity and change processes that occur within, between, and among individuals.

Further complexity, beyond multiple time scales and multiple, nested systems, comes from considering individual differences in how people respond to similar situations at similar points in development (Rothbart & Bates, 2006). To any given situation, different people bring different emotional or motivational tendencies, as well as different self-regulatory tendencies. These differences derive at least in part from early-appearing, biologically based, relatively stable traits that we call *temperament* or *basic personality* (Rothbart & Bates, 2006). However, individuals also change due a variety of factors including learning, biological development, and changes in environments (Patterson, Reid, & Dishion, 1992).

We think processes involving sleep can and should be considered in relation to the various components of the general systems models mentioned. The level at which one tackles various components of the system (e.g., neurological, behavioral, cultural) will be largely determined by the phenomena under study and the particular research question. For example, several studies have linked biological fluctuations in cortisol and napping in preschool children (Ward, Gay, Alkon, Anders, & Lee, 2008; Watamura, Donzella, Kertes, & Gunnar, 2004; Watamura, Kryzer, & Robertson, 2008). El-Sheikh and colleagues have extended the biological-sleep link to also include measures of physiological responding as well as family processes (El-Sheikh & Buckhalt, 2005; El-Sheikh & Erath, 2011; El-Sheikh, Buckhalt, Mize, & Acebo, 2006). There have even been studies of sleep in adulthood using computational models of the regulation of sleep–wake cycles, sleep deprivation and sustained attention, sleep and neurobehavioral performance, and the effects of fatigue on learning (Gonzalez, Best, Healy, & Kole, 2011; Gunzelmann, Gross, Gluck, & Dinges, 2009; Klerman & Hilaire, 2007; Postnova, Voigt, & Braun, 2009). Although these studies share the commonality of considering multiple system levels, much more research is needed to link multiple systems to intra- and inter-individual development.

Studying Sleep Developmentally

To study sleep developmentally requires a shift in theoretical perspective, different methods of data collection, and the addition of statistical methods designed to detect and explain processes of change. Sleep is a complex developmental phenomenon (van Geert, 2011) that undergoes periods of rapid change (e.g., shifting the longest sleep period to occur at night in the first weeks of life) and periods of stability. Much of the work done on changes in sleep across the lifespan has been through comparing age-group averages on sleep measures. From this research a clear picture is emerging of normative changes in sleep with consolidation of sleep into a single nighttime period by age five, a reduction in the number, frequency, and duration of nighttime awakenings, and considerable stability in the average amounts of nighttime sleep from toddlerhood through childhood (Staples & Bates, 2011). For example, in a prospective longitudinal study beginning at age one and continuing annually through age ten, parents reported child bedtimes, rise times, and amount of sleep during the day (Jenni, Molinari, Caflisch, & Largo, 2007). Similar to the charts used by pediatricians to track height and weight, there was a corresponding pattern of long-term rank order stability, in which children who slept less at one year of age tended to also sleep less through ten years of age. Although this type of research is a good example of a developmental approach to documenting normative patterns of sleep, there remain substantial questions—developmental questions—about *how* these changes occur, *why* these changes occur, and the consequences of these changes for other areas of development.

One area where there is progress in the study of normative changes of sleep and its possible consequences is in the area of slow wave sleep. Ringli and Huber (2011) provide an account of this area of research, the details of which are beyond the scope of this chapter. In brief, changes in slow wave sleep coincide with changes in synaptic density to such a strong degree that changes in slow wave sleep are hypothesized to occur because of changes in synaptic density. Furthermore, brain regions that show changes in slow wave sleep progress from the posterior to the anterior areas, which is consistent with increasing cognitive functioning from childhood through adolescence (Luna & Sweeney, 2004). It is also plausible that increases in synaptic density in early childhood followed by synaptic pruning in adolescence are influenced by the child's environment (e.g., nutrition, learning, family stress). It appears likely that there is a reciprocal relation between neurological development, developmental changes in sleep architecture, and contextual factors such as familial, social, and educational environments. Ultimately, developmental research that considers changes in slow wave sleep along with other measures such as cognition, language, and attention, may provide information about *why* we sleep and how sleep is related to and/or plays a causal role in development more broadly.

Another area that benefits from a developmental perspective is the study of sleep problems. Along with normative changes in sleep from infancy through adolescence, there is a sizeable minority of children who develop and maintain behavioral sleep problems, including difficulty falling asleep, difficulty staying asleep, and experiencing daytime fatigue (Mindell & Meltzer, 2008). For example, a recent study from a large national sample reported 25% of children between the ages of 6 and 11 and 39% of children between the ages of 12 and 17 did not get adequate sleep one or more nights in the preceding week according to parental reports (Smaldone, Honig, & Byrne, 2007). In addition, Smaldone and colleagues (2007) reported that children and adolescents who were not getting adequate sleep were also more likely to have trouble in school, emotional problems, and health problems. However, the cross-sectional nature of this and other studies (for a review, see Staples & Bates, 2011) makes it hard to establish the causal directions of associations between sleep and daytime functioning. In addition, the definition of poor sleep was based on the previous week, which does not address questions about possible differences between the consequences of short- and long-term sleep problems.

It is likely that short, infrequent periods of poor sleep like those during a brief illness, will have little impact on longer-term development. However, chronic or long-lasting periods of poor sleep during childhood and adolescence may have developmental consequences. Evidence from a variety of studies with children from infancy through adolescence have shown that sleep problems are associated with slower academic gains, increased negative affect, and higher rates of problem behavior (Staples & Bates, 2011). This is particularly evident in studies linking sleep disordered breathing with poorer academic outcomes, increased inattentiveness, difficulty regulating emotions, and increased daytime fatigue (Beebe, 2011; Beebe, Ris, Kramer, Long, & Amin, 2010). These findings of association between sleep problems and academic and behavioral outcomes point to the need to understand the contexts in which sleep problems occur, are maintained, and change. However, to date, much of the longitudinal research linking sleep with later developmental outcomes leaves questions about the directionality, timing, and magnitude of the association between sleep and development. Although we might prefer to attribute the outcomes to sleep based on sleep restriction and extension experiments, a few of which have been done with children (Carskadon, Harvey, & Dement, 1981; Fallone, Acebo, Arnedt, & Seifer, & Carskadon, 2001; Randazzo, Muehlbach, Schweitzer, & Walsh, 1998, Sadeh, Gruber, & Raviv, 2003), without a developmental analysis we lack a firm basis for this. We think of most common behavior problems as representing a social system's failure to solve smaller conflicts, and we think that chronic sleep deficits could impair children's and parents' efforts to effectively resolve these more minor, "building-block" conflicts, for example through efficiently stopping a child's coercive behavior (Patterson, Reid, & Dishion, 1992). Sleep restriction studies suggest that sleep deficits impair executive functioning (Walker & Stickgold, 2006), which would make it harder to regulate impulses and solve parent–child conflicts.

To understand sleep from a developmental perspective, one must consider questions of stability and change *within* an individual alongside questions of differences *between* individuals. For example, children show relative stability in being short or long sleepers from ages one to ten; however, children who were born in 1974 slept longer on average compared to children born in 1986 (Iglowstein, Jenni, Molinari, & Largo, 2003). The relation between intra-individual stability in conjunction with cohort differences in the amount of sleep highlight the need to study sleep as an "event in a context" (Kagan, 2007). Children are developing at particular rates and in particular families and in eras that could be socioculturally distinct.

Sleep is often considered as a solitary, nonsocial event, but how children transition from wakefulness to sleep, where that transition happens, and what is done if the child awakens at night is decidedly social and shows cultural variation (see Super and Harkness, Chapter 9). For example, parents of infants in the United States place less importance on both regular bedtimes and regular bedtime routines when compared to parents in Italy (Wolf, Lozoff, Latz, & Paludetto, 1996). Parents of infants in Japan place greater importance on a regular bedtime routine, but not a regular bedtime, compared to parents in the United States (Wolf et al., 1996). Understanding the importance parents place on regular bedtimes as well as regular bedtime routines may shed light on the relation between bedtime schedules and the development and/or maintenance of sleep problems. There are also wide variations in where the transition from wakefulness to sleep occurs, with both bed-sharing and room-sharing depending on the child's age and cultural context (Owens, 2008). One implication is that sleeping behaviors that may be problematic for one family may not be a problem for another, partially due to cultural differences (e.g., bedtime resistance in the United States, nighttime awakenings in Japan; Wolfson, 1996). In terms of development, it is important to understand how cultural factors may influence parental expectations and practices surrounding sleep-related behaviors, which may in turn have consequences for the development of both typical and atypical sleep behavior as well as typical and atypical daytime behavior.

Another difference in sleep that varies both with age and culture are naps. The transition to a single period of nighttime sleep is viewed as a developmental milestone in the United States, with most children no longer napping by age five (Staples & Bates, 2011). However, in Iceland, most children are no longer napping by age three (Owens, 2004). This difference suggests that the transition to a single period of sleep is likely to be a product of both biological forces and cultural practices. For example, in the United States there are large differences in napping between European-American and African-American children, with European-American children ceasing naps at an earlier age than African-American children. If researchers only account for nighttime sleep between the ages of three and five, it would appear that African-American children are getting much less sleep than European-American children (Owens, 2004). However, if the entire 24-hour period is taken into consideration, there is no difference in the amount of sleep between African- and European-American preschoolers. Thus, it appears that sleep development takes place in a larger context that considers familial and sociocultural factors (El-Sheikh, 2011). However, follow-on questions concern how familial and cultural differences arise and what impact they might have on later development. For example, how does earlier or later consolidation into a single period of sleep affect the development of sleep behavior and/or the development of other behaviors such as self-regulation, attention, or memory? One could ask if children who stop napping earlier also show corresponding advances in other regulatory areas such as motor development, emotion regulation, attentional flexibility, or learning. And if such consequences are found, are they common across all children or do they depend on the child's age (e.g., large differences between ages three and five, but not later) as well as their larger sociocultural environments (e.g., association of continued naps with lagging regulation occurs only in contexts where napping violates age norms)?

Variations in sleep that are associated with particular times in history, locations, and cultures typify the notion of an "event in context"; studying sleep developmentally also raises the issue of "response in context" (Kagan, 2007), where the same apparent behavior may mask different underlying causes. For example, the reasons why a child takes a long time to fall asleep are likely to differ if the child is three (perhaps they had a late or longer nap than usual) or thirteen (perhaps they are ruminating about an upcoming test or an earlier social interaction). Sleep disturbances, such as nightmares, may have different consequences for daytime functioning in young children (and their parents) compared to adolescents. Additionally, the same apparent behavior may evoke different responses. Not all parents view nighttime awakening as problematic and therefore their responses may differ, which could result in different outcomes. For example, parents who viewed their infant's nighttime crying as a sign of distress were more likely to intervene compared to parents who viewed the behavior as age-typical and not problematic (Erath & Tu, 2011). Intervening during nighttime awakenings during infancy has been associated with maintenance of sleep problems into toddlerhood and early childhood (Mindell & Meltzer, 2008). The interrelatedness between parent beliefs, child behavior, and parental response highlights the need for a developmental systems approach that considers not only the behavior, but also the behavior and response within a larger context.

In order to study sleep in a developmental-systems way, ideally one would measure sleep on more than one occasion. This asks a lot from both researchers and participating families. Choices must be made about the type of sleep measurement (questionnaire, diary, actigraphy, polysomnography, etc.), the number of measurements (daily, monthly, annually), and the breadth and depth of sleep behaviors (e.g., physiological, behavioral; see Spruyt, Chapter 18, and Horne and Biggs, Chapter 16). Several of these issues are discussed in depth in Part Three of this volume. From a developmental perspective, one of the central issues concerns the number of observations and their spacing.

An inescapable fact of research employing multiple measures is that the number of measurement occasions and the time between occasions limits the scope of the type of change that can be observed (Adolph, Robinson, Young, & Gill-Alvarez, 2008). In the simplest case of two measurement occasions, the only type of change that could be observed is that of linear change. At the other extreme, say, daily measurements for a year, larger trends may be masked by short-term variability. Achieving the balance between capturing the shape of change, maintaining a reasonably accurate measurement of the behavior, and not subjecting participants to undue burden, is not a trivial task. A more complete treatment of the issues concerning developmental research can be found in Laursen, Little, and Card (2012). One method that has been successfully used to balance within-person and between-person variability is the use of the burst measurement design. In this method, data are sampled in short bursts (e.g., daily for several weeks) separated by longer periods (e.g., 6-month intervals). This approach provides, among other things, a more stable estimate of within-person level at each burst occasion, which can then been linked to a longer-term trajectory of change (or stability). For example, in a recent study we measured sleep behaviors over seven consecutive nights followed by a laboratory assessment, which is repeated three times over the course of a year. These burst measurement occasions allow us to answer questions about whether the quality/quantity of sleep the night before, or the average of these variables over the preceding week, is more strongly related to the laboratory measures. In addition, we are able to answer questions about the relation between persistent or intermittent sleep problems and development over the course of a year.

A related issue concerns change versus development (Raeff, 2011). Imagine a situation in which a child who is sleeping through the night experiences several nights of poor sleep due to an illness and then returns to the previous pattern of sleeping. In this example, the child's sleep certainly *changed*, but there was no *development* per se. In general, developmental change occurs when there is a movement toward a more advanced form of development. This is not to say that there are not periods of growth followed by apparent periods of regression. Indeed, motor, language, cognitive, and emotional development in early childhood all show evidence of high variability in behavior during developmental transitions from earlier to later phases (Adolph et al., 2008; Hollenstein, Granic, Stoolmiller, & Snyder, 2004; Lewis, Koroshegyi, Douglas, & Kampe, 1997; van der Maas & Molenaar, 1992). Our expectation is that if sleep were studied on a daily basis for a sufficient period of time, it would show similar patterns of high variability in children's sleep during the transition from two daily sleep periods to a single period of sleep occurring at night. Developmentally, then, measurements must be sufficiently dense to separate meaningful change from normal variations in behavior. Of course, the time scale of observation would depend on the particular question of interest.

It is also possible that sleep may show increased variability during development in other domains (e.g., motor, cognitive, language). For example, a child who is beginning to crawl may experience a period of sleep disruption due to increased motor activity after falling asleep. In this example, changes in sleep during the later part of an infant's first year may be normative but not necessarily developmental. To date, there have been a handful of studies demonstrating greater nighttime awakenings in infants who are crawling/walking compared to infants who are not crawling/walking (Scher, 1996; 2005; Scher & Cohen, 2005). However, since each infant was assessed at only one time point, the relation between motor development and changes in sleep patterns may merely coincide due to some other factor. For example, it may be that children who are more active during the daytime crawl earlier and are also more active at nighttime compared to their less active peers. When the needed longitudinal data are collected, causal developmental-process associations between motor development and changes in sleep may be discovered.

Integrating Sleep and Developmental Research

Part of framing the integration of sleep and developmental research begins with the types of questions that require a developmental approach in research design, measurement, and analysis. For example, are the age-related changes in slow wave sleep that have been observed in studies with between-person designs also observed longitudinally within person? What person, context, and time variables are associated with or play a causal role in the reduction of slow wave sleep? Are variations in slow wave sleep preceded or followed by periods of learning? For example, do children show changes in slow wave sleep relative to the academic calendar? Is the relation between learning and sleep architecture the same in childhood and adolescence? Is there a longitudinal association between motor development and sleep development? Is there a longitudinal association between self-regulation development and regulation of the sleep-wake cycle? Is the association between regulation and sleep bidirectional, reciprocal, constant during development, or changing in sync with other developmental processes (e.g., synaptic development, motor development, puberty)? Each of these questions calls for research that considers process, person, context, and time to some degree. Preliminary answers to some of the questions can come from cross-sectional, multi-age samples, but we see the need ultimately for longitudinal designs that untangle within-person variability from between-person variability.

Another aspect of blending of sleep and developmental research areas is to ground the work in a larger theoretical milieu. While developmental systems theories provide guidance on *what* to consider, other theories will need to be utilized to explain *how* sleep and daytime behaviors mutually or directionally influence each other. The specific mechanistic hypothesis that one chooses will depend largely on the level at which the behaviors are observed. To date, sleep has been considered as part of a larger regulatory system that operates at the biological (Carskadon et al., 2004), neurological (Ringli & Huber, 2011), cognitive (Walker, 2009), and sociocultural levels (El-Sheikh, 2011). Each of these system levels are inherently interrelated, simultaneously active, going through periods of change and stability, thus providing a complex picture of the ways in which sleep and daytime behavior are inexorably linked.

In our research on the development of self-regulation in toddlerhood, we have posited three possible mechanisms for the role of naturally occurring sleep deficits. First, sleep deficits can be viewed as stressors (McEwen, 2007; Weissbluth, 1989) that produce dynamics in cortisol and other stress hormone levels that, in turn, can influence cognitive processing of information (Blair, Granger, & Peters Razza, 2005). Chronic sleep deficits, like chronic stress in general, would produce abnormal stress hormone dynamics with negative implications for cognitive processing and thus for self-regulation. Second, sleep deficits can more directly produce difficulties in cognition that impair behavioral and learning processes. In Dahl's (1996) terms, sleep deficits produce desynchronization of neuronal communication between brain centers, which, in complex high-challenge situations such as preschool, might lead to dysregulated affect and behavior. And third, sleep deficits diminish consolidation of learning, except for negative affect material (Walker, 2009). Thus, in addition to experiencing cognitive processing deficits due to hormonal and neural-network disruptions, the sleep-deprived child may fail to acquire sufficient knowledge from daily experience, especially in relation to amounts retained from negative emotional experiences. Each of these mechanisms require measurement of somewhat different systems and it is likely that until developmental data are available on all of these levels, we will not have a complete picture of how sleep plays a role in daytime functioning.

Framing questions of sleep developmentally and having a theory of how they are likely to relate then leads to questions of what to measure. The issues regarding measurement of sleep mentioned previously also apply to the selection of developmentally sensitive measures—what, how often, in what detail. As is always true of measurement, the answers depend upon the question. If one is interested in the relation between bedtime routines and the development of behavioral sleep problems during the transition from crawling to walking, then a burst measurement design that includes a 7- to 10-day assessment of sleep with daily diaries and actigraphy repeated at 4- to 6-weeks intervals seems appropriate. If one is interested in the relation between sleep and the development of behavior problems, choosing the instrument to measure behavior problems will depend upon on how often the assessments are repeated. For example, the widely used the *Child Behavior Checklist* (Achenbach, 1991) will be useful for studies examining changes that occur at semiannual or longer intervals, whereas the *Eyeberg Child Behavior Inventory* (Eyeberg & Pincus, 1999) may be more useful for assessments happening at more frequent intervals. Ultimately, the selection of measures will play a large role in whether a particular study is able to detect developmental change. If the measure selected is insensitive to change during the assessment period, then researchers may incorrectly conclude that there is no relation between sleep and the outcome variable. In contrast, if the measure shows wide variability with repeated assessments, then researchers may incorrectly conclude there is a relation between sleep and the outcome variable if other relevant factors such as parenting or cognitive development are not also assessed.

Similar issues arise when developmental researchers assess sleep. Some measures of sleep may be less sensitive to important sleep behaviors than others. For example, parents tend to underreport the number of times their child awakens at night (Tikotzky & Sadeh, 2001). Also, parents may underreport the presence of a sleep problem if they consider their child's sleep behavior (e.g., night awakening) to be age-normative and transitory (Lam, Hiscock, & Wake, 2003). Sleep problems in childhood often occur in conjunction with other issues such as medical problems, developmental disorders, and psychological and social relationship problems. Primary sleep disorders, such as sleep disordered breathing are associated with attention, emotion regulation, and academic performance problems (Beebe, 2006). Several recent reviews demonstrate sleep problems are often higher in children with a wide variety of conditions such as ADHD (Cortese, Faraone, Konofal, & Lecendreux, 2009), autistic spectrum disorder (Cortesi, Giannotti, Ivanenko, & Johnson, 2010), asthma (Bandla & Splaingard, 2004), anxiety, and depression (Dahl & Harvey, 2007). We would encourage developmental researchers, particularly those using normative community samples, to include health-related measures to better account for sleep problems that may be primarily physiological (e.g., sleep disordered breathing) and distinct from those that are primarily psychological and behavioral (e.g., nightmares or irregular parent management of bedtime).

Summary

In general, we have approached this chapter by asking what would it mean to view sleep from the perspective of developmental science. This was initially challenging for us because of our difficulty in imagining how sleep could be viewed from any other larger theoretical context. At its core, developmental science is the study of change throughout the lifespan. Why and by what mechanisms sleep is critical for human survival remains an open question. What is clear is that variations in sleep are related to learning, memory, information processing, motor coordination, decision making, emotion regulation, neural development, and other biological processes. How these variations in sleep come to be, the conditions under which variations in sleep are maintained or changed, and the consequences of variations in sleep for development are but a few ways that a developmental systems approach to understanding sleep can be informative.

Exciting advances will happen when sleep and human development are simultaneously considered.

Sleep research has made enormous strides toward a truly developmental perspective since 1978, when most our knowledge about the role of sleep in daytime functioning was based on studies of young, healthy men (Horne, 1978). Since then, studies have focused on sleep loss in adolescence (Wolfson & Carskadon, 1998; Acebo & Carskadon, 2002; Carskadon et al., 2004; Laberge, Petit, Simard, & Vitaro, 2001), normative changes in sleep patterns (Carno, Hoffman, Carcillo, & Sanders, 2003; S. Ottaviano, Giannotti, Cortesi, Bruni, & Ottaviano, 1996; Palmstierna, Sepa, & Ludvigsson, 2008), and the continuity and change in sleep problems from infancy into childhood and adolescence (Anders & Keener, 1985; Ednick et al., 2009; Gaylor, Burnham, Goodlin-Jones, & Anders, 2005; Iglowstein et al., 2003; Jenni et al., 2007). In the next decade there will likely be significant strides in our understanding of why we sleep and how sleep is necessary for human development.

How we approach the challenges of measuring individuals over time, and how often the assessments are made, will determine much of what is learned about sleep and development. The suggestion to measure behaviors in more than one domain is to explicitly direct researchers to consider that development does not happen uniformly across all areas of behavior, that development is shaped by biological, psychological, and social factors, and that understanding development in one domain will not be complete until it is placed within a larger developmental context.

Future Directions

From the perspective of developmental systems theories, future research needs to:

- Measure multiple aspects of sleep (e.g., behavioral, physiological, health-related)
- Follow individuals over time
- Take repeated measurements sufficiently close in time before, during, and after a period of developmental change
- Measure variables in more than one domain (e.g., sleep, cognition)
- Measure person and situation variables that are hypothesized not to change during the period under study (e.g., temperament, personality, housing)

References

Acebo, C., & Carskadon, M. (2002). Influence of irregular sleep patterns on waking behavior. In M. Carskadon (Ed.), *Adolescent Sleep Patterns: Biological, Social, and Psychological Influences* (pp. 220–235). Cambridge: Cambridge University Press.

Achenbach, T. M. (1991). *Child Behavior Checklist for Ages 4–18.* Burlington, VT: Achenback System of Empirically Based Assessment.

Adolph, K. E., & Robinson, S. R. (2008). In defense of change processes. *Child Development, 79*(6), 1648–1653.

Adolph, K. E., Robinson, S. R., Young, J. W., & Gill-Alvarez, F. (2008). What is the shape of developmental change? *Psychological Review, 115*(3), 527–543.

Anders, T. F., & Keener, M. (1985). Developmental course of nighttime sleep-wake patterns in full-term and premature infants during the first year of life. I. *Sleep, 8*(3), 173–192.

Bandla, H., & Splaingard, M. (2004). Sleep problems in children with common medical disorders. *Pediatric Clinics of North America, 51*(1), 203–227.

Beebe, D., & Gozal, D. (2002). Obstructive sleep apnea and the prefrontal cortex: Towards a comprehensive model linking nocturnal upper airway obstruction to daytime cognitive and behavioral deficits. *Journal of Sleep Research, 11*, 1–16.

Beebe, D. (2006). Neurobehavioral morbidity associated with disordered breathing during sleep in children: A comprehensive review. *Sleep: Journal of Sleep and Sleep Disorders Research, 29*(9), 1115–1134.

Beebe, D. W., Ris, M. D., Kramer, M. E., Long, E., & Amin, R. (2010). The association between sleep disordered breathing, academic grades, and cognitive and behavioral functioning among overweight subjects during middle to late childhood. *Sleep, 33*(11), 1447–1456.

Beebe, D. W. (2011). Cognitive, behavioral, and functional consequences of inadequate sleep in children and adolescents. *Pediatric Clinics of North America, 58*(3), 649–665.

Blair, C., Granger, D., & Peters Razza, R. (2005). Cortisol reactivity is positively related to executive function in preschool children attending head start. *Child Development, 76*(3), 554–557.

Bronfenbrenner, U., & Morris, P. A. (2006). The bioecological model of human development. In R. M. Lerner (Ed.), *Handbook of Child Psychology* (6th Edition. Vol. 1, pp. 793–828). Hoboken, NJ: John Wiley & Sons.

Cairns, R. B., Costello, E. J., & Elder, G. H. (2001). The making of developmental science. In R. B. Cairns, G. H. Elder, & E. J. Costello (Eds.), *Developmental Science* (pp. 223–234). Cambridge: Cambridge University Press.

Carno, M.-A., Hoffman, L. A., Carcillo, J. A., & Sanders, M. H. (2003). Developmental stages of sleep from birth to adolescence, common childhood sleep disorders: Overview and nursing implications. *Journal of Pediatric Nursing, 18*(4), 274–283.

Carskadon, M., Acebo, C., & Jenni, O. (2004). Regulation of adolescent sleep: Implications for behavior. *Annals of the New York Academy of Sciences, 1021*, 276–291.

Carskadon, M. A., Harvey, K., & Dement, W. C. (1981). Acute restriction of nocturnal sleep in children. *Perceptual and Motor Skills, 53*, 103–112.

Cicchetti, D. (2006). Development and psychopathology. In D. Cicchetti & D. J. Cohen (Eds.), *Developmental Psychopathology* (2nd Edition. Vol. 1, pp. 1–23). Hoboken, NJ: John Wiley & Sons.

Cortese, S., Faraone, S. V., Konofal, E., & Lecendreux, M. (2009). Sleep in children with attention-deficit/hyperactivity disorder: meta-analysis of subjective and objective studies. *Journal of the American Academy of Child and Adolescent Psychiatry, 48*(9), 894–908.

Cortesi, F., Giannotti, F., Ivanenko, A., & Johnson, K. (2010). Sleep in children with autistic spectrum disorder. *Sleep Medicine, 11*(7), 659–664.
Dahl, R. E. (1996). The regulation of sleep and arousal: Development and psychopathology. *Development and Psychopathology, 8*, 3–27.
Dahl, R. E., & Harvey, A. G. (2007). Sleep in children and adolescents with behavioral and emotional disorders. *Sleep Medicine Clinics, 2*(3), 501–511.
Ednick, M., Cohen, A. P., McPhail, G. L., Beebe, D., Simakajornboon, N., & Amin, R. S. (2009). A review of the effects of sleep during the first year of life on cognitive, psychomotor, and temperament development. *Sleep, 32*(11), 1449–1458.
El-Sheikh, M., & Buckhalt, J. A. (2005). Vagal regulation and emotional intensity predict children's sleep problems. *Developmental Psychobiology, 46*(4), 307–317.
El-Sheikh, M., Buckhalt, J., Mize, J., & Acebo, C. (2006). Marital conflict and disruption of children's sleep. *Child Development, 77*(1), 31–43.
El-Sheikh, M. (Ed.). (2011). *Sleep and Development: Familial and Socio-Cultural Considerations.* New York: Oxford University Press.
El-Sheikh, M., & Erath, S. A. (2011). Family conflict, autonomic nervous system functioning, and child adaptation: State of the science and future directions. *Development and Psychopathology, 23*(02), 703–721.
Erath, S. A., & Tu, K. M. (2011). The parenting context of children's sleep. In M. El-Sheikh (Ed.), *Sleep and Development: Familial and Socio-Cultural Considerations* (pp. 29–47). New York: Oxford University Press.
Eyeberg, S., & Pincus, D. (1999). *Eyeberg Child Behavior Inventory* and *Sutter-Eyeberg Student Behavior Inventory.* Lutz, FL: Psychological Assessment Resources.
Fallone, G., Acebo, C., Arnedt, T. J., Seifer, R., & Carskadon, M. A. (2001). Effects of acute sleep restriction on behavior, sustained attention, and response inhibition in children. *Perceptual and Motor Skills, 93(1),* 213–229.
Fogel, A. (1993). *Developing through relationships: Communication, self, and culture in early infancy.* Chicago, IL: The University of Chicago Press.
Ford, D. H., & Lerner, R. M. (1992). *Developmental systems theory: An integrative approach.* Thousand Oaks, CA: Sage Publications.
Gaylor, E., Burnham, M., Goodlin-Jones, B., & Anders, T. (2005). A longitudinal follow-up study of young children's sleep patterns using a developmental classification system. *Behavioral Sleep Medicine, 3*(1), 44–61.
Gonzalez, C., Best, B., Healy, A., & Kole, J. (2011). A cognitive modeling account of simultaneous learning and fatigue effects. *Cognitive Systems Research, 11*, 19–32.
Gunzelmann, G., Gross, J., Gluck, K., & Dinges, D. (2009). Sleep deprivation and sustained attention performance: Integrating mathematical and cognitive modeling. *Cognitive Science, 33*(5), 880–910.
Hollenstein, T., Granic, I., Stoolmiller, M., & Snyder, J. (2004). Rigidity in parent-child interactions and the development of externalizing and internalizing behavior in early childhood. *Journal of Abnormal Child Psychology, 32*(6), 595–607.
Horne, J. A. (1978). A review of the biological effects of total sleep deprivation in man. *Biological Psychology, 7*(1–2), 55–102.
Iglowstein, I., Jenni, O., Molinari, L., & Largo, R. (2003). Sleep duration from infancy to adolescence: Reference values and generational trends. *Pediatrics, 111*(2), 302–307.
Jenni, O. G., Molinari, L., Caflisch, J. A., & Largo, R. H. (2007). Sleep duration from ages 1 to 10 years: Variability and stability in comparison with growth. *Pediatrics, 120*(4), 769–776.
Kagan, J. (2007). The limitations of concepts in developmental psychology. In G. W. Ladd (Ed.), *Appraising the Human Developmental Sciences: Essays in Honor of Merrill-Palmer Quarterly* (p.30). Detroit: Wayne State University Press, *Project MUSE.*
Keller, E. F. (2005). DDS: Dynamics of developmental systems. *Biology & Philosophy, 20*(2–3), 409–416.
Klerman, E. B., & Hilaire, M. S. (2007). Review: On mathematical modeling of circadian rhythms, performance, and alertness. *Journal of Biological Rhythms, 22*(2), 91–102.
Laberge, L., Petit, D., Simard, C., & Vitaro, F. (2001). Development of sleep patterns in early adolescence. *Journal of Sleep Research, 10*(1), 59–67.
Lam, P., Hiscock, H., & Wake, M. (2003). Outcomes of infant sleep problems: A longitudinal study of sleep, behavior, and maternal well-being. *Pediatrics, 111*(3), 203–207.
Laursen, B., Little, T. D., & Card, N. A. (Eds.). (2012). *Handbook of Developmental Research Methods.* New York, NY: Guilford Press.
Lewis, M., Koroshegyi, C., Douglas, L., & Kampe, K. (1997). Age-specific associations between emotional responses to separation and cognitive performance in infancy. *Developmental Psychology, 33*, 32–42.
Luna, B., & Sweeney, J. A. (2004). The emergence of collaborative brain function: FMRI studies of the development of response inhibition. *Annals of the New York Academy of Sciences, 1021*, 296–309.
McEwen, B. S. (2007). Physiology and neurobiology of stress and adaptation: Central role of the brain. *Physiological Reviews, 87*, 873–904.
Mindell, J., & Meltzer, L. (2008). Behavioural sleep disorders in children and adolescents. *Annals Academy of Medicine Singapore, 37*(8), 722–727.
Ohayon, M., Carskadon, M., Guilleminault, C., & Vitiello, M. (2004). Meta-analysis of quantitative sleep parameters from childhood to old age in healthy individuals: developing normative sleep values across the human lifespan. *Sleep, 27*(7), 1255.
Ottaviano, S., Giannotti, F., Cortesi, F., Bruni, O., & Ottaviano, C. (1996). Sleep characteristics in healthy children from birth to 6 years of age in the urban area of Rome. *Sleep, 19*(1), 1–3.
Owens, J. A. (2004). Sleep in children: Cross-cultural perspectives. *Sleep and Biological Rhythms, 2*(3), 165–173.
Owens, J. A. (2008). Socio-cultural considerations and sleep practices in the pediatric population. *Sleep Medicine Clinics, 3*(1), 97–107.
Palmstierna, P., Sepa, A., & Ludvigsson, J. (2008). Parent perceptions of child sleep: A study of 10,000 Swedish children. *Acta Paediatrica, 97*(12), 1631–1639.
Patterson, G. R., Reid, J. B., & Dishion, T. J. (1992). *Antisocial Boys: A Social Interactional Approach* (Vol. 4). Eugene, OR: Castalia.
Postnova, S., Voigt, K., & Braun, H. A. (2009). A mathematical model of homeostatic regulation of sleep-wake cycles by hypocretin/orexin. *Journal of Biological Rhythms, 24*(6), 523–535.
Raeff, C. (2011). Distinguishing between development and change: Reviving organismic-developmental theory. *Human Development, 54*(1), 4–33.
Randazzo, A. C., Muehlbach, M. J., Schweitzer, P. K., & Walsh, J. K. (1998). Cognitive function following acute sleep restriction in children ages 10–14. *Sleep, 21(8),* 861–868.

Ringli, M., & Huber, R. (2011). Developmental aspects of sleep slow waves: Linking sleep, brain maturation and behavior. *Progress in Brain Research, 193*, 63–82.
Rothbart, M. K., & Bates, J. E. (2006). Temperament. In N. Eisenberg, W. Damon, & R. M. Lerner (Eds.), *Handbook of Child Psychology: Social, Emotional, And Personality Development* (6th Edition, Vol. 3, pp. 99–166). Hoboken, NJ: John Wiley & Sons.
Scher, A. (1996). The onset of upright locomotion and night wakings. *Perceptual and Motor Skills, 83*, 1122.
Sadeh, A., Raviv, A., & Gruber, R. (2000). Sleep patterns and sleep disruptions in school-age children. *Developmental Psychology, 36*(3), 291–300.
Sadeh, A., Gruber, R., & Raviv, A. (2003). The effects of sleep restriction and extension on school-age children: What a difference an hour makes. *Child Development, 74(2)*, 444–455.
Scher, A. (2005). Crawling in and out of sleep. *Infant and Child Development, 14*(5), 491–500.
Scher, A., & Cohen, D. (2005). Locomotion and nightwaking. *Child: Care, Health and Development, 31*(6), 685–691.
Simmering, V. R., & Spencer, J. P. (2008). Generality with specificity: The dynamic field theory generalizes across tasks and time scales. *Developmental Science, 11*(4), 541–555.
Smaldone, A., Honig, J. C., & Byrne, M. W. (2007). Sleepless in America: Inadequate sleep and relationships to health and well-being of our nation's children. *Pediatrics, 119*, 29–37.
Spencer, J. P., Perone, S., & Buss, A. T. (2011). Twenty years and going strong: A dynamic systems revolution in motor and cognitive development. *Child Development Perspectives, 5*(4), 260–266.
Staples, A. D., & Bates, J. E. (2011). Children's sleep deficits and cognitive and behavioral adjustment. In M. El-Sheikh (Ed.), *Sleep and Development: Familial and Socio-Cultural Considerations* (pp. 133–163). New York: Oxford University Press.
Steenbeek, H. (2007). A theory and dynamic model of dyadic interaction: Concerns, appraisals, and contagiousness in a developmental context. *Developmental Review, 27*(1), 1–40.
Thelen, E., & Smith, L. B. (1994). *A Dynamic Systems Approach to the Development of Cognition and Action*. Cambridge, MA: MIT Press.
Tikotzky, L., & Sadeh, A. (2001). Sleep patterns and sleep disruptions in kindergarten children. *Journal of Clinical Child Psychology, 30*(4), 581–591.
van der Maas, H. L., & Molenaar, P. C. (1992). Stagewise cognitive development: An application of catastrophe theory. *Psychological Review, 99*(3), 395–417.
van Geert, P. (2011). The contribution of complex dynamic systems to development. *Child Development Perspectives, 5*, 273–278.
Walker, M. (2009). The role of sleep in cognition and emotion. *Annals of the New York Academy of Sciences, 1156*, 168–197.
Walker, M. P., & Stickgold, R. (2006). Sleep, memory, and plasticity. *Annual Review of Psychology, 57*, 139–166.
Ward, T., Gay, C., Alkon, A., Anders, T., & Lee, K. (2008). Nocturnal sleep and daytime nap behaviors in relation to salivary cortisol levels and temperament in preschool-age children attending child care. *Biological Research For Nursing, 9*(3), 244.
Watamura, S. E., Donzella, B., Kertes, D. A., & Gunnar, M. R. (2004). Developmental changes in baseline cortisol activity in early childhood: Relations with napping and effortful control. *Developmental Psychobiology, 45*(3), 125–133.
Watamura, S. E., Kryzer, E. M., & Robertson, S. S. (2008). Cortisol patterns at home and child care: Afternoon differences and evening recovery in children attending very high quality full-day center-based child care. *Journal of Applied Developmental Psychology, 30*(4), 475–485.
Weissbluth, M. (1989). Sleep-loss stress and temperamental difficultness: Psychobiological processes and practical considerations. In G. A. Kohnstamm, J. E. Bates, & M. K. Rothbart (Eds.), *Temperament in Childhood*, (pp. 357–376). Chichester, England: John Wiley & Sons.
Wolf, A., Lozoff, B., Latz, S., & Paludetto, R. (1996). Parental theories in the management of young children's sleep in Japan, Italy, and the United States. In S. Harkness & C. Super (Eds.), *Parents' Cultural Belief Systems: Their Origins, Expressions, and Consequences* (pp. 364–384). New York: Guilford Press.
Wolfson, A. R. (1996). Sleeping patterns of children and adolescents: Developmental trends, disruptions and adaptations. *Child and Adolescent Psychiatric Clinics of North America, 5*(3), 549–568.
Wolfson, A. R., & Carskadon, M. A. (1998). Sleep schedules and daytime functioning in adolescents. *Child Development, 69*(4), 875–887.
Worthman, C. M., & Melby, M. K. (2002). Toward a comparative developmental ecology of human sleep. In M. A. Carskadon (Ed.), *Adolescent Sleep Patterns: Biological, Social, and Psychological Influences* (pp. 69–117). Cambridge, New York: Cambridge University Press.

CHAPTER

5 Developmental Changes in Sleep: Infancy and Preschool Years

Kurt Lushington, Yvonne Pamula, James Martin, *and* John Declan Kennedy

Abstract

The early years of childhood are characterized by rapid advances in growth, cognition and behavior. It is also the period of the human lifespan most occupied by sleep with correspondingly rapid changes in the structure, organization and regulation of sleep. The development and maturation of sleep during childhood is a dynamic process influenced by a range of physiological, genetic, biological, and psychosocial factors. Marked transformations are observed in sleep neurophysiology during the first few months of life, reflecting underlying central nervous system (CNS) growth and maturation while the emergence of circadian, homeostatic and ultradian regulatory processes modulate the timing and distribution of sleep-wake states. It is now well recognized that adequate sleep is essential for the health and well-being of children, with increasing evidence that sleep plays a crucial role in physical, psychological, and cognitive development. An improved understanding of normal sleep across the entire pediatric age range is therefore essential in understanding the role of sleep in child development and for the timely identification and treatment of sleep problems.

Key Words: sleep ontogeny, sleep EEG, circadian, infant, development

Ontogeny of Sleep EEG

> *"By age 2 years, the average child has spent 10,000 hours asleep and about 7,500 hours in all waking activities combined . . . by early school age, a typical child has spent more time asleep than in all social interactions, environmental explorations, eating, playing or any other waking activities" (Dahl, 1996, pp. 44–45).*

Despite the fact that we spend approximately one-third of our lives asleep, the functions of sleep remain largely unknown. Nevertheless, it is well recognized that adequate sleep is an essential requirement for normal physiological and psychological functioning and that sleep loss or disruption can result in a range of adverse health outcomes. The early years of childhood are characterized by rapid advances in growth, cognition and behavior. It is also the period of the human life span most occupied by sleep, with correspondingly rapid changes in sleep structure and organization. That early childhood cognitive and behavioral advancement parallels sleep development is not surprising given the substantial degree of central nervous system (CNS) growth and differentiation that occurs during this time (Casey, Tottenham, Liston, & Durston, 2005; Levitt, 2003; Segawa, 2006). However, sleep ontogenesis may be more than just a correlate of CNS development, as mounting evidence intimates reciprocal interactions between sleep and brain plasticity. In particular, sleep may play a role in two aspects of brain plasticity that underlie neurocognitive development: *(1)* brain growth and maturation and *(2)* memory consolidation (Graven, 2006; Maquet, Smith, & Stickgold, 2003; Miyamoto & Hensch, 2006; Peirano & Algarin, 2007; Sejnowski & Destexhe, 2000; Tarullo, Balsam, & Fifer, 2011).

Newborn infants spend approximately 60% of the 24-hour period sleeping, and while this percentage declines over childhood, children aged 4 to 5 years still sleep almost 12 hours a day (Galland, Taylor, Elder, & Herbison, 2012). Consequently, it is likely that a significant amount of early human development occurs during sleep (Sheldon, 1996). Conjecture of a more direct relationship between sleep and brain development was first advanced by Roffwarg, Muzio, and Dement (1966) following the unexpected finding that preschool children had more REM sleep than adults and the discovery of REM sleep in infants, suggesting that REM sleep had a functional role (see Sheldon, Chapter 2). Since this time, a growing body of evidence based on animal and human studies supports the view that sleep may play an important role in neural and cognitive development, with accumulating data suggesting that there may even be periods of brain development that are sensitive to sleep (Arditi-Babchuk, Feldman, & Eidelman, 2009; Aton et al., 2009; Bernier, Carlson, Bordeleau, & Carrier, 2010; Dionne et al., 2011; Frank, Issa, & Stryker, 2001; Holditch-Davis, Belyea & Edwards, 2005; Mirmiran & Ariagno, 2003; Mirmiran, Uylings & Corner, 1983; Ringli & Huber, 2011; Scher, 2005; Thomas et al., 2000; Touchette et al., 2007; Weisman, Magori-Cohen, Louzoun, Eidelman, & Feldman, 2011).

One of the putative mechanisms by which sleep may facilitate neural development is via endogenous stimulation arising from electroencephalographic (EEG) oscillations generated during sleep (particularly ponto-geniculo-occipital [PGO] waves, sleep spindles, and delta waves) or other sleep-related activities such as limb twitching (Blumberg, 2010; Denenberg & Thoman, 1981; Frank & Stryker, 2003; Jenni, Borbely, & Achermann, 2004; Marks, Shaffery, Oksenberg, Speciale, & Roffwarg, 1995; Roffwarg et al., 1966). The importance of endogenous neural activation in stimulating brain development is now well recognized, particularly with respect to neurogenesis, cell differentiation, neuronal migration, dendritic branching, apoptosis, and the formation of neural networks (Corner & Ramakers, 1992; Graven, 2006; Kilb, Kirischuk, & Luhmann, 2011; Penn & Shatz, 1999).

Given the above findings, there has been renewed interest in the development of sleep during infancy and childhood. A better understanding of the neural processes occurring during sleep, particularly during early human development, may elucidate and clarify the role of sleep in brain and cognitive development. The EEG provides a unique opportunity to study brain function and neural processes during sleep. Moreover, many aspects of the sleep EEG show predictable age-related changes, some of which are related to underlying brain reorganization and maturation, and thus the trajectory of sleep development can be used as a surrogate marker of CNS development and integrity (Feinberg & Campbell, 2010; Kohyama, 1998; Parmelee & Stern, 1972; Scher, 2011; Sheldon, 1996). The following section presents a brief outline of the general neurophysiological characteristics of sleep. This is followed by an overview of the development of the sleep EEG during infancy and early childhood.

The Electrophysiological Characteristics of Sleep

The human brain is distinguished by three main behavioral states: wake, non-rapid eye movement (NREM) sleep, and rapid eye movement (REM) sleep. These behavioral states are characterized by a recurring and relatively stable pattern of physiological and behavioral parameters that represent distinct modes of brain organization and function (Curzi-Dascalova, 2003; Parmelee & Stern, 1972; Prechtl, 1974). Conventionally, sleep–wake states are defined by the features of three major electrophysiological signals: the electroencephalograph (EEG), eye movements (electrooculargram, EOG) and chin muscle tone (submental electromyogram, EMG). In normal healthy children and adults these three parameters display a distinctive and concordant pattern of behavior that differs markedly between NREM and REM sleep, enabling highly reproducible sleep state identification. In the neonate and young infant, however, sleep structure and organization is comparatively immature and disorganized in the first few months of life as underlying brain structures and sleep regulatory systems are not yet fully developed. As a result, coherence between electrophysiological and behavioral parameters is quite variable in the neonatal period, making state identification more difficult. Additional parameters including behavioral observations and cardiorespiratory patterns are therefore used to assist in sleep–wake state identification. As the sleep EEG of newborns is also less differentiated than that of older children and adults, different terminology (*active sleep, quiet sleep*, and *indeterminate sleep*) is used to describe sleep states in early infancy. Over the first 3 to 6 months of life the characteristic features of NREM sleep gradually appear in the infant EEG, reflecting underlying CNS maturation and reorganization.

EEG Patterns

The EEG, when recorded from electrodes applied to the scalp, measures the summed electrical activity of numerous neurons, providing good temporal but poor spatial resolution. EEG activity is described by a number of standardized parameters including amplitude (or voltage, in microvolts), frequency (in cycles per second, hertz), and spatial distribution and patterning. EEG frequencies are conventionally grouped into four commonly used band widths: delta (<4 Hz), theta (4–7 Hz) alpha (8–13 Hz) and beta (>13 Hz). Distinct EEG waveforms and rhythms can also be seen over the background EEG activity and are described by their morphology and topography (the EEG electrode derivation in which they appear).

Additional topographical descriptors include whether EEG waveforms appear in homologous head regions (symmetrical versus asymmetrical) and, if symmetrical, whether their appearance is temporally synchronized. While at any given point in time the EEG comprises a mixture of frequencies, specific frequencies dominate particular sleep stages, and some EEG waveforms (e.g., sawtooth waves) are sleep-stage specific.

One of the most striking differences between wake and sleep is EEG activity. During wakefulness the EEG is characterized by relatively low-voltage, mixed-frequency activity, with alpha and beta (typically 18–25 Hz) frequencies dominating (Avidan, 2005). During relaxed wakefulness with eye closure, alpha rhythm (8–13 Hz) is very prominent, particularly in the occipital EEG derivations; this pattern is known as the *dominant posterior alpha rhythm.* In adults and older children, sleep onset begins with NREM sleep. Non-rapid eye movement sleep is further divided into four stages (1 to 4)[1] which approximate a continuum of sleep depth, with stage 1 being the lightest and stage 4 the deepest sleep and with arousal thresholds being correspondingly lowest in stage 1 and highest in stage 4 NREM sleep (Carskadon & Dement, 2011).

Stage 1 NREM sleep is characterized by a low-voltage mixed-frequency EEG background pattern with theta activity dominating. The EEG is generally slower than that observed during wake. Early in stage 1 sleep slow rolling eye movements may be observed, while vertex sharp waves may be seen in the latter stages. Stage 1 NREM sleep is a transitional sleep stage often following wake or gross body movements (Rechtschaffen & Kales, 1968). Stage 2 NREM sleep is characterized by two landmark EEG waveforms: sleep spindles and K-complexes. Sleep spindles and K-complexes show marked developmental changes during infancy and will be discussed in more detail later. In adults, sleep spindles appear as transient clusters of rhythmic activity with a mean frequency range of 12–14 Hz and often having a waxing and waning appearance. A K-complex is a transient biphasic EEG waveform comprising a large sharp negative EEG wave (upward deflection on the EEG trace) followed immediately by a slower positive (downward) component. K-complexes may appear spontaneously, in response to external stimuli, and may have sleep spindles as part of the complex (Rechtschaffen & Kales, 1968). Stages 3 and 4 NREM sleep are easily recognized by the appearance and predominance of slow, high-voltage delta waves (0.5–2 Hz). When combined, stages 3 and 4 NREM sleep are termed *slow wave sleep* (SWS). The very-high-voltage delta waves seen in SWS arise because the electrical activity of neuronal populations is very highly synchronized. Eye movements are generally absent in stage 2 and slow wave sleep, and chin EMG activity is reduced compared to wakefulness.

The EEG of REM sleep is very different from that of NREM sleep and is characterized by low-voltage, mixed-frequency (mostly theta) activity similar to that of wakefulness. Alpha activity is prominent in REM sleep but is typically 1–2 Hz slower than seen during wake (Rechtschaffen & Kales, 1968), and trains of sawtooth waves in the theta frequency range, having a characteristic triangular/serrated appearance, are commonly seen. Thus, during REM sleep the brain is significantly activated due to a high level of cortical activity. Two patterns of physiological behavior are seen in REM sleep: tonic and phasic. The tonic phase dominates REM sleep and is relatively quiescent, characterized by skeletal muscle atonia and the absence of eye movements. Phasic REM sleep is characterized by bursts of rapid, conjugate eye movements (REMS), transient muscle twitching, and irregularities in respiration and heart rate (Rama, Cho, & Kushida, 2005), while sleeping NREM and REM sleep periods alternate in a predictable cycle. The sequence, distribution and duration of sleep states across the night can be displayed visually as a sleep hypnogram. As with other aspects of sleep, sleep cycling shows marked developmental changes across the human lifespan.

The human sleep EEG undergoes significant ontogenetic changes, particularly in the first few years of life. In newborn infants the sleep EEG does not show the degree of differentiation and organization as described above but gradually develops into this pattern over the first 6 to 12 months. The following section broadly outlines sleep development in normal, healthy, term children from the time of birth to the early preschool years.

Development of the Sleep EEG

The structure and regulation of sleep in infants and children is significantly different from that of adults and in addition to showing a greater variety of EEG waveforms, infants and children often have higher EEG amplitudes (Scholle & Schafer, 1999). Furthermore, while sleep development in normal children follows an organized and predictable pattern of change, beginning during fetal development and continuing into adolescence, there is significant interindividual variation in the trajectory of sleep maturation (Hoppenbrouwers, Hodgman, Arakawa, Geidel, & Sterman, 1988; Sheldon, 1996). Thus variation is the rule rather than the exception. Sleep–wake states first emerge during fetal development. Cyclic periods of activity and rest become established after 24–28 weeks of gestation, with distinct cycling between REM-like and NREM-like sleep usually evident by 32 weeks of gestation (Curzi-Dascalova, 2003; Koos, 2008). Sleep–wake states in the premature infant will not be discussed here (see Andre et al., 2010; Vecchierini, André, & d'Allest, 2007), but have been well studied due to the extended period these infants spend in the neonatal intensive care unit where comprehensive and serial EEG monitoring is often performed.

The coordination and integration of physiological and behavioral activities by the CNS, including the generation of sleep, requires complex interactions between multiple interconnected neuronal networks. In the newborn infant neuronal networks are comparatively less developed, resulting in reduced concordance between the physiological and behavioral parameters that define behavioral states. With increasing postconceptional age physiological and behavioral variables become more coupled, leading to the emergence of more organized and sustained sleep–wake patterns. These developmental changes are believed to reflect maturation of the CNS, in particular the development of inhibitory and feedback control mechanisms in the brain (Parmelee & Stern, 1972). Maturation of sleep in the infant is reflected by the following features (Anders & Keener, 1985; Curzi-Dascalova & Challamel, 2000; Kohyama, 1998; Parmelee & Stern, 1972):

- increasing concordance among physiological and behavioral state parameters
- increasing quiescence and stability of several physiological processes (e.g., motor activity, respiration)
- the emergence of organized and stable between-state transitions
- increasing differentiation of the NREM sleep EEG including the disappearance and appearance of specific EEG waveforms and rhythms
- modification of the ultradian sleep cycle
- the emergence of a sleep circadian rhythm.

Sleep Organization and EEG Patterns in the Neonatal Period

The brain in developing infants is immature, and a degree of maturation is necessary before the classical behavioral states of NREM and REM sleep can be clearly differentiated. The sleep states in newborns, therefore, have some but not all the features of NREM and REM sleep. Three sleep states can be identified in the normal term infant: active sleep (AS), quiet sleep (QS) and indeterminate sleep (IS). While the precise mechanisms underlying the developmental progression of sleep are not yet fully understood, AS is believed to be the precursor of REM sleep while quiet sleep is believed to differentiate into the four NREM sleep stages (Anders, Emde, & Parmelee, 1971). Indeterminate sleep displays characteristics of both AS and QS and therefore does not unequivocally meet the criteria for either of these sleep stages. Within these behavioral states four major EEG patterns can be distinguished (Anders et al., 1971; Scher, 2006; Sheldon, 1996):

(1) A high-voltage, slow-frequency EEG pattern (HVS) dominated by continuous, moderately rhythmic delta activity and seen predominantly in QS.

(2) *Tracé alternant* (TA), a discontinuous EEG pattern seen only in QS. *Tracé alternant* typically comprises 3–8 second bilateral bursts of high-voltage, 0.5–3 Hz EEG waves that may have fast, low-voltage sharp waves superimposed. These high-voltage bursts are interspersed with low-voltage, mixed-frequency EEG activity of similar duration.

(3) A low-voltage irregular EEG pattern (LVI) seen in AS or when awake. The LVI pattern is characterized by a continuous, low-voltage, mixed-frequency EEG that is generally dominated by theta rhythms (especially when following QS) but

also contains significant amounts of delta activity (particularly if occurring at sleep onset).

(4) A mixed-frequency EEG pattern (M) that can be seen in wake and AS but is infrequently seen in QS. The mixed pattern consists of slow, moderate- to high-voltage delta activity and low-voltage mixed-frequency (theta, alpha, and beta) EEG components. The amplitude is usually lower than that seen in the HVS pattern.

Due to overlap of some of these EEG patterns across sleep–wake states and reduced concordance among state parameters (as discussed earlier) behavioral observations and cardiorespiratory patterns are important adjuncts to electrophysiological signals (EEG, EOG, submental chin EMG) in identifying behavioral states. Relevant behavioral observations include the type, pattern and frequency of eye movements, facial expressions, motor activity, and vocalizations (Thoman, 1990). With respect to cardiorespiratory behavior, irregularity in heart and respiratory rate and the presence of respiratory events such as sighs, apneas, and periodic breathing aid in sleep state identification (Anders et al., 1971; Sheldon, 1996).

Sleep in infants typically begins with AS, which can make sleep onset difficult to establish as the EEG of wakefulness and AS are not always easily differentiated. Sleep onset is therefore often behaviorally determined by the presence of sustained eye closure. The mixed (M) and LVI EEG pattern is seen in AS or, rarely, the HVS pattern, but TA does not occur (Anders et al., 1971). The background EEG voltage of AS is somewhat higher than seen in older children and adults (Hoban, 2005). Rapid eye movements (REMs) are usually observed, but slow rolling eye movements may also be present. Considerable motor activity occurs during AS (phasic periods), which is interspersed with periods of quiescence (tonic intervals). Facial movements commonly observed include sucking motions, twitches, smiles, frowns, and grimaces, and vocalizations (cries, whimpers and grunts) may be heard. Irregular and brief movement of digits and limbs is interspersed with more prolonged gross body movements. Body movements may be slow and writhing or sudden and jerky in nature and are more frequent and of longer duration than seen in older children and adults (Anders et al., 1971; Kahn, Dan, Groswasser, Franco, & Sottiaux, 1996; Sheldon, 1996). While muscle tone is reduced during AS there is frequent phasic activity and the pattern of the chin EMG can be quite variable and difficult to interpret, particularly if the infant is using a pacifier. During AS heart rate is quite variable and respiration is irregular, particularly during phasic periods. Episodes of tachypnea and bradypnea may be observed in addition to central apneas. Periodic breathing may also be present, particularly in preterm infants, although persistent periodic breathing in the neonatal period, or once the infant reaches conceptional age, suggests an underlying respiratory control problem (Sheldon, 1996). The generalized skeletal atonia which occurs during AS and a highly compliant chest wall seen in infants and young children can result in paradoxical breathing during AS.

Quiet sleep by contrast is characterized by an absence of body movements (except for occasional startles or twitches), regular and stable cardiorespiratory patterns, and an absence of REMs. The EEG shows the HSV, TA, or M pattern but not the LVI pattern (Anders et al., 1971). Indeterminate sleep does not unequivocally meet the criteria for AS or QS and can be seen interrupting an ongoing sleep state when the infant is aroused or occurring as a between-state transition (Anders et al., 1971; Curzi-Dascalova, 2003). Indeterminate sleep is more likely to occur when transitioning from AS to QS than when transitioning from QS to AS (Anders et al., 1971). There has been a tendency to disregard IS as little more than a transitional sleep state; however, IS represents a distinct and independent mode of CNS functioning (Curzi Dascalova, 2001) and excessive amounts or persistence of this sleep state in infancy may reflect a delay in CNS maturation (Anders et al., 1971; Gould, 1983; Ornitz, 1972).

Newborns spend approximately 15 hours of the 24-hour period sleeping (Galland et al., 2012), half of which is spent in AS. As stated previously the first sleep state typically seen in infants on entering sleep is AS, which is followed by a period of QS and then alternating episodes of AS and QS. The first episode of AS at sleep onset is often shorter than subsequent episodes (Roffwarg et al., 1966). Indeterminate sleep may or may not occur between episodes of AS and QS. Sleep is also punctuated by periods of wakefulness, particularly related to feeding. In newborns the transition between behavioral states is often quite rapid and the AS–QS cycle ranges between 30–70 minutes in duration (Scher, 2006; Sheldon, 1996).

Developmental Changes in the Sleep EEG During the First Twelve Months

During the first 3 months post-term, the sleep EEG gradually changes from the neonatal pattern to the infant pattern (de Weerd & van den Bossche, 2003). Two major changes in particular occur during this period: *(1)* the EEG begins to differentiate into the four NREM sleep stages and *(2)* the proportion of AS decreases. In normal term infants the *tracé alternant* pattern disappears between 3–4 weeks of age and is gradually replaced by high-voltage, slow-frequency EEG activity (Sheldon, 1996). Rudimentary sleep spindles emerge at around 4 weeks post-term but are often fragmentary and may be difficult to distinguish (Shibagaki, Kiyono, & Watanabe, 1982). Infant sleep spindles exhibit interhemispheric asymmetry and asynchrony (Sheldon, 1996) and have a different morphology (a spiky negative component with a rounded positive component), which gradually changes during the 9 months following birth (Jenni et al., 2004). By 8 to 12 weeks post-term, spindles are usually seen in most infants and are generally well formed, and this coincides with the emergence of a prominent peak in sigma activity in the EEG spectrum during QS (Ellingson, 1982; Jenni et al., 2004; Sankupellay et al., 2011; Sheldon, 1996). Spindle density and duration appears to be maximal at around 3 months of age with major developmental changes seen in topography, morphology, amplitude, and frequency over the first 12 months following birth (Dan & Boyd, 2006; Ellingson, 1982; Grigg-Damberger et al., 2007; Louis, Zhang, Revol, Debilly, & Challamel, 1992; Scholle & Schafer, 1999; Shibagaki, Kiyono, & Watanabe, 1982; Tanguay, Ornitz, Kaplan, & Bozzo, 1975). However, there is significant interindividual variation in development, and spindles may also show interhemispheric asynchrony up to 2 years of age (Dan & Boyd, 2006; Ellingson, 1982; Kahn et al., 1996). Sleep spindles are generated by synchronized activity of thalamocortical and thalamic reticular neurons (Destexhe, 2009), and the maturational changes seen in the first few months of life are believed to reflect developmental changes occurring in thalamocortical structures and in myelination and dendrite growth (Gould, 1983; Jenni et al., 2004; Louis et al., 1992). A reduction in spindle frequency and sigma activity has been reported in near-miss SIDS infants and infants at increased risk of SIDS (Gould, 1983; Guilleminault & Coons, 1983), while spindle abnormalities have also been found in children with CNS or neurodevelopmental disorders such as Down's syndrome (Sheldon, 1996; Shibagaki, Kiyono, & Watanabe, 1982; Shibagaki, Kiyono, Watanabe, & Hakamada, 1982). These findings may reflect delayed CNS maturation or more specific structural or functional abnormalities in the cerebral cortex or thalamus (Guilleminault & Coons, 1983; Gould 1983; Shibagaki, Kiyono, & Watanabe, 1982).

One of the most striking changes seen in sleep during human development is the marked decrease in AS/REM sleep. From birth through to adolescence there is an 80% reduction in REM sleep, most of which occurs during the first 5 years of life. In contrast, NREM sleep only declines by 25% (Roffwarg et al., 1966). The functional significance of this ontogenetic change has been the subject of much discussion (Garcia-Rill et al., 2003; Horne, 2000; Roffwarg et al., 1966). At conceptional term, AS comprises 50% of total sleep time which declines to between 35%–40% by 1 year of age (Anders & Keener 1985; Sheldon, 1996). This reduction in AS is paralleled by a concomitant increase in QS (Anders & Keener 1985; Hoppenbrouwers et al., 1988). In addition to the reduction in AS, sleep onset begins to gradually shift from AS to QS between 10–12 weeks post-term (Sheldon, 1996). The developmental changes in the distribution of AS and the proportion of AS to QS is sometimes viewed as an indicator of CNS maturation (Hoppenbrouwers et al., 1988; Ornitz, 1972). At both 6 weeks and 3 months of age, near-miss SIDS infants were found to have a significantly higher proportion of sleep onset via AS compared to control infants, which the authors concluded may reflect maturational delay or abnormalities in brain functioning (Guilleminault & Coons, 1983).

Three months of age appears to be a significant juncture for infant neurodevelopment, and the degree of sleep maturation at this time can be used as a surrogate benchmark for CNS organization (Sheldon, 1996). At 3 months post-term the EEG of QS has started to differentiate, and concordance between physiological and behavioral sleep–wake parameters is high (Kohyama, 1998). Coincident with these neurophysiological developments is the emergence during wake periods of attentive behaviors and social interactions. These maturational attainments are thought to reflect the development of inhibitory and feedback control mechanisms, particularly with respect to interactions between the brainstem and higher brain centers (Parmelee & Stern, 1972).

Significant changes in sleep organization and in the sleep EEG continue between 3–12 months post-term. Sleep gradually becomes consolidated into fewer but longer periods that occur mostly at night (Coons, 1987). Sleep onset is more common through QS after 3 months post-term, although episodes of AS onset can still be seen in normal infants up to 6–8 months of age (Sheldon, 1996). By 6 months of age the three major NREM sleep states (stage 1, stage 2 and SWS) can usually be identified in most infants. Over the course of the next 6–12 months the NREM EEG continues to become better differentiated, with changes in EEG amplitude and frequency enabling clearer delineation between stage 2 and SWS (Sheldon, 1996; Metcalf et al., 1971). Rudimentary vertex sharp waves can be seen in the neonatal EEG, and by 6 months of age they are generally well established and continue to undergo maturational changes in morphology, amplitude, frequency and duration throughout childhood, attaining the adult form by early adolescence (Grigg-Damberger et al., 2007; Sheldon, 1996). Clearly identifiable spontaneous K-complexes first appear in the infant EEG at around 6 months of age and undergo changes in morphology between the ages of 6 months and 2 years and again between the ages of 6 to 12 years (Metcalf *et al.*, 1971). Age-related changes are also seen in the frequency with which spontaneous K complexes are generated (Grigg-Damberger et al., 2007). The dominant posterior alpha rhythm emerges between 3–4 months of age and shows the following age-related increases in EEG frequency: 3–4 months: 3.5–4.5 Hz; 5–6 months: 5–6 Hz; 3 years: 8 Hz; 9–10 years: 9 Hz and 15 years: 10 Hz (Grigg-Damberger et al., 2007).

In summary, as the infant brain matures the relative amount of time spent in active sleep decreases while quiet sleep increases, and by the first year of life sleep has evolved into well-defined REM and NREM sleep (Louis, Cannard, Bastuji, & Challamel, 1997). In conjunction with the changes in quiet and active sleep, the amount of time spent asleep also decreases. Data from a large US survey suggests that sleep length decreases from up to 18 hours in newborns, to 14–18 hours in the first year of life, to 12–15 hours by the third year of life, and 11–13 hours by the fifth year of life (National Sleep Foundation, 2012). Much of this decrease is due to the reduction in active sleep. Sleep length and the distribution of active–quiet sleep demonstrate large interindividual differences and especially in the first year of life, with some newborns sleeping as few as 10 hours and others up to 18 hours per day, and active sleep accounting for as little as 30% and up to 70% of sleep time (e.g. Anders, Keener, & Kraemer, 1985; Iglowstein, Jenni, Molinari, & Largo, 2003). The preference for sleep length appears to remain consistent across childhood (Touchette et al., 2007) suggesting a genetic contribution to sleep length (He et al., 2009; Hor & Tafti, 2009).

Sleep EEG Development: One to Five years

Comparatively few studies have been undertaken to investigate sleep EEG development in normal children aged between 1 and 5 years. By 1 year of age sleep has attained a more mature pattern and changes in sleep architecture occur more slowly than seen in the first 12 months of life (Kahn et al., 1996; Sheldon, 1996). By 1 year of age the proportion of NREM sleep is greater than REM sleep, which is a reversal of the relationship seen at birth (Anders & Keener, 1985). The proportion of REM sleep continues to decline during early childhood, reaching the adult level of 20%–25% of total sleep time by 5 years of age (Sheldon, 1996). The distribution of NREM and REM sleep across the night changes, resulting in a preponderance of NREM sleep in the first third of the night and REM sleep toward the end of the night (Kahn et al., 1996). Sleep cycle length is approximately 60 minutes in duration at 2 to 3 years of age, which gradually increases to 90 minutes in duration by age five (Sheldon, 1996).

Changes in the sleep EEG are less prominent between the ages of 1 to 5 years. In general, background EEG frequencies are a little slower and EEG amplitudes are significantly higher than seen in adults (Scholle & Schafer, 1999; Sheldon, 1996). Prominent features of sleep–wake characteristics in early childhood are the EEG patterns of wakefulness and drowsiness, which are quite different compared to adults (Grigg-Damberger et al., 2007; Sheldon, 1996). Furthermore, a number of normal EEG patterns or variants can be seen during sleep in the pediatric age group that are not normally present in adults. These EEG patterns include anterior slow wave activity, hypnagogic hypersynchrony, hypersynchronous theta, post-arousal hypersynchrony, rhythmic anterior theta activity of drowsiness, and the frontal arousal rhythm. Discussion of these EEG patterns is beyond the scope of this chapter and the reader is referred to Westmoreland and Klass, (1990), Sheldon, (1996) and Grigg-Damberger et al. (2007) for a more comprehensive discussion.

Overview of Sleep Organization

The induction and maintenance of sleep is facilitated by multiple physiological and psychosocial factors. The most well accepted model for describing the regulation of sleep is Borbely's two-process model, where it is proposed that sleep propensity is dependent on the interaction between the (a) time spent awake (Process-S) and (b) time of day or circadian phase at which sleep is initiated (Process-C; Borbely, 1982). Process-S models the homeostatic drive that increases sleep need as a function of prior wakefulness, while Process-C models the cortically controlled circadian component that facilitates sleep at night and counteracts sleep during the day. The two-process model has been successfully used to predict sleep duration, sleep depth, and alertness based on timing and amount of prior wakefulness (Dijk & Lockley, 2002; Duffy, Kronauer, & Czeisler, 1996). It is thought that neuromodulating sleep-promoting substances that accumulate with increased wakefulness, such as adenosine, may underlie the homeostatic drive for sleep (Porkka-Heiskanen et al., 1997). Both the homeostatic drive for sleep and the dissipation of sleep pressure with sleep are greater in infants than adults. By contrast, the circadian influence on sleep is weaker in infants until relevant neural circuits reach maturity around 3 months of life (Rivkees, 2003).

Sleep and Process-S

The increased homeostatic drive for sleep and the dissipation of sleep pressure with sleep may partly account for the frequent cycling of sleep–wake bouts in infants and need for regular naps. Studies undertaken in older children and adolescents have revealed that sleep deprivation results in higher sleep pressure than that typically reported in adults (Jenni, Achermann, & Carskadon, 2005). The latter findings suggest that the homeostatic drive for sleep is higher in older children, and it is likely but untested that the response to sleep deprivation may be higher again in infancy. Indirect evidence for increased homeostatic drive for sleep in younger children is the high frequency of napping in that age group. A typical infant at 6 months of age may take two to three naps in a day of about 3–4 hours in duration, whereas by 12 months of age the typical infant may take two naps a day of 2–3 hours duration and by 18 months of age one nap during the day of about 1–2 hours duration (Acebo et al., 2005; Iglowstein et al., 2003; Sadeh et al., 1991).

Sleep and Process-C

The timing of sleep is regulated by the circadian system consisting of a biological clock and input and output pathways (see Crowley, Chapter 17). The "clock" component consists of specialized pacemaker cells located in the suprachiasmatic nucleus (SCN) of the anterior hypothalamus that oscillates with a periodicity slightly longer than 24 hours. This endogenous pacemaker facilitates the synchronization of internal body rhythms so that they are optimally timed with respect to each other. It also facilitates the synchronization of internal systems with the external environment such that an organism is optimally entrained to the day–night cycle. Animal studies suggest that the SCN regulates the timing and duration of sleep and wakefulness by facilitating the initiation and maintenance of wakefulness at night and by opposing a tendency to sleep that increases during the day (Gillberg, 1997). This "opponent model" of sleep/wake regulation is generally accepted for humans.

The phase of the circadian clock is synchronized to the day–night cycle by external time cues or "zeitgebers" (time givers). Apart from one exception, the circadian clock in humans is refractory to environmental, behavioral, or social cues, such as the timing of meals and rest/activity. The one exception is bright light, with the pacemaker cells differentially sensitive to light exposure at dawn and dusk (Duffy et al., 1996; Lowrey & Takahashi, 2000; Middleton, Arendt, & Stone, 1996). Light falling on the retinas is transduced via the retinohypothalamic tract to the SCN and other nonvisual brain regions (Edgar, Dement, & Fuller, 1993). As well as responsiveness to daylight, the SCN is sensitive to appropriately timed artificial bright light (Boivin, Duffy, Kronauer, & Czeisler, 1996; Czeisler et al., 1986; Duffy et al., 1996), thus making bright light exposure a useful tool for shifting phase in circadian-related sleep disorders (Czeisler et al., 1989). A high light intensity is thought necessary to shift phase, but exposure to normal room light has been reported to shift phase in young adults (Boivin & Czeisler, 1998), raising concerns as to the impact of excessive screen time and extended light exposure on sleep quality in children (Kohyama, 2011). When the phase-shifting response to light is plotted against the timing of light exposure, a characteristic phase-response curve (PRC) is produced (Honma & Honma, 1988; Minors, Waterhouse, & Wirz-Justice, 1991). The PRC to light has been plotted in adults but not in children. In adults who are normally entrained to the day–night cycle, exposure to bright light at dusk delays (i.e., shifts phase to a later time in subsequent cycles), while exposure at dawn advances (i.e., shifts phase to an earlier time in subsequent cycles), the circadian system. Between dusk and dawn is an inflection point separating the delay (dusk) and advance (dawn) portion of the PRC. The timing of the inflection point corresponds to the timing of the core body temperature minimum, approximately 0300–0500 h in entrained adults, and the closer the timing of the light exposure to the minimum, the greater the magnitude of the phase shift (Czeisler et al., 1989).

The effect of the circadian system on sleep–wake can also be studied by examining the response of an individual to the absence of entraining light, such as may occur naturally in the Antarctic winter and experimentally in specially constructed temporal isolation laboratories. Such studies have revealed that the circadian clock "free runs" with an endogenous rhythmic period (tau) greater than 24 hours (Czeisler et al., 1999). The slight discrepancy between the endogenous tau and the 24-hour terrestrial day permits for flexibility in clock timing but necessitates the daily resynchronization of the body clock with the external environment. As tau is longer than the length of a terrestrial day, the clock must be continually reset by light to maintain entrainment with the external environment; otherwise, with successive days it will drift progressively later in time or "free run."

The circadian system is not synchronized with the terrestrial day at birth. Indirect evidence from primate studies suggest that while the circadian system in human neonates may be sensitive to light (Hao & Rivkees, 1999), there is little evidence of a circadian rhythmicity in sleep–wake before 3 months of age (Meier-Koll, Hall, Hellwig, Kott, & Meier-Koll, 1978; Rivkees & Hao, 2000; Stern, Parmelee, Akiyama, Schultz, & Wenner, 1969). However, with neuronal development and exposure to the light–dark cycle, by 1 month of age wakefulness is greater during the day and sleep greater at night, and by at least 3 months of age, hormonal and sleep–wake cycles have begun to consolidate and show a regular 24-hour rhythm with characteristic peaks and troughs (de Weerd & van den Bossche, 2003; McMillen, Kok, Adamson, Deayton, & Nowak, 1991; Nishihara, Horiuchi, Eto, & Uchida, 2002) which remain stable until puberty (Kahn, Dan, Groswasser, Franco, & Sottiaux, 1996). The immaturity of the circadian system may explain the free-running rhythms observed in neonates with wake–activity plots revealing a progressive daily delay in the timing of the main sleep period, sometimes resulting in a reversal of normal sleep–wake timing with infants sleeping through the day but staying awake during the night (Kleitman & Engelmann, 1953; McGraw, Hoffmann, Harker, & Herman, 1999; Shimada et al., 1999; Weissbluth & Weissbluth, 1992). In addition to light–dark exposure, mother–infant interaction may further reinforce daily rhythm patterns and hence circadian rhythmicity (Ferber, Laudon, Kuint, Weller, & Zisapel, 2002).

In adults, sleepiness and hence the propensity for sleep also demonstrates a predictable circadian rhythmicity (Lack & Lushington, 1996; Lavie, 2001). Sleepiness gradually rises in the morning with a minor peak in the early afternoon (12:00–14:00 h), corresponding to the traditional siesta time, followed by a decline to a minimum in the early evening (19:00–22:00 h) (Carskadon & Dement, 1992; Monk, Buysse, Reynolds, & Kupfer, 1996). Sleepiness then increase throughout the evening to a major peak in the early morning (03:00–05:00 h), typically at the midpoint of the major nocturnal sleep period (Lack & Lushington, 1996). This pattern can be seen in the evolution of nap behavior from birth to early childhood with the establishment of a bimodal sleep pattern during daytime consisting of midafternoon and late evening sleeps, the midafternoon component of which, depending on culture practices, may be maintained until schooling is commenced (Iglowstein et al., 2003).

Sleep and Thermoregulation

The circadian rhythms of body temperature and sleep propensity are closely related. In adults, the two rhythms demonstrate an inverse reciprocal relationship (Lack, Gradisar, Van Someren, Wright, & Lushington, 2008), and of special note is that the magnitude of the pre-sleep increase in peripheral temperature and concomitant nocturnal decline in core body temperature is highly predictive of sleep onset and maintenance (Campbell & Broughton, 1994; Krauchi, Cajochen, Werth, & Wirz-Justice, 2000; Lushington, Dawson, & Lack, 2000; Van Someren, 2000). There is also extensive evidence that stimuli which raise core body temperature inhibit, while those that lower core body temperature facilitate, sleep (Bach et al., 2011; Krauchi & Deboer, 2010).

The relationship between the circadian rhythms of sleep and temperature are not well explored in infants. Nonetheless, available evidence suggests that by 3 months of age the circadian variation in body temperature coincides with the circadian variation in active sleep (Abe & Fukui, 1979; Glotzbach, Edgar, & Ariagno, 1995), with the core body temperature reaching a minimum about the midpoint of the nocturnal sleep period (Lodemore, Petersen, & Wailoo, 1992) and shifting to the last third of night, as in the adult, by 1 year of age (Glotzbach et al., 1995). It is likely that the emergence in infants of a robust core body temperature rhythm may facilitate sleep onset and maintenance. In support of this suggestion, there is preliminary evidence that lower core body temperature minimums are associated with longer mean sleep durations in 4-month-old infants (Lodemore, Petersen, & Wailoo, 1991).

Ultradian Rhythms

A third mechanism is also involved in the control sleep–wake behavior. Together with circadian variation, an ultradian rhythm (i.e., frequency < 24-hour) is also evident in many sleep parameters. Ultradian rhythms are evident at all levels of biological organization and are thought to provide the timekeeping for intracellular processes (Lloyd, 2008). An ultradian rhythm is evident in the cycling of NREM–REM sleep, which can be recognized from 4 to 6 weeks of age with cycles progressively lengthening from about 60 minutes at 1 month of age to 90 minutes by 5 years of age (Sheldon, 1996), with some groups reporting lengthening by 1 year of age (Hoppenbrouwers, 1992; Pace-Schott & Hobson, 2002). The sleep–wake rhythm itself also demonstrates ultradian variation. At birth, the sleep–wake rhythm cycles with a mean period of between 3–4 hours, but by 3 months of age a clear circadian sleep–wake rhythm has emerged (Meier-Koll et al., 1978; Peirano, Algarin, & Uauy, 2003).

Conclusion

During infancy and early childhood more time is spent sleeping than on any other activity. Congruent with all the other remarkable physical and behavioral changes that occur as a child grows and develops, sleep also undergoes striking developmental changes that are unparalleled in later adult life. The neurophysiological maturation of sleep is underpinned by structural and functional changes in CNS anatomy and physiology, while a complex interplay between physiological, biological, and psychosocial factors modulate sleep behavior. However, despite the central role that sleep occupies in early life much is still unknown about either the precise mechanisms underlying the development and regulation of sleep or of the role that sleep plays in infant and child development. This high proportion of time infants and young children spend sleeping corresponds to high levels of brain plasticity and sensitive periods of brain development, with mounting evidence suggesting that sleep plays a crucial and active role in the neurocognitive development of children.

Elucidating the role that sleep plays in brain development and, as a corollary, understanding the effects of sleep disturbance on neurocognitive development requires an improved understanding of normal sleep across the entire pediatric age range including the establishment of better normative data. Current normative data are limited largely to pioneering studies performed several decades ago. While these pioneering studies were seminal in establishing pediatric sleep medicine as a field in its own right, they have the usual shortcomings of early investigations including small biased samples that were restricted to certain age groups and a lack of standardization in methodology and data analysis. The advent of digital polysomnography (PSG), which has the ability to capture significantly more physiological data with relative ease, will extend the groundbreaking studies performed in the latter part of the last century and can provide a more comprehensive overview of normal sleep development.

Future Directions

There are many unanswered questions in relation to the development and regulation of sleep during infancy and childhood. Addressing the following questions may provide insights into the functions of sleep and may assist in identifying children who require clinical or behavioral interventions for sleep disorders:

- How does sleep architecture change with age? There is a need for longitudinal PSG data derived from normal, healthy children sampled at regular developmental periods.
- What is the relationship between sleep and brain development? That is, how does PSG data correlate with other measures of development such as motor skill, language, memory, social development, etc.?
- What are the genetic and epigenetic underpinning of sleep development?
- How do biopsychosocial factors influence sleep development?
- Does sleep intervention improve neurocognitive outcomes? For example, in children with neurodevelopmental disorders such as Down's or Asperger's Syndrome, which are often associated with significant sleep disturbance.

Notes

1. The traditional sleep stage terminology of Rechtschaffen and Kales (1968) is used throughout this chapter. See Carskadon and Dement (2011), with whom we concur, for a discussion on sleep nomenclature.

References

Abe, K., & Fukui, S. T. (1979). The individual development of circadian temperature rhythm in infants. *Journal of Interdisciplinary Cycle Research, 10*(3), 227–232.

Acebo, C., Sadeh, A., Seifer, R., Tzischinsky, O., Hafer, A., & Carskadon, M. A. (2005). Sleep/wake patterns derived from activity monitoring and maternal report for healthy 1- to 5-year-old children. *Sleep, 28*(12), 1568–1577.

Anders, T. F., Emde, R., & Parmelee Jr., A. (1971). *A Manual of Standardized Terminology, Techniques and Criteria for Scoring States of Sleep and Wakefulness in Newborn Infants.* Los Angeles: UCLA Brian Information Service, Neurological Information Network.

Anders, T. F., & Keener, M. A. (1985) Developmental course of nighttime sleep-wake patterns in full-term and premature infants during the first year of life I. *Sleep, 8*(3), 173–192.

Anders, T.F., Keener, M.A., & Kraemer, H. (1985). Sleep-wake state organization, neonatal assessment and development in premature infants during the first year of life II. *Sleep, 8*(3), 193–206.

Andre, M., Lamblin, M. D., d'Allest, A. M., Curzi-Dascalova, L., Moussalli-Salefranque, F., S., Nguyen, et al. (2010). Electroencephalography in premature and full-term infants. Developmental features and glossary. *Neurophysiologie Clinique 40*(2), 59–124.

Arditi-Babchuk, H., Feldman, R., & Eidelman, A. I. (2009). Rapid eye movement (REM) in premature neonates and developmental outcome at 6 months. *Infant Behavior & Development, 32*(1), 27–32.

Aton, S. J., Seibt, J., Dumoulin, M., Jha, S. K., Steinmetz, N., Coleman, T., et al. (2009). Mechanisms of sleep-dependent consolidation of cortical plasticity. *Neuron, 61*(3), 454–466.

Avidan, A. Y. (2005). Recognition of sleep stages and adult scoring technique. In S. Chokroverty, R. J. Thomas & M. Bhatt (Eds.), *Atlas of Sleep Medicine* (pp. 95–121). Philadelphia, PA: Elsevier.

Bach, V., Telliez, F., Chardon, K., Tourneux, P., Cardot, V., & Libert, J. P. (2011). Thermoregulation in wakefulness and sleep in humans. *Handbook of Clinical Neurology, 98*, 215–227.

Bernier, A., Carlson, S. M., Bordeleau, S., & Carrier, J. (2010). Relations between physiological and cognitive regulatory systems: Infant sleep regulation and subsequent executive functioning. *Child Development, 81*(6), 1739–1752.

Blumberg, M. S. (2010). Beyond dreams: Do sleep-related movements contribute to brain development? *Frontiers in Neurology, 1*(140), 1–10.

Boivin, D. B., Duffy, J. F., Kronauer, R. E., & Czeisler, C. A. (1996). Dose-response relationships for resetting of human circadian clock by light. *Nature, 379*(6565), 540–542.

Boivin, D. B., & Czeisler, C. A. (1998). Resetting of circadian melatonin and cortisol rhythms in humans by ordinary room light. *Neuroreport, 9*(5), 779–782.

Borbely, A. A. (1982). A two process model of sleep regulation. *Human Neurobiology, 1*(3), 195–204.

Campbell, S. S., & Broughton, R. J. (1994). Rapid decline in body temperature before sleep: Fluffing the physiological pillow? *Chronobiology International, 11*(2), 126–131.

Carskadon, M. A., & Dement, W. C. (1992). Multiple sleep latency tests during the constant routine. *Sleep, 15*(5), 396–399.

Carskadon, M. A., & Dement, W. C. (2011). Normal human sleep: An overview. In M. H. Kryger, T. Roth, & William C. Dement (Eds.), *Principles and Practice of Sleep Medicine* (5th edition, pp. 16–26). Philadelphia, PA: Saunders/Elsevier.

Casey, B. J., Tottenham, N., Liston, C., & Durston, S. (2005). Imaging the developing brain: What have we learned about cognitive development? *Trends in Cognitive Sciences, 9*(3), 104–110.

Coons, S. (1987). Development of sleep and wakefulness during the first 6 months of life. In C. Guilleminault (Ed.), *Sleep and Its Disorders in Children* (pp. 17–27). New York: Raven Press.

Corner, M. A., & Ramakers, G. J. (1992). Spontaneous firing as an epigenetic factor in brain development—physiological consequences of chronic tetrodotoxin and picrotoxin exposure on cultured rat neocortex neurons. *Developmental Brain Research, 65*(1), 57–64.

Curzi-Dascalova, L. & Challamel, M-J. (2000) Neurophysiological basis of sleep development. In G. M. Loughlin, J. L. Carroll, & C. L. Marcus (Eds.), *Sleep and Breathing in Children* (pp. 3–37). New York: Marcel Dekker, Inc.

Curzi Dascalova, L. (2001). Between-sleep states transitions in premature babies. *Journal of Sleep Research, 10*(2), 153–158.

Curzi-Dascalova, L. (2003). Developmental trend of sleep characteristics in premature and full-term infants In O. P. Mathew (Ed.), *Respiratory Control and Disorders in the Newborn* (pp. 149–182). New York: Marcel Dekker, Inc.

Czeisler, C. A., Allan, J. S., Strogatz, S. H., Ronda, J. M., Sanchez, R., Rios, C. D., et al. (1986). Bright light resets the human circadian pacemaker independent of the timing of the sleep-wake cycle. *Science, 233*(4764), 667–671.

Czeisler, C. A., Kronauer, R. E., Allan, J. S., Duffy, J. F., Jewett, M. E., Brown, E. N., et al. (1989). Bright light induction of strong (type 0) resetting of the human circadian pacemaker. *Science, 244*(4910), 1328–1333.

Czeisler, C. A., Duffy, J. F., Shanahan, T. L., Brown, E. N., Mitchell, J. F., Rimmer, D. W., et al. (1999). Stability, precision, and near-24-hour period of the human circadian pacemaker. *Science, 284*(5423), 2177–2181.

Dahl, R. E. (1996). The impact of inadequate sleep on children's daytime cognitive function. *Seminars in Pediatric Neurology, 3*(1), 44–50.

Dan, B., & Boyd, S. G. (2006). A neurophysiological perspective on sleep and its maturation. *Developmental Medicine and Child Neurology, 48*(9), 773–779.

de Weerd, A. W., & van den Bossche, R. A. (2003). The development of sleep during the first months of life. *Sleep Medicine Reviews, 7*(2), 179–191.

Denenberg, V. H., & Thoman, E. B. (1981). Evidence for a functional role for active (REM) sleep in infancy. *Sleep, 4*(2), 185–191.

Destexhe, A. (2009). Sleep oscillations. In L. R. Squire (Ed.), *Encyclopedia of Neuroscience* (pp. 1027–1034). Boston, MA: Elsevier.

Dijk, D. J., & Lockley, S. W. (2002). Integration of human sleep-wake regulation and circadian rhythmicity. *Journal of Applied Physiology, 92*(2), 852–862.

Dionne, G., Touchette, E., Forget-Dubois, N., Petit, D., Tremblay, R. E., Montplaisir, J. Y., et al. (2011). Associations between sleep-wake consolidation and language development in early childhood: a longitudinal twin study. *Sleep, 34*(8), 987–995.

Duffy, J. F., Kronauer, R. E., & Czeisler, C. A. (1996). Phase-shifting human circadian rhythms: Influence of sleep timing, social contact and light exposure. *Journal of Physiology, 495* (Pt 1), 289–297.

Edgar, D. M., Dement, W. C., & Fuller, C. A. (1993). Effect of SCN lesions on sleep in squirrel monkeys: Evidence for opponent processes in sleep-wake regulation. *Journal of Neuroscience, 13*(3), 1065–1079.

Ellingson, R. J. (1982). Development of sleep spindle bursts during the first year of life. *Sleep, 5*(1), 39–46.

Feinberg, I., & Campbell, I. G. (2010). Sleep EEG changes during adolescence: An index of a fundamental brain reorganization. *Brain and Cognition, 72*(1), 56–65.

Ferber, S. G., Laudon, M., Kuint, J., Weller, A., & Zisapel, N. (2002). Massage therapy by mothers enhances the adjustment of circadian rhythms to the nocturnal period in

full-term infants. *Journal of Developmental & Behavioral Pediatrics, 23*(6), 410–415.
Frank, M. G., Issa, N. P., & Stryker, M. P. (2001). Sleep enhances plasticity in the developing visual cortex. *Neuron, 30*(1), 275–287.
Frank, M. G., & Stryker, M. P. (2003). The role of sleep in the development of central visual pathways. In P. Maquet, C. Smith, & R. Stickgold (Eds.), *Sleep and Brain Plasticity* (pp. 189–206). Oxford; New York: Oxford University Press.
Galland, B. C., Taylor, B. J., Elder, D. E., & Herbison, P. (2012). Normal sleep patterns in infants and children: A systematic review of observational studies. *Sleep Medicine Reviews, 16*, 213–222.
Garcia-Rill, E., Kobayashi, T. & Good, C. (2003) The developmental decrease in REM sleep. *Thalamus & Related Systems, (2),*115–131.
Gillberg, M. (1997). Human sleep/wake regulation. *Acta Anaesthesiologica Scandinavica* (Suppl), *110*, 8–10.
Glotzbach, S. F., Edgar, D. M., & Ariagno, R. L. (1995). Biological rhythmicity in preterm infants prior to discharge from neonatal intensive care. *Pediatrics, 95*(2), 231–237.
Gould, J. B. (1983). SIDS—a sleep hypothesis. In J. T. Tildon, L. M. Roeder & A. Steinschneider (Eds.), *Sudden Infant Death Syndrome* (pp. 443–452). New York: Academic Press.
Graven, S. (2006). Sleep and brain development. *Clinics in Perinatology, 33*(3), 693–706, vii.
Grigg-Damberger, M., Gozal, D., Marcus, C. L., Quan, S. F., Rosen, C. L., Chervin, R. D., et al. (2007). The visual scoring of sleep and arousal in infants and children. *Journal of Clinical Sleep Medicine 3*(2), 201–240.
Guilleminault, C., & Coons, S. (1983). Sleep states and maturation of sleep: A comparative study between full-term normal controls and near-miss SIDS infants. In J. T. Tildon, L. M. Roeder, & A. Steinschneider (Eds.), *Sudden Infant Death Syndrome* (pp. 401–411). New York: Academic Press.
Hao, H., & Rivkees, S. A. (1999). The biological clock of very premature primate infants is responsive to light. *Proceedings of the National Academy of Science, USA, 96*(5), 2426–2429.
He, Y., Jones, C. R., Fujiki, N., Xu, Y., Guo, B., Holder Jr., J. L., et al. (2009). The transcriptional repressor DEC2 regulates sleep length in mammals. *Science, 325*(5942), 866–870.
Hoban, T. F. (2005). Pediatric polysomnography. In S. Chokroverty, R. J. Thomas, & M. Bhatt (Eds.), *Atlas of Sleep Medicine* (1st Edition, pp. 352–353). Philadelphia, PA: Elsevier.
Holditch-Davis, D., Belyea, M. & Edwards, L. J. (2005) Prediction of 3-year developmental outcomes from sleep development over the preterm period. *Infant Behavior & Development 28*:118–131.
Honma, K.I., & Honma, S. (1988). A human phase response curve for bright light pulses. *The Japanese Journal of Psychiatry and Neurology, 42*, 167–168.
Hoppenbrouwers, T., Hodgman, J., Arakawa, K., Geidel, S. A., & Sterman, M. B. (1988). Sleep and waking states in infancy: Normative studies. *Sleep, 11*(4), 387–401.
Hoppenbrouwers, T. (1992). *Ontogenesis of the Human Ultradian Rhythms*. London: Springer Verlag.
Hor, H., & Tafti, M. (2009). Physiology. How much sleep do we need? *Science, 325*(5942), 825–826.
Horne, J. A. (2000). REM sleep—by default? *Neuroscience and Biobehavioral Reviews, 24*(8), 777–797.
Iglowstein, I., Jenni, O. G., Molinari, L., & Largo, R. H. (2003). Sleep duration from infancy to adolescence: Reference values and generational trends. *Pediatrics, 111*(2), 302–307.
Jenni, O. G., Borbely, A. A., & Achermann, P. (2004). Development of the nocturnal sleep electroencephalogram in human infants. *American Journal of Physiology. Regulatory, integrative and comparative physiology, 286*(3), R528–R538.
Jenni, O. G., Achermann, P., & Carskadon, M. A. (2005). Homeostatic sleep regulation in adolescents. *Sleep, 28*(11), 1446–1454.
Kahn, A., Dan, B., Groswasser, J., Franco, P., & Sottiaux, M. (1996). Normal sleep architecture in infants and children. *Journal of Clinical Neurophysiology, 13*(3), 184–197.
Kilb, W., Kirischuk, S., & Luhmann, H. J. (2011). Electrical activity patterns and the functional maturation of the neocortex. *The European Journal of Neuroscience, 34*(10), 1677–1686.
Kleitman, N., & Engelmann, T. G. (1953). Sleep characteristics of infants. *Journal of Applied Physiology, 6*(5), 269–282.
Kohyama, J. (1998). Sleep as a window on the developing brain. *Current Problems in Pediatrics, 27*: 73–92.
Kohyama, J. (2011). Sleep health and asynchronization. *Brain and Development, 33*(3), 252–259.
Koos, B. J. (2008) Breathing and sleep states in the fetus and at birth. In: C. L. Marcus, J. L. Carroll, D. F. Donnelly, G. M. Loughlin (Eds.), *Sleep and Breathing in Children* (2nd Edition,pp. 1–17). New York: Informa Healthcare.
Krauchi, K., Cajochen, C., Werth, E., & Wirz-Justice, A. (2000). Functional link between distal vasodilation and sleep-onset latency? *American Journal of Physiology – Regulatory, Integrative and Comparative Physiology.*, *278*(3), R741–R748.
Krauchi, K., & Deboer, T. (2010). The interrelationship between sleep regulation and thermoregulation. *Frontiers in Bioscience, 15*, 604–625.
Lack, L. C., & Lushington, K. (1996). The rhythms of human sleep propensity and core body temperature. *Journal of Sleep Research, 5*(1), 1–11.
Lack, L. C., Gradisar, M., Van Someren, E. J., Wright, H. R., & Lushington, K. (2008). The relationship between insomnia and body temperatures. *Sleep Medicine Reviews, 12*(4), 307–317.
Lavie, P. (2001). Sleep-wake as a biological rhythm. *Annual Review of Psychology, 52*, 277–303.
Levitt, P. (2003). Structural and functional maturation of the developing primate brain. *The Journal of Pediatrics, 143* (4 Suppl), S35–S45.
Lloyd, David. (2008). *Ultradian Rhythms from Molecules to Mind.* New York: Springer.
Lodemore, M., Petersen, S. A., & Wailoo, M. P. (1991). Development of night time temperature rhythms over the first six months of life. *Archives of Disease in Childhood, 66*(4), 521–524.
Lodemore, M., Petersen, S. A., & Wailoo, M. P. (1992). Factors affecting the development of night time temperature rhythms. *Archives of Disease in Childhood, 67*(10), 1259–1261.
Louis, J., Zhang, J. X., Revol, M., Debilly, G., & Challamel, M. J. (1992). Ontogenesis of nocturnal organization of sleep spindles: A longitudinal study during the first 6 months of life. *Electroencephalography and Clinical Neurophysiology, 83*(5), 289–296.
Louis, J., Cannard, C., Bastuji, H., & Challamel, M. J. (1997). Sleep ontogenesis revisited: A longitudinal 24-hour home polygraphic study on 15 normal infants during the first two years of life. *Sleep, 20*(5), 323–333.
Lowrey, P. L., & Takahashi, J. S. (2000). Genetics of the mammalian circadian system: Photic entrainment, circadian

pacemaker mechanisms, and posttranslational regulation. *Annual Review of Genetics, 34*, 533–562.
Lushington, K., Dawson, D., & Lack, L. (2000). Core body temperature is elevated during constant wakefulness in elderly poor sleepers. *Sleep, 23*(4), 504–510.
Maquet, P., Smith, C., & Stickgold, R. (2003). *Sleep and Brain Plasticity*. Oxford; New York: Oxford University Press.
Marks, G. A., Shaffery, J. P., Oksenberg, A., Speciale, S. G., & Roffwarg, H. P. (1995). A functional role for REM sleep in brain maturation. *Behavioural Brain Research, 69*(1–2), 1–11.
McGraw, K., Hoffmann, R., Harker, C., & Herman, J. H. (1999). The development of circadian rhythms in a human infant. *Sleep, 22*(3), 303–310.
McMillen, I. C., Kok, J. S., Adamson, T. M., Deayton, J. M., & Nowak, R. (1991). Development of circadian sleep-wake rhythms in preterm and full-term infants. *Pediatric Research, 29*(4 Pt 1), 381–384.
Meier-Koll, A., Hall, U., Hellwig, U., Kott, G., & Meier-Koll, V. (1978). A biological oscillator system and the development of sleep-waking behavior during early infancy. *Chronobiologia, 5*(4), 425–440.
Metcalf, D.R., Mondale, J. & Butler, F. K. (1971) Ontogenesis of spontaneous K-complexes. *Psychophysiology, 8*(3), 340–347.
Middleton, B., Arendt, J., & Stone, B. M. (1996). Human circadian rhythms in constant dim light (8 lux) with knowledge of clock time. *Journal of Sleep Research, 5*(2), 69–76.
Minors, David S., Waterhouse, James M., & Wirz-Justice, A. (1991). A human phase-response curve to light. *Neuroscience Letters, 133*(1), 36–40.
Mirmiran, M., Uylings, H. B. M., & Corner, M. A. (1983) Pharmacological suppression of REM sleep prior to weaning counteracts the effectiveness of subsequent environmental enrichment on cortical growth in rats. *Developmental Brain Research, 7*, 102–105.
Mirmiran, M., & Ariagno, R. L. (Eds.). (2003). Role of REM sleep in brain development and plasticity. In P. Maquet, C. Smith, & R. Stickgold (Eds.), *Sleep and Brain Plasticity* (pp. 181–187). Oxford: Oxford University Press.
Miyamoto, H. & Hensch, T.K. (2006) Bidirectional interaction of sleep and synaptic plasticity: A view from visual cortex. *Sleep & Biological Rhythms, 4*, 35–43.
Monk, T. H., Buysse, D. J., Reynolds, C. F. 3rd, & Kupfer, D. J. (1996). Circadian determinants of the postlunch dip in performance. *Chronobiol International, 13*(2), 123–133.
National Sleep Foundation. 2004 Sleep in America poll. Available at: www.sleepfoundation.org/_content//hottopics/2004SleepPollFinalReport.pdf. Accessed Feb 22, 2012
Nishihara, K., Horiuchi, S., Eto, H., & Uchida, S. (2002). The development of infants' circadian rest-activity rhythm and mothers' rhythm. *Physiology & Behavior, 77*(1), 91–98.
Ornitz, E. M. (1972). Development of sleep patterns in autistic children. In C. D. Clemente, D. P. Purpura, & F. E. Mayer (Eds.), *Sleep and the Maturing Nervous System* (pp. 363–381). New York: Academic Press.
Pace-Schott, E. F., & Hobson, J. A. (2002). The neurobiology of sleep: Genetics, cellular physiology and subcortical networks. *Nature Reviews Neuroscience, 3*(8), 591–605.
Parmelee, A. H., & Stern, E. (1972). Development of states in infants. In C. D. Clemente, D. P. Purpura, & F. E. Mayer (Eds.), *Sleep and the Maturing Nervous System* (pp. 199–228). New York: Academic Press.
Peirano, P., Algarin, C., & Uauy, R. (2003). Sleep-wake states and their regulatory mechanisms throughout early human development. *The Journal of Pediatrics, 143*(4 Suppl), S70–S79.
Peirano, P., & Algarin, C. R. (2007). Sleep in brain development. *Biological Research, 40*(4), 471–478.
Penn, A. A., & Shatz, C. J. (1999). Brain waves and brain wiring: the role of endogenous and sensory-driven neural activity in development. *Pediatric Research, 45*(4 Pt 1), 447–458.
Porkka-Heiskanen, T., Strecker, R. E., Thakkar, M., Bjorkum, A. A., Greene, R. W., & McCarley, R. W. (1997). Adenosine: a mediator of the sleep-inducing effects of prolonged wakefulness. *Science, 276*(5316), 1265–1268.
Prechtl, H. F. (1974). The behavioural states of the newborn infant (a review). *Brain Research, 76*(2), 185–212.
Rama, A. N., Cho, S. C., & Kushida, C. A. (2005). NREM-REM sleep. In C. Guilleminault (Ed.), *Clinical Neurophysiology of Sleep Disorders; Handbook of Clinical Neurophysiology* (pp. 21–29). Edinburgh: Elsevier.
Rechtschaffen, A., & Kales, A. (1968). *A Manual of Standardized Terminology, Techniques, and Scoring Systems for Sleep Stages of Human Subjects*. Los Angeles: Brain Information/Brain Research Institute UCLA.
Ringli, M., & Huber, R. (2011). Developmental aspects of sleep slow waves: Linking sleep, brain maturation and behavior. *Progress in Brain Research, 193*, 63–82.
Rivkees, S. A., & Hao, H. (2000). Developing circadian rhythmicity. *Seminars in Perinatology, 24*(4), 232–242.
Rivkees, S. A. (2003). Developing circadian rhythmicity in infants. *Pediatrics, 112*, 373–381.
Roffwarg, H. P., Muzio, J. N., & Dement, W. C. (1966). Ontogenetic development of the human sleep-dream cycle. *Science, 152*(3722), 604–619.
Sadeh, A., Lavie, P., Scher, A., Tirosh, E., & Epstein, R. (1991). Actigraphic home-monitoring sleep-disturbed and control infants and young children: a new method for pediatric assessment of sleep-wake patterns. *Pediatrics, 87*(4), 494–499.
Sankupellay, M., Wilson, S., Heussler, H. S., Parsley, C., Yuill, M., & Dakin, C. (2011). Characteristics of sleep EEG power spectra in healthy infants in the first two years of life. *Clinical Neurophysiology 122*(2), 236–243.
Scher, A. (2005). Infant sleep at 10 months of age as a window to cognitive development. *Early Human Development, 81*(3), 289–292.
Scher, M. S. (2006) Electroencephalography of the newborn: Normal features. In: G. L. Holmes, H.R. Jones & S.L. Moshe (Eds) *Clinical Neurophysiology of Infancy, Childhood and Adolescence E-Book* (pp. 46–69). Philadelphia, PA: Elsevier.
Scher, M. S. (2011) Ontogeny of EEG sleep from neonatal through infancy periods. In P. Montagna & S. Chokroverty (Eds.), *Sleep Disorders I. Handbook of Clinical Neurology 98*,111–129. Amsterdam: Elsevier.
Scholle, S., & Schafer, T. (1999). Atlas of sleep and wakefulness in infants and children. *Somnologie 3*, 163–241.
Segawa, M. (2006). Epochs of development of the sleep–wake cycle reflect the modulation of the higher cortical function particular for each epoch. *Sleep and Biological Rhythms, 4*(1), 4–15.
Sejnowski, T. J., & Destexhe, A. (2000). Why do we sleep? *Brain Research, 886*(1–2), 208–223.
Sheldon, S. H. (1996). *Evaluating Sleep in Infants and Children*. Philadelphia: Lippincott-Raven.
Shibagaki, M., Kiyono, S., & Watanabe, K. (1982). Spindle evolution in normal and mentally retarded children: A review. *Sleep, 5*(1), 47–57.

Shibagaki, M., Kiyono, S., Watanabe, K., & Hakamada, S. (1982). Concurrent occurrence of rapid eye movement with spindle burst during nocturnal sleep in mentally retarded children. *Electroencephalography and Clinical Neurophysiology, 53*(1), 27–35.

Shimada, M., Takahashi, K., Segawa, M., Higurashi, M., Samejim, M., & Horiuchi, K. (1999). Emerging and entraining patterns of the sleep-wake rhythm in preterm and term infants. *Brain Development, 21*(7), 468–473.

Stern, E., Parmelee, A. H., Akiyama, Y., Schultz, M. A., & Wenner, W. H. (1969). Sleep cycle characteristics in infants. *Pediatrics, 43*(1), 65–70.

Tanguay, P. E., Ornitz, E. M., Kaplan, A., & Bozzo, E. S. (1975). Evolution of sleep spindles in childhood. *Electroencephalography and Clinical Neurophysiology, 38*(2), 175–181.

Tarullo, A. R., Balsam, P. D., & Fifer, W. P. (2011). Sleep and infant learning. *Infant and Child Development, 20*(1), 35–46.

Thoman, E. (1990) Sleeping and waking states in infants: A functional perspective. *Neuroscience and Biobehavioral Reviews, 14*(1), 93–107.

Thomas, A. J., Erokwu, B. O., Yamamoto, B. K., Ernsberger, P., Bishara, O., & Strohl, K. P. (2000). Alterations in respiratory behavior, brain neurochemistry and receptor density induced by pharmacologic suppression of sleep in the neonatal period. *Developmental Brain Research, 120*(2), 181–189.

Touchette, E., Petit, D., Seguin, J. R., Boivin, M., Tremblay, R. E., & Montplaisir, J. Y. (2007). Associations between sleep duration patterns and behavioral/cognitive functioning at school entry. *Sleep, 30*(9), 1213–1219.

Van Someren, E. J. W. (2000). More than a marker: Interaction between the circadian regulation of temperature and sleep, age-related changes, and treatment possibilities. *Chronobiology International, 17*(3), 313–354.

Vecchierini, M. F., André, M., & d'Allest, A. M. (2007). Normal EEG of premature infants born between 24 and 30 weeks gestational age: Terminology, definitions and maturation aspects. *Neurophysiologie Clinique/Clinical Neurophysiology, 37*(5), 311–323.

Weisman, O., Magori-Cohen, R., Louzoun, Y., Eidelman, A. I., & Feldman, R. (2011). Sleep-wake transitions in premature neonates predict early development. *Pediatrics, 128*(4), 706–714.

Weissbluth, M., & Weissbluth, L. (1992). Colic, sleep inertia, melatonin and circannual rhythms. *Medical Hypotheses, 38*(3), 224–228.

Westmoreland, B. F. & Klass, D. W. (1990) Unusual EEG patterns. *Journal of Clinical Neurophysiology, 7*(2), 209–228.

CHAPTER

6

The Relationship between Sleep and Daytime Cognitive/Behavioral Functioning: Infancy and Preschool Years

Kurt Lushington, Yvonne Pamula, A. James Martin, *and* John Declan Kennedy

Abstract

Sleep undergoes rapid and remarkable changes in structure and organization in the first few years of life. This is paralleled by similar changes in the brain. Evidence from studies in animals and, to a lesser extent infants, suggests that sleep plays a major role in cortical development, with sleep quality early in life predicting cognitive functioning later in life. Sleep is also important for cortical functioning. The most well-explored domain has been memory, with both REM and NREM sleep and possibly specific EEG frequencies within a sleep stage differentially affecting the formation and consolidation of differing memory types. Finally, sleep is important for optimal daytime functioning. Both sleep restriction and sleep pathology have negative and characteristic impacts on neuropsychological and behavioral functioning. Despite advances, however, our understanding of the role played by sleep in the interaction between gene expression and neural development, in neurocircuit formation, and, finally, on the interaction between sensory input and neural development remain to be more fully explored.

Key Words: sleep, infant, development, learning, memory, brain, neurocognitive, behavior

Sleep and the Developing Brain

Among the manifold functions of sleep is the role that it plays in cognitive development and especially memory and learning. The hypothesis that sleep is important for memory is thought to originate more than a century ago with the study of Ebbinghaus (1885), who found that memory of nonsense syllables was improved after sleep. Subsequent studies during the early part of the twentieth century have added credence to the proposal that sleep does play a role in memory. Until relatively recently, however, the general consensus was that the brain is quiet during sleep and memories could be consolidated without competing input from the external world. The discovery of rapid eye movement (REM) sleep in the early 1950s (Aserinsky & Kleitman, 1953) led to the recognition that sleep was not as homogenous as previously thought and a revaluation of the role of sleep in memory. In the late 1960s, Roffwarg, Muzio, and Dement (1966) proposed the prescient hypothesis that because young infants spend large amounts of time in REM sleep, and as infancy is a time of rapid brain development, then REM sleep might provide the internal source of brain stimulation necessary for ongoing structural maturation.

In the following decades the REM brain development hypothesis was tested in a series of animal studies examining the role of sleep in cortical development and especially that of the visual cortex. Two important findings to emerge from this period are, first, that brain weight and REM sleep increase in enriched environments (in the rat) and second, that the normal development of brain structures vital for the development of vision (e.g., lateral geniculate nucleus) are modulated by NREM sleep (Frank, 2011). In a separate but convergent area of investigation, researchers in the 1980s also began examining survival in premature infants and whether sleep–wake organization may predict cognitive development. Parallel to the findings in animals, infants with immature sleep electroencephalography (EEG) are more likely to demonstrate poorer development in later life (Anders, Keener, & Kraemer, 1985; Beckwith & Parmelee, 1986; Novosad, Freudigman, & Thoman, 1999; Richards, Parmelee, & Beckwith, 1986). Since the 1980s, and particularly in the past decade, the vital importance of sleep on cognition and particularly its effect on memory consolidation has been recognized. This has underpinned the rapid expansion in our knowledge of the electrophysiological and molecular mechanisms that subserve memory consolidation. What has also become clear is that if sleep is disrupted in a developing child, either by fragmentation or hypoxia, then there are concomitant effects on daytime function, particularly on attentional and behavioral domains. This chapter outlines aspects of this rapidly advancing area and highlights the relative lack of data on sleep and cognition in children relative to what is known in adults, along with the particular paucity of data in infants.

Normal Brain Development: A Role for Sleep?

Brain development in the fetus begins in the third week of gestation, continues into adolescence, and is dependent on three factors: *(1)* the influence of gene expression on neural development, *(2)* endogenous neural stimulation, and *(3)* sensory input from the environment. It is the dynamic interaction of these factors which leads to adaptation and the development of new neural circuits. Although Freud first highlighted the effect of early family experiences on the developing personality (Freud & Strachey, 1966), it is only with recent advances in statistical modeling that environmental factors—for example, auditory and visual input and quality of maternal care—have been shown to play a vital role in the pattern of brain gene expression (Lenroot & Giedd, 2011), thus demonstrating that the ontogeny of brain development is not solely driven by genetic influences.

The most rapid period of brain development occurs in the first few years of life, with the brain reaching approximately 90% of adult size by 6 years of age (Kennedy, Makris, Herbert, Takahashi, & Caviness, 2002; Reiss, Abrams, Singer, Ross, & Denckla, 1996). In the initial postnatal period, neural connectivity is greater than that of adults and is gradually pruned as the child matures (Lenroot & Giedd, 2011). In addition, synaptic connectivity during this developmental period demonstrates a high degree of plasticity, and recent studies have highlighted sleep's role in this process (Ribeiro, 2012). It does appear paradoxical that maximal brain growth should be so marked in the newborn period at a time when, purportedly, external sensory input is relatively limited—an observation that has prompted Dahl (1996) to propose that sleep is the single most important function of the developing brain, given that children spend over 50% of the first two years sleeping.

The Effect of REM and NREM on Brain Maturation and Function

The investigation of the role of different sleep states on brain maturation and function has been undertaken mainly in animals. The ontogenetic hypothesis proposes that REM sleep facilitates both normal brain development and experience-dependent synaptic plasticity (Roffwarg et al., 1966; Shaffery, Lopez, Bissette, & Roffwarg, 2006). This hypothesis is supported by studies in rats, where REM deprivation in the neonatal period is associated with reduced cortical and brainstem volume and altered neurotransmitter sensitivity (Mirmiran, Feenstra, Dijcks, Bos, & Van Haaren, 1988; Mirmiran, Uylings, & Corner, 1983). It may also have long-term impacts later in life. Adult rats who have been REM-deprived in the neonatal period also demonstrate reduced neural plasticity when put in an enriched environment, thereby suggesting that adult learning might be dependent on the neural plasticity mediated by REM sleep quality in infancy (Mirmiran, Scholtens, et al., 1983). Despite this evidence, however, a major criticism of REM deprivation studies is the problem of separating the effects of REM deprivation from the pharmacological effects of the REM-depressant drugs, which in and of themselves are known to alter monoaminergic neurotransmitters and, hence, mood and cognition (Herlenius & Lagercrantz, 2001).

Despite the focus on REM sleep, a possible role has also been reported for NREM sleep in cortical development. An experimental approach that avoids the problems associated with the pharmacological suppression of sleep has been to study the role of sleep in early life on the development of brain structures and especially visual pathways. Specifically, following a period of monocular deprivation, visual responses are known to move in favor of the non-obscured eye as indicated by changes in synaptic plasticity in key visual areas (e.g., lateral geniculate nucleus and the visual cortex; see Frank,

Issa, & Stryker, 2001). This transfer is augmented by NREM sleep (Frank, 2011). Thus, although the ontogenetic hypothesis emphasizes the primary role of REM sleep in brain development and plasticity, NREM sleep may also be important. Of note is that NREM maturation coincides with the development of thalamocortical and intracortical neural circuits and synaptic remodeling (Bear & Malenka, 1994; Cramer & Sur, 1995; Peirano & Algarin, 2007). Taking cortical development into account, and the potentially differing roles of REM and NMREM sleep, it is has been further hypothesized that REM sleep facilitates development of neural circuitry while NREM sleep consolidates changes in neural circuitry (Maquet, Smith, & Stickgold, 2003).

The Role of Sleep in Memory and Learning

The importance of sleep in processing and storing memory has become particularly evident over the past 25 years as an increasing number of studies have examined its effect on varying memory-related domains, including verbal learning, emotional memory, spatial recognition, and procedural memory (Payne, 2011). In the main, these studies have concentrated on animal and adult humans, but there is a growing literature that attests to sleep's importance in memory consolidation and learning in developing children.

The consensus view is that different sleep stages specifically benefit different types of memory (Payne, 2011). A compatible but more nuanced view is that the predominant EEG frequencies which occur within a specific sleep state may be the more important factor (Cheng, Williams, & Meck, 2008). NREM sleep is thought to be important for the consolidation of declarative and spatial memories (explicit memory), while REM sleep is thought to facilitate the encoding of procedural (implicit) and emotional memories (Payne, 2011). Different brain regions are also thought to be involved with the differing types of memory processing. Procedural memories are thought to be dependent on cortical and subcortical structures but independent of hippocampal structures, while implicit memories are served by the hippocampus and medial temporal regions and emotional memories are processed via the amygdala (Payne, 2011). As outlined by Walker (2010), there is considerable support for the suggestion that sleep also serves an overriding meta-level role in memory formation that extends beyond consolidation and recall by assimilating memories into the individual's cognitive matrix, thereby allowing a cohesive view of the individual's world to develop.

Memories also evolve over time, and this process involves not only the initial encoding of a fragile memory trace but also the subsequent consolidation, stabilization, and perhaps enhancement (Walker & Stickgold, 2006).

The Effect of Sleep and Its Individual Stages on Memory

The main conceptual model of the storage of memory is that neuronal circuits that were active during waking are reactivated off-line during sleep, thereby promoting long-lasting synaptic changes. One of the challenges of such a concept is how new memories can be formed without "overwriting" already stored memories. Another aspect of the storage of new information is that not all new memories are equally weighted, so some form of filtering with regard to importance is required. The model that has gained the greatest recognition to account for these aspects is the *Two Stage Model* of memory consolidation (Buzsaki, 1989). It proposes that memories are stored in both a temporary and more permanent storage site. For declarative memory, the areas of brain serving as these two storage sites are the hippocampus (temporary) and the neocortex (more permanent). The temporary store allows the rapid accumulation of memories but only maintains these memories for a short time, in contradistinction to the long-term store which accumulates at a slower rate. With initial memory encoding, both stores accumulate in parallel. But with repeated reactivation of the memory trace in the temporary store, or the hippocampus, long-term consolidation of the memory is facilitated in the neocortex by repeated stimulation of intracortical neural circuits. This repeated hippocampal–neocortical dialogue is thought to strengthen memory consolidation in the neocortex and to facilitate the insertion of new knowledge into a matrix of existing knowledge. Over time, these encoded neocortical memories become independent of the hippocampus, which then is capable of repeating the process with new learned experience (Diekelmann & Born, 2010). The current consensus is that these processes are thought to be facilitated by sleep, with individual sleep stages playing different roles. This model is supported by two lines of evidence. First, that declarative memories from a day's learning are more resistant to interference on the following day after a night's sleep (Ellenbogen, Hulbert, Stickgold, Dinges, & Thompson-Schill, 2006). Second, that sleep restriction after learning results in selective hippocampal deficits and disruption of the memory-strengthening hippocampal–neocortical dialogue resulting in impaired retention (Yoo, Hu, Gujar, Jolesz, & Walker, 2007).

In rat models, hippocampal–neocortical dialogue is facilitated by slow wave sleep (SWS) with the replaying of daytime spatial and novel experiences causing the same neural firing pattern in both hippocampus and neocortex that originally occurred during wakefulness (Dave & Margoliash, 2000; Ji & Wilson, 2007). The human brain response is thought to follow a similar pattern. For example, Rasch, Buchel, Gais, and Born (2007) report that when spatial learning was undertaken in the presence of a rose smell, reintroducing the same smell during subsequent SWS improved the consolidation of spatial memories.

A process that is integral to memory consolidation at a synaptic level is long-term potentiation (LTP). During this process, postsynaptic membrane depolarization occurs concomitantly with presynaptic action potentials, resulting in intracellular molecular changes and a resultant increase in synaptic strength, in other words synaptic consolidation. It is this lasting change in the strength of synaptic connections that underlies brain plasticity. It is thought that LTP may occur during the hippocampal slow wave oscillations and reactivations (Poe, Walsh, & Bjorness, 2010). A current hypothesis is that SWS could begin LTP and prime specific neuronal circuits for synaptic consolidation during later REM sleep (Diekelmann & Born, 2010). A counterargument suggests that NREM sleep results in a reduction in synapse strength, or synaptic downscaling. This would potentially allow the hippocampal synapses to depotentiate and thereby improve their potential to encode new declarative memories without overwhelming their inherent synaptic capacity.

As outlined earlier, specific EEG rhythms are thought to underlie memory consolidation and a number of signature events have been proposed including spindles, slow waves and sharp wave ripples in SWS and pontogeniculooccipital (PGO) waves and Theta rhythm in REM sleep. During SWS, large amplitude slow waves (delta) induce neural hyperpolarization (down-state) and depolarization (up-state). During depolarization there is an increase in neural firing, thereby facilitating hippocampal–neocortical dialogue and long-term storage of memories in the neocortex. Sleep spindles are thought to facilitate LTP, possibly by their faster stimulation frequency (Walker, 2010) and to prime cortical neural circuits to aid long-term memory storage in the neocortex (Diekelmann, Born, & Wagner, 2010), while hippocampal sharp-wave ripples are believed to facilitate specific synaptic potentiation in those circuits that were associated with an awake event (Born & Wilhelm, 2012). Thus, NREM ripples and spindles facilitate memory transfer from hippocampus to cortex during the depolarizing up-state of delta slow waves. During REM in the rat, PGO waves are thought to regulate synaptic plasticity in the amygdala and hippocampus (McCarley, 2007). Theta waves (4–8Hz) are also thought to induce LTP in hippocampal cells, but their specific role in memory formation remains to be fully elucidated (Walker, 2010). Walker (2010) suggests that over the early part of the night, when SWS predominates, hippocampal–neocortical crosstalk is maximal, while during stage 2 and REM intracortical crosstalk predominates. Recently attention has focused on the processing of emotional memories, which are thought to be REM-dependent, and it has been hypothesized that processing during successive REM periods allows the affective overlay of the memory to be disassociated. The latter is an area of great interest and potential, as it may be that emotional processing during sleep differs between children and adults. In 10–13-year-old children, positive compared to neutral emotions are reported to facilitate declarative but not procedural memory after sleep (Prehn-Kristensen et al., 2009). This is in contrast to adults, where positive emotional content is reported by some but not all studies to improve procedural memory after sleep, while negative memories are more resistant to decay and are enhanced by sleep (Walker, 2009). Exploration of the relationship between emotional valance, memory, and sleep in children is limited but offers the potential of gaining a better understanding the etiology and treatment of pediatric mental health problems.

The Effects of Sleep Disruption on Children's Neurocognitive and Behavioral Functioning

Over the past two decades there has been a rapid increase in our appreciation of the detrimental effects of sleep disruption on both adults and children. This has occurred *pari passu* as research attention has focused on the role of sleep in memory consolidation. However, in a recent review of childhood sleep disruption, O'Brien (2011) has pointed out that much of our knowledge of the effects of sleep disruption on young children is based on correlative or associative studies rather than those of robust experimental design. The picture in adults is somewhat clearer, as outlined by Lim and Dinges in their meta-analysis (2010), where there is good evidence that total sleep deprivation has a marked effect on adults' attention, a moderate effect on working memory and attention, and a lesser effect on short-term memory, while IQ and processing speed appear to be preserved, suggesting that compensatory mechanisms might be in play.

Can these results be extrapolated to children? There are several reasons for taking the view opining that "children are not small adults." Children's sleep duration and architecture change markedly between infancy and adolescence as does brain structure and functioning, with the prefrontal cortex reaching maturity in adolescence. In addition to the ethical and organizational limitations of undertaking sleep deprivation studies in children, there is the greater likelihood of confounding effects on results of socioeconomic factors such as different levels of attachment, childcare versus home care, parenting styles, split families, and schooling, thus making it difficult to isolate the specific impact of sleep disruption on neurocognitive and behavioral functioning (Beebe, 2011; also see O'Brien, Chapter 29). In addition, it is likely that there are "sensitive" periods of brain development when a potential insult will have a greater effect than at other times. Thus, the impact of sleep disruption on neurocognitive and behavioral functioning may vary with developmental age, making it difficult to draw conclusions that generalize across childhood. Gozal, Row, Schurr, and Gozal (2001) have recently demonstrated the impact of sleep disruption on functioning at sensitive periods in their study on the differential cerebral effects of hypoxia on rat pups of varying age. In summary, the extrapolation of sleep-deprivation findings in adults to children need to be treated with caution.

Although studies which have experimentally manipulated sleep in children are limited, sleep length is known to vary with cultural practice, an understanding of which could potentially inform our understanding of the association between sleep deprivation and daytime functioning. There is good evidence that children are sleeping less now than three decades ago (Matricciani, Olds, & Petkov, 2012), and in a recent study of Australian children between 1984 and 2004 it was found that children were sleeping up to 30 minutes less per night (attributable to later bed, not earlier rise times; see Dollman, Ridley, Olds, & Lowe, 2007). What remains unclear is whether this 5% reduction in sleep duration has had any appreciable impact on daytime functioning. It may be argued that the cumulative loss over many years of childhood is considerable, and even small reductions in sleep length may lead to significant daytime consequences. As a corollary, while survey data can tell us what is common practice regarding sleep habits (e.g., mean total sleep time for 4-year-olds in the community), the amount of sleep that children actually need for optimal daytime functioning is simply unknown. This gap in our understanding points to the need for empirically validated norms for parameters such as recommended sleep length according to age (Matricciani, Olds, Blunden, Rigney, & Williams, 2012).

A further approach to understanding the impact of sleep deprivation in children on daytime functioning is to examine children with problems that result in insufficient sleep (e.g., bedtime resistance, etc). Such sleep problems are common in young children, with a reported prevalence rate as high as 38% in the first years of life (Anders, Halpern, & Hua, 1992; Gaylor, Burnham, Goodlin-Jones, & Anders, 2005; Gaylor, Goodlin-Jones, & Anders, 2001; Lam, Hiscock, & Wake, 2003; Quach, Hiscock, & Wake, 2012; Wake et al., 2006; Zuckerman, Stevenson, & Bailey, 1987). Findings from longitudinal studies typically suggest that insufficient sleep in young children is associated with increased internalized problematic behaviors such as anxiety and depression and, to a lesser extent, externalized problematic behaviors such as aggressive behavior and hyperactivity (Astill, Van der Heijden, Van Ijzendoorn, & Van Someren, 2012; Beebe, 2011).

While studies have examined sleep restriction in children and its impact on daytime functioning, most have focused on sleep quantity and relatively less attention has been paid to sleep quality. Where researchers have examined sleep quality, to date most have focused on sleep disordered breathing (SDB) with its associated hypoxia and sleep fragmentation. A substantial number of studies and reviews have now been undertaken confirming decrements in daytime behavior and cognition in children with SDB (e.g., Beebe, 2006; Kheirandish & Gozal, 2006; Kohler, Lushington, & Kennedy, 2010). The behavioral domains reported to be most consistently affected by SDB include somatic complaints, depression, and social problems; neurocognitive domains include intelligence, attention, and executive function and, less commonly, deficits in memory, visual–spatial ability, language skills, and sensorimotor functioning (Kohler et al., 2010). Neurocognitive deficits also seem to be evident in early life in children with SDB. Our group has demonstrated that children who snore within the first month of life (on parental report) have reduced cognitive development at 6 and

12 months of age (Piteo, Kennedy, et al., 2011; Piteo, Lushington, et al., 2011). Montgomery-Downs and Gozal (2006) report that snoring-associated arousals are also associated with reduced cognitive development in healthy 8-month-old children without SDB. Despite the consensus that sleep disruption secondary to hypoxia or arousals in children with SDB is linked with daytime deficits, the parameters currently measured on standard polysomnography do not correlate strongly with these deficits. The lack of support for an association between SDB severity and daytime deficits is concerning, and current research is focused on more subtle analysis of the sleep EEG, such as cyclic alternating pattern analysis and power spectral analysis and its association to daytime functioning (e.g., Bruni et al., 2012). Finally, while the focus has been on children with SDB, other occult sleep disorders have been examined. For example, children with periodic limb movement disorder are reported to have a higher frequency of ADHD, while fragmented sleep in children with eczema predicts ADHD and oppositional behavior (Camfferman et al., 2010), further underlining the pivotal importance of normal sleep architecture (Crabtree, Ivanenko, O'Brien, & Gozal, 2003).

In very broad terms, research examining the effect of sleep disruption on children has mainly focused on infants or school-aged participants, with less analysis of its effect on toddlers and the kindergarten age groups. In addition, the majority of studies have been cross-sectional in design. Finally, much of the research on infant sleep and daytime functioning has been preoccupied with the hypothesis that the organization of sleep architecture early in life reflects brain maturity and thus the finding of disruption of the normal pattern of sleep in early life will predict later developmental deficits. As succinctly noted by Scher, "…infant sleep becomes a window to later cognitive development" (2005). The impetus for the development of such predictive factors was the survival of increasing numbers of premature infants during the 1980s.

In one of the first studies of its kind, Anders, Keener, and Kraemer (1985) evaluated the sleep–wake organization of 24 premature infants (mean gestational age = 31 weeks and range = 27–35 weeks) with video somnograms at term and subsequently on seven occasions up to 1 year of age. They report that mental performance was predicted by the "holding index," or long quiet sleep periods early in the night, while at 1 year it was predicted by the stability of the longest sleep period uninterrupted by wakefulness. Consistent with Ander's findings, Beckwith and Parmelee (1986) report that premature infants who had less *tracé alternant* on their sleep EEG at term had lower developmental scores at intervals up to 8 years of age. However, an exception was those children reared in an enriched environment where, despite having less *tracé alternant*, by 24 months their scores were equal to those with greater *tracé alternant*, thereby highlighting the buffering effect of family environment. Similar modulating effects of an enriched environment have been noted by Gertner, Greenbaum, Sadeh, Dolfin, Sirota, and Ben-Nun (2002) who found in healthy premature infants that a rich home environment together with lower time spent asleep and higher nocturnal activity at 32–36 weeks gestational age was associated with higher cognitive development at 6 months. Highlighting the importance of sleep architecture, Scher (1996) found in a combined group of healthy premature and term infants that fewer arousals, lower REMs per minute, and shorter sleep latencies from awake to active sleep at term were associated with lower cognitive development at 1 and 2 years —findings echoed by Arditi-Babchuk, Feldman, and Eidelman (2009). Scher (2005), in a study of 50 healthy term infants evaluated at 10 months, noted that greater motor activity (at 10 months) and a more fragmented sleep pattern were also associated with lower developmental index scores. Dearing, McCartney, Marshall, and Warner (2001) report that regular sleep patterns at 7 and 19 months were positively associated with higher cognitive developmental scores at 24 months and language scores at 36 months of age. Van den Bergh and Mulder (2012) report that when monitoring three sleep parameters (heart rate, body movements, and rapid eye movements) in fetuses of 36–38 weeks gestation, the time taken to pass from quiet to active sleep (i.e., within 3 minutes) was associated with a higher level of effortful control at 8–9 and 14–15 years of age. The authors suggest that this supports the concept that interfetal differences in brain development underpin some of the variability seen in children's response to their environment and, moreover, that those fetuses with more advanced sleep state patterns have more balanced reactivity and regulation with more efficient modulation of cognition and emotions. In summary, the current literature suggests an association between sleep and subsequent developmental attainment, but as studies are correlational, causality has not been proven (Beebe, 2011). As outlined above, the influence of family environment, attachment, rearing practices, and genetic vulnerability will potentially all play a significant moderating role in the child's eventual development.

There is a general consensus that children with poor sleep patterns have adverse behavioral outcomes (Minde et al., 1993; Smedje, Broman, & Hetta, 2001; Stein, Mendelsohn, Obermeyer, Amromin, & Benca, 2001; Zuckerman et al., 1987). Moreover, these deficits are reversible with improvements in sleep patterns paralleling those in behavioral functioning (e.g., Minde, Faucon, & Falkner, 1994). There is also strong evidence that sleep quality makes a unique contribution to problematic behavior over and above that attributable to other causes. Results from structural equation modeling have revealed that sleep problems, after controlling for other predictors, account for a significant proportion of the variance in problematic externalizing and internalizing behaviors (Bates, Viken, Alexander, Beyers, & Stockton, 2002; Calhoun et al., 2012; Reid, Hong, & Wade, 2009; Weinraub et al., 2012). It is also likely that the relationship between sleep and behavior is bidirectional with behavioral deficits influencing sleep quantity and quality.

Given the findings of experimental sleep restriction in adults, with its adverse effects on attention and memory, pediatric researchers have focused on sleep duration as a modulator of childhood neurobehavioral outcomes. As has been previously noted, sleep duration has not been experimentally manipulated in the majority of studies of young children, and authors have relied either on parental report or sleep–wake activity (e.g., actigraphy) to assess sleep. Touchette and colleagues (2007) reported that in a cohort of 1492 children followed from age 5 months to 6 years, those who slept one hour less up to the age of 41 months (and who normalized their sleep duration thereafter) had increased hyperactivity-impulsivity scores and lower receptive vocabulary and nonverbal intellectual skills at 6 years. The authors suggested that there is a critical period in early childhood where shortened sleep duration has a long-term adverse effect. Support for the effect of sleep on language development in young children is also provided by Dionne et al. (2011), who found in their longitudinal study that better sleep consolidation in the first 2 years of life was associated with better language skills up to three years later. O'Callaghan et al. (2010) followed children prospectively to teenage years and reported that those children who often had sleep problems as reported by parents when aged 2–4 years had attention difficulties when assessed at both 5 and 14 years.

Several recent studies have focused on sleep problems in preschool children and have noted that cognitive/behavioral outcomes during early school years is subsequently delayed. Ravid et al. (2009) report that children with shorter sleep durations, higher number of nocturnal awakenings, and lower sleep efficiency had worse cognitive/behavioral performance, while Paavonen, Porkka-Heiskanen, and Lahikainen (2009) report that shorter sleep duration and sleep difficulties in general were related to both a higher frequency of inattention and externalizing symptoms. Liu and colleagues (2012), in a large cohort of 1385 5-year-old Chinese children, noted that those with sleep problems scored 2–3 points lower on IQ testing. The unanswered question is whether this deficit is cumulative or whether some children with sleep problems are more susceptible to adverse neuropsychological outcomes, especially if affected during putative "sensitive" periods (see O'Brien, Chapter 29).

While the consensus in the literature is that pediatric sleep difficulties do adversely affect development, a note of caution needs to be struck. In a meticulous and landmark meta-analysis of the effect of sleep quantity on cognition and behavior in children aged 5–12 years, Astill and colleagues (2012) evaluated 86 studies involving 35,936 children. They found a significant positive association between sleep duration and several (cognitive capacity, executive functioning, and school performance) but not all (sustained attention, declarative or procedural memory, and intelligence) neurocognitive measures. By contrast, they found little evidence of an association between sleep efficiency and neurocognitive measures (sustained attention and executive functioning). The findings for behavioral functioning were also mixed and where significant the relationships were weak. Astill et al. report a significant relationship between shorter sleep and the frequency of problematic behavior (both internalized and externalized) but not for sleep efficiency. Further and contrary to the domains most commonly reported to be affected in adults, they report little evidence for an association between both sleep duration and sleep efficiency and either sustained attention or memory. Finally, despite the lack of evidence for an association between sleep duration and intelligence, nonetheless school performance and multiple-domain measures of cognitive functioning were compromised in children with shorter sleep. In a cogent discussion of developmental differences between children's and adults' brain structure, Astill and colleagues suggest that children may be less sensitive to the impact of sleep restriction because their neuronal networks are less well-developed, and this is further mitigated by a more efficient memory system.

Conclusion

Evidence from experimental studies in animals and, to a lesser extent, experimental studies and studies investigating the impact of sleep pathology on daytime functioning in infants all clearly indicate that sleep plays a major role in brain development and especially the development of long-term or permanent neurocircuits. In addition to changes at the neurophysiological level, there is clear evidence that sleep quality impacts neurocognitive performance, with memory being the best explored to date in infants and young children. Preliminary evidence suggests that some but not all of the sleep and memory relationships observed in adults are present in children, with the role of sleep on emotional valance being the least well-explored. Despite current advances, we are only at the threshold of understanding the role that sleep plays in the interaction between gene expression and neural development, the formation of neurocircuits, and the interplay between sensory input and neural development.

Future Directions

There are many unanswered questions in relation to the role that sleep plays in brain development. Insights into the how sleep moderates the brain during development and the consequences for behavioral and cognitive functioning will help us develop new treatment strategies and better identify children at risk. Key areas for future research in children include:

- The development of experimental methodologies that will allow us to ethically investigate the impact of sleep restriction on daytime functioning
- Empirically validated norms for parameters such as recommended sleep length according to age
- Longitudinal studies that examine the role of sleep during "sensitive" developmental periods
- Observational and experimental studies that examine the relationship between emotional valance, memory, and sleep in children and the relationship of sleep to mental well-being

References

Anders, T. F., Keener, M. A., & Kraemer, H. (1985). Sleep-wake state organization, neonatal assessment and development in premature infants during the first year of life. II. *Sleep, 8*(3), 193–206.

Anders, T. F., Halpern, L. F., & Hua, J. (1992). Sleeping through the night: A developmental perspective. *Pediatrics, 90*(4), 554–560.

Arditi-Babchuk, H., Feldman, R., & Eidelman, A. I. (2009). Rapid eye movement (REM) in premature neonates and developmental outcome at 6 months. *Infant Behavior & Development, 32*(1), 27–32.

Aserinsky, E., & Kleitman, N. (1953). Regularly occurring periods of eye motility, and concomitant phenomena, during sleep. *Science, 118*(3062), 273–274.

Astill, R. G., Van der Heijden, K. B., Van Ijzendoorn, M. H., & Van Someren, E. J. (2012). Sleep, cognition, and behavioral problems in school-age children: A century of research meta-analyzed. *Psychological Bulletin, 138(6), 1109–1138.*

Bates, J. E., Viken, R. J., Alexander, D. B., Beyers, J., & Stockton, L. (2002). Sleep and adjustment in preschool children: Sleep diary reports by mothers relate to behavior reports by teachers. *Child Development, 73*(1), 62–74.

Bear, M. F., & Malenka, R. C. (1994). Synaptic plasticity: LTP and LTD. *Current Opinion in Neurobiology, 4*(3), 389–399.

Beckwith, L., & Parmelee, A. H., Jr. (1986). EEG patterns of preterm infants, home environment, and later IQ. *Child Development, 57*(3), 777–789.

Beebe, D. W. (2006). Neurobehavioral morbidity associated with disordered breathing during sleep in children: A comprehensive review. *Sleep, 29*(9), 1115–1134.

Beebe, D. W. (2011). Cognitive, behavioral, and functional consequences of inadequate sleep in children and adolescents. *Pediatric Clinics of North America, 58*(3), 649–665.

Born, J., & Wilhelm, I. (2012). System consolidation of memory during sleep. *Psychological Research, 76*(2), 192–203.

Bruni, O., Kohler, M., Novelli, L., Kennedy, D., Lushington, K., Martin, J., et al. (2012). The role of NREM sleep instability in child cognitive performance. *Sleep, 35*(5), 649–656.

Buzsaki, G. (1989). Two-stage model of memory trace formation: A role for "noisy" brain states. *Neuroscience, 31*(3), 551–570.

Calhoun, S. L., Fernandez-Mendoza, J., Vgontzas, A. N., Mayes, S. D., Tsaoussoglou, M., Rodriguez-Munoz, A., et al. (2012). Learning, attention/hyperactivity, and conduct problems as sequelae of excessive daytime sleepiness in a general population study of young children. [Research Support, N.I.H., Extramural]. *Sleep, 35*(5), 627–632.

Camfferman, D., Kennedy, J. D., Gold, M., Martin, A. J., Winwood, P., & Lushington, K. (2010). Eczema, sleep, and behavior in children. *Journal of Clinical Sleep Medicine, 6*(6), 581–588.

Cheng, R. K., Williams, C. L., & Meck, W. H. (2008). Oscillatory bands, neuronal synchrony and hippocampal function: Implications of the effects of prenatal choline supplementation for sleep-dependent memory consolidation. *Brain Research, 1237*, 176–194.

Crabtree, V. M., Ivanenko, A., O'Brien, L. M., & Gozal, D. (2003). Periodic limb movement disorder of sleep in children. *Journal of Sleep Research, 12*(1), 73–81.

Cramer, K. S., & Sur, M. (1995). Activity-dependent remodeling of connections in the mammalian visual system. *Current Opinion in Neurobiology, 5*(1), 106–111.

Dahl, R. E. (1996). The impact of inadequate sleep on children's daytime cognitive function. *Semininars in Pediatric Neurology, 3*(1), 44–50.

Dave, A. S., & Margoliash, D. (2000). Song replay during sleep and computational rules for sensorimotor vocal learning. *Science, 290*(5492), 812–816.

Dearing, E., McCartney, K., Marshall, N. L., & Warner, R. M. (2001). Parental reports of children's sleep and wakefulness: Longitudinal associations with cognitive and language outcomes. *Infant Behavior and Development, 24*(2), 151–170.

Diekelmann, S., & Born, J. (2010). The memory function of sleep. *Nature Reviews Neuroscience, 11*(2), 114–126.
Diekelmann, S., Born, J., & Wagner, U. (2010). Sleep enhances false memories depending on general memory performance. *Behavioural Brain Research, 208*(2), 425–429.
Dionne, G., Touchette, E., Forget-Dubois, N., Petit, D., Tremblay, R. E., Montplaisir, J. Y., et al. (2011). Associations between sleep-wake consolidation and language development in early childhood: A longitudinal twin study. *Sleep, 34*(8), 987–995.
Dollman, J., Ridley, K., Olds, T., & Lowe, E. (2007). Trends in the duration of school-day sleep among 10- to 15-year-old South Australians between 1985 and 2004. *Acta Paediatrica, 96*(7), 1011–1014.
Ebbinghaus, H. (1885). *Über das Gedächtnis. Untersuchungen zur experimentellen Psychologie*. Leipzig: Duncker & Humblot.
Ellenbogen, J. M., Hulbert, J. C., Stickgold, R., Dinges, D. F., & Thompson-Schill, S. L. (2006). Interfering with theories of sleep and memory: Sleep, declarative memory, and associative interference. *Current Biology, 16*(13), 1290–1294.
Frank, M. G., Issa, N. P., & Stryker, M. P. (2001). Sleep enhances plasticity in the developing visual cortex. *Neuron, 30*(1), 275–287.
Frank, M. G. (2011). Sleep and developmental plasticity: Not just for kids. In E. J. W. Van Someren, Y. D. van der Werf, P.R. Roelfsema, H.D. Mansvelder, & F. H. L. Da Silva Fernando (Eds.), *Progress in Brain Research* (Vol. 193, Chapter 14, pp. 221–232): Elsevier.
Freud, S., & Strachey, J. (1966). *The Complete Introductory Lectures on Psychoanalysis*. New York: W. W. Norton.
Gaylor, E. E., Goodlin-Jones, B. L., & Anders, T. F. (2001). Classification of young children's sleep problems: A pilot study. *Journal of the American Academy of Child and Adolescent Psychiatry, 40*(1), 61–67.
Gaylor, E. E., Burnham, M. M., Goodlin-Jones, B. L., & Anders, T. F. (2005). A longitudinal follow-up study of young children's sleep patterns using a developmental classification system. *Behavioral Sleep Medicine, 3*(1), 44–61.
Gertner, S., Greenbaum, C. W., Sadeh, A., Dolfin, Z., Sirota, L., & Ben-Nun, Y. (2002). Sleep-wake patterns in preterm infants and 6 month's home environment: Implications for early cognitive development. *Early Human Development, 68*(2), 93–102.
Gozal, E., Row, B. W., Schurr, A., & Gozal, D. (2001). Developmental differences in cortical and hippocampal vulnerability to intermittent hypoxia in the rat. *Neuroscience Letters, 305*(3), 197–201.
Herlenius, E., & Lagercrantz, H. (2001). Neurotransmitters and neuromodulators during early human development. *Early Human Development, 65*(1), 21–37.
Ji, D., & Wilson, M. A. (2007). Coordinated memory replay in the visual cortex and hippocampus during sleep. *Nature Neuroscience, 10*(1), 100–107.
Kennedy, D. N., Makris, N., Herbert, M. R., Takahashi, T., & Caviness, V. S. (2002). Basic principles of MRI and morphometry studies of human brain development. *Developmental Science, 5*(3), 268–278.
Kheirandish, L., & Gozal, D. (2006). Neurocognitive dysfunction in children with sleep disorders. *Developmental Science, 9*(4), 388–399.
Kohler, M., Lushington, K., & Kennedy, J.D. (2010). Neurocognitive performance and behavior before and after treatment for sleep-disordered breathing in children. *Nature and Science of Sleep, 2,* 159–185.
Lam, P., Hiscock, H., & Wake, M. (2003). Outcomes of infant sleep problems: A longitudinal study of sleep, behavior, and maternal well-being. *Pediatrics, 111*(3), e203–e207.
Lenroot, R. K., & Giedd, J. N. (2011). Annual research review: Developmental considerations of gene by environment interactions. *Journal of Child Psychology and Psychiatry and Allied Disciplines, 52*(4), 429–441.
Lim, J., Tan, J.C., Parimal, S., Dinges, D.F., & Chee, M.W. (2010). Sleep deprivation impairs object-selective attention: a view from the ventral visual cortex. *PloS one, 5*(2), e9087.
Liu, J., Zhou, G., Wang, Y., Ai, Y., Pinto-Martin, J., & Liu, X. (2012). Sleep problems, fatigue, and cognitive performance in Chinese kindergarten children. *The Journal of Pediatrics, 161(3), 520–525.*
Maquet, P., Smith, C., & Stickgold, R. (2003). *Sleep and Brain Plasticity*. Oxford; New York: Oxford University Press.
Matricciani, L. A., Olds, T., & Petkov, J. (2012). In search of lost sleep: Secular trends in the sleep time of school-aged children and adolescents. *Sleep Medicine Reviews, 16*(3), 203–211.
Matricciani, L. A., Olds, T. S., Blunden, S., Rigney, G., & Williams, M. T. (2012). Never enough sleep: A brief history of sleep recommendations for children. *Pediatrics, 129*(3), 548–556.
McCarley, R. W. (2007). Neurobiology of REM and NREM sleep. *Sleep Medicine, 8*(4), 302–330.
Minde, K., Popiel, K., Leos, N., Falkner, S., Parker, K., & Handley-Derry, M. (1993). The evaluation and treatment of sleep disturbances in young children. *Journal of Child Psychology and Psychiatry and Allied Disciplines, 34*(4), 521–533.
Minde, K., Faucon, A., & Falkner, S. (1994). Sleep problems in toddlers: Effects of treatment on their daytime behavior. *Journal of the American Academy of Child and Adolescent Psychiatry, 33*(8), 1114–1121.
Mirmiran, M., Scholtens, J., van de Poll, N. E., Uylings, H. B., van der Gugten, J., & Boer, G. J. (1983). Effects of experimental suppression of active (REM) sleep during early development upon adult brain and behavior in the rat. *Brain Research, 283*(2–3), 277–286.
Mirmiran, M., Uylings, H. B., & Corner, M. A. (1983). Pharmacological suppression of REM sleep prior to weaning counteracts the effectiveness of subsequent environmental enrichment on cortical growth in rats. *Brain Research, 283*(1), 102–105.
Mirmiran, M., Feenstra, M. G., Dijcks, F. A., Bos, N. P., & Van Haaren, F. (1988). Functional deprivation of noradrenaline neurotransmission: Effects of clonidine on brain development. *Progress in Brain Research, 73,* 159–172.
Montgomery-Downs, H. E., & Gozal, D. (2006). Snore-associated sleep fragmentation in infancy: Mental development effects and contribution of secondhand cigarette smoke exposure. *Pediatrics, 117*(3), e496–e502.
Novosad, C., Freudigman, K., & Thoman, E. B. (1999). Sleep patterns in newborns and temperament at eight months: A preliminary study. *Journal of Developmental and Behavioral Pediatrics, 20*(2), 99–105.
O'Brien, L. M. (2011). The neurocognitive effects of sleep disruption in children and adolescents. *Sleep Medicine Clinics, 6*(1), 109–116.
O'Callaghan, F. V., Al Mamun, A., O'Callaghan, M., Clavarino, A., Williams, G. M., Bor, W., et al. (2010). The link between sleep problems in infancy and early childhood and attention problems at 5 and 14 years: Evidence from a birth cohort study. *Early Human Development, 86*(7), 419–424.

Paavonen, E. J., Porkka-Heiskanen, T., & Lahikainen, A. R. (2009). Sleep quality, duration and behavioral symptoms among 5–6-year-old children. *European Child & Adolescent Psychiatry, 18*(12), 747–754.

Payne, J. D. (2011). Learning, memory, and sleep in humans. *Sleep Medicine Clinics, 6*(1), 15–30.

Peirano, P. D., & Algarin, C. R. (2007). Sleep in brain development. *Biological Research, 40*(4), 471–478.

Piteo, A. M., Kennedy, J. D., Roberts, R. M., Martin, A. J., Nettelbeck, T., Kohler, M. J., et al. (2011). Snoring and cognitive development in infancy. *Sleep Medicine, 12*(10), 981–987.

Piteo, A. M., Lushington, K., Roberts, R. M., Martin, A. J., Nettelbeck, T., Kohler, M. J., et al. (2011). Parental-reported snoring from the first month of life and cognitive development at 12 months of age. *Sleep Medicine, 12*(10), 975–980.

Poe, G. R., Walsh, C. M., & Bjorness, T. E. (2010). Cognitive neuroscience of sleep. *Progress in Brain Research, 185*, 1–19.

Prehn-Kristensen, A., Göder, R., Chirobeja, S., Breßmann, I., Ferstl, R., & Baving, L. (2009). Sleep in children enhances preferentially emotional declarative but not procedural memories. *Journal of Experimental Child Psychology, 104*(1), 132–139.

Quach, J., Hiscock, H., & Wake, M. (2012). Sleep problems and mental health in primary school new entrants: Cross-sectional community-based study. *Journal of Paediatrics and Child Health, 48(12), 1076–1081.*

Rasch, B., Buchel, C., Gais, S., & Born, J. (2007). Odor cues during slow-wave sleep prompt declarative memory consolidation. *Science, 315*(5817), 1426–1429.

Ravid, S., Afek, I., Suraiya, S., Shahar, E., & Pillar, G. (2009). Sleep disturbances are associated with reduced school achievements in first-grade pupils. *Developmental Neuropsychology, 34*(5), 574–587.

Reid, G. J., Hong, R. Y., & Wade, T. J. (2009). The relation between common sleep problems and emotional and behavioral problems among 2- and 3-year-olds in the context of known risk factors for psychopathology. *Journal of Sleep Research, 18*(1), 49–59.

Reiss, A. L., Abrams, M. T., Singer, H. S., Ross, J. L., & Denckla, M. B. (1996). Brain development, gender and IQ in children. A volumetric imaging study. *Brain: A Journal of Neurology, 119* (Pt. 5), 1763–1774.

Ribeiro, S. (2012). Sleep and plasticity. *Pflugers Archiv: European Journal of Physiology, 463*(1), 111–120.

Richards, J. E., Parmelee, A. H., Jr., & Beckwith, L. (1986). Spectral analysis of infant EEG and behavioral outcome at age five. *Electroencephalography and Clinical Neurophysiology, 64*(1), 1–11.

Roffwarg, H. P., Muzio, J. N., & Dement, W. C. (1966). Ontogenetic development of the human sleep-dream cycle. *Science, 152*(3722), 604–619.

Scher, A. (2005). Infant sleep at 10 months of age as a window to cognitive development. *Early Human Development, 81*(3), 289–292.

Shaffery, J. P., Lopez, J., Bissette, G., & Roffwarg, H. P. (2006). Rapid eye movement sleep deprivation revives a form of developmentally regulated synaptic plasticity in the visual cortex of post-critical period rats. *Neuroscience Letters, 391*(3), 96–101.

Smedje, H., Broman, J. E., & Hetta, J. (2001). Associations between disturbed sleep and behavioural difficulties in 635 children aged six to eight years: a study based on parents' perceptions. *European Child & Adolescent Psychiatry, 10*(1), 1–9.

Stein, M. A., Mendelsohn, J., Obermeyer, W. H., Amromin, J., & Benca, R. (2001). Sleep and behavior problems in school-aged children. *Pediatrics, 107*(4), E60.

Touchette, E., Petit, D., Seguin, J. R., Boivin, M., Tremblay, R. E., & Montplaisir, J. Y. (2007). Associations between sleep duration patterns and behavioral/cognitive functioning at school entry. *Sleep, 30*(9), 1213–1219.

Van den Bergh, B. R., & Mulder, E. J. (2012). Fetal sleep organization: a biological precursor of self-regulation in childhood and adolescence? *Biological Psychology, 89*(3), 584–590.

Wake, M., Morton-Allen, E., Poulakis, Z., Hiscock, H., Gallagher, S., & Oberklaid, F. (2006). Prevalence, stability, and outcomes of cry-fuss and sleep problems in the first 2 years of life: Prospective community-based study. *Pediatrics, 117*(3), 836–842.

Walker, M. P., & Stickgold, R. (2006). Sleep, memory, and plasticity. *Annual Review of Psychology, 57*, 139–166.

Walker, M. P. (2009). The role of sleep in cognition and emotion. *Annals of the New York Academy of Sciences, 1156*, 168–197.

Walker, M. P. (2010). Sleep, memory and emotion. *Progress in Brain Research, 185*, 49–68.

Weinraub, M., Bender, R. H., Friedman, S. L., Susman, E. J., Knoke, B., Bradley, R., et al. (2012). Patterns of developmental change in infants' nighttime sleep awakenings from 6 through 36 months of age. *Developmental Psychology, 48(6), 1511–1528.*

Yoo, S. S., Hu, P. T., Gujar, N., Jolesz, F. A., & Walker, M. P. (2007). A deficit in the ability to form new human memories without sleep. *Nature Neuroscience, 10*(3), 385–392.

Zuckerman, B., Stevenson, J., & Bailey, V. (1987). Sleep problems in early childhood: Continuities, predictive factors, and behavioral correlates. *Pediatrics, 80*(5), 664–671.

CHAPTER

7 Postpartum Sleep: Impact of Infant Sleep on Parents

Robyn Stremler

Abstract

Sleep for parents in the first postpartum year is affected by nighttime care of and interactions with the infant. Women experience decreases in subjective sleep quality and increased nighttime awakenings. Limited research on fathers' sleep in the postpartum suggests they too undergo changes in their sleep, but to a lesser degree. Decisions around infant feeding and sleep location, and parent cognitions related to infant sleep, have effects on parental sleep in the postpartum but more research is needed to elucidate these relationships. Much of the evidence that interventions to improve infant sleep result in improvements in parental sleep is limited by methodological problems, and evaluations of interventions aimed at improving parental sleep are few. This chapter examines what is known about the quality and quantity of sleep for parents in the postpartum and the factors that influence parental sleep. Parental interactions with the infant with effects on parental sleep are discussed, including feeding method, infant sleep location, responses to nighttime infant needs, and parent cognitions around sleep. Postpartum depression, decreased relationship satisfaction, and postpartum weight retention are explored as consequences of disturbed sleep. Finally, evidence of effectiveness of interventions to improve sleep for parents in the postpartum is summarized, and recommendations for future research are proposed.

Key Words: sleep, infant, maternal, paternal, breastfeeding, bed sharing, postpartum depression

Introduction

Although postpartum is defined as the period "immediately following childbirth," adaptation to life with a baby occurs over much of the first year of the child's life. Sleep for parents in the first postpartum year is influenced by their care of and interactions with the infant, whose sleep initially is distributed across the 24-hour day and marked with frequent nighttime awakenings. Much more is known about maternal sleep than paternal sleep, but sleep disturbance in the postpartum has effects on important outcomes for families and has led to the development of interventions to improve sleep.

Parental Sleep in the Postpartum

Both self-report and actigraphy studies have shown that mothers have disturbed sleep after the birth of their baby and experienced more nighttime awakenings during the first few postpartum weeks in comparison to the end of pregnancy and later postpartum months (Nishihara & Horiuchi, 1998; Signal et al., 2007; Swain, O'Hara, Starr, & Gorman, 1997; Wolfson, Crowley, Anwer, & Bassett, 2003). Several studies have demonstrated that more time was spent napping and women had later wake times in the first month postpartum, presumably to compensate for these nighttime sleep disruptions (Nishihara & Horiuchi, 1998; Signal et al., 2007; Swain et al., 1997; Wolfson et al., 2003). Along with changes in sleep, maternal fatigue levels were high in the first three months postpartum compared to prepregnancy reports (Lee & Zaffke, 1999; Troy, 2003).

Actigraphy and self-report estimates of nocturnal sleep time in the first 2 months postpartum have ranged from 6.15–7.18 hours (Quillin, 1997; Stremler et al., 2013; Stremler et al., 2006; Thomas & Foreman, 2005; Yamazaki, 2007). A longitudinal examination of sleep using actigraphy in the first four postpartum months revealed that maternal nocturnal sleep time was within recommended limits (mean 7.2 hours) and did not significantly change across time, but was highly fragmented (Montgomery-Downs, Insana, Clegg-Kraynok, & Mancini, 2010). Sleep fragmentation decreased through the first several months postpartum, with a subsequent improvement in sleep efficiency (from 80% to 90%).

When maternal sleep was studied using polysomnography, increases in slow wave sleep and decreases in stage 1 and 2 sleep were observed in the first postpartum month (Coble et al., 1994; Driver & Shapiro, 1992; Lee & Zaffke, 1999; Lee, Zaffke, & McEnany, 2000; Nishihara & Horiuchi, 1998). These differences may be related to the action of prolactin, as it has been observed that breastfeeding women have less stage 1 and stage 2 sleep, fewer arousals, and more slow wave sleep, when compared to non-lactating postpartum women (Blyton, Sullivan, & Edwards, 2002).

Women and their infants experience low ambient daytime light levels in the early postpartum months (Tsai, Barnard, Lentz, & Thomas, 2009), likely due to heavy infant-care demands, which limit activity outside the home. Changes in melatonin secretion patterns may influence subsequent sleep quality via alterations to circadian rhythms, yet few studies have examined the influence of circadian rhythm disruption on sleep disturbance or fatigue in the postpartum. A comparison of urinary 6-sulfatoxymelatonin levels and timing of release in women at 4–10 weeks postpartum and nonpregnant nulliparous women suggests that postpartum women have higher baseline and lower percent rise in melatonin levels (Thomas & Burr, 2006). These differences suggest altered circadian rhythm, and may contribute to sleep disruption in the postpartum period.

Few studies have examined both maternal and paternal sleep and related outcomes in the postpartum. Wrist actigraphy was used to objectively measure sleep in 72 couples over two days and nights in the last month of pregnancy and the first month postpartum (Gay, Lee, & Lee, 2004). Fathers' sleep did not significantly change from pregnancy to postpartum, while mother's nighttime sleep changed significantly with an average of 41 minutes less sleep per night in the postpartum. Amount of nighttime sleep and fatigue in the postpartum did not differ between mothers and fathers, but mothers self-reported significantly greater sleep disturbance. Another sample of 21 couples underwent actigraphy over one week at 3–8 weeks postpartum. In this sample women obtained more nighttime sleep than their partners, but that sleep included a greater number of awakenings and more time awake (Insana & Montgomery-Downs, 2012). No differences on self-reported sleep quality or fatigue were found between partners, but men had increased sleepiness compared to their partners. Significant fatigue was observed in a small sample of mothers and fathers of twins in the early postpartum months (Damato & Burant, 2008), and greater increases in fatigue from pregnancy to postpartum were seen in a group of fathers as compared to their partners (n = 44) (Elek, Hudson, & Fleck, 2002). It may be that these variations between studies in performance on measures of sleep, sleep quality, and fatigue can be attributed to variation in infant sleep, the unknown variable in these studies.

The belief that parental sleep is directly influenced by infant sleep is reasonable, yet unsupported by empirical evidence. Sinai and Tikotzky (2012) correlated infants' sleep measures with mothers' and fathers' sleep as recorded in sleep logs at between 4 and 5 months postpartum. Night wakings and time spent awake at night for infants were both significantly positively correlated with both mothers' and fathers' outcomes on these measures; however, associations were stronger for mothers. In general, mothers woke more times and spent more time awake at night, likely reflecting a greater role in nighttime parenting for mothers.

Influence of Parental Interaction with Infant

INFANT FEEDING METHOD

A great deal of parent–infant interaction at night is related to infant feeding, so an understanding of its influence on sleep in the postpartum is essential. In a cross-sectional study of 37 women at 4 to 10 weeks postpartum, sleep diaries were used to record maternal and infant sleep over a 24-hour period (Thomas & Foreman, 2005). Total amount of maternal sleep achieved was related to the length of infant feedings, and the length of the longest maternal sleep period was directly related to the length of the longest infant sleep period. Thirty of the participants were exclusively breastfeeding their infants, but analysis for differences based on infant feeding method were not conducted. Provision of guidance to families around how frequently their infant should be fed at various ages, and advice on how to make feedings efficient, such as by utilizing skin-to-skin contact to promote alertness during feeding, may maximize sleep opportunities for parents.

In a study of the effects of infant feeding method on sleep at 3 months postpartum, parental sleep was measured actigraphically and averaged over 2 nights, and feeding method was reported by sleep diary (Doan, Gardiner, Gay, & Lee, 2007). Sleep for parents whose infants were exclusively breastfed across the 2-day period (n = 89) was compared to that for parents whose infants received a combination of breast milk and formula or exclusively formula (n = 44). Mothers who exclusively breastfed their infants slept an average of 40 minutes longer (7.2 ± 1.3 hours vs. 6.4 ± 1.3 hours, $p = 0.008$) than women whose infants received formula. No group differences in amount of sleep achieved over the monitoring period were noted for fathers. Interestingly, self-reported sleep disturbance did not differ for mothers or fathers in the two groups in spite of the relatively large differences in nighttime sleep. When comparisons were made with parents grouped by feeding type in the evening (18:00–23:59) and the night (00:00– 06:00), differences in both mothers' and fathers' sleep were apparent with significantly more sleep across the whole night if exclusive breastfeeding occurred in either the evening or the night. The authors suggest that time taken for preparation of formula feeds at night may explain greater sleep for families choosing to breastfeed, and that mothers may awaken for their infants' feeding even if the father is taking responsibility for the evening or nighttime feeds. Frequency and length of feeds and infant sleep outcomes were not reported in this study, so the influence of these variables cannot be determined.

An examination of maternal sleep measured with actigraphy, subjective sleep reports, fatigue, and sleepiness for postpartum women (n = 80) across weeks 2 to 12 after birth found no differences on any measures between women who exclusively breastfed, exclusively formula fed, or combined both feeding methods (Montgomery-Downs, Clawges, & Santy, 2010). This study did not collect corresponding infant sleep data or infant feeding episode characteristics. Similar results were found in a group of first-time parents whose 1-month-old infants were exclusively breastfed (n = 46) or received formula (n = 14) (Gay et al., 2004). The only difference found on objective sleep measures obtained by actigraphy and self-reported sleep disturbance and fatigue was that exclusively breastfeeding mothers had more time awake after sleep onset; however, this did not result in any differences in total sleep time at night.

There is evidence, collected via sleep diaries in the fourth week postpartum, that breastfed infants sleep less at night and wake more frequently than those who are formula fed, and mothers of breastfed infants wake more often than those of formula-fed infants (n = 44) (Quillin, 1997). Other studies have established via parent report, in 9-month-old infants (n = 41; DeLeon & Karraker, 2007) and in preterm or low birth weight infants at 4 months postterm (n = 128; Schwichtenberg & Poehlmann, 2009) that breastfeeding is associated with more infant night wakings and less total sleep time at night; however, parental sleep was not measured.

Lack of consistency in methods and findings among these studies makes it difficult to draw conclusions on the relationship between infant feeding method and parental sleep. Studies employing objective measures of sleep have found either no difference (Gay et al., 2004; Montgomery-Downs, Clawges, et al., 2010) or preservation of sleep (Lee & Zaffke, 1999) for parents whose infants are breastfed. Although it stands to reason that parents who are waking less and sleeping more have infants that are doing the same, none of the studies employing actigraphy measured infant sleep, and details of frequency and length of feeds were not reported. An examination of the influence of these variables is needed to elucidate the mechanism behind any differential effects of feeding method. While several studies have included one or more of objective measures of infant and parental sleep, subjective reports of sleep quality or satisfaction, and length, frequency, and type of feedings, none have included all these measures. It may be that all these elements require examination in a single, prospective, longitudinal cohort to best determine the interplay between parent and infant sleep, feeding, and another variable of importance, infant sleep location. Videography in combination with objective measures of sleep outcomes in the home environment may be needed to best characterize infant feeding episodes, parent–infant interactions, and infant proximity at night.

While the available evidence related to the amount of and characteristics of parent and infant sleep is conflicting, promotion of breastfeeding is recommended in order to optimize many other important infant and maternal health outcomes (World Health Organization, 2002). Since supplementation of breastfeeding with formula is often perceived as a means by which to increase infant sleep at night, parents should be made aware that the research literature does not support a recommendation of formula feeding as a means to improve sleep. It may also help women planning to breastfeed to know that no studies that have asked parents to report on the quality of their sleep found any differences between parents with breastfed versus formula-fed infants.

INFANT SLEEP LOCATION

Parents may bed-share (i.e., infant sleeps in the same bed as parents) or room-share (i.e., infant sleeps in the same room but in a separate bed from parents) with their infant or have their infant sleep alone (i.e., in a separate room in a separate bed). Few studies exist that have examined the effects of infant sleep location on maternal sleep, and none have examined fathers' sleep. The following summary of evidence related to infant sleep location is focused on effects on sleep for parents (see also Burnham, Chapter 12).

Women and their infants, 20 of whom were routinely (>4 hours/night, >5 days/week) bed sharing, and 15 of whom routinely slept in separate rooms (<1 night/week with bed sharing), spent two nights in a sleep lab undergoing polysomnography (Mosko, Richard, & McKenna, 1997). On one night the mother–infant dyads slept in their usual sleep conditions and on the other, they slept in the alternate condition; order of nights was randomly assigned. Although sleep parameters were within normal range on all nights, on the bed-sharing night all mothers spent a slightly larger portion (4% more) of the night in Stage 1–2 NREM sleep and a slightly smaller portion (4% less) in Stage 3–4 NREM sleep, regardless of usual infant sleep location. No change in amount of REM sleep was found. Arousals from sleep to wake were more frequent during bed sharing regardless of usual infant sleep location; mean increase was 3.6 arousals per hour. Although arousals were more frequent during bed sharing, total time awake at night did not increase, indicating the arousals were brief. Since differences in sleep architecture were noted regardless of usual infant sleep location, women may not "get used to" bed sharing. Women who routinely had their infant sleep in a separate room rated their sleep quality as lower on the assigned bed-sharing night, indicating that occasional bed sharing may be more disruptive to self-reported sleep quality than routine bed sharing. Synchronous arousals with the infant also were more frequent on bed-sharing nights. More frequent arousals and lighter sleep may allow mothers to better monitor their infants while bed sharing, but any protective effect on infants' health of this alteration in maternal sleep has yet to be established.

In another study examining infant–parent interaction, 40 routinely bed-sharing infants aged 5–27 weeks were matched for age with infants who routinely slept on a separate surface in their parents' bedroom (Baddock, Galland, Bolton, Williams, & Taylor, 2006). Overnight video recordings of these families over 2 nights determined infant sleep time and number of feeding interactions and parental "checks" on the infant. Bed-sharing parents looked at or touched their infants significantly more frequently than did room-sharing parents (median 11 vs. 4 times per night; $p<0.0001$), but given that these interactions were only visually observed, the extent and length of arousal or awakening and impact on parental sleep quantity and subjective sleep quality was not evaluated. Presumably, checking on the infant during bed sharing occurs in a shorter time and with less arousal than checking on an infant on a separate sleep surface, even if they are in close proximity. Given that many families who choose to bed-share do so as a means to obtain more sleep or be less disrupted by having to get out of bed to care for the infant, the impact on parental sleep quantity and quality of breastfeeding and checking on the infant merit further exploration. It remains unknown what is preferable to maximize sleep quantity or quality—multiple brief awakenings with an infant in close proximity, or fewer, more alerting interactions with an infant in a separate sleep location.

First-time mothers ($n = 246$) provided information regarding planned and actual infant sleep location at 6 and 12 weeks postpartum (Stremler et al., in press). Actigraphy provided objective evaluation of sleep, and subjective maternal sleep disturbance was also measured. Women were classified as "usually bed sharing," "usually room sharing" or "usually solitary sleeping" if they indicated the infant spent the whole night or most of the night in the indicated sleep location. Room sharing was the most common usual sleeping arrangement, with 46% of infants doing so at 6 weeks and 39% at 12 weeks. At 6 weeks, 17% of families were usually bed sharing; rates decreased to 12% at 12 weeks postpartum. At 6 weeks, usually bed-sharing mothers had shorter stretches of sleep than those usually solitary sleeping (130 mins vs. 156 mins; $p = 0.03$) and more awakenings than those usually room sharing and solitary sleeping (11 vs. 9 vs. 8; $p = 0.001$). At 12 weeks, usually room-sharing mothers had shorter stretches of uninterrupted sleep than those usually solitary sleeping (164 mins vs. 192 mins; $p = 0.04$). There were no significant differences between infant sleep location groups on maternal subjective sleep disturbance. Given the variation in infant sleep location choice, and evidence that infant sleep location has effects on objective maternal sleep outcomes, further prospective, longitudinal research is needed on the effects of infant sleep location on a broad range of health outcomes for infant, mother, and partner across the first postpartum year. Such studies would need to account for parents' experiences with the infant, as parental responses to infant feeding, crying, or sleeping behaviors may shape where the infant sleeps.

INFANT CARE RESPONSIBILITIES

Patterns of women's sleep and women's responses to sleep disruption (Hislop & Arber, 2003) are affected by the nature of women's roles and responsibilities. Despite increased participation in paid work, women still bear primary responsibility for childcare (Statistics Canada, 2011), including physical and emotional care for young children at night (Tikotzky, Sadeh, & Glickman-Gavrieli, 2011). This work at night can be viewed as an additional "shift" where women's sleep needs are subjugated to those of other family members (Venn, Arber, Meadows, & Hislop, 2008). In a qualitative study (Kennedy, Gardiner, Gay, & Lee, 2007), women during pregnancy and postpartum used naps as a way of coping with sleep loss at night; however, paid work demands and partner availability for childcare coverage determined if naps could occur.

For women still on maternity leave from work (around 4 months postpartum in the country of study, Israel), greater parenting stress was associated with more infant wake time at night, shorter infant daytime naps, and more maternal night wakings; these relationships did not hold true for women who had returned to work (Sinai & Tikotzky, 2012). The authors suggest that women on leave from paid employment do not find opportunities to nap, and that women who return to work perhaps experience less stress due to more control over their own schedule and having breaks from continuous caregiving. Given variations in length of maternity leave for employed women (e.g., typically 6 weeks in the United States, 12 months in Canada), differences in families' experiences of sleep and fatigue based on time of return to work merits further examination.

A study of 51 mothers of 3-month-old infants examined factors related to mothers' decisions to take naps (Cottrell & Karraker, 2002). Nap taking was predicted by maternal perceptions of sleep disturbance rather than by actual amount of sleep or infant wake time at night. Mothers who were engaged in more hours of employment or who had more children at home reported less nap taking. Almost half of the women took no naps at all over the 3-day recording period, and of those who did nap the average length was 30 minutes. Similarly, actigraphic evidence determined that after postpartum week 2, fewer than 50% of women napped at least one time per week, and those who did nap did so only an average of two times each week (Montgomery-Downs, Insana, et al., 2010). Given that few postpartum women nap during the day, and there is little evidence of its contribution to improved sleep outcomes, it may be time to dispense with the age-old advice to "sleep when the baby sleeps."

COGNITIONS AROUND INFANT SLEEP

Evidence suggests that maternal cognitions around limit-setting, anger at the infant's demands at night, and doubts around parenting ability are associated with infant sleep problems (Morrell, 1999; Morrell & Steele, 2003) and that those cognitions influence nighttime parenting behavior (Sadeh, Flint-Ofir, Tirosh, & Tikotzky, 2007; Teti & Crosby, 2012; Tikotzky & Sadeh, 2009). Links between maternal behaviors and infant sleep also seem to be bidirectional; that is, infants with sleep difficulties require greater maternal involvement, but maternal involvement in infant sleep can also serve to shape infant sleep abilities (Tikotzky & Sadeh, 2009). No examinations of these relationships have measured parental sleep—again, likely because the assumption is that if the infant is waking at night, so is the parent. Since parent involvement in sleep may be influenced by the amount and nature of parent sleep at night, these relationships merit further examination. Since it is unknown if parent cognitions about infant sleep are related to parent cognitions about their own sleep, it may be revelatory to evaluate the influence of parent cognitions around sleep in general and their influence on sleep behavior. Parents who have their own difficulty with sleep may find that this radically alters their behaviors with their child, perhaps leading to more interaction at night given their own wakefulness, or more anger toward the child if the child's wakefulness exacerbates the parent's existing sleep disturbance.

Consequences of Disturbed Postpartum Sleep

POSTPARTUM DEPRESSION

Onset of depression frequently occurs during the childbearing years, affecting approximately 13%

of postpartum women (Gale & Harlow, 2003). Maternal depression adversely affects maternal–infant relationships, parenting practices, family functioning, and general well-being (Gale & Harlow, 2003; Yonkers et al., 2009). Sleep disturbance is associated with depression in nonpregnant populations (Breslau, Roth, Rosenthal, & Andreski, 1996; Buysse et al., 2008), and there is evidence to suggest a relationship between sleep disturbance and maternal depression in the postpartum, although directionality of this relationship has not been determined.

Associations are consistently reported between maternal sleep disturbances, presumably due to the disruptive nature of infant sleep at night, and maternal depression. Depressive symptoms and self-reported sleep quantity have been found to be associated in the early postpartum period (Huang, Carter, & Guo, 2004; Lee & Zaffke, 1999; Swain et al., 1997). In a cross-sectional study of 2830 women in Norway at 6–19 weeks postpartum, depression was associated with low sleep quality even when adjusting for other risk factors such as previous depression, poor partner relationship, and depression during pregnancy (Dorheim, Bondevik, Eberhard-Gran, & Bjorvatn, 2009). Postpartum mothers' increased time awake during the night and poor sleep quality were strongly associated with increased negative daytime mood, particularly in the first four weeks after delivery (Quillin, 1997; Wolfson et al., 2003). Frequency of night awakenings detected by polysomnography was related to negative mood at one month postpartum for women who reported higher levels of depressed mood (Lee, McEnany, & Zaffke, 2000).

There are few longitudinal, prospective examinations of childbearing women's sleep and relationship to depression. In a population-based postpartum depression study (n = 505), mothers exhibiting major depressive symptoms at 4 and 8 weeks postpartum were significantly more likely to report having received <6 hours of sleep in a 24-hour period over the previous week and being awakened by their baby three or more times between 10 pm and 6 am (Dennis & Ross, 2005). Self-reported sleep disturbance and depressive symptoms were associated in late pregnancy and at 1, 2, and 3 months postpartum in 124 primiparous women; however, the ability to predict depressive symptoms based on sleep disturbance scores was not assessed (Goyal, Gay, & Lee, 2007).

Since most studies employed maternal report of maternal sleep disturbance and infant sleep problems, the possibility exists that depressed mothers may perceive their own or their infant's sleep more negatively than nondepressed mothers, or be more likely to report sleep problems whether they exist or not. However, there is evidence that treatment of infant sleep problems results in decreased incidence of maternal depression. Two randomized, controlled trials of brief behavioral interventions to decrease infant sleep problems significantly decreased maternal report of an infant sleep problem and reduced maternal symptoms of depression (Hiscock & Wake, 2001, 2002). Similarly, Wolfson and colleagues demonstrated that parent training focused on developing healthy infant sleep patterns improves parental competence and marital satisfaction and decreases parents' stress (Wolfson, Lacks, & Futterman, 1992).

Little is known about the relationship between infant sleep and paternal depression in the postpartum period. A one-group, pre/post intervention study (n = 71 mothers, 60 fathers) found decreases in problematic infant behaviors and decreases in depression scores in both mothers and fathers. However, analysis was not conducted based on type of behavior problem (i.e., crying, sleeping, feeding), so these findings are only suggestive of a possible relationship between treatment of infant sleep problems and improvement in paternal mood (Smart & Hiscock, 2007).

RELATIONSHIP WITH PARTNER

Given the effects of sleep disturbance on mood and cognition, it is plausible that postpartum sleep disturbance could contribute to a decline in partner relationships in the first year as parents. With the arrival of a child comes the physical and emotional work of caretaking and new roles and responsibilities for parents to take on and negotiate. Indeed, women have described sleep itself as a negotiated behavior that requires balancing the infant's needs, the woman's own sleep needs, and relying upon support from the partner and others to allow the woman time to sleep uninterrupted (Kennedy et al., 2007).

Marital satisfaction for both mothers and fathers diminished across the first year postpartum in a study of 107 first-time parent couples (Meijer & van den Wittenboer, 2007). Marital satisfaction was measured before birth and at 2 weeks, 7 weeks, and 1 year after birth, when parents also reported amount of infant sleep, number of nighttime awakenings, and degree of parental insomnia (defined as problems with initiating, maintaining, or nonrestorative sleep). The steepest rate of decline in marital satisfaction occurred between 7 weeks and 1 year postpartum. There were no direct effects of the infant's sleep on maternal or paternal insomnia or marital satisfaction. Interestingly, over time, fathers' insomnia appeared to contribute to mothers' insomnia and vice versa. These findings may indicate that parents' abilities to cope with or support each other through the challenges of infant sleep—for example, the ability to initiate sleep when the opportunity presents or to return to sleep once awakened—may be more important than any disruptive effects of infant sleep alone.

In a study of 72 first-time parent dyads, no significant associations were found between parent-reported length of uninterrupted infant nighttime sleep and marital satisfaction when the infant was 3 months old (Loutzenhiser & Sevigny, 2008). As parents were asked to report on infant sleep in only one way, the effects of total amount of infant sleep and the number of awakenings across the night could not be evaluated. To better elucidate the effects of infant sleep on marital satisfaction, future research should objectively measure length and continuity of both infant and parent sleep and evaluate subjective sleep quality for parents along with marital satisfaction.

POSTPARTUM WEIGHT RETENTION

Short sleep duration in the postpartum is linked to greater retention of weight in the postpartum. Sleep deprivation results in alteration in the production of appetite-regulating hormones leptin and ghrelin (Dzaja et al., 2004; Mullington et al., 2003), which may contribute to overeating and weight gain. Prospective examinations of self-reported usual sleep duration at 6 months and 1 year postpartum found an association between short sleep duration (<5 hours per night) and substantial postpartum weight retention (>5 kg above pregravid weight) at 1 year postpartum (Gunderson et al., 2008), and higher adiposity at 3 years postpartum (Taveras et al., 2011). These findings were independent of potential confounders, including prepregnancy body mass index, gestational weight gain, and parity. Researchers evaluating the effectiveness of interventions to improve infant and parent sleep should consider inclusion of postpartum weight retention as a study outcome, given the potential contribution of postpartum weight retention to the development of obesity in women.

Interventions to Improve Postpartum Sleep

Interventions to improve postpartum sleep for parents have typically focused on changing the infant's sleep by preventing infant sleep problems in the early postpartum or by treating infant sleep problems in infants in the second half of the first postpartum year (see Gruber, Constantin, Cassoff, and Michaelsen, Chapter 39). Randomized controlled trials (RCTs) of interventions aimed at promoting infant sleep in the first few postpartum months (Kerr, Jowett, & Smith, 1996; Pinilla & Birch, 1993; St James-Roberts, Sleep, Morris, Owen, & Gillham, 2001; Symon, Marley, Martin, & Norman, 2005; Wolfson et al., 1992) have provided parents with basic education on infant sleep and training in strategies aimed at limiting the development of unwanted sleep associations, increasing the infant's self-soothing ability, and facilitating day-night entrainment. All these trials used parent report of infant sleep and found longer, more consolidated sleep periods for infants who received the experimental intervention. Although none of these studies examined the effects of the intervention on parental sleep outcomes, presumably assuming that if infant sleep improved so too must parent sleep, one author did examine effects on parents' stress (Wolfson et al., 1992). Using the Hassles and Uplifts Scales (Kanner, Coyne, Schaefer, & Lazarus, 1981), Wolfson et al. (1992) measured life stressors and positive experiences before the baby's birth and at 6–9 and 16–20 weeks after delivery. Although no differences between groups were observed with respect to positive experiences, parents who received training related to infant sleep reported significantly fewer hassles than parents in the control group when the infant was 6–9 weeks old. Parents in the sleep training group also did not experience an increase in hassles over the course of the study, as was observed in the control group parents.

RCTs conducted with older infants (Hiscock et al., 2007; Hiscock & Wake, 2002; Mindell et al., 2011a; Mindell, Telofski, Wiegand, & Kurtz, 2009) aimed to provide information regarding negative sleep associations and the importance of self-soothing ability. Strategies to decrease night feeding and waking were also recommended, including use of a bedtime routine, controlled crying and gradual removal of parental presence at sleep onset. No advice related to parents' sleep was offered. Three of the studies (Hiscock et al., 2007; Hiscock & Wake, 2002; Mindell et al., 2011a) included maternal sleep outcomes and found reductions in problematic infant sleep behaviors and a concomitant improvement in maternal report of sleep outcomes using select items from, or the entire, Pittsburgh Sleep Quality Index (PSQI; Buysse, Reynolds, Monk, Berman, & Kupfer, 1989).

Using two items from the PSQI, sleep quality at 2 months post-intervention was evaluated in the final 57 women enrolled in an RCT, not the total sample (total n = 156; Hiscock & Wake, 2002). Women in the intervention group were significantly more likely than those in the control group to rate their sleep quality as "very good" and less likely to rate it as "very bad." Women assigned to the intervention group were also more likely to report they had "enough" sleep and less likely to have "not enough sleep." PSQI total scores were not reported. When sleep quality was evaluated at the 4-month post-intervention assessment, group differences were not maintained.

Hiscock et al.'s (2007) cluster RCT with 328 mothers at maternal–child health centers found statistically significant differences between groups, with more control than intervention mothers reporting poor sleep quality at 3 months (72% vs. 63%) and 5 months (63% vs. 52%) post-randomization. More women assigned to the control group reported insufficient sleep than women who received the intervention (45% vs. 34%), but only at the 5-month post-randomization assessment. The PSQI items used for these assessments were not reported. Although participants were followed to 17 months and 6 years post-randomization, no maternal sleep quality data were reported at follow-up (Hiscock, Bayer, Hampton, Ukoumunne, & Wake, 2008; Price, Wake, Ukoumunne, & Hiscock, 2012).

An RCT of an Internet-based intervention that included infants and toddlers (age range 6–36 months) reported improvements on the PSQI for maternal sleep onset latency, total sleep time, number of night awakenings, time spent awake at night, and sleep efficiency for women assigned to the intervention groups at 1 and 2 weeks post-intervention (Mindell et al., 2011a). However, analyses were presented as within-group, one-way repeated measures ANOVAs rather than as between-group comparisons, thereby eliminating the benefits conferred by randomization to group. Although improvement within groups (including the control group) was demonstrated over time, improvements in sleep outcomes cannot be attributed to experimental condition given the presentation of data. Total PSQI scores were analyzed across groups, and at 2 weeks post-intervention fewer control group participants (25%) were good sleepers (PSQI total score <5) as compared to either of the intervention group participants (33.3% intervention; 47.6% intervention plus routine); these differences were statistically significant. Sleep was reassessed 1 year post-intervention (Mindell et al., 2011b) using a single item from the PSQI to evaluate global sleep quality. Again, these follow-up data were examined within groups only and showed improvement in sleep quality compared to baseline, although at lower ratings than 2 weeks post-intervention.

Only one study of an intervention to decrease infants' behavioral sleep problems has evaluated both maternal and paternal subjective sleep quality (Hall, Clauson, Carty, Janssen, & Saunders, 2006). Using a one-group, pretest/post-test design with 39 couples, statistically significant improvements were found on PSQI total scores from baseline to 6 weeks post-intervention (2.2 point decrease). Unfortunately, data were presented in aggregate form so effects of gender were not reported. Although sleep quality was also measured at 16 weeks post-intervention, those data were not included, so longer-term maintenance of sleep quality improvement is unknown.

Overall, the strength of evidence from these studies of sleep interventions in older infants is limited; only one uncontrolled study examined fathers' sleep, none used objective measures of sleep, and all had methodological or reporting problems. There is also little evidence of improved sleep outcomes for parents beyond the immediate post-intervention study period.

Given that infant and parent sleep are presumed to affect one another, it is surprising that few examinations of strategies to improve parents' sleep exist. Three RCTs (Lee & Gay, 2011; Stremler et al., 2013; Stremler et al., 2006) tested interventions aimed at improving parents' sleep, independent from the infant's.

Two samples of parents were enrolled in a RCT of a modified sleep hygiene intervention to reduce parental nighttime disruption (Lee & Gay, 2011). All advice focused on the nighttime sleep environment; no advice related to behavioral modification of infant sleep was given. Parents in the experimental groups were seen in the last month of pregnancy and were instructed to have the infant close to the maternal bedside for care at night, reduce noise from the infant through use of a white noise machine, and use a night light to ensure low lighting in the maternal bedroom. The environmental sleep recommendations were expected to make infant care more convenient and less arousing, thereby decreasing parent awakenings due to intermittent infant noise and facilitating parents' return to sleep when awakened. The two samples of first-time expectant parents included women and their partners in stable relationships (n = 118) recruited from fee-based childbirth classes, and women (n = 122) recruited from free prenatal classes and clinics serving low-income women. Parents' sleep was measured over a 48-hour period at 1 and 3 months postpartum using actigraphy and self-report of sleep disturbance. In the socioeconomically advantaged sample, bedroom environment modifications alone did not improve sleep, as there were no differences between groups on any sleep outcomes. In the sample of low-income women, those in the intervention group attained more nocturnal sleep (7.1 hours vs. 6.5 hours), better sleep efficiency (80% vs. 75%), and less wake time after sleep onset (19% vs. 23%) than women in the control group at 3 months postpartum; these differences reached statistical significance. Number of night awakenings was not reported, although the intervention was described as focused on reducing the frequency of arousals in addition to their duration. Sleep disturbance scores did not differ between groups in either sample. While the intervention was acceptable to both samples, low fidelity of use of the interventions in the experimental groups (particularly the white noise machine) and contamination with intervention strategies in the control groups likely limited ability to detect differences in sleep outcomes between groups. It may be that women and their partners from socioeconomically advantaged backgrounds are better able to access advice related to maternal and infant sleep, and to acquire material resources to modify the bedroom environment, than are women with limited income. The home environments of the less advantaged sample also may have been less conducive to sleep (e.g., noisier, more crowded) so that the modifications made to the bedroom in the experimental group were more impactful.

A pilot RCT (n = 30) tested a behavioral-educational intervention designed to increase nighttime sleep and sleep continuity for both mother and infant in the early postpartum (Stremler et al., 2006). First-time mothers in the intervention group received a 45-minute meeting with a nurse in the immediate postpartum in-hospital, a written booklet, and weekly phone contact to reinforce information and problem-solve. Topics covered included maternal sleep hygiene, strategies to make maternal sleep a priority, maternal relaxation techniques (e.g., progressive muscle relaxation, deep breathing), discussion of the challenges of sleep deprivation and parenting, information on what to expect from infant sleep and sleep cues, strategies for infant sleep promotion (e.g., stretching length between feedings, bedtime routine), and strategies for promoting infant night–day entrainment and self-soothing. Control group participants received a 10-minute meeting to discuss only maternal sleep hygiene and basic information about infant sleep. Based on actigraphy data, statistically significant differences between groups were found. Infants in the intervention group woke less often and had longer stretches of sleep, and women in the intervention group achieved more sleep (433 vs. 376 minutes) compared to the control group. Significantly fewer mothers in the intervention group rated their sleep as a problem at 6 weeks.

In follow-up to this pilot work, a large-scale RCT (n = 246) was conducted to be adequately powered to detect differences on a greater number of maternal and infant sleep and other health outcomes, to enroll a more diverse sample, and to examine outcomes at 12 weeks postpartum (Stremler et al., 2013). The group conditions were slightly modified: control group participants received no information about maternal or infant sleep, and telephone contacts were made to both groups at 1, 2, and 4 weeks postpartum instead of weekly. No statistically significant differences between groups were found on any outcomes at 6 or 12 weeks postpartum. Although women in the larger trial were ethnically diverse (63% Caucasian, 20% Asian, 7% Black), they were overwhelmingly partnered (97%), educated at the postsecondary level (90%), and had a mean age of 32 years. These high levels of socioeconomic status and support may explain lack of effect of the intervention. Furthermore, many women in both the intervention and control groups (61%) independently sought out information about sleep, and may have been able to implement maternal and infant sleep strategies on their own. It also may be that the newborn period is too early to implement maternal and infant sleep strategies, or that the early postpartum period is such a period of great change, role adjustment, and sleep debt for families that planning for and consistently implementing sleep strategies is not feasible or is not a priority.

The few examinations of interventions to improve parent sleep provide little support for such strategies in late pregnancy or the early postpartum. Socially disadvantaged families may benefit most from advice regarding infant and maternal sleep, and future interventions should be tested in this population. An exploration of parents' beliefs around infant and parent sleep, and their experience of barriers, facilitators, and motivations related to implementing sleep strategies, would provide insight for development and testing of future intervention studies at points farther along in the first postpartum year.

Conclusion

Women experience decreases in subjective sleep quality, changes in sleep architecture, and increased nighttime awakenings with the arrival of a new baby. Limited research on fathers' sleep experiences in the postpartum suggests that they too experience changes in their sleep, but to a lesser degree than mothers. Few studies have linked infant sleep outcomes to parental sleep outcomes; rather, a direct relationship between the two is assumed given the need for care of the infant at night. The effects of feeding method on parental sleep are unclear, except to say that there is likely no benefit conferred by offering formula at night. Similarly, there is no one infant sleep location that clearly preserves sleep for parents. A more comprehensive approach to the study of sleep within the family, including important variables such as infant feeding method, infant sleep location, parental cognitions around sleep, employment status, and division of infant care responsibilities would lend greater insight on the mechanisms of sleep disturbance in the postpartum and better allow for development of interventions and recommendations for parents. Future research on sleep in the postpartum should be longitudinal in design across the first postpartum year; examine infant, maternal, and paternal sleep; and include important related health outcomes such as depression and breastfeeding rates.

Future Directions

Inclusion of men in studies of sleep in the postpartum is needed to characterize the impact of infant sleep on fathers.

Studies that concurrently measure, with objective methods, infant sleep and parental sleep are necessary to define the relationship between infant and parent sleep, which is assumed but as yet is not definitively demonstrated.

Examinations of infant and parental sleep should include measurements across the first postpartum year with attention to the influence of infant feeding method, infant sleep location, infant care activities and responsibilities, and parental cognitions around sleep.

References

Baddock, S. A., Galland, B. C., Bolton, D. P., Williams, S. M., & Taylor, B. J. (2006). Differences in infant and parent behaviors during routine bed sharing compared with cot sleeping in the home setting. *Pediatrics, 117*, 1599–1607.

Blyton, D. M., Sullivan, C. E., & Edwards, N. (2002). Lactation is associated with an increase in slow-wave sleep in women. *Journal of Sleep Research, 11*, 297–303.

Breslau, N., Roth, T., Rosenthal, L., & Andreski, P. (1996). Sleep disturbance and psychiatric disorders: A longitudinal epidemiological study of young adults. *Biological Psychiatry, 39*, 411–418.

Buysse, D. J., Reynolds, C. F., Monk, T. H., Berman, S. R., & Kupfer, D. J. (1989). The Pittsburgh Sleep Quality Index: a new instrument for psychiatric practice and research. *Psychiatry Research, 28*, 193–213.

Buysse, D. J., Angst, J., Gamma, A., Ajdacic, V., Eich, D., & Rossler, W. (2008). Prevalence, course, and comorbidity of insomnia and depression in young adults. *Sleep, 31*, 473–480.

Coble, P. A., Reynolds, C. F. 3rd, Kupfer, D. J., Houck, P. R., Day, N. L., & Giles, D. E. (1994). Childbearing in women with and without a history of affective disorder. II. Electroencephalographic sleep. *Comprehensive Psychiatry, 35*, 215–224.

Cottrell, L., & Karraker, K. H. (2002). Correlates of nap taking in mothers of young infants. *Journal of Sleep Research, 11*, 209–212.

Damato, E. G., & Burant, C. (2008). Sleep patterns and fatigue in parents of twins. *Journal of Obstetrical Gynecological and Neonatal Nursing, 37*, 738–749.

DeLeon, C. W., & Karraker, K. H. (2007). Intrinsic and extrinsic factors associated with night waking in 9-month-old infants. *Infant Behavior and Development, 30*, 596–605.

Dennis, C. L., & Ross, L. (2005). Relationships among infant sleep patterns, maternal fatigue, and development of depressive symptomatology. *Birth, 32*, 187–193.

Doan, T., Gardiner, A., Gay, C. L., & Lee, K. A. (2007). Breastfeeding increases sleep duration of new parents. *Journal of Perinatal and Neonatal Nursing, 21*, 200–206.

Dorheim, S. K., Bondevik, G. T., Eberhard-Gran, M., & Bjorvatn, B. (2009). Sleep and depression in postpartum women: a population-based study. *Sleep, 32*, 847–855.

Driver, H. S., & Shapiro, C. M. (1992). A longitudinal study of sleep stages in young women during pregnancy and postpartum. *Sleep, 15*, 449–453.

Dzaja, A., Dalal, M. A., Himmerich, H., Uhr, M., Pollmacher, T., & Schuld, A. (2004). Sleep enhances nocturnal plasma ghrelin levels in healthy subjects. *American Journal of Physiology -Endocrinology and Metabolism, 286*, E963–E967. Elek, S. M., Hudson, D. B., & Fleck, M. O. (2002). Couples' experiences with fatigue during the transition to parenthood. *Journal of Family Nursing, 8*, 221–240.

Gale, S., & Harlow, B. L. (2003). Postpartum mood disorders: A review of clinical and epidemiological factors. *Journal of Psychosomatic Obstetrics and Gynaecology, 24*, 257–266.

Gay, C. L., Lee, K. A., & Lee, S. Y. (2004). Sleep patterns and fatigue in new mothers and fathers. *Biological Research for Nursing, 5*, 311–318.

Goyal, D., Gay, C. L., & Lee, K. A. (2007). Patterns of sleep disruption and depressive symptoms in new mothers. *Journal of Perinatal and Neonatal Nursing, 21*, 123–129.

Gunderson, E. P., Rifas-Shiman, S. L., Oken, E., Rich-Edwards, J. W., Kleinman, K. P., Taveras, E. M., & Gillman, M. W. (2008). Association of fewer hours of sleep at 6 months postpartum with substantial weight retention at 1 year postpartum. *American Journal of Epidemiology, 167*, 178–187.

Hall, W. A., Clauson, M., Carty, E. M., Janssen, P. A., & Saunders, R. A. (2006). Effects on parents of an intervention to resolve infant behavioral sleep problems. *Pediatric Nursing, 32*, 243–250.

Hiscock, H., & Wake, M. (2001). Infant sleep problems and postnatal depression: A community-based study. *Pediatrics, 107*, 1317–1322.

Hiscock, H., & Wake, M. (2002). Randomised controlled trial of behavioural infant sleep intervention to improve infant sleep and maternal mood. *British Medical Journal, 324(7345)*, 1062–1065.

Hiscock, H., Bayer, J., Gold, L., Hampton, A., Ukoumunne, O. C., & Wake, M. (2007). Improving infant sleep and maternal mental health: A cluster randomised trial. *Archives of Disease in Childhood, 92*, 952–958.

Hiscock, H., Bayer, J. K., Hampton, A., Ukoumunne, O. C., & Wake, M. (2008). Long-term mother and child mental health effects of a population-based infant sleep intervention: Cluster-randomized, controlled trial. *Pediatrics, 122*, e621–e627.

Hislop, J., & Arber, S. (2003). Sleepers wake! The gendered nature of sleep disruption among mid-life women. *Sociology–The Journal of the British Sociological Association, 37*, 695–711.

Huang, C. M., Carter, P. A., & Guo, J. L. (2004). A comparison of sleep and daytime sleepiness in depressed and non-depressed mothers during the early postpartum period. *Journal of Nursing Research, 12*, 287–296.

Insana, S. P., & Montgomery-Downs, H. E. (2012). Sleep and sleepiness among first-time postpartum parents: A field- and laboratory-based multimethod assessment. *Developmental Psychobiology.*

Kanner, A. D., Coyne, J. C., Schaefer, C., & Lazarus, R. S. (1981). Comparison of two modes of stress measurement: daily hassles and uplifts versus major life events. *Journal of Behavioral Medicine, 4*, 1–39.

Kennedy, H. P., Gardiner, A., Gay, C., & Lee, K. A. (2007). Negotiating sleep: A qualitative study of new mothers. *Journal of Perinatal and Neonatal Nursing, 21*, 114–122. Kerr, S. M., Jowett, S. A., & Smith, L. N. (1996). Preventing sleep problems in infants: A randomized controlled trial. *Journal of Advanced Nursing, 24*, 938–942.

Lee, K. A., & Zaffke, M. E. (1999). Longitudinal changes in fatigue and energy during pregnancy and the postpartum period. *Journal of Obstetrical, Gynecological and Neonatal Nursing, 28*, 183–191.

Lee, K. A., McEnany, G., & Zaffke, M. E. (2000). REM sleep and mood state in childbearing women: Sleepy or weepy? *Sleep, 23*, 877–885.

Lee, K. A., Zaffke, M. E., & McEnany, G. (2000). Parity and sleep patterns during and after pregnancy. *Obstetrics and Gynecology, 95*, 14–18.

Lee, K. A., & Gay, C. L. (2011). Can modifications to the bedroom environment improve the sleep of new parents? Two randomized controlled trials. *Research in Nursing and Health, 34*, 7–19.

Loutzenhiser, L., & Sevigny, P. (2008). Infant sleep and family functioning in first-time parents of three-month old infants. *Fathering, 6*, 2–19.

Meijer, A. M., & van den Wittenboer, G. L. H. (2007). Contribution of infants' sleep and crying to marital relationship of first-time parent couples in the 1st year after childbirth. *Journal of Family Psychology, 21*, 49–57.

Mindell, J. A., Telofski, L. S., Wiegand, B., & Kurtz, E. S. (2009). A nightly bedtime routine: Impact on sleep in young children and maternal mood. *Sleep, 32*, 599–606.

Mindell, J. A., Du Mond, C. E., Sadeh, A., Telofski, L. S., Kulkarni, N., & Gunn, E. (2011a). Efficacy of an internet-based intervention for infant and toddler sleep disturbances. *Sleep, 34*, 451–458.

Mindell, J. A., Du Mond, C. E., Sadeh, A., Telofski, L. S., Kulkarni, N., & Gunn, E. (2011b). Long-term efficacy of an internet-based intervention for infant and toddler sleep disturbances: One year follow-up. *Journal of Clinical Sleep Medicine, 7*, 507–511. Montgomery-Downs, H. E., Clawges, H. M., & Santy, E. E. (2010). Infant feeding methods and maternal sleep and daytime functioning. *Pediatrics, 126*, e1562–e1568. Montgomery-Downs, H. E., Insana, S. P., Clegg-Kraynok, M. M., & Mancini, L. M. (2010). Normative longitudinal maternal sleep: The first 4 postpartum months. *American Journal of Obstetrics and Gynecology, 203*, 465 e461–e467.

Morrell, J. M. (1999). The role of maternal cognitions in infant sleep problems as assessed by a new instrument, the Maternal Cognitions About Infant Sleep questionnaire. *Journal of Child Psychology and Psychiatry, 40*, 247–258.

Morrell, J. M., & Steele, H. (2003). The role of attachment security, temperament, maternal perception, and care-giving behavior in persistent infant sleeping problems. *Infant Mental Health Journal, 24*, 447–468.

Mosko, S., Richard, C., & McKenna, J. (1997). Maternal sleep and arousals during bedsharing with infants. *Sleep, 20*, 142–150.

Mullington, J. M., Chan, J. L., Van Dongen, H. P., Szuba, M. P., Samaras, J., Price, N. J., et al. (2003). Sleep loss reduces diurnal rhythm amplitude of leptin in healthy men. *Journal of Neuroendocrinology, 15*, 851–854.

Nishihara, K., & Horiuchi, S. (1998). Changes in sleep patterns of young women from late pregnancy to postpartum: Relationships to their infants' movements. *Perceptual and Motor Skills, 87*, 1043–1056.

Pinilla, T., & Birch, L. L. (1993). Help me make it through the night: Behavioral entrainment of breast-fed infants' sleep patterns. *Pediatrics, 91*, 436–444.

Price, A. M., Wake, M., Ukoumunne, O. C., & Hiscock, H. (2012). Outcomes at six years of age for children with infant sleep problems: Longitudinal community-based study. *Sleep Medicine.*

Quillin, S. I. (1997). Infant and mother sleep patterns during 4th postpartum week. *Issues in Comprehensive Pediatric Nursing, 20*, 115–123.

Sadeh, A., Flint-Ofir, E., Tirosh, T., & Tikotzky, L. (2007). Infant sleep and parental sleep-related cognitions. *Journal of Family Psychology, 21*, 74–87.

Schwichtenberg, A. J., & Poehlmann, J. (2009). A transactional model of sleep-wake regulation in infants born preterm or low birthweight. *Journal of Pediatric Psychology, 34*, 837– 849. Signal, T. L., Gander, P. H., Sangalli, M. R., Travier, N., Firestone, R. T., & Tuohy, J. F. (2007). Sleep duration and quality in healthy nulliparous and multiparous women across pregnancy and post-partum. *Australia New Zealand Journal of Obstetrics and Gynaecology, 47*, 16–22.

Sinai, D., & Tikotzky, L. (2012). Infant sleep, parental sleep and parenting stress in families of mothers on maternity leave and in families of working mothers. *Infant Behavior and Development, 35*, 179–186.

Smart, J., & Hiscock, H. (2007). Early infant crying and sleeping problems: A pilot study of impact on parental well-being and parent-endorsed strategies for management. *Journal of Paediatric and Child Health, 43*, 284–290.

St James-Roberts, I., Sleep, J., Morris, S., Owen, C., & Gillham, P. (2001). Use of a behavioural programme in the first 3 months to prevent infant crying and sleeping problems. *Journal of Paediatric and Child Health, 37*, 289–297.

Statistics Canada. (2011). *General social survey - 2010: Overview of the time use of Canadians.* (Catalogue no. 89–647-X). Ottawa: Statistics Canada.

Stremler, R., Hodnett, E., Lee, K., MacMillan, S., Mill, C., Ongcangco, L., & Willan, A. (2006). A behavioral-educational intervention to promote maternal and infant sleep: A pilot randomized, controlled trial. *Sleep, 29,* 1609–1615.

Stremler, R., Hodnett, E., Kenton, L., Lee, K., Macfarlane, J., Weiss, S. J., et al. (2013). Effect of a behavioural-educational intervention on sleep for primiparous women and their infants in the early postpartum: multisite randomised controlled trial. *British Medical Journal, 346,* f1164.

Stremler, R., Hodnett, E., Kenton, L., Lee, K. A., Macfarlane, J., Weiss, S., et al. (in press). Infant sleep location: Bed sharing, room sharing and solitary sleeping at 6 and 12 weeks postpartum. *The Open Sleep Journal.*

Swain, A. M., O'Hara, M. W., Starr, K. R., & Gorman, L. L. (1997). A prospective study of sleep, mood, and cognitive function in postpartum and nonpostpartum women. *Obstetrics and Gynecology, 90,* 381–386.

Symon, B. G., Marley, J. E., Martin, A. J., & Norman, E. R. (2005). Effect of a consultation teaching behaviour modification on sleep performance in infants: A randomised controlled trial. *Medical Journal of Australia, 182,* 215–218.

Taveras, E. M., Rifas-Shiman, S. L., Rich-Edwards, J. W., Gunderson, E. P., Stuebe, A. M., & Mantzoros, C. S. (2011). Association of maternal short sleep duration with adiposity and cardiometabolic status at 3 years postpartum. *Obesity, 19,* 171–178.

Teti, D. M., & Crosby, B. (2012). Maternal depressive symptoms, dysfunctional cognitions, and infant night waking: The role of maternal nighttime behavior. *Child Development, 83,* 939–953.

Thomas, K. A., & Foreman, S. W. (2005). Infant sleep and feeding pattern: Effects on maternal sleep. *Journal of Midwifery and Women's Health, 50,* 399–404.

Thomas, K. A., & Burr, R. L. (2006). Melatonin level and pattern in postpartum versus nonpregnant nulliparous women. *Journal of Obstetrical, Gynecological and Neonatal Nursing, 35,* 608–615.

Tikotzky, L., & Sadeh, A. (2009). Maternal sleep-related cognitions and infant sleep: A longitudinal study from pregnancy through the 1st year. *Child Development, 80,* 860–874.

Tikotzky, L., Sadeh, A., & Glickman-Gavrieli, T. (2011). Infant sleep and paternal involvement in infant caregiving during the first 6 months of life. *Journal of Pediatric Psychology, 36,* 36–46.

Troy, N. W. (2003). Is the significance of postpartum fatigue being overlooked in the lives of women? *MCN American Journal of Maternal and Child Nursing, 28,* 252–257.

Tsai, S. Y., Barnard, K. E., Lentz, M. J., & Thomas, K. A. (2009). Twenty-four hours light exposure experiences in postpartum women and their 2–10-week-old infants: An intensive within-subject design pilot study. *International Journal of Nursing Studies, 46,* 181–188.

Venn, S., Arber, S., Meadows, R., & Hislop, J. (2008). The fourth shift: exploring the gendered nature of sleep disruption among couples with children. *British Journal of Sociology, 59,* 79–97.

Wolfson, A., Lacks, P., & Futterman, A. (1992). Effects of parent training on infant sleeping patterns, parents' stress, and perceived parental competence. *Journal of Consulting and Clinical Psychology, 60,* 41–48.

Wolfson, A. R., Crowley, S. J., Anwer, U., & Bassett, J. L. (2003). Changes in sleep patterns and depressive symptoms in first-time mothers: Last trimester to 1-year postpartum. *Behavioral Sleep Medicine, 1,* 54–67.

World Health Organization. (2002). The optimal duration of exclusive breastfeeding: Report of an expert consultation. http://www.who.int/nutrition/publications/optimal_duration_of_exc_bfeeding_report_eng.pdf

Yamazaki, A. (2007). Family synchronizers: Predictors of sleep-wake rhythm for Japanese first-time mothers. *Sleep and Biological Rhythms, 5,* 218–225.

Yonkers, K. A., Wisner, K. L., Stewart, D. E., Oberlander, T. F., Dell, D. L., Stotland, N., et al (2009). The management of depression during pregnancy: A report from the American Psychiatric Association and the American College of Obstetricians and Gynecologists. *General Hospital Psychiatry, 31,* 403–413.

CHAPTER

8 Developmental Changes in Circadian Timing and Sleep: Adolescence and Emerging Adulthood

Mary A. Carskadon *and* Leila Tarokh

Abstract

A common feature of adolescent development is a change in the timing of sleep: most teens seem to need the same amount of sleep they did as preadolescents, yet they show a strong preference to fit their sleep into a later temporal niche, going to bed and waking up at much later times. This tendency is fueled by biological and psychosocial factors. Sleep bioregulatory processes—circadian timing and sleep homeostasis—show evidence of pronounced changes across adolescent development. The circadian system moves to a delayed phase position, and the sleep homeostatic system shows slower buildup of sleep pressure in the daytime, although the recuperative process does not change across adolescence. The lives of teens and emerging adults reflect these bioregulatory changes primarily in later bedtimes, where the biology also catches the wave of enticing twenty-first century technologies that add to late-night arousal and light exposure. Problems arise because social pressures—in particular the start of the school day—result in early mornings that cut short the amount of sleep. Short sleep on school days and long and late sleep on weekends result in a pattern of insufficient and irregular sleep that may have consequences for physical, emotional, and mental health.

Key Words: adolescents, sleep EEG, two-process model, circadian rhythms, sleep homeostasis, sleep patterns, puberty

Introduction

One of the most accepted generalities about sleep patterns is the change that occurs during adolescent development, a time when bedtimes in particular get later and later. Reports about sleep patterns in teenagers from the North and South America, Europe, Australia, Asia, and Africa are consistent in this regard (Yang, Kim, Patel, & Lee, 2005; Park, Matsumoto, Seo, Kang, & Nagashima, 2002; Arakawa et al., 2001; Gau & Soong, 2003; Andrade & Menna-Baretto, 2002; National Sleep Foundation, 2006; Carskadon, 1990; Wolfson & Carskadon, 1998; Gibson et al., 2006; Laberge et al., 2001; Saarenpaa-Heikkila, Rintahaka, Laippala, & Koivikko, 1995; Iglowstein, Jenni, Molinary, Largo, 2003; Strauch & Meier, 1988; Thorleifsdottir, Bjornsson, Benediktsdottir, Gislaso, & Kristbjarnarson, 2002; Bearpark & Michie, 1987; Dorofaeff & Denny, 2006; Reid, Maldonado, & Baker, 2002). The specifics may be culturally informed—for example, in South Korean youth for whom academic pressure pushes bedtimes later than in most other samples (Yang et al., 2005)—but the underlying trend for sleep timing to delay across the second decade is a robust occurrence. Accumulated scientific evidence points to a growing momentum that is accelerating this phenomenon as society adapts to the trappings of twenty-first century technology (see Gradisar and Short, Chapter 11).

Among the important considerations that one needs to keep in mind is that human sleep–wake behaviors evolve from a complex set of factors that are based in biology, social circumstances, and cultural norms (see Super and Harkness, Chapter 9).

Furthermore, the interactions among these factors are intricate, though with predictable associations. Most important for understanding sleep patterns of adolescents and emerging young adults are biological (bioregulatory) factors that may drive the sleep–wake behavior problems and the ways that behavior feeds back on the maturing biological milieu. This chapter will examine the maturational patterns of sleep–wake bioregulatory systems and then discuss how behavior patterns can affect the biology.

2-Process Model of Sleep Regulation

The starting point for this undertaking is the core theoretical model for sleep regulation, the two-process model (Borbely, 1982; Daan, Beersma, & Borbely, 1984). This model was derived primarily from studies of sleep in nonhuman mammals, in which the patterning of sleep and the quantifiable EEG slow wave activity (SWA) of sleep were used to predict and model responses to experimental perturbations of sleep. Responses to extended wakefulness or reduced time for sleep identify a homeostatic process in which sleep amount and intensity (EEG SWA) vary in a predictable manner: the longer one is awake, the longer is subsequent sleep and the greater the amount of SWA. Sleep–wake homeostasis (also known as *Process S*), therefore, describes the compensatory system the brain uses to keep these factors in balance. The second regulatory process is the central timing system (circadian rhythms, i.e., *Process C*) that favors sleeping and waking at different times of day.

Adolescent Development and Process S

We note that the sleep EEG comprising SWA provides a metric for Process S; however, one of the most visible changes that occurs to sleep across adolescence is an overall reduction (by at least 40%) of this feature of sleep (Jenni & Carskadon, 2004; Carskadon, 1982; Campbell et al., 2011; Feinberg, Higgins, Khaw, & Campbell, 2006; Tarokh & Carskadon, 2010). This phenomenological change is marked by a reduction in the amount of sleep identified as slow wave sleep (stages 3 and 4 of NREM sleep; N3) (Carskadon, 1982; Jenni & Carskadon, 2004; Karacan, Anch, Thornby, Okawa, & Williams, 1975; Tarokh, Van Reen, LeBourgeois, Seifer, & Carskadon, 2011; Williams, Karacan, Hursch, & Davis, 1972), in the amplitude of the EEG signal (Jenni & Carskadon, 2004; Carskadon, 1982; Campbell et al., 2011; Feinberg et al., 2006; Tarokh & Carskadon, 2010), and in the quantity of SWA. Figure 8.1 illustrates this difference in the sleep EEG of a prepubertal 9.4-year-old girl and the same child 30 months later when she was postpubertal. As striking as this phenomenon appears, and as strong a developmental signal it provides, the changes in EEG appear to bear little functional relation to the maturational changes in sleep regulation. Instead, they are commonly thought to be a passive reflection of a programmed reduction in cortical synapses that accompanies adolescent maturation (Feinberg, 1982; Feinberg, Thode, Chugani, & March, 1990).

Our group and others have examined whether components of Process S change during adolescence by examining the dissipation of sleep pressure (Process S) across the night, by fitting a model to the SWA during sleep before and after a night of sleep deprivation to examine the accumulation of Process S, and by assessing the speed of falling asleep after prolonged waking. In the first place, data collected from a cross-sectional sample of pre- and postpubertal adolescents (Jenni, Achermann, & Carskadon, 2005) and two longitudinal samples (Campbell et al., 2011; Tarokh, Carskadon, & Achermann, 2012), were unable to detect a difference in the decay rate (recovery rate) for SWA during sleep. We have interpreted this finding to indicate that

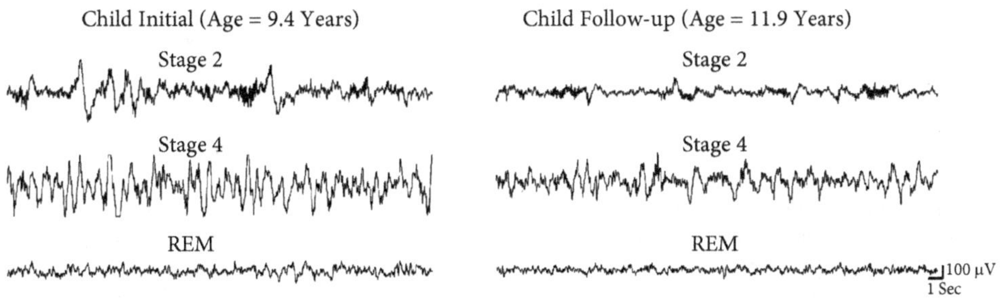

Figure 8.1 Thirty seconds of exemplary sleep EEG tracings from a girl whose sleep was recorded when she was 9.4 years old (left column) and again at age 11.9 years (right column). The amplitude of the signal is diminished at the follow-up recording session in all sleep stages. This decline is thought to reflect the cortical synaptic pruning that occurs in healthy adolescents.

perhaps the rate of functional recovery—possibly a measure of sleep need—may not change during adolescence (Carskadon, 2012).

On the other hand, the rate of accumulation of Process S with extended wake shows evidence of becoming slower as adolescents mature (Jenni et al., 2005). Another way to look at this phenomenon is to measure how fast one falls asleep when staying awake for a long time using a method called the *multiple sleep latency test* (MSLT). The MSLT measures speed of falling asleep under standardized conditions at 2-hour intervals (Carskadon et al., 1986). Taylor and colleagues (2005) examined Process S in this way in prepubertal and postpubertal adolescents and showed that the speed of falling asleep was significantly faster in the prepubertal group after 14.5 and 16.5 hours of wakefulness, as shown in Figure 8.2. We interpret these findings to indicate that the pressure to fall asleep builds up more slowly during adolescent development and, therefore, staying awake longer gets easier for teens (Carskadon, 2012). Jenni and LeBourgeois (2006) suggest that this pattern is an extension of a maturational process that begins in early childhood, where the reduced rate of Process S accumulation during waking accompanies the dropout of napping. The importance of this change in adolescence may be most relevant as "permissive" of late-night behaviors that interdict early bedtimes for teenagers.

Adolescent Development and Process C

The circadian timing system has a simple outcome—daily cycling—that comes with complex components that inform the system (see Crowley, Chapter 17, and Auger and Crowley, Chapter 23). Figure 8.3 shows a simple diagram identifying important parts of the circadian system. The central pacemaker for circadian timing in mammals is located in small paired nuclei, the *suprachiasmatic nuclei* (SCN), located in the hypothalamus above the optic chasm and straddling the third ventricle (Dunlap, Loros, & DeCoursey, 2004). Neurons in this region receive light information through a nonvisual retinal hypothalamic (RHT) pathway. Retinal light is integrated from rods and cones through specialized retinal ganglion (ipRTG) cells that themselves are intrinsically photosensitive to light in shorter (blue) wavelengths (Berson, Dunn, & Takao, 2002). The outputs of the SCN are conveyed through many circuits to impact thousands of physiological processes, including activity/rest and sleep/wake, as well as such things as hormone release and metabolic processes. Running wheel activity is the classic circadian rhythm used by rodent circadian biologists. Melatonin release—timed to occur during darkness—is a prominent circadian rhythm often used as a marker of the internal system in human studies. Biologists have found that neurons in other brain regions, as well as cells in other organs, are capable of sustaining daily rhythms. The SCN output, however, is thought to give the daily cue to all these cells, keeping the many rhythms in appropriate synchrony with one another.

An important feature of this mechanism is its response to light signals from the environment, which are the most important synchronizing

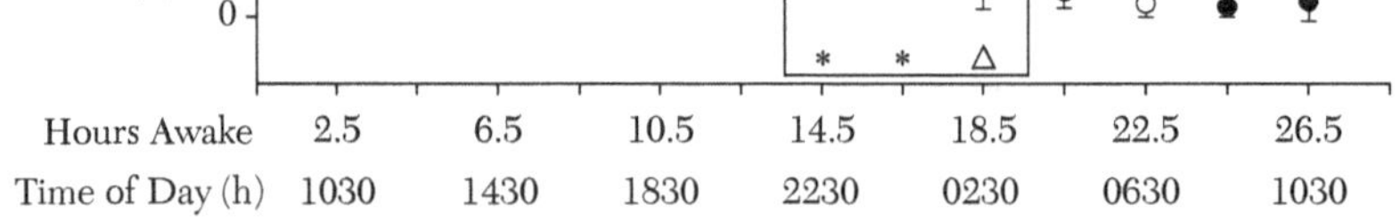

Figure 8.2 The speed of falling asleep as measured by multiple sleep latency tests (MSLT) is shown for prepubertal (Tanner 1) and postpubertal (Tanner 5) adolescents who were kept awake for over 24 hours. All had been well slept beforehand with a sleep–wake schedule of 10:00 pm bedtime and 8:00 am rise time for over one week. Participants were given a 20-minute opportunity every 2 hours to fall asleep under controlled conditions. The three time points indicated by the box show where the pre- and postpubertal sleep latencies diverged at 14.5, 16.5, and 18.5 hours after waking, when the postpubertal participants took a few minutes longer to fall asleep. We interpret this finding, along with changes to the function describing the accumulation of process-S across wakefulness in older adolescents, as evidence for a "permissive" process in which it becomes "easier" to stay awake longer. [* $p<.01$; Δ $p<.05$] (Redrawn with permission from Taylor et al, 2005.)

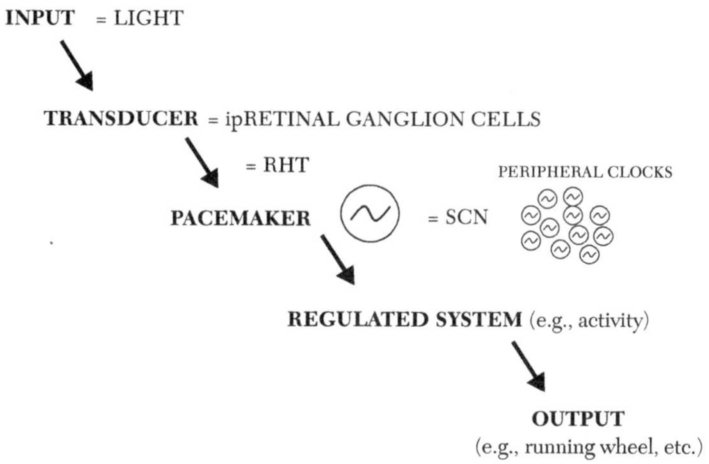

Figure 8.3 Features of the mammalian circadian timing system are portrayed in this schematic diagram. The central portion of the figure shows the mammalian master clock, the suprachiasmatic nuclei (SCN) of the hypothalamus, and indicates that many cells in the periphery also contain cellular elements of the circadian timing system. For the SCN, light is the principal environmental entraining stimulus, and the light signals are transduced by retinal photoreceptors including newly described, intrinsically photosensitive retinal ganglion cells (ipRGC). This photic signal is transmitted to the SCN neurons over a retinal hypothalamic tract (RHT) that is separate from the visual light pathways. The signal from the SCN goes to regulated systems (including those with peripheral oscillators that are entrained by the SCN signal). Finally, circadian activity is observed by examining the output of the regulated system, such as running wheel activity or the secretory pattern of hormones. The most commonly used hormonal clock output signal is melatonin, which rises in the nighttime of the brain and is suppressed in the daytime.

time cues. (Such other events as restricted timing of feeding or activity are able to cue the clock in experimental studies; external substances, such as melatonin, can also influence clock timing.) The clock's response to light depends on the phase when the light signal is received. In general, light signals that occur in the evening and first half of nighttime provide a "push" that puts the timing back, called a delay. Light signals that occur in the second half of the night or early morning provide a "pull" that moves the timing earlier, an advance. It should be clear, therefore, that circadian timing can be influenced by behaviors that affect the timing of light.

Another important feature of the circadian timing system is the "speed" of the daily clock mechanism. Although the control clock provides daily timing signals to synchronize rhythms, the clock itself requires environmental input to run at 24 hours. Thus the term *circadian* is meant literally: *circa* = about; *dies* = day. The intrinsic period of this clock can only be measured under specific environmental circumstances, such as *constant conditions* (as in a rodent placed in a continuously dark cage) or an experimental paradigm called *forced desynchrony* (as in placing the animal on a 28-hour or 20-hour day length). In either circumstance, the rhythms run free of the environment and express their intrinsic period. A longer intrinsic period is associated with later phase under normal lighting conditions; a shorter intrinsic period is associated with earlier phase.

With these features of the circadian timing system in mind, we can make several predictions of developmental changes that would produce later sleep–wake timing in adolescents.

- Phase preference is later
- Phase position is later
- Intrinsic period is longer
- Phase response to light signals change

The majority of evidence for developmental changes in circadian timing comes from data in humans, although several other mammalian species show changes in the juvenile period, as reviewed by Hagenauer and colleagues (2009).

A seminal finding in 1993 (Carskadon et al.) documented a significantly later phase preference (i.e., preferred timing for such behaviors as studying, rise time, exercise) in sixth-grade girls who rated themselves as farther along in pubertal development compared to prepubertal girls. Others have confirmed this trend in teens (girls and boys), most notably Roenneberg and colleagues (2004) using a measure of chronotype, that is, midpoint of sleep time, on weekends (see Figure 8.4). Circadian phase, measured by dim light melatonin onset (DLMO) time is also later in teens living in normal uncontrolled circumstances (Carskadon,

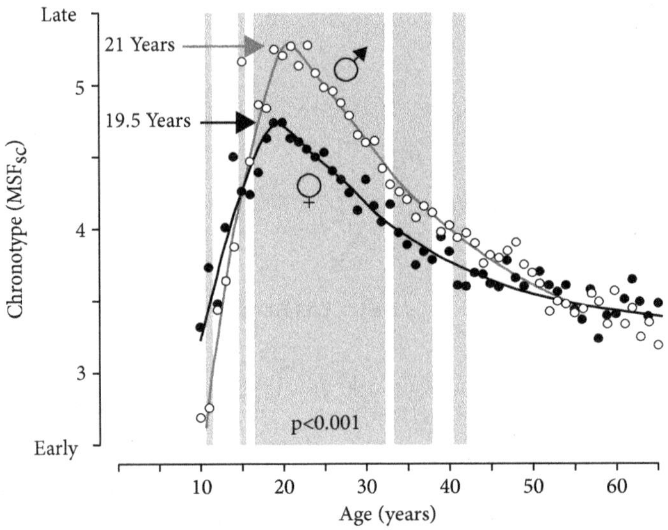

Figure 8.4 The Munich ChronoType Questionnaire (MCTQ) was administered to approximately 25,000 individuals ages 10 to 70 years to measure chronotype. The distribution of chronotype as a function of age is depicted. A progressive shift toward later chronotypes was found until the age of 20 years, at which point the pattern reversed favoring an advance in chronotype. Women reached the maximal delay earlier (19.5 years) than men (20.9 years). Roenneberg and colleagues suggest that the transition from delaying to advancing may mark the end of adolescence. (Redrawn with permission from Roenneberg et al., 2004.)

Richardson, Tate, & Seifer, 1997). This finding was confirmed using biological measures in adolescents who slept on identical schedules (i.e., with similar light–dark exposures); adolescents with greater pubertal development measured by Tanner stage (Tanner, 1962) had later phase measured by DLMO (Carskadon, Acebo, & Jenni, 2004).

As mentioned, measuring circadian period requires special methodology, and while it is a challenge in adults it is especially so in children and adolescents (see Crowley, Chapter 17). Our group has made these assessments using a 28-hour forced desynchrony protocol, however in too few participants (it takes 3 weeks full time in the lab to measure the variable) to examine the developmental hypothesis (Carskadon, Labyak, Acebo, & Seifer, 1999). On the other hand, when intrinsic period of adolescents is compared to adults measured in the same way, intrinsic period is slightly and significantly longer in adolescents (Carskadon & Acebo, 2005). This finding provides evidence to support the hypothesis that the adolescent phase delay may be due in part to long intrinsic period.

Evidence for an adolescent developmental change in the phase response to light is unclear at this time. To support a phase delay, one would expect that the (delaying) phase response to light in the evening might become more sensitive in older adolescence and/or that the (advancing) phase response to light in the early morning might become less sensitive. We found a small difference in response to morning light in adolescence, but not large enough to support the hypothesis (Carskadon et al., 2002). On the other hand, a cross sectional study of adult and juvenile mice found a marked increase in the delaying effects of evening light in the juveniles versus adults (Weinert & Kompauerova, 1998).

Although the occurrence of a developmental change in the light phase response is unclear at this time, we can identify ways that adolescent behavior may affect this mechanism and facilitate later circadian timing. Thus, when youngsters stay awake late and encounter light (and perhaps especially the short light wave lengths common to computer screens) late into the evening, this is a signal to the clock that can delay the circadian phase. When adolescents block light in the morning, either through sleeping in or using heavy curtains or eye shades to avoid morning light, then they block the phase advancing effects of light.

Sleep Behavior during Adolescent Development and Emerging Adulthood

The typical pattern of sleep across adolescence includes a delay in the timing of bedtime and—on free days—of rise time, too. Issues arise, however, when societal pressures, most often an early start time for school, requires teens with late bedtimes to rise well before they can get sufficient sleep. Thus, many teens live their lives in a sleep-deprived state, with risks for behavior problems, mood disorders, metabolic issues and weight gain, and impaired learning (Carskadon, 2012). Many school districts in the USA have considered the possibility of moving school to a later time for older adolescents in response to the compelling data about insufficient sleep in teens, especially the growing evidence that sleep *per se* aids learning (c.f., Carskadon, 2011; see Au, Appleman, and Stavitsky, Chapter 38). These issues may be even greater in other cultures. For example, Yang et al (2005) reported that S. Korean teens were obtaining over an hour less sleep on school nights than students in the USA.

Given developmental changes in the sleep-wake regulatory system, which seem to "permit" staying awake longer (though still needing as much sleep), and in the circadian regulatory system, which seem to push sleep timing later, it is no surprise that teenagers in the 21st century in developed countries cannot seem to get adequate sleep. They no longer receive light exposure tied to the natural environment to help reset and perhaps advance their daily clocks; indeed, they schedule their light and dark exposures to give their clocks phase delaying cues and to block phase advancing cues. Teens are able to take advantage of the "permissive" sleep-wake system by engaging in arousing activities in the evening, most prominently electronic communication (often also with evening light exposure). Fifty years ago, by contrast, teens did not have a television set in the bedroom, nor a computer monitor with Internet access around-the-clock, much less cellular phones and smart phones (see Gradisar and Short, Chapter 11). Indeed, even the trend for early school start in the USA arose primarily in the 1970s with the energy crisis.

Sleep-wake behavior in emerging adulthood is not nearly as well studied as in adolescence (see Thacher, Chapter 40). A few groups have examined sleep of college students. Miller et al., (Miller & Shattuck, 2005), for example, showed that first-year cadets at the US Military Academy were sleeping only about 5 hours per night on school nights and about 6.5 hours on weekend nights. We have recently reported a link between a short sleep (<7 hr/night during 8 weeks) and depressed mood phenotype with serotonin transporter genotype (short alleles of 5-HTTLPR in the SLC6A4 gene) in first-year university students (Carskadon, Sharkey, Knopik, & McGeary, 2012). Such data indicate that—at least for late adolescents who continue to further education—schoolday sleep patterns remain late and short and problematic.

A study by Roenneberg and colleagues (Roenneberg et al., 2004) used the chronotype measure as a "biological marker for the end of adolescence." As shown in Figure 8.4 presenting data from a large epidemiologic European sample, the strong tendency for the midpoint of "free (i.e., weekend) sleep" to delay occurred at the start of the second decade. Whether this inflection point is driven entirely by intrinsic biological timing mechanisms or also reflects behavioral changes, perhaps associated with work schedules, the pattern of change is compelling. By the same token, across late adolescence and early adulthood, the substantial delay of weekend sleep relative to earlier school or workday sleep patterns results in two important issues that are thought to pose important consequences for physical and mental well-being. In the first place, late and short sleep on weekdays can lead to insufficient sleep and consequent problems. The variable weekend and weekday sleep schedules with, as Roenneberg termed it "social jet lag," has now also been associated with, for example, an increased susceptibility to obesity (Roenneberg et al., 2012; see Harvey, Alfano, and Clarke, Chapter 35).

Conclusion

In summary, many teens' sleep patterns are delayed, leading to too little sleep on weekdays and great variability of weekday and weekend sleep patterns. Erratic and insufficient sleep have consequences to physical and emotional health, as well as learning and memory. Although the findings are clear and disturbing, the trends toward less and later sleep in teens does not appear to be moderating, with the exception of families where parents are helping teens manage their sleep and communities where school bells are no longer ringing before 8:30 am.

Future Directions

- Cross-sectional data indicate that the intrinsic circadian period lengthens in adolescent development: can this be confirmed with longitudinal studies?
- Data from juvenile mice indicate that the phase response curve to light is different from adult mice: can we confirm this finding in humans?
- Can we identify teenagers most at risk for adverse consequences of inadequate and irregular sleep patterns?
- Can we identify and test interventions to minimize development of poor sleep patterns in adolescents?
- Do sleep habits constitute an "environmental exposure" that interacts with genotype leading

to functional genetic changes? Will epigenetic approaches help identify such interactions?

• Can longitudinal monitoring across late childhood into adolescence of sleep behavior in conjunction with longitudinal monitoring of the sleeping EEG help to identify whether sleep timing and/or amount affect cortical brain structure and functional pathways in this important developmental period?

Acknowledgments

We thank the National Institutes of Health for support of our research summarized in this chapter: MH52415, MH01358, MH45945, MH58879, HL71120, MH076969, MH079179, AA13252. We also acknowledge our colleagues, fellows, students, staff, and participants who make important contributions to our research.

References

Andrade, M., & Menna-Baretto, L. (2002). Sleep patterns of high school students living in Sao Paulo, Brazil. In M. A. Carskadon (Ed.), *Adolescent Sleep Patterns: Biological, Social, and Psychological Factors* (pp. 118–131). New York: Cambridge University Press.

Arakawa, M., Taira, K., Tanaka, H., Yamakawa, K., Toguchi, H., Kadekaru, H., et al. (2001). A survey of junior high school students' sleep habit and lifestyle in Okinawa. *Psychiatry and Clinical Neurosciences, 55*(3), 211–212.

Bearpark, H. M., & Michie, P. (1987). Prevalance of sleep-wake distrubances in Sydney adolescents. *Journal of Sleep Research, 16*, 304.

Berson, D. M., Dunn, F. A., & Takao, M. (2002). Phototransduction by retinal ganglion cells that set the circadian clock. *Science, 295*(5557), 1070–1073.

Borbely, A. A. (1982). A two process model of sleep regulation. *Human Neurobiology, 1*(3), 195–204.

Campbell, I. G., Darchia, N., Higgins, L. M., Dykan, I. V., Davis, N. M., de Bie, E., et al. (2011). Adolescent changes in homeostatic regulation of EEG activity in the delta and theta frequency bands during NREM sleep. *Sleep, 34*(1), 83–91.

Carskadon, M. A. (1982). The second decade. In C. Guilleminault (Ed.), *Sleep and Waking Disorders: Indications and Techniques* (pp. 99–125). Menlo Park: Addison Wesley.

Carskadon, M. A., Dement, W. C., Mitler, M. M., Roth, T., Westbrook, P. R., & Keenan, S. (1986). Guidelines for the multiple sleep latency test (MSLT): A standard measure of sleepiness. *Sleep, 9*(4), 519–524.

Carskadon, M. A. (1990). Patterns of sleep and sleepiness in adolescents. *Pediatrician, 17*(1), 5–12.

Carskadon, M. A., Vieira, C., & Acebo, C. (1993). Association between puberty and delayed phase preference. *Sleep, 16*(3), 258–262.

Carskadon, M. A., Acebo, C., Richardson, G. S., Tate, B. A., & Seifer, R. (1997). An approach to studying circadian rhythms of adolescent humans. *Journal of Biological Rhythms, 12*(3), 278–289.

Carskadon, M. A., Labyak, S. E., Acebo, C., & Seifer, R. (1999). Intrinsic circadian period of adolescent humans measured in conditions of forced desynchrony. *Neuroscience Letters, 260*(2), 129–132.

Carskadon, M. A., Acebo, C., & Arnedt, J. T. (2002). Failure to identify pubertally-mediated melatonin sensitivity to light in adolescents. *Sleep, 25* (Suppl.), A191.

Carskadon, M. A., Acebo, C., & Jenni, O. G. (2004). Regulation of adolescent sleep: Implications for behavior. *Annals of the New York Academy of Sciences, 1021*, 276–291.

Carskadon, M. A., & Acebo, C. (2005). Intrinsic circadian period in adolescents versus adults from forced desynchrony. *Sleep, 28* (Suppl.), A71.

Carskadon, M. A. (2011). Sleep's effects on cognition and learning in adolescence. *Progress in Brain Research, 190*, 137–143.

Carskadon, M. A. (2012). Sleep in adolescents: the perfect storm. *Pediatric Clinics of North America, 58*(3), 637–647.

Carskadon, M. A., Sharkey, K. M., Knopik, V. S., & McGeary, J. E. (2012). Short sleep as an environmental exposure: a preliminary study associating 5-HTTLPR genotype to self-reported sleep duration and depressed mood in first-year university students. *Sleep, 35*(6), 791–796.

Daan, S., Beersma, D. G., & Borbely, A. A. (1984). Timing of human sleep: Recovery process gated by a circadian pacemaker. *American Journal of Physiology, 246*(2 Pt 2), R161–R183.

Dorofaeff, T. F., & Denny, S. (2006). Sleep and adolescence. Do New Zealand teenagers get enough? *Journal of Paediatrics and Child Health, 42*(9), 515–520.

Dunlap, J. C., Loros, J. J., & DeCoursey, P. J. (2004). *Chronobiology: Biological Timekeeping*. Sunderland: Sinauer Associates.

Feinberg, I. (1982). Schizophrenia: Caused by a fault in programmed synaptic elimination during adolescence? *J Psychiatr Res, 17*(4), 319–334.

Feinberg, I., Thode, H. C., Jr., Chugani, H. T., & March, J. D. (1990). Gamma distribution model describes maturational curves for delta wave amplitude, cortical metabolic rate and synaptic density. *Journal of Theoretical Biology, 142*(2), 149–161.

Feinberg, I., Higgins, L. M., Khaw, W. Y., & Campbell, I. G. (2006). The adolescent decline of NREM delta, an indicator of brain maturation, is linked to age and sex but not to pubertal stage. *American Journal of Physiology – Regululatory, Integrative and Comparative Physiology, 291*(6), R1724–R1729.

Foundation, N. S. (2006). *2006 Sleep In America Poll Summary Findings*. Retrieved July 12, 2010, from http://www.sleepfoundation.org/sites/default/files/2006_summary_of_findings.pdf.

Gau, S. F., & Soong, W. T. (2003). The transition of sleep-wake patterns in early adolescence. *Sleep, 26*(4), 449–454.

Gibson, E. S., Powles, A. C., Thabane, L., O'Brien, S., Molnar, D. S., Trajanovic, N., et al. (2006). "Sleepiness" is serious in adolescence: Two surveys of 3235 Canadian students. *BMC Public Health, 6*, 116.

Hagenauer, M. H., Perryman, J. I., Lee, T. M., & Carskadon, M. A. (2009). Adolescent changes in the homeostatic and circadian regulation of sleep. *Developmental Neuroscience, 31*(4), 276–284.

Iglowstein, I., Jenni, O. G., Molinari, L., & Largo, R. H. (2003). Sleep duration from infancy to adolescence: Reference values and generational trends. *Pediatrics, 111*(2), 302–307.

Jenni, O. G., & Carskadon, M. A. (2004). Spectral analysis of the sleep electroencephalogram during adolescence. *Sleep, 27*(4), 774–783.

Jenni, O. G., Achermann, P., & Carskadon, M. A. (2005). Homeostatic sleep regulation in adolescents. *Sleep, 28*(11), 1446–1454.

Jenni, O. G., & LeBourgeois, M. K. (2006). Understanding sleep-wake behavior and sleep disorders in children: The value of a model. *Current Opinion in Psychiatry, 19*(3), 282–287.

Karacan, I., Anch, M., Thornby, J. I., Okawa, M., & Williams, R. L. (1975). Longitudinal sleep patterns during pubertal growth: Four-year follow up. *Pediatric Research, 9*(11), 842–846.

Laberge, L., Petit, D., Simard, C., Vitaro, F., Tremblay, R. E., & Montplaisir, J. (2001). Development of sleep patterns in early adolescence. *Journal of Sleep Research, 10*(1), 59–67.

Miller, N. L., & Shattuck, L. G. (2005). Sleep patterns of young men and women enrolled at the United States Military Academy: Results from year 1 of a 4-year longitudinal study. *Sleep, 28*(7), 837–841.

Park, Y. M., Matsumoto, K., Seo, Y. J., Kang, M. J., & Nagashima, H. (2002). Changes of sleep or waking habits by age and sex in Japanese. *Perceptual and Motor Skills, 94*(3 Pt 2), 1199–1213.

Reid, A., Maldonado, C. C., & Baker, F. C. (2002). Sleep behavior of South African adolescents. *Sleep, 25*(4), 423–427.

Roenneberg, T., Allebrandt, K. V., Merrow, M., & Vetter, C. (2012). Social jetlag and obesity. *Current Biology, 22*(10), 939–943.

Roenneberg, T., Kuehnle, T., Pramstaller, P. P., Ricken, J., Havel, M., Guth, A., et al. (2004). A marker for the end of adolescence. *Current Biology, 14*(24), R1038–R1039.

Saarenpaa-Heikkila, O. A., Rintahaka, P. J., Laippala, P. J., & Koivikko, M. J. (1995). Sleep habits and disorders in Finnish schoolchildren. *Journal of Sleep Research, 4*(3), 173–182.

Strauch, I., & Meier, B. (1988). Sleep need in adolescents: A longitudinal approach. *Sleep, 11*(4), 378–386.

Tanner, J. (1962). *Growth at Adolescence*. Oxford: Blackwell.

Tarokh, L., & Carskadon, M. A. (2010). Developmental changes in the human sleep EEG during early adolescence. *Sleep, 33*(6), 622–634.

Tarokh, L., Van Reen, E., LeBourgeois, M., Seifer, R., & Carskadon, M. A. (2011). Sleep EEG provides evidence that cortical changes persist into late adolescence. *Sleep, 34*(10), 1385–1393.

Tarokh, L., Carskadon, M. A., & Achermann, P. (2012). Dissipation of sleep pressure is stable across adolescence. *Neuroscience, 216*, 167–177.

Taylor, D. J., Jenni, O. G., Acebo, C., & Carskadon, M. A. (2005). Sleep tendency during extended wakefulness: Insights into adolescent sleep regulation and behavior. *Journal of Sleep Research, 14*(3), 239–244.

Thorleifsdottir, B., Bjornsson, J. K., Benediktsdottir, B., Gislason, T., & Kristbjarnarson, H. (2002). Sleep and sleep habits from childhood to young adulthood over a 10-year period. *Journal of Psychosomatic Research, 53*(1), 529–537.

Weinert, D., & Kompauerova, V. (1998). Light induced phase and period responses of circadian activity rhythms in laboratory mice of different age. *Zoology, 101*, 45–52.

Williams, R. L., Karacan, I., Hursch, C. J., & Davis, C. E. (1972). Sleep patterns of pubertal males. *Pediatric Research, 6*(8), 643–648.

Wolfson, A. R., & Carskadon, M. A. (1998). Sleep schedules and daytime functioning in adolescents. *Child Development, 69*(4), 875–887.

Yang, C. K., Kim, J. K., Patel, S. R., & Lee, J. H. (2005). Age-related changes in sleep/wake patterns among Korean teenagers. *Pediatrics, 115*(1 Suppl), 250–256.

PART 2

Complexity of Issues and Factors Influencing Sleep

CHAPTER

9

Culture and Children's Sleep

Charles M. Super *and* Sara Harkness

Abstract

The cultural model for infants' and children's sleeping arrangements familiar to most sleep researchers is highly unusual in global perspective, and it is a relatively recent addition to the human scene. This has limited our understanding. A broader examination reveals that, for example, the pattern of associations between co-sleeping during infancy and other variables (such as sleep problems) is culturally constructed—although commonly found, or assumed, in US and other Western samples, it is not generally found where co-sleeping is normative. We know little, however, about how sleep itself, including its internal architecture, is influenced by the developmental niche. The available evidence suggests that the development of sleep, like that of all biologically driven, universal behaviors, is culturally regulated, and therefore it shows interesting and important variation across cultural and ecological environments.

Key Words: culture, co-sleeping, customary practices, developmental niche, long-term effects, parental ethnotheories, SIDS, sleep architecture, sleep problems

Sleep seems inherently such a solitary, biologically driven, and universal behavior, one might easily ask: What does culture have to do with it? Briefly, the answer is that the development of sleep, like that of all biologically driven, universal behaviors, is culturally regulated, and therefore it shows interesting and sometimes important variation across cultural and ecological environments. This brief answer, however, rests on surprisingly few and recent reports. We know much more about how the general behavior of "sleeping" is integrated into the cultural life of children and families around the world than we do about cultural variation in sleep itself.

The Ecology of Children's Sleep

Discovering Variation

For the first half-century of anthropology—Western science's exploration of other peoples' ways of life—sleep was not a topic of note except on occasions when it related to something else of interest; for example, Malinowski's (1929) observation that changes in sleeping patterns of young adults mark new bonds affecting interfamily relations. As anthropologists began to focus on the psychological significance of customary behaviors and rituals, especially from a developmental point of view, the social ecology of sleeping arrangements took on greater significance in its own right. Of particular interest to psychological anthropologists was the frequently observed combination of three aspects of cultural life: exclusive mother–infant sleeping arrangements near the mother, a prolonged postpartum sex taboo, and circumcision rites for adolescent boys (Whiting, Kluckhohn, & Anthony, 1958). Whiting (1977) used a psychoanalytic framework to tie together these and other observations into a "psycho-cultural model," and the more general compilation of ethnographic reports from this era—"cross-cultural research" in the original sense—has proven a lasting resource. The most complete and widely cited report involving sleeping arrangements, by Barry and Paxson (1971), used a sample of 143 independent, nonindustrial societies. They found that among the 90 cases with reliable data on the topic, mothers and infants slept in the same bed in 46% of the societies, in the same room with bed unspecified in 33%, and in the same room in separate beds in the remaining 21%. This finding subsequently proved to be an important contribution to another discussion, concerning Sudden Infant Death Syndrome, as discussed later in this chapter. Other studies from the cross-cultural tradition have explored the relationship of cultural variation in sleeping arrangements in childhood to aspects of the social structure, psychological functioning, economy, and climate (Munroe &Munroe, 1987; Whiting & Edwards, 1988; Whiting & Whiting, 1975; Whiting, 1964, 1981).

Exploring Origins

More recently anthropologists have examined the evolutionary ecology of human sleep (Worthman, 2006; Worthman & Melby, 2002), and the emerging picture is informative, particularly as it expands the narrow question of co-sleeping to a broader understanding of the variations developed by our species. Worthman and Melby (2002) reviewed both old and new ethnographic material on a worldwide range of traditional forager, pastoralist, horticulturist, and agriculturalist communities to shed light on early human sleep ecology. Three of their observations are particularly striking and relevant to this chapter. The first is that sleep in these groups is essentially a social activity—no one healthy ever sleeps alone. Second, the immediate environment is often sensory-rich, not just due to co-sleepers but also to the soft voices of nearby conversation and to the smells and rustlings of domestic animals and the surrounding forests or savannahs. Third, the circadian pattern is not rigidly monophasic. In groups that routinely use nighttime fires for protection or heat, for example, "sleepers rouse frequently in the night to monitor the fire and replenish it as necessary" (Worthman & Melby, 2002, p. 75). In trying to understand the variety of contemporary environments for the development of sleep and their possible consequences, these three features can serve as useful reference points.

Exploring Variation

In the late twentieth century—a hundred years after the establishment of psychology, sociology, and anthropology as the triumvirate of Western social science (Super, 2005)—a new kind of literature on culture and children's sleep began to appear. Prompted by the general globalization of science and the more specific realization that behavioral science knowledge rests on distinctly unrepresentative samples (e.g., Arnett, 2008), more psychologists and medically trained researchers became involved in the cross-cultural study of sleep. Two characteristics of this new wave of reports stand out. First, because sleep-related behaviors are a primary interest, the reports often contain much greater detail on behavior than do the older ethnographic studies, which ranged more broadly in their coverage. Second, new researchers may bring valuable new perspectives, but by the same token they do not always share the intellectual heritage of a systematic approach to culture that is characteristic of the anthropological work. The emerging literature shows substantial contemporary variation in where and with whom infants and children sleep, in customary and changing practices surrounding bedtime and sleeping, and in the way parents think about children's sleep as an aspect of their development. These three interconnected systems—settings, customs, and beliefs—together form a "developmental niche," the culturally constructed context of child development (Harkness & Super, 1992; Super & Harkness, 1986, 2002). This theoretical framework provides a basis for analyzing the specific environment of growth and adaptation for a child or, more generally, for the typical child in an identifiable cultural community.

PHYSICAL AND SOCIAL SETTINGS

There is ample evidence of diversity in the contemporary settings of children's sleep, both within and across societies. Without overlooking possible contributions of the physical environment—see Whiting's (1981) example of average winter temperature and infant carrying/caching—a brief review highlights the cultural nature of the settings for infant sleep.

Morelli and colleagues document what is probably the most familiar contrast, between a northern, urban, Western sample and a tropical, rural, agricultural one (Morelli, Rogoff, Oppenheim, & Goldsmith, 1992). Comparing infant sleeping arrangements among Mayan farmers in highland Guatemala and middle-class Euro-American families, the authors found that all the Guatemalan infants slept in their mother's bed at night, sometimes with the father and/or siblings, well into toddlerhood. Beyond that, they slept with siblings or other relatives until nearing adolescence. Among the US infants, over three-quarters were sleeping in their own room by six months. Other broad contrasts are reviewed by Jenni and O'Connor (2005) and Giannotti and Cortesi (2009).

Substantial differences can also be found within a single geographic area and climate zone. Hewlett and colleagues observed infant life in two neighboring but quite distinct ethnic groups in Central Africa, the foraging Aka and agrarian Ngandu (Hewlett, Lamb, Shannon, Leyendecker, & Schölmerich, 1998). Although their quantitative data cover 12 daylight hours and thus no night sleep, the daytime data for 3–4- and 9–10-month-olds demonstrate that the amount of daytime sleep was about the same in both ethnic groups (about 41% at the younger age, 23% older). For the older Aka infants, virtually all of this sleep was while being held by a caretaker; the comparable figure among the Ngandu is 66%, with the remaining 33% spent alone, lying on a mat or other surface. At night, the Aka infants slept with siblings and parents; the Ngandu babies slept with the mother.

Considerable variation in the settings for children's sleep has also been noted among industrialized societies. The dominant Western model of parents in one bed and child in a separate bed and room is familiar to most sleep researchers, and documented by reports such as that by Morelli and colleagues (1992). In Japan, however, the typical arrangement is for parents and children to sleep next to each other on a futon or mattress (Fukumizu, Kaga, Kohyama, & Hayes, 2005). A large-scale, Internet-based survey by Mindell and colleagues found that in five English-speaking countries, the majority of infants (birth–36 months) slept in their own room, especially after the first few months; among 12 Asian sites, this arrangement was in the minority and in most cases rare (Mindell, Sadeh, Wiegand, How, & Goh, 2010).

Cross-cultural variability in sleeping arrangements is also evident in multiethnic societies. In New Zealand, Abel and colleagues found that bed sharing was a dominant practice among Maori and other Pacific Island groups, but not among those of European background (Abel, Park, Tipene-Leach, Finau, & Lennan, 2001). Landrine and Klonoff (1996) present data that indicate African Americans in California participate in bed sharing more than other ethnic groups there, even when controlling for economic status.

CUSTOMARY PRACTICES

It is evident from these last examples that whatever environmental features shaped child-rearing traditions, many practices are carried over in the context of migration or social change (Greenfield & Cocking, 1994; Moscardino, Nwobu, & Axia, 2006; Raghavan, Harkness, & Super, 2010). Thus the practice of separate infant or child sleeping quarters has been maintained within the Anglo-European diaspora from Canada to New Zealand, and for ex–colonial minorities in such places as India, Kenya, and Hong Kong; the same can be said for co-sleeping among African-heritage families in the United States and Pacific Islanders in New Zealand. Likewise, the custom of bed sharing on a floor mat persists in Japan and Korea despite dramatic changes in the ecology of daily life over the last 50 and 100 years.

Yet, sometimes customs change rapidly in new physical and social ecologies. Yovsi and Keller (2007) provide an example in their study of co-sleeping among Nso subsistence farmers in Cameroon and wage-earning Nso who live in town, a few kilometers away. In both samples infants slept with their mothers. Among the traditional farmers, however, bed sharing was exclusively mother and infant—the father slept elsewhere. Among the wage-earning families, living in town, the father often slept in the same bed with mother and infant. In addition, urban Nso families practiced particular bedtime routines including bathing and a specific hour for sleep; these were absent in the farming families. Green and Smith (2007) report a related but slower transition across three generations of Emirati mothers, all of whom co-slept with their infants and young children, but have moved the child to its own room at a progressively younger age, from 10 to 6 to 4 years.

Bedtime routines are among the most evident customs in the lives of infants and young children. In rural (and some urban) areas of Africa, South and Central America, and South Asia, infants and young children typically do not have a set bedtime and tend to fall asleep on their own, both during the day and in the evening. In Africa, this is often while in a caretaker's arms or strapped to a caretaker's back (Konner, 1976; Super & Harkness, 1982). In Korea (Harkness et al., 2007) and Japan (Caudill & Weinstein, 1969), the transition to sleep is more likely a deliberate and time-consuming process in which the mother holds the baby in her arms until the baby falls asleep. Among Western groups there is often comparatively less physical closeness, but soothing routines (such as an evening bath) and "sleep aids" (a favorite toy, soothing music) may be provided (Valentin, 2005). As the older infant or toddler is moved into her own room, the responsibility for going to sleep lies increasingly with the child (Milan, Snow, & Belay, 2007; New & Richman, 1996).

The use of a "security blanket" or other object to provide comfort during the transition from wake to sleep has attracted particular attention by cross-cultural researchers, in part for its presumptive implications for individuation and attachment. Gaddini (1970), a psychoanalyst, was probably the first to explore this issue, using three samples: Italians from a rural town, Italians in Rome, and foreign, largely Anglo-Saxon families residing in Rome. The results were striking: 6% of the rural infants used a blanket or equivalent for the transition to sleep, 31% of the Roman Italian infants, and 61% among the Anglo-Saxon babies. This gradient corresponded inversely to group differences in rocking, co-sleeping, and breastfeeding, leading the author to conclude that low maternal contact and proximity led to the use of a "transitional object" for comfort at bedtime. Other studies, both within a single population and cross-culturally, have replicated this basic finding. Hong and Townes (1976), for example, surveyed native Euro-American and native Korean mothers of children ranging from 7 months to 8 years, as well as comparable Korean mothers living in the United States. They found co-sleeping was highest and attachment to transitional objects lowest among the Korean children; the reverse was true among the US children; and both measures were intermediate among the Korean mothers in the United States. These and other studies (e.g., Harlow & Suomi, 1970; Hayes, Fukumizu, Troese, Sallinen, & Gilles, 2007; Marvin, VanDevender, Iwanaga, LeVine, & LeVine, 1977; Wolf & Lozoff, 1989) make a strong case that attachment to a soft blanket or equivalent at bedtime is the cultural product of a particular style of customary infant care.

PSYCHOLOGY OF THE CARETAKERS

By and large, parents are aware of what they are doing, and within their own frame of reference they can justify most of their customary practices. In the Morelli and Rogoff comparison of US and Guatemalan parents, for example, the US families were focused on promoting autonomy and independence in their child. "I think that he would be more dependent," one mother indicated, "if he was constantly with us [when sleeping]." The Mayan parents, in contrast, explained their practices in terms of the emotional value of closeness with their infants. Harwood and colleagues found a similar contrast between Anglo-US and Puerto Rican mothers, with the former valuing and promoting independence more than the latter (Feng, Harwood, Leyendecker, & Miller, 2001; Harwood, Schölmerich, Schulze, & Gonzalez, 1999). Interestingly, white Appalachian mothers in the United States, whose practices in this regard are more like the Mayans' and Puerto Ricans' than their Euro-American compatriots', convey some of the same thinking regarding the value of closeness during infancy and the promotion of emotional bonds through bed sharing, "How can you expect to hold on to them later in life if you begin their lives by pushing them away?" (Slone, 1978, p. 60, quoted in Abbott, 1992, p. 34).

As one might infer from these brief quotations, the meaning of "physical closeness" with infants and young children is culturally nuanced. The issue was investigated directly by Rothbaum and colleagues through semistructured interviews with Euro-American and Chinese immigrant families (Rothbaum, Morelli, Pott, & Liu-Constant, 2000). They found a number of important differences, including more bed sharing in the Chinese immigrant families. The meanings associated with such closeness, coded from the interviews, were captured by two themes contrasting (1) "growing apart" vs. "growing (up) with," and (2) celebrating vs. not celebrating the individual distinctiveness of the child. Overall, 40% of the Euro-American parents endorsed the "apart" and "distinctive" positions, compared to 3% in the Chinese immigrant sample; the reverse proportions (5% and 40%) endorsed the "growing up together" and "not celebrating distinctiveness" poles. Shwalb and Shwalb (1996) report a related contrast from interviewing Japanese mothers about infant temperament, and the same can be seen to underlie some of the differences in bedtime routines reviewed above (e.g., Caudill & Weinstein, 1969; Harkness et al., 2007)

A more indirect indication of differences in parental beliefs was found by Nakagawa and Sukigara (2005) as they developed a Japanese version of the Infant Behavior Questionnaire (Gartstein & Rothbart, 2003). Discovering that original (US) factor structure did not completely replicate in Japan, they asked Japanese mothers to assign each of the questionnaire items to one of the 14 original dimensional categories. Of the 16 infant behaviors relating to sleeping in the original category "Distress to Limitations" (e.g., fussing at bedtime), nearly half (7) were not considered by the Japanese mothers to belong in that group. The authors interpret this result to mean that sleeping is not seen as a confining or distressing situation. This is consistent with the soothing and comforting co-sleeping customs reported elsewhere for Japanese society (Caudill & Plath, 1966; Latz, Wolf, & Lozoff, 1999; Wolf, Lozoff, Latz, & Paludetto, 1996).

Distinctive patterns of belief (and practice) can be found between neighboring groups often clustered together as "Western European." Middle-class Swedish families in the International Study of Parents, Children and Schools, for example, provided separate bedrooms for their children, as did all the other Western samples studied (Harkness et al., 2011; Super, Welles-Nyström et al., 2012; Welles-Nyström, 2005). Increasingly over the first three years of life, however, the majority of Swedish children (unlike the other groups) were found to "night wander" and come into the parents' bed in the early morning hours. Their parents tolerated and even encouraged such behavior, in part from a conviction that their children had a right to physical closeness with their parents "at any time of day or night" (Welles-Nyström, 2005, p. 357). The need for closeness was mutual, however; as one mother expressed it, "We see so little of the children during the day that we all want to fill up our tanks with love at night sleeping together" (Welles-Nyström, 2005, p. 358).

Another distinctive pattern was found in the Netherlands, where the "three Rs" of childrearing (*rust, regelmaat,* and *reinheid,* or rest, regularity, and cleanliness) has been an officially endorsed formula for over a century (van Hulst, 1905) and remains evident in the childcare literature of today. The official "baby book" provided to new mothers by the Dutch National Health Service warns against overstimulation and gives suggestions for achieving rest and regularity (Super et al., 1996; Ten Hoopen, 2005, pp. 23, 25, 54). Harkness, Super, and their colleagues found that the "three R's" were frequently mentioned by the Dutch parents they interviewed (Harkness et al., 2007), and instantiation of the beliefs in practice was found in the Dutch parents' regulation of their children's day (Harkness & Super, 1999; Super et al., 1996).

Identifying Culture in Development

The Developmental Niche

It is evident from this review that the three components of the developmental niche are not independent categories: parental belief systems underlie most customary practices, and these practices are carried out in specific, often deliberately chosen settings. As we have written elsewhere at greater length (Harkness & Super, 1992; Super & Harkness, 1986, 1999, 2002), the three components are in continuous mutual adaptation, acting as subsystems of the larger system of the niche. They share the common function of mediating the individual's developmental experience within the larger culture, with homeostatic mechanisms promoting consonance among them. Parents try not to put their children in settings they think inappropriate, for example; and as a family's ecology changes with a move to urban life, some customs become difficult to maintain. Regularities in the subsystems provide material from which the child abstracts the physical, social, affective, and cognitive rules of the culture, much as the rules of grammar are abstracted from the regularities of the speech environment. It is through such reinforcing patterns that culture has its most immediate and powerful influence. In addition, thematic continuity of the niche's central regularities from one developmental stage to the next provides a second, often more symbolic, source of cultural learning.

Even while the three components of the niche operate as a system of mutually influencing parts, they also interact with other features of the larger culture and ecology. That is, the developmental niche is an "open system" in the formal sense (von Bertalanffy, 1968). Parents' ideas are influenced by the informal networks of family and friends; by more formal routes of advice from teachers, medical staff, and religious leaders (Harkness & Super, 1996); and, more broadly, by education and cultural change (Cervera & Méndez, 2006). The settings of care reflect, among other factors, the physical ecology and economic base of the community (Barry, Child, & Bacon, 1959; Whiting & Edwards, 1988). Customary practices represent the behavioral tools received from earlier generations, as well as adaptations to changing technologies and values. This openness of the niche can be seen to operate in studies of change in children's sleeping arrangements, several of which are described above: Yovsi and Keller's (2007) comparison of farming and wage-earning families in Cameroon; Hong and Townes' (1976) report on Korean mothers in the United States; Caudill and Frost's on Japanese-American families (1974); and Green and Smith's three-generation comparison of Emirati mothers (2007). The story of how a Peace Corps volunteer in Togo adapted traditional African back-carrying to invent the "Snugli" in 1969, which met with immediate commercial success in the changing US culture, provides another interesting example (About.com, 2008).

Finally, the child at the "center" of the niche (see Figure 9.1) and the niche itself are also in a continuous (but often incomplete) process of mutual adaptation. The infant or child is adapting to and learning from the environment, to be sure, but the niche accommodates as well to the particular age, gender, temperament, and other characteristics of the child (including, perhaps, as yet unidentified genetic or epigenetic contributions to sleep behavior). Some aspects of bedtime routines have been noted as "reactive," that is, responding to the child's behavior rather than coming *de novo* from the parents; this seems to be the case for physically closer, more involved routines in some middle-class US (Hayes et al., 2007) and German (Valentin, 2005) families, groups where bed sharing is not normative.

The Uses of "Culture" in Sleep Research

It should be evident that the concept of "culture" used in the developmental niche framework is a complex, organic one, drawing heavily from anthropological traditions of ethnography and empiricism. Within that discipline, culture has been given many divergent definitions, but there is general agreement among anthropologists who study children and families on several key features (Harkness, Super, Mavridis, Barry, & Zeitlin, 2013). The most relevant here are:

1. Culture is shared among members of an interacting community, and it organizes meanings and actions across widely diverse domains (LeVine, 1984).
2. Culture exists both externally in the environment and also in the minds of individuals (Handwerker, 2002). As with language, there is a constant process of transaction between the mind of the individual participant and the common social environment.
3. Culturally based beliefs exist in a variety of forms, from the specifications of law to the implicit, "taken-for-granted" ideas about the nature of the world and the right and natural way to do things.
4. All cultures are unique, but none is completely different from all others. Rather, cultural communities tend to share some characteristics with other communities, due in part to common historical roots, the diffusion of ideas and technologies, and similar challenges and opportunities for living.
5. Understanding any particular cultural group necessarily involves a more complex, multimethod strategy than is typical of behavioral research in which the multidimensionality of culture is not considered (Weisner, 1996).

This approach can be contrasted to simpler, monodimensional studies that have been used by some more psychologically oriented researchers. Perhaps the most frequent of these in studies of child development draws a contrast between individualism and collectivism (I/C). Originally developed as one of several dimensions differentiating middle-level managers in IBM's worldwide operations, (Hofstede, 1980), the I/C contrast

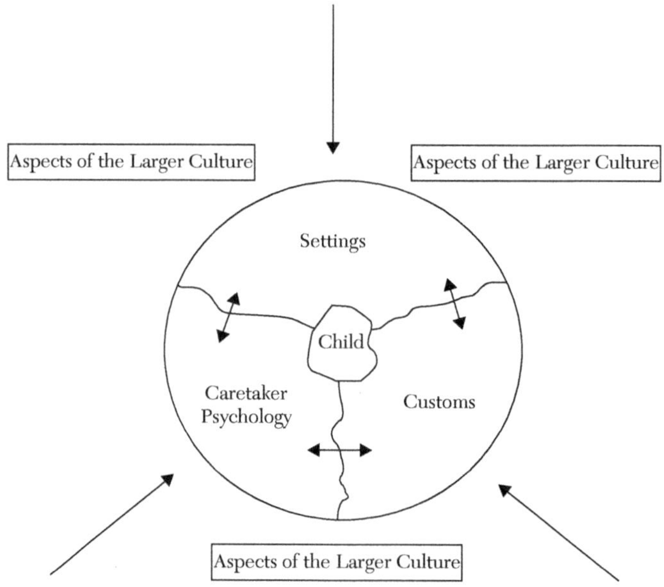

Figure 9.1 The Developmental Niche

(sometimes referred to as independence and interdependence) has frequently been taken as a primary measure of culture in developmental research. In that context, the dimension does capture something important about educated urban Western childrearing compared to that found in rural farming families in low- and middle-income countries. By itself, however, the concept fails to make use of the rich complexity of cultures, and many researchers have found it does not sufficiently map onto their empirical findings (e.g., Harkness, Super, & van Tijen, 2000; Javo, Ronning, & Heyerdahl, 2004; Kağitçibaşi, 2007; Keller et al., 2004; Leyendecker, Harwood, Lamb, & Schölmerich, 2002). As examples used above indicate, the degree of variation in important aspects of child rearing—including sleep routines—within any one "type" of society is substantial. Examining the developmental niche is an essential step in understanding the dynamics of sleep routines and their variants in any particular place.

Culture in Developmental Research

The relationship of developmental and cultural research on any given topic usually has four phases. First, investigators explore the parameters of a behavior of interest (sleep, walking, logical reasoning, etc.) in their local environment (traditionally North America or Europe). It is common in this phase to assume that the basic structure and timing of developmental growth found at home is essentially universal.

The second phase involves a search for developmental or behavioral variation in other locales. Traditionally this was done by anthropologists (Kilbride & Kilbride, 1975; Mead, 1928), later joined by others with interdisciplinary training (Konner, 1972; New & Richman, 1996; Super, 1976; Weisner & Gallimore, 1977), and now, in the global twenty-first century, by both Western investigators from varied disciplinary backgrounds and also increasingly by trained researchers in their non-Western home countries. This phase is marked by the discovery of "strong" and "weak" universals (Dasen, Lavalée, & Retschitzki, 1979), interesting variations in timing (Jahoda, 1983; Kilbride & Kilbride, 1975), and the occasional discovery of something quite novel (Shweder & LeVine, 1975).

Phase 3, achieved in various eras for separate domains, involves "unpacking" (Whiting, 1976) the culture to identify the causal networks behind the cross-cultural findings (that is, delineating the developmental niche). Thus the study of infant motor behavior was explored in detail by Americans McGraw (1932) and Shirley (1931) in the 1930s; it was taken overseas two decades later by Géber (1956) and others, who reported significant variation; then, after another two decades, it was the subject of focused ethnographic study to understand its cultural regulation (Kilbride & Kilbride, 1975; Super, 1976).

A final phase (Phase 4) may occur when the insights from cross-cultural work are brought back to the originating cultures (usually the United States or Western Europe), where they contribute to innovative paradigms in the clinic (Field, 2002) or research laboratory (Zelazo, Zelazo, Cohen, & Zelazo, 1993).

The developmental study of behaviors surrounding sleep—bed sharing, sleep aids, bedtime routines—is well established in Phase 2, as the variations described above demonstrate, and there are some beginnings of Phase 3. The study of sleep itself, however, has barely entered the age of discovery of variation. How does culture contribute to the shape and frequency of sleep problems? Are there differences in how much children sleep, or in the diurnal pattern of nighttime sleep and daytime napping? Do the internal phases of sleep develop at the same ages everywhere, and are they evident in the same proportion? Are unconsciousness and arousal always differentiated at the same pace and integrated into daily life the same way? We have partial answers to some of these questions, but puzzles far outnumber the resolutions.

Sleep Problems

DIFFERENCES IN RATE

There are two aspects of children's sleep problems that invite cross-cultural comparison. The first is the question of rate or incidence. Although it is tempting to simply compare various reports, there are a number of issues that complicate such comparisons—including specification of the cultural community sampled, ages studied, definition of terms, sources of information (parent, professional, or direct measurement), and the format and psychological context of data collection. Fortunately, there are a few reports that draw comparisons within a single study. Some of these yield no differences, for example Scher and colleagues' (1995) study of Israeli Jewish mothers of various origins—Ashkenazi (European or American in origin) and Sephardim (from North Africa or Asia)—regarding children's night waking and other sleep characteristics. Others studies, however, have identified large differences. In the United Kingdom, Rona and colleagues found that 5-year-olds with a family background in the Indian subcontinent suffered nearly twice the rate of sleep problems as did those of native British (white) origin (Rona, Li,

Gulliford, & Chinn, 1998). Liu and colleagues collected large samples of parental reports for elementary school children in southeastern New England (United States) and eastern China (Jinan), using the same questionnaire, and found significantly higher levels of sleep problems in the Chinese sample.

Teasing out the cause of such reported differences can be difficult but rewarding. LeBourgeois and colleagues surveyed over 1300 adolescents in Rome (Italy) and Hattiesburg (Mississippi, USA) about both the quality of their sleep and their "sleep hygiene," meaning sleep habits such as avoiding (or not) emotionally or physiologically arousing behavior shortly before bed (LeBourgeois, Giannotti, Cortesi, Wolfson, & Harsh, 2005). Although substantial differences in sleep quality were found between the two groups, the cultural difference nearly disappeared when sleep habits were statistically controlled. That is to say, the two cultural samples had different patterns of behavior surrounding sleep, and those sleep habits differentiated the groups to about the same degree as the nominal cultural category did. How those "hygiene" differences are integrated into the developmental niche now stands out as an important possibility for future research.

There are also occasional descriptions of sleep difficulties that may not be familiar to most (Western) readers, but are not difficult to understand once the researcher explains essential details of the children's environment. Why would the major predictor of sleep disturbance in 7–12-year-old children involve fear of death and death squads? Dollinger, Molina, and Monteiro (1996, p. 255), who report this finding, indicate that in the poor neighborhoods of Brazil where they carried out their research, "children are likely to know about and have anxieties associated with incidents of rioting or the occurrence of explosions, as well as anxieties associated with the death squads (believed by many to be off-duty police officers)." Around the world, children encounter an array of traumatic circumstances—war, drought, domestic violence, hurricanes—and we know that dramatic or enduring stress may be disruptive of sleep (Spilsbury, 2009; see Spilsbury, Chapter 14).

DIFFERENCES IN PATTERN

More interesting and complex than comparisons of rate are studies that demonstrate different *patterns* of association between the same variables in different settings. Latz and colleagues specifically compared the relationship of co-sleeping to sleep problems (Latz et al., 1999). In their US sample, regular co-sleeping (15% of the sample) was significantly associated with bedtime struggles, night waking, and a summary measure of stressful sleep problems (see also Blader, Koplewicz, Abikoff, & Foley, 1997). In Japan, where co-sleeping was four times more frequent, only night waking was related. This divergence of associations probably reflects, at least in part, US parents' adaptive response to bedtime resistance (see Hayes et al., 2007; Valentin, 2005), whereas in Japan the co-sleeping is normative, not reactive.

Comparing separate studies, which engages a host of familiar methodological problems, presents a mixed picture. In Japan, Fukumizu and colleagues (2005) found a complex set of associations suggesting that in infancy night crying was connected to co-sleeping, but at older ages it was not. Co-sleeping in a Singapore sample (where, again, it is common) is not correlated with children's sleep problems (Chng, 2008); but in Taiwan, Wu and colleagues attributed a high rate of sleep problems in young children to the high rate of bed sharing (Wu et al., 2012). In Finland, too, there is an association of co-sleeping and young children's sleep problems (Sourander, 2001). Li and colleagues report patterns of bed sharing and room sharing that may be uniquely Chinese in their determinants (Li et al., 2009); both kinds of sharing were associated with sleep problems (Li et al., 2008). Overlooking for the moment methodological differences among all these studies, one can ask: If Japan and Singapore show little or no relationship between co-sleeping and sleep problems, why do Taiwan and China, where co-sleeping is also common (Jiang et al., 2007), not present the same picture? Mindell, Sadeh, Kohyama, and How (2010), reporting on their 17-site Internet study, suggest that parental involvement in sleep onset mediates the relationship between co-sleeping and sleep outcome, and it is therefore more likely the actual cause of sleep differences: in culture areas where co-sleeping is common (primarily Asia), and it bears no correlation with sleep disturbance, a parent is usually present at bedtime regardless of the location of the child's bed. In contrast, in areas where co-sleeping is not common (primarily Western European in origin), young children fall asleep alone if their bed is in a separate room, whereas a parent may be present if the location is not separate. Thus, the authors conclude, co-sleeping per se does not account for differences in sleep outcome; rather, the relationship is mediated by parental behavior. Elaborating this idea is the finding by Teti and colleagues in a US sample that maternal emotional availability at bedtime may be more important for infant sleep quality than any particular practice (Teti, Kim, Mayer, & Countermine, 2010).

We have few studies of sleep disturbance that include analysis of the developmental niche sufficient to understand specific pathways of association. Recent studies of co-sleeping, as reviewed above, illustrate the potential of more detailed or multivariate investigation of how the niche defines the behavioral and psychological parameters of young children's sleep.

SUDDEN INFANT DEATH SYNDROME

Studies of infant sleeping arrangements, especially in nonindustrial societies, have played a central role in the complex discussion of co-sleeping, sleeping position, and Sudden Infant Death Syndrome (SIDS). The core of this discussion concerns how best to understand the relationship of the contemporary Western model, in which the infant sleeps separately from the mother, to the dominant model for the thousands of years when modern humans were evolving. Briefly, "the evidence suggests that infant–parent co-sleeping represents the species-wide pattern of sleep in which human infant physiology evolved" (McKenna et al., 1993, p. 263).

That conclusion does not by itself indicate that mothers and infants should always co-sleep, however, in part because "co-sleeping" has several separable components. First, there is a set of complex adaptations and sensory exchanges between mother and co-sleeping infant: there are frequent mutual micro-arousals, and thermoregulation is easily achieved. These and other effects, McKenna and others argue, may contribute to a reduction in the risk of SIDS (McKenna, Mosko, Richard, & Drummond, 1994; McKenna, Ball, & Gettler, 2007; McKenna & Fleming, 1994; Mosko, Richard, McKenna, & Drummond, 1996). Further, co-sleeping infants usually lie supine (on their backs), a position that minimizes the risk of suffocation on soft bedding materials; this may be of particular importance for infants with compromised reflexes or underdeveloped neck muscles.

Nevertheless, there is circumstantial evidence that co-sleeping, as evidenced in non-Western societies, is associated with lower rates of SIDS (Farooqi, Perry, & Beevers, 1993; Konner & Super, 1987). Paradoxically, it was also found that in some Western urban samples infants born of mothers belonging to immigrant (i.e., non-Western) or minority groups typically used sleeping arrangements thought to create a higher risk for SIDS than did non-minority mothers (e.g., Corwin et al., 2003; Schlaud et al., 1999). Still, in the mid-1990s the argument was deemed sufficient to warrant public information campaigns to alter the way parents put their infants to bed, and the prone position was the most common target. A number of programs (such as "back to sleep") proved successful in reducing the incidence of SIDS (e.g., Wennergren et al., 1997).

Effective application of culturally related insights to public health policy, however, is complex and requires local knowledge: because co-sleeping is differentially associated in different locales with particular bedding materials, sleep clothing, and sleeping positions (prone, etc.), public health campaigns need to be tailored to the specific community targeted (Fleming, 1994; Nelson et al., 2001; Nelson, Taylor, & Weatherall, 1989; Schluter, Paterson, & Percival, 2007; see Burnham, Chapter 12).

Information about the developmental niche, especially in contrasting examples, helps us to focus on the causal pathways underlying the paradoxical minority/majority differences. In Thailand, bed sharing with young infants is a common practice, and nearly a third of the 3692 infants studied by Anuntaseree and colleagues (2008) were placed in a prone position; contrary to Western findings, the rate of SIDS is relatively low. Part of the explanation appears to be that older, high-SES mothers in Thailand were the most likely to bed-share and to put the infant in a prone position, whereas the young, poor mother of a low-weight infant was less likely to engage in these high-risk behaviors—exactly the opposite pattern reported for most Western countries. The authors attribute the pattern to some unidentified aspect of culture, but we can presume it includes customary practices and parental ethnotheories, as well as the risks associated with lower birth weight.

In Haifa (Israel), Inbar and colleagues identified two minority groups who had low risk for SIDS after a brief informational intervention, but for different reasons (Inbar et al., 2005). First, mothers who had been born in the former Soviet Union and immigrated to Israel after 1990 routinely put their babies to sleep in a back or side position, prior to the intervention; thus their customary behavior and the thinking behind it were already a protective factor. Second, Israeli-born Arab mothers, compared to Israeli-born Jewish mothers, were generally more disposed to follow the advice of the high-status medical personnel; thus they were more likely to alter their behavior to produce a relatively low-risk situation. In this case, the psychology of the caretakers, in interaction with the larger environment of support and advice, led to a protective change in maternal behavior.

Variations in the pattern of associations with sleep problems, ranging from night waking to SIDS, may be puzzling, but for that very reason they can also be illuminating. The "packages" of behavior, risk, and outcome that are found—or seem obvious—in one cultural setting may not hold together in another. By highlighting the cultural construction of risk factors, comparative studies can lead us to reexamine familiar findings from the commonly surveyed settings.

Sleep Duration

One curious characteristic of human sleep, as Worthman (2006) has elaborated, is the high degree of plasticity in the amount that is "needed." Individuals can relatively easily adapt to longer or shorter amounts of sleep, at least on a short-term basis, depending on contextual demands. In addition, there is now reason to believe that there are chronic differences between various cultural groups in the amount of sleep during infancy and childhood.

The methodological problems in comparing sleep times reported in different studies are substantial. Traditional issues in self- and parent-report data (Sadeh, 1996), combined with variations in procedure and sampling, as well as possibly subtle cultural differences in defining the thresholds of "sleep," make any two-study comparison difficult to interpret with confidence. Nevertheless, the relatively large number of reports now available permits a broad examination. A meta-analysis of adolescent sleep studies in 23 countries found strong evidence that total sleep time in Asian settings (China, India, Japan, Korea, and Taiwan) averages up to one hour less than in North America, and two hours less than in Europe, on both school days and non–school days (Olds, Blunden, Petkov, & Forchino, 2010). The first of these generalizations is illustrated by the more stringent comparison by Liu and colleagues, who carried out parallel data collection on elementary school children in China and the United States and reported averages, respectively, of 9.25 and 10.15 hours, a difference of just under 1 hour (Liu, Liu, Owens, & Kaplan, 2005). Several authors have pointed to strong pressure for homework and academic success in many Asian countries as a possible cause of children's shorter sleep time in China, Japan, Korea, and other Asian countries (Ouyang et al., 2009).

Among infants and young children, several comparative studies also suggest overall differences in total sleep. Ethnic differences have been demonstrated in the United States (Kentucky), with young African-American children getting less sleep than Euro-Americans (independent of SES), primarily due to later bedtimes (McLaughlin Crabtree et al., 2005). Kohyama and colleagues (Kohyama, Mindell, & Sadeh, 2011), using a subset of data from a large Internet study (Mindell, Sadeh, Wiegand et al., 2010), found that Japanese infants and toddlers slept less than those in other Asian countries, at least after 3 months of age. Shorter sleep times are also reported for infants in Shanghai (Jiang et al., 2007). Within Europe, the large-scale IDEFICS study has identified significant national differences in parental report of weekday nocturnal sleep for children from 2 to 9 years, ranging from an average of 9.5 hours in Estonia to 11.2 hours in Belgium (Hense, Barba, Pohlabeln, De Henauw, Marild, Molnar, et al., 2011).

Almost all of these studies rely on parents' recall of their children's sleep, a method known to bias toward overestimateion, at least in populations with little bed sharing (Sadeh, 1996). In contrast, Super and colleagues collected infant sleep data using both parental diaries (not recall) and actigraph measures; although the two methods yielded different absolute measures, both indicated approximately 2 hours more sleep in Dutch samples than in samples from the northeast United States (Blom, Super, & Harkness, 2012; Super, Blom, Harkness, Ranade, & Londhe,, 2012; Super et al., 1996; Super, Welles-Nyström et al., 2012). An examination of the infants' respective developmental niches documents strong differences in parents' ethnotheories, customary practices, and the settings of everyday life that would support such a divergence in sleep development (Blom et al., 2012; Harkness et al., 2007; Super, Blom et al., 2012; Super et al., 1996; Super, Welles-Nyström et al., 2012).

One report from rural Kenya (Super & Harkness, 1982), using time logs kept by a family member, suggests that these Kipsigis infants slept less than any other reported group: about 11 hours at 8 months, compared to about 12 hours in Japan (Kohyama et al., 2011) and the United States (Super, Blom et al., 2012), and nearly 14 hours in Zurich, Switzerland (Iglowstein, Jenni, Molinari, & Largo, 2003). The Kipsigis infants were often cared for, and entertained, by their older siblings, which may have reduced their opportunities for sleep (Super & Harkness, 1994).

Despite some methodological limitations, then, we can conclude that variations in the developmental niche can produce significant differences in the amount of sleep that infants, children, and adolescents typically have. We are just beginning, however, to see the parameters of plasticity in sleep duration during development. The younger such differences are found, the more it challenges the idea that early sleep development is invariant, at least in this regard, driven solely by the forces of maturation.

Sleep Timing

We know a great deal about variations in when children around the world sleep. There are substantial differences in how regular their bedtime is, how early or late they go to bed at night, and how much of their total sleep is, in fact, nocturnal.

Regularity of bedtime is one element of what has come to be called "sleep hygiene" (Zarcone, 2002), and it is generally found to contribute to sleep quality and high functioning during the day (Acebo, Carskadon, & Achenbach, 2002). It can be noted, however, that in the populations and age groups studied for this purpose, regularity of daytime functioning is also common—school and work hours are fixed, set externally and independently of individual sleep behavior. For infants and young children, or in nonindustrial societies where activities during the day may not be so structured by the clock, there is no evidence of contemporaneous negative consequences to irregular bedtimes. Flexibility in when (and often, where) young humans sleep is the norm among hunter-gathering and most agrarian groups (Hewlett et al., 1998; Konner, 1976; Super, 1981). None of the nonindustrial groups reviewed by Worthman and Melby (2002) had regular bedtimes. Young children, especially, may sleep when drowsy but when evening activities are interesting they remain awake and engaged. To a lesser degree, this pattern of flexible bedtimes for the young is also seen in many Mediterranean and tropical cultures. New and Richman (1996) contrast the scheduled life of infants in a middle-class US community to the relatively adaptable time of transitions in an Italian town near Rome, where young infants frequently stayed with other members of the family and fell asleep before being put to bed. Wolf and colleagues (1996), however, found significantly more Italian than US families reporting regular bedtimes for their sample of toddlers from Naples—a clear reminder that we rarely know the limits of generalization for our samples of convenience. Puerto Rican families in the United States frequently continue their customary (flexible) bedtime pattern for infants and preschoolers with no untoward contemporary consequences (Feng et al., 2001; Korn & Gannon, 1983). When these children begin school, however, those who are not able to quickly adapt to the new and rigid schedule are likely to encounter at least transient difficulty (Thomas & Chess, 1977).

In general, in communities where children do not have a fixed bedtime, they tend to stay up later and nap more during the day, compared to children with more scheduled routines. This is certainly true in the large contrast of nonindustrial societies vs. modern urban groups (Worthman & Melby, 2002). In modern communities where midday napping is common, usually related to daytime heat, napping by children and infants fits easily into the ecology of family life (Reimão, De Souza, & Gaudioso, 1999; Reimão et al., 2000; Reimão, De Souza, P., Medeiros, & Almirão, 1998; Worthman & Brown, 2007). The connection between naps and nighttime sleep is not necessarily a straightforward one, however. In the Dutch sample that showed great attention to regular bedtimes, for example, infants took more and slightly longer daytime naps than did the US infants studied; further, it was the daytime sleep that accounted for almost all of the total sleep difference of 1.5 hours (Super, Blom et al., 2012). Within modern urban societies, there are substantial differences in napping among different ethnic groups. Forty percent of African-American 8-year-olds in Mississippi studied by Crosby and colleagues, for example, regularly took daytime naps, compared to 5% of Euro-Americans in the same community; the ethnic difference could not be accounted for by other common demographic variables (Crosby, LeBourgeois, & Harsh, 2005). Notably, the total weekly sleep duration was nearly identical for the two groups, and napping was not related to psychosocial functioning.

Sleep Architecture

There has been almost no attention to sleep architecture (the timing and sequence of sleep stages) in divergent natural settings, but the few reported findings are intriguing. Quan and colleagues (2003) recorded one night of unattended, home polysomnography in US children ages 6 to 11 years, and report more stage 2 sleep and less deep sleep among Hispanics than Caucasian children. This bears some resemblance to an earlier report of higher REM density among Hispanic adtults (Rao, Poland, Lutchmansingh, Ott, McCracken, & Keh-Ming, 1999), but given a large number of unknown, potential ecological differences, it is difficult to draw any firm conclusions. Petre-Quadens, Hussain, and Balaratnam (1975) carried out polygraphic recordings on two young adults from the Teminar tribe living in the rainforests of Malaysia. They found few differences from the familiar Western pattern, but did note that the REM densities were consistently low by established standards.

Compared to the rainforests of Malaysia, the ecologies of middle-class Dutch and US families seem very similar. Nevertheless, the Dutch infants we studied engaged in significantly more quiet sleep than did our US sample, as estimated by Sadeh's algorithm (Sadeh, Acebo, Seifer, & Aytur, 1995) applied to actigraph recordings (Super, Blom et al., 2012; see Horne and Biggs, Chapter 16). This finding is consistent with the strong emphasis in Dutch ethnotheories, customs, and settings on the "three R's" of "rest, regularity, and cleanliness," and the US emphasis on early stimulation for cognitive development (Harkness et al., 2007; Super et al., 1996). It may be that the US and Dutch developmental niches for these infants are so divergent with regard to the level of activation during waking time that they produce divergence in sleep architecture.

Developmental Consequences and Sleep After Childhood

It is almost universally true that meaningful differences in the context or content of early development are followed by thematically or structurally related differences in childhood and beyond. It is therefore virtually impossible to examine *independent* effects of early experience of the sort discussed in this chapter. Nevertheless, it remains of profound importance, for both theoretical and diagnostic reasons, to understand to what degree differences in early sleep can carry through and contribute to later functioning. Three kinds of possibilities seem evident.

First, situations at the extreme of known variation could set the stage for particular kinds of dysfunction. One question, for example, is whether infants who are "overstimulated" and get relatively limited sleep will show effects parallel to sleep deprivation in adulthood: increased levels of cortisol, lowered carbohydrate tolerance, elevation of sympathovagal balance, and changes in key hormones that regulate metabolism and appetite (Copinschi, 2005; Spiegel et al., 2004); and, by extension, whether they will show effects regarding the regulation of arousal, activity, appetite, body weight, and emotionality (Meaney, Aitken, Bhatnagar, Van Derkel, & Sapolsky, 1988; Susman, 2006; Weissbluth, 1989).

A second kind of consequence of early sleep patterns might be found in communities where there is a disjuncture between the habits of infancy and early childhood, on the one hand, and the ecological requirements that follow—cases similar to Thomas and Chess' Puerto Rican sample in New York (Korn & Gannon, 1983; Thomas & Chess, 1977). This pattern is most likely in groups where the traditions of early child care were developed in an ecology distinctly different from their current situation, and can be seen in a variety of immigrant populations. The opposite case—reared to a regular, monophasic rhythm but now trying to function in a "siesta culture" (Webb & Dinges, 1989)—is probably far less common, and certainly less well documented.

Finally, there is the observation that differences in childhood sleep and sleep routines may constitute anticipatory socialization and promote the early development of particular dispositions and skills. Some instances of this are immediately evident, for example in the life-long continuities of social density at night, as Worthman and Brown (2007) describe for Egyptian families. We accept and come to rely on familiar ways. More profoundly, however, developmental science has just begun to address important questions about the socialization of arousal and self-regulation. Infants who are carried by a family member all day experience going in and out of sleep surrounded by voices and the noise of family work, as well as the rhythms and jounces of the caretaker's body. Do they learn skills of sleeping despite these distractions, just as US infants learn to sleep alone in silence? Do those skills get further advanced in maturity?

Margaret Mead advances one interesting example. Part of what attracted her to work in Bali was a film she had seen of child trance, and the idea of an institutionalized dissociative state, as was reported for adults, fit her theoretical interest and curiosity at that time (Jacknis, 1988). In the main report on that project, Mead and Macgregor (1951) describe infants' and young children's ability to sleep under any circumstances, including those involving intense emotion, an ability that is apparently elaborated in adolescence and adulthood. Suddenly falling into a deep sleep when frightened or anxious is a named phenomenon in Bali: *tadoet poeles,* "fear sleep." They write (p. 51): "As children and later as adults, Balinese go to sleep in situations that are threatening or dangerous, and sleep so soundly that they have to be shaken awake. A thief falls asleep while his case is being decided; servants fall asleep if they have broken or lost something; a child at a delivery will sleep soundly on the platform bed on which the birth is taking place." As the authors comment, these are situations in which most Europeans and Americans would exhibit heightened alertness, not sleep. Exactly what the neuroregulatory systems were doing in the Balinese case is not known (is it related to narcolepsy?), but the phenomenon suggests a systemic state change that does not come easily to those not reared into it. Clearly the behavior was normative and institutionalized in Bali, integrated with other spiritual beliefs and activities; its origins in early socialization are less clear, although Mead and Macgregor draw attention to the flow of arousal and sleep in infants as they are carried during the daily activities of parents and siblings.

A second interesting example of continuity in state behavior is the dream work found among the Senoi of Malaysia. The primary ethnographic source for this activity is the work of Stewart (Stewart, 1951; 1954a, 1954b), who visited the Senoi in the 1930s (and whose work was swept up in the "human potential" movement in the 1960s). In Stewart's description, dreams among the Senoi were a major avenue of individual creativity and mental health, and when they were incorporated into community affairs they became a source of problem solving, dispute resolution, and social harmony. The Senoi learned to manage their dreams, and the learning of this skill was a family affair: "The Senoi parent inquires of his child's dream at breakfast, praises the child for having the dream, and discusses the significance of it. He asks about past incidences and tells the child how to change his behavior and attitude in future dreams. He also recommends certain social activities or gestures which the dream makes necessary or advisable" (Stewart, 1954a, p. 396). Although Stewart's work, and especially the use that was later made of it, has come under sharp criticism, there is some confirmation of his basic ethnographic observations (Domhoff, 2003). We can also note that *Senoi* refers to a group of tribes in the rainforests of Malaysia, one of which is also called *Teminar*, the affiliation of the two young men in whom Petre-Quadens and colleagues (1975) found evidence of unusual REM states.

Conclusion and Future Directions

We spend one-third of our life in sleep; during our infancy and early childhood, it is fully half. There is no reason to think that what happens during that time, or surrounding our transitions in and out, is unimportant. This much is taken for granted by sleep researchers. An article of developmental faith—"You can't understand where you are if you don't know how you got there"—is increasingly accepted by sleep researchers as well. What does the cultural perspective have to offer beyond all that?

Most immediately, it lets us see that the cultural model of sleeping arrangements for infants and children most familiar to most sleep researchers is highly unusual in global perspective, and it is a relatively recent addition to the human scene. Despite that, it is the paradigm on which most sleep research is carried out, and we are just learning the degree to which it has shaped our infant discipline. Thus, for example, the pattern of associations between co-sleeping during infancy and other variables (such as sleep problems) is culturally constructed; this pattern is not generally found where co-sleeping is normative. Other phenomena, both normative and clinically germane, will benefit from careful examination of patterns in multiple contexts, and an essential component of that examination is a delineation of the developmental niche. With a better understanding of the variation in the settings, customs, and cultural beliefs that shape the context of early sleep, we will be in a better position to see and to make sense of culturally induced differences in sleep itself.

We can conclude, therefore, that our understanding of normal sleep and sleep disturbances during infancy and childhood will be particularly advanced by two kinds of research:

- *Multi-site studies of divergent cultural communities*, whether within or across nations. Because monocultural studies necessarily yield ambiguous results—Is there something about this context that yields this pattern of behavior and its causal pathways?—the identification of patterns in multiple sites is an essential step toward a science for our species. This is true for both clinical and normative research. Multisite designs highlight a particular burden of measurement equivalence, but that is ultimately necessary for making sense of comparative findings.
- *An empirical focus on the developmental niche.* There are proven methods to measure children's physical and social settings, the customary practices followed in their families and communities, and the beliefs and attitudes of their caretakers. Without systematic data on these elements of the niche, it is extremely difficult to make reliable interpretations of patterns—whether varying or invariant.

References

Abbott, S. (1992). Holding on and pushing away: Comparative perspectives on an Eastern Kentucky child-rearing practice. *Ethos, 20*, 33–65.

Abel, S., Park, J., Tipene-Leach, D., Finau, S., & Lennan, M. (2001). Infant care practices in New Zealand: a cross-cultural qualitative study. *Soc Sci Med, 53*(9), 1135–1148.

About.com. (2008). *Ann Moore—Snugli.* Retrieved March 20, 2013, from http://inventors.about.com/library/inventors/bl_Ann_Moore.htm.

Acebo, C., Carskadon, M. A., & Achenbach, T. M. (2002). Influence of irregular sleep patterns on waking behavior. In M. A. Carskadon (Ed.), *Adolescent Sleep Patterns: Biological, Social, and Psychological Influences* (pp. 220–235). New York: Cambridge University Press.

Anuntaseree, W., Mo-Suwan, L., Vasiknanonte, P., Kuasirikul, S., Ma, A. L. A., & Choprapawon, C. (2008). Factors associated with bed sharing and sleep position in Thai neonates. *Child: Care, Health and Development, 34*(4), 482–490.

Arnett, J. J. (2008). The neglected 95%: Why American psychology needs to become less American. *American Psychologist, 63*(7), 602–614.

Barry, H. III, & Paxson, L. (1971). Infancy and early childhood: Cross-cultural codes. *Ethnology, 10,* 466–508.

Barry, H. I., Child, I. L., & Bacon, M. K. (1959). Relation of child training to subsistence economy. *American Anthropologist, 61,* 51–63.

Blader, J. C., Koplewicz, H. S., Abikoff, H., & Foley, C. (1997). Sleep problems of elementary school children. A community survey. *Archives of Pediatric & Adolescent Medicine, 151*(5), 473–480.

Blom, M. J. M., Super, C. M., & Harkness, S. (2012). Culturally regulated environmental cues and sleep development in Dutch and U.S. infants. *Submitted for publication.*

Caudill, W., & Plath, D. W. (1966). Who sleeps by whom? Parent-child involvement in urban Japanese families. *Psychiatry, 29*(4), 344–366.

Caudill, W., & Weinstein, H. (1969). Maternal care and infant behavior in Japan and America. *Psychiatry, 32,* 12–43.

Caudill, W., & Frost, L. (1974). A comparison of maternal care and infant behavior in Japanese-American, American, and Japanese families. In *Mental Health Research in Asia and the Pacific: Youth, Socialization, and Mental Health.* (Vol. 2, pp. 4–15). Oxford, England: University Press of Hawaii.

Cervera, M. D., & Méndez, R. M. (2006). Temperament and ecological context among Yucatec Mayan children. *International Journal of Behavioral Development, 30*(4), 326–337.

Chng, S. Y. (2008). Sleep disorders in children: The Singapore perspective. *Annals of the Academy of Medicine, Singapore, 37*(8), 706–709.

Copinschi, G. (2005). Metabolic and endocrine effects of sleep deprivation. *Essential Psychopharmacology, 6*(6), 341–347.

Corwin, M., Lesko, S., Heeren, T. C., Vezina, R., Hunt, C., Mandell, F., et al. (2003). Secular changes in sleep position during infancy: 1995–1998. *Pediatrics, 111,* 52–60.

Crosby, B., LeBourgeois, M. K., & Harsh, J. (2005). Racial differences in reported napping and nocturnal sleep in 2- to 8-year-old children. *Pediatrics, 115*(1 Suppl), 225–232.

Dasen, P. R., Lavalée, M., & Retschitzki, J. (1979). Training conservation of quantity (liquids) in West African (Baoulé) children. *International Journal of Psychology, 14,* 57–68.

Dollinger, S. J., Molina, B. S., & Monteiro, J. M. C. (1996). Sleep and anxieties in Brazilian children: The role of cultural and environmental factors in child sleep disturbance. *American Journal of Orthopsychiatry, 66*(2), 252–261.

Domhoff, G. W. (2003). *Senoi Dream Theory: Myth, Scientific Method, and the Dreamwork Movement,* from http://dreamresearch.net/Library/senoi.html. Accessed May 22, 2013.

Farooqi, S., Perry, I. J., & Beevers, D. G. (1993). Ethnic differences in infant-rearing practices and their possible relationship to the incidence of sudden infant death syndrome (SIDS). *Paediatric and Perinatal Epidemiology, 7*(3), 245–252.

Feng, X., Harwood, R. L., Leyendecker, B., & Miller, A. M. (2001). Changes across the first year of life in infants' daily activities and social contacts among middle-class Anglo and Puerto Rican families. *Infant Behavior & Development, 24*(3), 317–339.

Field, T. (2002). Massage therapy. *The Medical Clinics of North America, 86*(1), 163–171.

Fleming, P. J. (1994). Understanding and preventing sudden infant death syndrome. *Current Opinion in Pediatrics, 6*(2), 158–162.

Fukumizu, M., Kaga, M., Kohyama, J., & Hayes, M. J. (2005). Sleep-related nighttime crying (yonaki) in Japan: a community-based study. *Pediatrics, 115*(1 Suppl), 217–224.

Gaddini, R. (1970). Transitional objects and the process of individuation: A study in three different social groups. *Journal of the American Academy of Child Psychiatry, 9*(2), 347–365.

Gartstein, M. A., & Rothbart, M. K. (2003). Studying infant temperament via the Infant Behavior Questionnaire. *Child Development, 26*(1), 64–86.

Géber, M. (1956). Développement psycho-moteur de l'enfant africain. *Courrier, 6,* 17–29.

Giannotti, F., & Cortesi, F. (2009). Family and cultural influences on sleep development. *Child and Adolescent Psychiatric Clinics of North America, 18*(4), 849–861.

Green, K. E., & Smith, D. E. (2007). Change and continuity: Childbirth and parenting across three generations of women in the United Arab Emirates. *Child: Care, Health and Development, 33*(3), 266–274.

Greenfield, P. M., & Cocking, R. R. (Eds.). (1994). *Cross-Cultural Roots of Minority Child Development.* Hillsdale, New Jersey: Lawrence Erlbaum.

Handwerker, W. P. (2002). The construct validity of cultures: Cultural diversity, culture theory, and a method for ethnography. *American Anthropologist, 104*(1), 106–122.

Harkness, S., & Super, C. M. (1992). The developmental niche: A theoretical framework for analyzing the household production of health. *Social Science and Medicine, 38*(2), 217–226.

Harkness, S., & Super, C. M. (1996). Introduction. In S. Harkness & C. M. Super (Eds.), *Parents' Cultural Belief Systems: Their Origins, Expressions, and Consequences* (pp. 1–23). New York: Guilford.

Harkness, S., & Super, C. M. (1999). From parents' cultural belief systems to behavior: Implications for the development of early intervention programs. In L. Eldering & P. Lesemen (Eds.), *Effective Early Education: Cross-Cultural Perspectives* (pp. 67–90). New York: Falmer Press.

Harkness, S., Super, C. M., & van Tijen, N. (2000). Individualism and the "Western mind" reconsidered: American and Dutch parents' ethnotheories of children and family. In S. Harkness, C. Raeff & C. M. Super (Eds.), *Variability in the Social Construction of the Child (New Directions for Child and Adolescent Development)* (Vol. 87, pp. 23–39). San Francisco: Jossey-Bass.

Harkness, S., Super, C. M., Moscardino, U., Rha, J.-H., Blom, M. J. M., Huitrón, B., et al. (2007). Cultural models and developmental agendas: Implications for arousal and self-regulation in early infancy. *Journal of Developmental Processes, 1*(2), 5–39.

Harkness, S., Zylicz, P. O., Super, C. M., Welles-Nyström, B., Ríos Bermúdez, M., Bonichini, S., et al. (2011). Children's activities and their meanings for parents: A mixed-methods

study in six Western cultures. *Journal of Family Psychology, 25*(6), 799–813.
Harkness, S., Super, C. M., Mavridis, C. J., Barry, O., & Zeitlin, M. (2013). Culture and early childhood development: Implications for policy and programs. In P. R. Britto, P. Engle & C. M. Super (Eds.), *Oxford Handbook of Early Childhood Development and Its Impact on Global Policy (pp. 142–160).* [A joint UNICEF-SRCD publication]. New York: Oxford.
Harlow, H. F., & Suomi, S. J. (1970). Nature of love: Simplified. *American Psychologist, 25*(2), 161–168.
Harwood, R. L., Schölmerich, A., Schulze, P. A., & Gonzalez, Z. (1999). Cultural differences in maternal beliefs and behaviors: A study of middle-class Anglo and Puerto Rican mother-infant pairs in four everyday situations. *Child Development, 70*(4), 1005–1016.
Hayes, M. J., Fukumizu, M., Troese, M., Sallinen, B. A., & Gilles, A. A. (2007). Social experiences in infancy and early childhood co-sleeping. *Infant and Child Development, 16*(4), 403–416.
Hense, S., Barba, G., Pohlabeln, H., De Henauw, S. Marild, S., Molnar, D., Moreno, L. A., Hadjigeorgiou, C., Viedebaum, T., & Ahrens, W. (2011). Factors that influence weekday sleep duration in European children. *Sleep, 34(5)*, 633–639.
Hewlett, B. S., Lamb, M. E., Shannon, D., Leyendecker, B., & Schölmerich, A. (1998). Culture and early infancy among central African foragers and farmers. *Developmental Psychology, 34*(4), 653–661.
Hofstede, G. H. (1980). *Culture's Consequences: International Differences in Work-Related Values.* Beverly Hills, CA: Sage.
Hong, K. M., & Townes, B. D. (1976). Infants' attachment to inanimate objects: A cross-cultural study. *Journal of the American Academy of Child Psychiatry, 15*(1), 49–61.
Iglowstein, I., Jenni, O. G., Molinari, L., & Largo, R. H. (2003). Sleep duration from infancy to adolescence: Reference values and generational trends. *Pediatrics, 111*(2), 302.
Inbar, Z., Meibar, R., Shehada, S., Irena, V., Rubin, L., & Rishpon, S. (2005). "Back to sleep": parents compliance with the recommendation on the most appropriate sleeping position of infants, Haifa District, Israel, 2001. *Preventive Medicine: An International Journal Devoted to Practice and Theory, 40*(6), 765–768.
Jacknis, I. (1988). Margaret Mead and Gregory Bateson in Bali: Their use of photography and film. *Cultural Anthropology, 3*(2), 160–177.
Jahoda, G. (1983). European "lag" in the development of an economic concept: A study in Zimbabwe. *British Journal of Developmental Psychology, 1*(2), 113–120.
Javo, C., Ronning, J. A., & Heyerdahl, S. (2004). Child-rearing in an indigenous Sami population in Norway: A cross-cultural comparison of parental attitudes and expectations. *Scandinavian Journal of Psychology, 45*(1), 67–78.
Jenni, O. G., & O'Connor, B. B. (2005). Children's sleep: An interplay between culture and biology. *Pediatrics, 115*(1 Suppl), 204–216.
Jiang, F., Shen, X., Yan, C., Wu, S., Jin, X., Dyken, M., et al. (2007). Epidemiological study of sleep characteristics in Chinese children 1–23 months of age. *Pediatrics International, 49*(6), 811–816.
Kağitçibaşi, Ç. (2007). *Family, Self, and Human Development Across Cultures: Theory and Applications* (2nd Edition). Mahwah, NJ: Erlbaum.
Keller, H., Lohaus, A., Kuensemueller, P., Abels, M., Yovsi, R., Voelker, S., et al. (2004). The bio-culture of parenting: Evidence from five cultural communities. *Parenting: Science and Practice, 4*(1), 25–50.
Kilbride, J. E., & Kilbride, P. L. (1975). Sitting and smiling behavior of Baganda infants: The influence of culturally constituted experience. *Journal of Cross-Cultural Psychology, 6*, 88–107.
Kohyama, J., Mindell, J. A., & Sadeh, A. (2011). Sleep characteristics of young children in Japan: Internet study and comparison with other Asian countries. *Pediatrics International, 53*(5), 649–655.
Konner, M. J. (1972). Aspects of the developmental ethology of a foraging people. In N. G. Blurton Jones (Ed.), *Ethological Studies of Child Behavior.* Cambridge, England: Cambridge University Press.
Konner, M. J. (1976). Maternal care, infant behavior and development among the !Kung. In R. Lee & I. DeVore (Eds.), *Kalahari Hunter-Gatherers* (pp. 218–245). Cambridge, MA: Harvard University Press.
Konner, M. J., & Super, C. M. (1987). Sudden infant death syndrome: An anthropological hypothesis. In C. M. Super (Ed.), *The Role of Culture in Developmental Disorder* (pp. 95–109). New York: Academic Press.
Korn, S. J., & Gannon, S. (1983). Temperament, cultural variation and behavior disorder in preschool children. *Child Psychiatry and Human Development, 13*(4), 203–212.
Landrine, H., & Klonoff, E. A. (1996). Traditional African-American family practices: Prevalence and correlates. *Western Journal of Black Studies, 20*(2), 59–62.
Latz, S., Wolf, A. W., & Lozoff, B. (1999). Cosleeping in context: Sleep practices and problems in young children in Japan and the United States. *Archives of Pediatrics and Adolescent Medicine, 153*(4), 339–346.
LeBourgeois, M. K., Giannotti, F., Cortesi, F., Wolfson, A. R., & Harsh, J. (2005). The relationship between reported sleep quality and sleep hygiene in Italian and American adolescents. *Pediatrics, 115*(1 Suppl), 257–265.
LeVine, R. A. (1984). Properties of culture. In R. A. Shweder & R. L. LeVine (Eds.), *Culture theory: Essays on Mind, Self, and Emotion* (pp. 67–87). New York: Cambridge University Press.
Leyendecker, B., Harwood, R. L., Lamb, M. E., & Schölmerich, A. (2002). Mothers' socialisation goals and evaluations of desirable and undesirable everyday situations in two diverse cultural groups. *International Journal of Behavioral Development, 26*(3), 248–258.
Li, S., Jin, X., Yan, C., Wu, S., Jiang, F., & Shen, X. (2008). Bed- and room-sharing in Chinese school-aged children: Prevalence and association with sleep behaviors. *Sleep Medicine, 9*(5), 555–563.
Li, S., Jin, X., Yan, C., Wu, S., Jiang, F., & Shen, X. (2009). Factors associated with bed and room sharing in Chinese school-aged children. *Child: Care, Health, Development, 35*(2), 171–177.
Liu, X., Liu, L., Owens, J. A., & Kaplan, D. L. (2005). Sleep patterns and sleep problems among schoolchildren in the United States and China. *Pediatrics, 115*(1 Suppl), 241–249.
Malinowski, B. (1929). *The Sexual Life of Savages in North-Western Melanesia.* London: Routledge & Sons. Excerpted in R. A. LeVine and R. New (Eds.). (2008). *Anthropology and Child Development: A Cross-Cultural Reader* (pp. 28–33). Malden, MA: Blackwell.
Marvin, R. S., VanDevender, T. L., Iwanaga, M. I., LeVine, S. E., & LeVine, R. A. (1977). Infant-caregiver attachment among the Hausa of Nigeria. In H. McGurk (Ed.), *Ecological Factors*

in Human Development (pp. 247–260). Amsterdam: North Holland.

McGraw, M. B. (1932). From reflex to muscular control in the assumption of an erect posture and ambulation in the human infant. *Child Development, 3*, 291–297.

McKenna, J., Mosko, S., Richard, C., & Drummond, S. (1994). Experimental studies of infant-parent co-sleeping: Mutual physiology and behavioral influences and their relevance to SIDS (sudden infant death syndrome). *Early Human Development, 38*(3), 187–201.

McKenna, J. J., Thoman, E. B., Anders, T. F., Sadeh, A., Schechtman, V. L., & Glotzbach, S. F. (1993). Infant-parent co-sleeping in an evolutionary perspective: Implications for understanding infant sleep development and the sudden infant death syndrome. *Sleep, 16*(3), 263–282.

McKenna, J. J., & Fleming, P. J. (1994). Ethnicity and the sudden infant death syndrome: Important clues from anthropology. *Archives of Disease in Childhood, 70*(5), 450.

McKenna, J. J., Ball, H. L., & Gettler, L. T. (2007). Mother-infant cosleeping, breastfeeding and sudden infant death syndrome: What biological anthropology has discovered about normal infant sleep and pediatric sleep medicine. *American Journal of Physical Anthropology, Suppl 45*, 133–161.

McLaughlin Crabtree, V., Beal Korhonen, J., Montgomery-Downs, H. E., Faye Jones, V., O'Brien, L. M., & Gozal, D. (2005). Cultural influences on the bedtime behaviors of young children. *Sleep Medicine, 6*(4), 319–324.

Mead, M. (1928). Samoan children at work and play. *Natural History*, November/December, 103–104. Reprinted in R. A. LeVine and R. New (Eds.). (2008). *Anthropology and Child Development: A Cross-Cultural Reader* (pp. 2022–2024). Malden, MA: Blackwell

Mead, M., & Macgregor, F. C. (1951). *Growth and Culture.* New York: Putnam.

Meaney, M., Aitken, D. H., Bhatnagar, S., Van Derkel, C., & Sapolsky, R. M. (1988). Postnatal handling attenuates neuroendocrine, anatomical, and cognitive impairments related to the aged hippocampus. *Science, 238*, 766–768.

Milan, S., Snow, S., & Belay, S. (2007). The context of preschool children's sleep: Racial/ethnic differences in sleep locations, routines, and concerns. *Journal of Family Psychology, 21*(1), 20–28.

Mindell, J. A., Sadeh, A., Kohyama, J., & How, T. H. (2010). Parental behaviors and sleep outcomes in infants and toddlers: A cross-cultural comparison. *Sleep Medicine, 11*(4), 393–399.

Mindell, J. A., Sadeh, A., Wiegand, B., How, T. H., & Goh, D. Y. T. (2010). Cross-cultural differences in infant and toddler sleep. *Sleep Medicine, 11*(3), 274–280.

Morelli, G. A., Rogoff, B., Oppenheim, D., & Goldsmith, D. (1992). Cultural variation in infants' sleeping arrangements: Questions of independence. *Developmental Psychology, 28*(4), 604–613.

Moscardino, U., Nwobu, O., & Axia, G. (2006). Cultural beliefs and practices related to infant health and development among Nigerian immigrant mothers in Italy. *Journal of Reproductive and Infant Psychology, 24*(3), 241–255.

Mosko, S., Richard, C., McKenna, J., & Drummond, S. (1996). Infant sleep architecture during bedsharing and possible implications for SIDS. *Sleep, 19*(9), 677–684.

Munroe, R. L., & Munroe, R. H. (1987). The couvade and male pregnancy symptoms. In Ç. Kağitçibaşi (Ed.), *Growth and Progress in Cross-Cultural Psychology: Selected papers from the eighth International Conference of the International Association for Cross-Cultural Psychology held at Istanbul, Turkey, July 6–10, 1986* (pp. 394–402). Berwyn, PA, US: Swets North America.

Nakagawa, A., & Sukigara, M. (2005). How are cultural differences in the interpretation of infant behavior reflected in the Japanese Revised Infant Behavior Questionnaire? *Japanese Journal of Educational Psychology, 53*(4), 491–503.

Nelson, E. A., Taylor, B. J., & Weatherall, I. L. (1989). Sleeping position and infant bedding may predispose to hyperthermia and the sudden infant death syndrome. *Lancet, 1*(8631), 199–201.

Nelson, E. A., Taylor, B. J., Jenik, A., Vance, J., Walmsley, K., Pollard, K., et al. (2001). International Child Care Practices Study: Infant sleeping environment. *Early Human Development, 62*(1), 43–55.

New, R. S., & Richman, A. L. (1996). Maternal beliefs and infant care practices in Italy and the United States. In S. Harkness & C. M. Super (Eds.), *Parents' Cultural Belief Systems: Their Origins, Expressions, and Consequences.* (pp. 385–404). New York: Guilford Press.

Olds, T., Blunden, S., Petkov, J., & Forchino, F. (2010). The relationships between sex, age, geography and time in bed in adolescents: A meta-analysis of data from 23 countries. *Sleep Medicine Reviews, 14*(6), 371–378.

Ouyang, F., Lu, B. S., Wang, B., Yang, J., Li, Z., Wang, L., et al. (2009). Sleep patterns among rural Chinese twin adolescents. *Sleep Medicine, 10*(4), 479–489.

Petre-Quadens, O., Hussain, H., & Balaratnam, C. (1975). Paradoxical sleep characteristics and cultural environment. *Acta Neurologica Belgica, 75*(2), 85–92.

Quan, S. F., Goodwin, J. L., Babar, S. I., Kaemingk, K. L., Enright, P. L., Rosen, G. M., et al. (2003). Sleep architecture in normal Caucasian and Hispanic children aged 6–11 years recorded during unattended home polysomnography: Experience from the Tucson Children's Assessment of Sleep Apnea Study (TuCASA). *Sleep Medicine, 4*(1), 13–19.

Raghavan, C. S., Harkness, S., & Super, C. M. (2010). Parental ethnotheories in the context of immigration: Asian Indian immigrant and Euro-American mothers and daughters in an American town. *Journal of Cross-Cultural Psychology, 41*(4), 617–632.

Rao, U., Poland, R. E., Lutchmansingh, P., Ott, G. E., McCracken, J. T., & Keh-Ming, L. (1999). Relationship between ethnicity and sleep patterns in normal controls: Implications for psychopathology and treatment. *Journal of Psychiatric Research, 33*(5), 419–426.

Reimão, R., De Souza, J. C., P., C. R., Medeiros, M. M., & Almirão, R. I. (1998). Sleep habits in native Brazilian Terena children in the state of Mato Grosso do Sul, Brazil. *Arquivos de Neuro-Psiquiatria, 56*(4), 703–707.

Reimão, R., De Souza, J. C., & Gaudioso, C. E. (1999). Sleep habits in native Brazilian Bororo children. *Arquivos de Neuro-Psiquiatria, 57*(1), 14–17.

Reimão, R., De Souza, J. C., Gaudioso, C. E. V., Guerra, H. d. C., Alves, A. d. C., Oliveira, J. C. F., et al. (2000). Siestas among Brazilian native Terena adults: A study of daytime napping. *Arquivos de Neuro-Psiquiatria, 58*(1), 39–44.

Rona, R. J., Li, L., Gulliford, M. C., & Chinn, S. (1998). Disturbed sleep: Effects of sociocultural factors and illness. *Archives of Disease in Childhood, 78*(1), 20–25.

Rothbaum, F., Morelli, G., Pott, M., & Liu-Constant, Y. (2000). Immigrant-Chinese and Euro-American parents' physical closeness with young children: Themes of family relatedness. *Journal of Family Psychology, 14*(3), 334–348.

Sadeh, A. (1996). Evaluating night wakings in sleep-disturbed infants: A methodological study of parental reports and actigraphy. *Sleep, 19*(10), 757–762.

Sadeh, A., Acebo, C., Seifer, R., & Aytur, S. (1995). Activity-based assessment of sleep-wake patterns during the 1st year of life. *Infant Behavior & Development, 18*(3), 329–337.

Scher, A., Tirosh, E., Jaffe, M., Rubin, L., Sadeh, A., & Lavie, P. (1995). Sleep patterns of infants and young children in Israel. *International Journal of Behavioral Development, 18*(4), 701–711.

Schlaud, M., Eberhard, C., Trumann, B., Kleemann, W. J., Poets, C. F., Tietze, K. W., et al. (1999). Prevalence and determinants of prone sleeping position in infants: Results from two cross-sectional studies on risk factors for SIDS in Germany. *American Journal of Epidemiology, 150*(1), 51–57.

Schluter, P. J., Paterson, J., & Percival, T. (2007). Infant care practices associated with sudden infant death syndrome: Findings from the Pacific Islands Families study. *Journal of Paediatrics and Child Health, 43*(5), 388–393.

Shirley, M. (1931). The sequential method for the study of maturing behavior patterns. *Psychological Review, 38*(6), 507–528.

Shwalb, D. W., & Shwalb, B. J. (1996). *Japanese Child Rearing: Two Generations of Scholarship.* New York: Guilford Press.

Shweder, R. A., & LeVine, R. A. (1975). Dream concepts of Hausa children: A critique of the "doctrine of invariant sequence" in cognitive development. *Ethos, 3*(2), 209–230.

Slone, V. M. (1978). *Common Folks.* Pippa Passes, KY: Alice Lloyd College.

Sourander, A. (2001). Emotional and behavioural problems in a sample of Finnish three-year-olds. *European Child and Adolescent Psychiatry, 10*(2), 98–104.

Spiegel, K., Leproult, R., L'Hermite-Baleriaux, M., Copinschi, G., Penev, P. D., & Van Cauter, E. (2004). Leptin levels are dependent on sleep duration: Relationships with sympathovagal balance, carbohydrate regulation, cortisol, and thyrotropin. *Journal of Clinical Endocrinology and Metabolism, 89*(11), 5762–5771.

Spilsbury, J. C. (2009). Sleep as a mediator in the pathway from violence-induced traumatic stress to poorer health and functioning: A review of the literature and proposed conceptual model. *Behavioral Sleep Medicine, 7*(4), 223–244.

Stewart, K. (1951). Dream theory in Malaya. *Complex, 6*, 21–33.

Stewart, K. (1954a). Mental hygiene and world peace. *Mental Hygiene, 38*, 387–407.

Stewart, K. (1954b). *Pygmies and Dream Giants.* New York: Norton.

Super, C. M. (1976). Environmental effects on motor development: The case of African infant precocity. *Developmental Medicine and Child Neurology, 18*, 561–567.

Super, C. M. (1981). Behavioral development in infancy. In R. H. Munroe, R. L. Munroe & B. B. Whiting (Eds.), *Handbook of Cross-Cultural Human Development* (pp. 181–270). New York: Garland Press.

Super, C. M., & Harkness, S. (1982). The infant's niche in rural Kenya and metropolitan America. In L. L. Adler (Ed.), *Cross-Cultural Research at Issue* (pp. 47–56). New York: Academic Press.

Super, C. M., & Harkness, S. (1986). The developmental niche: A conceptualization at the interface of child and culture. *International Journal of Behavioral Development, 9*, 545–569.

Super, C. M., & Harkness, S. (1994). The cultural regulation of temperament-environment interactions. *Researching Early Childhood, 2*(1), 59–84.

Super, C. M., Harkness, S., van Tijen, N., van der Vlugt, E., Dykstra, J., & Fintelman, M. (1996). The three R's of Dutch child rearing and the socialization of infant arousal. In S. Harkness & C. M. Super (Eds.), *Parents' Cultural Belief Systems: Their Origins, Expressions, and Consequences.* (pp. 447–466). New York: Guilford Press.

Super, C. M., & Harkness, S. (1999). The environment as culture in developmental research. In T. Wachs & S. Friedman (Eds.), *Measurement of the Environment in Developmental Research* (pp. 279–323). Washington, DC: American Psychological Association.

Super, C. M., & Harkness, S. (2002). Culture structures the environment for development. *Human Development, 45*(4), 270–274.

Super, C. M. (2005). The globalization of developmental psychology. In D. Pillemer & S. H. White (Eds.), *Developmental Psychology and Social Change: Research, History, and Policy* (pp. 11–33). Cambridge: Cambridge University Press.

Super, C. M., Blom, M. J. M., Harkness, S., Ranade, N., & Londhe, R. (2012). Cultural and sleep: A study in the Netherlands and the U.S. *Submitted for publication.*

Super, C. M., Welles-Nyström, B., Bermúdez, M. R., Carrasco-Zylicz, A., Bonichini, S., & Harkness, S. (2012). Sleep as a cultural activity. *Submitted for publication.*

Susman, E. J. (2006). Psychobiology of persistent antisocial behavior: Stress, early vulnerabilities and the attenuation hypothesis. *Neuroscience & Biobehavioral Reviews, 30*(3), 376–389.

Ten Hoopen, E. (2005). *Groeiboek.* Den Hague: Gemeente Den Haag

Teti, D. M., Kim, B.-R., Mayer, G., & Countermine, M. (2010). Maternal emotional availability at bedtime predicts infant sleep quality. *Journal of Family Psychology, 24*(3), 307–315.

Thomas, A., & Chess, S. (1977). *Temperament and Development.* New York: Brunner/Mazel.

Valentin, S. R. (2005). Commentary: Sleep in German infants—the "cult" of independence. *Pediatrics, 115*(1 Suppl), 269–271.

van Hulst, A. G. (1905). *Reinheid, rust en regelmaat: Een beknopte uiteenzetting, hoe moeders hare zuigelingen op de minst omslachtige wijzie goed kunnen verzorgen.* [Cleanliness, rest, and regularity: A brief statement concerning how mothers may provide good care for their infants in the most straightforward manner.]. Harlingen: Provinciale Friesche Groene-Kruis Fonds.

von Bertalanffy, L. (1968). *General Systems Theory (Revised. Ed.).* New York: George Braziller.

Webb, W. B., & Dinges, D. F. (1989). Cultural perspectives on napping and the siesta. In D. F. Dinges & R. J. Broughton (Eds.), *Sleep and Alertness: Chronobiological, Behavioral and Medical Aspects of Napping* (pp. 247–265). New York: Raven.

Weisner, T. S., & Gallimore, R. (1977). My brother's keeper: Child and sibling caretaking. *Current Anthropology, 18*(2), 169–190.

Weisner, T. S. (1996). Why ethnography should be the most important method in the study of human development. In A. Colby, R. Jessor & R. Shweder (Eds.), *Ethnography and Human Development: Context and Meaning in Social Inquiry* (pp. 305–324). Chicago: University of Chicago Press.

Weissbluth, M. (1989). Sleep-loss stress and temperamental difficultness: Psychobiological processes and practical considerations. In G. A. Kohnstamm, J. E. Bates, & M. K. Rothbart

(Eds.), *Temperament in childhood* (pp. 357–375). Chichester, UK: Wiley.

Welles-Nyström, B. (2005). Co-sleeping as a window into Swedish culture: Considerations of gender and health care. *Scandinavian Journal of Caring Sciences, 19*(4), 354–360.

Wennergren, G., Alm, B., Oyen, N., Helweg-Larsen, K., Milerad, J., Skjaerven, R., et al. (1997). The decline in the incidence of SIDS in Scandinavia and its relation to risk-intervention campaigns: Nordic Epidemiological SIDS Study. *Acta Paediatrica, 86*(9), 963–968.

Whiting, B. B., & Whiting, J. W. M. (1975). *The Children of Six Cultures: A Psychocultural Analysis.* Cambridge, Mass: Harvard University Press.

Whiting, B. B. (1976). The problem of the packaged variable. In K. F. Riegel & J. A. Meacham (Eds.), *The Developing Individual in a Changing World* (Vol. 1, pp. 303–309). The Hague: Mouton.

Whiting, B. B., & Edwards, C. P. (1988). *Children of Different Worlds: The Formation of Social Behavior.* Cambridge, MA.: Harvard University Press.

Whiting, J. W. M., Kluckhohn, R., & Anthony, A. A. (1958). The function of male initiation ceremonies at puberty. In E. E. Maccoby, T. M. Newcomb & E. L. Hartley (Eds.), *Readings in Social Anthropology* (pp. 359–370). New York: Holt.

Whiting, J. W. M. (1964). Effects of climate on certain cultural practices. In W. H. Goodenough (Ed.), *Explorations in Cultural Anthropology: Essays in Honor of George Peter Murdock* (pp. 511–544). New York: McGraw-Hill.

Whiting, J. W. M. (1977). A model for psychocultural research. In P. H. Leiderman, S. R. Tulkin & A. Rosenfeld (Eds.), *Culture and Infancy: Variations in the Human Experience (pp. 29–48).* New York: Academic Press.

Whiting, J. W. M. (1981). Environmental constraints on infant care practices. In R. H. Munroe, R. L. Munroe & B. B. Whiting (Eds.), *Handbook of Cross-Cultural Human Development* (pp. 155–181). New York: Garland.

Wolf, A. W., & Lozoff, B. (1989). Object attachment, thumb-sucking, and the passage to sleep. *Journal of the American Academy of Child and Adolescent Psychiatry, 28,* 287–292.

Wolf, A. W., Lozoff, B., Latz, S., & Paludetto, R. (1996). Parental theories in the management of young children's sleep in Japan, Italy, and the United States. In S. Harkness & C. M. Super (Eds.), *Parents' Cultural Belief Systems: Their Origins, Expressions, and Consequences (pp. 364–384).* New York: Guilford Press.

Worthman, C. M., & Melby, M. (2002). Toward a comparative developmental ecology of human sleep. In M. A. Carskadon (Ed.), *Adolescent Sleep Patterns: Biological, Social, and Psychological Influences* (pp. 69–117). New York: Cambridge University Press.

Worthman, C. M. (2006). After dark: The evolutionary ecology of human sleep. In W. R. Trevathan, E. O. Smith & J. McKenna (Eds.), *Evolutinary Medicine and Health: New Perspectives* (pp. 291–313). Oxford: Oxford University Press.

Worthman, C. M., & Brown, R. A. (2007). Companionable sleep: Social regulation of sleep and cosleeping in Egyptian families. *Journal of Family Psychology, 21*(1), 124–135.

Wu, Y.-T., Chen, W. J., Hsieh, W.-S., Chen, P.-C., Liao, H.-F., Su, Y.-N., et al. (2012). Maternal-reported behavioral and emotional problems in Taiwanese preschool children. *Research in Developmental Disabilities, 33*(3), 866–873.

Yovsi, R. D., & Keller, H. (2007). The architecture of cosleeping among wage-earning and subsistence farming Cameroonian Nso families. *Ethos, 35*(1), 65–84.

Zarcone, V. (2002). Sleep hygiene. In M. H. Kryger & W. C. Dement (Eds.), *Principles and Practice of Sleep Medicine* (3rd ed., pp. 657–661). Philadelphia, PA: W. B. Saunders.

Zelazo, N. A., Zelazo, P. R., Cohen, K. M., & Zelazo, P. D. (1993). Specificity of practice effects on elementary neuromotor patterns. *Developmental Psychology, 29*(4), 686–691.

CHAPTER

10 Social Determinants of Children's Sleep

Lauren Hale, Victoria Parente, *and* Gwendolyn K. Phillips

Abstract

An emerging literature has identified consistencies across the social patterning of sleep behaviors and disorders among adult and child populations. This chapter provides an overview of the social characteristics of sleep patterns among youth. In particular, we investigate three dimensions of the social patterning of sleep—ethnicity, household composition, and neighborhood of residence. For each category, we review what is known in the literature from infancy through adolescence. While there are still gaps in the scientific understanding of the social determinants of child and adolescent sleep, several clear patterns emerged. Low socioeconomic status (SES), minority ethnic background, family conflict, and neighborhood disadvantage predict negative sleep outcomes in children and adolescents, although the strength of these associations varies by age. Given the importance of sleep for healthy development of children, these findings suggest sleep is a possible contributor to health and developmental disparities and highlight the importance of improving sleep in efforts to promote well-being for all persons.

Key Words: social determinants of sleep, infants, toddlers, children, adolescents

Introduction

Social epidemiologists and demographers strive to understand how social and demographic factors are associated with health and mortality patterns. Typically, they use population-based datasets to statistically investigate a range of associations between social and demographic characteristics with health and mortality outcomes, while adjusting for behavioral and health factors that may confound any observed association. The data show, time and again, that important social variables such as SES (measured by income, education, and occupation), neighborhood advantage, social cohesion, and ethnicity are important predictors of health among children and adults (Adler et al., 1999; Berkman & Kawachi, 2000; Currie, Shields, & Price, 2007; Kawachi & Berkman, 2003). Generally speaking, these associations fall along lines of social disadvantage, such that racial minorities and those in low-income households have worse health outcomes (Berkman & Kawachi, 2000; Adler et al., 1999). These findings are critical for understanding and addressing social disparities in health.

Sleep is embedded in a social context and influenced by a range of social processes, although research on the social and demographic determinants of sleep in children and adolescents is a relatively new area of inquiry. Among adults, analyses of nationally representative datasets reveal that sleep patterns correspond to social factors such as ethnicity, employment, education, marital status, and neighborhood context (Hale, 2005; Hale & Do, 2006; Hale & Do, 2007; Hale, Hill, & Burdette, 2010; Krueger & Friedman, 2009; Lauderdale et al., 2006). However, it is not clear when differentials in adults' sleep begin in the life course. Unlike among adults where there may be a bidirectional association between socioeconomic status (SES) and sleep (e.g., poor sleep may impair job performance, job insecurity may disrupt sleep), children's social status, which is often measured by characteristics of their parents, is less likely to be affected by children's inadequate sleep. In this chapter, we draw upon the contributions of previous scholars about the social, demographic, and community predictors of child and adolescent sleep. Understanding the social context is necessary to identify target populations and develop effective, culturally sensitive interventions for improving sleep and well-being.

Ethnicity

Ethnicity is a known predictor of health and well-being, with health differences between ethnic groups appearing early in life. For example, Black children are more likely to be born of low birth weight, have reduced access to health care, and are more likely to grow up in a disadvantaged neighborhood (Conley, Strully, & Bennett, 2003; Smedley, Stith, & Nelson, 2003; Smedley & Syme, 2000). While less frequently investigated, sleep patterns also differ by ethnicity.

Ethnicity and Infant Sleep

The vast majority of studies on infant sleep have investigated among White women and children (DeLeon & Karraker, 2007) and, therefore, relatively little is known about how patterns of infant sleep vary by ethnicity. However, the few studies with substantial representation of minority women and infants suggest that sleep behaviors vary by ethnicity as early as 6 months of age. One study found Black infants sleep approximately 1 hour less per day than White children at ages 6 months and 1 year, even after adjusting for other potentially confounding characteristics (Nevarez, Rifas-Shiman, Kleinman, Gillman, & Taveras, 2010). Hispanic infants sleep approximately 30 minutes less per day than White infants at ages 6 months and 1 year (Nevarez et al., 2010). However, Nevarez et al. (2010) found that while Black and Hispanic infants slept less than White infants at night, they tended to sleep more during daytime naps. Variations in parenting style and expectations among different cultures may contribute to increased parental perception of sleep problems, decreased sleep duration, and later bedtimes in infants (Mindell, Sadeh, Wiegand, How, & Goh, 2010). Although these few studies suggest an association between ethnicity and sleep behavior of infants, more research is needed to investigate diverse samples of the US population and how they compare to the sleep patterns of infants in ethnic populations around the world.

Ethnicity and Toddler and Preschooler Sleep

More evidence exists of ethnic differences in sleep patterns among toddlers and preschoolers than among infants (Lozoff, Askew, & Wolf, 1996; Nevarez et al., 2010). At age 2, Black and Hispanic children sleep approximately 1 hour less per night than non-Hispanic White children (Nevarez, et al., 2010). Black and Hispanic children have later bedtimes with similar rise times, resulting in shorter total sleep hours even after controlling for SES and family structure (Hale, Berger, LeBourgeois, & Brooks-Gunn, 2009; McLaughlin Crabtree et al., 2005; Milan, Snow, & Belay, 2007). Moreover, sleep duration varies by ethnicity and day of the week; while Black children sleep less than non-Hispanic White children during the weekdays, they sleep more on the weekends (Crosby, LeBourgeois, & Harsh, 2005). Napping behaviors may also differ by ethnicity; Black children are significantly more likely to nap past age 2 than non-Hispanic White children (Crosby et al., 2005). However, whether these differential sleep patterns by ethnicity in toddlers and preschoolers translate to increased daytime sleepiness remains unclear. Again, while these findings are attenuated when controlling for socioeconomic factors, they remain statistically significant. In one study, Black parents are more likely to report their child is excessively sleepy during the day, while another study found non-Hispanic White parents are more likely to do so (McLaughlin Crabtree et al., 2005; Milan et al., 2007).

Familial habits surrounding sleep behaviors also differ by ethnicity. Minority children are less likely to have a regular bedtime or bedtime routine than non-Hispanic White children. This association remains statistically significant even after adjusting for socioeconomic status, family structure, and sleeping location (Hale et al., 2009; Milan et al., 2007). Non-Hispanic White children are most likely to sleep in their own bedroom, Black children are most likely to sleep with a sibling, and Latino children are most likely to sleep with a parent (Milan et al., 2007). Similarly, another study found that bed sharing during toddlerhood is more common among Black and Hispanic children than among non-Hispanic White children in a sample of low-income families (Barajas, Martin, Brooks-Gunn, & Hale, 2011). These ethnic differences persist after accounting for socioeconomic status, which may affect where the child commonly sleeps. Ethnicity may also play a role in how parents perceive their children's sleep patterns. For example, non-Hispanic White mothers are more likely to report distress about their child's sleep and view it as problematic than are Black mothers (Lozoff et al., 1996; Milan et al., 2007), even after adjusting for other sociodemographic variables.

Finally, prevalence of sleep-related disorders varies by ethnicity among toddlers and preschoolers. An initial study by Redline, Tishler, et al. (1999) found that Black children aged 2–18 are more likely to have sleep disordered breathing (SDB), even after controlling for obesity, respiratory problems, smoking, and neighborhood of residence. Subsequent studies confirmed these findings specifically in preschoolers and demonstrated that SDB is also more common among Black children after controlling for maternal education (Bonuck et al., 2011; Brouillette, Horwood, Constantin, Brown, & Ross, 2011; Montgomery-Downs, Jones, Molfese, & Gozal, 2003; Redline et al., 1999). Recently, Brouillette, Horwood, et al. (2011) found that Black children were more than three times as likely to have obstructive sleep apnea (OSA) compared to children of other ethnic backgrounds. Furthermore, while non-Hispanic White parents report more noisy breathing during sleep, Black and Hispanic parents are significantly more likely to report their child snores, which may reflect a difference in breathing or parental reporting (Goldstein et al., 2011; Gottlieb et al., 2003). Studies examining snoring rates in Asian children and comparing this to children of other ethnic groups have found conflicting results. (Gottlieb, et al., 2003; Kuehni, Strippoli, Chauliac, & Silverman, 2008). Thus, more research is needed to better understand sleep in this population.

Ethnicity and School-Aged Children's Sleep

Ethnic disparities in sleep persist in school-age children. Black children have more problematic sleep patterns, fewer hours of sleep, and later bedtimes than White children, even after controlling for SES (Adam, Snell, & Pendry, 2007; Buckhalt, El-Sheikh, & Keller, 2007; Goodwin et al., 2007; McLaughlin Crabtree et al., 2005; Smaldone, Honig, & Byrne, 2007). Studies have also found that non-Hispanic White children sleep for roughly 23 minutes longer than Black children and 21 minutes longer than Hispanic children per night (Buckhalt et al., 2007).

Multiple explanations have been put forth to help understand observed ethnic differences in sleep. For example, Black school-aged children have later bedtimes, earlier school start times, spend more time traveling to school, and spend more time watching television (Adam et al., 2007; Buckhalt et al., 2007; Kieckhefer, Ward, Tsai, & Lentz, 2008; Spilsbury et al., 2004). Similarly, Hispanic children also have later bedtimes and spend more time traveling to school (Adam et al., 2007; Kieckhefer et al., 2008). Another contributor to sleep differences by ethnicity may be that African-American and Hispanic children are more likely to share a bedroom than non-Hispanic White children, even after controlling for other sociodemographic factors (Adam et al., 2007; Buckhalt et al., 2007).

Napping behaviors also vary by ethnicity, and may in fact reduce ethnic differences in weekly sleep duration between non-Hispanic White and minority children (Crosby et al., 2005). While napping declines with age, Black and Hispanic school-aged children are more likely to nap than non-Hispanic White children (Buckhalt et al., 2007; Crosby et al., 2005; Goodwin et al., 2007; Kieckhefer et al., 2008). One study of Black children suggests increased napping is only on the weekends (Buckhalt et al., 2007), while another study of Black children found napping occurs on more days per week (Crosby et al., 2005). Importantly, adjustment for sociodemographic characteristics did not fully explain this association (Crosby et al., 2005). Hispanic children are also more likely to nap than non-Hispanic White children at ages 6–8, but by 9–11 years of age, there is not a significant difference (Goodwin et al., 2007).

As is true among younger children, prevalence of sleep disorders varies between Black and non-Hispanic White children. Black school-aged children are significantly more likely to have SDB (Bixler et al., 2009; Boss, Smith, & Ishman, 2011; Calhoun et al., 2010; Chervin et al., 2003; Hibbs et al., 2008; Pinto et al., 2011; Redline et al., 1999; Rosen et al., 2003; Rudnick, Walsh, Hampton, & Mitchell, 2007). Moreover, among children who have SDB, Black children are more likely suffer from more severe symptoms (Chervin et al., 2003; Rosen et al., 2003). The differences remain significant after adjusting for other respiratory problems and obesity, which elevate the risk of SDB (Redline et al., 1999); however, more research is needed on SES in relation to SDB. Other potential explanations for a link between ethnicity and SDB are preterm birth and upper airway characteristics. Preterm birth is more common among Black children and is also a risk factor for SDB (Rosen, Larkin et al., 2003). On the other hand, while neuromotor function and upper airway characteristics often trigger SDB, one study suggests physiological differences cannot explain these ethnic disparities (Pinto et al., 2011).

Non-Black minority children also experience differences in sleep compared to non-Hispanic

White children; however, research on sleep in other minority populations is limited. One study suggests Asian children sleep less than non-Hispanic White children (Adam et al., 2007), whereas another study found no difference (Biggs et al., 2010). Both studies found that Asian children spend more time on homework, which may delay bedtime (Adam et al., 2007; Biggs et al., 2010). Asian parents are more likely than non-Hispanic White parents to report that homework is more important than sleep, and are less likely to believe their child needs more sleep (Biggs et al., 2010). Asian parents are also more likely to report that "snoring is a healthy sign" than White parents (Biggs et al., 2010). Furthermore, compared to youths in countries composed mostly of Caucasian families, children from countries predominantly composed of Asian families are more likely to stay up later, sleep for shorter amounts of time, have parents who believe their children have a sleep disturbance, and share a bed with either parents or other children (Mindell et al., 2010; Sadeh, Mindell, & Rivera, 2011). Adam, Snell, and Pendry (2007) found that socioeconomic factors had only a mild impact on any of their findings and did not affect the significance of their results, while Biggs et al. (2010) found no difference in SES between the Caucasian and Asian groups.

Hispanic children may not sleep as deeply as non-Hispanic White children; using polysomnography data, Hispanic children are found to have less stage 3 and 4 sleep, and more stage 2 sleep than the non-Hispanic White children (Quan et al., 2003). These results were not affected by parental education (Quan et al., 2003). One study also suggested that Hispanic parents are more likely to witness an episode of sleep apnea compared to non-Hispanic White parents, though the potential effects of SES were not examined in this study (Goodwin, Babar, et al., 2003). However, there is no evidence for ethnic differences between Hispanics and non-Hispanics in the rates of sleep disorders including SDB, sleepwalking, sleep talking, or sleep terrors (Goodwin, Kaemingk, et al., 2003).

Ethnicity and Adolescent Sleep

Several studies have documented disparities in sleep by ethnicity among adolescents (Adam, et al., 2007; Knutson & Lauderdale, 2009; Moore, Kirchner, Drotar, Johnson, Rosen, & Redline, 2011; Roberts, Roberts, & Chan, 2006). For example, national data from the United States indicate that Black and female adolescents are most at risk of having inadequate sleep duration (Eaton et al., 2010). Adam and colleagues, in a study of 1187 adolescents, found that African-American teens slept, on average, about 25 minutes less than non-Hispanic White teens per night (Adam et al., 2007). This discrepancy has been attributed to later bedtimes with similar wake times in African-American adolescents resulting in less total sleep (Roberts et al., 2006), as well as social factors such as greater time spent traveling to school (Adam et al., 2007). Furthermore, minority status has been associated not only with decreased total sleep time compared to non-minorities but also with increased night-to-night variability in hours of sleep (Moore, Kirchner, et al., 2011).

While differences in sleep patterns exist by ethnicity, the extent to which this relationship is genetically versus socioculturally determined is unknown. In one study, controlling for SES eliminated differences in ethnic variation of insomnia symptoms (Roberts et al., 2006). This suggests that sleep differences by ethnicity may be manifestations of socioeconomic disparities rather than genetic differences. Using data on twins, Moore et al. found that in 10–17-year-olds, only 30% of sleep variation is attributable to heritable factors, which is far less than in younger children. (Moore, Slane, Mindell, Burt, & Klump, 2011). Hence, it is likely that racial differences in sleep patterns are primarily due to social and environmental factors.

Household Characteristics

Household characteristics are important predictors of children's health and well-being (Case & Paxson, 2006; Currie & Lin, 2007). In this section, we investigate how these characteristics vary by sleep across childhood from infancy through adolescence.

Household Characteristics and Infant Sleep

Household and parental characteristics, such as household income and parental education, are relatively understudied determinants of infant sleep patterns. One study reveals poorer sleep behaviors among infants of mothers with lower education and income (Nevarez et al., 2010). These differences may be due to parenting behaviors. For example, upper-middle-class parents tend to give their children more structured daily schedules, whereas low-income and working-class parents place more emphasis on providing comfort, food, and shelter. Studies have shown that higher SES women are more likely to focus on sleep schedules than those of lower SES, which influences infant sleep behavior (Fouts, Roopnarine, & Lamb, 2007; Leyendecker, Lamb, Scholmeric, & Fracasso, 1995). In addition, parental behaviors such as bed sharing, nursing to sleep, putting infants to bed already asleep, irregular bedtime routines, and exposure to television are potentially modifiable habits that increase risk for infant sleep problems and vary by SES (Burnham, Goodlin-Jones, Gaylor, & Anders, 2002; DeLeon & Karraker, 2007; Sadeh, Mindell, Luedtke, & Wiegand, 2009; Touchette et al., 2005).

Household characteristics such as family structure also predict infant sleep behavior. For example, infants who have single parents, have divorced parents, or have fathers that do not participate in infant care are at increased risk of sleep problems (Nevarez et al., 2010; Tikotzky, Sadeh, & Glickman-Gavrieli, 2011). In a pre–birth cohort study of 1676 mother–infant pairs, Nevarez et al. found in bivariate analyses that infants whose mothers were not married, had lower incomes, or had less education reported their infants slept less per day compared to those whose mothers were married or cohabitating, had higher incomes, or more education (Nevarez et al., 2010). Additionally, the authors reported that SES significantly attenuated the relationship between maternal smoking and less infant sleep documented in other studies. While several studies have looked at the influence of maternal behaviors on infant sleep, few have looked at paternal actions. However, one study that investigated paternal infant care and sleep found greater paternal involvement was associated with more consolidated sleep (i.e., less nighttime waking; Tikotzky et al., 2011). Thus, evidence supports that family structure and household characteristics can begin to influence children's sleep as early as infancy.

Household Characteristics and Toddler and Preschooler Sleep

Household and parenting characteristics are also relevant for toddlers' and preschoolers' sleep. SES and education of the parents are associated with sleep behaviors among toddlers and preschoolers. For example, children who come from households with lower incomes have later bedtimes than children from higher-income households (Hale et al., 2009). Sleep disorders are also related to SES of the household; toddlers and preschoolers from lower SES households are more likely to snore and to have OSA (Bonuck et al., 2011; Brouillette et al., 2011; Goldstein et al., 2011; Kuehni et al., 2008). In addition, parental employment characteristics, such as late time leaving and returning home, are associated with shorter sleep duration due to later bedtimes and more irregular sleep (Komada et al., 2011). Low maternal education is also associated in young children with fewer sleep routines, being overly tired, and difficulty falling asleep (Milan et al., 2007).

In addition, parents who have anxiety problems or depression are more likely to have children who wake up frequently at night (Atkinson, Vetere, & Grayson, 1995). The association may begin prenatally; O'Conner et al. (2007) found that mothers with higher levels of anxiety and depression during gestation are more likely to have a child with sleep disturbances at 18 and 30 months. Another study indicates that parental depression is associated with negative parenting, which may trigger sleep disturbances in children (Reid, Hong, & Wade, 2009).

Parental smoking behavior is also associated with sleep disorders in this age range. In children aged 6 months to just less than 7 years old, maternal smoking is associated with SDB (Bonuck et al., 2011). In addition, smoking by one or both parents is associated with snoring in children ages 1 to 4 (Kuehni et al., 2008).

Finally, as seen with infants, family structure may be an important predictor of toddler and preschooler sleep habits. Children who have a single mother are less likely to have a bedtime routine and more likely to snore or have OSA (Brouillette et al., 2011; Hale et al., 2009; Kuehni et al., 2008). Preschoolers who live in large households are less likely to use bedtime routines than those who live in small households (Hale et al., 2009). In addition, when housing is inadequate, either due to overcrowding or homelessness, the likelihood that parents report their toddler or preschooler is overly tired or has SDB also increases (Bonuck et al., 2011; Milan et al., 2007). Parents or caregivers of only children are less likely to report their child has a sleep problem or SDB compared to children who have siblings (Bonuck et al., 2011; Sadeh et al., 2011). Moreover, parents of toddlers and preschoolers who bed-share are more likely to report their children have sleep disturbances, wake up frequently at night, and complain about going to bed (Kataria, Swanson, & Trevathan, 1987; Lozoff et al., 1996). Finally, children who do not fall asleep in their own beds are more likely to have sleep problems than those who do (Atkinson et al., 1995).

Household Characteristics and School-Aged Children's Sleep

Among school-aged children, higher levels of parental education are associated with increased sleep duration, falling asleep faster, and decreased risk of snoring (Goodwin et al., 2007; Li et al.,

2010; Smaldone et al., 2007; Urschitz et al., 2004). Parental education moderates the association between measures of poor sleep and academic success (Buckhalt, El-Sheikh, Keller, & Kelly, 2009). Low parental education increases the likelihood that a child will have poor academic performance after disturbed sleep (Buckhalt et al., 2009). Parental unemployment is also associated with insomnia in children; however, paternal employment may be a stronger predictor of insomnia in children than maternal employment (Zhang et al., 2009).

The marital status of parents may also impact sleep in school-aged children. Children who have single mothers are more likely to have SDB, even after controlling for ethnicity, a known risk factor for SDB (Hibbs, Johnson et al. 2008). Similarly, children of unmarried parents are more likely to be excessively tired during the day and co-sleep with parents (Cortesi, Giannotti, Sebastiani, & Vagnoni, 2004; Hibbs et al., 2008; Yolton et al., 2010). Among children of married parents, El-Sheikh et al. (2007) found that, although marital conflict was not directly associated with sleep disruptions (assessed by actigraphy), a third variable, children's emotional insecurity about the relationship, mediated the relationship between parental conflict and sleep disruptions (El-Sheikh, Buckhalt, Cummings, & Keller, 2007). Thus, children who were emotionally aroused or behaviorally dysregulated by their parents' arguments were more likely to have disrupted sleep than children who simply witnessed the conflict and had minimal response (El-Sheikh et al., 2007). This emotional response/sleep disruption combination also led to a decline in the child's academic performance (El-Sheikh et al., 2007).

Bed-sharing behaviors vary depending on family and cultural context. For example, Worthman and Brown (2007) found that Egyptians co-sleep with 1 to 4 people around 69% of the time.

Parental physical health also influences children's sleep. This may be partially due to parental behaviors that directly impact a developing child; for example, maternal smoking during pregnancy is associated with habitual snoring during middle childhood (Li et al., 2010). Another study found that parents who snore are more likely to have children with insomnia, even after controlling for environmental and sociodemographic similarities (Zhang et al., 2009). There may also be indirect effects that lead to sleep disruption. Among children in elementary school, those with fathers in fair or poor physical health are more likely to have inadequate sleep compared to children with healthier parents (Smaldone et al., 2007).

Poor parental mental health affects children's sleep duration, increases sleep disruption, and leads to excessive daytime sleepiness (Smaldone et al., 2007; Yolton et al., 2010). Conversely, parents who connect with their children in a positive way are more likely to have children who get adequate sleep (Adam et al., 2007). One study found that the emotional health of the father is more strongly related to sleep outcomes than the emotional health of the mother (Smaldone et al., 2007).

Low SES is related to the frequency with which children wake up during the night, snore habitually, have adequate sleep duration, are tired during the day, sleep with parents, experience parasomnias, and have noisy sleep (Buckhalt et al., 2007; Chervin et al., 2003; Cortesi et al., 2004; Li et al., 2010, Smaldone et al., 2007; Stein, Mendelsohn, Obermeyer, Amromin, & Benca, 2001; Yolton et al., 2010). Finally, several studies have indicated that SES is associated with SDB (Calhoun et al., 2010; Chervin et al., 2003). However, other studies did not find a persistent association between SES and sleep disturbances. One study found that the severity of breathing problems during sleep is not associated with SES (Kohler et al., 2008). Another study of Portuguese children found that there were no SES differences between children who snored loudly and those who did not snore (Ferreira et al., 2000). A third study found that the association between SES and SDB disappeared after adjusting for BMI of the child (Chervin et al., 2003).

Finally, physical and social aspects of the home environment are associated with sleep outcomes in children (see Gradisar and Short, Chapter 11). Having a television in the child's bedroom is associated with elevated rates of disrupted sleep in school-aged children (Owens et al., 1999; Taveras, Hohman, Price, Gortmaker, & Sonneville, 2009). In addition, children are more likely to experience insomnia when they are living in public housing or when their homes are noisy (Zhang et al., 2009). Surprisingly, one study showed that greater number of people living in the house compared to the number of bedrooms (higher density), or an increased number of siblings, is associated with decreased rates of SDB in children with asthma (Yolton et al., 2010). Asthmatic children who are exposed to secondhand smoke in the house are also more likely to have sleep disruptions including delayed sleep onset, parasomnias, SDB, feeling tired during the day, and total sleep disruption (Yolton et al., 2010). In separate studies, sharing a room is not associated with poor sleep outcomes; however, sharing a bed is associated with greater tiredness in a population of healthy children (Liu, Liu, & Wang, 2003; Stein et al., 2001). Furthermore, at the household level, research indicates that children in households with marital instability are more likely to exhibit sleep disturbances (El-Sheikh et al., 2007; Mannering et al., 2011). Indeed, children from families that shout, argue in a heated way, hit each other, or throw things during disagreements experience inadequate sleep (Smaldone et al., 2007). Furthermore, the likelihood that a child will experience sleep problems is elevated in families where there is child abuse or other forms of family violence (see Spilsbury, Chapter 14; McFarlane, Groff, O'Brien, & Watson, 2003). Certain types of past exposure to violence can also cause sleep disturbances. For example, having a grandparent that died violently (even before the child was born), a parent that was tortured, or a father that scolds frequently are associated with sleep disruptions in refugee children arriving in Denmark (Montgomery & Foldspang, 2001).

Household Characteristics and Adolescent Sleep

US adolescents sleep approximately 2 hours less on weekday nights than the recommended 9 hours per night (Knutson & Lauderdale, 2009; NSF, 2006). The inability of adolescents to meet their sleep needs can be attributed to a range of increased societal demands. Many of these demands are affected by household-level behaviors and beliefs. Teenagers have a range of time-consuming activities and behaviors (e.g., homework, extracurricular activities, after-school jobs, computer use and television viewing) that can interfere with sleep timing and quality. These time spent in each of these activities may vary by several household characteristics including parental education and income, parenting style, and family cultural values (see Gradisar and Short, Chapter 11).

Several studies have indicated that adolescents at both ends of the socioeconomic continuum report worse sleep (Knutson & Lauderdale, 2009; McHale, Kim, Kan, & Updegraff, 2011). Due to the importance of sleep to executive functioning in adolescents, poor sleep among low SES teens may contribute to inequalities in academic performance by SES. In fact, low SES teens, when reporting sleepiness, may be particularly "susceptible" to poor executive functioning (Anderson, Storfer-Isser, Taylor, Rosen & Redline, 2009). One recent study by Marco et al. investigated the influence of a wide range of SES-related factors and sleep in young adolescents assessed through 1 week of actigraphy (Marco, Wolfson, Sparling & Azuaje, 2011). They found that living in a multiunit building and having a lower household income put youths at risk for less consistent sleep on school nights and poorer sleep schedules on the weekends. Additionally, they reported an association between greater inconsistency in school and weekend-night sleep schedules, and lower household incomes and single parent family structures (Marco et al., 2011). However, only a handful of studies have included or studied sufficient numbers of disadvantaged youths. More research is needed to investigate the barriers to adequate sleep in this at-risk population and the potential negative consequences of poor sleep in contributing to other health, educational, or social disparities.

In addition to teens from lower SES families, those from families of higher SES are also at risk for poor sleep. Consistent with this finding, parental acculturation, a variable associated with upward mobility and higher incomes, is associated with less time sleeping at night and more time spent napping during the day (McHale et al., 2011). Acculturation and higher income of parents may affect youth sleep by fostering increased pressure for individual achievement that requires a youth's daily routines to include several extracurricular activities, such that youth have reduced opportunity for sleep. Supporting this hypothesis, Carskadon et al. found that high school students spending >20 hours per week or more involved in extracurricular activities had less total sleep time and significantly later bedtimes (Carskadon, 1990). Moreover, increased personal access to Internet and television by more advantaged teens may also negatively impact sleep behavior (Adam et al., 2007).

The interpersonal relationships and dynamics between family members may also contribute to the quantity or quality of sleep of adolescents within the household. While several studies have found relationships between high marital conflict and poor sleep in younger children, the results in adolescents have not been as consistent (Adam et al., 2007; El-Sheikh, Buckhalt, Mize & Acebo, 2006; McHale et al., 2011). For example, one study reported that measures of family dynamics that predicted sleep in younger children —such as parental warmth, parenting stress, or family conflict—did not significantly relate to adolescent sleep (Adam et al., 2007). However, a different study suggests parental conflict does affect adolescent sleep. A study that used teen reports of conflict rather than parental reports did find marital conflict to contribute to poorer nighttime sleep in adolescents (El-Sheikh et al., 2006).

Additionally, the importance of parental warmth and parental rules on child sleep may be influenced by the age of the child. Parental warmth may be more influential in the sleep of younger children, while presence of parental rules may more predictive of sleep in older youths and teens (Adam et al., 2007). Parental warmth may play a role in sleep in younger children by promoting feelings of safety, which may not be as important to adolescent sleep. Rather, in the teen years, boundaries and rules may be more important to enforce early bedtimes for adolescents, who experience both peer and physiologic pressure toward later bedtimes. Moreover, regular family activities such as meal time, which strengthen relationships between family members, are beneficial for adolescents' sleep (Adam et al., 2007).

Neighborhood Characteristics and Sleep

People who live in disadvantaged neighborhoods are more likely to experience negative health outcomes than those who live in more affluent areas. Living in a neighborhood that is noisy, dilapidated, and has a high crime rate may interfere with the ability to fall asleep or stay asleep (Hale & Do, 2007; Hale et al., 2010; Hill, Burdette & Hale, 2009). While ethnic and income characteristics often direct people to live certain neighborhoods, the effects of environment on sleep persist even after controlling for these demographic traits. In this section we discuss neighborhood influences on sleep among children of different ages.

Neighborhood Characteristics and Infant Sleep

The neighborhood in which an infant lives may also affect behavior and development. The majority of studies assessing the relationship between environment and infant sleep have been conducted in the neonatal intensive care unit (NICU). Indeed, environmental stimuli such as loud noise levels or bright lights interrupt infant sleep–wake cycles and stimulate the stress response (Peng et al., 2009). Limited research exists outside of the NICU investigating how neighborhood noise, lights, or violence affect infant sleep. One study did find that traumatic events in infancy may lead to sleep disturbances similar to post-traumatic stress disorder in adults (Bogat, DeJonghe, Levendosky, Davidson, & von Eye, 2006). However, the association between neighborhood environment and infant sleep cycles has yet to be formally investigated.

Neighborhood Characteristics and Toddler and Preschooler Sleep

Several studies support the association between neighborhood disadvantage and disordered sleep, even among toddlers and preschoolers. For example, children who reside in neighborhoods with higher levels of disadvantage and higher population density are more likely to have OSA compared to children from less populated and more economically privileged areas (Brouillette et al., 2011). McLaughlin and colleagues began using residential zip codes in conjuction with sleep data and found that living in a low-income neighborhood is also associated with having shorter nighttime sleep duration, even after adjusting for ethnic disparities (McLaughlin Crabtree et al., 2005). Finally, areas with higher levels of car traffic are associated with greater frequency of snoring in this young-age population (Kuehni et al., 2008).

Neighborhood Characteristics and School-Aged Children Sleep

Although there are only few studies examining the association between neighborhood characteristics and sleep in school-aged children, the literature suggests that an association exists. Using census tracts to measure SES, children aged 2–11 with OSA are more likely to live in poor neighborhoods compared to those without OSA (Brouillette et al., 2011; Spilsbury et al., 2006). These associations are still significant after adjusting for ethnicity, obesity of the children, premature birth, and household-level SES, which are all important predictors of sleep disruption (Brouillette et al., 2011; Spilsbury et al., 2006). The effects of neighborhood may be partly related to feelings of safety. Inadequate sleep is more commonly found among school-aged children whose parents are fearful for their child's safety than in children whose parents feel they are safe (Smaldone et al., 2007).

Neighborhood Characteristics and Adolescent Sleep

Negative neighborhood characteristics such as high crime rates may influence the sleep of adolescents living in those environments. Inner-city Black teens are at increased risk for sleep disturbances when more "bad things happened to a family member or friend" within their neighborhood (Umlauf, Bolland & Lian, 2011). Furthermore, the researchers found that increased sleep disturbance is associated with aggressive behaviors in youth, increased worry, and quick-temperedness, and is negatively related to warmth toward the mother. Reports of negative neighborhood sentiments or distress over neighborhood have also been shown to predict reduced sleep duration, increased daytime napping, and increased variability in sleep duration (McHale et al., 2011; Moore, Kirchner, et al., 2011). Residence in an urban compared to rural setting has also been associated with adolescent sleep in a study performed in Taiwan; urban children had more sleep problems than their rural counterparts (Yen, King, & Chang, 2010).

Conclusion: Implications for Health Disparities

Sleep and sleep-related behaviors are important factors in understanding the emergence and persistence of health disparities. While social epidemiologists and other social scientists have observed wide disparities in health outcomes by SES at all ages (Adler et al., 1999), very few scholars (Hale, Peppard, & Young, 2006; Moore, Adler, Williams, & Jackson, 2002; Sickel, Moore, Adler, Williams, & Jackson, 1999) have included sleep (a basic biological need) as a predictor, mediator, or moderator in their models of disparities. This is surprising given that sleep is a powerful mechanism driving behavioral, cognitive, emotional, and physiological development (Bates, Viken, Alexander, Beyers, & Stockton, 2002; Carskadon, Acebo, & Jenni, 2004; Lavigne et al., 1993; Minde et al., 1993; Richman, Stevenson, & Graham, 1975; Sadeh, Gruber, & Raviv, 2003). Gregory and O'Connor (2002) were the first to study sleep in children longitudinally, and they found that poor sleep at age 4 predicts the onset of emotional problems in later childhood and adolescence. These results could largely be explained by psychosocial risk factors during childhood (Gregory, Eley, et al. 2004). Furthermore, data show associations between children's sleep timing and school readiness (Crosby et al., 2006), an early source of socioeconomic disparities. Buckhalt (2011) analyzes how the cognitive, behavioral, and emotional impacts of poor sleep may partially explain the academic achievement gap seen between children of different ethnicities and SES. To date, however, little research has investigated how sleep environments and sleep-related behaviors learned early in life may set children on divergent sleep, cognitive, and health trajectories, especially up through young adulthood. We hypothesize that sleep-related behaviors taught by caregivers in early childhood may have long-lasting influences on the sleep behaviors of children, adolescents, and adults. Furthermore, social and environmental factors beyond individual or familial control have profound influences on child sleep and, therefore, health outcomes. In this chapter, we systematically reviewed three levels of influence—ethnicity, household factors, and neighborhood factors—on the social determinants of sleep during childhood.

Table 10.1 summarizes whether disparities in sleep exist across ethnicity, household characteristics, and neighborhood advantage in children from infancy through adolescence. As shown, in nearly every period of childhood, sleep disparities line up with ethnic, household, and neighborhood characteristics. From this table it is apparent that social determinants of sleep begin early in life and continue throughout childhood and adolescence. The table also indicates that more research is needed to analyze whether there is an association between neighborhood factors and sleep during infancy, which is the only category that currently lacks evidence of an association between social context and sleep. Future work on sleep disparities in children is also needed to better understand the underlying sources of poor sleep among children of all ages, in addition to whether and how these factors are modifiable.

Table 10.1 Summary of Overview of the Literature regarding Disparities in Sleep Across Childhood and Adolescents by Ethnicity, Household Characteristics, and Neighborhood Characteristics

	Ethnicity	Household Characteristics	Neighborhood Characteristics
Infant	Yes	Yes	Unknown
Toddlers and Preschoolers	Yes	Yes	Yes
School-Aged Children	Yes	Yes	Yes
Adolescents	Yes	Yes	Yes

Note: "Yes" indicates that disparities in sleep are observed for this population by the social determinant category described across the top. "Unknown" indicates there is not enough evidence to draw a conclusion.

Evidence indicates strong associations between social characteristics and sleep in children and adolescents, as summarized in Table 10.1. While social determinants of sleep are important in both young children and teens, social and demographic predictors of sleep may be different in adolescents compared with younger children. Furthermore, while the vast majority of research on sleep and sleep-related behaviors of children in the United States has studied populations that are primarily non-Hispanic White and/or from higher SES families (Crowell, Keener, Ginsburg, & Anders, 1987; Okami, Weisner, & Olmstead, 2002; Sadeh, Mindell, Luedtke, & Wiegand, 2009; Wolfson & Carskadon, 1998), understanding the determinants of sleep in disadvantaged or minority youth remains a critical area for future research.

In addition, despite the growing knowledge on the social determinants of sleep, nearly all of this research has been conducted in industrialized nations in the Western hemisphere. In fact, 71% of the primary journal articles cited in this chapter relied upon data from the United States. An additional 18% recruited their participants from the United Kingdom, Australia, Canada (English and French-speaking), Germany, Italy, Portugal, Denmark, and Finland. The remaining studies were conducted in non-Western countries: Since 2009, there have been eight studies examining the impact of sociodemographic characteristics on child and adolescent sleep in Asian countries, two of which were cross-cultural comparisons of sleep behaviors and attitudes (Mindell et al., 2010; Sadeh et al., 2011). In addition, two studies have been conducted in Israel—one looking at paternal involvement in infant sleep and another at school-aged children's sleep duration (Sadeh et al., 2003; Tikotzky et al., 2011). Finally, Worthman and Brown (2007) conducted a study in Egypt looking the prevalence of familial bed sharing and how this affects sleep duration and quality. The paucity of international research on social differences in children's sleep highlights a need for future research in the area.

Understanding the determinants of poor sleep in at-risk populations will allow for the development, design, intervention, and evaluation of programs and policies that may improve the sleep and well-being of children.

Future Directions

- Future research on the social determinants of children's sleep should seek to design studies that include longitudinal data, experimental study designs (when possible), and multiple methods of sleep measurement (i.e., self-report or parent report and actigraphy).
- Researchers should be oriented toward thinking about how social disparities in sleep might be reduced. What effect would this have on overall health and health disparities?
- Currently, the research does not adequately address the mechanisms through which social factors (ethnicity, parental, household, neighborhood) translate into sleep disparities.
- More research is needed on understanding sleep in different cultures around the world.
- Research needs to better understand when different patterns of sleep in children emerge. For example, do social disparities in sleep begin during gestation? How do social and neighborhood factors affect infant sleep?

References

Adam, E. K., Snell, E. K., & Pendry, P. (2007). Sleep timing and quantity in ecological and family context: A nationally representative time-diary study. *Journal of Family Psychology, 21*(1), 4–19.

Adler, N. E., Marmot, M., McEwen, B. S., & Stewart, J. (1999). *Socioeconomic Status and Health in Industrial Nations: Social, Psychological, and Biological Pathways* (Vol. 896). New York: Annals of the New York Academy of Sciences.

Anderson, B., Storfer-Isser, A., Taylor, H. G., Rosen, C. L., & Redline, S. (2009). Associations of executive function with sleepiness and sleep duration in adolescents. *Pediatrics, 123*(4), e701–e707.

Atkinson, E., Vetere, A., & Grayson, K. (1995). Sleep disruption in young children. The influence of temperament on the sleep patterns of pre-school children. *Child: Care, Health and Development, 21*(4), 233–246.

Barajas, R. G., Martin, A., Brooks-Gunn, J., & Hale, L. (2011). Mother-child bed-sharing in toddlerhood and cognitive and behavioral outcomes. *Pediatrics, 128*(2), e339–e347.

Bates, J. E., Viken, R. J., Alexander, D. B., Beyers, J., & Stockton, L. (2002). Sleep and adjustment in preschool children: Sleep diary reports by mothers relate to behavior reports by teachers. *Child Development, 73*(1), 62–74.

Berkman, L. F., & Kawachi, I. o. (2000). *Social Epidemiology*. New York: Oxford University Press.

Biggs, S. N., Pizzorno, V. A., van den Heuvel, C. J., Kennedy, J. D., Martin, A. J., & Lushington, K. (2010). Differences in parental attitudes towards sleep and associations with sleep-wake patterns in Caucasian and Southeast Asian school-aged children in Australia. *Behavioral Sleep Medicine, 8*(4), 207–218.

Bixler, E. O., Vgontzas, A. N., Lin, H. M., Liao, D., Calhoun, S., Vela-Bueno, A., et al. (2009). Sleep disordered breathing in children in a general population sample: Prevalence and risk factors. *Sleep, 32*(6), 731–736.

Bogat, G. A., DeJonghe, E., Levendosky, A. A., Davidson, W. S., & von Eye, A. (2006). Trauma symptoms among infants exposed to intimate partner violence. *Child Abuse & Neglect, 30*(2), 109–125.

Bonuck, K. A., Chervin, R. D., Cole, T. J., Emond, A., Henderson, J., Xu, L., et al. (2011). Prevalence and persistence of sleep disordered breathing symptoms in young children: A 6-year population-based cohort study. *Sleep, 34*(7), 875–884.

Boss, E. F., Smith, D. F., & Ishman, S. L. (2011). Racial/ethnic and socioeconomic disparities in the diagnosis and treatment of sleep-disordered breathing in children. *International Journal of Pediatric Otorhinolaryngology, 75*(3), 299–307.

Brouillette, R. T., Horwood, L., Constantin, E., Brown, K., & Ross, N. A. (2011). Childhood sleep apnea and neighborhood disadvantage. *Journal of Pediatrics, 158*(5), 789–795 e781.

Buckhalt, J. A., El-Sheikh, M., & Keller, P. (2007). Children's sleep and cognitive functioning: race and socioeconomic status as moderators of effects. *Child Development, 78*(1), 213–231.

Buckhalt, J. A., El-Sheikh, M., Keller, P. S., & Kelly, R. J. (2009). Concurrent and longitudinal relations between children's sleep and cognitive functioning: The moderating role of parent education. *Child Development, 80*(3), 875–892.

Buckhalt, J. A. (2011). Insufficient Sleep and the Socioeconomic Status Achievement Gap. *Child Development Perspectives, 5*(1), 59–65.

Burnham, M. M., Goodlin-Jones, B. L., Gaylor, E. E., & Anders, T. F. (2002). Nighttime sleep-wake patterns and self-soothing from birth to one year of age: A longitudinal intervention study. *Journal of Child Psychology and Psychiatry, 43*(6), 713–725.

Calhoun, S. L., Vgontzas, A. N., Mayes, S. D., Tsaoussoglou, M., Sauder, K., Mahr, F., et al. (2010). Prenatal and perinatal complications: Is it the link between race and SES and childhood sleep disordered breathing? *Journal of Clinical Sleep Medicine, 6*(3), 264–269.

Carskadon, M. A. (1990). Patterns of sleep and sleepiness in adolescents. *Pediatrician, 17*(1), 5–12.

Carskadon, M. A., Acebo, C., & Jenni, O. G. (2004). Regulation of adolescent sleep: Implications for behavior. *Annals of the New York Academy of Sciences, 1021*, 276–291.

Case, A., & Paxson, C. (2006). Children's health and social mobility. *The Future of Children, 16*(2), 151–173.

Chervin, R. D., Clarke, D. F., Huffman, J. L., Szymanski, E., Ruzicka, D. L., Miller, V., et al. (2003). School performance, race, and other correlates of sleep-disordered breathing in children. *Sleep Medicine, 4*(1), 21–27.

Conley, D., Strully, K., & Bennett, N. (2003). *Starting Gate: Birth Weight and Life Chances.* Berkeley: University of California Press.

Cortesi, F., Giannotti, F., Sebastiani, T., & Vagnoni, C. (2004). Cosleeping and sleep behavior in Italian school-aged children. *Journal of Developmental & Behavioral Pediatrics, 25*(1), 28–33.

Crosby, B., LeBourgeois, M. K., & Harsh, J. (2005). Racial differences in reported napping and nocturnal sleep in 2- to 8-year-old children. *Pediatrics, 115*(1 Suppl), 225–232.

Crosby, B. M., Gryczkowski, M., LeBourgeois, M. K., Olmi, D., Rabian, B., & Harsh, J. (2006). Mid-sleep time and school readiness in black and white preschool children. *Sleep, 30*, A78.

Crowell, J., Keener, M., Ginsburg, N., & Anders, T. (1987). Sleep habits in toddlers 18 to 36 months old. *Journal of the American Academy of Child and Adolescent Psychiatry, 26*(4), 510–515.

Currie, A., Shields, M. A., & Price, S. W. (2007). The child health/family income gradient: Evidence from England. *Journal of Health Economics, 26*(2), 213–232.

Currie, J., & Lin, W. (2007). Chipping away at health: More on the relationship between income and child health. *Health Affairs (Millwood), 26*(2), 331–344.

DeLeon, C. W., & Karraker, K. H. (2007). Intrinsic and extrinsic factors associated with night waking in 9-month-old infants. *Infant Behavior and Development, 30*(4), 596–605.

Eaton, D. K., McKnight-Eily, L. R., Lowry, R., Perry, G. S., Presley-Cantrell, L., & Croft, J. B. (2010). Prevalence of insufficient, borderline, and optimal hours of sleep among high school students—United States, 2007. *Journal of Adolescent Health, 46*(4), 399–401.

El-Sheikh, M., Buckhalt, J. A., Mize, J., & Acebo, C. (2006). Marital conflict and disruption of children's sleep. *Child Development, 77*(1), 31–43.

El-Sheikh, M., Buckhalt, J. A., Mark Cummings, E., & Keller, P. (2007). Sleep disruptions and emotional insecurity are pathways of risk for children. *Journal of Child Psychology and Psychiatry, 48*(1), 88–96. xxx

Ferreira, A. M., Clemente, V., Gozal, D., Gomes, A., Pissarra, C., Cesar, H., et al. (2000). Snoring in Portuguese primary school children. *Pediatrics, 106*(5), E64.

Fouts, H. N., Roopnarine, J. L., & Lamb, M. E. (2007). Social experiences and daily routines of African American infants in different socioeconomic contexts. *Journal of Family Psycholology, 21*(4), 655–664.

Goldstein, N. A., Abramowitz, T., Weedon, J., Koliskor, B., Turner, S., & Taioli, E. (2011). Racial/ethnic differences in the prevalence of snoring and sleep disordered breathing in young children. *Journal of Clinical Sleep Medicine, 7*(2), 163–171.

Goodwin, J. L., Babar, S. I., Kaemingk, K. L., Rosen, G. M., Morgan, W. J., Sherrill, D. L., et al. (2003). Symptoms related to sleep-disordered breathing in white and Hispanic children: the Tucson Children's Assessment of Sleep Apnea Study. *Chest, 124*(1), 196–203.

Goodwin, J. L., Kaemingk, K. L., Fregosi, R. F., Rosen, G. M., Morgan, W. J., Sherrill, D. L., et al. (2003). Clinical outcomes associated with sleep-disordered breathing in Caucasian and Hispanic children—the Tucson Children's Assessment of Sleep Apnea study (TuCASA). *Sleep, 26*(5), 587–591.

Goodwin, J. L., Silva, G. E., Kaemingk, K. L., Sherrill, D. L., Morgan, W. J., & Quan, S. F. (2007). Comparison between reported and recorded total sleep time and sleep latency in 6- to 11-year-old children: the Tucson Children's Assessment of Sleep Apnea Study (TuCASA). *Sleep Breath, 11*(2), 85–92.

Gottlieb, D. J., Vezina, R. M., Chase, C., Lesko, S. M., Heeren, T. C., Weese-Mayer, D. E., et al. (2003). Symptoms of sleep-disordered breathing in 5-year-old children are associated with sleepiness and problem behaviors. *Pediatrics, 112*(4), 870–877.

Gregory, A. M., & O'Connor, T. G. (2002). Sleep problems in childhood: a longitudinal study of developmental change and association with behavioral problems. *Journal of the American Academy of Child and Adolescent Psychiatry, 41*(8), 964–971.

Gregory, A. M., Eley, T. C., O'Connor, T. G., & Plomin, R. (2004). Etiologies of associations between childhood sleep and behavioral problems in a large twin sample. *Journal of the American Academy of Child and Adolescent Psychiatry, 43*(6), 744–751.

Hale, L. (2005). Who has time to sleep? *Journal of Public Health (Oxford), 27*(2), 205–211.

Hale, L., & Do, D. P. (2006). Re: "Objectively measured sleep characteristics among early-middle-aged adults: The Cardia Study". *American Journal of Epidemiology, 15*(165), 231–232.

Hale, L., Peppard, P. E., & Young, T. (2006). Does the demography of sleep contribute to health disparities? In D. Leger & S. R. Pandi-Perumal (Eds.), *Sleep Disorders: Their Impact on Public Health* (1st edition, pp. 1–19): Informa Healthcare.

Hale, L., & Do, D. P. (2007). Racial differences in self-report of sleep duration in a population-based study. *Sleep, 30*(9), 1092–1099.

Hale, L., Berger, L. M., LeBourgeois, M. K., & Brooks-Gunn, J. (2009). Social and demographic predictors of preschoolers' bedtime routines. *Journal of Developmental & Behavioral Pediatrics, 30*(5), 394–402.

Hale, L., Hill, T. D., & Burdette, A. M. (2010). Does sleep quality mediate the association between neighborhood disorder and self-rated physical health? *Preventive Medicine, 51*(3–4), 275–278.

Hibbs, A. M., Johnson, N. L., Rosen, C. L., Kirchner, H. L., Martin, R., Storfer-Isser, A., et al. (2008). Prenatal and neonatal risk factors for sleep disordered breathing in school-aged children born preterm. *Journal of Pediatrics, 153*(2), 176–182.

Hill, T. D., Burdette, A. M., & Hale, L. (2009). Neighborhood disorder, sleep quality, and psychological distress: Testing a model of structural amplification. *Health Place, 15(4), 1006–1013.*

Kataria, S., Swanson, M. S., & Trevathan, G. E. (1987). Persistence of sleep disturbances in preschool children. *Journal of Pediatrics, 110*(4), 642–646.

Kawachi, I., & Berkman, L. F. (2003). *Neighborhoods and Health.* Oxford; New York: Oxford University Press.

Kieckhefer, G. M., Ward, T. M., Tsai, S. Y., & Lentz, M. J. (2008). Nighttime sleep and daytime nap patterns in school age children with and without asthma. *Journal of Developmental & Behavioral Pediatrics, 29*(5), 338–344.

Knutson, K. L., & Lauderdale, D. S. (2009). Sociodemographic and behavioral predictors of bed time and wake time among US adolescents aged 15 to 17 years. *Journal of Pediatrics, 154*(3), 426–430, 430 e421.

Kohler, M., Lushington, K., Couper, R., Martin, J., van den Heuvel, C., Pamula, Y., et al. (2008). Obesity and risk of sleep related upper airway obstruction in Caucasian children. *Journal of Clinical Sleep Medicine, 4*(2), 129–136.

Komada, Y., Abe, T., Okajima, I., Asaoka, S., Matsuura, N., Usui, A., et al. (2011). Short sleep duration and irregular bedtime are associated with increased behavioral problems among Japanese preschool-age children. *The Tohoku Journal of Experimental Medicine, 224*(2), 127–136.

Krueger, P. M., & Friedman, E. M. (2009). Sleep duration in the United States: a cross-sectional population-based study. *American Journal of Epidemiology, 169*(9), 1052–1063.

Kuehni, C. E., Strippoli, M. P., Chauliac, E. S., & Silverman, M. (2008). Snoring in preschool children: Prevalence, severity and risk factors. *European Respiratory Journal, 31*(2), 326–333.

Lauderdale, D. S., Knutson, K. L., Yan, L. L., Rathouz, P. J., Hulley, S. B., Sidney, S., et al. (2006). Objectively measured sleep characteristics among early-middle-aged adults: The CARDIA study. *American Journal of Epidemiology, 164*(1), 5–16.

Lavigne, J. V., Binns, H. J., Christoffel, K. K., Rosenbaum, D., Arend, R., Smith, K., et al. (1993). Behavioral and emotional problems among preschool children in pediatric primary care: Prevalence and pediatricians' recognition. Pediatric Practice Research Group. *Pediatrics, 91*(3), 649–655.

Leyendecker, B., Lamb, M. E., Scholmeric, A., & Fracasso, M. (1995). The social worlds of 8-month old and 12-month old infants: Early experiences in two subcultural contexts. *Social Development*(4), 194–208.

Li, S., Jin, X., Yan, C., Wu, S., Jiang, F., & Shen, X. (2010). Habitual snoring in school-aged children: Environmental and biological predictors. *Respiratory Research, 11,* 144.

Liu, X., Liu, L., & Wang, R. (2003). Bed sharing, sleep habits, and sleep problems among Chinese school-aged children. *Sleep, 26*(7), 839–844.

Lozoff, B., Askew, G. L., & Wolf, A. W. (1996). Cosleeping and early childhood sleep problems: Effects of ethnicity and socioeconomic status. *Journal of Developmental & Behavioral Pediatrics, 17*(1), 9–15.

Mannering, A. M., Harold, G. T., Leve, L. D., Shelton, K. H., Shaw, D. S., Conger, R. D., et al. (2011). Longitudinal associations between marital instability and child sleep problems across infancy and toddlerhood in adoptive families. *Child Development, 82*(4), 1252–1266.

Marco, C. A., Wolfson, A. R., Sparling, M., & Azuaje, A. (2011). Family socioeconomic status and sleep patterns of young adolescents. *Behavioral Sleep Medicine, 10*(1), 70–80.

McFarlane, J. M., Groff, J. Y., O'Brien, J. A., & Watson, K. (2003). Behaviors of children who are exposed and not exposed to intimate partner violence: An analysis of 330 black, white, and Hispanic children. *Pediatrics, 112*(3 Pt 1), e202–e207.

McHale, S. M., Kim, J. Y., Kan, M., & Updegraff, K. A. (2011). Sleep in Mexican-American adolescents: Social ecological and well-being correlates. *Journal of Youth and Adolescence, 40*(6), 666–679.

McLaughlin Crabtree, V., Beal Korhonen, J., Montgomery-Downs, H. E., Faye Jones, V., O'Brien, L. M., & Gozal, D. (2005). Cultural influences on the bedtime behaviors of young children. *Sleep Medicine, 6*(4), 319–324.

Milan, S., Snow, S., & Belay, S. (2007). The context of preschool children's sleep: racial/ethnic differences in sleep locations, routines, and concerns. *Journal of Family Psychology, 21*(1), 20–28.

Minde, K., Popiel, K., Leos, N., Falkner, S., Parker, K., & Handley-Derry, M. (1993). The evaluation and treatment of sleep disturbances in young children. *Journal of Child Psychology and Psychiatry, 34*(4), 521–533.

Mindell, J. A., Sadeh, A., Wiegand, B., How, T. H., & Goh, D. Y. (2010). Cross-cultural differences in infant and toddler sleep. *Sleep Medicine, 11*(3), 274–280.

Montgomery, E., & Foldspang, A. (2001). Traumatic experience and sleep disturbance in refugee children from the Middle East. *European Journal of Public Health, 11*(1), 18–22.

Montgomery-Downs, H. E., Jones, V. F., Molfese, V. J., & Gozal, D. (2003). Snoring in preschoolers: Associations with sleepiness, ethnicity, and learning. *Clinical Pediatrics (Philadelphia), 42*(8), 719–726.

Moore, M., Kirchner, H. L., Drotar, D., Johnson, N., Rosen, C., & Redline, S. (2011). Correlates of adolescent sleep time and variability in sleep time: the role of individual and health related characteristics. *Sleep Medicine, 12*(3), 239–245.

Moore, M., Slane, J., Mindell, J. A., Burt, S. A., & Klump, K. L. (2011). Genetic and environmental influences on sleep problems: a study of preadolescent and adolescent twins. *Child: Care, Health and Development, 37*(5), 638–641.

Moore, P. J., Adler, N. E., Williams, D. R., & Jackson, J. S. (2002). Socioeconomic status and health: the role of sleep. *Psychosomatic Medicine, 64*(2), 337–344.

Nevarez, M. D., Rifas-Shiman, S. L., Kleinman, K. P., Gillman, M. W., & Taveras, E. M. (2010). Associations of early life risk factors with infant sleep duration. *Academic Pediatrics, 10*(3), 187–193.

NSF. (2006). *2006 Sleep in America Poll: America's Sleepy Teens.* Washington DC: National Sleep Foundation.

O'Connor, T. G., Caprariello, P., Blackmore, E. R., Gregory, A. M., Glover, V., & Fleming, P. (2007). Prenatal mood disturbance predicts sleep problems in infancy and toddlerhood. *Early Human Development, 83*(7), 451–458.

Okami, P., Weisner, T., & Olmstead, R. (2002). Outcome correlates of parent-child bedsharing: an eighteen-year longitudinal study. *Journal of Developmental & Behavioral Pediatrics, 23*(4), 244–253.

Owens, J., Maxim, R., McGuinn, M., Nobile, C., Msall, M., & Alario, A. (1999). Television-viewing habits and sleep disturbance in school children. *Pediatrics, 104*(3), e27.

Peng, N. H., Bachman, J., Jenkins, R., Chen, C. H., Chang, Y. C., Chang, Y. S., et al. (2009). Relationships between environmental stressors and stress biobehavioral responses of preterm infants in NICU. *Journal of Perinatal and Neonatal Nursing, 23*(4), 363–371.

Pinto, S., Huang, J., Tapia, I., Karamessinis, L., Pepe, M., Gallagher, P. R., et al. (2011). Effects of race on upper airway dynamic function during sleep in children. *Sleep, 34*(4), 495–501.

Quan, S. F., Goodwin, J. L., Babar, S. I., Kaemingk, K. L., Enright, P. L., Rosen, G. M., et al. (2003). Sleep architecture in normal Caucasian and Hispanic children aged 6–11 years recorded during unattended home polysomnography: experience from the Tucson Children's Assessment of Sleep Apnea Study (TuCASA). *Sleep Medicine, 4*(1), 13–19.

Redline, S., Tishler, P. V., Schluchter, M., Aylor, J., Clark, K., & Graham, G. (1999). Risk factors for sleep-disordered breathing in children. Associations with obesity, race, and respiratory problems. *American Journal of Respiratory Critical Care Medicine, 159*(5 Pt 1), 1527–1532.

Reid, G. J., Hong, R. Y., & Wade, T. J. (2009). The relation between common sleep problems and emotional and behavioral problems among 2- and 3-year-olds in the context of known risk factors for psychopathology. *Journal of Sleep Research, 18*(1), 49–59.

Richman, N., Stevenson, J. E., & Graham, P. J. (1975). Prevalence of behaviour problems in 3-year-old children: an epidemiological study in a London borough. *Journal of Child Psychology and Psychiatry, 16*(4), 277–287.

Roberts, R. E., Roberts, C. R., & Chan, W. (2006). Ethnic differences in symptoms of insomnia among adolescents. *Sleep, 29*(3), 359–365.

Rosen, C. L., Larkin, E. K., Kirchner, H. L., Emancipator, J. L., Bivins, S. F., Surovec, S. A., et al. (2003). Prevalence and risk factors for sleep-disordered breathing in 8- to 11-year-old children: Association with race and prematurity. *Journal of Pediatrics, 142*(4), 383–389.

Rudnick, E. F., Walsh, J. S., Hampton, M. C., & Mitchell, R. B. (2007). Prevalence and ethnicity of sleep-disordered breathing and obesity in children. *Otolaryngology – Head and Neck Surgery, 137*(6), 878–882.

Sadeh, A., Gruber, R., & Raviv, A. (2003). The effects of sleep restriction and extension on school-age children: What a difference an hour makes. *Child Development, 74*(2), 444–455.

Sadeh, A., Mindell, J. A., Luedtke, K., & Wiegand, B. (2009). Sleep and sleep ecology in the first 3 years: A web-based study. *Journal of Sleep Research, 18*(1), 60–73.

Sadeh, A., Mindell, J., & Rivera, L. (2011). "My child has a sleep problem": A cross-cultural comparison of parental definitions. *Sleep Medicine, 12*(5), 478–482.

Sickel, A. E., Moore, P. J., Adler, N. E., Williams, D. R., & Jackson, J. S. (1999). The differential effects of sleep quality and quantity on the relationship between SES and health. In N. Adler, M. Marmot, B. S. McEwen & J. Stewart (Eds.), *Socioeconomic Status and Health in Industrial Nations: Social Psychological and Biological Pathways* (Vol. 896, pp. 431–434). New York: New York Academy of Sciences.

Smaldone, A., Honig, J. C., & Byrne, M. W. (2007). Sleepless in America: Inadequate sleep and relationships to health and well-being of our nation's children. *Pediatrics, 119* (Suppl 1), S29–S37.

Smedley, B. D., Syme, S. L., & Institute of Medicine (U.S.). Committee on Capitalizing on Social Science and Behavioral Research to Improve the Public's Health. (2000). *Promoting Health: Intervention Strategies from Social and Behavioral Research.* Washington, DC: National Academy Press.

Smedley, B. D., Stith, A. Y., Nelson, A. R., & Institute of Medicine (U.S.). Committee on Understanding and Eliminating Racial and Ethnic Disparities in Health Care. (2003). *Unequal Treatment: Confronting Racial and Ethnic Disparities in Health Care.* Washington, DC: National Academy Press.

Spilsbury, J. C., Storfer-Isser, A., Drotar, D., Rosen, C. L., Kirchner, L. H., Benham, H., et al. (2004). Sleep behavior in an urban US sample of school-aged children. *Archives of Pediatrics & Adolescent Medicine, 158*(10), 988–994.

Spilsbury, J. C., Storfer-Isser, A., Kirchner, H. L., Nelson, L., Rosen, C. L., Drotar, D., et al. (2006). Neighborhood disadvantage as a risk factor for pediatric obstructive sleep apnea. *Journal of Pediatrics, 149*(3), 342–347.

Stein, M. A., Mendelsohn, J., Obermeyer, W. H., Amromin, J., & Benca, R. (2001). Sleep and behavior problems in school-aged children. *Pediatrics, 107*(4), E60.

Taveras, E. M., Hohman, K. H., Price, S., Gortmaker, S. L., & Sonneville, K. (2009). Televisions in the bedrooms of racial/ethnic minority children: How did they get there and how do we get them out? *Clinical Pediatrics (Philadelphia), 48*(7), 715–719.

Tikotzky, L., Sadeh, A., & Glickman-Gavrieli, T. (2011). Infant sleep and paternal involvement in infant caregiving during the first 6 months of life. *Journal of Pediatric Psychology, 36*(1), 36–46.

Touchette, E., Petit, D., Paquet, J., Boivin, M., Japel, C., Tremblay, R. E., et al. (2005). Factors associated with fragmented sleep at night across early childhood. *Archives of Pediatrics & Adolescent Medicine, 159*(3), 242–249.

Umlauf, M. G., Bolland, J. M., & Lian, B. E. (2011). Sleep disturbance and risk behaviors among inner-city African-American adolescents. *Journal of Urban Health, 88*(6), 1130–1142.

Urschitz, M. S., Guenther, A., Eitner, S., Urschitz-Duprat, P. M., Schlaud, M., Ipsiroglu, O. S., et al. (2004). Risk factors and natural history of habitual snoring. *Chest, 126*(3), 790–800.

Wolfson, A. R., & Carskadon, M. A. (1998). Sleep schedules and daytime functioning in adolescents. *Child Development, 69*(4), 875–887.

Worthman, C. M., & Brown, R. A. (2007). Companionable sleep: Social regulation of sleep and cosleeping in Egyptian families. *Journal of Family Psychology, 21*(1), 124–135.

Yen, C. F., King, B. H., & Chang, Y. P. (2010). Factor structure of the Athens Insomnia Scale and its associations with demographic characteristics and depression in adolescents. *Journal of Sleep Research, 19*(1 Pt 1), 12–18.

Yolton, K., Xu, Y., Khoury, J., Succop, P., Lanphear, B., Beebe, D. W., et al. (2010). Associations between secondhand smoke exposure and sleep patterns in children. *Pediatrics, 125*(2), e261–e268.

Zhang, J., Li, A. M., Kong, A. P., Lai, K. Y., Tang, N. L., & Wing, Y. K. (2009). A community-based study of insomnia in Hong Kong Chinese children: Prevalence, risk factors and familial aggregation. *Sleep Medicine, 10*(9), 1040–1046.

CHAPTER

11 Sleep Hygiene and Environment: Role of Technology

Michael Gradisar *and* Michelle A. Short

Abstract

Technological devices have become more affordable, multifunctional, and portable over recent years. Not only have the number of devices increased in families' households, but also increasingly more evidence documents that children and adolescents keep these devices in their bedrooms. On a related note, the percentage of youth who use technology before bed is remarkably high, and emerging evidence shows technology is now being used during the night. This chapter reviews the effects of various technological devices (TVs, computers/Internet, video games, cell phones, music players) on the sleep of children and adolescents. Possible mechanisms explaining these effects (including displacing bedtime, arousal, light and electromagnetic transmission, and nighttime sleep disruption) are discussed, as well as potential modifying factors of age, gender, socioeconomic status, and parental involvement. Directions for future research and recommendations for families and health professionals are provided in order to continue to improve the sleep hygiene of our youth.

Key Words: children, adolescents, technology, media, sleep

Introduction

Sleep hygiene is commonly known as a collection of behaviors that promote healthy sleep (Hauri, 1977) and is often imbedded as a treatment component within a larger multicomponent treatment for sleep problems (e.g., cognitive behavior therapy for insomnia). However, it is likely that many parents will seek information about "healthy sleep tips" prior to seeking professional help. This may lead families to reduce stimulation close to bedtime and promote a bedroom environment that is optimal for relaxation and sleep. Reducing caffeine intake, avoiding evening exercise, and ensuring their child's bedroom is quiet and dark are some examples of improving sleep hygiene. Possibly the most challenging sleep hygiene issue confronting parents of late is the presence and use of technology in their child's bedroom—but what is the current evidence?

Despite widespread discussion on the effect of technology on sleep, very few studies have directly examined this relationship and still fewer have done so using longitudinal or experimental methodologies. Indeed, this research area is challenging because the pace of technological change often outstrips that of the research process. As such, much of the current research covers "older" technologies. A number of studies have examined the impact of particular items on sleep, including television (TV), music, gaming, computers and laptops, and fixed and cellular phones (e.g., NSF, 2011; Tan, 2004; van den Bulck, 2000; 2003; 2007). Increasingly, the functionality of these different technologies is being combined within one portable unit. For example, modern cell phones or so-called "smart phones" can be used to send, read, and receive text and picture messages and emails, access the Internet, play and record audio and music files, play and record video files, take photos, play computer games—and even make and receive calls—enabling access to a broad range of technologies in the one device. These rapid changes pose a challenge to researchers and to parents in managing any risks associated with media use in a rapidly changing technological landscape.

The present chapter will review the literature in this field, discussing the impact of technology use on sleep, different aspects of sleep that may be affected (and the possible mechanisms for this), and highlighting the many unanswered questions and future research directions.

The Relationship between Technology Use and Sleep

Watching Television

Television viewing has become part of the culture of many households in developed and developing countries (van den Bulck, 2000). One study of US children found that 42% of children aged 2–18 yrs live in homes where the TV is on "most of the time," and 58% of children have meals with the TV on (Roberts, Foehr, Rideout & Brodie, 1999). School-aged children have been reported to spend as much time watching television every week as they do going to school (approximately 25 hours per week; Owens, Maxim, McGuinn, Nobile & Msall, 1999). This pattern of TV viewing does not appear restricted to North American children. In India, children aged 3–10 yrs were reported to spend an average of 18.5 hours per week watching TV (Gupta, Saini, Acharya & Miglani, 1994), while Turkish children in the 2nd and 3rd grades spend an average of 17.3 hours per week watching television (Toyran, Ozmert & Yurdakok, 2002).

Not only is TV part of the household milieu, it is an increasing presence in the bedrooms of children and adolescents. The number of 6th-grade children with a TV in their bedroom has increased from 6% in 1970 to 77% in 1999 (Roberts et al., 1999), and has since plateaued (76%; Kaiser Family Foundation [KFF], 2010). The proportion of children with a TV in their bedroom also increases with increasing child age (Owens et al., 1999; Mindell, Meltzer, Carskadon & Chervin, 2009). However, even very young children are being immersed in technology. One study found that 17% of toddlers had a TV in their bedroom (Mindell et al., 2009). The effects of this in contributing to poor sleep hygiene are clear, with children and adolescents with a TV in their bedroom spending more time, on average, watching TV (KFF, 2010; Oka, Suzuki & Inoue, 2008; Owens et al., 1999; Shochat, Flint-Bretler & Tzischinsky, 2010), obtaining less sleep (Mindell et al., 2009; Shochat et al., 2010; van den Bulck, 2004), and having later bedtimes (Oka et al., 2008; Shochat et al., 2010; van den Bulck, 2004), later wake times on weekends (van den Bulck, 2004), and increased sleep disturbance (Owens et al., 1999).

As well as the location of TV viewing, the time spent TV viewing is associated with a raft of sleep concerns in children and adolescents, including later bedtimes on school nights (Adam, Snell & Pendry, 2007; Eggermont & van den Bulck, 2006; Tynjala, Kannas & Valimaa, 1993; van den Bulck, 2004), and weekends (Oka et al., 2008; van den Bulck, 2004), less school night sleep (Adam et al., 2007; Mindell et al., 2009; van den Bulck, 2004), less weekend sleep (Eggermont & van den Bulck, 2006), difficulty initiating sleep (Eggermont & van den Bulck, 2006; Gaina, Sekine, Kanayama, Sengoku, Yamagami & Kagamimori, 2005; Li, Jin, Wu, Jiang, Yan & Shen, 2007; Tynjala et al., 1993; van den Bulck, 2000), lower sleep efficiency (Dworak, Schierl, Bruns & Struder, 2007), increased nighttime awakening (Owens et al., 1999), greater likelihood of sleep disturbance (Li et al., 2007; Mistry, Minkovitz, Strobino & Borzekowski, 2007; Mitrofan, Paul & Spencer, 2009; Owens et al., 1999; Paavonen, Pennonen, Roine, Valkonen & Lahikainen, 2006), and daytime sleepiness or tiredness (Saarenpaa-Heikkila, Laippala & Koivikko, 2000; van den Bulck, 2004). TV viewing also affects diurnal sleep, with infants aged 4–35 months experiencing irregular napping (Thompson & Christakis, 2005). While most research has relied upon cross-sectional associations, one longitudinal study found associations between TV viewing and subsequent sleep problems (Johnson, Cohen, Kasen, First & Brook, 2004). Johnson and colleagues (2004) followed a cohort of 759 mothers and their children from early adolescence (~14 years), across middle adolescence (~16 years) and emerging adulthood (~22 years). They found that increased TV viewing at age 14 predicted difficulties of sleep onset, sleep maintenance, and having one or more sleep problems at 16 years and 22 years, after controlling for age, sex, prior sleep problems, psychiatric disorders, neglect, parental education and income, and parent psychiatric problems. In addition, Johnson et al. found that adolescents who reduced their TV viewing to less than 1 hour per day significantly reduced their risk of developing subsequent sleep problems.

Worth noting at this point is that not all studies have found deleterious consequences associated with the quantity of TV viewing. A recent study of 14,782 adolescents in the United States found that watching 4 or more hours of TV per school day *increased* the likelihood of "sufficient sleep," defined as at least 8 hours of sleep on school nights (Foti, Eaton, Lowry & McKnight-Ely, 2011). This may suggest that TV watching on school days is a sedentary behavior for adolescents which helps to de-arouse them in preparation for sleep. In a separate study of Finnish adolescents, TV viewing of 2 or more hours a day did not predict the development or maintenance of excessive daytime sleepiness (Saarenpaa-Heikkila, Rintahaka, Laippala & Koivikko, 2000), which may be due to the study being underpowered to detect even small effects when incorporating several predictors' variables (i.e., two small samples were used; N = 68 and N = 75).

In addition to the location and quantity of TV viewing, the timing and content of TV viewing may affect sleep. Children and adolescents who watched TV at night reported later wake times on school mornings (Adam et al., 2007;Thorleifsdottir, Bjornsson, Benediktsdottir, Gislason, & Kristbjarnarson, 2002) and weekends (Oka et al., 2008), as well as later bedtimes (Thorleifsdottir et al., 2002) and increased sleep disturbances including bedtime resistance, sleep onset delay, sleep anxiety, and shortened total sleep (Owens et al., 1999). Among a group of Finnish children, aged 5–6 years, watching TV at bedtime was associated with greater likelihood of sleep–wake transition disorders and disorders of excessive somnolence, while children who watch TV by themselves were more likely to have difficulties initiating and maintaining sleep (Paavonen et al., 2006). At the other end of the sleep period, children who watched TV programs that were aired early on weekend mornings were found to wake earlier on weekends (Thorleifsdottir et al., 2002). This may be a protective factor, especially in adolescents, as it may prevent the delay of the circadian rhythm that may lead to sleep–wake transition issues. This study also raises another issue in that, despite parental concerns around TV viewing and poor sleep, one study of children and adolescents aged 2–20 years estimated that half of all children and adolescents had no rules around the content of their TV viewing (Roberts et al., 1999). While the content of weekend morning TV programs may be developmentally appropriate for children, this is unlikely to be the case for late-night TV program content.

In summary, TV ownership and use is one of the most studied forms of technology use in relation to sleep. The most consistent evidence is *(1)* that TV watching is consuming a large proportion of children and adolescent's waking time, and *(2)* that the bedroom presence and use of TVs is associated with later bedtimes, difficulties initiating sleep, and less nocturnal sleep. This is somewhat alarming in that, compared to other forms of technology yet to be reviewed, TVs are less portable, are mainly unifunctional, and possess some element of the "knowledge of time" (i.e., when TV programs cease).

Computer and Internet Use

Very few studies have examined the relationship between computer use and sleep in a pediatric population. While computers and laptops have become more commonplace in many homes (Roberts et al., 1999), as well as in many children's bedrooms (Li et al., 2007), there is suggestion that children currently spend less time in front of this form of technology than they do in front of the television (Olds, Ridley & Dollman, 2006; Roberts et al., 1999). Increased computer use has been associated with shorter sleep duration (Foti et al., 2011; Fuligni & Hardway, 2006; Punamaki, Wallenius, Nygard, Saarni & Rimpela, 2007; Shochat et al., 2010), more variable sleep timing (Fuligni & Hardway, 2006), and greater tiredness during the day (Punamaki et al., 2007). Adolescents who use a computer at night report worse sleep quality, increased daytime sleepiness, and more sleep disorders (Mesquita & Reimao, 2007). One study of 19,299 Chinese children aged 5–11 years found that having a computer in the bedroom, but not time spent on the computer, predicted bedtime resistance and sleep anxiety after controlling for child and parent demographic variables (Li et al., 2007).

One difficulty with these studies is that it remains unclear whether computer use includes time spent on the Internet. Shochat and colleagues (2010) were able to observe this specific behavior, with Israeli adolescents (age 14 years) spending more time using the computer for the Internet as opposed to gaming. Furthermore, computer usage was higher if the adolescent had a computer in his or her bedroom (Shochat et al., 2010). Among children aged 6–16 years, greater Internet use as well as Internet use before bed were associated with later bedtimes on weekdays and weekends, less total sleep time on weekdays, later wake times on weekends (Oka et al., 2008; van den Bulck, 2004), and more tiredness (van den Bulck, 2004). Among these groups, very few of the children (Oka et al., 2008) and none of the adolescents (van den Bulck, 2004) had Internet access in their bedrooms. Yet, recent data from the United States shows 33% of 8–18-year-olds have access to the Internet in their bedroom (Kaiser Family Foundation, 2010). At the extreme, greater Internet addiction among Taiwanese adolescents was associated with short sleep duration and increased subjective insomnia (Yen, Ko, Yen & Cheng, 2008). More recently, the 2011 National Sleep Foundation's (NSF) *Sleep in America Poll* found that adolescents (13–18 years) were much more likely to use computers and laptops in the hour before the sleep attempt compared to adults over 30 years old, with 61% of adolescents using computers or laptops in the hour before sleep at least a few nights a week (NSF, 2011). Most commonly, computers and laptops were being used to access the Internet (53%), send or receive emails (37%), watch videos (20%), or use a word-processing or spreadsheet program. These adolescents were significantly less likely to report a good night's sleep, were more likely to be classified as sleepy on the Epworth Sleepiness Scale (Johns, 1991), and more likely to drive drowsy (NSF, 2011).

In summary, the evidence suggests that computer and/or Internet presence and use is consistently related to reduced nocturnal sleep and some form of daytime impairment (i.e., sleepiness or tiredness). How sleep is becoming restricted in response to computer/Internet use is yet to be elucidated (i.e., later bedtimes, longer sleep latency, or both). Understanding these effects is made more difficult due to the variability in how computers are used. One of the longstanding uses of computers—video gaming—is emerging as one of the most clinically detrimental forms of technology in our youth.

Video Gaming

Studies of school-aged children and adolescents have reported that between one-quarter and one-third use video games in the hour before bed (NSF, 2011; Oka et al., 2008), and a sizeable proportion have video game consoles in their bedrooms (Oka et al., 2008). While video gaming does not appear to consume as much time as television viewing in this age group (Olds et al., 2006; Roberts et al., 1999), playing video games and using the Internet before bed have been argued as having a larger negative impact on the sleep of children and adolescents than either watching TV or using cell phones (Oka et al., 2008). Indeed, Internet addiction treatment centers exist in China, South Korea, Taiwan, the United States, England, and the Netherlands (King, Delfabbro, Griffiths & Gradisar, 2011), with online gaming being a significant issue.

Cross-sectional research has shown that children with video games in their bedrooms spent more time playing video games and have later school night bedtimes and less sleep (Oka et al., 2008; van den Bulck, 2004). Increased time spent using video games is also associated with later bedtimes on school nights (Adam et al., 2007; Eggermont & van den Bulck, 2006; Oka et al., 2008; van den Bulck, 2004) and weekends (Adam et al., 2007; van den Bulck, 2004), longer sleep onset times (Dworak et al., 2007; Gaina, Sekine, Hamanishi, Chen, Kanayama, Yamagami et al., 2006; Gaina et al., 2005; Weaver, Gradisar, Dohnt, Lovato & Douglas, 2010), less total sleep (Adam et al., 2007; BaHammann, Bin Saeed, Al-Faris & Shaikh, 2006; Eggermont & van den Bulck, 2006; Foti et al., 2011; Oka et al., 2008; van den Bulck, 2004), later wake times on weekdays (Adam et al., 2007) and weekends (Oka et al., 2008; van den Bulck, 2004), more daytime sleepiness (Eggermont & van den Bulck, 2006; van den Bulck, 2004), and heightened physiological arousal (Anderson & Bushman, 2001). Adam and colleagues (2007) used a time-use diary to examine the relationship between video gaming and sleep in 2454 children and adolescents aged 5–19 years. They found that each hour spent playing video games was associated with a loss of 10 minutes of sleep in children (aged 5–12 yrs) and 14 minutes in adolescents (aged 12–19 yrs), mainly due to later bedtimes (Adam et al., 2007). A number of these studies reported gender differences in video gaming; however, we address these issues later (see *Moderating Factors*).

Unlike prior research examining the effect of children's TV and computer use on sleep, which overwhelmingly relied upon cross-sectional associations, the effect of video gaming on sleep has received more attention in experimental paradigms. Dworak and colleagues (2007) compared the sleep of 11 young adolescents across three nights including video gaming (i.e., playing the racing game *Need for Speed*), video watching, and no technology, in randomized order. Sleep was monitored using home polysomnography and self-report. Video game playing resulted in a longer time taken to fall asleep, increased "light" sleep (stage 2), and less deep sleep (stages 3 and 4). Sleep onset latencies (SOLs) increased from 11 minutes on the control night to 33 minutes after video game playing. The authors also observed significant individual differences in participants' responses to the game. This could indicate that some children and adolescents may be at greater risk for negative sleep-related consequences of video gaming before bed. Indeed, recent evidence has demonstrated that "naïve gamers" (≤1 hour/day) may be more susceptible to the arousing effects of video gaming compared to "experienced gamers" (≥ 3 hours/day), with a near-doubling of sleep latency for the naïve gamers (SOL ≈ 40 minutes) compared to the experienced gamers (SOL ≈ 20 minutes) after playing a violent video game (Ivarsson, personal communication). Furthermore, naïve gamers reported worse sleep quality overall.

However, meaningful changes to sleep following video game play are not consistently found. For instance, 19 Swedish boys (aged 12–15 years) played a violent video game (*Manhunter*), a non-violent video game, and a no video game control between 8pm and 10pm in a randomized order across three nights (Ivarsson, Anderson, Akerstedt & Lindblad, 2009). No significant differences in sleep were found despite an increase in heart rate variability following the violent video game. In contrast, Weaver and colleagues (2010) found 13 adolescent boys (aged 14–18 years) showed no differences in heart rate when playing a violent video game (*Call of Duty 4*), compared to a slow-paced documentary (*March of the Penguins*). A statistical increase in sleep onset latency was found (3 minutes following the documentary; 7.5 minutes following the video game); however this difference is not meaningful. Furthermore, no differences in sleep architecture were found between the two conditions.

In summary, evidence is accumulating for a relationship between video gaming and later bedtimes, longer sleep latencies, and less nocturnal sleep. This may likely be due to the stimulating nature of video games creating longer sleep latencies, alongside this technology's lack of "time knowledge" that may delay bedtimes. However, replication of these findings is lacking in controlled laboratory studies. In addition, few studies have examined the effects of online gaming on sleep (Lemola et al., 2011), which may delay bedtimes, advance rise times in order to play with other gamers in a different time zones, or result in sleep disruption in order to check online gaming progress in 24/7 online games. All of these behaviors would result in sleep loss, which could demonstrate observable daytime impairments to significant others (teachers, parents) if performed on consecutive nights over weeks, if not months.

Using Cell Phones

Cell phones are becoming more commonplace among children and adolescents, and are possibly the most multifunctional and portable device. This results in very high access to and use of cell phones by youth. Astonishingly, in Sweden, 99.6% of adolescents aged 15–19 years reported access to a cell phone (Soderqvist, Carlberg & Hardell, 2008), and in Japan, 84% of adolescents reported using a cell phone *every day* (Munezawa et al., 2011). In relation to sleep, the 2011 National Sleep Foundation's Sleep in America Poll reported that 72% of adolescents bring their cell phones into their bedrooms and use them when they are attempting to fall asleep. In the hour before the sleep attempt, 56% of adolescents sent, read, or received text messages *every night or almost every night*. This proportion was significantly higher among adolescents than older age groups. Texting in the hour before the sleep attempt at least *a few nights per week* was associated with less likelihood of reporting a good night's sleep, unrefreshing sleep, more sleepiness, and greater likelihood of driving drowsy (NSF, 2011). Similar cross-sectional relationships have been found between mobile phone use and sleep disturbances (Munezawa et al., 2011), less total sleep (Harada, Morikuni, Yoshii, Yamashita & Takeuchi, 2002; Munezawa et al., 2011; Punamaki et al., 2007), poor sleep quality (Munezawa et al., 2011), insomnia symptoms (Munezawa et al., 2011), irregular sleep (Punamaki et al., 2007), later wake times and more evening circadian typology (Harada et al., 2002), and daytime sleepiness or tiredness (Munezawa et al., 2011; Punamaki et al., 2007; van den Bulck, 2007). One study of 1656 Belgian adolescents found that among those adolescents who reported being very tired, 35% of cases were attributed to mobile phone use (van den Bulck, 2007).

More than any other device, however, cell phones are the greatest technological culprit to create wakings from sleep. In the United States, 28% of adolescents reported sleeping with their cell phones in their bedrooms with the ringer turned on during the night, and 18% of adolescents reported being woken up by phone calls, text messages, or emails at least *a few nights per week* (NSF, 2011). Due to their portability, the evidence suggests cell phones are likely to be used in the bedroom after the lights are turned off. The evidence shows that daytime impairments associated with cell phone use are common—even in the long term.

Listening to Music

Listening to music rarely comes to mind when considering pediatric technology use; however, media devices are frequently used by children and adolescents to play, record, and share music (Cain & Gradisar, 2010; NSF, 2011). Sixty-four percent of adolescents report using an electronic media device to listen to music in the hour before sleep attempt, with 59% using computers and laptops and 42% using a mobile phone to listen to music (Hamblin & Wood, 2002). Using these devices to listen to music has been associated with increased sleepiness, less likelihood of having a good night's sleep, and greater likelihood of driving drowsy. In a Belgian study of 2546 7th- and 10th-grade adolescents, over 60% reported using music as a sleep aid. Far from aiding sleep, though, its use was associated with later bedtimes, less total sleep time, and increased tiredness (Eggermont & van den Bulck, 2006).

The effect that music listening has on sleep is likely to depend, at least in part, on the type of music. One experimental study of 86 elementary school children in Taiwan found that listening to sedative music (60 to 80 beats per minute) was associated with improved sleep. Children were randomly assigned to either a music listening group or a no-music control group. The music group listened to music for 45 minutes every day before naptime and bedtime. Compared to controls, the music-listening group had improved sleep quality, better sleep efficiency, and longer sleep duration (Tan, 2004). Unfortunately, the music group was also instructed to use breathing and muscle relaxation techniques when attempting to sleep, so it is unclear to what extent any sleep improvements can be ascribed to the music. Another experimental study found that toddlers and preschool-aged children who were randomly assigned to listen to classical music during the sleep attempt had shorter latencies to sleep onset than those who did not (Field, 1999).

Despite prolific use of music prior to sleep in the studies reviewed here, much more evidence is needed to understand the positive (e.g., distraction from worries) and negative (e.g., extending the sleep onset process) influence of music on sleep. This will be challenging and complicated, as listening to music can be performed not just in the typical "hour before bed," but also after lights-out. This can introduce measurement error for researchers when attempting to assess sleep latency. Specifically, the beginning of the sleep onset process may not be when lights-out occurred, but the time when the child/adolescent decides to attempt sleep. As this may occur while listening to music, it may be very difficult to estimate—it may even be unknown.

Multimedia Use and Screen Time

While the majority of studies have examined particular media devices, very few have examined the collective effect of technology use, often referred to as "screen time" (Drescher, Goodwin, Silva & Quan, 2011; Olds et al., 2006). While this does not allow the examination of unique effects of particular devices, it does overcome the issue of how to measure media use at a time when children and adolescents use portable products with multimedia capabilities within one device (e.g., cell phones, iPads, and laptops).

Just over 1000 Australian children aged 10–13 years completed a multimedia activity recall diary for 24 hours on two to four occasions (Olds et al., 2006). They reported that a median of 27% of their waking hours were spent using electronic media. On school days, an average of 3 hours and 10 minutes per day was spent on electronic media and 4 hours and 20 minutes on non-school days. Of the media used, television constituted 73% of all screen time, 19% was video games, 6% was non-game computer use, and 2% was cinema going. Every extra 1 hour of screen time was associated with a decline of 10 minutes of sleep per night. This may seem negligible if only one hour of screen time is obtained; however, the impact holds greater significance after several hours of screen time, especially if conducted on a regular basis over weeks and months of a school term.

Another study found an association between electronic screen time (incorporating TV, Internet, computer use, and video games) and less total sleep among 10–17-year-olds according to parent report or polysomnography (Drescher et al., 2011). Among 100 adolescents from the United States, those who spent more time using electronic media between 9pm and 6am obtained less total sleep, took longer to fall asleep, drank more caffeinated beverages, had more daytime sleepiness, and were more likely to fall asleep in class. Among these adolescents, 66% had a TV in their bedroom, 30% had a computer, 90% had a cell phone, and 79% had an MP3 digital audio player. Around 1–2 hours/night was spent after 9pm using electronic media (Calamaro, Mason & Ratcliffe, 2009)

Limitations of Prior Research

The primary limitation of much prior work is that it has relied upon cross-sectional methodologies and thus causation cannot be determined. A host of other factors may influence both technology use and sleep (e.g., poor parental limit-setting, depression), thus it is possible that this relationship may be much more complex. Some studies controlled for other demographic and family factors, while others did not. Alternatively, reverse causation may be occurring, whereby children and adolescents who cannot sleep (evidenced by later bedtimes and/or longer sleep onset latencies) use technology to fill in this time. For example, among Belgian adolescents, a surprising 28% of boys and 15% of girls used video games as a "sleep aid"—that is, to replace lying in bed awake (possibly worrying about the present and next day's events; Gregory et al., 2010) with video gaming (Eggermont & van den Bulck, 2006). A second limitation is the lack of uniformity in how both sleep and technology use has been operationalized. For example, measurement of sleep patterns varied from polysomnography to a single self-report item asking subjects what their average sleep was over the past month (e.g., Adam et al., 2007; Drescher et al., 2011; NSF, 2011; Weaver et al., 2010), and between parent report and self-report (e.g., Drescher et al., 2011; Munezawa et al., 2011; Owens et al., 1999). Many studies have revealed a small effect size, or have not considered the clinical or practical significance of any statistical differences. Translating the true meaning of these research findings to the community is important, considering the topical nature of this area. Lastly, as we have highlighted in this section, the relationship between technology use and sleep may not be so intuitive. The field requires a framework in which to understand the complexities of this relationship, which may help to inform future investigations and potential "treatments" of this aspect of sleep hygiene.

Theoretical Implications

A 2010 review of electronic media use and sleep in school-aged children and adolescents found that the most consistent research finding was a relationship between media use and later bedtimes and less total sleep (Cain & Gradisar, 2010). However as previously mentioned, the relationship between technology and pediatric sleep is likely to be complex and to vary according to different factors. Here we expand upon the model proposed by Cain and Gradisar (2010) so as to incorporate new evidence and perspectives.

Moderating Factors

The indirect effect of the bedroom presence of electronic media, as well as the direct effects of daytime and evening use of technology, has already been reviewed in this chapter. Relationships between technology use and the child's age, gender, socioeconomic status (SES), and parenting factors have been reported and demonstrate the complexities involved when examining effects on sleep.

First, a number of studies report gender differences in the type or quantity of technology use (Eggermont & van den Bulck, 2006; Gaina et al., 2006; Mesquita & Reimao, 2007; Munezawa et al., 2011; NSF, 2006; Olds et al., 2006; Punamaki et al., 2007; Roberts et al., 1999; Soderqvist et al., 2008). Boys have been reported as more likely to use video games as a sleep aid (Eggermont & van den Bulck, 2006), have a video game console in their bedroom (Eggermont & van den Bulck, 2006), play video games (NSF, 2006; Olds et al., 2006; Punamaki et al., 2007; Roberts et al., 1999), use the Internet (Punamaki et al., 2007), watch TV (NSF, 2006; Olds et al., 2006; Roberts et al., 1999), use computers (Gaina et al., 2006), and have more screen time (Olds et al., 2006; Roberts et al., 1999) than girls. Girls are more likely to listen to music (Eggermont & van den Bulck, 2006; Roberts et al., 1999), read books (Eggermont & van den Bulck, 2006; NSF, 2006), use cell phones (Munezawa et al., 2011; NSF, 2006; Punamaki et al., 2007; Soderqvist et al., 2008), and use a computer (Mesquita & Reimao, 2007; Olds et al., 2006).

Second, older children and adolescents are more likely to use TV and music as a sleep aid (Eggermont & van den Bulck, 2006), listen to music (Eggermont & van den Bulck, 2006), use cell phones every day (NSF, 2006; Soderqvist et al., 2008) and use cell phone after lights-out (NSF, 2011), have more devices in their bedroom (NSF, 2006), be woken by incoming text messages (van den Bulck, 2003), and have more screen time (Olds et al., 2006) than younger children. Younger children, however, are more likely to use books to help them to fall asleep (Eggermont & van den Bulck, 2006).

Third, socioeconomic status (SES) has been operationalized in different ways across different studies; however, consistent associations between higher SES and decreased media use have been found. Children from higher SES backgrounds are less likely to use TVs or computers as a sleep aid (Eggermont & van den Bulck, 2006), yet more likely to read books (Eggermont & van den Bulck, 2006). They also watch less TV (Mistry et al., 2007; Owens et al., 1999), are less likely to have a TV in their bedroom (Calamaro, Mason & Ratcliffe, 2009; Owens et al., 1999), are less likely to fall asleep regularly in front of the television (Owens et al., 1999), and have less overall screen time (Olds et al., 2006). As higher SES has also been associated with better sleep patterns, including more total sleep and greater ease of initiating sleep (NSF, 2006), SES presents an important factor to include in any study of media use and sleep. Researchers need to be mindful, though, that families from lower SES backgrounds may differ in the types of technological devices owned compared to families from higher SES backgrounds (i.e., laptops, tablets, etc.).

Lastly, both technology use and sleep may co-vary with parenting factors (Eggermont & van den Bulck, 2006; Paavonen et al., 2006). Although parents' level of education has been found to be related to adolescents' use of TV and video gaming before lights out (Eggermont & van den Bulck, 2006), this does not inform of specific parental behaviors that moderate their children's evening technology use. More direction is provided from a study of young children (aged 2.5–5.5 years), where "parental involvement" in children's activities was associated with less TV watching and less likelihood of having a TV in the bedroom (Mistry et al., 2007). Children of single parents have been reported as watching more TV, more likely to have a TV in the bedroom, and less likely to have rules about watching TV (Roberts et al., 1999). Indeed, the American Academy of Pediatrics (AAP, 2001) has recommended that parents discourage children under 2 years of age from watching TV and that children older than 2 years limit their screen time to 1–2 hours per day of quality programming (i.e., educational, pro-social content, etc.). In relation to sleep hygiene, the AAP (2001) has also recommended that TVs are not present in children's bedrooms, yet this is often ignored. Such position statements are also present in other countries (e.g., Canada; Ford-Jones & Nieman, 2003), yet lacking from peak pediatric bodies in other countries (e.g., Australia, United Kingdom). However, the most common parenting factor asserted as affecting technology use is parental limit-setting (Anderson & Bushman, 2001; Eggermont & van den Bulck, 2006; Owens et al., 1999). It has been argued that diminished parental limit-setting may lead to increased or inappropriate technology use as well as increased sleep problems such as bedtime resistance, later bedtimes, and less sleep (Eggermont & van den Bulck, 2006; Owens et al., 1999). Eggermont and van den Bulck (2006) argued that parents who do not control or have any regard for children's media use might also be less likely to control or have regard for their bedtimes.

In summary, the type and quantity of technology used is likely to vary according to age, gender, socioeconomic status, and parenting factors. We recommend that these variables be assessed in future research—especially parenting factors, which will eventually help to inform best practices for families of children of varying age, gender, and socioeconomic backgrounds. Rather than simply controlling for these factors, a more developed understanding of the mechanisms explaining the relationship between technology use and sleep would also help to unify the current research, and hopefully give some account to divergent findings.

Potential Mechanisms

Several mechanisms have been proposed as explaining the relationship between technology use and sleep. These have included sleep displacement, arousal, light exposure, electromagnetic field exposure, and sleep interruption. While many studies discuss possible mechanisms, few directly test these relationships. It is probably likely that more than one mechanism is responsible for the effect of technology use on sleep, and that the mechanism is likely to vary according to variables pertaining to the technology use (type, timing, quantity) and variables pertaining to the individual (age, parental influences, SES, etc.).

Displacement

The displacement hypothesis states that technology use affects sleep by displacing the time that the child or adolescent would usually spend asleep (Eggermont & van den Bulck, 2006; Gupta et al., 1994; Olds et al., 2006; van den Bulck, 2000; 2004). That is, using technology before one's typical bedtime results in delaying bedtime. It is argued that technological activities are more likely to displace sleep than structured activities that have a clear beginning and end (e.g., sports practice; van den Bulck, 2004). This notion is consistent with findings of later bedtimes and less sleep associated with technology use. However, it does not give an account for why technology use would prolong sleep latencies. While there is some debate about whether technology use displaces sleep (van den Bulck, 2004), displaces physical activity (Olds et al., 200), or simply displaces other activities that may be part of unstructured leisure time (Gupta et al., 1994), this issue has only been tested retrospectively (i.e., gauging differences in bedtimes when using different devices). Therefore, prospective empirical research (i.e., assessing bedtimes before and after a technological device is provided) is needed to further support this mode of action.

Arousal

Physiological, cognitive, and emotional arousal are frequently put forward as possible mechanisms explaining the relationship between technology use and sleep in children and adolescents. It is argued that media with stimulating content is likely to result in heightened arousal, which then impedes sleep onset and potentially shortens sleep (Anderson & Bushman, 2001; Denot-Ledunois, Vardon, Perruchet & Gallego, 1998; Eggermont & van den Bulck, 2006; Fleming & Rickwood, 2001; Ivarsson et al., 2009; Munezawa et al., 2011; Oka et al., 2008; Wang & Perry, 2006; Weaver et al., 2010). Particularly among younger children, developmentally inappropriate violent or adult content may result in emotional arousal and then bedtime resistance, long sleep onset latencies, and nightmares (Mistry et al., 2007; Owens et al., 1999; Paavonen et al., 2006; Thompson & Christakis, 2005). For example, among 297 Finnish children aged 5–6 years, the content of TV programs was the most important predictor of sleeping problems, compared to quantity of TV viewing and quantity of exposure to TV (Paavonen et al., 2006). Just over 1 in 10 boys and nearly 1 in 4 girls aged 16–18 years reported difficulty falling asleep after watching a suspenseful program on TV at night (van den Bulck, 2000). The experimental work that has been done in this area has focused upon arousal following video game playing.

Experimental paradigms that have compared pre-bed violent video gaming to either a nonviolent video game (Fleming & Rickwood, 2001; Ivarsson et al., 2009) or a non-video control condition (Ivarsson et al., 2009; Wang & Perry, 2006; Weaver et al., 2010) have found video games to result in increased heart rate (Fleming & Rickwood, 2001; Ivarsson et al., 2009; Wang & Perry, 2006), decreased subjective sleepiness (Fleming & Rickwood, 2001; Weaver et al., 2010), increased sleep onset latency (Weaver et al., 2010; Ivarsson, personal communication), heightened cognitive alertness (measured as alpha power; Weaver et al., 2010), higher systolic and diastolic blood pressure, increased ventilation and respiratory rate, increased oxygen consumption and increased energy expenditure (Wang & Perry, 2006) in children and adolescents aged 7–18 years. These results mirror those found among adults (Hebert, Beland, Dionne-Fournelle, Crete & Lupien, 2005; Higuchi, Motohashi, Liu & Maeda, 2005). Research examining a nonviolent video game highlighted that the content of the video game may result in differential effects (Denot-Ledinois et al., 1998). A further illustration was demonstrated with 10 children (aged 9 years) while playing the puzzle game *Tetris* (Denot-Ledinois et al., 1998). Playing this game did not result in any increases to heart rate or cortisol. Breathing frequency decreased from baseline, possibly as a response to the increased attention required to deal with unpredictable stimuli. These results further highlight the effect of video game playing is likely to depend on the type of game played.

Light

Light is an important *zeitgeber* (time giver), and helps to entrain the individual to the 24-hour circadian rhythm, especially in the morning. However, exposure to light at night increases the risk of shifting circadian rhythms later, a risk already heightened during adolescence due to maturational factors (Taylor, Jenni, Acebo & Carskadon, 2005). While a number of studies of technology use in children and adolescents refer to light exposure as a mechanism that affects sleep (Eggermont & van den Bulck, 2006; Johnson et al., 2004; Oka et al., 2008; Thompson & Christakis, 2005), researchers have not directly examined this process. Studies of adults have shown that low-intensity light (100lux) can suppress melatonin secretion and shift circadian rhythm timing (Boivin, Duffy, Kronauer & Czeisler, 1996; Cajochen, Zeitzer, Czeisler & Dijk, 2000; Zeitzer, Dijk, Kronauer, Brown & Czeisler, 2000). The answer to whether or not light from technology devices can exert any effect is likely to be complex and depend on the intensity, timing, and duration of light, as well as the wavelength of light. Light has a stronger delaying effect at greater intensities two hours prior to the endogenous circadian temperature minimum (often occurring around 5am; Crowley, Acebo, & Carskadon, 2007; Minors, Waterhouse, & Wirz-Justice, 1991). Yet, the evidence for adolescents is nonexistent. The closest study to date is of young adults (mean age 24.7 years) playing video games with either a dark display (15lux) or bright display (45lux) between 11pm and 1:45am. No significant differences were found between the two light displays and their effect on sleep (Higuchi et al., 2005), possibly due to the bright light display not being bright enough. Technology devices tend to radiate low-intensity light (Eggermont & van den Bulck, 2006). Whether or not light exposure from technological devices is of sufficient brightness, duration, and proximity to the circadian nadir is a subject for further research (Lasko, Kripke & Elliot, 1999).

Electromagnetic Fields

Exposure to electromagnetic fields emitted from cell phones has been proposed as a possible mechanism which could interfere with sleep (Hamblin & Wood, 2002; Loughran, Wood, Barton, Croft, Thompson & Stough, 2005; Munezawa et al., 2011; Wood, Loughran & Stough, 2006), either through the effect of emissions on sleep architecture, on melatonin secretion, or both. Previous findings have been inconsistent and performed on adults (Hamblin & Wood, 2002); however, enhanced electroencephalogram (EEG) spectral power in the alpha-wave band has been reported in several studies of human and animals (Hamblin & Wood, 2002). One study compared a group of 55 adults who received one night of 30 minutes of exposure to cell phone emissions and one night of 30 minutes of sham exposure, in randomized order (Wood et al., 2006). Total melatonin metabolite output was not significantly different between conditions; however melatonin output at bedtime was significantly reduced following cell phone exposure, indicating possible changes to melatonin onset time (a marker of circadian rhythm timing) following exposure. When considering individual responses to exposure, the results were suggestive of a small number of responders in the group. This is after only 30 min exposure, which is likely to be less than the average amount of time spent on such a device in the hours before bed. In a similar experimental protocol, Loughran and colleagues (2005) found a transitory increase in EEG spectral power in the sleep spindle frequency and reduced rapid eye movement (REM) sleep latency, but no significant changes to sleep quality or melatonin secretion following exposure. Inconsistent findings in adults, coupled with a lack of pediatric studies, mean that the contribution of electromagnetic emissions to sleep changes following mobile phone use is unclear.

Sleep Interruption

While the pre-bedtime period is a time when technology is often used and is likely to influence the timing and onset of sleep, the impact of technology *during* the sleep period may also be an important contributor—particularly among adolescents, and mainly with the ubiquitous cell phone. One study reported that while most cell phone use occurred immediately after lights out, 20.3% of teens text and 17.3% make calls between midnight and 3am. An additional 18.6% who send text messages and 20.2% who make calls after lights-out report using their mobile phone at *any time* of the night (van den Bulck, 2007). Among older adolescents (aged 15–17 years), 1 in 5 reported being woken by an incoming text message between one and three times per month, 1 in 10 were woken at least once per week by text messages, while 8.9% were woken several times per week and 2.9% reported being woken *every day* (van den Bulck, 2003). Thus, it would appear that a number of teens are being roused from sleep by cell phone calls and messages. Eighteen percent of adolescents (13–18 yrs) in the NSF 2011 Sleep in America Poll reported that they were woken *at least a few nights per week* by calls, text messages, or emails on their mobile phone. Over one-quarter of those teens slept with their cell phone in their bedroom with the ringer switched on. Whether this suggests that "Generation Z'ers" (13–18 years) expect to be available 24/7 is yet to be determined. Emerging evidence is suggesting the socialization and formation of new friendships is a form of enjoyment via technology use despite poorer sleep quality (e.g., Smyth, 2007).

The NSF (2011) also asked participants about the activities they perform during periods when they are awake during the night. Of the 35% of adolescents who reported waking during the night, 32% reported watching TV during wake periods, 14% use the Internet, 35% send, read, or receive text messages, 32% listen to music on a portable music device (such as an MP3 player or iPod), 8% play video games, 16% talk on the phone, and 11% watch videos on a computer, laptop, or mobile phone. These statistics suggest these teens had easy access to all of these devices during the night. Clearly, engaging with these devices (and each other) is likely to extend the period of wakefulness during the night, thus reducing their sleep obtained. These results also highlight the importance of considering technology use *during* the sleep period, as well as obtaining information about wake periods after sleep onset, in order to draw casual conclusions.

Moving Forward

Directions for Future Research

We propose here areas where future research efforts may be directed in order to keep a current understanding of the influences of technology use on sleep, as well as understanding how these effects occur:

- Large-scale surveys of children's and adolescents' use of technology are needed on a regular basis to keep up with the rapid advances in technological devices and their capabilities. Similarly, prospective studies of cohorts will inform of concurrent changes in sleep and technology use.
- For large-scale surveys, ideally, standardized measures of sleep should be used that capture

bedtimes, sleep latency, number of awakenings, wake after sleep onset, and total sleep time on school nights and weekends (e.g., School Sleep Habits Survey; Wolfson et al., 2003).

- In relation to the above, researchers are asked to pay particular attention to measuring the moderating influences of age, gender, SES and, most importantly, parental involvement when conducting large-scale surveys.
- Experimental studies are also required to understand the mechanisms of how technology use affects sleep. Currently, most empirical research has been tested with video gaming. We recommend researchers also investigate other devices, particularly cell phones.
- Researchers are also asked to look at their data for individual differences. That is, which children and adolescents are showing the largest responses to technology use? Why them?
- Finally, if a child's or adolescent's sleep is affected by technology use, then we should expect some negative consequence of this in order for it to be a problem. Thus, we recommend investigating possible impairments (e.g., tiredness, sleepiness, etc.) in both large-scale surveys and experimental paradigms.

Recommendations for Families and Professionals

Trends indicate the number of technological devices in families' homes will continue to grow, and the exponential growth of the number of children and adolescents who use these devices before bed will begin to plateau as it reaches the ceiling of 100%. Although the suite of technological activities is not considered addictive (with the exception of online gaming; King et al., 2011), we nevertheless provide a range of suggestions based on the principle of harm reduction (Marlatt & Witkiewitz, 2002)—that is, allowing use of technology yet also setting limits to reduce the effects on sleep. These suggestions are based on the evidence reviewed in this chapter, as well as the model presented in Figure 11.1:

- Broadly, we recommend parents remain involved and knowledgeable about the types of technology that their children and adolescents are using. This will help parents and caregivers to be aware of the content of the media that is being accessed. The AAP already has advice and policies with regard to children's media use, and we recommend families familiarize themselves with these (http://www2.aap.org/healthtopics/mediause.cfm).
- Despite the few studies investigating the content of media use, we nevertheless recommend parents use available tools to restrict inappropriate content. Many TVs have content filters with which parents can restrict programs according to their classification. Parent-controlled timers exist on some TVs and video game consoles that restrict the times they can be used, or how long they can

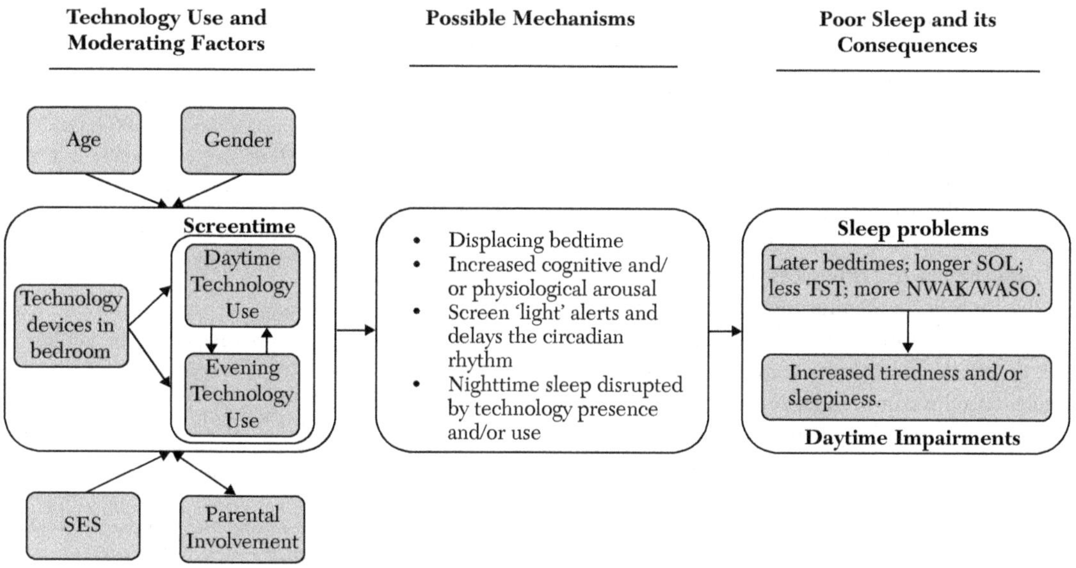

Figure 11.1 Proposed model of the effects of technology use on the sleep of children and adolescents.

Abbreviations: SES = socioeconomic status; SOL= sleep onset latency; TST = total sleep time; NWAK = number of awakenings; WASO = wake after sleep onset.

be played. Content filters are beneficial on all devices that have Internet capabilities, and can be introduced at the router or application level, so content may be restricted at or away from home, respectively.

- Parents will inevitably have difficultly removing technological devices from their children's bedrooms, but the emerging evidence suggests that of all devices, cell phones and other portable devices (e.g., iPods, iPads) should be removed near and/or at bedtime. This action should protect against longer sleep latencies and sleep disruption, as well as the proposed effects of light and electromagnetic transmission.
- In recognition of the possibility that adolescents may use media as a "sleep aid," the evidence suggests parents encourage their children to exchange at least some of the time using technological devices for reading printed books before bed.

Conclusion

In the past couple of decades, we have seen (among others) Captain Kirk's communicator become a reality (i.e., cell phones), families exchange information across the globe with remarkable speed (i.e., the Internet), and the ability to manipulate information with a simple touch, swipe, or pinch of our fingertips (i.e., multi–touch screen technology). Short of intending to make our lives "easier," and notwithstanding the educational benefits of using such tools, current technological devices are primarily providing a highly stimulating and entertaining experience. In moderation, technology use can enhance our lives. However, "technological stimulation" is in opposition to the relaxation necessary for healthy, uninterrupted sleep. It is clear from the evidence that too many children and adolescents are "technologically stimulated" too close to the time needed for sleep. While TVs are the most commonly researched technological device thus far, we view the mobility and multitasking of cell phones as the most disruptive to healthy sleep in youth. What the sleep community requires is to provide evidence-based recommendations to families about safe limits (i.e., how much use, the type of activity/device, and when to stop) of technology use for their children. Future investigations of *(1)* the effects of each activity and total "screentime," *(2)* the mechanisms involved, and *(3)* the characteristics of children and adolescents whose sleep is most affected by technology use are needed in order to promote healthy sleep hygiene.

Note

This chapter concentrated on technological aspects of sleep hygiene. For other aspects (e.g., caffeine, drugs, alcohol) we refer the reader to Chapter 36—Substance Use: Caffeine, Alcohol, and Other Drugs.

References

Adam, E. K., Snell, E. K., & Pendry, P. (2007). Sleep timing and quantity in ecological and family context: A nationally representative time-diary study. *Journal of Family Psychology, 21*, 4–19.

American Academy of Pediatrics Committee on Communications. (1995). Media violence. *Pediatrics, 95*, 949–951.

American Academy of Pediatrics Committee on Public Education. (2001). Children, adolescents, and television. *Pediatrics, 107*, 423–426.

Anderson, C. A., & Bushman, B. J. (2001). Effects of violent video games on aggressive behaviour, aggressive cognition, aggressive affect, physiological arousal, and prosocial behaviour: A meta-analytic review of the scientific literature. *Psychological Science, 12*, 353–359.

BaHammam, A., Bin Saeed, A., Al-Faris, E., & Shaikh, S. (2006). Sleep duration and its correlates in a sample of Saudi elementary school children. *Singapore Medical Journal, 47*, 875–881.

Boivin, D. B., Duffy, J. F., Kronauer, R. E., & Czeisler, C. A. (1996). Dose-response relationships for resetting of human circadian clock by light. *Nature, 379*, 540–542.

Cain, N., & Gradisar, M. (2010). Electronic media use and sleep in school-aged children and adolescents: A review. *Sleep Medicine, 11*, 735–742.

Cajochen, C., Zeitzer, J. M., Czeisler, C. A., & Dijk, D-J. (2000). Does-response relationship for light intensity and ocular and electroencephalographic correlates of human alertness. *Behavioural Brain Research, 115*, 75–83.

Calamaro, C. J., Mason, T. B. A., & Ratcliffe, S.J. Adolescents living the 24/7 lifestyle: Effects of caffeine and technology on sleep duration and daytime functioning. *Pediatrics* [serial online] 2009 [cited June 22, 2009];*123*:e1005–e1010.

Crowley, S. J., Acebo, C., & Carskadon, M. A. (2007). Sleep, circadian rhythms, and delayed phase in adolescence. *Sleep Medicine, 8*, 602–612.

Denot-Ledunois, S., Vardon, G., Perruchet, P., & Gallego, J. (1998). The effect of attentional load on the breathing pattern in children. *International Journal of Psychophysiology, 29*, 13–21.

Drescher, A. A., Goodwin, J. L., Silva, G. E., & Quan, S. F. (2011). Caffeine and screen time in adolescence: Associations with short sleep and obesity. *Journal of Clinical Sleep Medicine, 7*, 337–342.

Dworak, M., Schierl, T., Bruns, T., & Struder, H. K. (2007). Impact of singular excessive computer game and television exposure on sleep patterns and memory performance of school-aged children. *Pediatrics, 120*, 978–985.

Eggermont, S., & Van den Bulck, J. (2006). Nodding off or switching off? The use of popular media as a sleep aid in secondary-school children. *Journal of Paediatrics and Child Health, 42*, 428–433.

Field, A. R. (1999). Music enhances sleep in preschool children. *Early Child Development and Care, 150*, 65–68.

Fleming, M. J., & Rickwood, D. J. (2001). Effects of violent versus non-violent video games on children's arousal, aggressive mood, and positive mood. *Journal of Applied Social Psychology, 31*, 2047–2071.

Ford-Jones, A., & Nieman, P. (2003). Impact of media use on children and youth. *Paediatrics & Child Health, 8,* 301–306.

Foti, K. E., Eaton, D.K., Lowry, R., & McKnight-Ely, L. R. (2011). Sufficient sleep, physical activity and sedentary behaviors. *American Journal of Preventative Medicine, 41,* 596–602.

Fuligni, A. J., & Hardway, C. (2006). Daily variation in adolescents' sleep, activities, and psychological well-being. *Journal of Research on Adolescence, 16,* 353–378.

Gaina, A., Sekine, M., Kanayama, H., Sengoku, K., Yamagami, T., & Kagamimori, S. (2005). Short and long sleep latency and associated factors in Japanese junior high school children. *Sleep and Biological Rhythms, 3,* 162–165.

Gaina, A., Sekine, M., Hamanishi, S., Chen, X., Kanayama, H., Yamagami, T., et al. (2006). Epidemiological aspects of self-reported sleep onset latency in Japanese junior high school children. *Journal of Sleep Research, 15,* 266–275.

Gregory, A. M., Noone, D. M., Eley, T. C., & Harvey, A. G. (2010). Catastrophizing and symptoms of sleep disturbances in children. *Journal of Sleep Research, 19,* 175–182.

Gupta, R. K., Saini, D. P., Acharya, U., & Miglani, N. (1994). Impact of television on children. *Indian Journal of Pediatrics, 61,* 153–159.

Hamblin, D. L., & Wood, A. W. (2002). Effects of mobile phone emissions on human brain activity and sleep variables. *International Journal of Radiation Biology, 78,* 659–669.

Harada, T., Morikuni, M., Yoshii, S., Yamashita, Y., & Takeuchi, H. (2002). Usage of mobile phone in the evening or at night makes Japanese students evening-typed and night sleep uncomfortable. *Sleep and Hypnosis, 4,* 149–153.

Hauri, P. J. (1977). *Current Concepts: The Sleep Disorders.* Kalamazoo, MI: Upjohn.

Hebert, S., Beland, R., Dionne-Fournelle, O., Crete, M., & Lupien, S. J. (2005). Physiological stress response to video-game playing: the contribution of built-in music. *Life Sciences, 76,* 2371–2380.

Higuchi, S., Motohashi, Y., Liu, Y., & Maeda, A. (2005). Effects of playing a computer game using a bright display on presleep physiological variables, sleep latency, slow wave sleep and REM sleep. *Journal of Sleep Research, 14,* 267–273.

Ivarsson, M., Anderson, M., Akerstedt, T., & Lindblad, F. (2009). Playing a violent television game affects heart rate variability. *Acta Paediatrica, 98,* 166–172.

Johns. M. W. (1991). A new method for measuring daytime sleepiness: The Epworth sleepiness scale. *Sleep, 14,* 540–545.

Johnson, J. G., Cohen, P., Kasen, S., First, M. B., & Brook, J. S. (2004). Association between television viewing and sleep problems during adolescence and early adulthood. *Archives of Pediatric and Adolescent Medicine, 158,* 562–568.

Kaiser Family Foundation. (2010). *Generation M2: Media in the lives of 8- to 18-year-olds.* Menlo Park, California: Henry J Kaiser Family Foundation.

King, D. L., Delfabbro, P. H., Griffiths, M. D., & Gradisar, M. (2011). Assessing clinical trials of Internet addiction treatment: A systematic review and CONSORT evaluation. *Clinical Psychology Review, 31,* 1110–1116.

Lasko, T. A., Kripke, D. F., & Elliot, J. A. (1999). Melatonin suppression by illumination of upper and lower visual fields. *Journal of Biological Rhythms, 14,* 122–125.

Lemola, S., Brand, S., Vogler, N., Perkinson-Gloor, N., Allemand, M., & Grob, A. (2011). Habitual computer game playing at night is related to depression symptoms. *Personality and Individual Differences, 51,* 117–122.

Li, S., Jin, X., Wu, S., Jiang, F., Yan, C., & Shen, X. (2007). The impact of media use on sleep patterns and sleep disorders among school-aged children in China. *Sleep, 30,* 361–367.

Loughran, S. P., Wood, A. W., Barton, J. M., Croft, R. J., Thompson, B., & Stough, C. (2005). The effect of electromagnetic fields emitted by mobile phones on human sleep. *Neuroreport, 16,* 1973–1976.

Marlatt, G. A., & Witkiewitz, K. (2002). Harm reduction approaches to alcohol use: Health promotion, prevention, and treatment. *Addictive Behaviors, 27,* 867–886.

Mesquita, G., & Reimao, R. (2007). Nightly use of computer by adolescents: Its effect on quality of sleep. *Arquivos de Neuro-Psiquiatria, 65,* 428–432.

Mindell, J. A., Meltzer, L. J., Carskadon, M. A., & Chervin, R. D. (2009). Developmental aspects of sleep hygiene: Findings from the 2004 National Sleep Foundation "Sleep in America Poll." *Sleep Medicine, 10,* 771–779.

Minors, D. S., Waterhouse, J. M., & Wirz-Justice, A. (1991). A human phase-response curve to light. *Neuroscience Letters, 133,* 36–40.

Mistry, K. B., Minkovitz, C. S., Strobino, D. M., & Borzekowski, D. L. G. (2007). Children's television exposure and behavioural and social outcomes at 5.5 years: Does timing of exposure matter? *Pediatrics, 120,* 762–769.

Mitrofan, O., Paul, M., & Spencer, N. (2009). Is aggression in children with behavioural and emotional difficulties associated with television viewing and video game playing? A systematic review. *Child: Care, Health and Development, 35,* 5–15.

Munezawa, T., Kaneita, Y., Osaki, Y., Kanda, H., Minowa, M., Suzuki, K., et al. (2011). The association between use of mobile phones after lights out and sleep disturbances among Japanese adolescents: A nationwide cross-sectional survey. *Sleep, 34,* 1013–1020.

National Sleep Foundation (2006). *2006 Sleep in America Poll.* Washington, DC: National Sleep Foundation.

National Sleep Foundation (2011). *2011 Sleep in America Poll.* Washington, DC: National Sleep Foundation.

Oka, Y., Suzuki, S., & Inoue, Y. (2008). Bedtime activities, sleep environment, and sleep/wake patterns of Japanese elementary school children. *Behavioral Sleep Medicine, 6,* 220–233.

Olds, T., Ridley, K., & Dollman, J. (2006). Screenieboppers and extreme screenies: The place of screen time in the time budgets of 10–13 year-old Australian children. *Australian and New Zealand Journal of Public Health, 30,* 137–142.

Owens, J., Maxim, R., McGuinn, M., Nobile, C., & Msall, M. Television-viewing habits and sleep disturbance in school children. *Pediatrics* [serial online] 1999 [cited May 13, 2008];*104*:e27. Available from: www.pediatrics.org/cgi/content/full/104/3/e27.

Paavonen, E. J., Pennonen, M., Roine, M., Valkonen, S., & Lahikainen, A. R. (2006). TV exposure associated with sleep disturbances in 5- to 6-year-old children. *Journal of Sleep Research, 15,* 154–161.

Punamaki, R.-L., Wallenius, M., Nygard, C.-H., Saarni, L., & Rimpela, A. (2007). Use of information and communication technology (ICT) and perceived health in adolescence: the role of sleeping habits and waking-time tiredness. *Journal of Adolescence, 30,* 569–585.

Roberts, D. F., Foehr, U. G., Rideout, V. J., & Brodie, M. (1999). *Kids and Media @ the New Millennium.* Kaiser Family Foundation: Washington D.C.

Saarenpaa-Heikkila, O., Laippala, P., & Koivikko, M. (2000). Subjective daytime sleepiness in schoolchildren. *Family Practice*, *17*, 129–133.

Saarenpaa-Heikkila, O. A., Rintahaka, P. J., Laippala, P. J., & Koivikko, M. J. (2000). Subjective daytime sleepiness and related predictors in Finnish schoolchildren. *Sleep and Hypnosis*, *2*, 139–146.

Shochat, T., Flint-Bretler, O., & Tzischinsky, O. (2010). Sleep patterns, electronic media exposure and daytime sleep-related behaviours among Israeli adolescents. *Acta Paediatrica*, *99*, 1396–1400.

Smyth, J. M. (2007). Beyond self-selection in video game play: An experimental examination of the consequences of massively multiplayer online role-playing game play. *Cyberpsychology & Behavior*, *10*, 717–721.

Soderqvist, F., Carlberg, M., & Hardell, L. Use of wireless telephones and self reported health symptoms: A population-based study among Swedish adolescents aged 15–19 years. *Environmental Health* [serial online] 2008 [cited June 22, 2009];7. Available from: http://www.ehjournal.net/content/7/1/18.

Tan, L. P. (2004). The effects of background music on quality of sleep in elementary school children. *Journal of Music Therapy*, *41*, 128–150.

Taylor, D. J., Jenni, O. G., Acebo, C., & Carskadon, M. A. (2005). Sleep tendency during extended wakefulness: Insights into adolescent sleep regulation and behavior. *Journal of Sleep Research*, *14*, 239–244.

Thompson, D. A., & Christakis, D. A. (2005). The association between television viewing and irregular sleep schedules among children less than 3 years of age. *Pediatrics*, *116*, 851–856.

Thorleifsdottir, B., Bjornsson, J.K., Benediktsdottir, B., Gislason, T., & Kristbjarnarson, H. (2002). Sleep and sleep habits from childhood to young adulthood over a 10-year period. *Journal of Psychosomatic Research*, *53*, 529–537.

Toyran, M., Ozmert, E., & Yurdakok, K. (2002). Television viewing and its effect on physical health of school-age children. *Turkish Journal of Pediatrics*, *44*, 94–203.

Tynjala, J., Kannas, L., & Valimaa, R. (1993). How young Europeans sleep. *Health Education Research*, *8*, 69–80.

Van den Bulck, J. (2000). Is television bad for your health? Behavior and body image of the adolescent "couch potato." *Journal of Youth and Adolescence*, *29*, 273–288.

Van den Bulck, J. (2003). Text messaging as a cause of sleep interruption in adolescents, evidence from a cross-sectional study. *Journal of Sleep Research*, *12*, 263.

Van den Bulck, J. (2004). Television viewing, computer game playing, and internet use and self-reported time to bed and time out of bed in secondary-school children. *Sleep*, *27*, 101–104.

Van den Bulck, J. (2007). Adolescent use of mobile phones for calling and for sending text messages after lights out: Results from a prospective cohort study with a one-year follow-up. *Sleep*, *30*, 1220–1223.

Wang, X., & Perry, A.,C. (2006). Metabolic and physiologic responses to video game play in 7- to 10-year old boys. *Archives of Pediatric and Adolescent Medicine*, *160*, 411–415.

Weaver, E., Gradisar, M., Dohnt, H., Lovato, N., & Douglas, P. (2010). The effect of pre-sleep video game playing on adolescent sleep. *Journal of Clinical Sleep Medicine*, *6*, 184–189.

Wolfson, A. R., Carskadon, M. A., Acebo, C., Seifer, R., Fallone, G., Labyak, S.E., et al. (2003). Evidence for the validity of a sleep habits survey for adolescents. *Sleep*, *26*, 213–216.

Wood, A. W., Loughran, S. P., & Stough, C. (2006). Does evening exposure to mobile phone radiation affect subsequent melatonin production? *International Journal of Radiation Biology*, *82*, 69–76

Yen, C. F., Ko, C. H., Yen, J. Y., & Cheng, C. P. (2008). The multidimensional correlates associated with short nocturnal sleep duration and subjective insomnia among Taiwanese adolescents. *Sleep*, *31*, 1515–1525.

Zeitzer, J. M., Dijk, D-J., Kronauer, R. E., Brown, E. N., & Czeisler, C. A. (2000). Sensitivity of the human circadian pacemaker to nocturnal light: Melatonin phase resetting and suppression. *Journal of Physiology*, *526*, 695–702.

CHAPTER

12 Co-sleeping and Self-soothing during Infancy

Melissa M. Burnham

Abstract

This chapter explores the contextualized nature of the constructs of co-sleeping and self-soothing. Definitions and relevant theoretical frameworks are considered first, followed by a review of the relevant literature. Self-soothing and co-sleeping are regarded as components of an infant's developmental niche and as transactional. That is, one cannot understand or judge the effectiveness of either self-soothing or co-sleeping outside of the parenting, familial, racial/ethnic, and cultural contexts within which they occur. It is equally important to consider that infant characteristics are likely to play a role in the development of self-soothing and family sleep arrangement choices. This chapter reviews the controversies and research base behind each perspective on co-sleeping and self-soothing to present a balanced perspective. It concludes with recommendations for future research.

Key Words: co-sleeping, bed sharing, self-soothing, infant sleep, contextual factors, developmental niche

The regulation of infant sleep across the first year of life is arguably one of the greatest apprehensions for new parents, given that sleep concerns are among the top worries brought to the attention of pediatricians (Lozoff, Wolf, & Davis, 1985). Sleep is uniquely situated within a number of embedded contexts, from the macro level of one's cultural, ethnic, and/or societal norms to the micro level of one's family norms and preferences, and the individual characteristics of the infant herself. Parents in modern, postindustrial societies are barraged with an immense volume of often conflicting information regarding establishing healthy sleep habits in their infants. From the neighbor next door whose infant slept through the night from the time he arrived home from the hospital, to the pediatrician who insists that sleep regulation can only occur by following a rigid plan, to the multitude of books written by "experts" with their own unique strategies, to their own feelings regarding what is right based on their upbringing and family norms, it is no wonder that modern parents face unease with regard to infant sleep regulation. The topics of this chapter are particularly timely, given the American Academy of Pediatrics Task Force on Sudden Infant Death Syndrome's (2011) recently revised policy statement on safe sleeping environments and the media attention given to a public service announcement published by the Milwaukee Health Department, equating co-sleeping to sleeping next to a butcher knife. The Milwaukee Health Department ad displays an angelic sleeping baby on a bed with a butcher knife lying next to her, in an attempt to warn parents of the dangers of co-sleeping (Herzog & Stephensen, 2011). These recent events add to the growing body of information on successfully managing the development of sleep regulation that postmodern parents face.

The purpose of this chapter is to summarize what is known about co-sleeping and self-soothing in infancy from the research literature, with a particular emphasis on the importance of considering the contexts within which they emerge and develop. This chapter will define co-sleeping and self-soothing, identify important theoretical frameworks that illustrate the contextual nature of these constructs, and finally discuss the research that has been conducted on co-sleeping and self-soothing with an emphasis on work that has been conducted over the past 5 years. Although much has been learned, there is a great need for further research to develop a greater understanding and more consistent, deliberate recommendations for parents that recognize and support contextual variability.

Defining the Constructs

Co-Sleeping

Co-sleeping is a practice that is inclusive of a number of different sub-practices, each of which involves some form of social sleeping environment. Although some equate co-sleeping with parents sharing the same bed with their infants, the more specific term for this sub-practice is "bed sharing." The term *bed sharing* distinguishes itself from other social sleep situations, such as sleeping in the same room but on a different sleep surface, or sleeping with a different member of the family, which would both fall under the broader category of co-sleeping (c.f., Burnham & Gaylor, 2011). Using this broad definition, the American Academy of Pediatrics actually endorses a form of co-sleeping, namely, room sharing, over the infant's first year of life (American Academy of Pediatrics Task Force on Sudden Infant Death Syndrome, 2011). Despite the existence of more specific terminology, the popular definition of co-sleeping equates it as bed sharing; this chapter will adopt the inclusive definition. When discussing specific studies, however, terminology will be clarified in an attempt to maintain consistency and facilitate understanding of what is being discussed.

Self-Soothing (AKA "sleeping through the night")

Self-soothing is simply the ability of an infant to self-regulate from a more active or distressed state into a quieter one. In the context of sleep regulation, self-soothing specifically refers to moving from an awake state into a sleep state without assistance from or the presence of another person (Anders, 1979). The ability to self-regulate develops gradually across the first year of life; parental emotional availability and specific parenting practices that allow infants the space to practice this skill are thought to assist in its development (e.g., Burnham, Goodlin-Jones, Gaylor, & Anders, 2002; Teti, Kim, Mayer, & Countermine, 2010). Once self-soothing emerges, infants are capable of putting themselves to sleep at night and putting themselves back to sleep after nighttime awakenings. In fact, most infants do continue to wake up during the night across the first year of life; it is the ability to self-soothe that develops in some infants which leads parents to believe that the infant is sleeping through the night.

Context & Parental Expectations

Consistent with viewing development as embedded within a "niche" (Super & Harkness, 1986), context is important when considering self-soothing and co-sleeping. According to Super and Harkness, viewing child development as decontextualized and universal ignores the rich complexity and individual differences that occur due to differences in physical and social settings, culturally regulated customs of child care and child rearing, and the psychology of caretakers, which comprise the child's "developmental niche." The culture in which one lives, along with one's socioeconomic status and ethnicity, greatly impacts what is considered "normal" with regard to expectations regarding sleep habits, sleep locations, and whether sleep is considered a solitary or social experience, among others (Latz, Wolf, & Lozoff, 1999; Lozoff, Askew, & Wolf, 1996; Morelli, Rogoff, Oppenheim, & Goldsmith, 1992; Rothrauff, Middlemiss, & Jacobson, 2004; Wolf, Lozoff, Latz, & Paludetto, 1996). Beyond developments that appear universal, such as the tendency for infants to sleep for longer bouts during the night across the first year of life, sleep experiences and expectations differ greatly across cultures and, indeed, within cultures across parents. Thus, talking about what is considered "normal" with regard to co-sleeping or self-soothing is problematic at best. What is normal for one family in one context may be completely irrelevant to another family in a different context, both within and across cultures.

Another important aspect to consider in relation to the developmental niche framework is the implications for immigrant families (Meléndez, 2005). In effect, immigrant families may experience what could be considered a niche within a niche, the two of which may not be compatible. For example, an immigrant family from a culture in which active parental soothing and co-sleeping were considered normative, indeed, essential, for healthy growth and development may find it challenging to integrate into a culture where such practices are frowned upon and may experience dissonance. This mismatch "holds the potential for conflict and increases the need for cultural sensitivity and competence in those working with families and young children" (Meléndez, 2005, p. 136). Immigrant families potentially experience judgment from the host society with regard to their practices. Moreover, their practices, co-sleeping in particular, may be viewed as dangerous, deviant, and in need of modification (Meléndez, 2005). Meléndez emphasizes the need for practitioners to be sensitive and understanding when interacting with immigrant families and sharing research-based information from their own culture.

The transactional model discussed by Sadeh and Anders (1993) and Anders (1994) proposes bidirectional influences between infant sleep characteristics and contextual factors such as parental beliefs, culture, and so forth. This model has been empirically supported by the work of Tikotsky and Sadeh (2009), which showed that maternal cognitions specific to sleep predicted the sleep characteristics of their infants at 12 months. Moreover, infant sleep characteristics at 6 months predicted maternal cognitions at 12 months, supporting the notion that bidirectional influences exist. Specifically, infants who woke more at 6 months had mothers who endorsed the need for limits regarding sleep at 12 months, possibly indicating that the poor sleep of their infants influenced their cognitions about the need for limit-setting. These authors also found that maternal cognitions related to feeling that their infants experienced distress during the night led to more nighttime interventions and ultimately poorer sleep in their infants. Tikotsky and Sadeh conclude "parents of sleep disturbed infants may experience an internal discrepancy between the knowledge of what is the 'right' approach and their inability to follow this line of action with their own child" (p. 871). Data presented by Burnham et al. (2002) also provide support for the transactional model, with variables related to the infant, the sleeping context, and the parent all contributing to the development of self-soothing at 12 months of age. Thus, there is empirical support for viewing the development of sleep characteristics and the choice of sleep environments using a perspective that acknowledges the importance of both proximal and distal bidirectional contexts. Considering the contexts within which they occur is essential for any analysis or understanding of self-soothing and co-sleeping.

Co-Sleeping: Prevalence, Controversies, and Research

Prevalence

The prevalence of co-sleeping is challenging to pinpoint, partly due to factors related to how co-sleeping is defined and partly because of the likely tendency of parents' self-report to underestimate prevalence, especially in societies where co-sleeping is viewed as dangerous and/or aberrant. Data on prevalence must be considered in light of these qualifications. In general, prevalence has been considered to be higher in cultures which place high value on interdependence as a child socialization goal compared to cultures which place more value on independence (e.g., Asian vs. Western cultures; Nelson, Taylor, et al., 2001), although the independent–interdependent distinction may be an oversimplification. Wolf and colleagues (1996), for example, found that both White and Black American families in their sample valued fostering independence with their 6- to 48-month-old infants. However, 58% of Black families co-slept regularly, while only 19% of White families did so. Indeed, the prevalence of co-sleeping among Black families in their sample was similar to that reported of Japanese families by Latz and colleagues (1999), despite cultural differences between these two groups. Co-sleeping rates within the United States have been reported to be higher for African Americans, single parents, teenage parents, and among parents with lower levels of education, indicating that co-sleeping has multiple determining factors, culture being only one (Brenner, Simons-Morton, Bhaskar, Revenis, Das, & Clemens, 2003; Weimer, Dise, Evers, Ortiz, Welldaregay, & Steinmann, 2002; Willinger, Ko, Hoffman, Kessler, & Corwin, 2003). Thus, differences found in sleep environment prevalence cannot be fully attributed to overarching cultural values. Further, research does not support a link between the degree of preschoolers' independent behaviors and solitary sleeping history (Keller & Goldberg, 2004). Indeed, these researchers found more independent behaviors among preschoolers who had a history of early co-sleeping. Both proximal and distal variables contribute to prevalence rates of co-sleeping, and there does not appear to be an influence on children's degree of independence based on whether or not they experience a social sleeping environment.

In perhaps the largest study to examine sleeping arrangements in the United States to date, Hauck and colleagues (2008) examined data from the Infant Feeding Practices Study II, an investigation that included regular questionnaire assessments of mothers of infants between 2 weeks and 12 months of age (sample sizes ranged from 2353 at 2 weeks to 1778 at 12 months). Bed-sharing rates were reported as 41.5% at 2 weeks, 34% at 3 months, 31% at 6 months, 28% at 9 months, and 27% at 12 months. These relatively high rates were found despite the fact that the sample underrepresented ethnic minorities and mothers with lower socioeconomic status (Hauck, Signore, Fein, & Raju, 2008). The rates also were similar to those reported in a sample from England, where 47% of neonates had shared a bed with a parent at least once (Blair & Ball, 2004) and a sample of Australian infants, 41% of which bed-shared between 2 and 12 weeks (Rigda, McMillen, & Buckley, 2000). It should be underscored that the relatively high rates of bed sharing reported by Hauck and colleagues occurred within the United States, a country where co-sleeping is not recommended by authorities such as the American Academy of Pediatrics or the Consumer Products Safety Commission.

Bed-sharing rates are generally even higher for 3-month-olds in other countries (e.g., China: 88%, Sweden: 65%, Chile: 64%) when compared to rates within the United States (Nelson, Taylor, et al., 2001). When co-sleeping is more broadly defined and includes room-sharing, Nelson and colleagues report even higher prevalence rates (e.g., 100% in Beijing, China, 88% in Florence, Italy, and 91% in Copenhagen, Denmark with 3-month-old infants). It is clear that, in the United States and across the world, co-sleeping is quite prevalent, especially when infants are younger. A notable exception to this general finding of higher prevalence with younger infants comes from a longitudinal study conducted by Jenni and colleagues (2005). Jenni et al. found that regular bed-sharing rates were low (less than 10%) in the first year of life and peaked between 3 and 5 years of age (38%) in their sample of Swiss children. Thus, although most studies have reported higher rates of co-sleeping with younger infants, this finding is not uniform and deserves further investigation with longitudinal, cross-cultural samples that extend beyond the first two years of life.

Controversies

DANGERS

Despite its prevalence within the United States and worldwide, co-sleeping is highly controversial, especially in light of several reports of the dangers of co-sleeping in modern, Western beds and the ensuing position statements of the American Academy of Pediatrics (AAP; most recently, AAP Task Force on Sudden Infant Death Syndrome, 2011). The controversy, which began brewing in the 1990s, was heightened with the publication of a US Consumer Products Safety Commission (CPSC) Safety Alert (1999), which cautioned parents against placing babies in adult beds for sleep due to risks of suffocation and entrapment. An article reviewing and analyzing data collected by the CPSC on adult bed hazards was published in the same year (Nakamura, Wind, & Danello, 1999). In sum, these authors warned of the risks of overlying, entrapment, and suffocation, which resulted in an average of 64 deaths per year for infants sleeping on adult beds. Other research was published around the same time, warning of an increased risk of Sudden Infant Death Syndrome (SIDS) associated with co-sleeping (e.g., Blair et al., 1999; Carroll-Pankhurst & Mortimer, 2001; Kemp et al., 2000; Thogmartin, Siebert, & Pellan, 2001). A more recent meta-analysis confirmed a relationship between bed sharing and SIDS risk (Vennemann et al., 2012). These publications spurred reactions from both contextual sleep researchers and the American Academy of Pediatrics, with the former outraged at the seeming one-sided nature of the admonitions against co-sleeping and the latter spurred to develop a policy statement on safe sleeping environments. A full review of the multiple iterations of the AAP's policy statements extends beyond the scope of this chapter. Instead, the most recent policy statement will be discussed in detail.

The most recent iteration of the AAP's policy statement on safe infant sleeping environments was published in 2011. While earlier iterations had focused on the risk of SIDS from adult–infant bed sharing, the 2011 iteration rightfully expands the risk to Sudden unexpected infant death (SUID), a broader term that encompasses SIDS as well as any sudden and unexpected death in infancy, whether explained or unexplained (AAP Task Force on Sudden Infant Death Syndrome, 2011). According to this policy statement, the subset of sleep-related SUIDs includes SIDS, sleep-related suffocation, asphyxia, and entrapment. This term is more appropriate, given that it is difficult to distinguish whether an infant death during co-sleeping is caused by SIDS or is called SIDS but actually may have been caused by suffocation, asphyxia, or entrapment. Further, death scene reports appear to be highly variable in classifying causes as SIDS, accidental suffocation and strangulation in bed, and/or a combination of factors (Shapiro-Mendoza, Tomashek, Anderson, & Wingo, 2006). Although earlier research focused on links between SIDS and co-sleeping, the more appropriate link includes this wider variety of causes. The recommendations made in the AAP's policy statement (2011) that are specific to infant sleep practices include the following:

1. Back to sleep for every sleep by every caregiver until 1 year;
2. Use a firm sleep surface;
3. Room-sharing without bed-sharing is recommended;
4. Keep soft objects and loose bedding out of the crib to reduce the risk of SIDS, suffocation, entrapment, and strangulation;
5. Breast feeding is recommended;
6. Consider offering a pacifier at naptime and bedtime; and
7. Avoid overheating (AAP Task Force on Sudden Infant Death Syndrome, 2011, pp. 1031–1034).

Notably, although the AAP actively discourages bed sharing, the 2011 policy statement includes a list of specific circumstances that "substantially increase the risk of SIDS or suffocation while bed-sharing" (AAP Task Force on Sudden Infant Death Syndrome, 2011, p. 1033). In effect, although they are not recommending any bed sharing as appropriate, they do provide a list of situations in which bed sharing should absolutely be avoided, thereby indirectly including a list of considerations for safe bed sharing. These include: (a) infant age under 3 months, (b) bed sharing with a current smoker, (c) with someone who is extremely tired, (d) with someone using medications or substances that reduce arousal, (e) with anyone other than one's own parent, (f) with multiple people, (g) on a soft surface, and (h) on a surface with soft bedding (AAP Task Force on Sudden Infant Death Syndrome, 2011, p. 1033). This list indirectly addresses the concerns of some sleep professionals who found the "just don't do it" recommendations of 2000 and 2005 a bit myopic (e.g., McKenna & McDade, 2005; Morgan, Groer, & Smith, 2006; Wailoo, Ball, Fleming, & Platt, 2004). As stated by Morgan and colleagues (2006), "to simply admonish parents not to sleep with their infants, ever, under any circumstances, is unrealistic, quite possibly unethical, and does not provide the optimum in nutrition and sleep physiology for infants" (p. 686).

ALTERNATIVE VIEWPOINTS

The AAP position statements, CPSC warnings, and variety of epidemiological research finding links between SIDS (or, more appropriately SUIDs) and co-sleeping fueled controversy among a variety of groups, particularly among those endorsing breastfeeding, acknowledging the evolutionary context within which infant sleep developed, endorsing attachment theory, and acknowledging the pervasiveness of co-sleeping worldwide. Co-sleeping has been endorsed as a method of maximizing breastfeeding opportunities during the night. Indeed, McKenna and colleagues (1997) reported that infants who were routine bed-sharers breastfed three times longer than infants who were routine solitary sleepers in their laboratory investigation. Ball (2006) also reported a longer duration of breastfeeding for infants sleeping with their mothers on a postnatal ward compared to infants sleeping in a standalone crib (80 minutes vs. 30 minutes, respectively). Similar, Tollenaar and colleagues (2012) reported that both partial and full co-sleeping infants in the first 2 months of life received more breastfeeding when compared to solitary-sleeping infants. Baddock and colleagues (2006) reported breastfeeding as 3.7 times more frequent in bed-sharing infants compared to those who slept separately. Thus, co-sleeping does appear to increase the opportunity for breastfeeding during the night.

Further, co-sleeping proponents often cite the fact that infant sleep "grew up" in the evolutionary context of close body contact with another adult, and thus co-sleeping promotes optimal infant sleep development (McKenna & Mosko, 1993; Morgan, Horn, & Bergman, 2011). A recent investigation by Morgan and colleagues (2011) lends support for this theoretical argument. These researchers found a 176% increase in autonomic activity (measured by heart rate variability) for 2-day-old infants sleeping separately from their mothers compared to when the same infants slept in skin-to-skin contact. Morgan et al. (2011) also reported an 86% decrease in quiet sleep and a longer latency to quiet sleep for separated neonates. These findings suggest that separation in the human neonate is an autonomically stressful experience and that skin-to-skin contact may facilitate greater autonomic regulation and perhaps brain development, through its association with increased levels of quiet sleep. Although this investigation included a small sample size, the results support the argument that close contact between mothers and neonates after birth facilitates optimal physiologic regulation, and thus is most likely the condition under which neonatal physiology evolved (Morgan et al., 2011).

Research by Tollenaar and colleagues (2012) provides further support for the argument that co-sleeping (defined as either bed sharing or room sharing) facilitates physiologic regulation. Tollenaar et al. (2012) found increased cortisol reactivity in response to a mild stressor (bathing) for solitary-sleeping 5-week-old infants compared to co-sleeping infants of the same age. This relationship held despite the authors' controlling for breastfeeding, quality of maternal caregiving behavior, infant night awakenings, and sleep duration. The authors hypothesize that co-sleeping facilitates greater parental contact and thus more external stress regulation, thus decreasing infants' cortisol reactivity during the first 2 months of life (Tollenaar et al., 2012). These findings are indeed controversial, given the AAP's absolute discouragement of bed sharing for infants under 3 months old. They do illustrate, however, that the AAP recommendations against co-sleeping are not uniformly supported by research. Incidentally, there is not universal agreement in research on cortisol reactivity and co-sleeping. Lucas-Thompson and colleagues (2009) reported increased cortisol reactivity to inoculation in both 6- and 12-month-old co-sleeping infants compared to their same-age solitary-sleeping peers. As Tollenaar et al. (2012) point out, these different findings may be due to differences in sleep data collection methods (daily diary vs. questionnaire), different definitions of co-sleeping, possible differences in reasons for co-sleeping at different ages, or possible age-dependent effects on cortisol reactivity of co-sleeping at different ages. Larger longitudinal samples of a wider age range of infants (e.g., starting in the first month and continuing through the first year) with a greater number of cortisol collection points throughout the day and consistent definitions and methods of data collection are needed in order to resolve this discrepancy.

Some co-sleeping advocates also endorse an attachment theory perspective, in which sensitive, responsive caregiving during the first year of life is thought to influence the development of secure attachments between infants and their parent(s). From this perspective, nighttime caregiving that promotes sensitive responsiveness would facilitate the development of secure attachment relationships. To the extent that proximity makes parental nighttime responsiveness to infants more likely, both room sharing and bed sharing would promote secure attachment. Indeed, maternal responsiveness at night (i.e., active soothing) is related to security of attachment, with mothers of securely attached infants more often picking up and soothing their infants during nighttime awakenings (Higley & Dozier, 2009). Further, Teti and colleagues (2010) found that maternal emotional availability during the bedtime routine predicted quality of infant sleep in their sample of 1- to 24-month-old infants. Although not focusing on bed sharing per se, the sample in this investigation did include 13 infants who co-slept with their parent(s), 5 of whom were bed sharing. Co-sleeping mothers and infants in this sample did experience more close contact during the night than did solitary-sleeping pairs (Teti, Kim, Mayer, & Countermine, 2010). Interestingly, but consistent with Tollenaar et al. (2012), emotional availability did not differ between solitary and co-sleeping mothers, although the unequal comparison groups and small sample of co-sleeping mothers limit the generalizability of this finding. Thus, though the evidence is largely indirect, it does point to the possibility that co-sleeping may contribute to parental behaviors that facilitate security of attachment.

Admonishing parents against co-sleeping also ignores the cultural or ethnic context by which the family abides. As noted earlier in framing this chapter, co-sleeping cannot be understood detached from its context. McKenna and McDade (2005) note that "the traditional habit of labeling one sleeping arrangement as being superior to another without an awareness of family, social, and ethnic context is not only wrong but possibly harmful" (p. 134). Co-sleeping supporters also often cite the fact that separate sleep is a Western, industrialized phenomenon. In most cultures around the world with ethnographic descriptions of nighttime sleep environments, mothers and their infants sleep in close physical contact during nighttime sleep (McKenna & McDade, 2005). Further, evidence does not always support a universal negative impact on infants from bed sharing. Wailoo and colleagues (2004), for example, point out that one of the largest and most sophisticated epidemiological investigations found no association between infant death and bed sharing among nonsmoking families. Although the risk was clear for parents who were smokers, there was no relationship between bed sharing per se and infant death for nonsmoking families. In addition, although epidemiological research points to the increased likelihood of suffocation in bed-sharing situations due to airway covering, Ball (2009) found no effect of airway covering during bed sharing on either infants' oxygen saturation levels or heart rate. Thus, although Ball did confirm that airway covering did regularly occur for the majority of infants when parents and infants shared the same bed, she did not find a physiologic effect. Barajas and colleagues (2011) also did not find a relationship between bed sharing and later cognitive or behavioral outcomes in children, once child and mother characteristics were controlled. Given the varying evidence, on the one hand, showing a link between SUIDs and co-sleeping and on the other, showing links between breastfeeding, physiologic regulation, and co-sleeping and its ubiquity worldwide, it seems premature to uniformly endorse one form of sleeping arrangement over another for all families. The controversy will remain unresolved until more sophisticated epidemiological research shows more definitive results.

Self-Soothing: Prevalence, Research, and Controversies

Prevalence

As defined above, self-soothing refers to the capacity of the human infant to move from a more alert to a less alert behavioral state on his/her own. In the context of developmental sleep research, the focus is on the capacity of the infant to fall asleep at bedtime by him/herself and the capacity to put him/herself back to sleep following nighttime awakenings. For the most part, in Western societies, this capacity is viewed as an important milestone, and Western parents often seek to maximize the chance that their infants will develop it. What has been acknowledged for some time is that infants are not "sleeping through the night," as once commonly thought. Instead, many infants continue to wake up throughout the first year of life; it is the capacity to self-soothe that develops in some, leading parents to believe that their infants are sleeping through (e.g., Burnham, et al., 2002). Using objective video observations of nighttime sleep–wake behaviors, these authors found that self-soothing increased linearly from 1 month to 12 months of age in their longitudinal, nonclinical sample, with 1-month-old infants self-soothing after 28% and 12-month-olds self-soothing after 46% of awakenings. Surprisingly, more than half of awakenings at 12 months did require parental intervention. Similar results were found by the same authors with a cross-sectional sample (Goodlin-Jones, Burnham, Gaylor, & Anders, 2001). Thus, although self-soothing is often thought to be viewed by parents as the ultimate goal for their infants, at least half of infants in nonclinical samples still require nighttime intervention at 1 year of age.

In a large, cross-cultural comparison of parent behaviors and sleep characteristics of over 29,000 infants and toddlers in 17 different countries, Mindell, Sadeh, Kohyama, and How (2010) found that self-reported parenting behaviors at sleep onset and following nighttime awakenings differed significantly between primarily Caucasian (P-C) and primarily Asian (P-A) populations. Although these researchers did not study self-soothing directly, self-soothing behavior can be surmised based on whether or not parents intervened at night. The majority of parents in both groups reported that they intervened in some way at sleep onset and following nighttime awakenings, indicating that self-soothing is not common in infants worldwide. Just 23% of infants in the entire sample were reported to fall asleep on their own, whereas 31% most commonly fell asleep in their parents' bed with their parents present (Mindell et al., 2010). However, these percentages differed when viewed by P-A vs. P-C groups. Fifty-seven percent of infants in P-C countries were reported to fall asleep in their own crib by themselves, whereas this pattern was reported for only 4% of P-A infants. Falling asleep with a parent in the parents' bed was reported for 38% of P-A infants but only 11% of P-C infants. Following nighttime awakenings, the most commonly reported intervention for the entire sample was nursing or bottle-feeding (30%), whereas only 6% of parents reported allowing the child to cry him or herself back to sleep. These results were relatively similar across groups, with 29% and 25% of parents reporting nursing back to sleep, respectively, for example. The most striking difference was in the percentage of parents reporting allowing the child to cry, with only 2% of P-A parents endorsing this technique compared to 16% of P-C parents. Thus, although the techniques parents use tend to differ, most 0- to 36-month-old infants worldwide are reported to receive assistance both at bedtime and after nighttime awakenings.

Self-Soothing Research

Other research on self-soothing focuses not only on prevalence but also on the predictors, correlates, and outcomes of self-soothing behaviors. As discussed above in the section on co-sleeping, Teti et al. (2010) studied the relative impact of maternal emotional availability vs. specific maternal bedtime behaviors on infant sleep and self-soothing characteristics, using nighttime video observations.

These researchers found that emotional availability of mothers during the bedtime routine predicted infant sleep quality more than did specific bedtime behaviors such as close contact, quiet activities, and nursing. That is, the quality of maternal–infant interactions at bedtime predicted infants' ability to self-soothe during the night, while the specific techniques used did not. Infants of mothers with lower emotional availability scores tended to both wake up more during the night and require additional interventions at bedtime beyond the first attempt. The authors conclude that, "whatever bedtime practices parents decide to use, the emotional quality of these practices will bear importantly on infants' ability to settle to sleep and to regulate their sleep behavior throughout the night" (Teti et al., 2010, p. 314). These findings, however, do contradict extant research, which has reported correlations between bedtime soothing strategies and infant sleep characteristics (e.g., Burnham et al., 2002; Tikotsky & Sadeh, 2009). Perhaps soothing practices have acted as a proxy for emotional quality in previous research. Regardless, emotional quality of bedtime interactions appears to be an important variable to include in future research on infant self-soothing.

Interestingly, Teti and colleagues (2010) also found that emotional availability of mothers was inversely correlated with infant age. That is, mothers' bedtime interactions were rated as less sensitive with infants older than 12 months, compared to younger infants. This is consistent with the findings of Tikotsky and Sadeh (2009), who found that mothers become less responsive with infant age. This decrease is most likely due to a complex interplay of infants' own physiological regulatory capacity, the increasing tendency of toddlers to resist bedtime and thus require more directive strategies, and mothers' attempts to try different strategies as infants grow older.

In their work on nighttime maternal responsiveness and infant attachment, Higley and Dozier (2009) found that maternal sensitivity during nighttime awakenings was related to security of attachment, with secure infants having mothers who consistently and sensitively responded to their signaled awakenings. There were no differences in the number of nighttime awakenings between securely and insecurely attached infants. Previous research has indicated that "extensive" soothing techniques at bedtime and during the night are related to infant sleep disturbances (e.g., Morrell & Cortina-Borja, 2002). One could argue that picking up and actively soothing an infant following a nighttime awakening, and/or feeding or actively soothing the infant at bedtime would qualify as "extensive" strategies. Thus, it is somewhat surprising that the recent observational work of both Teti and colleagues (2010) and Higley and Dozier (2009) have found that the quality of the implementation of these strategies is more important than the strategies per se. The differences in findings may be attributable to different methodologies. Morrell and Cortina-Borja (2002) used self-report questionnaires on soothing strategies used and perception of infant sleep problems, while both of the latter studies used video observations, so were able to analyze the quality of parent–infant interactions. It is intriguing to consider that parental behaviors once thought to be predictive of night waking and self-settling problems are not the only determinants in a complex web of potential causal factors. These recent findings indicate that the sensitivity and responsiveness qualities of these nighttime interactions are more important to infant sleep characteristics than the fact that they occur. Simple prescriptions for parents to reduce nighttime interaction, then, may not be warranted. Perhaps health care providers and educators should also focus on the quality of these interactions.

An intriguing new line of work has brought focus to the potential sequelae of self-soothing and nighttime sleep for infants. Most pediatric research to date has focused on the consequences of sleep disturbances for school-age children (e.g., Sadeh, Gruber, & Raviv, 2002), thus leaving the potential daytime impact of infant sleep and self-soothing characteristics largely unknown. To date, those studying the development of sleep and self-soothing in infancy have focused on delineating characteristics, and perhaps impact on parents. However, the "so what" question, in terms of daytime consequences, has yet to be answered. Bernier and colleagues (2010) have initiated a line of research examining sleep regulation and executive functioning in 12- to 26-month-old infants, thus beginning to fill the extant gap. These researchers' measures of executive functioning assessed working memory (18 months), impulse control (26 months), and a combination of working memory, set shifting, and inhibitory control (26 months). Sleep at 12 and 18 months was measured through 3-day, 24-hour parent diaries. Most interesting in relation to self-soothing was that sleep fragmentation (i.e., number of night awakenings that parents were aware of) did not relate to measures of executive functioning at either 18 or 26 months. Instead, the only consistent relationship with executive functioning emerged for percent of sleep occurring at night at both 12 and 18 months (Bernier et al., 2010). Children obtaining more nighttime sleep (i.e., less time napping during the day) had higher scores, especially on the measure relating to impulse control, even when controlling for socioeconomic status and general cognitive ability. The line of research focusing on daytime correlates of infant sleep characteristics provides a rich foundation for future work. Thus far, there is no direct evidence that non-self-soothing is detrimental to infants' daytime functioning, at least with regard to executive functioning.

Controversies

Similar to the controversy with regard to co-sleeping, a comparable controversy exists with regard to whether or not the development of self-soothing should be encouraged in infants during the first year of life. A commonly prescribed technique to promote self-soothing is extinction, which involves eliminating or gradually reducing parental responsiveness to infants' signaling behavior at night (Jenni & O'Connor, 2005). Ramos and Youngclarke's (2006) review of parenting advice books found that 61% of books surveyed endorsed an extinction method. However, extinction methods are not universally sanctioned, most notably by proponents of attachment theory who believe that consistent sensitive responsiveness is important for the parent–infant relationship. It is largely recognized that if an infant's non-self-soothing and continued awakenings are not a problem for parents, then they are not a problem that needs to be "fixed" (e.g., Germo, Goldberg, & Keller, 2009; Jenni & O'Connor, 2005; Wolf et al., 1996). Indeed, this notion is supported by the work of Bernier and colleagues (2010), who found no relationship between sleep fragmentation and executive functioning. However, whether or not parents should encourage self-soothing during the first year is still highly contested.

On the one hand, many parenting advice books and well-intentioned, but mostly not sleep-trained, Western clinicians appear to support a "self-soothing is best" platform (Jenni & O'Connor, 2005). Pediatric sleep clinicians see parents who suffer the effects of their infants' non-self-soothing, and thus recommend strategies to help the infant learn to self-soothe. The focus of these techniques is to change infant behavior and thus improve parental well-being. Both parental expectations regarding infants' sleeping through the night and demands of the daytime work environment may combine to create the "perfect storm" for parental distress. Focusing on reducing the number of nighttime interventions necessary has been shown to improve parental feelings of well-being (e.g., Sadeh, Mindell, & Owens, 2011; Wolfson, Lacks, & Futterman, 1992). Clinicians often point out that if non-self-soothing is a problem for parents, then it is a problem that deserves attention. According to Sadeh and colleagues (2011), "... it is certainly in the best interests of the infant to have healthy, well-rested and ultimately more responsive parents" (p. 335). There is some indication that sleep during the first year does relate to cognitive and psychomotor infant development, although the relationships are much more clearly defined in older children and adults, and there is no research to date that suggests the relationship is causal in infancy (Ednick, Cohen, McPhail, Beebe, Simakajornboon, & Amin, 2009). Thus, in promoting self-soothing during infancy, clinicians on this side of the debate focus on (a) the impact on parents of infant non-self-soothing, and (b) the research pointing to correlations between sleep characteristics and daytime function.

On the other hand, many developmental sleep researchers point to the complexity and contextualized nature of self-soothing, and thus do not endorse a one-size-fits-all approach. Indeed, not all parents place a high value on the development of their infants' ability to self-soothe (Germo et al., 2009). Germo et al. found that parents who began bed sharing during the first year and beyond tended to place a lower importance on their infants' ability to sleep through the night, compared to parents who maintained solitary sleeping arrangements. Not surprisingly, these parents also reported less difficulty in helping their child to sleep through the night than did mothers who endorsed solitary sleeping and self-soothing. Thus, parenting values and expectations, once again, are found to be important correlates to infants' sleep and self-soothing characteristics. Other researchers have pointed out that parental expectations regarding infant sleep are influenced by culture and race/ethnicity, such that parents who anticipate self-soothing as "normal" are more distressed by non-self-soothing, and thus bring these concerns to clinicians and seek intervention techniques (Jenni & O'Connor, 2005; Milan, Snow, & Belay, 2007). Milan et al. (2007) found that a significantly greater percentage of White mothers in the United States reported that their infants' sleep was troublesome compared to African-American and Latina mothers. The sense of distress that parents feel by non-self-soothing is summarized best in one mother's response during an interview on sleep practices: "She doesn't go to sleep by herself and that means she's never going to be an independent person" (Rowe, 2003, p. 188). Thus, there is a complex interplay between culture, parenting values, parental expectations, and race/ethnicity and viewing infant sleep behaviors as problematic.

Further, as discussed above, Higley and Dozier (2009) have reported a relationship between mother–infant attachment and infant self-soothing at 12 months. Specifically, securely attached infants did tend to signal for their mothers during the night, with 63% being classified as clear signalers. Perhaps more importantly, these researchers found a strong relationship between attachment style (secure/insecure) and mothers' patterns of nighttime interactions. Mothers of securely attached infants picked up and soothed their infants during nighttime awakenings significantly more than did mothers of insecurely attached infants; however, there was no difference in frequency of responding between the two groups. Further, consistent with previous nighttime observational research (e.g., Burnham et al., 2002), about half of 12-month-olds, regardless of attachment status, were placed into their cribs already asleep. According to Higley and Dozier, "the interactions most characteristic of secure dyads involved infants signaling their awakenings with fussing or crying and mothers responding quickly by picking up and soothing the baby" (p. 357). Although directionality cannot be inferred, the correlation between sensitive and responsive interactions at night and infant–mother attachment security warrants further attention.

A recent theoretical review also calls into question the universal endorsement of extinction approaches to nighttime sleep training (Blunden, Thompson, & Dawson, 2011). These researchers point out that disregarding an infant's cry, arguably his/her only method of communicating distress, requires parents to ignore "their emotional and instinctive drives" (p. 328). Blunden et al. further note that extinction methods are gauged "successful" if they result in a decrease in nighttime crying and parental interventions; however, it is unknown how the infant interprets and experiences the lack of responsiveness to his/her attempts at communicating distress. In their conclusion, Blunden and colleagues encourage researchers "to consider that 'desirable' infant sleep behavior is... morally and culturally defined" (p. 332) (see Moore and Mindell, Chapter 37). As self-identified challengers of the status quo, Blunden and colleagues raise to awareness a number of interesting points that are worthy of discussion rather than outright dismissal.

Conclusion

Although much has been learned about co-sleeping and self-soothing through the rigorous work of sleep and development researchers over the past decade, there is clearly more work to be done. Further research into both co-sleeping and self-soothing is sorely needed, particularly that which includes an analysis of a rich variety of contextual factors (e.g., culture, race/ethnicity, parenting values) and a measure of the quality of nighttime parenting interactions rather than only the behaviors themselves. Epidemiological research on the correlates of SUIDS should include a wide variety of potential variables, including both bed sharing and independent sleep arrangements, along with covariates such as race/ethnicity, in order to disentangle the relationships previously found between bed sharing and SUIDS. Further, this research should consider a detailed account of the death scene, such that other factors (e.g., parental intoxication, bedding) can be included in analyses. Research designs should be longitudinal wherever possible to examine the same infants and parents across time, and sleep and nighttime interaction measures should be objective (e.g., in the form of actigraphy, video, or a combination thereof). While correlational research is helpful in determining relationships between variables, experimental designs would greatly enrich the field and allow for analysis of causal relationships. Finally, research should continue along the path initiated by Bernier and colleagues (2010), analyzing the daytime impact of sleep regulation during infancy. It is only through careful attention to sleep development across infancy, analyzed within its developmental niche, that we will be capable of disentangling the complex web of influential factors.

If anything, this chapter illuminates the fact that co-sleeping and self-soothing in infancy are complex phenomena. They must be understood in the familial and cultural contexts within which they occur. Safety factors must be an added consideration in relation to co-sleeping. Two ultimate recommendations are suggested: First, we need to continue the rich lines of research begun in these two areas, particularly with family context and quality of parenting considered. Second, parents would benefit from receiving valid, reliable, consistent, research-based information on both co-sleeping and self-soothing so that they can make informed decisions. Although it would be impossible, and perhaps not even desirable, to eliminate the vast number of parenting advice books written by sleep "experts" with diverging opinions on what is necessary or "best," it may behoove the actual experts (i.e., the researchers and clinicians studying these phenomena) to provide consistent, research-based information to families, with pros and cons of different strategies noted objectively. Additionally, families would benefit from advice on how to be objective, informed consumers of media on self-soothing and co-sleeping so they can make decisions that work best within their unique contexts. What is true to date is that we do not have sufficient evidence to fully endorse or reject any strategy for all people. Sleep and its development are highly contextual and must be recognized as such. It would seem beneficial, then, for real sleep experts to disseminate this balanced approach to parents. Perhaps more sleep would be had by all if a more balanced view was more widely recognized.

Future Directions

While there is a growing body of research into co-sleeping and self-soothing, more questions remain. The following questions present some of the difficult problems that deserve attention in the field of sleep and development:

- Do sleeping environments and soothing styles have a direct impact on child development or children's daytime behavior? If so, under what contexts, for which children, and at what age(s)?
- What specific aspects define the quality of nighttime parenting interactions and how can these best be studied both reliably and validly? Is quality defined differently for different ages of infants?
- Using objective measures, which aspects of infants' daytime behavior are correlated with sleep regulation or sleep environment differences?
- Through experimental manipulation and a longitudinal design, can a causal relationship be established between infants' sleep regulation and daytime behavior or functioning? Under what contexts, for which children, and at what age(s)?

References

American Academy of Pediatrics Task Force on Sudden Infant Death Syndrome. (2011). SIDS and other sleep-related infant deaths: Expansion of recommendations for a safe infant sleeping environment. *Pediatrics, 128,* 1030–1039.

Anders, T. F. (1979). Night waking in infants during the first year of life. *Pediatrics, 63,* 860–864.

Anders, T. F. (1994). Infant sleep, nighttime relationships, and attachment. *Psychiatry: Interpersonal and Biological Processes, 57,* 11–21.

Baddock, S. A., Galland, B. C., Bolton, D. P. G., Williams, S. M., & Taylor, B. J. (2006). Differences in infant and parent behaviors during routine bed sharing compared with cot sleeping in the home setting. *Pediatrics, 117,* 1599–1607.

Ball, H. L. (2006). Bed sharing on the postnatal ward: Breastfeeding and infant sleep safety. *Paediatrics and Child Health, 11*(Suppl A): 43A–46A.

Ball, H. (2009). Airway covering during bed-sharing. *Child: Care, Health, and Development, 35,* 728–737.

Barajas, R. G., Martin, A., Brooks-Gunn, J., & Hale, L. (2011). Mother-child bed-sharing in toddlerhood and cognitive and behavioral outcomes. *Pediatrics, 128,* e339–e347.

Bernier, A., Carlson, S. M., Bordeleau, S., & Carrier, J. (2010). Relations between physiological and cognitive regulatory systems: Infant sleep regulation and subsequent executive functioning. *Child Development, 81,* 1739–1752.

Blair, P. S., Fleming, P. J., Smith, I. J., Platt, M. W., Young, J., Nadin, P., et al., & the CESDI SUDI Research Group. (1999). Babies sleeping with parents: Case-control study of factors influencing the risk of the sudden infant death syndrome. *British Medical Journal, 319,* 1457–1462.

Blair, P. S., & Ball, H. L. (2004). The prevalence and characteristics associated with parent-infant bed-sharing in England. *Archives of Disease in Childhood, 89,* 1106–1110.

Blunden, S. L., Thompson, K. R., & Dawson, D. (2011). Behavioural sleep treatments and night time crying in infants: Challenging the status quo. *Sleep Medicine Reviews, 15,* 327–334.

Brenner, R. A., Simons-Morton, B. G., Bhaskar, B., Revenis, M., Das, A., & Clemens, J. D. (2003). Infant-parent bed sharing in an inner-city population. *Archives of Pediatric and Adolescent Medicine, 157,* 33–39.

Burnham, M. M., Goodlin-Jones, B. L., Gaylor, E. E., & Anders, T. F. (2002). Nighttime sleep-wake patterns and self-soothing from birth to one year of age: A longitudinal intervention study. *Journal of Child Psychology & Psychiatry, 43,* 713–725.

Burnham, M. M., & Gaylor, E. E. (2011). Sleep environments of young children in post-industrial societies. In M. El-Sheikh (Ed.), *Sleep and Development: Familial and Socio-Cultural Considerations* (pp. 195–217). New York: Oxford University Press.

Carroll-Pankhurst, C., & Mortimer, E. A. (2001). Sudden infant death syndrome, bedsharing, parental weight, and age at death. *Pediatrics, 107,* 530–536.

Consumer Products Safety Commission (1999). *CPSC Cautions Caregivers about Hidden Hazards for Babies on Adult Beds* (Report No. 5091). Retrieved from http://www.cpsc.gov/cpscpub/pubs/5091.pdf. http://www.cpsc.gov/PageFiles/112793/5091.pdf Last accessed: 7/17/13

Ednick, M., Cohen, A. P., McPhail, G. L., Beebe, D., Simakajornboon, N., & Amin, R. S. (2009). A review of the effects of sleep during the first year of life on cognitive, psychomotor, and temperament development. *Sleep, 32,* 1449–1458.

Germo, G. R., Goldberg, W. A., & Keller, M. A. (2009). Learning to sleep through the night: Solution or strain for mothers and young children? *Infant Mental Health Journal, 30*(3), 223–244.

Goodlin-Jones, B. L., Burnham, M. M., Gaylor, E. E., & Anders, T. F. (2001). Night waking, sleep-wake organization, and self-soothing in the first year of life. *Journal of Developmental and Behavioral Pediatrics, 22*(4), 226–233.

Hauck, F. R., Signore, C., Fein, S. B., & Raju, T. N. K. (2008). Infant sleeping arrangements and practices during the first year of life. *Pediatrics, 122*, S113–S120.

Herzog, K., & Stephensen, C. (November 9, 2011). Ad campaign unveiled as another co-sleeping death is announced. *Journal Sentinel Online*. Retrieved from http://m.jsonline.com/topstories/133552808.htm. http://www.jsonline.com/news/milwaukee/ad-campaign-unveiled-as-another-cosleeping-death-is-announced-s030073-133552808.htmlLastaccessed: 7/17/13

Higley, E., & Dozier, M. (2009). Nighttime maternal responsiveness and infant attachment at one year. *Attachment and Human Development, 11*, 347–363.

Jenni, O. G., Fuhrer, H. Z., Iglowstein, I., Molinari, L., & Largo, R. H. (2005). A longitudinal study of bed sharing and sleep problems among Swiss children in the first 10 years of life. *Pediatrics, 115*, 233–240.

Jenni, O. G., & O'Connor, B. B. (2005). Children's sleep: An interplay between culture and biology. *Pediatrics, 115*, 204–216.

Keller, M. A., & Goldberg, W. A. (2004). Co-sleeping: Help or hindrance for young children's independence? *Infant and Child Development, 13*(5), 369–388.

Kemp, J. S., Unger, B., Wilkins, D., Psara, R. M., Ledbetter, T. L., Graham, M. A., et al. (2000). Unsafe sleep practices and an analysis of bedsharing among infants dying suddenly and unexpectedly: Results of a four-year, population-based, death-science investigation study of Sudden Infant Death Syndrome and related deaths. *Pediatrics, 106*, e41.

Latz, S., Wolf, A. W., & Lozoff, B. (1999). Cosleeping in context: Sleep practices and problems in young children in Japan and the United States. *Archives of Pediatric and Adolescent Medicine, 153*, 339–346.

Lozoff, B., Wolf, A. W., & Davis, N.S. (1985). Sleep problems seen in pediatric practice. *Pediatrics, 75*, 477–483.

Lozoff, B., Askew, G. L., & Wolf, A. W. (1996). Cosleeping and early childhood sleep problems: Effects of ethnicity and socioeconomic status. *Developmental and Behavioral Pediatrics, 17*, 9–15.

Lucas-Thompson, R., Goldberg, W. A., Germo, G. R., Keller, M. A., Davis, E. P., & Sandman, C. A. (2009). Sleep arrangements and night waking at 6 and 12 months in relation to infants' stress-induced cortisol responses. *Infant and Child Development, 18*, 521–544.

McKenna, J. J., & Mosko, S. (1993). Evolution and infant sleep: An experimental study of infant-parent co-sleeping and its implications for SIDS. *Acta Paediatrica Supplement, 389*, 31–36.

McKenna, J. J., Mosko, S. S., & Richard, C. A. (1997). Bedsharing promotes breastfeeding. *Pediatrics, 100*, 214–219.

McKenna, J. J., & McDade, T. (2005). Why babies should never sleep alone: A review of the co-sleeping controversy in relation to SIDS, bedsharing, and breast feeding. *Paediatric Respiratory Reviews, 6*, 134–152.

Meléndez, L. (2005). Parental beliefs and practices around early self-regulation: The impact of culture and immigration. *Infants and Young Children, 18*, 136–146.

Milan, S., Snow, S., & Belay, S. (2007). The context of preschool children's sleep: Racial/ethnic differences in sleep locations, routines, and concerns. *Journal of Family Psychology, 21*, 20–28.

Mindell, J. A., Sadeh, A., Kohyama, J., & How, T. H. (2010). Parental behaviors and sleep outcomes in infants and toddlers: A cross-cultural comparison. *Sleep Medicine, 11*, 393–399.

Morelli, G. A., Rogoff, B., Oppenheim, D., & Goldsmith, D. (1992). Cultural variation in infants' sleeping arrangements: Questions of independence. *Developmental Psychology, 28*, 604–613.

Morrell, J., & Cortina-Borja, M. (2002). The developmental change in strategies parents employ to settle young children to sleep, and their relationship to infant sleeping problems, as assessed by a new questionniare: The Parental Interactive Bedtime Behaviour Scale. *Infant and Child Development, 11*, 17–41.

Morgan, B. E., Horn, A. R., & Bergman, N. J. (2011). Should neonates sleep alone? *Biological Psychiatry, 70*, 817–825.

Morgan, K. H., Groer, M. W., & Smith, L. J. (2006). The controversy about what constitutes safe and nurturant infant sleep environments. *Journal of Obstetric, Gynecologic, and Neonatal Nursing, 35*, 684–691.

Nakamura, S., Wind, M., & Danello, M. A. (1999). Review of hazards associated with children placed in adult beds. *Archives of Pediatrics and Adolescent Medicine, 153*, 1019–1023.

Nelson, E. A. S., Taylor, B. J., & the Infant Child Care Practices Study Group. (2001). International Child Care Practices Study: Infant sleeping environment. *Early Human Development, 62*, 43–55.

Ramos, K. D., & Youngclarke, D. M. (2006). Parenting advice books about child sleep: Cosleeping and crying it out. *Sleep, 29*, 1616–1623.

Rigda, R. S., McMillen, I. C., & Buckley, P. (2000). Bed sharing patterns in a cohort of Australian infants during the first six months after birth. *Journal of Paediatrics and Child Health, 36*, 117–121.

Rothrauff, T., Middlemiss, W., & Jacobson, L. (2004). Comparison of American and Austrian infants' and toddlers' sleep habits: A retrospective, exploratory study. *North American Journal of Psychology, 6*(1), 125–144.

Rowe, J. (2003). A room of their own: The social landscape of infant sleep. *Nursing Inquiry, 10*(3), 184–192.

Sadeh, A., & Anders, T. (1993). Infant sleep problems: Origins, assessment, intervention. *Infant Mental Health Journal, 14*, 17–34.

Sadeh, A., Gruber, R., & Raviv, A. (2002). Sleep, neurobehavioral functioning, and behavior problems in school-age children. *Child Development, 73*, 405–417.

Sadeh, A., Mindell, J. A., & Owens, J. (2011). Why care about sleep of infants and their parents? *Sleep Medicine Reviews, 15*, 335–337.

Shapiro-Mendoza, C. K., Tomashek, K. M., Anderson, R. N., & Wingo, J. (2006). Recent national trends in sudden, unexpected infant deaths: More evidence supporting a change in classification or reporting. *American Journal of Epidemiology, 163*, 762–769.

Super, C. M., & Harkness, S. (1986). The developmental niche: A conceptualization at the interface of child and culture. *International Journal of Behavioral Development, 9*, 545–569.

Teti, D. M., Kim, B-R., Mayer, G., & Countermine, M. (2010). Maternal emotional availability at bedtime predicts infant sleep quality. *Journal of Family Psychology, 24*(3), 307–315.

Thogmartin, J. R., Siebert, C. F., & Pellan, W. A. (2001). Sleep position and bed-sharing in sudden infant deaths: An examination of autopsy findings. *Journal of Pediatrics, 138*, 212–217.

Tikotsky, L., & Sadeh, A. (2009). Maternal sleep-related cognitions and infant sleep: A longitudinal study from pregnancy through the first year. *Child Development, 80*, 860–874.

Tollenaar, M. S., Beijers, R., Jansen, J., Riksen-Walraven, J. M. A., & de Weerth, C. (2012). Solitary sleeping in young infants is associated with heightened cortisol reactivity to a bathing session but not to a vaccination. *Psychoneuroendocrinology, 37*, 167–177.

Vennemann, M. M., Hense, H-W., Bajankowski, T., Blair, P. S., Complojer, C., Moon, R. Y., & Kierchl-Kohlendorfer, U. (2012). Bed sharing and the risk of Sudden Infant Death Syndrome: Can we resolve the debate? *The Journal of Pediatrics, 160*, 44–48.

Wailoo, M., Ball, H., Fleming, P., & Platt, M. W. (2004). Infants bed-sharing with mothers. *Archives of Disease in Childhood, 89*, 1082–1083.

Weimer, S. W., Dise, T. L., Evers, P. B., Ortiz, M. A., Welldaregay, W., & Steinmann, W. C. (2002). Prevalence, predictors, and attitudes toward cosleeping in an urban pediatric center. *Clinical Pediatrics, 41*, 433–438.

Willinger, M., Ko, C-W., Hoffman, H. J., Kessler, R. C., & Corwin, M. J. (2003). Trends in infant bed sharing in the United States, 1993–2000: The national infant sleep position study. *Archives of Pediatric and Adolescent Medicine, 157*, 43–49.

Wolf, A. W., Lozoff, B., Latz, S., & Paludetto, R. (1996). Parental theories in the management of young children's sleep in Japan, Italy, and the United States. In S. Harkness & C. M. Super (Eds.), *Parents' Cultural Belief Systems: Their Origins, Expressions, and Consequences* (pp. 364–404). New York: Guilford.

Wolfson, A., Lacks, P., & Futterman, A. (1992). Effects of parent training on infant sleeping patterns, parents' stress, and perceived parental competence. *Journal of Consulting and Clinical Psychology, 60*, 41–48.

CHAPTER

13 The Impact of Pediatric Chronic Illness on Caregiver Sleep and Daytime Functioning

Lisa J. Meltzer *and* Colleen M. Walsh

Abstract

While sleep disruptions are common for parents of typically developing children, caring for a child with a chronic illness often goes above and beyond typical parenting. This chapter reviews the impact of pediatric chronic illness on caregiver sleep and daytime functioning, including the prevalence, potential causes, and consequences of caregiver sleep disruption. Detailed knowledge of potential causes and consequences of sleep disruption in parental caregivers is limited. Possible sources of parent sleep disruption include nighttime medical caregiving, frequent monitoring of illness symptoms or required technology, child sleep disruptions, and emotional stress. In turn, sleep disruptions may impact caregiving as well as parental psychological distress, health, cognitive daytime functioning, interpersonal relationships, and quality of life. Longitudinal and intervention studies are needed that address the limitations of the existing literature, focusing on relationships among child and caregiver sleep disturbance, child disease-related symptoms, and consequences for caregiver daytime functioning.

Key Words: caregivers, children, pediatric, chronic illness, parents, sleep

Introduction

Sleep disruptions are common among parents of typically developing children, and have been associated with excessive sleepiness (Boergers, Hart, Owens, Streisand, & Spirito, 2007), increased fatigue, and impairment of mood and daytime functioning (Meltzer & Mindell, 2007). However, sleep disturbance experienced by caregivers of children with pediatric chronic illnesses often results in a greater overall negative impact, particularly on caregiver daytime functioning (Cottrell & Khan, 2005; Meltzer & Mindell, 2006; Moore, David, Murray, Child, & Arkwright, 2006).

Caregiving goes beyond the requirements of normal parenting, requiring a parent or guardian to provide medical care within the home. Though not universally defined, pediatric chronic illness is commonly characterized as a health condition lasting or expected to endure for at least 12 months (Perrin, Bloom, & Gortmaker, 2007). In the United States, between five and nine million children have a pediatric chronic illness, including asthma, diabetes, and cystic fibrosis (Child and Adolescent Health Measurement Initiative, 2005; Perrin et al., 2007). Compared to parents of healthy children, parents of children with chronic illnesses often have worsened functioning compared to before their child's diagnosis (Kazak, 2001), including reported elevated levels of parenting stress (Gallagher, Phillips, & Carroll, 2010), anxiety during and after the child's treatment (Best, Streisand, Catania, & Kazak, 2001), and poorer health (Raina et al., 2005). Along with the demands and stress of being a medical caregiver for the child, parental sleep disruptions provide another underlying mechanism that contributes to these negative outcomes (Meltzer & Mindell, 2006). Further, daytime consequences of sleep disruption may adversely impact parents' ability to provide the best possible care to their child. Despite the prevalence of pediatric chronic illness and increased interest in this area, detailed knowledge of the potential causes and consequences of sleep disruption in the caregiving population is not widely recognized. Traditionally, caregiver research has placed little emphasis on parental caregivers, with the focus primarily on caregivers of adults with dementia or cancer.

This chapter reviews the current literature regarding the impact of pediatric chronic illness (from infancy through adolescents) on caregiver sleep and daytime functioning, with a focus on the prevalence, potential causes, and consequences of caregiver sleep disruption. For the remainder of this chapter, unless otherwise stated, the term *caregiver* includes parents or other family members (e.g., grandparents, foster parents) who are responsible for all aspects of the day-to-day care of the child. We will begin with a description of general sleep disruptions commonly reported by parents of typically developing children, as well as children with a chronic illness. We will then review potential sources and causes of sleep disruption for these caregivers, as well as the consequences of sleep disruption for specific areas of caregiver functioning. Finally, the limitations of the current literature, recommendations for future research, and clinical implications will be addressed.

Sleep Disruptions in Parents of Typically Developing Children

It is common for parents of all children to experience sleep disruptions (Boergers et al., 2007; Meltzer & Mindell, 2006). A common culprit for parental sleep disruptions is the child, whose own disrupted sleep often results in the child seeking parental attention. Young children may experience developmentally appropriate, though undesirable, sleep issues such as night terrors, bedwetting, and trouble falling asleep alone, which may require the presence of the parent and result in sleep disruptions for both parent and child.

Interestingly, a recent study has suggested that parents may frequently underestimate the sleep needs of children while overestimating the adequacy of sleep experienced by them. When surveying parents on their current knowledge and beliefs about sleep practices, Owens and Jones (2011) found that compared to typical recommendations, 76% of parents of young children (N = 184) underestimated the sleep needs of their children, while a mere 8% noted their children's sleep duration to be inadequate.

The sleep issues of a typically developing child not only impact the parents' sleep, but also areas of parental daytime functioning. Frequent sleep disturbance, particularly among mothers, may result in detriments to health and mood, and contribute to stress and fatigue (Boergers et al., 2007; Martin, Hiscock, Hardy, Davey, & Wake, 2007; Meltzer & Mindell, 2007). Due to the unique challenges of the caregiver role, parental caregivers are likely to report similarly deleterious experiences on yet another level, with a multitude of sources of sleep disruptions and more serious challenges and implications.

Caregiving: Above and Beyond Parenting

The demands of informal caregiving, where a parent or guardian often becomes a medical provider within the home, go above and beyond typical parenting. In addition to performing typical day-to-day parenting activities (e.g., preparing meals, bathing, etc.), at any given time the caregiver must be ready to administer medical care, manage the child's disease symptoms, attend medical appointments or hospitalizations, and assist in treatment delivery (Brown et al., 2008). While allowing the caregiver to play an important and rewarding role in the child's health care, the strain of these added, uncompensated responsibilities may present challenging situations and negatively impact various realms of the caregiver's life, such as daytime functioning, marital relationship, and employment (George, Vickers, Wilkes, & Barton, 2008). For example, it may be necessary for the caregiver to use sick time or modify working arrangements in order to attend the child's medical visits, possibly leading to financial stress and workplace tension (Brown et al., 2008; Diette et al., 2000; George et al., 2008). In addition, caregiver stress is often exacerbated by high medical bills, costs of treatment equipment, and other out-of-pocket expenses.

In some cases, caring for a child with a chronic illness also has a detrimental effect on the marital relationship, with studies reporting parents' descriptions of changes in marital satisfaction, decline in sexual interactions, and general feelings of carrying a burden (Brown et al., 2008; Coffey, 2006). Similarly affected are single parents and lone caregivers of a child or adolescent with a chronic illness (Brown et al., 2008). While the literature is severely limited, there is evidence of higher levels of psychological distress, predominantly among single mothers, immediately following the child's diagnosis (Dolgin et al., 2007).

An additional challenge often faced by caregivers is the need to deal with pediatric conditions that require specialized care during the night (George et al., 2008). In particular, technology-dependent children, such as those needing ventilator-assistance, may require additional caregiving support from trained home–health care medical professionals, such as home-care nurses or respite providers (Meltzer, Boroughs, & Downes, 2010). However, it is regularly left to the caregiver to fill this role, often at a moment's notice and particularly at nighttime when there is a shortage of available trained professionals. Due to prohibitive costs and nursing shortage, caregivers often receive inconsistent home nursing coverage or no nighttime assistance at all (Meltzer et al., 2010; Quint, Chesterman, Crain, Winkleby, & Boyce 1990).

Finally, most caregivers report having no significant issues with daytime functioning prior to their child's diagnosis; however, following diagnosis and treatment, parental caregivers may be at risk for post-traumatic stress symptoms (PTSS; Best et al., 2001; Kazak et al., 2004), as well as poorer health-related quality of life (Klassen et al., 2008), more distress (Bonner, Hardy, Willard, & Hutchinson, 2007; Reiter-Purtill et al., 2008), and more sleep disturbances (Gedaly-Duff, Lee, Nail, Nicholson, & Johnson, 2006).

Yet, despite the above-mentioned challenges and hazards of being a pediatric caregiver, surprisingly little is known about the interplay between a child's chronic illness, the caregiver's own sleep, and the resulting impact on caregiver daytime functioning (Meltzer & Moore, 2008).

Prevalence of Sleep Disruptions among Caregivers

In a review of the available literature through 2007, prevalence rates of sleep disruptions (e.g., poor sleep quality, insufficient sleep quantity) among pediatric caregivers ranged from 15% to 86% (Meltzer & Moore, 2008). Much of the wide variance may be explained by the different definitions of sleep disruptions, the large variety of pediatric chronic illnesses—which include asthma, atopic dermatitis, diabetes, cancer, epilepsy, and ventilator-dependency, among many others—and by different design methodologies, which are largely qualitative or mixed methods. Few studies have compared the prevalence of sleep disruptions among caregivers across pediatric illnesses or a similar comparison group, such as parents of healthy, typically developing children. However, the prevalence of sleep disruptions and need for parental nighttime caregiving is high among children with physical disabilities (Hemmingsson, Stenhammar, & Paulsson, 2008; Wright, Tancredi, Yundt, & Larin, 2006), cerebral palsy (Newman, O'Regan, & Hensey, 2006), and eczema (Reid & Lewis-Jones, 1995). Further, caregivers of these children reported experiencing significantly greater sleep disturbances than those reported by parents of healthy, typically developing children in the same age group (Newman et al., 2006; Wright et al., 2006).

Potential Causes of Sleep Disruptions for Caregivers

Pediatric caregivers have reported experiencing elevated rates of sleep disruption in comparison to caregivers of typically developing children (Meltzer & Mindell, 2006; Meltzer & Moore, 2008). While they may experience sleep disruptions commonly reported by most parents of young children, a multitude of additional potential sources or causes of sleep disruption exist due to the unique experience of the caregiver role.

Medical Management Responsibilities

Caregivers are often tasked with the responsibility of managing their child's medical care. However, some medical management responsibilities, such as illness symptom monitoring (Williams et al., 2000) and nighttime caregiving (Gedaly-Duff et al., 2006), may necessitate vigilance or administration at intervals throughout the night. For example, caregivers of children with type 1 diabetes, one of the most common pediatric chronic illnesses, may regularly monitor nighttime blood glucose levels for hypoglycemia (Monaghan, Hilliard, Cogen, & Streisand, 2009; Sullivan-Bolyai, Deatrick, Gruppuso, Tamborlane, & Grey, 2002). Similarly, the caregiver of a young child with epilepsy may worry about the timing of the next unpredictable seizure, particularly if the child is newly diagnosed (Modi, 2009). This places the burden of medical responsibility directly on the caregiver, as in some cases the consequences of infrequently monitoring the child's condition and symptoms may result in medical complications, errors, unintended injuries, or fatalities.

Further, studies have demonstrated that sleep problems and nighttime caregiving needs may vary among diagnoses and are dependent on specific symptoms and frequency or type of treatment administration (Hemmingsson et al., 2008). Evidence exists that certain types of treatment for the child's condition, such as medication, may negatively impact the child's sleep, in turn possibly impacting caregiver sleep (Lewandowski, Ward, & Palermo, 2011). For example, there is evidence for increased tiredness, fatigue, and significant sleep disturbances including night wakings among pediatric cancer patients using corticosteroids (Drigan, Spirito, & Gelber, 1992; Harris et al., 1986; Sanford et al., 2008). During certain phases of cancer treatment, patients cycle on and off oral and intravenous corticosteroids, with interim side effects including higher levels of mood disturbance (Stuart, Segal, & Keady, 2005) and increased pain (Gaynon & Siegel, 2002).

Finally, caregiver's sleep may be disrupted as a result of false monitor alarms, specifically for technology-dependent children such as those assisted by a mechanical ventilator (Heaton et al., 2006; Meltzer & Mindell, 2006; Meltzer et al., 2010).

Location of the Child's Care

The location at which the child receives the majority of care may affect the caregiver's sleep as much as the child's prognosis. Both hospitalization and home care can lead to caregiver sleep disruption, whether as a result of anxieties pertaining to the child's inpatient experience or needing to provide medical care throughout the night in one's home. Caregivers of a child staying in a hospital are not only given the opportunity to remain at the bedside overnight, but are also often encouraged and even expected to room-in with the child (Stremler, Wong, & Parshuram, 2008). Given the limited privacy, overcrowding, and general distress associated with a typical hospital visit, caregiver's sleep while at the bedside is easily disrupted (Dudley & Carr, 2004; Stremler et al., 2008). Equally, caregivers of children whose conditions require home health care provision, such as those dependent upon technology, may be required to fill the role typically performed by trained home health care professionals (Quint et al., 1990). As a consequence of inconsistent home nursing coverage or lack of any overnight assistance, caregivers often forego nights of uninterrupted sleep in order to monitor, administer, and provide care for their child throughout the night (Meltzer et al., 2010).

Disturbance of the Child's Sleep

Not surprisingly, the disturbed sleep of the child is often a major cause of sleep disruption for the caregiver. While this correlation is true for nearly all parents and caregivers, it is heightened among chronically ill children when they experience disturbed sleep resulting from their medical conditions or symptoms related to their diagnoses, such as pain (Hinds et al., 2007) or side effects from medications (Zupanec, Jones, & Stremler, 2010), which in turn may require nighttime attention by the caregiver. For example, compared to healthy children, children with cancer are reported to have more night wakings requiring parental attention (Gedaly-Duff et al., 2006; Hinds et al., 2007; Meltzer & Moore, 2008).

Similar to typically developing children, sleep disturbance in children with chronic illnesses has also been associated with the presence of the child in the caregiver's bed (Sullivan-Bolyai, Knafl, Deatrick, & Grey, 2003). However, in contrast to parents of healthy, typically developing children, co-sleeping with children who have chronic illness may result from heightened vigilance of illness symptoms, caregiving requirements during the night, pain complaints from the child, or child sleep onset difficulties, where the child needs the parent present in order to fall asleep (Meltzer & Moore, 2008). Among caregivers of children with physical disabilities such as cerebral palsy, muscular dystrophy, and spina bifida, the need for parental nighttime attention is also high, as pain experienced by the child is associated with sleep problems and the need for parental support during the night (Hemmingsson et al., 2008; Wright et al., 2006).

Emotional Stress

Additionally, pediatric caregivers may experience emotional stress, worries, and anxieties about the child's illness or treatment as a common source of sleep disturbance (Ferrell, Rhiner, Shapiro, & Dierkes, 1994). In some studies, caregivers have reported pervasive uncertainty regarding the child's illness (Stewart & Mishel, 2000), psychological distress (Bonner et al., 2007), and worry about the future (Murphy, Christian, Caplin, & Young, 2006). They may be hypervigilant during the night, monitoring the child's illness due to worry or fear for the future (Williams et al., 2000), or experience frequent night wakings themselves due to stress related to the child's health issues (Meltzer & Mindell, 2006).

Thus, because of caregiving demands and the child's disrupted sleep, a number of different causes may contribute to the sleep disturbance of the caregiver, with consequences that should not go unnoticed.

Consequences of Sleep Disruptions on Daytime Functioning in Caregivers

While parents of most healthy, typically developing children may report experiencing unwanted consequences of repeated sleep disruption, the disturbed sleep of caregivers of children with pediatric chronic illnesses often results in a greater overall negative impact on various areas of daytime functioning and has strong implications for caregiving ability. Two of the most common complaints associated with sleep disruption are excessive daytime sleepiness (the tendency to fall asleep when the individual would otherwise be awake and alert) and fatigue (a general lack of physical and/or cognitive energy not relieved by increased sleep).

Daytime Functioning and Caregiving Ability

Sleepiness, a common side effect of frequent sleep disruption, has often been associated with risk of injury among adults, particularly in work-related incidents (Ayas et al., 2006), motor vehicle accidents (Connor, Whitlock, Norton, & Jackson, 2001), and medical errors (Balas, Scott, & Rogers, 2006; Gold et al., 1992; Owens, 2001). Both chronic partial sleep deprivation (or insufficient sleep) and fragmented sleep can contribute to excessive daytime sleepiness. For example, it has been shown that after 14 nights of chronic restriction of sleep to 6 hours per night, adult performance was equivalent to 2 nights of total sleep deprivation (Van Dongen, Maislin, Mullington, & Dinges, 2003). Even if sleep duration is sufficient, highly fragmented sleep can also contribute to negative daytime functioning. For example, one study found that the duration of sleep in mothers of newborn infants does not significantly change; however, the sleep of postpartum mothers is highly fragmented (Montgomery-Downs, Insana, Clegg-Kraynok, & Mancini, 2010), contributing to significant daytime dysfunction.

These studies have important implications for parental caregivers who provide a significant amount of care at home during the night. For example, caregivers of ventilator-assisted children must frequently provide nighttime care, often covering overnight nursing shifts without any assistance (Heaton, Noyes, Sloper, & Shah, 2006). One study found that caregivers who received limited or no overnight nursing support reported an average of 6 or fewer hours of sleep per night (Meltzer et al., 2010), a number associated with significant impairment of daytime performance (Dinges et al., 2005). Our recent work shows that caregivers may not be experiencing significant shorter sleep duration, but they do have sleep that is highly fragmented (Meltzer & Avis, 2011). Studies examining the level of injury risk or medical errors associated with caregiver sleep loss are needed.

Sleep Quality

Caregivers who report frequent vigilance and caregiving during the night have reported reduced total sleep time as well as diminished sleep quality (Ferrell et al., 1994; Meltzer et al., 2010). Frequent worrying about the child's condition can also result in difficulty falling asleep, shorter sleep quantity, and lack of restful sleep, which may also contribute to increased daytime tiredness and fatigue in parents (Ferrell et al., 1994; Gallagher et al., 2010; Gedaly-Duff et al., 2006; Meltzer & Mindell, 2006). As previously described, parents may be hypervigilant during the night, monitoring the child's illness, which leads to increased night wakings, decreased sleep quality and sleep efficiency, and increased sleep onset latency due to worry or fear for the future. Poor sleep quality may even adversely affect immune functioning and stress responses among caregivers (Lee et al., 2004) and result in poorer health (Cottrell & Khan, 2005; Raina et al., 2005).

Our recent work has shown that not only do some caregivers experience shortened or disrupted sleep, but may be affected by "chronobiotic chaos" (see Figure 13.1 for examples of actigraphic recordings) as a result of inconsistent sleep schedules (Meltzer & Avis, 2011). Similar to shift workers or those who have a circadian rhythm sleep disorder, the often unpredictable demands of caregiving, including whether or not families have additional support such as nursing care, can result in a highly variable bedtime, wake time, and total sleep duration. In fact, variability in sleep duration within this population was associated with more depressive symptoms, more daytime fatigue, and poorer executive functioning (Meltzer, 2009). These inconsistencies in timing and duration of sleep can, in turn, contribute to poor sleep quality, especially when a caregiver's sleep opportunity is not in sync with his or her circadian rhythm.

Emotional and Psychological Distress

Caregivers often report experiencing parenting stress as a consequence of sleep disruption due to fears and anxieties regarding their ability to provide the proper care for the child's immediate symptoms (Monaghan et al., 2009) and worry about what is yet to come, including experiencing anxiety during and

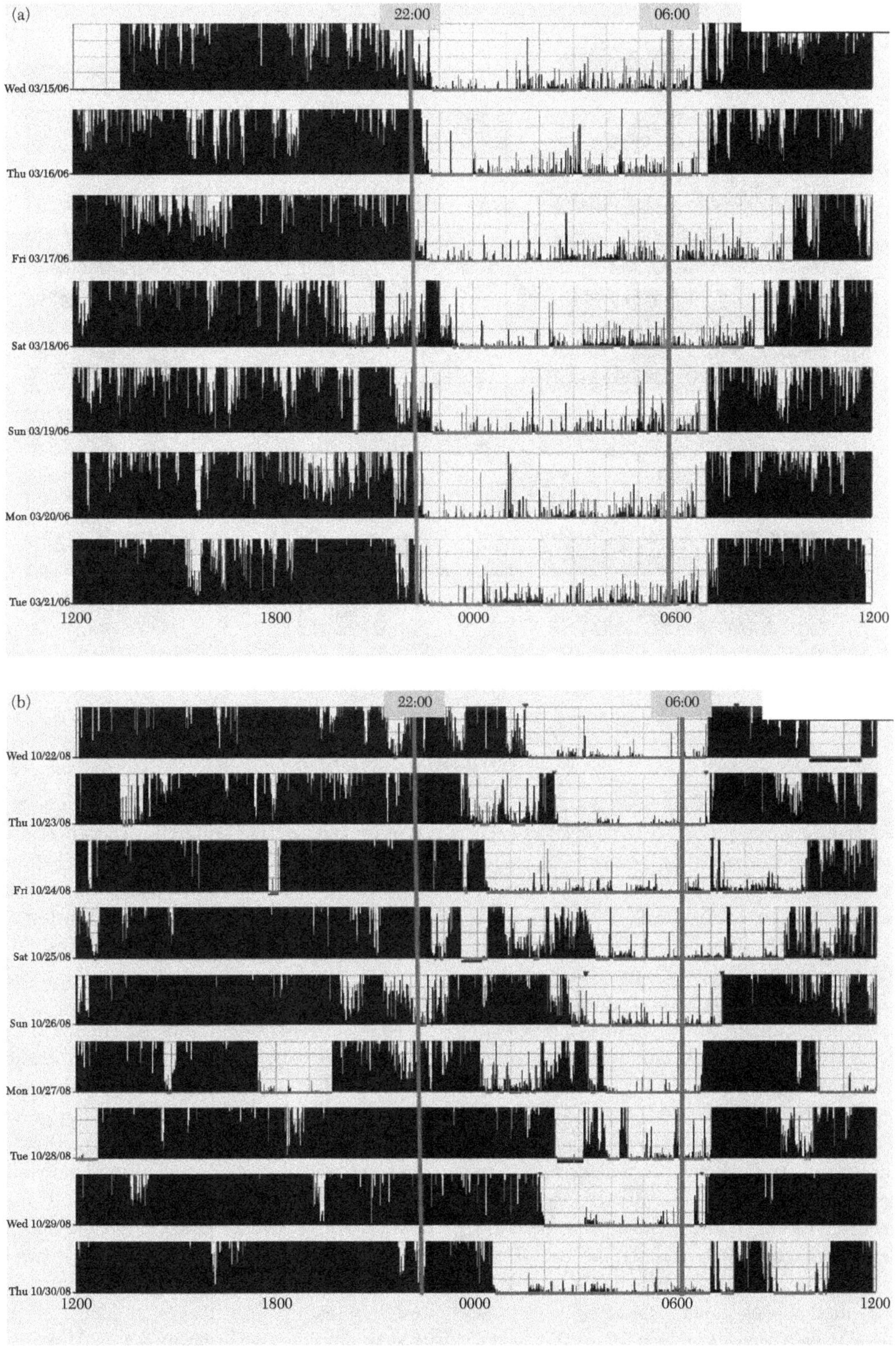

Figure 13.1 Examples of actigraphic studies for parents of children with and without chronic illness. Each horizontal timeline represents 24 hours. The date for each timeline is on the left and the time of day is across the bottom, starting at noon, with midnight in the middle. The black vertical lines on each timeline are when the actigraph interpreted the parent's movement as a period of wake. The sections underlined in grey are when the actigraph interpreted the lack of movement to indicate that the parent was asleep. (a)Relatively stable sleep schedule for a mother of a healthy, typically developing 9-year-old child. (b)"Chronobiotic chaos," or an inconsistent sleep schedule in a mother of a 9-year-old ventilator-assisted child. (c) "Chronobiotic chaos," or an inconsistent sleep schedule in a father of a 7-year-old ventilator-assisted child.

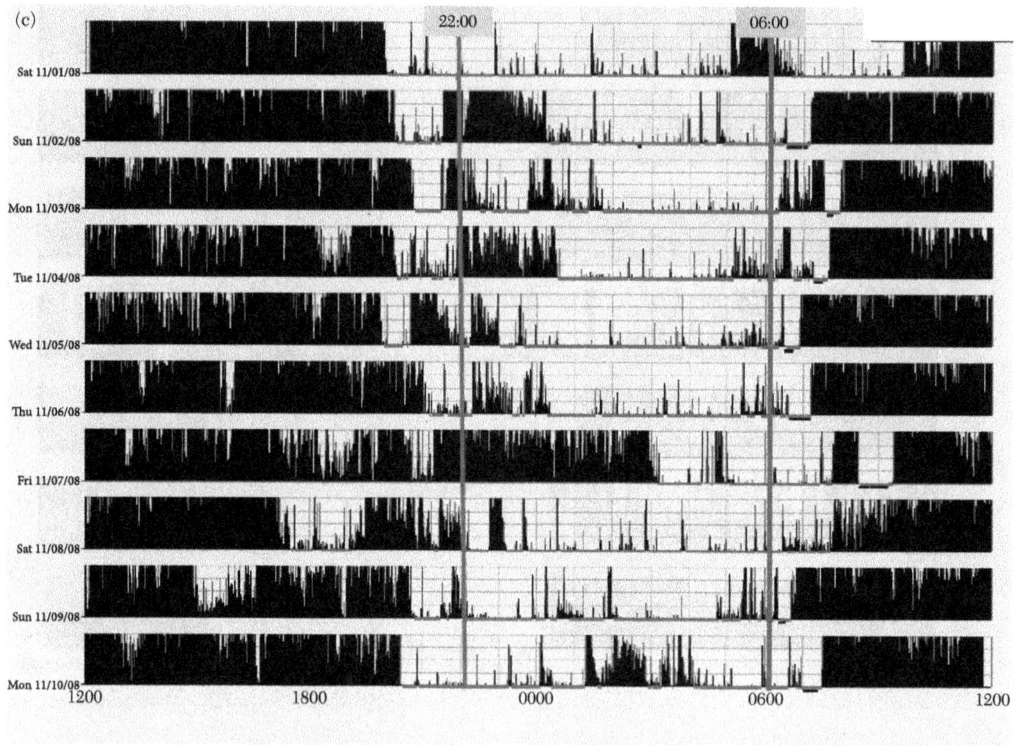

Figure 13.1 Continued

after the child's treatment (Best et al., 2001). Several studies have demonstrated correlations between caregiver sleep disturbance and parental stress or anxiety among caregivers of children with type 1 diabetes (Monaghan et al., 2009; Sullivan-Bolyai, Knafl, Deatrick, & Grey, 2003), cystic fibrosis (Meltzer & Mindell, 2006), developmental disabilities (Gallagher et al., 2010), and epilepsy (Modi, 2009; Wirell, Blackman, Barlow, Mah, & Hamiwka, 2005). For conditions such as these, caregivers often become hypervigilant, continually monitoring the child's symptoms throughout the night, which further contributes to poor quality or disrupted sleep.

Additionally, studies have found evidence for an association between sleep and depression among parental caregivers of children with autism spectrum disorders (Meltzer, 2011), eczema (Moore et al., 2006), and asthma (Yuksel et al., 2007), as well as negative mood among parents caring for a ventilator-assisted child (Meltzer & Mindell, 2006).

The limited knowledge about the dynamic interaction between sleep loss due to caregiving and adverse daytime outcomes suggest more research is needed that focuses on the relationship between child illness, caregivers' sleep, and caregiver functioning (Meltzer & Moore, 2008). The consequences of sleep disturbance may have important implications for caregivers of children with a chronic illness on many levels, including the fact that parents are often the primary and most comprehensive source of insight for healthcare providers regarding symptoms and progression of the child's illness.

Conclusion

Many parents commonly experience sleep disruptions. Although the impact of sleep disruptions has been shown to significantly impair the sleep, stress, and daytime functioning among parents of healthy, typically developing children, these negative outcomes are even greater among parental caregivers of children with a chronic illness. Caring for a child with a chronic illness often requires a level of care above and beyond that of typical parenting, such as medication administration, nighttime care, and monitoring for changes in illness symptoms or side effects, in addition to the usual demanding parental responsibilities. In general, sleep disruptions experienced by children with chronic illness may require caregiver attention during the night, resulting in further disruption of the caregiver's sleep and causing further daytime impairment to caregiver functioning. This vicious cycle places an added burden on caregivers who may already be coping with exceptional circumstances.

In the current literature, pediatric caregivers have reported negative impacts on health, mood, and daytime functioning, including depression, anxiety, fatigue, and decreased executive functioning. While parents of healthy, typically developing children might also experience many of these consequences, there are important clinical implications for caregivers of children with chronic illness. Namely, a negative impact on the caregiver's ability to properly provide the child with necessary care, medical management, and treatment may result in medical errors, increased symptomology, or an overall worsened condition for the child.

Despite the prevalence of pediatric chronic illness, detailed knowledge of potential causes and consequences of sleep disruption in the caregiving population is limited. This highlights the need for additional longitudinal and intervention research to better understand the relationship between child and caregiver sleep, as well as the impact of the child's illness on caregiver sleep and general functioning. In addition, targeted interventions for caregivers should focus on increasing parent knowledge of positive sleep practices, as well as awareness of the impact of insufficient sleep on caregiver and child mood, health, and general daytime functioning. Ultimately, the literature should better equip health and medical professionals with an understanding of the relationship and impact of the child's illness on caregiver's sleep and functioning, and provide tools to the caregiver to combat sources of sleep disruption and to achieve a better night's sleep.

Future Directions

Given the overall prevalence of pediatric chronic illness and negative impact on general functioning among parental caregivers, additional research is needed on both the impact of child illness on caregiver's sleep and the benefit of interventions to improve caregiver sleep. Together these will serve to inform and guide health professionals who work with families of children with chronic illnesses. Specific recommendations include:

- Longitudinal studies to help disentangle the potential causes and consequences of caregiver sleep disruption, as well as to better understand the dynamic relationship between child illness, child sleep, and parent sleep.
- The utilization of appropriate comparison groups in research, including parents of children with different chronic illnesses and/or parents of typically developing children.
- The development and evaluation of interventions that directly benefit caregiver sleep, including behavioral and medical interventions to improve child sleep and reduce stress related to caregiving.
- The evaluation of targeted interventions for caregivers that focus on increasing parent knowledge of positive sleep practices, as well as awareness of the impact of insufficient sleep on caregiver and child mood, health, and general daytime functioning. Further, studies are needed examining the level of injury risk or medical errors associated with caregiver sleep loss.

References

Ayas, N. T., Barger, L. K., Cade, B. E., Hashimoto, D. M., Rosner, B., Cronin, J. W., et al. (2006). Extended work duration and the risk of self-reported percutaneous injuries in interns. *Journal of the American Medical Association, 296*, 1055–1062.

Balas, M. C., Scott, L. D., & Rogers, A. E. (2006). Frequency and type of errors and near errors reported by critical care nurses. *Canadian Journal of Nursing Research, 38*, 24–41.

Best, M., Streisand, R., Catania, L., & Kazak, A. E. (2001). Parental distress during pediatric leukemia and posttraumatic stress symptoms (PTSS) after treatment ends. *Journal of Pediatric Psychology, 26*(5), 299–307.

Boergers, J., Hart, C., Owens, J. A., Streisand, R., & Spirito, A. (2007). Child sleep disorders: Associations with parental sleep duration and daytime sleepiness. *Journal of Family Psychology, 21*(1), 88–94.

Bonner, M. J., Hardy, K. K., Willard, V. W., & Hutchinson, K. C. (2007). Brief report: Psychosocial functioning of fathers as primary caregivers of pediatric oncology patients. *Journal of Pediatric Psychology, 32*(7), 851–856.

Brown, R. T., Wiener, L., Kupst, M. J., Brennan, T., Behrman, R., Compas, B. E., et al. (2008). Single parents of children with chronic illness: An understudied phenomenon. *Journal of Pediatric Psychology, 33*(4), 408–421.

Child and Adolescent Health Measurement Initiative. (2005). National survey of children's health. *Data Resource Center on Child and Adolescent Health Website.* Retrieved May 12, 2010, from www.childhealthdata.org.

Coffey, J. S. (2006). Parenting a child with chronic illness: A metasynthesis. *Pediatric Nursing, 32*, 51–59.

Connor, J., Whitlock, G., Norton, R., & Jackson, R. (2001). The role of driver sleepiness in car crashes: A systematic review of epidemiological studies. *Accident Analysis and Prevention, 33*, 31–41.

Cottrell, L., & Khan, A. (2005). Impact of childhood epilepsy on maternal sleep and socioemotional functioning. *Clinical Pediatrics, 44*, 613–616.

Diette, G. B., Markson, L., Skinner, E. A., Nguyen, T. T. H., Algatt-Bergstrom, P. A., & Wu, A.W. (2000). Nocturnal asthma in children affects school attendance, school performance, and parents' work attendance. *Archives of Pediatric Adolescent Medicine, 154*, 923–928.

Dinges, D. F., Rogers, N. L., & Baynard, M. D. (2005). Chronic sleep deprivation. In M. H. Kryger, T. Roth, & W. C. Dement (Eds.), *Principles and Practice of Sleep Medicine* (4th edition, pp. 67–76). Philadelphia, PA: Elsevier Saunders.

Dolgin, M., Phipps, S., Fairclough, D., Sahler, O. J., Askins, M., Noll, R., et al. (2007). Trajectories of adjustment in mothers of children with newly diagnosed cancer: A natural history investigation. *Journal of Pediatric Psychology, 32*, 771–782.

Drigan, R., Spirito, A., & Gelber, R. D. (1992). Behavioral effects of corticosteroids in children with acute lymphoblastic leukemia. *Medical and Pediatric Oncology, 20*, 13–21.

Dudley, S. K., & Carr, J. M. (2004). Vigilance: The experience of parents staying at the bedside of hospitalized children. *Journal of Pediatric Nursing, 19*, 267–275.

Ferrell, B. R., Rhiner, M., Shapiro, B., & Dierkes, M. (1994). The experience of pediatric cancer pain, part I: Impact of pain on the family. *Journal of Pediatric Nursing, 9*, 368–379.

Gallagher, S., Phillips, A. C., & Carroll, D. (2010). Parental stress is associated with poor sleep quality in parents caring for children with developmental disabilities. *Journal of Pediatric Psychology, 35*(7), 728–737.

Gaynon, P. S., & Siegel, S. E. (2002). Childhood acute lymphoblastic leukemia. In E. S. Henderson, T. A. Lister, & M. F. Greaves (Eds). *Leukemia* (7th edition, Chapter 26). Philadelphia: Saunders.

Gedaly-Duff, V., Lee, K. A., Nail, L., Nicholson, H. S., & Johnson, K. P. (2006). Pain, sleep disturbance, and fatigue in children with leukemia and their parents: A pilot study. *Oncology Nursing Forum, 33*, 641–646.

George, A., Vickers, M. H., Wilkes, L., & Barton, B. (2008). Working and caring for a child with chronic illness: Challenges in maintaining employment. *Employee Responsibilities and Rights Journal, 20*, 165–176.

Gold, D. R., Rogacz, S., Bock, N., Tosteson, T. D., Baum, T. M., Speizer, F. E., & Czeisler, C. A. (1992). Rotating shift work, sleep, and accidents related to sleepiness in hospital nurses. *American Journal of Public Health, 82*(7), 1011–1014.

Harris, J. C., Carel, C. A., Rosenberg, L. A., Joshi, P., & Leventhal, B. G. (1986). Intermittent high dose corticosteroid treatment in childhood cancer: Behavioral and emotional consequences. *Journal of American Academy of Child Psychiatry, 25*, 120–124.

Heaton, J., Noyes, J., Sloper, P., & Shah, R. (2006). The experiences of sleep disruption in families of technology-dependent children living at home. *Children and Society, 20*, 196–208.

Hemmingsson, H., Stenhammar, A. M., & Paulsson, K. (2008). Sleep problems and the need for parental night-time attention in children with physical disabilities. *Child: Care, Health and Development, 35*(1), 89–95.

Hinds, P. S., Hockenberry, M., Rai, S. N., Zhang, L., Razzouk, B. I., McCarthy, K., et al. (2007). Nocturnal awakenings, sleep environment interruptions, and fatigue in hospitalized children with cancer. *Oncology Nursing Forum, 34*, 393–402.

Kazak, A. E. (2001). Comprehensive care for children with cancer and their families: A social ecological framework guiding research, practice, and policy. *Children's Services Social Policy, Research, and Practice, 4*, 217–233.

Kazak, A. E., Alderfer, M., Rourke, M. T., Simms, S., Streisand, R., & Grossman, J. R. (2004). Posttraumatic stress disorder (PTSD) and posttraumatic stress symptoms (PTSS) in families of adolescent childhood cancer survivors. *Journal of Pediatric Psychology, 29*(3), 211–219.

Klassen, A. F., Klaassen, R., Dix, D., Pritchard, S., Yanofsky, R., O'Donnell, M., Scott, A., & Sung, L. (2008). Impact of caring for a child with cancer on parents' health-related quality of life. *Journal of Pediatric Oncology Nursing, 26*(36), 5884–5889.

Lee, K., Cho, M., Miaskowski, C., & Dodd, M. (2004). Impaired sleep and rhythms in persons with cancer. *Sleep Medicine Reviews, 8*, 199–212.

Lewandowski, A. S., Ward, T. M., & Palermo, T. M. (2011). Sleep problems in children and adolescents with common medical problems. *Pediatric Clinics of North America, 58*, 699–713.

Martin, J., Hiscock, H., Hardy, P., Davey, B., & Wake, M. (2007). Adverse associations of infant and child sleep problems and parent health: An Australian population study. *Pediatrics, 119*(5), 947–955.

Meltzer L. J., & Mindell, J. A. (2006). Impact of a child's chronic illness on maternal sleep and daytime functioning. *Archives of Internal Medicine, 166*, 1749–1755.

Meltzer, L. J., & Mindell, J. A. (2007). Relationship between child sleep disturbances and maternal sleep, mood, and parenting stress: A pilot study. *Journal of Family Psychology, 21*, 67–73.

Meltzer, L. J., & Moore, M. (2008). Sleep disruptions in parents of children and adolescents with chronic illnesses: Prevalence, causes, and consequences. *Journal of Pediatric Psychology, 33*(3), 279–291.

Meltzer, L. J. (2009). *Sleep and Daytime Functioning in Parents of Children with Chronic Illness.* Poster session presented at the annual convention of the American Psychological Association, Toronto.

Meltzer, L. J., Boroughs, D. S., & Downes, J. J. (2010). The relationship between home-nursing coverage, sleep, and daytime functioning in parents of ventilator-assisted children. *Journal of Pediatric Nursing, 25*, 250–257.

Meltzer, L. J. (2011). Factors associated with depressive symptoms in parents of children with autism spectrum disorders. *Research in Autism Spectrum Disorders, 5*, 361–367.

Meltzer, L. J. & Avis, K. (2011). Impact of chronobiotic chaos on sleep and daytime functioning in parents of ventilator-assisted children. *Sleep, 34*, A284.

Modi, A. C. (2009). The impact of a new pediatric epilepsy diagnosis on parents: Parenting stress and activity patterns. *Epilepsy & Behavior, 14*, 237–242.

Monaghan, M. C., Hilliard, M. E., Cogen, F. R., & Streisand, R. (2009). Nighttime caregiving behaviors among parents of young children with Type 1 diabetes: Associations with illness characteristics and parent functioning. *Families, Systems, & Health, 27*(1), 28–38.

Montgomery-Downs, H. E., Insana, S. P., Clegg-Kraynok, M. M., & Mancini, L. M. (2010). Normative longitudinal maternal sleep: The first four postpartum months. *American Journal of Obstetrics and Gynecology, 203(5)*, 465.e1–465.e7.

Moore, K., David, T. J., Murray, C. S., Child, F., & Arkwright, P. D. (2006). Effect of childhood eczema and asthma on parental sleep and well-being: A prospective comparative study. *British Journal of Dermatology, 154*, 514–518.

Murphy, N. A., Christian, B., Caplin, D. A., & Young, P. C. (2006). The health of caregivers for children with disabilities: Caregiver perspectives. *Child: Care, Health, and Development, 33*(2), 180–187.

Newman, C. J., O'Regan, M., & Hensey, O. (2006). Sleep disorders in children with cerebral palsy. *Developmental Medicine and Child Neurology, 48*, 564–568.

Owens, J. A. (2001). Sleep loss and fatigue in medical training. *Current Opinion in Pulmonary Medicine, 7*, 411–418.

Owens, J. A., & Jones, C. (2011). Parental knowledge of healthy sleep in young children: Results of a primary care clinic survey. *Journal of Developmental and Behavioral Pediatrics, 32*(6), 447–453.

Perrin, J. M., Bloom, S. R., & Gortmaker, S. L. (2007). The increase of childhood chronic conditions in the United States. *Journal of the American Medical Association, 297*(24), 2755–2759.

Quint, R. D., Chesterman, E., Crain, L. S., Winkleby, M., & Boyce, W. T. (1990). Home care for ventilator-dependent children. *American Journal of Diseases of Children, 144*, 1238–1241.

Raina, P., O'Donnell, M., Rosenbaum, P., Brehaut, J., Walter, S. D., Russell, D., et al. (2005). The health and well-being of caregivers of children with cerebral palsy. *Pediatrics, 115*, e626–e636.

Reid, P., & Lewis-Jones, M. S. (1995). Sleep difficulties and their management in preschoolers with atopic eczema. *Clinical and Experimental Dermatology, 20*, 38–41.

Reiter-Purtill, J., Schorry, E. K., Lovell, A. M., Vannatta, K., Gerhardt, C. A., et al. (2008). Parental distress, family functioning, and social support in families with and without a child with neurofibromatosis 1. *Journal of Pediatric Psychology, 33*(4), 422–434.

Sanford, S. D., Okuma, J. O., Pan, J., Srivastava, D. K., West, N., Farr, L., & Hinds, P. S. (2008). Gender differences in sleep, fatigue, and daytime activity in a pediatric oncology sample receiving dexamethasone. *Journal of Pediatric Psychology, 33*(3), 298–306.

Stewart, J. L., & Mishel, M. H. (2000). Uncertainty in childhood illness: A synthesis of the parent and child literature. *Scholarly Inquiry for Nursing Practice: An International Journal, 14*(4), 299–319.

Stremler, R., Wong, L., & Parshuram, C. (2008). Practices and provisions for parents sleeping overnight with a hospitalized child. *Journal of Pediatric Psychology 33*(3), 292–297.

Stuart, F. A., Segal, T. Y., & Keady, S. (2005). Adverse psychological effects of corticosteroids in children and adolescents. *Archives of Disease in Childhood, 90*, 500–506.

Sullivan-Bolyai, S., Deatrick, J., Gruppuso, P., Tamborlane, W., & Grey, M. (2002). Mothers' experiences raising young children with Type 1 diabetes. *Journal for Specialists in Pediatric Nursing, 7*, 93–103.

Sullivan-Bolyai, S., Knafl, K., Deatrick, J., & Grey, M. (2003). Maternal management behaviors for young children with Type 1 diabetes. *American Journal of Maternal Child Nursing, 28*, 161–166.

Van Dongen, H. P., Maislin, G., Mullington, J. M., & Dinges, D. F. (2003). The cumulative cost of additional wakefulness: Dose-response effects on neurobehavioral functions and sleep physiology from chronic sleep restriction and total sleep deprivation. *Sleep, 26*, 117–126.

Williams, J., Lange, B., Sharp, G., Griebel, M., Edgar, T., Haley, T., et al. (2000). Altered sleeping arrangements in pediatric patients with epilepsy. *Clinical Pediatrics, 39*, 635–642.

Wirell, E., Blackman, M., Barlow, K., Mah, J. & Hamiwka, L. (2005). Sleep disturbances in children with epilepsy compared with their nearest-aged sibling. *Developmental Medicine and Child Neurology, 47*, 754–759.

Wright, M., Tancredi, A., Yundt, B. & Larin, H. (2006). Sleep issues in children with physical disabilities and their families. *Physical and Occupational Therapy in Pediatrics, 26*, 55–72.

Yuksel, H., Sogut, A., Yilmaz, O., Demet, M., Ergin, D., & Kirmaz, C. (2007). Evaluation of sleep quality and anxiety-depression parameters in asthmatic children and their mothers. *Respiratory Medicine, 101*, 2550–2554.

Zupanec, S., Jones, H., & Stremler, R. (2010). Sleep habits and fatigue of children receiving maintenance chemotherapy for ALL and their parents. *Journal of Pediatric Oncology Nursing, 27*(4), 217–228.

CHAPTER

14 Children's Sleep in Violent Environments

James C. Spilsbury

Abstract

Millions of children worldwide live in environments of collective and interpersonal violence. Living in such settings profoundly affects many children's sleep, with effects sometimes persisting for substantial periods of time. The relevant scientific literature, coming mainly from the field of traumatic stress, has focused primarily on the presence of insomnia and nightmares—core diagnostic criteria of traumatic stress disorders. However, studies examining other sleep parameters, particularly those few using objective measures of sleep, also show negative effects in a range of sleep indices. Also, though understudied, the available literature indicates that violent settings may alter the sleep environment itself, as children and families move (or are forced to move) to other, often "makeshift," environments. Families may also modify the sleep environment to try to increase their safety, make the environment more conducive to sleep, or both. Directions for future research are given to better understand how violent environments shape children's sleep and how best to mitigate these effects.

Key Words: children, adolescents, collective violence, interpersonal violence, sleep, environment

Introduction

The subject of this chapter is children's sleep in violent environments or settings. For the purposes of this chapter, violence is defined as "the intentional use of physical force or power, threatened or actual, against oneself, another person, or against a group or community, that either results in or has a high likelihood of resulting in injury, death, psychological harm, maldevelopment or deprivation" (World Health Organization, 1996). Using a recently developed typology (Krug, Dahlberg, Mercy, Zwi, & Lozano, 2002), the chapter focuses on settings involving two major types of violence: *(1) collective violence*, which is generally perpetrated by large groups of individuals or states for political, social, and economic reasons (e.g., war, state-sponsored torture, genocide, ethnic cleansing, terrorism); and *(2) interpersonal violence*, consisting of family violence (e.g., abuse, intimate-partner violence, sibling violence), and community violence (e.g., violence between unrelated individuals, often taking place outside the home, random acts of violence, violence in institutional settings). Two additional forms of violence, *self-directed* (e.g., suicidal, self-abusive, self-mutilatory behavior) and *structural* (harm inflicted upon others via the manner in which society itself is structured) are certainly relevant to sleep but are beyond the scope of the present chapter.

Collective and interpersonal violence permeate much of our world. The number of children living in settings of one or both of these forms of violence is staggering. Although precise numbers are difficult to come by, international organizations estimate that in the previous decade wars killed or severely injured approximately eight million children, orphaned one million children, and dislocated 14 million children from their homes (United Nations, 1996, 2005). The estimate of the number of children worldwide who witness domestic violence each year is 133–275 million (United Nations, 2006). Moreover, an estimated 150 million girls and 73 million boys are victims of sexual violence involving physical contact (United Nations, 2005), and results of some population-based surveys indicate that between 25%–50% of children in some locations are victims of frequent, severe physical abuse, such as being beaten, kicked, or tied up by their parents (Krug et al., 2002).

In the United States, an estimated 15.5 million children live in households with intimate partner violence, and nearly half of them have observed forms of severe partner violence, such as an adult being hit with an object, beaten up, bitten, choked, burned, or threatened with a knife or gun (McDonald, Jouriles, Ramisetty-Mikler, Caetano, & Green, 2006). Moreover, though rates have declined over the past decade, over 100,000 cases of substantiated or indicated child physical abuse and 70,000 cases of child sexual abuse still occur annually (Child Trends, 2011). Furthermore, results of a recent nationally representative survey of 3614 US adolescents revealed that 38% of adolescents witnessed at least one form of community violence (Zinzow et al., 2008). Results of several smaller studies suggest that anywhere from 50%–75% of children in selected US urban areas have been exposed to community violence (Kupersmidt, Shahinfar, & Voegler-Lee, 2002; Singer, Menden Anglin, Song, & Lunghofer, 1995).

Most of our knowledge about the relationship between violence and sleep derives from the scientific literature on traumatic stress, including post-traumatic stress disorder (PTSD) and acute stress disorder (ASD). Sleep disturbances and traumatic stress are clearly intertwined; insomnia and nightmares are considered core criteria of these two disorders (American Psychiatric Association: *Diagnostic and Statistical Manual of Mental Disorders, Fourth Edition, Text Revision*, 2000). There are several excellent publications specifically reviewing the sleep disturbances that arise from traumatic experiences such as violence (Glod, 2011; Caldwell & Redeker, 2005; Harvey, Jones, & Schmidt, 2003; Lavie, 2001; Pillar, Malhotra, & Lavie, 2000; Singareddy & Balon, 2002). Other relevant information comes from studies of the effects of violence on child development—recently reviewed by Masten & Narayan (2012), and Carpenter & Stacks (2009)—and on mental health in general.

The traumatic stress literature represents a rich source of information regarding the sleep of children who have experienced violence. Articles that provide details on children's traumatic symptomatology often include sleep characteristics, typically reporting frequencies of the individual sleep-related items comprising the traumatic stress measures used by the investigators. However, on the whole, the literature understandably focuses on the sleep-related criteria for diagnosing ASD or PTSD; namely, sleep onset or sleep maintenance insomnia and nightmares. Less information is provided about other sleep parameters. Moreover, there is the tendency for studies to investigate and report information on nonspecific "sleep disturbances" or "sleep problems" without further information about the specific nature of the these phenomena. The intent of this chapter is to expand the discussion from insomnia, nightmares, and unspecified "sleep disturbances" to other sleep parameters when the literature allows, including what the literature and our own pilot work involving children in the greater Cleveland, Ohio area reveal about children's sleep environments in settings of violence. The chapter first addresses children's sleep in settings of collective violence, followed by sleep in environments of interpersonal violence. Within each section, results are grouped by the type of sleep measure utilized by the investigators: persons' perceptions of sleep, or indices derived from objective measures of sleep. The chapter then moves to the topic of sleep environments of children in settings of violence and concludes with recommendations for future research. The chapter focuses on children, here defined as individuals 18 years of age or younger.

Sleep of Children in Environments of Collective Violence—Subjective Measures

Although there may be considerable variability in what any individual child experiences in a setting of collective violence, the traumatic-stress literature has documented the millions of children living in environments of war, ethnic cleansing, and terrorism who are killed or injured, who witness fighting with diverse weaponry, who experience the death or injury of relatives and nonrelatives, as well as the destruction of their homes and communities (e.g., Dyregrov, Gupta, Gjestad, & Mukanoheli, 2000; Kamphuis, Tuin, Timmermans, & Punamäki, 2008; Qouta, Punamäki, & El Sarraj, 2003; Somasundaram & Jamunanantha, 2002; Sadeh, Hen-Gal, & Tikotzky, 2008). Children living in settings of collective violence may also routinely witness scenes of death and destruction via the mass media (Thabet, Abed, & Vostanis, 2001; Wang et al., 2006).

Frequently, collective violence also brings dislocation or migration, as persons are forcibly removed from their homes or as they flee violent zones to other, presumably safer, areas of their country or to other countries altogether. Besides the stressors experienced directly in the war setting, the transit experience itself may be perilous as persons move through war zones or other areas of social unrest or upheaval (Perez Foster, 2001). Transit may also involve dangerous modes of transportation, as well as high risk of sexual violence, forced labor, confinement, or imprisonment. Also, persons in refugee camps and detention centers may be at risk of physical and sexual violence from other refugees, staff, or both. Once in the host country, refugees or undocumented migrants may have limited economic resources and therefore live in disadvantaged areas with elevated rates of violence and crime. The stress of life in a new sociocultural environment, particularly with diminished material and social resources, can be traumatic and may heighten risk of family violence (Midlarsky, Venkataramani-Kothari, & Plante, 2006; Pumariega, Rothe, & Pumariega, 2005). Indeed, parsing out the effects of war on sleep from the effects resulting from the transit/migration experience and its consequences can be difficult.

In light of what people have experienced in environments of collective violence, as victim, witness, or both, it is unsurprising that these experiences may be traumatic and influence sleep. Numerous studies have investigated the effects of this exposure on the psychological health of children. Many investigations include information about sleep problems, usually based on subjective assessment of specific characteristics or qualities of sleep made by child, parent, or practitioner.

War and Displacement

Cross-sectional studies investigating sleep of children living in settings of collective violence or those recently departed from such settings (e.g., displaced persons or refugees) have generally reported substantial numbers of children of all ages experiencing sleep problems: "sleep disturbances" or "sleep difficulties" ranging from 32%–77% in school-age children and adolescents (Somasundaram & Jamunanantha, 2002; Thabet, Abed, & Vostanis, 2004; Tišinović, 2000; Zeidner, 2005) and 29%–48% among preschool children (Somasundaram & Jamunanantha, 2002; Thabet, Karim, & Vostanis, 2006); frequent nightmares or dreams with violent confrontations ranging from 22%–59% in adolescents (Khamis, 2005; Zeidner, 2005) and from 13%–75% in preschool and school-age children (Chimienti, Nasr, & Khalifeh, 1989; Masalha, 1993; Thabet & Vostanis, 1999); insomnia ranging from 20%–57% in samples of school-age children and adolescents (Khamis, 2005; Montgomery & Foldspang, 2001; Thabet, Abed, & Vostanis, 2001); and enuresis/encopresis prevalence of approximately 15% among school-age children (Chimienti et al., 1989). Several cross-sectional studies of displaced or refugee children undertaken 1 year or more after departing a war zone report substantial numbers of children still experiencing sleep disturbances or problems, insomnia, or nightmares/unpleasant dreams (Ajdukovic, 1998, Angel, Hjern, & Ingleby, 2001; Dyregrov et al., 2000; Hjern, Angel, & Hojer, 1991; Realmuto et al., 1992).

Two cross-sectional studies in particular asked respondents to compare current sleep with sleep before exposure to war. Obradović, Kanazir, Zališevskij, Popadić, and Simić's (1993) study of 102 Bosnia-Herzegovinian and Croatian refugees 8–19 years of age, who had lived in a war-affected area 1–5 months before leaving the war zone for Serbia, found that 78% of these adolescents reported sleep disturbances since the war began, while only 40% reported that disturbances occurred before the war. Similarly, in Sadeh and colleagues' recent (2008) study of 74 Israeli children 2–7 years of age who were relocated to a safety camp during the second Israel–Lebanon War, parents reported that substantial numbers of children exhibited new sleep-related problems since the start of the conflict: 10% excessive sleep, 43% enuresis/encopresis, 50% fear or problems falling asleep, and 52% nightmares.

Although studies incorporating use of a comparison group in their designs generally show worse sleep among children exposed to violence, this isn't always the case. In one early study, Rofé and Lewin (1982) compared the sleep behavior of 216 Israeli adolescents living in a border town subjected to repeated acts of collective violence to that of 270 adolescents living in a non-border town. Interestingly, based on self-completed sleep journals, the border town teens reported earlier bedtimes (21:59 vs. 22:27, $p < .001$), time when falling asleep (22:30 vs. 22:54, $p < .001$), rise times (06:39 vs. 06:49, $p < .05$) and slightly greater sleep duration (8.2 vs. 7.9 hrs, $p < .05$) than did their peers away from the violence. The investigators suggested that sleep patterns of the teens in the border towns were linked to a repressive personality dimension, which led to decreased worry among these teens or efforts to avoid thinking about war-related danger by sleeping. In subsequent research, Al-Eissa (1995) compared the sleep of 106 Kuwaiti refugee children from the first Iraq War to a comparison group consisting of a school-based sample of similarly aged Saudi schoolchildren approximately 1–2 months after the invasion. He found, based on parent report, that a greater number of the refugee children experienced difficulty sleeping (35% vs. 7%, $p < .001$), nightmares (37% vs. 9%, $p < .001$), and enuresis (24% vs. 13%, $p < .05$) compared to the non-refugees, respectively. Similarly, Paardekooper, De Jong, and Hermanns' (1999) study of 193 Sudanese refugee school-age children revealed a greater number of the refugees experiencing a range of sleep problems "sometimes" or "often" compared to a similarly aged school-based group of 80 children in host country Uganda: 46% vs. 15% can't sleep ($p < .001$), 56% vs. 20% nightmares of a traumatic event ($p < .001$), 53% vs. 15% cannot sleep because of worry or memories ($p < .001$). Punamäki, Ali, Ismahil, and Nuutinen (2005) compared the dreams of 65 war-displaced Kurdish orphans 9–17 years of age living in Iraqi Kurdistan to those of 57 nondisplaced, non-orphan children living in a nearby school. The investigators found that being an orphan affected only characteristics of dream structure: orphan's dreams were more narrative (effect size = .13), less vivid (effect size = .07), and less interrupted by nightmares (effect size = .15). Increased trauma exposure (orphan or not) was associated with an increase in unpleasant dreams (e.g., themes of death and destruction, negative feelings, and hostility) and dream-interrupting nightmares, effect sizes ranging from .05–.12.

Longitudinal research involving children's sleep in settings of collective violence has mainly involved displaced or refugee children. However, two studies investigated children's sleep *in situ*. First, Lavie, Amit, Epstein, and Tzischinsky (1993) compared the sleep behavior of 61 Israeli preschool children 5 months before the first Gulf War versus 10 days after the war. Results, based on parent report, revealed that before the war 93% of children slept during the day, compared to 68% after the war ($p < .001$). However, the investigators found no change over time in sleep duration, bedtime, wake-up time, sleep location, difficulties settling to sleep, night wakings, or the number of children sleeping too little.

In the second study, Thabet and Vostanis (2000) investigated parent- and teacher-reported sleep characteristics of 234 Palestinian (Gaza) school-age children "representative of the general population" at baseline and 12 months after the Second Intifada. Results showed a decrease in reported nightmares from 13.1% to 8.5% at the 12-month follow-up. Sleep disturbances similarly declined from 3% at baseline to 1.8% at follow-up.

Longitudinal research of displaced or refugee children also reports decreases in nonspecified sleep problems or disturbances over time, but with troublesome percentages of persons reporting problems months or even years later. For example, Ajdukovic and Ajdukovic's (1998) study of a convenience study of 110 mostly Croatian children 18 years of age or less, receiving services from a displaced person/refugee center's clinic in Croatia, showed a decline in both "sleep disturbances" (1.8% before displacement, 16.4% at 6 months after displacement, 9.8% at 12 months after displacement) and nightmares (2.7% before displacement, 22.7% at 6 months after displacement, and 9.8% at 12 months after displacement). Similarly, Almqvist and Brandell (1997) reported a decrease from 43% to 29% of sleep disorders in a sample of 50 Iranian refugees 1 year versus 2.5 years after resettlement in Sweden. In one of the longer follow-up periods, Hjern and Angel (2000) reported decreases in "sleep disturbances" among a community-based sample of 63 school-age Bosnian refugees from the initial baseline assessment 4–6 months after arrival in Stockholm compared to follow-up at 17–19 months and 6–7 years post-arrival: 60% at baseline, 42% at 17–19 months, and 16% at 6–7 years after arrival.

Terrorist Attacks

Studies conducted after terrorist attacks such as those in New York City and Washington, DC on September 11, 2001, or the 1998 bombing of the American Embassy in Nairobi, Kenya, suggest that such attacks may have a substantial, persistent effect on some children's sleep. In the case of September 11, a survey of a nationally representative sample of 570 US adults conducted 3 to 5 days after the attacks indicated that 10% of the homes with children 5–18 years of age had at least one child who had trouble falling or staying asleep since the day of the attacks, and 6% had a child experiencing nightmares (Schuster et al., 2001). A second web-based survey of a nationally representative survey of 2273 adults conducted 1 to 2 months after the attacks revealed that 61% of households in the New York metropolitan area, 57% of other metropolitan areas, and 48% of the rest of the United States had at least one child who was still "upset" by the attacks, and 28% of these upset children were having trouble sleeping according to the parent (Schlenger et al., 2002).

Smaller cross-sectional surveys were undertaken in the attacked cities at later time points. For example, approximately 3 months after the attacks, over 20% of a sample of 47 public-school 4th–6th graders in Washington, DC self-reported nightmares, and their parents reported that over 10% of the children still had problems falling or staying asleep and over 10% were having nightmares (Phillips, Prince, & Schiebelhut, 2004). Of note, self-reported sleep problems were more frequent among children who reported watching substantial television coverage of the attacks versus children who watched little or no coverage (42% vs. 11%, $p < .05$). DeVoe, Bannon, and Klein's (2006) survey of 156 children 0–5 years of age in daycare facilities in the greater New York City area revealed that 43% of the children had difficulty going to sleep based on parent report up to 3 months after the events.

Other surveys of community (usually school) based samples of schoolchildren in cities in the US midwest (Hock, Hart, Kang, & Lutz, 2004) and west coast (Kennedy, Charlesworth, & Chen, 2004; Lengua, Long, Smith, & Meltzoff, 2005), undertaken anywhere from 1 week to 3 months after the September 11 attacks, reported 12%–25% of children experiencing nightmares or bad dreams, 10%–19% having sleep disturbances or trouble sleeping, and 3% bedwetting. Moreover, levels of child-reported anxiety (Lengua et al., Hock et al.), parents' worry about their child's safety (Hock et al.), and parent-reported conduct problems (Lengua et al.), all measured before September 11, predicted children's PTS symptoms following the attack.

Hoven et al.'s (2004) study of a representative sample of 8326 4th–12th graders in the New York City public school system 6 months after the attacks revealed that 21% of the children reported having had "a lot" of bad dreams or nightmares the previous 4 weeks and 26% reported often wanting to have a parent nearby in order to fall asleep. Pfefferbaum et al.'s (2006) survey of 156 Kenyan 10–12-year-old children who knew someone killed in the 1998 bombing of the American embassy in Nairobi revealed that 8–14 months after the bombing, nearly half (46%) of the children reported still having dreams about the event "sometimes" or "often," and 41% reported having trouble falling asleep or staying asleep "sometimes" or "often." Of note, the authors noted that substantial numbers of children had been exposed to a range of other potentially traumatic events after the bombing.

Finally, Chemtob, Nomura, and Abramovitz (2008) conducted a study of a convenience sample of 116 children recruited from schools and other social services institutions in lower Manhattan, who were 5 years of age or younger during the September 11 attacks. The children were assessed 1.5–4.5 years after the attacks. The investigators collected information from the parents about the child's exposure to high-intensity World Trade Center events (e.g., saw people jumping out of the building, saw dead bodies, saw a tower collapse), lifetime exposure to a wide range of traumatic events other than the September 11 attacks (e.g., natural disasters, serious accidents or injuries, interpersonal loss, animal attacks, other war or terrorist acts), and behavior problems using well-established, psychometrically sound instruments. Results of logistic regression adjusted for the effects of child age, socioeconomic status (maternal educational level), time since the attack, and lifetime history of other traumatic events showed that the children exposed to high-intensity World Trade Center events were nearly 10 times more likely to have sleep problems than those children without exposure to high-intensity events (adjusted odds ratio [aOR] = 9.7, 95% CI 1.9 – 50.2).

In summary, studies based on subjective reports of children's sleep in environments of collective violence suggest that substantial numbers of children experience sleep problems, including nightmares and insomnia, core criteria for PTSD and ASD. Although these disturbances may decrease over time, they remain in a troublesome number of children. Moreover, the studies involving terrorist acts indicate that children need not reside in the location of a terrorist attack to be affected. Generally, studies utilizing a comparison-group design show greater problems among children experiencing community violence than those not in such environments.

Sleep of Children in Environments of Collective Violence—Objective Measures

Lavie and colleagues (1993) studied the effects of discrete acts of collective violence, namely, nighttime Scud missile attacks, on a sample of 55 school-aged Israeli children during the first Gulf War. To my knowledge, this is the only study to use an objective measure of sleep—actigraphy—during a period of ongoing collective violence. A wrist actigraph is small, noninvasive, device that is worn like a wristwatch. It contains a small microchip that electronically records arm movement. After it is worn, actigraph data are downloaded into a computer algorithm program that translates recorded movement into valid estimates of sleep/wake status (Morgenthaler et al., 2007). The actigraph permits investigators to obtain valid, objective estimates of sleep parameters such as sleep duration and sleep efficiency (proportion of time in bed when an individual is actually asleep) in the child's home environment. Lavie and colleagues found that children's sleep efficiency significantly decreased on the nights when missile attacks occurred after bedtime compared to nights when the attacks occurred before bedtime (91.2% vs., 88%, $p < .008$). Data suggested that during a post-bedtime missile attack, children were initially awakened by the alarm warning citizens of the incoming missiles but then resumed sleep shortly after the "all-clear" was sounded, with no noticeable difficulty. Moreover, comparison of the study children's sleep characteristics during nights without a missile attack with those of 64 similarly-aged children recorded 1 year before the war revealed no significant differences in time of sleep onset, sleep duration, or sleep efficiency. Thus, besides the immediate response to the missile attack, the actigraphy-derived indices of sleep seemed minimally affected.

The Sleep of Children in Environments of Interpersonal Violence—Subjective Measures

Interpersonal violence includes numerous actions such as physical and sexual abuse, intimate partner violence, and community violence. Children's sleep in settings of these forms of interpersonal violence is discussed below.

Physical and Sexual Abuse

Compared to other forms of interpersonal violence, a larger number of studies involving the effects of child maltreatment have examined sleep. In a cross-sectional study, Wolfe, Sas, and Wekerle's (1994) sample of 90 young Canadian adolescents participating in a child abuse assessment and court preparation project revealed that 58% reported that nightmares about the sexual abuse occurred "sometimes" or "a lot," and the same percentage reported trouble falling asleep because of intrusive thoughts of the events.

Since the 1980s, several studies utilizing a comparison-group design have reported differences in sleep characteristics of mainly agency-based or clinic-based samples of children and adolescents who experienced physical and/or sexual abuse compared to non-abused peers. For example, Janus, McCormack, Burgess, and Hartman (1987) compared the prevalence of dreams about physical abuse, insomnia, and nonspecified "sleep problems" in a shelter-based sample of 58 adolescents in Toronto, Canada, who left home because of physical abuse versus 76 adolescents who ran away for other reasons. Results showed that the physically abused runaways reported significantly greater dreams about abuse (53% vs. 32%, $p < .01$), and unspecified "sleep problems" (76% vs. 40%, $p < .001$), but not trouble falling or staying asleep (52% vs. 38%). Goldston, Turnquist, and Knutson (1989) performed a chart review of the sleep disturbances of 195 girls 2–18 years of age (mean age 10.1, standard deviation not reported) who were consecutively admitted to one of three mental health services in a midwestern US city. The investigators found that greater numbers of sexually abused girls had sleep disturbances compared to similarly aged non-abused girls (37% vs. 18.6% among the 2–11-year-old girls and 20.7% vs. 8.3% among 12–18-year-old girls), but these differences were not statistically significant.

Sadeh et al. (1994) conducted retrospective chart reviews of 100 children 2–13 years of age consecutively admitted to a psychiatric inpatient facility in Providence, Rhode Island. Forty-nine of these children had a history of sexual abuse, 23 had been physically abused, and 28 had no documented history of either physical or sexual abuse. Analyses controlling for child age revealed that a significantly greater number of sexually abused children exhibited parasomnias (e.g., sleep terrors, sleepwalking, partial arousal disorders) compared to either the physically abused or non-abused children (20.4%, 4.4%, and 3.7%, respectively [$p < .05$]). No differences were observed for sleep onset, night walking, enuresis, or encopresis. Kelly and Ben-Meir (1993) compared a clinic-based convenience sample of 55 sexually abused California adolescents matched on age and sex to 37 non-abused children recruited through a school who were experiencing "excessive or unreasonable fears." Analyses revealed that more sexually abused children reported nightmares (34% vs. 0%, $p < .001$) and trouble getting to sleep at night (21% vs. 0%) than the non-abused children. Finally, in a retrospective chart review of patients treated over a 5-year period at a Washington State public psychiatric hospital, McCellan, Adams, Douglas, McCurry, and Storck (1995) found over twice the odds of nightmares ($OR = 2.27$, $p < .0001$) among 273 sexually abused 5–18-year-old children and adolescents versus 226 similar non-abused patients.

Of note, differences are not always detected for every sleep-related problem. For example, Famularo, Kinscherff, and Fenton's (1992) case-control study of a US urban, court-based sample of 61 severely maltreated 5–10-year-old children found no difference in either child or parent report of enuresis or encopresis compared to a control group of 35 non-maltreated children. These investigators found similar results in a subsequent study of a court-based sample of school-age children with and without PTSD (Famularo, Fenton, Kinscherff, & Augustyn, 1996).

Concerning longitudinal study of abused children's sleep, Calam, Horne, Glasgow, and Cox (1998) examined 99 cases of sexually or physically abused children living in Liverpool City, UK, who had been reported as suffering from alleged/suspected child abuse over a 12-month period. Children were 1–16 years of age at baseline and were followed at 4 weeks, 9 months, and 2 years after initiation of the case. Results based on social worker report showed that at 4 weeks, 20% of the 65 children for whom data were available exhibited sleep problems. Nine months later, 57 of the 99 children were examined and 34% experienced sleep problems. Two years after baseline, 66 of the original 99 children were assessed and 33% exhibited sleep problems. Unfortunately, changes in the sample composition over time make interpretation of the reported results difficult.

In a more recent study, Noll, Trickett, Susman, and Putnam (2006) investigated self-reported sleep disturbances (as assessed by a 12-item composite measure) and sleep duration of a greater Washington, DC clinical sample of 78 sexually abused girls 6–16 years of age who were assessed approximately 10 years after disclosure of the sexual abuse. Results adjusted for age showed that the abused girls reported significantly more sleep disturbances compared to a convenience sample of 69 similarly aged non-abused girls recruited from the same neighborhoods of residence as the abused girls (Z scores 0.22 ± 1.06 vs. -0.24 ± 0.90, respectively, $p = .009$). Moreover, abuse status significantly predicted sleep disturbances even after adjusting for depression and PTSD symptoms.

Other research has investigated whether sleep disturbances among abused children differ by type or chronicity of abuse, chronicity of PTSD, or co-occurrence of other disorders. For example, Noll et al. (2006) reported that after adjusting for the effects of age, PTSD, and depression, only study participants victimized by single-perpetrator abuse reported significantly greater sleep disturbances than a non-abused comparison group (Z scores 0.79 ± 1.11 vs. -0.18 ± 0.91, respectively, $p < .05$). However, sleep disturbances of participants who were victimized by multiple perpetrators (Z score = 0.18 ± 1.07) or by their biological fathers (Z score = 0.23 ± 0.98) were not significantly different from the non-abused comparison group. Adjusted results also showed that a greater percentage of participants victimized by a single perpetrator reported less than 7 hours of nightly sleep compared to the participants victimized by multiple perpetrators (37.7% vs. 13.2%, $p < .05$). No other differences among groups in the percentages of participants sleeping 7 hours or fewer were detected. Noll and colleagues indicate that the link between higher sleep disturbance and single perpetrator victimization may be due to the fact that this was a relatively less severe form of abuse compared to abuse by multiple perpetrators or by the participants' fathers, perhaps resulting in less intensive treatment than was actually needed to address later disturbances.

McCellan et al.'s (1995) retrospective chart review study of 5–18-year-old patients at the psychiatric hospital described above found greater odds of nightmares (OR = 1.63, $p < .005$) among 150 chronically abused patients than in 123 patients with isolated or intermittent abuse. Runyon, Faust, and Orvaschel's (2002) study of PTSD symptom patterns in a US clinic-based sample of 34 children diagnosed with PTSD, compared to 27 children with dual diagnosis of PTSD and major depressive disorder, revealed greater trouble sleeping and bad dreams among the children with the dual diagnosis (64% vs. 29%, $p < .01$). Famularo, Kinscherff, and Fenton (1990) studied traumatic stress symptoms in a US clinic-based sample of 5–13-year-old children and reported more frequent nightmares and difficulty falling asleep among the 10 children with acute PTSD versus the 14 children with chronic PTSD.

Intimate Partner Violence

Published research on the sleep of children living in settings of intimate partner violence appears limited to cross-sectional studies. In Smaldone, Honig, and Byrne's (2009) secondary analysis of data from 68,418 parents or caregivers of children aged 6–17 years who participated in the 2003 US National Survey of Children's Health, the authors combined three survey questions to create a variable that classified families as having one of three conflict styles: violent disagreements, heated disagreements, or calm. Results of multivariable logistic regression adjusting for the effects of numerous child, family, and environment variables revealed that compared to families with a calm conflict style, families with a violent disagreement conflict style had nearly twice the odds (aOR = 1.91, 95% confidence interval = 1.45–2.50) of a child with severely inadequate sleep, defined as sleeping well 2 nights per week or fewer.

Three smaller cross-sectional studies have also provided data relating to the proportion of children experiencing sleep disturbances in families with intimate partner violence. Graham-Berman and Levendosky's (1998) investigation of a shelter-based convenience sample of 64 children 7–12 years of age living in Michigan cities revealed that 9% of the children reported dreams or nightmares occurring at least once per month that were specific to violence they observed, and 13% reported sleep disturbances, trouble falling asleep, or trouble staying asleep occurring at least once per month since the violent event(s) that led the children to a shelter.

In a second study, Levendosky, Huth-Bocks, Semel, and Shapiro's (2002) investigation of an agency-based convenience sample of 62 children 3–5 years of age living in a midwestern US city revealed that 21% of the children experienced either an increased number of frightening dreams, or nightmares about past violent events, which occurred at least once per month based on maternal report. Three percent of children reported having difficulty going to sleep for at least 1 month in duration since the violent event. Finally, Humphreys and Lee (2006) studied a convenience sample of 43 San Francisco Bay area children 2–18 years of age whose mothers were battered and who were living with their mothers in transitional housing for a minimum of 3 weeks. The study revealed via parent report that 40% of the children resisted going to bed, 30% had difficulty falling asleep, 36% were never or rarely easy to wake in the morning. Moreover, the mothers reported that 36% of the children experienced restless sleep, 38% experienced excessive movement during sleep, and 37% of the children had awakened their mother four or more times during the previous week. Nineteen percent of the children, mostly boys, were bedwetting. Night terrors were rare (5%), but 18% of the children experienced nightmares 4 or more nights per week. Moreover, the authors reported that nearly three-quarters of the children did not meet established sleep requirements for their ages.

Community Violence

Several studies have provided cross-sectional data on sleep characteristics of children living in settings with elevated levels of community violence. Fitzpatrick and Boldizar's (1993) study of a convenience sample of 221 children living in a large, south-central US city, with presumed chronic exposure to community violence, reported that over 50% of the children experienced bad dreams/nightmares, and 37% reported difficulty sleeping. In a smaller study of 64 adolescents 16–18 years of age living in a mid-Atlantic US city, Cooley-Quille and Lorion (1999) assessed via self-report participants' lifetime exposure to community violence and their sleep difficulties the previous week using a 5-item investigator-developed questionnaire. No significant sex or age differences were found for either violence exposure or sleep disturbances. However, sleep disturbances and exposure to community violence categorized as low, medium, or high were significantly and positively related, in a clear dose-response manner.

In a similar study involving younger children, Nordstrom Bailey et al. (2005) examined the associations between child-reported difficulties going to sleep and exposure to community violence as both witness and victim in a clinic-derived birth cohort of 268 urban US children, who were 6–7 years of age at the time of assessment. Children who reported being victimized by community violence had nearly twice the odds of difficulty sleeping compared to children who were not victimized, after adjusting for the effects of numerous individual and family demographic and health factors ($OR = 1.94$, $p < .01$). Similarly, children at or above the median level of witnessing violence had a 79% increased risk of difficulty sleeping ($p < .05$) compared to children below the median.

Stewart et al.'s (2004) study of an agency-based convenience sample of 374 homeless adolescents in greater Seattle revealed that 83% had been victimized after leaving home. Moreover, 17% of participants' self-reported bad dreams and nightmares at least once per week, and 25% reported trouble sleeping at least once per week.

Concerning longitudinal research, Pynoos and colleagues conducted a series of studies of traumatic stress symptoms of US elementary school children following a school shooting (Nader, Pynoos, Fairbanks, & Frederick, 1990; Pynoos, Frederick, et al., 1987; Pynoos, Nader, Frederick, Gonda, & Stuber, 1987). Approximately one month post-shooting, a cross-sectional survey of 157 of these children's parents revealed that 46% of the children were experiencing sleep disturbances and that the proportion of children with sleep disturbances increased based on the children's location during the shooting: 77% of those on the playground where the shooting occurred, 56%

of those in school but not on the playground, 42% of those not in school that day, and 24% of those who were on vacation ($p < .001$). Moreover, 46% of all children had bad dreams following the shooting, with similar decrease in percentage the farther away a child was from the site of the shooting (e.g., 63% of children who were on the playground that day vs. 33% who were on vacation ($p < .01$).

In a 1-year follow-up study of 251 of the children present at the school during the shooting, Pynoos, Nader, et al. (1987) showed that 11% still reported dreams about the shooting. Significantly greater percentages of children reported these dreams if *(1)* they knew the victim "well" (e.g., 25% who knew victim well vs. 5% who knew the victim "not at all") and *(2)* if they were located on the playground the day of the shooting (24% who were on the playground vs. 8% in school not on playground vs. 6% not in school the day of the shooting). A 14-month follow-up of the schoolchildren showed that these associations continued: 18% of all children reported sleep disturbances (42% who were on the playground that day) and 20% of all children reported nightmares, with 42% of children who were on the playground doing so (Nader et al., 1990). Similar findings were reported in a clinical sample consisting of 64 children 5–14 years of age following a shooting in another US school (Schwartz & Kowalski, 1991): 8–14 months after the event, 30% of children reported recurrent distressing dreams at least "some of the time," and 30% complained of insomnia at least "some of the time."

Mixed Forms

Several studies have examined subjective reports of sleep disturbances involving samples of children exposed to mixed forms of interpersonal violence. Three small (i.e., 10–55 participants), clinic-based studies of US children collectively 3–18 years of age, exposed to their parents' sexual assault (Pynoos & Nader, 1988) or murder (Malmquist, 1986; Eth & Pynoos, 1994), revealed 80%–100% of the children reported nightmares of the event at least once per week, and preschool children displayed more sleep disturbances associated with deeper sleep (e.g., sleep walking, sleep talking, night terrors) than adolescents (Eth & Pynoos, 1994).

In Linares et al.'s (2001) cross-sectional study of a randomized clinic-based sample of 160 children 3–5 years of age living in high-crime Boston neighborhoods, parents disclosed that 31% of children reported nightmares of violence, 15% experienced trouble sleeping, 29% woke up at night, 41% were afraid to sleep alone, and 49% were afraid of the dark. Unfortunately, the duration of time between the reported violent event(s) and the assessment were not provided. Carrion, Weems, Ray, and Reiss (2002) conducted a similar clinic-based, cross-sectional study of 59 US school-age children and found that 64% of the children reported distressing dreams and 59.3% reported sleep problems. In one of the better studies in terms of sample size (representative nationwide of over 8000 students) and control for potentially confounding factors, a case-control study of French adolescents found that after adjusting for the effects of sex and age, the odds of adolescent victims experiencing nightmares "fairly often" or "very often" was 3.2 (95% CI 1.4–7.2) times that of non-victimized teenagers matched on sex, age, school district, and school level (Choquet, Darves-Bornoz, Ledoux, Manfredi, & Hassler, 1997).

In summary, the available literature indicates that sleep problems are commonly reported among children and adolescents living in environments with various forms of interpersonal violence, and typically occur in greater frequency compared to peers not exposed to violence. Similar to community violence, longitudinal research suggests that these problems may persist for years in some cases.

The Sleep of Children in Environments of Interpersonal Violence—Objective Measures

Sexual Abuse

Two studies have used objective sleep measures to examine clinical samples of sleep characteristics of abused children. In the first study, Sadeh et al. (1995) compared several actigraphy-derived indices (e.g., sleep duration, sleep onset, sleep efficiency) in three groups of 7–14-year-old children who were inpatients at a Providence, Rhode Island hospital: 12 children with sexual and physical abuse, 8 children with physical abuse only, 7 with sexual abuse only, and 12 children with no history of abuse. Actigraphy data were collected during one to three evenings. Analyses revealed that the physically abused children exhibited less sleep efficiency than the non-abused or sexually abused children ($89.2 \pm 4.8\%$, $93.1 \pm 3.7\%$, $93.9 \pm 1.4\%$, respectively, $p < .05$). Moreover, the children victimized by physical abuse, with ($58.5 \pm 10.3\%$) or without sexual abuse ($58.3 \pm 7.1\%$), spent less time in quiet, motionless sleep than the children who were sexually abused only ($67.3 \pm 10.1\%$) or the non-abused children ($67.8 \pm 9.7\%$). Other sleep parameters did not differ across groups.

Glod, Teicher, Hartman, and Harakal (1997) conducted a similar actigraphy study utilizing a clinical sample of 19 abused US children (sexually, physically, or both) compared to 10 children with clinically diagnosed depression and 15 children neither abused nor depressed. Actigraphy data from 3 consecutive nights were collected. Analyses revealed that compared to the non-abused, non-depressed group of children, the abused group had twice the nocturnal activity (104.7 ± 51.3 vs. 52.6 ± 13.9, $p<.001$), twice the percentage of nocturnal activity (7.4 ± 3.1 vs. 3.6 ± 1.1, $p<.0001$), three times the sleep latency (33.9 ± 27.2 minutes vs. 11.0 ± 8.8 minutes, $p<.005$), and less sleep efficiency (91.6 ± 5.1 vs. 96.1 ± 1.6, $p<.005$). The abused group also showed significantly greater nocturnal activity, percent nocturnal activity, and sleep latency than the group of non-abused children with depressive disorders.

Intimate Partner Violence.

To my knowledge, El-Sheikh, Buckhalt, Mize, and Acebo (2006) have conducted the only published study examining the association between objectively measured children's sleep characteristics and marital conflict. In this study, a school-based sample of 54 3rd-grade children from a southeastern US city wore actigraphs for 7 days. Psychometrically validated instruments were used to measure parent-reported and child-reported levels of marital conflict, as well as child-reported daytime sleepiness. Results showed that after adjusting for the effects of child age, sex, ethnicity, and BMI, increased child-reported marital conflict in families significantly predicted decreased total sleep time, decreased sleep percent (akin to percentage of minutes of actual sleep during the period of time between the onset of sleep time and the end of sleep time) and increased nighttime activity while in bed. Also, increased parent-reported marital conflict was significantly associated with increased child-reported daytime sleepiness.

In summary, a handful of studies have used objective measures of sleep to detect alterations in sleep among children exposed to various forms of interpersonal violence. Collectively, the research has generally documented poorer sleep quantity, quality, or both among these children compared to unexposed children.

Children's Sleep Environments in Settings of Violence

Most of the existing knowledge about violence and sleep focuses on the sleep-related symptoms of traumatic stress children experience; for example, insomnia, nightmares, and nonspecific sleep "disturbances" or "problems." Less studied is how living in violent settings influences actual sleep environments. Most of our knowledge about this topic comes from qualitative research or case studies that typically involve adult report (e.g., Berman, 2000; Groves, 2001; Howard, Kaljee, Rachuba, & Cross, 2003; Humphreys, Lowe, & Williams, 2009; Lowe, Humphreys, & Williams, 2007). Information from children's perspectives is less common. Moreover, several ethnographic-like works that provide detailed accounts of children's lives in violence-prone areas have included information pertaining to the sleep environment (e.g., Kotlowitz, 1991; Kozol, 1995; Raymond & Raymond, 2000).

One common theme that emerges from the available literature on the sleep environment in settings of violence is displacement out of the area, which may lead to profound changes in the sleep environment. Perhaps the most drastic example of such displacement is in cases involving collective violence, where families literally flee or are forced from their countries because of the occurrence or threat of violence. For example, recent accounts of both Croatian and Ugandan children trying to escape the collective violence that encompassed their towns and that killed their parents and other family members described how the children avoided their homes and slept for substantial periods of time in the forest (Amone-P'Olak, Garnefski, & Kraaij, 2007; Raymond & Raymond, 2000). Displaced persons and refugees may stay for weeks, months, or even years in shelters, detention or sorting camps, or centers. Although some facilities may provide a reasonable standard of living for residents (Sadeh et al., 2008), others may be overcrowded, have substandard facilities, and be dangerously violent in their own right. Accounts of sleeping arrangements in some of the published scientific literature speak to the difficult conditions. For example, consider the experience of a young Bosnian refugee, child "E":

> E, 5 years old, her parents, and older brother reached southern Sweden by bus and were immediately placed in a temporary sorting camp 1000 miles north. E's parents described barrack life as unexpectedly and harshly primitive: 14 persons of all ages were crowded into a single room. Adult war veterans smoked and paced the floor all night, infants screamed. The only help the nurse had to offer was earplugs. (Goldin, Levin, Persson, & Hägglöf, 2001, p. 37)

Of course, displacement is not limited to war, terrorism, and ethnic cleansing but may also occur in settings of interpersonal violence. Sex and/or physical abuse at home compels children and adolescents to flee their homes and live (and sleep) on the street or in shelters or other forms of transitory housing (Janus et al., 1987). Similarly, intimate partner violence and community violence may force parents to leave their homes with their children. Such parents may initially resort to emergency shelters, which may be crowded and limited in their ability to adequately house families.

Families may also seek refuge at transitional housing or the residences of family members and friends. We have conducted pilot longitudinal research on the sleep of 46 children 8–16 years of age exposed to family and/or community violence that involved police intervention and who were referred to our study by a community-based program that provides counseling and other services to children who witness violence (Drotar et al., 2003). As part of this study, we have directly observed and collected information from participants on their current sleep environment(s) shortly after the event that brought police intervention and then conducted a follow-up visit approximately 3 months later to collect additional information. One striking finding was that nearly one-third of families changed residence *within three months* of the violent event that generated a referral to the community-based program, and three families moved twice over the course of the study (Spilsbury, Frame, & Winfield, 2010). Participants indicated that violence, particularly domestic violence, often compelled the families to move for numerous reasons: *(1)* safety concerns; *(2)* loss of income and subsequent inability to afford current housing because of the perpetrator's absence or incarceration; *(3)* psychological need to leave the house where violence occurred; *(4)* death of caretaker(s) and transfer of children to new caretaker.

In such situations, as pilot study families moved to another household—typically moving in with friends or relatives as a less expensive alternative—observed sleep arrangements were often makeshift. In six cases, multiple children slept on the living room floor or shared a sofa or chair. In another nine cases, children shared a bed with 1–2 other children. These new sleeping arrangements were difficult for several participants. For example, 12-year-old "Mary" and her mother left their home to stay at a family friend's already cramped apartment. Mary and her mother slept in the apartment's living room each night, Mary on the sofa and her mother on a mattress on the floor. Mary complained that after she lay on the sofa to sleep for the night, people would enter the living room and turn on the overhead light. Also, her brothers frequently played video games on the living room TV after Mary's bedtime, and her mother watched TV into the early hours of the next day. Mary's mother instructed her daughter to turn over and face the wall instead of the TV. Sometimes Mary would take a blanket and pillow and try to sleep on the floor at the far end of the living room, the point farthest from the TV, but she explained that people would step on her and wake her up. Clearly, this makeshift arrangement was not "sleep friendly" to Mary.

The literature also reveals efforts made by families to improve their perceived safety in cases where they remain in their residence. In accounts of children living in war zones, families might move to the basement of homes to sleep during bombardments or avoid exterior rooms that would be targeted by snipers (Raymond & Raymond, 2000). Similar actions have been noted in violence-prone inner cities, where families may move beds away from windows, sleep in central rooms, or even sleep in bathtubs to avoid intruders or stray bullets (Kotlowitz, 1991; Kozol, 1995). Families may also keep bedroom windows shut even in homes without air conditioning during the hot summer months (Klinenberg, 2002).

A series of two articles (Humphreys et al., 2009; Lowe et al., 2007) based on a focus-group study of 17 UK women survivors of domestic violence (14 of whom were mothers of 28 children) has provided a fascinating and terrifying window into the nature of sleep in settings of domestic violence, where fear is the "organizing principle" (Lowe et al., 2007, p. 550). The mothers reported frequent disruptions to their children's sleep—trouble settling at night, nightmares, and night terrors. Several of the women reported that their children developed enuresis because of the violence, in some cases because they felt their children were literally too scared to get out of bed at night. A case study of children's sleep in domestic violence settings similarly echoed children's fear to get out of bed or make a sound in their bedrooms lest it upset the perpetrator of violence (Berman, 2000).

Participants in the Lowe and Humphreys studies described several strategies employed to maximize their safety, which included changing their sleeping location to avoid sleeping in their bedroom next to the violent partner and sleeping elsewhere in the house, such as on a sofa or in their children's bedrooms. Even after the perpetrator was no longer present, some women reported sleeping downstairs where they could watch the front door or be alerted to sounds of someone breaking into the house.

A number of case studies in the medical literature have included information pertaining to changes in sleep routines in response to the experience of violence that subsequently change environmental "features" or introduce new objects into the sleep environment. Many of these changes are related to efforts to improve perceived safety. For example, Kaufman, Birmaher, Clayton, Retano, and Wongchaowart (1997) reported that a young girl who had been victimized by sexual abuse began taking a toy dog and duck to bed with her every evening. She reported sleeping with the dog to prevent further attacks because, according to the girl, the perpetrator was afraid of dogs. Similarly, other studies have reported that children may take weapons to bed with them in order to protect themselves in the event of an attack (Pynoos & Nader, 1988). Other children may sleep in their street clothes to facilitate escaping from an attack (Dawes, Tredoux, & Feinstein, 1989). Families may place bars or extra locks on bedroom windows, lock doors and windows, or make sure they are locked before retiring each night (Groves, 2001; Howard et al., 2003; Pynoos & Nader, 1988). Children may change sleeping location to sleep nearby or with others to increase their perceived safety (Gaffney, 2006; Gorham, 1997; Kaplow, Saxe, Putnam, Pynoos, & Lieberman, 2006; Spencer, Dobbs, & Swanson, 1988).

Similarly, in our pilot study in Cleveland, we observed families modifying the household environment to improve perceived safety: relocating to a siblings' or mother's bedroom to sleep with someone, padlocking bedroom doors at night, blocking nearby entryways with large appliances (e.g., refrigerators) to restrict movement within the domicile, or keeping windows shut, even in rooms without air conditioning during hot weather, to keep out unwanted intruders. We also observed some caregivers altering the sleep environment specifically to improve children's sleep: moving children's beds away from noisy walls, adding curtains to block unwanted light, reducing unwanted TV noise, providing additional (comfortable) bedding materials. Moreover, the family of one 11-year-old boy who had witnessed his mother assaulted by her partner installed a dimmer switch for the light in his bedroom so he could adjust light levels to enhance comfort, perceived safety, or both.

Sleep and Exposure to Virtual Environments of Violence

Nighttime use of televisions, computers, and video games contribute to poorer sleep among children and adolescents wherever studied (reviewed by Cain & Gradisar, 2010; Van den Buick 2010). Moreover, substantial numbers of children and adolescents spend considerable time watching television with violent content, playing violent video games, or both. The violent content of these media may be especially concerning in regard to sleep problems: use of violent video games has been linked to increased arousal and other physiological alterations in players' cardiovascular and respiratory systems (Ivarsson, Anderson, Åkerstedt, & Lindblad, 2009; also reviewed by Anderson & Bushman, 2001). Of note, a recent study of the differential effects on sleep of content and timing of television, video game, and computer use revealed that both daytime media use with violent content and evening media use were independently associated with increased sleep problems among a randomized sample of 612 US preschool children taking part in a controlled trial to promote healthy media (Garrison, Liekweg, & Christakis, 2011).

Conclusion

The scientific literature indicates that substantial numbers of children and adolescents living in settings of collective and interpersonal violence experience sleep disturbances, including nightmares and insomnia, as assessed by parent or child report. Similarly, the small number of studies using objective measures of sleep (actigraphy) generally reported links between poor sleep quantity, sleep quality, and increased nighttime activity with increased exposure to violence. Although one of the actigraphy-based studies (Sadeh et al., 1995) suggested that sleep effects may differ by form of violence (physical abuse vs. sexual abuse), the collective literature on sleep–violence linkages seems to suggest that the effects of different forms of violence on sleep are more similar than they are different.

Collectively, the few longitudinal studies available indicate that although the number of children with sleep problems or disturbances declines over time, the effects of violence on sleep may persist in a substantial number of children and adolescents for a considerable length of time, even for years in some cases. To the best of my knowledge, the currently available longitudinal research consists entirely of sleep as assessed by parent, child, adolescent, or provider perceptions of sleep quantity and quality. No longitudinal studies have been published involving an objective measure of sleep.

Research on the sleep environment in settings of violence show notable similarities regardless of the specific form of violence. First, violence often brings dislocation, which may well entail profound changes in the sleep environment. These new environments may be "makeshift," inadequate, and dangerous in their own right. Second, families living in settings of collective or interpersonal violence take steps to increase the safety of the sleep environment. Such steps might include physically moving to a part of the dwelling "out of the line of fire," or sleeping with or nearby others. Families may also take action to make the sleep environment as conducive to sleep as possible, even in makeshift situations.

Although the existing research has made significant strides in our understanding of the relationship between sleep and violence, limitations are apparent. First, most of the literature on the sleep of children exposed to violence has examined subjective perceptions of sleep problems or disturbances. Information about such basic sleep parameters as bedtime, wake time, nightly sleep duration, sleep efficiency, or daily napping behavior is scant. Second, research using objective measures of children's sleep in violent settings is rare, limited to a handful of actigraphy-based studies. Published research involving polysomnographic data on children or adolescents living in violent environments is apparently nonexistent. Third, most of the studies conducted with child and adolescent participants to date are cross-sectional in nature, so the trajectory of sleep over time is unclear in this population. Fourth, studies have been uneven in their effort to distinguish the effects of violence from those of other factors that may be related to or even caused by violence. Children living in a violent environment may experience multiple forms of violence, traumatic events unrelated to violence (e.g., car accident), migration or dislocation from one's home, the death of a loved one, or substandard housing, to name but a few factors or conditions that might influence sleep. Some investigations have noted (e.g., Pfefferbaum et al., 2006) or even accounted for (e.g., Chemtob et al., 2008) the presence of other traumatic events in their study populations in their analyses. Unfortunately, not all studies collect such information and the tendency to misattribute symptoms of distress to specific violent acts has been noted (Wilson & Spenciner, 2004). In light of these limitations, the next section highlights suggested future directions.

Future Directions

- *Investigate sleep more broadly.* To fully understand the effects of violence on children's sleep behavior, research is needed that incorporates a wider range of sleep characteristics, including those obtained by objective methods such as actigraphy and polysomnography. Polysomnographic studies would generate data on the sleep architecture of children and adolescents living in violent environments, thereby providing a more complete picture of violence's influence on sleep and perhaps provide clues for interventions. Likewise, expanding the investigative gaze to include children's sleep environments would provide information potentially invaluable for interventions.
- *Conduct longitudinal studies of sleep in children exposed to violence and include nonclinical populations.* Results of the small number of extent longitudinal studies on violence and sleep indicate that the effects of violence on sleep may persist for substantial periods of time. More longitudinal studies are needed to fully characterize violence-induced changes in sleep behavior and the sleep environment, including identification of potential moderators and mediators of observed effects. Ideally, such research would also take into account changes in children's exposure to violence over time. Also, to better understand the effects of violence on sleep, more research is needed with nonclinical community samples of children and adolescents, particularly in the domain of interpersonal violence.
- *Distinguish the effects of violence from effects of other factors.* Future research should develop strategies to better parse the effects of violence from the effects of co-occurring factors or the sequelae of violence. Understanding the relative contributions of multiple factors that shape sleep is important in order to identify the best factors to target for intervention.
- *Investigate sleep in children and adolescents who are being exposed to virtual environments of violence through their use of the mass media and video games.* Of course, when such sobering numbers of children and adolescents are exposed to real environments of violence and suffering, the viewpoint that (precious) resources spent on virtual violence could be better used elsewhere is understandable. However, given the wide use of these media and the growing evidence of their influence on children and adolescents, further research on the effects of virtual violence on sleep quantity and quality, including changes in the timing of sleep, is merited.

• *Interventions to improve sleep of children living in violent environments.* Surely, the most effective way to decrease the number of children whose sleep is adversely affected by violence is to remove violence from the living environment—a daunting task that leads us instead to focus on other strategies. Although sleep characteristics—notably insomnia and nightmares—are typically addressed in psychological treatment of traumatic stress disorder, evidence-based, sleep-focused interventions for children who are exposed to violence are rare. Sadeh and colleagues' (2008) "Huggy Puppy" intervention for preschool children represents one of the few publications providing efficacy data on such an intervention. More research is needed in this direction. Along these lines, further research is needed to identify effective methods to incorporate sleep into the work of social workers and other providers serving children and families in violent settings. Clearly, issues around safety are first priority, but these frontline workers have the opportunity to directly observe sleep environments and discuss sleep problems or concerns with families. Putting sleep more firmly "on the radar screen" of social workers may provide an effective avenue to improve families' sleep.

References

Ajdukovic, M. (1998). Displaced adolescents in Croatia: Sources of stress and posttraumatic stress reaction. *Adolescence, 33,* 209–217.

Ajdukovic, M., & Ajdukovic, D. (1998). Impact of displacement on the psychological well-being of refugee children. *International Review of Psychiatry, 10,* 186–195.

Al-Eissa, Y. A. (1995). The impact of the Gulf armed conflict on the health and behavior of Kuwaiti children. *Social Science and Medicine, 41,* 1033–1037.

Almqvist, K., & Brandell-Forsberg, M. (1997). Refugee children in Sweden: Post-traumatic stress disorder in Iranian preschool children exposed to organized violence. *Child Abuse & Neglect, 21,* 351–366.

American Psychiatric Association (2000). *Diagnostic and Statistical Manual of Mental Disorders, Fourth Edition, Text Revision.* Washington, DC: American Psychiatric Association.

Amone-P'Olak, K., Garnefski, N., & Kraaij, N. (2007). Adolescents caught between fires: Cognitive emotion regulation in response to war experiences in Northern Uganda. *Journal of Adolescence, 30,* 655–669.

Anderson, C. A., & Bushman, B. J. (2001). Effects of violent video games on aggressive behavior, aggressive cognition, aggressive affect, physiological arousal, and prosocial behavior: A meta-analytic review of the scientific literature. *Psychological Science, 12,* 353–359.

Angel, B., Hjern, A., & Ingleby, D. (2001). Effects of war and organized violence on children: A study of Bosnian refugees in Sweden. *American Journal of Orthopsychiatry, 71,* 5.

Berman, H. (2000). The relevance of narrative research with children who witness war and children who witness woman abuse. (2000). *Journal of Aggression, Maltreatment, and Trauma, 3,* 107–125.

Cain, N., & Gradisar, M. (2010). Electronic media use and sleep in children and adolescents: A review. *Sleep Medicine, 11,* 735–742.

Calam, R., Horne, L., Glasgow, D., & Cox, A. (1998). Psychological disturbance and child sexual abuse: A follow-up study. *Child Abuse & Neglect, 22,* 901–913.

Caldwell, B. A., & Redeker, N. (2005). Sleep and trauma: An overview. *Issues in Mental Health Nursing, 26,* 721–738.

Carpenter, G. L., & Stacks, A. M. (2009). Developmental effects of exposure to intimate partner violence in early childhood: A review of the literature. *Children and Youth Services Review, 31,* 831–839.

Carrion, V. G., Weems, C. F., Ray, R., & Reiss, A. L. (2002). Toward an empirical definition of pediatric PTSD: The phenomenology of PTSD symptoms in youth. *Journal of the American Academy of Child and Adolescent Psychiatry, 41,* 166–173.

Chemtob, C. M., Nomura, Y., & Abramovitz, R. A. (2008). Impact of conjoined exposure to the World Trade Center attacks and to other traumatic events on the behavioral problems of preschool children. *Archives of Pediatrics and Adolescent Medicine, 162,* 126–133.

Child Trends. (March 1, 2011). *Child Maltreatment.* Retrieved October 24, 2011 from http://www.childtrendsdatabank.org/sites/default/files/40_Child_Maltreatment.pdf.

Chimienti, G., Nasr, J. A., & Khalifeh, I. (1989). Children's reactions to war-related stress. *Social Psychiatry and Psychiatric Epidemiology, 24,* 282–287.

Choquet, M., Darves-Bornoz, J. M., Ledoux, S., Manfredi, R., & Hassler, C. (1997). Self-reported health and behavioral problems among adolescent victims of rape in France: Results of a cross-sectional survey. *Child Abuse & Neglect, 21,* 823–832.

Cooley-Quille, M., & Lorion, R. (1999). Adolescents' exposure to community violence: Sleep and physiological functioning. *Journal of Community Psychology, 27,* 367–375.

Dawes, A., Tredoux, C., & Feinstein, A. (1989). Political violence in South Africa: Some effects on children of the violent destruction of their community. *International Journal of Mental Health, 18,* 16–43.

DeVoe, E. R., Bannon, W. M., & Klein, T. P. (2006). Post 9/11 helpseeking by New York City parents on behalf of highly exposed young children. *American Journal of Orthopsychiatry, 76,* 167–175.

Drotar, D., Flannery, D., Day, E., Friedman, S., Creeden, R., Gartland, H., et al. (2003). Identifying and responding to the mental health service needs of children who have experienced violence: A community-based approach. *Clinical Child Psychology and Psychiatry, 8,* 198–203.

Dyregrov, A., Gupta, L., Gjestad, R., & Mukanoheli, E. (2000). Trauma exposure and psychological reactions to genocide among Rwandan children. *Journal of Traumatic Stress, 13,* 1.

El-Sheikh, M., Buckhalt, J. A., Mize, J., & Acebo, C. (2006). Marital conflict and disruption of children's sleep. *Child Development, 77,* 31–43.

Eth, S., & Pynoos, R. S. (1994). Children who witness the homicide of a parent. *Psychiatry, 57,* 287–306.

Famularo, R., Kinscherff, R., & Fenton, T. (1990). Symptom differences in acute and chronic presentation of childhood post-traumatic stress disorder. *Child Abuse & Neglect, 14,* 439–444.

Famularo, R., Kinscherff, R., & Fenton, T. (1992). Psychiatric diagnoses of maltreated children: Preliminary findings. *Journal of the American Academy of Child and Adolescent Psychiatry, 31*, 863–867.

Famularo, R., Fenton, T., Kinscherff, R., & Augustyn, M. (1996). Psychiatric comorbidity in childhood posttraumatic stress disorder. *Child Abuse & Neglect, 20*, 953–961.

Fitzpatrick, K. M., & Boldizar, J. P. (1993). The prevalence and consequences of exposure to violence among African American youth. *Journal of the American Academy of Child and Adolescent Psychiatry, 32*, 424–430.

Gaffney, D. A. (2006). The aftermath of disaster: Children in crisis. *Journal of Clinical Psychology: In Session, 62*, 1001–1016.

Garrison, M. M., Liekweg, K., & Christakis, D. A. (2011). Media use and child sleep: The impact of content, timing, and environment. *Pediatrics, 128*, 29–35.

Glod, C. (2011). Effects of trauma on children's sleep. In M. El-Sheikh (Ed.), *Sleep and Development: Familial and Socio-Cultural Considerations* (pp. 99–111). New York: Oxford University Press.

Glod, C. A., Teicher, M. H., Hartman, C. R., & Harakal, T. (1997). Increased nocturnal activity and impaired sleep maintenance in abused children. *Journal of the American Academy of Child and Adolescent Psychiatry, 36*, 1236–1243.

Goldin, S., Levin, L., Persson, L. Ä., & Hägglöf, B. (2001). Stories of pre-war, war and exile: Bosnian refugee children in Sweden. *Medicine, Conflict, and Survival, 17*, 25–47.

Goldston, D. B., Turnquist, D. C., & Knutson, J. F. (1989). Presenting problems of sexually abused girls receiving psychiatric services. *Journal of Abnormal Psychology, 98*, 314–317.

Gorham, E. L. (1997). Sixteen-step strategic family therapy for the treatment of child sexual abuse: A treatment adaptation and case example. *Psychotherapy in Private Practice, 16*, 21–37.

Graham-Berman, S. A., & Levendosky, A. A. (1998). Traumatic stress symptoms in children of battered women. *Journal of Interpersonal Violence, 13*, 111–128.

Groves, B. (2001). When home isn't safe: Children and domestic violence. *Smith College Studies in Social Work, 71*, 183–207.

Harvey, A. G., Jones, C., & Schmidt, D. A. (2003). Sleep and posttraumatic stress disorder: A review. *Clinical Psychology Review, 23*, 377–407.

Hjern, A., Angel, B., & Hojer B. (1991). Persecution and behavior: A report of refugee children from Chile. *Child Abuse & Neglect, 15*, 239–248.

Hjern, A., & Angel, B. (2000). Organized violence and mental health of refugee children in exile: A six-year follow-up. *Acta Paediatrica, 89*, 722–727.

Hock E., Hart, M., Kang, M. J., & Lutz, W. J. (2004). Predicting children's reactions to terrorist attacks: The importance of self-reports and preexisting characteristics. *American Journal of Orthopsychiatry, 74*, 253–362.

Hoven, C. W., Duarte, C. S., Wu, P., Erickson, E. A., Musa, G. J., & Mandell, D. J. (2004). Exposure to trauma and separation anxiety in children after the WTC attack. *Applied Developmental Science, 8*, 172–183.

Howard, D. E., Kaljee, L., Rachuba, L. T., & Cross, S. I. (2003). Coping with youth violence: Assessments by minority parents in public housing. *American Journal of Health Behavior, 27*, 483–492.

Humphreys, C., Lowe, P., & Williams, S. (2009). Sleep disruption and domestic violence: Exploring the interconnections between mothers and children. *Child and Family Social Work, 14*, 4.

Humphreys, J. C., & Lee, K. A. (2006). Sleep of children of abused women in transitional housing. *Pediatric Nursing, 32*, 311–316.

Ivarsson, M., Anderson, M., Åkerstedt, Torbjörn, M., & Lindlad, F. (2009). Playing a violent television game affects heart rate variability. *Acta Paediatrica, 98*, 166–172.

Janus, M., McCormack, A., Burgess, A. W., & Hartman, C. (1987). *Adolescent Runaways: Causes and Consequences*. Lexington, MA: Lexington Books.

Kamphuis, J. H., Tuin, N., Timmermans, M., & Punamäki, R. (2008). Extending the Rorschach Trauma Content Index and aggression indexes to dream narratives of children exposed to enduring violence: An exploratory study. *Journal of Personality Assessment, 90*, 578–584.

Kaplow, J. B., Saxe, G. N., Putnam, F. W., Pynoos, R. S., & Lieberman, A. F. (2006). The long-term consequences of early childhood trauma: A case study and discussion. *Psychiatry, 69*, 362–375.

Kaufman, J., Birmaher, B., Clayton, S., Retano, A., & Wongchaowart, B. (1997). Case study: Trauma-related hallucinations. *Journal of the American Academy of Child and Adolescent Psychiatry, 36*, 1602–1605.

Kelly, R. J., & Ben-Meir, S. (1993). Emotional effects. In Waterman, J., Kelly, R. J., Oliveri, M. K., & McCord, J. (Eds.), *Behind the Playground Walls* (pp. 106–119). New York: Guilford Press.

Kennedy, C., Charlesworth, A., & Chen, J. L. (2004). Disaster at a distance: Impact of 9.11.01 televised news coverage on mothers' and children's health. *Journal of Pediatric Nursing, 19*, 329–339.

Khamis, V. (2005). Post-traumatic stress disorder among school age Palestinian children. *Child Abuse & Neglect, 29*, 81–95.

Klinenberg, E. (2002). *Heat Wave: A Social Autopsy of Disaster in Chicago*. Chicago, IL: University of Chicago Press.

Kotlowitz. A. (1991). *There Are No Children Here: The Story of Two Boys Growing Up in The Other America*. New York: Anchor Books.

Kozol, J. (1995). *Amazing Grace*. New York: Crown Publishers, Inc.

Krug, E. G., Dahlberg, L. L., Mercy, J. A., Zwi, A. B., & Lozano, R. (Eds.). (2002). *World Report on Violence and Health*. Geneva: World Health Organization.

Kupersmidt, J. B., Shahinfar, A., & Voegler-Lee, M. E. (2002). Children's exposure to community violence. In A. M. LaGreca (Ed.), *Helping Children Cope with Disasters and Terrorism* (pp. 381–401). Washington, DC: American Psychological Association.

Lavie, P., Amit, Y., Epstein, R., & Tzischinsky, O. (1993). Children's sleep under the threat of attack by ballistic missiles. *Journal of Sleep Research, 2*, 34–37.

Lavie, P. (2001). Sleep disturbance in the wake of traumatic events. *New England Journal of Medicine, 345*, 1825–1832.

Lengua, L. J., Long, A. C., Smith, K. I., & Meltzoff, A. N. (2005). Pre-attack symptomatology and temperament as predictors of children's responses to the September 11 terrorist attacks. *Journal of Child Psychology and Psychiatry, 46*, 631–645.

Levendosky, A. A., Huth-Bocks, A. C., Semel, M. A., & Shapiro, D. L. (2002). Trauma symptoms in preschool-age children exposed to domestic violence. *Journal of Interpersonal Violence, 17*, 150–164.

Linares, L. O., Heeren, T., Bronfman, E., Zuckerman, B., Augustyn, M., & Tronick, E. (2001). A mediational model for the impact of exposure to community violence on early child behavior problems. *Child Development, 72*, 639–652.

Lowe, P., Humphreys, C., & Williams, S. J. (2007). Night terrors: Women's experiences of (not) sleeping where there is domestic violence. *Violence Against Women, 13*, 549–561.

Malmquist, C. P. (1986). Children who witness parental murder: Posttraumatic aspects. *Journal of the American Academy of Child Psychiatry, 25*, 320–325.

Masalha S. (1993). The effect of prewar conditions on the psychological reactions of Palestinian children to the Gulf War. In L. A. Leavitt & N. A. Fox (Eds.), *The Psychological Effects of War and Violence on Children* (pp. 131–142). Hillsdale, NJ: Lawrence Erlbaum Associates.

Masten, A. S., & Narayan, A. J. (2012). Child development in the context of disaster, war, and terrorism: Pathways of risk and resilience. *Annual Review of Psychology, 63*, 227–257.

McCellan, J., Adams, J., Douglas, D., McCurry, C., & Storck, M. (1995). Clinical characteristics related to severity of sexual abuse: A study of seriously mentally ill youth. *Child Abuse & Neglect, 19*, 1245–1254.

McDonald, R., Jouriles, E. N., Ramisetty-Mikler, S., Caetano, R., & Green C. E. (2006). Estimating the number of American children living in partner-violent families. *Journal of Family Psychology, 20*, 137–142.

Midlarsky E., Venkataramani-Kothari, A., Plante, M. (2006). Domestic violence in the Chinese and South Asian Immigrant Communities. *Annals of the New York Academy of Sciences, 1087*, 279–300.

Montgomery, E., & Foldspang, A. (2001). Traumatic experience and sleep disturbance in refugee children from the Middle East. *European Journal of Public Health, 11*, 18–22.

Morgenthaler, T., Alessi, C., Friedman, L., Owens, J., Kapur, V., Boehlecke, B., et al. (2007). Practice parameters for use of actigraphy in the assessment of sleep and sleep disorders: An update for 2007. *Sleep, 30*, 519–529.

Nader, K., Pynoos, R., Fairbanks, L., & Frederick, C. (1990). Children's PTSD reactions one year after a sniper attack at their school. *The American Journal of Psychiatry, 147*, 1526–1530.

Noll, J. G., Trickett, P. K., Susman, E. J., & Putnam, F. W. (2006). Sleep disturbances and childhood sexual abuse. *Journal of Pediatric Psychology, 31*, 469–480.

Bailey, B. N., Delaney-Black, V., Hannigan, J. H., Ager, J., Sokol, R. J., & Covington, C. Y. (2005). Somatic complaints in children and community violence exposure. *Developmental and Behavioral Pediatrics, 26*, 341–348.

Obradović, B., Kanazir, V., Zališevskij, G., Popadić, K., & Simić, I. (1993). A threat to mental health of children and young people in exile. *Psihijatrija danas, 25*, 91–98.

Paardekooper, B., De Jong, J. T. V. M., & Hermanns, J. M. A. (1999). The psychological impact of war and the refugee situation on South Sudanese children in refugee camps in Northern Uganda: An exploratory study. *Journal of Child Psychology and Psychiatry, 40*, 529–536.

Perez Foster, R. (2001). When immigration is trauma: Guidelines for the individual and family clinician. *American Journal of Orthopsychiatry, 71*, 153–170.

Pfefferbaum, B., North, C. S., Doughty, D. E., Pfefferbaum, R. L., Dumont, C. E., & Pynoos, R. S. (2006). Trauma, grief, and depression in Nairobi children after the 1998 bombing of the American embassy. *Death Studies, 30*, 561–577.

Phillips, D., Prince, S., Schiebelhut, L. (2004). Elementary school children's responses 3 months after the September 11 terrorist attacks: A study in Washington, DC. *American Journal of Orthopsychiatry, 74*, 509–528.

Pillar, G., Malhotra, A., & Lavie, P. Post-traumatic stress disorder and sleep—what a nightmare! (2000). *Sleep Medicine Review, 4*, 183–200.

Pumariega, A. J., Rothe, E., Pumariega, J. B. (2005). Mental health of immigrants and refugees. *Community Mental Health Journal, 41*, 581–597.

Punamäki, R. L., Ali, K. J., Ismahil, H., & Nuutinen, J. (2005). Trauma, dreaming, and psychological distress among Kurdish children. *Dreaming, 15*, 178–194.

Pynoos, R. S., Frederick, C., Nader, K., Arroyo, W., Steinberg, A., Eth, S., et al. (1987). Life threat and posttraumatic stress in school-age children. *Archives of General Psychiatry, 44*, 1057–1063.

Pynoos, R. S., Nader, K., Frederick, C., Gonda, L., & Stuber, M. (1987). Grief reactions in school age children following a sniper attack at school. *Israeli Journal of Psychiatry and Related Sciences, 24*, 53–63.

Pynoos, R. S. & Nader, K. (1988). Children who witness the sexual assaults of their mothers. *Journal of the American Academy of Child and Adolescent Psychiatry, 27*, 567–572.

Qouta, S., Punamäki, R. L., & El Sarraj, E. (2003). Prevalence and determinants of PTSD among Palestinian children exposed to military violence. *European Child and Adolescent Psychiatry, 12*, 265–272.

Raymond, A., & Raymond, S. (2000). *Children in War*. New York: TV Books, LLC.

Realmuto, G. M., Masten, A., Carole, L. F., Hubbard, J., Groteluschen, A., & Chhun, B. (1992). Adolescent survivors of massive childhood trauma in Cambodia: Life events and current symptoms. *Journal of Traumatic Stress, 5*, 589–599.

Rofé, Y., & Lewin, I. (1982). The effect of war environment on dreams and sleep habits. In Spielberger, C. D., & Sarason, I. G. (Eds.), *Stress and Anxiety* (pp. 67–79). Washington, DC: Hemisphere Publishing Corporation.

Runyon, M. K., Faust, J., & Orvaschel, H. (2002). Differential symptom pattern of post-traumatic stress disorder (PTSD) in maltreated children with and without concurrent depression. *Child Abuse & Neglect, 26*, 39–53.

Sadeh A., Hayden, R. M., McGuire J. P. D., Sachs, H. & Civita, R. (1994). Somatic, cognitive, and emotional characteristics of abused children in a psychiatric hospital. *Child Psychiatry and Human Development, 24*, 191–200.

Sadeh, A., McGuire, J. P. D., Sachs, H., Seifer, R., Tremblay, A., Civita, R., et al. (1995). Sleep and psychological characteristics of children on a psychiatric inpatient unit. *Journal of the American Academy of Child and Adolescent Psychiatry, 34*, 813–819.

Sadeh, A., Hen-Gal, S., & Tikotzky, L. (2008). Young children's reactions to war-related stress: A survey and assessment of an innovative intervention. *Pediatrics, 121*, 46–53.

Schlenger, W. E., Caddell, J. M., Ebert, L., Jordan, B. K., Rourke, K. M., Wilson, D., et al. (2002). Psychological Reactions to Terrorist Attacks: Findings from the National Study of Americans' Reactions to September 11. *Journal of the American Medical Association*, 288, 581–588.

Schuster, M. A., Stein, B. D., Jaycox, L. H., Collins, R. L., Marshall, G. N., Elliott, M. N., et al. (2001). A national survey of stress reactions after the September 11, 2001 terrorist attacks. *New England Journal of Medicine, 345*, 1507–1512.

Schwartz, E. D., & Kowalski, J. M. (1991). Malignant memories: PTSD in children and adults after a school shooting. *Journal of the American Academy of Child and Adolescent Psychiatry, 30,* 936–944.

Singareddy, R. K., & Balon, R. (2002). Sleep in posttraumatic stress disorder. *Annals of Clinical Psychiatry, 14,* 183–190.

Singer, M. I., Menden Anglin, T., Song, L. Y., & Lunghofer, L. (1995). Adolescents' exposure to violence and the association of psychological trauma. *Journal of the American Medical Association, 273,* 477–482.

Smaldone, A., Honig, J. C., & Byrne, M. W. (2009). Does sleep inadequacy across its continuum inform associations with child and family health? *Journal of Pediatric Health Care, 23,* 394–404.

Somasundaram, D., & Janumanantha, C. S. (2002). Psychosocial consequences of war: Northern Sri Lankan experience. In J. DeJong (Ed.), *Trauma, War, and Violence: Public Mental Health in Socio-Cultural Context* (pp. 205–258). New York: Kluwer Academic/Plenum Publisher.

Spencer, M. B., Dobbs, B., & Swanson, D. P. (1988). African American adolescents: Adaptational processes and socioeconomic diversity in behavioural outcomes. *Journal of Adolescence, 11,* 117–137.

Spilsbury, J. C., Frame, J., & Winfield, M. (2010). Violence and children's sleep environments. *Sleep, 33*(Abstract Suppl.), A324.

Stewart, A. J., Steiman, M., Cauce, A. M., Cochran, B. N., Whitbeck, L. M., & Hoyt, D. R. (2004). Victimization and posttraumatic stress disorder among homeless adolescents. *Journal of the American Academy of Child and Adolescent Psychiatry, 43,* 325–331.

Thabet, A. A., & Vostanis, P. (1999). Post-traumatic stress reactions in children of war. *Journal of Child Psychology and Psychiatry, 40,* 385–391.

Thabet, A.A., & Vostanis, P. (2000). Posttraumatic stress disorder reactions in children of war: A longitudinal study. *Child Abuse & Neglect, 24,* 291–298.

Thabet, A. A., Abed, Y., & Vostanis, P. (2001) Effect of trauma on the mental health of Palestinian children and mothers in the Gaza strip. *Eastern Mediterranean Health Journal, 7,* 413–421.

Thabet, A. A., Abed, Y., & Vostanis, P. (2004). Comorbidity of PTSD and depression among refugee children during war conflict. *Journal of Psychology and Psychiatry, 45,* 533–542.

Thabet, A. A., Karim, K., & Vostanis, P. (2006). Trauma exposure in pre-school children in a war zone. *British Journal of Psychiatry, 188,* 154–158.

Tišinović, S. (July 7–8, 2000). War through children's eyes a year after the NATO bombing. In S. Powell & E. Durakovic-Belko (Eds.), *Sarajevo 2000: The Psychological Consequences of War* (pp. 232–233). Presentations from a Symposium held at the Faculty of Philosophy in Sarajevo, July 7 and 8, 2000. Sarajevo: UNICEF.

United Nations (2006). *Behind Closed Doors: The Impact of Domestic Violence on Children.* Retrieved January 10, 2012 from http://www.unicef.org/protection/files/BehindClosedDoors.pdf.

United Nations. (1996). *State of the World's Children: Children in War.* Retrieved January 10, 2012 from http://www.unicef.org/sowc96/contents.htm.

United Nations. (September 7, 2005). *Report of the Special Representative of the Secretary-General for Children and Armed Conflict.* Retrieved January 10, 2012 from http://www.unicef.org/emerg/files/report_SRSG_cac.pdf.

Van den Buick, J. (2010). The effects of media on sleep. *Adolescent Medicine State of the Art Reviews, 21,* 418–429.

Wang, Y., Nomura, Y., Pat-Horenczyk, R., Doppelt, O., Abramovitz, R. Brom, D., et al., (2006). Association of direct exposure to terrorism, media exposure to terrorism, and other trauma with emotional and behavioral problems in preschool children. *Annals of the New York Academy of Sciences, 1094,* 363–368.

Wilson, W. C., & Spenciner, B. (2004). Psychological effects of attack on the World Trade Center: Analysis before and after. *Psychological Reports, 94,* 587–606.

Wolfe, D. A., Sas, L., & Wekerle, C. (1994). Factors associated with the development of posttraumatic stress disorder among child victims of sexual abuse. *Child Abuse & Neglect, 18,* 37–49.

World Health Organization. Global Consultation on Violence and Health. (1996). *Violence: A Public Health Priority* (WHO/EHA/SPI.POA.2). Geneva. World Health Organization.

Zeidner, M. (2005). Contextual and personal predictors of adaptive outcomes under terror attack: The case of Israeli adolescents. *Journal of Youth and Adolescence, 34,* 459–479.

Zinzow, H. M., Ruggiero, K. J., Hanson R. F., Smith, D. W., Saunders, B. E., & Kilpatrick, D. G. (2008). Witnessed community and parental violence in relation to substance use and delinquency in a national sample of adolescents. *Journal of Traumatic Stress, 22,* 525–533.

PART 3

Assessment of Sleep and Sleep Problems

CHAPTER

15 Functional Behavioral Analysis of Sleep in Infants and Children

Neville M. Blampied

Abstract

Behavior analysis is the scientific study of those interactions between individuals and their environment responsible for behavior change. Behavioral assessment and functional analysis are procedures that identify and quantify the causal and outcome variables in the behavior change process. This chapter summarizes a behavior analysis model of sleep in infants and children and discusses behavioral assessment and functional analysis as applied in family contexts to understanding and treating children's sleep problems. It explains some key attributes of behavior analysis as a domain within psychology, shows how behavior analysis provides insight into the moment-by-moment interactional processes that contribute to the origin and maintenance of children's sleep problems, and supplies a rationale for intervention guided by functional behavioral assessment and analysis.

Key Words: behavior analysis, discriminated operant, interviews, questionnaires, direct observations, reinforcement, pediatric sleep disturbance

To juxtapose words involving "function" and "sleep" in a title invites a supposition that what will be dealt with is the central mystery of sleep, namely, "Why do we sleep?" (Siegel,2005). Or, it might lead to an expectation that the matter discussed will be the contribution sleep makes to our well-being and functioning in everyday life (e.g., Giallo, Rose, & Vittorino, 2011; Mitchel & Kelly, 2008; Sarsour, van Brunt, Johnston, Foley, Morin, & Walsh, 2010; Verster, Pandi-Perumel, & Streiner, 2008). This chapter will address neither of these issues. It is concerned with the application of behavior analysis and the science of behavior change to issues of sleep in infants and children, and with behavioral assessment and functional analysis as applied in family contexts to understanding and treating children's sleep problems. It will briefly explain some key attributes of behavior analysis as a domain within psychology, show how behavior analysis provides insight into the moment-by-moment interactional processes that contribute to the origin and maintenance of children's sleep problems and difficulties, and supply a rationale for intervention guided by functional behavioral assessment and analysis.

Behavior Analysis

Behavior analysis is a domain of behavioral science associated with B. F. Skinner (1904–1990), although Skinner acknowledged the influence of the earlier research of Pavlov, Thorndike, and Watson, the epistemology of the physicist-philosopher Mach, and the evolutionary biology of Darwin (Boakes, 1984; Moxley, 1992; 2005; Skinner, 1979). It studies those interactions between individuals and their environment that bring about behavior change. Following Skinner's inspiration, behavior analysis is unwaveringly committed to psychology as a natural science of behavior and rejects explanatory appeals to dualist, mentalist, or other nonmaterial entities. It is also suspicious of explanatory reductionism, believing that we should study behavior as a phenomenon in its own right (Delprato & Midgley, 1992).

Skinner was a pragmatist, emphasizing prediction and control of phenomena as the primary aim of science (Moxley, 1992). This led quite early to the application of behavior analysis to human problems, in the field now called *applied behavior analysis* (Baer, Wolf, & Risley, 1968; 1987; Kazdin, 1978; Skinner, 1953). Also, behavior analysis research was ideographic in character from the outset, focused on the individual behaving organism; later researchers developed Skinner's initial procedures into systematic single-case research designs (Barlow, Hayes, & Nelson, 1984; Barlow, Nock, & Hersen, 2004; Hersen & Barlow, 1976; Sidman, 1960) that stand in marked contrast to the group-averaging, null-hypothesis testing paradigm of mainstream psychology (Blampied, 1999; 2013; J. Cohen, 1994; Rucci & Tweney, 1980).

Single-case research involves the intensive study of individuals and the gathering of extensive, repeated, quantitative data about one or more of their behaviors. An initial period of observation is called *baseline*, and the stability of the data—assessed in terms of its level (relative to the measurement scale and possible maxima and minima), its trend over time, and its variability—must be established before any further investigation. Variability is treated as part of the behavioral phenomenon to be investigated and controlled experimentally, not as "error" to be disposed of statically (Sidman, 1960). Once a stable baseline is established, a treatment phase may be instituted and observations continued. The data are typically graphed and visual analysis via inspection of the graphs is used, by way of within- and between-phase comparisons, to determine if any change occurred coincident with the introduction of the independent (treatment) variable. Visual analysis is typically dismissed as highly inferior to inferential statistical analysis using null-hypothesis tests, but visual analysis is, in fact, a powerful analysis technique when employed appropriately by properly trained researchers (Parker & Hagen-Burke, 2007).

To conclude that the treatment caused any observed change requires that baseline-treatment phases be repeated and the observed change in behavior replicated (Schmidt, 2009) if it is to be inferred (tentatively) that the treatment caused the change. This may be done by within-subject or between-subject replications, and different replication procedures yield different kinds of single-case research designs (Hersen & Barlow, 1976; Kratochwill et al., 2010). Additional direct, systematic, and clinical replications may strengthen conclusions about the effects of treatment (Barlow et al., 1984). Single-case research designs have been widely used in the evaluation of interventions for children's sleep problems, up to and including randomized-controlled trials of different kinds of interventions (France & Blampied, 2005) and placebo-controlled, double-blind analyses of sedative drugs (France, Blampied, & Wilkinson, 1999).

The purpose of Skinner's pragmatic and ideographic experimentation, which he called *functional analysis,* was to establish *functional relations*. These are systematic, and ideally parametric, demonstrations of how a behavioral response (the dependent variable) changes as a result of changes in some environmental variable (the independent variable). "Functional analysis yields functional relations that are the basic facts of a science of behaviour." (Delprato & Midgley, 1992, p. 1509).

Skinner was among the first to clearly distinguish between Pavlovian behavior (i.e., based on reflexes) and instrumental or, using Skinner's term, *operant behavior,* a term chosen to emphasize the function of the behavior in operating on (i.e., changing) the environment (Skinner, 1937). For Skinner, Pavlovian (he called it *respondent behavior* to reflect its elicited nature) and operant behavior constituted the fundamental building blocks of each individual's behavior repertoire (Delprato & Midgley, 1992). Although Skinner acknowledged the importance of respondent behavior, the primary focus of his research, and of behavior analysis since, has been on operant behavior.

In studying operant behavior in behavior analysis, the unit of analysis is not the target response per se, as in the description or analysis of the form or topography of the behavior, but is on the *discriminated operant* (Thompson, 2007). This specifies a unit that embraces the environmental context (which supplies antecedent stimuli) within which the response occurs, the response, and the consequences of the response (i.e., its effects on the environment). Skinner termed this relationship *the three-term contingency* (Skinner, 1974). This unit is dynamic and reciprocally transactive (Morris, 1988), in that the effect of behavior at one moment in time is to change the environment, and such changes create new contexts for the behavior stream so that the behavior stream is embedded within and is part of a stream of contexts which it both changes and is changed by.

Behavior analysis also recognizes that particular stimuli in a context may have multiple functions with respect to behavior at any moment in time (Cooper, Heron, & Heward, 2007). For instance, a baby's cry may function for the mother as a Pavlovian *conditioned stimulus* eliciting a *conditioned response* of milk let-down in her breasts. At the same time the cry may be a *discriminative stimulus* that exerts what behavior analysis terms *stimulus control* over an operant response, such as picking the baby up and beginning to nurse it, with that response, in turn, generating some environmental changes, such as cessation of the crying and pleasure in the nursing. Although the discriminative stimulus is spoken of as "controlling" the operant response, the relationship between the stimulus and the response is different between the Pavlovian and operant cases. The Pavlovian stimulus elicits an automatic, reflex response over which the individual has no voluntary control. But in the case of the operant response, the stimulus changes the probability of the response occurring because of a prior history of reinforcement in the context of the stimulus; however, the response is not compelled to occur (Cooper et al., 2007). Other stimuli will concurrently control other elements of the behavior repertoire, so that any particular discriminated operant always occurs as a result of a momentary choice among alternatives, with the alternative chosen reflecting the momentary relative strength of that response (Herrnstein, 1970).

This conceptualization of the unit of analysis as the discriminated operant is a subtle but important feature of behavior analysis. It means that behavior of the same form or topography may be the behavioral element in many different discriminated operants. For instance, a child's cry occurring in the context of darkness, being alone in bed, and perhaps in discomfort from a wet diaper, may be the behavioral component of a discriminated operant where the context is the bed environment and the wet diaper, and the consequence is that a parent appears and removes the discomfort (one class of consequences), or one where the consequence is that a parent appears and provides social stimulation and food (another class of consequence; see below). Despite the common environmental context (bed, darkness, dampness) and form of the behavior (crying) these are separate discriminated operants because the consequences are different. Equally, a child may cry and experience the consequence of parent-provided attention when waking in the cot in darkness at night or when in a car seat in a moving car in daylight. Again, these are different discriminated operants, because while the behavior and the consequences are the same, the context is different. Where a different context has stimuli that are similar to or overlap with those for a learned discriminated operant, the process of *stimulus generalization* may change the probability of the associated operant response (Cooper et al., 2007) with orderly changes in the response (the *generalization gradient*) indexing the extent of similarity or difference in the contexts.

Note, also, that a cry may be an unconditioned or conditioned Pavlovian response elicited by a painful stimulus or a stimulus predictive of pain/discomfort, as well as an operant response strengthened by its consequences. Parents may, with time, get quite good at discriminating these different kinds of cries, since they have subtly different physical properties (Zeifman, 2001; Zeskind & Lester, 2001). The task of determining what class of behavior (Pavlovian or operant) one is dealing with, and what the key environmental stimuli and behavioral consequences are for any discriminated operant, is what behavioral assessment and functional analysis (in the applied sense; see below) are for.

One of the legacies inherited by behavior analysis was Thorndike's Law of Effect (Thorndike, 1911). This postulated that certain consequences of behavior act to strengthen behavior and make it more likely to occur in the future, while other consequences make the behavior less likely to occur. The Law of Effect has been subsumed within the study of "the contingencies of reinforcement" (Skinner, 1969), involving the detailed analysis of the consequences of responding. Initially, behavior analysts refined Thorndike's formulation by re-labeling the process that strengthened behavior as *reinforcement*, while the process that weakens behavior is termed *punishment*. Then they drew further distinctions based upon careful analysis of the nature of the change in the environment that occurs as a consequence of a response (Cooper et al., 2007).

In the case of reinforcement, when the response consequence is to now experience something that was not present prior to the response, that contingency is called *positive reinforcement* (so long as the long-term effect is demonstrably to strengthen behavior). The term *positive* refers to the additive nature of the change occurring as a consequence of the response, while *reinforcement* reflects the strengthening effect of the experience. However, if the strengthening consequence of the response is such that something that was experienced prior to the response is now not experienced, because it is removed or prevented from occurring, this is termed *negative reinforcement*—negative referring, of course, to the subtraction of stimuli from what was being experienced. In the examples above, when the child's cry is followed by the removal of the discomfort of a wet diaper, that is an example of negative reinforcement (for the child), and when the cry results in parental attention and food, that is positive reinforcement (again, for the child). For the parent, escape from hearing the child cry—whether produced by changing the diaper, providing attention and food, or both—yields negative reinforcement for caregiving. Such reciprocity of interactions and effects must always be recognized in behavioral analysis by acknowledging the embeddedness of behavior in reciprocal social interactions of all kinds (Heiby & Haynes, 2004; Patterson & J. Reid, 1973).

Positive reinforcement can be thought of generally as strengthening and maintaining approach and engagement and negative reinforcement as strengthening and maintaining escape and avoidance. In neither case do the terms *positive* and *negative* refer to the hedonic properties of the consequences experienced, though of course these often do have hedonic value—in general, we like things that function as positive reinforcers and dislike the events we escape and avoid. And, of course, both positive and negative reinforcement contingencies may be experienced simultaneously and, in such cases, the behavior may be strengthened particularly effectively and may be hard to change. Returning to the example given above, since it is hard to change a diaper without providing attention, the cry in that case is likely to be both positively and negatively reinforced. Note that there is a parallel definitional scheme for positive and negative punishment, not considered further here (see Cooper et al., 2007).

Some reinforcing events are termed *primary* (or unlearned or unconditioned) reinforcers because they emerge for almost all individuals in the course of development and are closely linked to primary motivational states of the organism (Michael, 2000). In addition to obvious things such as food, water, warmth, and so on, physical proximity to a parent, touch, and benign facial expressions may all be primary reinforcers for infants and children, as are infants' smiles for parents (Bijou, 1993; Cooper et al., 2007). *Secondary* (or learned or conditioned) reinforcers also play important roles in strengthening behavior. These are stimuli that acquire reinforcing properties by a history of being paired with primary reinforcers (B. Williams, 1994). Verbal praise and star charts are examples (Cooper et al., 2007). The moment-by-moment potency of both kinds of reinforcers is influenced by motivating operations such as deprivation and satiation (Michael, 2000). When reinforcers for a previously reinforced response are withdrawn and no longer occur, the procedure is called *extinction*, and its longer-term effect is to reduce the strength of the behavior so that it is performed infrequently or not at all (Lerman & Iwata, 1996). The immediate effect of extinction is often to produce brief intensification of the behavior, called *post-extinction response bursts*, a side-effect that necessitates care in the use of extinction and sometimes rules it out as a treatment (Lerman & Iwata, 1995).

Important changes have also occurred in how behavior analysts conceptualized the environmental/stimulus side of the three-term contingency. Skinner was never an S-R theorist (contra Chomsky, 1959; see MacCorquodale, 1970; Palmer, 1998; Skinner, 1974) and as behavior analysis has developed, it has become more and more contextual (Morris, 1988; 1992) since "context gives behavior its meaning (i.e., its function)" (Morris, 1988, p. 299). Operant behaviors are conceived of as occurring within complex and multidimensional contexts/environments (Schlinger, 1992). In principle, these contexts extend over time, so that the way the environment has changed over time may need to be examined in any functional analysis. Indeed, in behavior analysis the environment is conceived of as extending back in time from the present moment through the ontogenetic history of the individual into the phylogenetic history of the individual's species. This makes it possible, in principle, for behavioral analysis to incorporate genes, epigenetic effects, gestational and perinatal events, and anything else that has occurred in the course of the individual's developmental history (Skinner, 1966; Bijou, 1993; Morris, 1988; Gewirtz & Peláez-Nogueras, 1992) as explanatory factors. However, because we cannot change the past, only the present and the future, behavior analysis pragmatically emphasizes the role of recent and contemporary events rather than the more distant past, and focuses assessment on these.

Furthermore, Skinner, unlike the methodological behaviorists such as Watson and Hull, accepted private events into his science (Anderson, Hawkins, Freeman, & Scotti, 2000; Skinner, 1974), hence the adoption of the term *radical behaviorism* as the name of his position (Schneider & Morris, 1987). This has many important ramifications for behavior analysis, but for now it is sufficient to note that it means that internal physical states of the organism (such as pain) may also contribute to the environment that specifies a discriminated operant and that private events such as thinking, perceiving, and emoting (i.e., cognition and affect) may be considered to be behaviors and their internal effects as behavioral consequences, thereby embracing such phenomena within the three-term contingency (J. Moore, 1984; Skinner, 1974; Thompson, 2007), as is recognized in the development of cognitive-behavior therapy (O'Donohue & Krasner, 1995).

Contemporary behavior analysis is regarded as containing four different strands of scholarship, research, and application (Hawkins & Anderson, 2002; J. Moore & Cooper, 2003), and some scholars suggest a fifth strand, *translational behavior analysis* (Lerman, 2003). The foundation strand is called *conceptual behavior analysis* and involves the continuous development of the philosophy of radical behaviorism and the concepts and methods used within the field (Skinner, 1974). The second strand is the *experimental analysis of behavior* (Skinner, 1938). This conducts basic laboratory research investigating behavioral phenomena (Madden, 2012). Subjects used are often species such as rats and pigeons, but sometimes humans participate (Bijou, 1996; Lattal & Perone, 1998).

The third and fourth strands lie within *applied behavior analysis* (Baer et al., 1968, 1987; J. Moore & Cooper, 2003). Strand three is applied behavior analysis as an applied science:

> Applied behavior analysts conduct experiments aimed at discovering and clarifying functional relations between *socially significant behavior* and its controlling variables, with which they can contribute to the further development of a humane and effective technology of behavior change. (Cooper et al., 2007, p. 20; emphasis added).

It is the focus on socially significant behavior, not the methodology of the science, that distinguishes applied from experimental analysis (Baer et al., 1968). The final strand is known variously as *clinical behavior analysis* (Thyer, 1999) or *behavior-analytic service delivery* (J. Moore & Cooper, 2003), and is a professional activity analogous to medical practice or engineering (Johnston, 1996) in which individuals, trained in the science base of the conceptual, experimental, and applied analysis of behavior and often licensed or regulated (J. Moore & Shook, 2001), provide evidence-based services to clients in a wide range of settings and for a wide range of problems.

Problems and difficulties associated with getting to sleep and maintaining sleep of satisfactory depth and duration are frequently encountered across the life span from infancy to old age and impact adversely on quality of life and health (Verster et al., 2008). Pediatric sleep disturbances/difficulties (PSD) are in themselves challenging to the health and well-being of the child and the family when they occur, and predictive of other difficulties later in life. They are, therefore, socially significant phenomena and ones to which applied behavior analysis should give attention. This is the topic of the next section.

Behavior Analysis of Infant and Child Sleep

The application of behavior analysis to PSD (indeed, to sleep across the life span; see Blampied & Bootzin, 2013) is based on several key assumptions. The first of these, paradoxically, was the realization that sleep is *not* a behavior (Blampied & France, 1993). If sleep were a behavior then it either could be elicited by a Pavlovian unconditioned stimulus or be strengthened by reinforcement, and problems of sleep initiation and maintenance would easily be solved, but they are not. Rather, sleep is a state of the organism (Becker & Thoman, 1983; Thoman, 1990), distinctive because it is associated with the strong inhibition of overt behavior, although high rates of metabolic and neural activity continue. Humans, from birth, cycle between states of waking and sleeping and each of these states has its own distinctive structure and developmental trajectory (see Chapter 5 this volume). Further, sleep is a biological necessity, and individuals are motivated to enter sleep, with that motivation increasing with prior deprivation (Borbély, 1982). Understanding this leads behavior analysts to focus on the key transitions between waking and sleep and sleep and waking, recognizing that behavior plays key roles in these transitions (Blampied & France, 1993).

The second key insight was provided by Bootzin (1977), who identified "falling asleep" as a key operant behavior in the wake-to-sleep transition, with the behavior being reinforced by entering sleep. Furthermore, Bootzin (1977) noted that since falling asleep is operant behavior, it must be under stimulus control (i.e., it must be a discriminated operant) and that appropriate stimulus control is the key to good sleep, while inadequate or inappropriate stimulus control may account for insomnia. This is the basis for his highly effective stimulus control therapy for adult insomnia (Bootzin, Smith, Franzen, & Shapiro, 2010). Specifically in the case of infants and children, Anders and colleagues (Anders, Halpern & Hua, 1992; Goodlin-Jones, Burnham, Gaylor, & Anders, 2001) have identified a capacity for *self-soothing* as a critical component of the "falling asleep" behavior. Self-soothing may involve the overt use of comfort objects such as soft toys, blankets, thumb-sucking, and so forth, but it may also involve less obvious behaviors, especially in older individuals, such as postural adjustments, relaxing, and turning attention away from sources of stimulation.

Building on these initial insights, France, Blampied and colleagues (Blampied & France, 1993; France & Blampied, 1999; France, Blampied, & Henderson, 2003) developed an account of PSD that incorporated both a developmental and a behavior analytic perspective in an integrated explanation of the child and parent factors and interactions that account for both the development and maintenance of good sleep and of common forms of PSD; for example, bed resistance, settling problems, delayed sleep onset, and persistent night waking. This is a holistic model in which the same developmental and learning process are seen at work across the spectrum of PSDs (France & Blampied, 1999), but it is useful, for explanatory purposes, first to discuss bedtime and initial sleep onset and then subsequent wakings (i.e., to differentiate between wake–sleep and sleep–wake transitions).

Going to Bed and Falling Asleep

If an individual is successfully to go to sleep, he or she must pass through a state transition from waking to sleep (Thoman, 1990). This transition requires the attainment and maintenance of a state of behavioral quietude; in other words, the reduction of overt motor activity, covert cognitive activity, and perceptual stimulation to a low level. The necessary duration of this period of quietude before the individual enters the first stages of sleep is a function of many variables, and these variables change over the life span and from day to day; nevertheless, some period of behavioral quietude is needed for the transition to be made. Motivation to make the transition grows with fatigue, and when sleep is achieved this acts as a primary reinforcer. Viewed this way, the behavioral quietude that immediately precedes sleep onset can be viewed as a consummatory response, analogous to eating food when hungry—it is the response that consumes the reinforcer of sleep (Blampied & France, 1993).

This consummatory response must be a discriminated operant, but what are the discriminative stimuli? There are a number that potentially might control falling asleep. These include interoceptive stimuli such as fatigue, proprioceptive stimuli arising from posture and body orientation, and exteroceptive stimuli arising from the physical environment and social context in which the wake–sleep transition occurs. Time of day is also important and may be both an interoceptive and external stimulus. As Bootzin (1977) was the first to note, when a distinctive set of stimuli have a history of consistently being associated with the behavior of falling asleep and the reinforcement of sleep, then the process comes under strong stimulus control; and when the stimuli are present, the behavior is highly likely to occur. Disrupt the stimuli—try to sleep when not fatigued, at odd times, in unusual postures, in novel places, and with unfamiliar persons—and sleep onset will be difficult, perhaps impossible. Infants and children have a high need for sleep and their motivation to enter sleep is high, and so they may tolerate more variability in the antecedent stimuli for sleep than adults do (i.e., their sleep-onset generalization gradient is wider); nevertheless, the more consistent the antecedent stimuli which infants and children experience in going to sleep the stronger the stimulus control of sleep will be, the more established the discriminated operant of falling asleep will be in their behavior repertoire, and the easier it will be for them to get to sleep.

Discriminated operants that function as consummatory responses do not normally stand alone; they are part of larger organizational units—for example, food, before it can be chewed and swallowed, must be located, prepared, and placed in the mouth. So it is with falling asleep. These larger units of behavior are termed *behavior chains* (Cooper et al., 2007). Each link in the behavior chain is a separate discriminated operant, but what is distinctive about behavior chains is that for each link except the last (called the *terminal link* because it contains the consummatory response that consumes the primary reinforcer) the stimuli produced as a consequence of each response serve a dual function; they are secondary reinforcers of the response that precedes them, and simultaneously discriminative stimuli for the response that follows them (Cooper et al., 2007). Understanding this widens the scope of our analysis to incorporate the sequences of behavior that precede the final falling asleep response; in other words, the full bed-preparation sequence. Establishing regular bed preparation routines ensures that chains of behavior are under strong stimulus control, and so the whole chain is emitted as a behavioral unit leading reliably to the terminal link and sleep. Positive bedtime routines incorporating a consistent bedtime are a well-established intervention for children's bed delay, resistance, and refusal (Adams & Rickert,

1989; Ferber, 1985; Mindell, 1999) and are key features of sleep hygiene at all ages (Stepanski & Wyatt, 2003).

Another important insight follows from the recognition that getting to sleep involves a behavior chain. As noted above, all operant behavior occurs in a context of choice (Grace & Hucks, 2013) and so at any moment, while emitting one chain of behavior, individuals have choices and may switch from the current chain to another. These choices are controlled by the different discriminative stimuli present in the environment and the secondary and primary reinforcers associated with the behaviors linked historically with those stimuli. This alerts us to the fact that there is nothing inevitable about the completion of a chain of behavior. Choice, distraction, disruption—shifts to other behavior chains—is always possible. When the stimuli associated with these alternative responses are highly salient, and the reinforcers associated are immediate or highly attractive (as they typically are for bedtime tantrums and other forms of delay and resistance), while the reinforcer for completing the chain and going to sleep is delayed, the likelihood of choice of the alternative is high and, therefore, so is the likelihood of disruption of the bed-preparation chain. So, as Bootzin (1977) presciently argued, we need to identify and remove from the sleep environment those stimuli that control behavior options that have the potential to disrupt progress to falling asleep. For older children (and adolescents and adults) this may require restriction of access to entertainment and communication technology that is now commonly found in bedrooms (Van den Bulck, 2007). With toddlers now using iPads and similar devices, this is an area urgently needing more research (see Chapter 11, this volume).

Infants and young children are highly dependent on their parents and caregivers for establishing bed-preparation routines and for managing sources of distraction and disruption. In advising parents about appropriate bedtime routines, therapists need to emphasize the need for consistency of the routines and the need to attend to possible competing stimuli and behaviors, especially those that increase arousal and divert from the bed-preparation routine. Parents must also understand the need to eliminate reinforcement (such as their own social attention) for distracting and disruptive behavior while positively reinforcing bed-preparation behaviors (J.A. Owens & Mindell, 2005).

There is a second, and important, reason to consider the things that parents do in interaction with their infant or child during the bedtime period. Parents and their actions are salient parts of the stimulus context within which their child's bed-preparation and falling asleep behavior chain is completed. Parent actions and instructions are highly likely to be the stimuli that initiate the sequence for infants and young children, and even older children. Everything known from research on parenting is clinically relevant in assisting parents with the use of appropriate and effective instructions, including the use (from an appropriate age) of descriptive praise for compliance with instructions (J. A. Owens & Mindell, 2005; Sanders, 1992). It is highly desirable, though, that parent-supplied stimuli become less salient toward the end of the bed preparation and falling asleep chain, especially right at the end. Stimuli present at this point will become associated with the consummatory transition to sleep and the natural reinforcer of sleep. Parent-provided stimuli, arising from their actions or just their presence, if they overshadow the natural stimuli of the bed environment and become controlling stimuli for falling asleep, will then have to be provided every time if the child is to go to sleep. This may be acceptable during infancy, but parents may find this burdensome as their child grows older (Ferber, 1985). To avoid this, parent-associated stimuli should be withdrawn from the last phase of the bedtime routine as the child grows, leaving naturally occurring bed cues to control the final discriminated operants in the chain (Blampied & France, 1993).

Researchers and clinicians have documented a wide variety of bedtime rituals which parents learn to perform because they appear necessary to getting their child to sleep. These may range from breast-feeding or bottle-feeding the child to sleep, to more elaborate and prolonged activities of rocking, singing, patting, walking the child about, driving about in cars, co-sleeping, and abandoning any attempt at putting the child to bed at all and allowing them to fall asleep in the midst of family activities (Teng, Bartle, Sadeh, & Mindell, 2012). When these rituals have developed they are clinically challenging to deal with, since even slight changes to the discriminative stimuli within the chain disrupt progress to sleep onset. Establishing positive routines and supporting parents through the distress and disruption that accompanies implementing them is one intervention (Adams & Rickert, 1989; France, 1994; France et al., 1996) used in such cases.

An alternative is the parental presence procedure of Sadeh (1994; also known as extinction with parental presence; see Chapter 22, this volume). This involves the dissociation of the parent's actions and interactions at bedtime from their properties as a stimulus. In this procedure, at the end of the bedtime routine the child is placed in bed, and then the parent remains in the room with the child until the child falls asleep—sitting on a chair or lying on another bed, in view of the child—but does not further interact with them. Once the child is reliably falling asleep the parent ceases the practice, often after about a week. This procedure is very effective (France & Blampied, 2005; Mindell, 1999; Selim, France, Blampied, & Liberty, 2006; Wilson, 2013). Sadeh (1994) provided a rationale in attachment theory terms, while France and Blampied (2005) suggested additionally that the parent's presence (as a stimulus) might be acting as a Pavlovian safety signal (see Blampied & Bootzin, 2013 for a fuller explanation of this idea). All agree that the cessation of parent interactions with the child constitutes an extinction procedure for sleep-incompatible behavior performed by the child.

Another important point emerges from this analysis, which is the necessity of placing the infant or child into bed awake. If they have gone to sleep in some other context, then the stimuli of that context, not those associated with the bed, will potentially become the controlling discriminative stimuli for falling asleep. If this happens routinely, then the bed-associated stimuli never have the opportunity to become discriminative stimuli for falling asleep. Research has consistently shown that whether infants are placed in bed awake or asleep is a strong predictor of later sleep outcomes, with being placed down awake predictive of better sleep outcomes (Adair, Bauchner, Philipp, Levenson, & Zuckerman, 1991).

Given that initially in early childhood and at times thereafter the bed environment and separation from parents may evoke fear and anxiety in infants and children (Sadeh et al., 2010), parents need to ensure that the environment is modified as much as possible to reduce this potential to induce fear and distress. Exposure to novel and/or fear-evoking stimuli does typically result in habituation, in time, and this may be enhanced by gradual exposure. But the child must be conscious if habituation and adaptation is to occur. Sadeh's parental presence procedure may work, in part, because it facilitates habituation by the awake infant to the bed environment while minimizing separation anxiety.

Night Waking

The importance of bed-associated cues in controlling sleep becomes even more evident when the factors affecting night waking are considered (Blampied & France, 1993). Many children who go to bed and fall asleep without difficulty do chronically wake during the night. Indeed, it is normative for infants to wake to be fed during the first months of their life, but even when sleep has consolidated into long continuous periods (Henderson, France, Owens, & Blampied, 2010; Henderson, France, & Blampied, 2011), evidence from studies of the maturation of sleep indicate that infants will enter at least the early stage of the sleep–wake transition a number of times per night (Ferber & Boyle, 1983). At each of these times, two outcomes are possible: The child may return to sleep without evidence of overt arousal and without expression of distress, or the child may wake and exhibit distress and arousal. Which course is followed depends on the presence or absence in their behavior repertoire of self-soothing/falling asleep responses and the stimulus control of these or competing behaviors.

The response of self-soothing/falling asleep is one that, once acquired, gives those who possess it the ability to fall asleep again if and when they wake after initially falling asleep. For the infant or child who has learned to go to sleep under the discriminative control of bed-associated cues, these cues are also present if they wake later. The presence of these cues makes it likely that self-soothing and falling asleep will again occur, and be reinforced by the transition back into sleep. For these individuals, sleep may be said to be "self-regulated" (Henderson et al., 2010).

If, however, these skills have not been acquired, or if sleep is under the control of discriminative stimuli that are different from those encountered in the bed environment on later waking, and/or if other- rather than self-soothing is required to get to sleep, then any night waking is likely to be associated with arousal and distress. If parent-supplied stimuli were required to go to sleep initially, then the parents will need to return to supply them again. The child is likely to continue to cry and signal that they are awake until the parent responds and engages in their standard rituals for getting the child back to sleep (Ferber, 1985). But, as noted above, parent attention is also likely to be reinforcing of the behavior it follows, so arousal and crying and calling out get strengthened. This is a classic behavior trap (Patterson & J. Reid, 1973). The child's crying is aversive to the parent, and the parent acts to produce cessation of the crying and thereby escapes it but, in doing so, positively reinforces the child with attention, thus making the child's behavior more likely to occur (Patterson, 1982). At the same time, the parent's behavior in terminating the crying is negatively reinforced. Child and parent are both more likely to behave this way again.

Since parent-supplied reinforcement is seen as the key variable maintaining the crying and calling out, extinction via the withdrawal (or at least reduction to a minimum) of parent attention (France & Blampied, 1999; C. Williams, 1959) is the key to remedying the problem (Blampied & France, 1993; France & Hudson, 1990; Richman et al., 1985). There is now a large body of outcome research confirming the effectiveness of extinction-based procedures for PSD, and exploring various modifications to make the procedures less stressful and more acceptable to parents (e.g., C. Lawton, France, & Blampied, 1991; Rolider & van Houten, 1984; Healey et al., 2009). There is also excellent evidence that they cause no long-term harm to children's emotional development or mental health (France, 1992; Price, Wake, Ukoumunne, & Hiscock, 2012).

The behavior analysis of the development of infant and child sleep has systematically identified a number of important variables; notably, the antecedent context and associated discriminative stimuli, the behaviors, and the reinforcers that constitute chains of behavior that either facilitate or disrupt sleep during transitions into and out of sleep. It has also shown how intimately reciprocal the behaviors of parents and infants and children are in the processes that lead either to good or poor sleep (for both parties). For both research and clinical purposes, these variables need identification and careful assessment. How this is achieved is considered next.

Behavioral Assessment and Applied Functional Analysis

Behavioral assessment and functional analysis within behavioral analysis emerged from a tradition that can be traced back to Lightner Witmer (1867–1956), the founder of clinical psychology (Blampied, 2013; McReynolds, 1997; Witmer, 1996, original work 1907) and even earlier (Ollendick, Alvarez, & Greene, 2004). Witmer defined clinical psychology as in essence involving the determination of the "status of an individual mind... by observation and experiment" and the provision of "treatment... to effect a change" (Witmer, 1996, p. 251), which, with some changes in terminology, could stand as a general description of applied or clinical behavior analysis/cognitive-behavior therapy today. From this beginning in Witmer's clinic, psychological assessment developed thus:

> [Its] intent is description and prediction [for] planning, executing, and evaluating therapeutic interventions and predicting future behavior. Any of numerous techniques can be used, singly or in combination, depending on the orientation of the clinician and the specific questions for which answers are sought. Thus, interviews with the client or with others; observation in natural or contrived situations; or the use of tests of different functions, varying in breadth, objectivity, psychometric refinement, and inference might all be included. The immediate goal may be the relatively precise measurement of a particular psychological function or the construction of a "working image or model of the person." (Korchin & Schuldberg, 1981, p. 1147).

As many commentators (e.g., Heiby & Haynes, 2004; Korchin & Schuldberg, 1981; Weiner, 2003) note, while behavioral assessment (by which they mean clinical assessment as undertaken by those with a behavioral or cognitive-behavioral orientation) fits within the wider and historically older framework of psychological assessment, it has a number of distinctive features. Among these is the important fact that behavioral assessment is not much (or perhaps ever) concerned with formal typological categorization and diagnosis; nor is it typically concerned with normative comparisons to the population or some reference group using standardized psychometric instruments, although this may happen where there is concern for the social validity (Wolf, 1978) of the treatment outcome. For instance, recent research into early intensive behavioral interventions for children with autism spectrum disorder has used standardized tests of intelligence to relate changes in clients' IQ to published norms (e.g., Howard, Sparkman, H. Cohen, Green, & Stanislaw, 2005). In the case of infants' sleep, there is now good contemporary data on the development of sleep consolidation from birth to 36 months (Henderson et al., 2010; Teng et al., 2012) which can be used to inform parents and assess therapy outcomes.

Further, behavioral assessment is focused on recent and contemporary events, not the past. Behavioral assessment is also distinctive in that it normally makes repeated measures and observations of each individual throughout baseline and treatment phases, consistent with the idiographic, outcome-focused, single-case approach described above. There are, therefore, both differences and continuities across assessment practices in psychological and behavioral assessment, with underlying theories and conceptual foundations being the source of the major differences (Ollendick et al., 2004; Weiner, 2003).

Behavioral assessment has shifted at various times between focusing more on the "form" and sometimes more on the "function" of behavior (O'Brien & Carhart, 2011; O'Brien, McGrath, & Haynes, 2003; Ollendick et al., 2004), and in the period when behavioral therapies were initiated the emphasis was on "topographical analysis" (i.e., form; O'Brien et al., 2003) using operations designed to accurately characterize problem behaviors and identify their consequences. Over this time the term *functional analysis* has taken on many shades of meaning (O'Brien et al., 2003), such that the terms *behavioral assessment, functional assessment* and *functional analysis* have sometimes been used interchangeably (Carr & LeBlanc, 2003). There has been a recent shift (Drossel, Rummel, & Fisher, 2009; O'Brien et al., 2003), however, to now focus on both form **and** function of behavior rather than form alone. Behavior assessment and applied functional analysis as defined in this chapter, therefore, means directing attention to the entire discriminated operant—antecedent context, behavior, consequences, inclusive of form and function. To this end, behavioral assessment shares techniques with psychological assessment, but applied functional analysis procedures require quantitative, time-series data obtained by direct observation.

In undertaking the behavioral assessment and functional analysis of PSD it is essential to separate out the assessment of the sleep state per se from the assessment of sleep difficulties that are behavioral in origin. Analysis and assessment of sleep states is an important domain of sleep science but its purpose is often for description or diagnosis (as in the *International Classification of Sleep Disorders, Revised*; American Academy of Sleep Medicine, 2001) and for screening for research, diagnostic, or treatment purposes. These objectives are not ones to which behavioral analysis contributes (see above; Blampied & Bootzin, 2013). Rather, behavior assessment focuses on the events and contexts leading up to the transition into and out of sleep, consistent with the behavior analysis of sleep (see the section Behavior Analysis of Infant and Child Sleep above).

Behavioral Assessment

The process of behavioral assessment benefits from multiple methods and multiple sources of information, some indirect and some direct (e.g., Eifert & Feldner, 2004; Fernández-Ballesteros, 2004; O'Brien et al., 2003; Ollendick et al., 2004; J. Reid, Patterson, & Snyder, 2002). Further, in the investigation of PSD a holistic focus must be maintained that includes the infant/child, other siblings, parents and caregivers, and possibly other family members as well (Chadez & Nuris, 1987; Dahl & El-Sheik, 2007). This requires the use of a range of methods suited for individuals at very different ages and states of development. The field is dominated by parent reports about their children and themselves, rather than reports from the target child her/himself or other observers, with the exception of psychophysiological measures, which normally come directly from the child by way of professionally supervised recordings. Since psychophysiological measurements such as polysomonography and actigraphy are covered in other chapters (see Chapters 5 and 16, this volume) they will not be discussed further here.

Indirect methods of assessment include interviews, ratings and checklists, and parent-completed questionnaires (or self-completed by older children), while direct functional analysis methods require behavioral observations. Most indirect measures are retrospective, in that they ask about the past. Observations are prospective in that they record events as they occur in time from the point where the assessment was initiated.

Indirect Methods

INTERVIEWS

Interviews are the mainstay of behavioral assessment (Cooper et al., 2007; Ollendick et al., 2004), as they are of psychological assessment generally. The form of the interview is structured to yield information useful for behavior analysis: "The goal of a behavioral interview is to obtain clear and objective information about the problem behaviors, antecedents, and consequences" (Cooper et al., 2007, p. 510). To this end, questions are focused on describing each target behavior in its range of form, intensity, and frequency, and clarifying when, in what settings, and with whom it occurs. The interviewer probes to establish the settings and contexts typically associated with the occurrence and the non-occurrence of the behavior and what typically happens after the behavior (i.e., its consequences). The interviewer should also ask about thoughts, feelings and emotions, preferences, and concerns, and discover what if any prior attempts at problem-solving and behavior change have previously been made (Diden, Curfs, van Driel, & de Moor, 2002; France, 1994; Sadeh & Tikotzky, & Scher, 2010).

Because there are not otherwise many forms of assessment procedure that will yield relevant knowledge, the interview is also the place to investigate the possibility that Pavolvian stimuli and responses, especially those expressed in fear, anxiety, or other forms of strong arousal, are contributing to sleep problems (Blampied & Bootzin, 2013). This means asking questions about possible unconditioned and conditioned stimuli that may elicit fear, anxiety, (dis)stress, and arousal for the infant/child and other family members (e.g., see Diden, Curfs, Sikkema, & de Moor, 1998). If the interview discloses life events that might have functioned as occasions for the conditioning of such behavior to occur (e.g., traumatic events, illnesses and treatments, sudden events or changes in circumstances) then these need to be probed for the potential that conditioned responses have developed that affect sleep or adjustment in the child or other family members (King, Ollendick, & Tonge, 1997). Unfortunately, the role of Pavlovian processes in PSD remains underinvestigated (Blampied & Bootzin, 2013).

Ollendick et al. (2004) stress the importance of using traditional clinical interviewing skills to establish rapport with the interviewee(s), build a relationship between therapist and client(s), and build a common understanding of goals and outcome expectations. Where infant and children's sleep difficulties are the focus, the primary informants in the interview will be parents and possibly other caregivers, although older children should be interviewed as their social and cognitive skills allow (Barbour & Davison, 2004). A careful developmental history must be taken covering the child's life from the prenatal period onward; parents' beliefs, expectations about, and knowledge of the development of infant and child sleep must be explored, and information about sleep clearly communicated (France, 1994; France, Henderson, & Hudson, 1996).

Interview-style information gathering remains important throughout the assessment and therapy process. Sanders and J. Lawton (1993) describe what they term a *Guided Participation Model,* embedded in an interview or series of interviews that should be used to give parents and children feedback incorporating information from the whole assessment process. It is particularly important to be aware of cultural, ethnic, and language differences between clinician and client throughout the assessment process, and extra care, time, training, and external support may be required where such differences are encountered (Barbour & Davison, 2004).

RATINGS, CHECKLISTS, SELF-REPORT MEASURES

Informants, who are usually significant others in the life of the person whose behavior is the target of investigation, can use rating scales and checklists to provide overall descriptions of behaviors, settings, and consequences, often at broad levels of analysis and high levels of generality. Response formats vary (see Spruyt & Gozal, 2011a). These methods are regarded as convenient and cost-effective (Cooper et al., 2007; Ollendick et al., 2004) but have considerable limitations, particularly lack of specificity, bias, and often poor psychometric quality (Cooper et al., 2007; Spruyt & Gozal, 2011a, b).

QUESTIONNAIRES

In considering self-report questionnaires a broad classification can be imposed: those concerned with the child, particularly his/her sleep but also including developmental stage, temperament and other attributes, and mostly filled out by parents/caregivers; and those concerned with the parents' health, well-being, and opinions about the problem or its treatment, almost always completed by the adults involved. In the field of pediatric sleep there are many questionnaires available. Those for general use have been comprehensively reviewed by Lewandowski, Toliver-Sokol, and Palermo (2011) and Spruyt and Gozal (2011b) and those for children with developmental delays by Bonuck, Hyden, Ury, Barnett, Ashkinaze, and Briggs (2011) [see also Chapter 18, this volume]. All these authors agree that the psychometric qualities of these instruments are generally poor (Spruyt & Gozal, 2011a, b), but Lewandowski et al. (2011) identify six that meet criteria developed by the Society of Pediatric Psychology Assessment Taskforce (L. Cohen, La Greca, Blount, Kazak, Holmbeck, & Lemanek, 2008) as being evidence-based. The majority of these cover child age ranges that that begin somewhere in middle childhood and extend (for three of the six) into adolescence. Only one, the Brief Infant Sleep Questionnaire (BISQ, Sadeh, 2004; see also Sadeh, Mindell, Luedtke, & Wiegand, 2009), can be used with infants under 12 months of age and one other, the Infant Sleep Questionnaire (ISQ, Morell, 1999), covers 12- to 18-month-old infants. These questionnaires are useful for screening, for problem identification and specification, and may identify aspects of contexts or consequences that warrant closer attention, but they are not sufficient of themselves to be the basis of a functional analysis.

For the assessment of parent/caregiver health, well-being, and other attributes, there are many self-report questionnaires of varying psychometric quality that purport to assess almost every domain of psychological functioning. Examples of those used in intervention research for PSD include the Beck Depression Inventory (BDI, Beck, Ward, Mendelson, Mock, & Erbaugh, 1961; e.g., Mindell & Durand, 1993), the Dyadic Adjustment Scale (DAS, Spanier, 1976; e.g., Hiscock & Wake, 2002; Mindell & Durand, 1993), The Depression, Anxiety and Stress Scale-Short Form (DASS-21, Henry & Crawford, 2005; e.g., Price, et al., 2012), The General Health Questionnaire (GHQ, Goldberg, 1978; e.g., Scott & Richards, 1989), The Profile of Mood States (POMS, McNair, Lorr, & Droppleman, 1971; e.g., Mindell, Telofski, Weigand, & Kurtz., 2009), and the State-Trait Anxiety Inventory (STAI, Speilberger, 1983; e.g., C. Lawton, Blampied, & France, 1995). Researchers also use parent-completed measures of child temperament, behavior, and well-being as part of both baseline and outcome assessment. Examples include the Child Behavior Checklist (CBCL, Achenbach & Ruffle, 2000; e.g., Lam, Hiscock, & Wake, 2003), the Child Behavior Characteristics Scale Revised (CBC-R, Borgatta & Fanshel, 1970; e.g., France, 1992), the Flint Infant Security Scale (FIS, Flint, 1974; e.g., France, 1992), the Pediatric Quality of Life Inventory (PedsQL 4.0, Varni, Seid, & Kurtin, 2001; e.g., Price, et al., 2012), and the Strengths and Difficulties Questionnaire (SDQ, Goodman, 1997; e.g., Hiscock, Canterford, Ukoumunne, & Wake, 2007).

Measures of this kind can be important in several ways. First, parent/caregiver and child factors may be epidemiologically important as correlates or markers of sleep difficulties in children, and useful, then, in predicting the scope or magnitude of the problem. They may also be prognostic with respect to the likely outcomes achieved by particular interventions (Francis & Chorpita, 2004).

Second, the psychological state, temperament, or disposition of a parent or child may be functionally important as part of the context within which sleep difficulties develop and are maintained. They may act as moderator variables in the relationship between the antecedent context, the behavior, and its consequences (Heiby & Haynes, 2004). Finally, showing that general child, parent, and family health and well-being improve (or at least do not deteriorate) after treatment is an important part of demonstrating the generality of therapeutic effects and the social validity of the outcomes (Price, et al., 2012; Wolf, 1978). Consistent with concern for the acceptability and social validity of treatments and outcomes, some investigators (e.g., Bramble, 1996; Healey et al., 2009; C. Lawton et al., 1991) have systematically used brief self-report measures of various kinds to assess consumer satisfaction with the interventions used, and this practice is strongly encouraged.

Direct Functional Analysis

Direct functional analysis requires the acquisition of real-time observational data. For infant and child sleep, collecting such data can be a challenge because it mostly has to be collected at night, in the privacy of people's homes (Richman, Douglas, Hunt, Lansdown, & Levere, 1985). It has sometimes been collected by trained observers, almost always staff in residential institutions using observation schedules over 24-hour periods (e.g., Piazza & Fisher, 1991), and parents have also been trained in this technique (Ashbaugh & Peck, 1998; Rolider & Van Houten, 1984). Also, in-home audio (or video) recordings may be made by parents at bedtime and later analyzed by trained observers (e.g., B. Moore, Friman, Fruzetti, & MacAleese, 2007).

The most common method for getting data about infant and child sleep is through parent/caregiver daily sleep diaries (Richman et al., 1985). The ubiquity of this method is shown in Mindell (1999), where 32 out of the 34 reviewed studies report using parent diaries as the primary or sole source of sleep data. Parent/caregiver diaries may cover all episodes of sleep, including daytime naps (Ward, Gay, Anders, Alkon, & Lee, 2007) or just night sleep, depending on the age of the child and the nature of the problem being investigated. There is no standard diary in general use, and investigators and clinicians typically design their own forms, but there is a high degree of commonality in the information recorded. To be useful in functional analysis diaries should record the timing of events, such as the beginning of bed-preparation activities, actually going to bed, and any subsequent wakes; the duration of such events; and the actions of both parents and child as they interact throughout the period being recorded.

Parents are instructed in the use of the diary, usually face-to-face as part of the initial interview, and it is common to follow up with phone calls and sometimes further face-to-face contact to ensure that parents are consistently completing the diary (e.g., M. Reid, Walter, & O'Leary, 1999). Richman (1985) developed the Sleep Behavior Scale as a way of summarizing data from diary records, typically over 5–7 days. This composite measure is useful to characterize baseline levels of sleep disturbance (France & Blampied, 2005) and as a way of estimating the size of overall therapy effects (e.g., France et al., 1999).

The accuracy of parent sleep diaries has been evaluated against all-night video recordings (videosomnography, Anders & Sostek, 1976; e.g., Minde, Faucon, & Falkner, 1994), actigraph records (e.g., Sadeh, 1994), mechanical devices that record parent activities near the crib (France & Hudson, 1990), and sometimes a second diary kept by another parent or family member (McGarr & Hovell, 1980; Ronen, 1991). The conclusion from these procedures is that parent diaries typically achieve satisfactory levels of accuracy (interobserver agreement typically exceeds 75%), not inferior to that achieved by parent records of many kinds of child behavior (Blampied & France, 1993), although they commonly underestimate the frequency of night waking that is not accompanied by crying or other disturbance (e.g., Sadeh, 1994). Videosomnography (Anders & Sostek, 1976) is the "gold standard" for assessment of the accuracy of sleep diaries (Blampied & Bootzin, 2013) because it captures not only sleep states and transitions, but also actual child and parent behavior in the bedroom (e.g., Healey et al., 2009). Such videos do not, however, typically capture events during the lead-up to going to bed, when functionally important things also happen.

There are at least two other methods of functional analysis that might be used in the assessment of PSD. The first involves various forms of conditional probability and correlation analyses. O'Brien (O'Brien & Carhart, 2011, O'Brien et al., 2003) provides a general introduction to the use of conditional probability in functional assessment, and Patterson and colleagues (Patterson, 1982; J. Reid et al., 2002) identified antecedents and consequences by way of lag-correlational analyses of time-series parent–child interaction data. No actual instances of these kinds of functional analyses of sleep data seem to exist.

The second method involves the use of analogue experimental functional analysis of the kind developed by Iwata and colleagues (Iwata & Worsdell, 2005) for the functional analysis of challenging behavior (Cooper et al., 2007). For individuals with developmental disabilities these methods have become highly standardized, with routines designed to reveal particular classes of possible antecedents or reinforcements applied in analogue rather than natural settings (Carr & LeBlanc, 2003), and typically with trained observers rather than parents. Although advocated for use in the development of interventions for child sleep problems (Brown & Piazza, 1999), these analogue functional analysis methods have not been used either, at least not directly in connection with sleep problems, but there are examples of analogue functional analysis of the influence of chronic sleep deprivation on daytime problem behavior (Kennedy & Meyer, 1996; O'Reilly, 1995). The existing standard methods are unsuited to the analysis of night sleep and there are major problems of privacy, practicality, ethics, and acceptability standing in the way of extending these analogue experimental functional analysis procedures to sleep problems, although it may be that some aspects of them could be adapted for problems affecting daytime naps.

Behavioral Case Formulation

Behavioral case formulation integrates the information from behavior assessment and functional analysis into a coherent, but often tentative, account of the client's problems and links this with a treatment plan (Godoy & Haynes, 2011; Haynes & A. Williams, 2003). A behavioral formulation is constructed within behavior analysis parameters, but the formulation must also draw on a profound understanding of child development (Bijou, 1993), must be ecological in orientation, and view the child and the family as a system embedded in larger systems (Holmbeck, Devine, & Bruno, 2010; Mash & Lee, 1993). There are a number of general guides to the process (e.g., Page & Golden, 2009; Drossel et al., 2009), and Sanders (Sanders & Dadds, 1993, Sanders & J. Lawton, 1993) provides a specific guide when working with families.

It is critical that the target problem behavior(s) be clearly identified and quantitatively specified. For there to be a "problem" somebody must complain about it (Baer et al., 1968), but complaints are open to interpretation. Psychoeducation or cognitive reframing for the complainer is an option always to consider. This is where comprehensive developmental knowledge is essential, so that, for instance, parents can be helped to understand the typical trajectories of infant sleep development and appraise the sleep of their own child in that context. Sociocultural factors may play an important role in this as well.

Given that the clients and the clinician concur that there is a problem, the next step in the case formulation is to consider the context in all its ecological complexity. This may embrace the whole (extended) family, the parents individually and as they relate to each other, siblings, and the target child (or children). Temperaments, cognitions, emotions, past behaviors, and social and material circumstances all need consideration (France & Blampied, 1999; Sadeh et al., 2010). It can be helpful to organize this along a continuum of distal to proximal variables. Distal (and unmodifiable) variables may need to be factored in as mediators and moderators of any causal factors (tentatively) identified, while proximal, modifiable variables offer scope for intervention. Sleep diary records provide important information about common patterns of parent–child interaction and the discriminative stimuli occurring before and during sleep, and this is a major source informing causal hypotheses and treatment plans.

Sleep diaries are also critical sources of information about potential reinforcers. Reciprocity in parent–child interaction patterns means attention must be paid to what reinforces both parties, recalling that preventing (avoiding) things may be as potent a source of (negative) reinforcement as getting something (positive reinforcement). Parents' pre-bed rituals are often strongly negatively reinforced and supported by beliefs about their rightness or necessity, and strong emotional disquiet may be expressed at suggestions they be changed or abandoned. Equally, if stimuli in the child's environment evoke fear or anxiety, behavior that replaces these with other stimuli, especially those bringing comfort and companionship, will be negatively reinforced and probably positively reinforced as well. These sources of distress need careful modification (King et al., 1997).

All this information guides the planning of interventions, drawing on the factors identified in the functional analysis. This may involve changing the antecedent context, as in using positive routines, or changing the reinforcing consequences, as in using an extinction-based intervention, or some form of positive reinforcement, as in star charts, or modifying both antecedents and consequences (as in the parental presence procedure). Empirical reviews of the various behavioral interventions for infant and child sleep difficulties are provided by Kuhn and Elliot (2003), Mindell (1999), and J. Owens, Palermo, and Rosen (2002) (see Chapter 22, this volume). Empirically validated interventions constitute *default technologies* (Cooper et al., 2007), which can be matched to particular problems via functional analysis and then feature in clinicians' recommendations to parents, allowing parents choice where possible (France, 1994; France et al., 1996; Sanders & J. Lawton, 1993).

The pragmatic test of any case formulation is to see what happens when the treatment is implemented. Assessment, at least in the form of continued observations of the target behavior, must continue and be closely monitored to see if behavior changes in the predicted way. If it does not, given sufficient time, then the case formulation must be revisited, perhaps additional assessment undertaken and a modified treatment implemented and evaluated, until success is achieved.

The need to support parents through the implementation process is strongly emphasized (France, 1994; France et al., 1996), especially in the initial phases where phenomena such as post-extinction response bursts may be common (France & Hudson, 1990; Lerman & Iwata, 1995). Compliance with treatment procedures may be a problem, especially with more complex ones (C. Lawton et al., 1991; Healey et al., 2009), and information from the parent diaries should be closely examined to check that parents are implementing the treatment as planned. Evidence shows that parents commonly modify treatments, usually to make them easier to use (Healey et al., 2009). A maintenance phase in which parents and child consolidate the gains made and new practices become integrated into everyday life are essential, and there should be a follow-up to ensure that gains are maintained and any relapse or residual problems attended to. Finally, measures of acceptability and consumer satisfaction should be gathered (Kazdin, 1980; Wolf, 1978).

Conclusion

The goal of applied behavior analysis is to develop humane and effective technologies for addressing socially significant behavior problems (Cooper et al., 2007). For PSD this goal has been substantively met, and there are empirically valid behavioral interventions available to tackle common sleep problems throughout the life span (Blampied & Bootzin, 2013). For children, there are also well-established behavioral interventions for other sleep-disruptive problems such as nighttime fears (Pincus, Weiner, & Friedman, 2012; see Chapter 24, this volume) and nocturnal enuresis (M. Brown, Pope, & E. Brown, 2011; see Chapter 26, this volume). What is now needed is systematic and programmatic research to establish the generality of the effects of behavioral interventions over the age range from mid-childhood to adolescence, for families with special needs (Doran, Harvey & Horner, 2006), and across a wide range of family sociocultural diversity. Pioneering research into prevention of PSD by Wolfson and colleagues (Wolfson, Lacks, & Futterman, 1992) needs to be extended (see Chapter 39, this volume). Showing that there are general and continuing benefits of intervention to general health and well-being should also be a research priority.

There is little doubt that interviews and sleep diaries will remain the mainstay of behavioral assessment for PSD, but as Lewandowski et al (2011) note, technology, especially widespread access to mobile devices and the Internet, is likely to change how data are collected. Some form of focused experience sampling (e.g., ecological momentary assessment; Buysse et al., 2007) via mobile devices could enhance information gathering about interactions at bedtime, while mobile phone apps could be developed to gather data as events happen at any time. The rapid development of unobtrusive, highly sensitive digital cameras opens the way, via the Internet, to realtime videosomnography with computer algorithms for pattern recognition yielding both sleep-state and behavioral data, while providing reassurance to parents that their child is not endangered by their nonintervention during some treatment phases.

Finally, there are, of course, other ways of viewing the sleep problems of infants and children than one based on behavior analysis. Should these other perspectives be given more weight? One of the eminent founders of applied behavior analysis has this advice:

> Do not postulate a more complex, longer, less observable, and less manageable explanation until you have exhausted the behavior-analytic ones. When they are sufficient they are also more parsimonious... that makes them better science. (Baer, 1988, p. 288).

Future Directions

- Extend behavioral intervention research to more comprehensively cover sleep problems in older children and adolescents.
- Do much more prevention research.
- Investigate the impact of behavioral interventions on general family health and well-being over the long term.
- Systematically explore the generality of behavioral interventions for individuals with special needs and for socioculturally diverse families.
- Explore ways to use mobile and Internet technology to enhance behavioral assessment and functional analysis.

Author note

This chapter was written in the aftermath of the Canterbury earthquakes, which began on September 4, 2010, and continued with destructive force throughout 2011 and into 2012. I am very appreciative of the many expressions of concern and support I received from friends and colleagues worldwide during this time. I also gratefully acknowledge the productive sharing of ideas about children's sleep that has occurred in collaboration with two friends and colleagues: Dr. Karyn France, who began the Canterbury Sleep Project more than two decades ago, and Dr. Jacki Henderson. Thank you both for your invaluable help—past, present, future. I dedicate this chapter to my parents, Morris and Glenny Blampied, who lovingly cared for a baby son who was a chronic night waker for the first two years of his life, and to my daughter Meredith, who learned to sleep like a baby but only after a judicious bit of planned ignoring.

References

Achenbach, T. M., & Ruffle, T. M. (2000). The Child Behavior Checklist and related forms for assessing behavioral/emotional problems and competencies. *Pediatric Review, 21*, 265–271.

Adams, L. A., & Rickert, V. I. (1989). Reducing bedtime tantrums: Comparison between positive routines and graduated extinction. *Pediatrics, 84*, 756–761.

Adair, R., Bauchner, H., Philipp, B., Levenson, S., & Zuckerman, B. (1991). Night waking during infancy: Role of parental presence at bedtime. *Pediatrics, 87*, 500–504.

American Academy of Sleep Medicine. (2001). *International Classification of Sleep Disorders, Revised: Diagnostic and Coding Manual.* Westchester, IL: Author.

Anders, T.F., & Sostek, A.M. (1976). The use of time lapse video recording of sleep-wake behavior in human infants. *Psychophysiology, 13*, 155–158.

Anders, T. F., Halpern, L. F., & Hua, J. (1992). Sleeping through the night: A developmental perspective. *Pediatrics, 90*, 554–560.

Anderson, C. M., Hawkins, R. P., Freeman, K. A., & Scotti, J. R. (2000). Private events: Do they belong in a science of human behavior? *The Behavior Analyst, 23*, 1–10.

Ashbaugh, R., & Peck, S. M. (1998). Treatment of sleep problems in a toddler: A replication of the faded bedtime with response cost protocol. *Journal of Applied Behavior Analysis, 31*, 127–129.

Baer, D. M., Wolf, M. M., & Risley, T. R. (1968). Some current dimensions of behavior analysis. *Journal of Applied Behavior Analysis, 1*, 91–97.

Baer, D. M., Wolf, M. M., & Risley, T. R. (1987). Some still current dimensions of behavior analysis. *Journal of Applied Behavior Analysis, 20*, 313–327.

Baer, D. M. (1988). Guest Editor's note. *Journal of Experimental Child Psychology, 46*, 287–288.

Barbour, K. A., & Davison, G. C. (2004). Clinical interviewing. In S. N. Haynes & E. M. Heiby (Eds.), *Comprehensive Handbook of Psychological Assessment, Vol. 3, Behavioral Assessment* (pp. 194–221). Hoboken, NJ: Wiley.

Barlow, D. H., Hayes, S. C., & Nelson, R. O. (1984). *The Scientist Practitioner: Research and Accountability in Clinical and Educational Settings*. New York, NY: Pergamon.

Barlow, D. H., Nock, M. K., & Hersen, M. (2004). *Single-case Experimental Designs: Strategies for Studying Behavior Change*. Boston, MA: Pearson.

Beck, A. T., Ward, C. H., Mendelson, M., Mock, J., & Erbaugh, J. (1961). An inventory for measuring depression. *Archives of General Psychiatry, 4*, 564–571.

Becker, P. T., & Thoman, E. B. (1983). Organization of sleeping and waking states in infants: Consistency across contexts. *Physiology & Behavior, 31*, 405–410.

Bijou, S. W. (1993). *Behavior Analysis of Child Development*. Reno, NV: Context Press.

Bijou, S. W. (1996). Reflections on some early events related to behavior analysis of child development. *The Behavior Analyst, 19*, 49–60.

Blampied, N. M. (1999). A legacy neglected: restating the case for single-case research in cognitive-behaviour therapy. *Behaviour Change, 16*, 89–104.

Blampied, N. M. (2013). Single-case research designs and the scientist-practitioner ideal in applied psychology. In G. Madden (Editor-in-Chief), *Handbook of Behavior Analysis, Vol. 1. Methods and Principles* (pp. 177–197). Washington, DC: American Psychological Association.

Blampied, N. M., & Bootzin, R. R. (2013). Sleep: A behavioral account. In G. Madden (Editor-in-Chief), *Handbook of Behavior Analysis, Vol. 2. Translating Principles into Practice* (pp. 425–453). Washington, DC: American Psychological Association.

Blampied, N. M., & France, K. G. (1993). A behavioral model of infant sleep disturbance. *Journal of Applied Behavior Analysis, 26*, 477–492.

Boakes, R. (1984). *From Darwin to Behaviorism*. Cambridge, UK: Cambridge University Press.

Bonuck, K. A., Hyden, C., Ury, G., Barnett, J., Ashkinaze, H., & Briggs, R. D. (2011). Screening for sleep problems in early intervention and early childhood special education. *Infants & Young Children, 24*, 295–308.

Bootzin, R. R., (1977). Stimulus control treatment for insomnia. In R. Stuart (Ed.), *Behavioral Self-management Strategies and Outcomes* (pp. 176–195). New York, NY: Brunner-Mazel.

Bootzin, R. R., Smith, L. J., Franzen, P. L., & Shapiro, S. L. (2010). Stimulus control therapy. In M. J. Sateia & D. J. Buysse (Eds.), *Insomnia: Diagnosis and Treatment* (pp. 268–276). London, UK: Informa Healthcare.

Borbély, A. A. (1982). A two process model of sleep regulation. *Human Neurobiology, 1*, 195–204.

Borgatta, E. F., & Fanshel, D. (1970). The Child Behavior Characteristics (CBC) form: Revised age-specific forms. *Multivariate Behavioral Research, 5*, 49–81.

Bramble, D. (1996). Consumer opinion concerning the treatment of a common sleep problem. *Child: Care, Health and Development, 22*, 355–366.

Brown, K. A., & Piazza, C. C. (1999). Commentary: Enhancing the effectiveness of sleep treatments: Developing a functional approach. *Journal of Pediatric Psychology, 24*, 487–489.

Brown, M. L., Pope, A. W., & Brown, E. L. (2011). Treatment of primary nocturnal enuresis in children: A review. *Child: Care, Health and Development, 37*, 153–160.

Buysse, D. J., Thompson, W., Scott, J., Franzen, P. L., Germain, A., Hall, M.... Kupfer, D.J. (2007). Daytime symptoms in primary insomnia: A prospective analysis using ecological momentary assessment. *Sleep Medicine, 8*, 198–208.

Carr, J. E., & LeBlanc, L. A. (2003). Functional analysis of problem behaviour. In W. O'Donohue, J. E. Fisher, & S. C. Hayes (Eds.), *Cognitive Behavior Therapy: Applying Empirically Supported Techniques in Your Practice* (pp. 167–175). Hoboken, NJ: Wiley.

Chadez, L. H., & Nuris, P. S. (1987). Stopping bedtime crying: Treating the child and the parents. *Journal of Clinical Child Psychology, 16*, 212–217.

Cohen, J. (1994). The earth is round ($p < .05$). *American Psychologist, 49*, 997–1003.

Cohen, L. L., La Greca, A. M., Blount, R. L., Kazak, A. E., & Holmbeck, G. N., & Lemanek, K. L. (2008). Introduction to special issue: Evidence-based assessment in pediatric psychology. *Journal of Pediatric Psychology, 33*, 911–915.

Cooper, J. O., Heron, T. E., & Heward, W. L. (2007). *Applied Behavior Analysis* (2nd Edition). Upper Saddle River, NJ: Pearson.

Chomsky, N. (1959). *Verbal Behavior*. By B. F. Skinner. *Language, 35*, 26–58.

Dahl, R. E., & El-Sheik, M. (2007). Considering sleep in a family context: Introduction to the Special Issue. *Journal of Family Psychology, 21*, 1–3.

Delprato, D. J., & Midgley, B. D. (1992). Some fundamentals of B.F. Skinner's behaviorism. *American Psychologist, 47*, 1507–1520.

Diden, R., Curfs, L. M. G., Sikkema, S. P. E., & de Moor, J. (1998). Functional assessment and treatment of sleeping problems with developmentally disabled children: Six case studies. *Journal of Behavior Therapy & Experimental Psychiatry, 29*, 85–97.

Diden, R., Curfs, L. M. G., van Driel, S., & de Moor, J. M. H. (2002). Sleep problems in children and young adults with developmental disabilities: Home-based functional assessment and treatment. *Journal of Behavior Therapy & Experimental Psychiatry, 33*, 49–58.

Doran, S. M., Harvey, M. T., & Horner, R. H. (2006). Sleep and developmental disabilities: Assessment, treatment, and outcome measures. *Mental Retardation, 44*, 13–27.

Drossel, C., Rummel, C., & Fisher, J. E. (2009). Assessment and cognitive behavior therapy: Functional analysis as key process. In W. O'Donohue & J. E. Fisher (Eds.), *General Principles and Empirically Supported Techniques of Cognitive Behavior Therapy* (pp. 15–41). Hoboken, NY: Wiley.

Eifert, G. H., & Feldner, M. T. (2004). Conceptual foundations of behavioral assessment strategies: From theory to assessment. In S. N. Haynes & E. M. Heiby (Eds.), *Comprehensive Handbook of Psychological Assessment, Vol. 3, Behavioral Assessment* (pp. 94–107). Hoboken, NJ: Wiley.

Ferber, R., & Boyle, M. P. (1983). Sleeplessness in infants and toddlers: Sleep initiation difficulty masquerading as sleep maintenance insomnia. *Sleep Research, 12*, 240.

Ferber, R. (1985). *Solve Your Child's Sleep Problems.* New York, NY: Simon & Schuster.

Fernández-Ballesteros, R. (2004). Self-report questionnaires. In S. N. Haynes & E. M. Heiby (Eds.), *Comprehensive Handbook of Psychological Assessment, Vol. 3, Behavioral Assessment* (pp. 194–221). Hoboken, NJ: Wiley.

Flint, B. M. (1974). *The Flint Infant Security Scale.* Toronto: University of Toronto Press.

France, K. G. (1992). Behavior characteristics and security in sleep-disturbed infants treated with extinction. *Journal of Pediatric Psychology, 17,* 467–475.

France, K. G. (1994). Handling parents' concerns regarding the behavioural treatment of infant sleep disturbance. *Behaviour Change, 11,* 71–109.

France, K. G., & Blampied, N. M. (1999). Infant sleep disturbance: Description of a problem behavior process. *Sleep Medicine Reviews, 3,* 265–280.

France, K. G., & Blampied, N. M. (2005). Modifications of systematic ignoring in the management of infant sleep disturbances: Efficacy and infant distress. *Child & Family Behavior Therapy, 27,* 1–16.

France, K. G., Blampied, N. M., & Henderson, J. M. T. (2003). Infant sleep disturbance. *Current Pediatrics, 13,* 241–246.

France, K. G., Blampied, N. M., & Wilkinson, P. (1999). A multiple-baseline, double-blind evaluation of the effects of trimeprazine tartrate on infant sleep disturbance. *Experimental & Clinical Psychopharmacology, 7,* 502–513.

France, K. G., Henderson, J. M. T., & Hudson, S. M. (1996). Fact, act, tact: A three stage approach to treating sleep problems of infants and young children. *Child & Adolescent Psychiatric Clinics of North America, 5,* 581–599.

France, K. G., & Hudson, S. M. (1990). Behavior management of infant sleep disturbance. *Journal of Applied Behavior Analysis, 23,* 91–98.

Francis, S. E., & Chorpita, B. F. (2004). Behavioral assessment of children in outpatient settings. In S. N. Haynes & E. M. Heiby (Eds.), *Comprehensive Handbook of Psychological Assessment, Vol. 3, Behavioral Assessment* (pp. 291–319). Hoboken, NJ: Wiley.

Gewirtz, J. L., & Peláez-Nogueras, M. (1992). B.F. Skinner's legacy to human infant behavior and development. *American Psychologist, 47,* 1411–1422.

Giallo, R., Rose, H., & Vittorino, R. (2011). Fatigue, wellbeing, and parenting in mothers of infants and toddlers with sleep problems. *Journal of Reproductive and Infant Psychology, 29,* 236–249.

Godoy, A., & Haynes, S. N. (2011). Clinical case formulation: Introduction to the Special Section. *European Journal of Psychological Assessment, 27,* 1–3.

Goldberg, D. (1978). *Manual of the General Health Questionnaire.* Windsor, UK: NFER.

Goodlin-Jones, B. L., Burnham, M. M., Gaylor, E. E., & Anders, T. F. (2001). Night waking, sleep-wake organization, and self-soothing in the first year of life. *Journal of Developmental & Behaviour Pediatrics, 22,* 226–233.

Goodman, R. (1997). The Strength and Difficulties Questionnaire: A research note. *Journal of Child Psychology & Psychiatry, 38,* 581–586.

Grace, R. C., & Hucks, A. D. (2013). The allocation of operant behavior. In G. Madden (Editor-inChief), *Handbook of Behavior Analysis, Vol 1, Methods and Principles* (pp. 307–337. Washington, DC: American Psychological Association.

Hawkins, R. P., & Anderson, C. M. (2002). On the distinction between science and practice: A reply to Thyer and Adkins. *The Behavior Analyst, 25,* 115–119.

Haynes, S. N., & Williams, A. E. (2003). Case formulation and design of behavioral treatment programs. *European Journal of Psychological Assessment, 19,* 164–174.

Healey, D., France, K. G., & Blampied, K. G. (2009). Treating sleep disturbance in infants: What generalizes? *Behavioral Interventions, 23,* 1–19.

Heiby, E. M., & Haynes, S. N. (2004). Introduction to behavioral assessment. In S. N. Haynes & E. M. Heiby (Eds.), *Comprehensive Handbook of Psychological Assessment, Vol 3, Behavioral Assessment* (pp. 3–18). Hoboken, NJ: Wiley.

Henderson J. M. T, France, K. G., & Blampied, N. M. (2011). The consolidation of infants' nocturnal sleep across the first year of life. *Sleep Medicine Reviews, 15,* 210–222.

Henderson, J. M. T., France, K. G., Joseph L. Owens, J. L., & Blampied, N. M. (2010). Sleeping through the night: The consolidation of self-regulated sleep across the first year of life. *Pediatrics, 126,* e1081–1087.

Henderson, J. M. T., France, K. G., Owens, J. L., & Blampied, N. M. (2012). The development of infant sleep: Predictors of self-regulated sleep across the first year of life. Under review.

Henry, J. D., & Crawford, J. R. (2005). The short-form version of the Depression, Anxiety, Stress Scales (DASS-21): Construct validity and normative data in a large non-clinical sample. *British Journal of Clinical Psychology, 44,* 227–239.

Herrnstein, R. J. (1970). On the law of effect. *Journal of the Experimental Analysis of Behavior, 13,* 243–266.

Hersen, M., & Barlow, D. H. (1976). *Single-case Experimental Designs: Strategies for Studying Behavior Change.* Oxford, UK: Pergamon.

Hiscock, H., & Wake, M. (2002). Randomised controlled trial of behavioural sleep intervention to improve infant sleep and maternal mood. *British Medical Journal, 324,* 1062.

Hiscock, H., Canterford, L., Ukoumunne, O. C., & Wake, M. (2007). Adverse associations of sleep problems in Australian preschoolers: National population study. *Pediatrics, 119,* 86–93.

Holmbeck, G. N., Devine, K. A., & Bruno, E. F. (2010). Developmental issues and considerations in research and practice. In J. R., Weiz & A. E. Kazdin (Eds.), *Evidence-based Psychotherapies for Children and Adolescents* (pp. 28–39). New York, NY: Guilford.

Howard, J. S., Sparkman, C. R., Cohen, H. G., Green, G., & Stanislaw, H. (2005). A comparison of intensive behavior analytic and eclectic treatments for young children with autism. *Research in Developmental Disabilities, 26,* 359–383.

Johnston, J. M. (1996). Distinguishing between applied research and practice. *The Behavior Analyst, 19,* 35–47.

Iwata, B. A., & Worsdell, A. S. (2005). Implications of functional analysis methodology for the design of intervention programs. *Exceptionality, 13,* 25–34.

Kazdin, A. E. (1978). *History of Behavior Modification: Experimental Foundations of Contemporary Research.* Baltimore, MD: University Park Press.

Kazdin, A. E. (1980). The acceptability of alternative treatments for deviant child behavior. *Journal of Applied Behavior Analysis, 13,* 259–273.

Kennedy, C. H., & Meyer, K. A. (1996). Sleep deprivation, allergy symptoms, and negatively reinforced problem behavior. *Journal of Applied Behavior Analysis, 29,* 133–135.

King, N., Ollendick, T. H., & Tonge, B. J. (1997). Children's nighttime fears. *Clinical Psychology Review, 17*, 431–443.

Korchin, S. J., & Schuldberg, D. (1981). The future of clinical assessment. *American Psychologist, 36*, 1147–1158.

Kratochwill, T. R., Hitchcock, J., Horner, R. H., Levin, J. R., Odom, S. L., Rindskopf, D. M., & Shadish, W. R. (2010). *Single-case designs technical documentation.* What Works Clearing House, http://ies.ed.gov/ncee/wwc/pdf/wwc_scd.pdf. Accessed 8th July, 2010.

Kuhn, B. R., & Elliot, A. J. (2003). Treatment efficacy in behavioral pediatric sleep medicine. *Journal of Psychosomatic Research, 54*, 587–597.

Lam, P., Hiscock, H., & Wake, M. (2003). Outcomes of infant sleep problems: A longitudinal study of sleep, behavior, and maternal wellbeing. *Pediatrics, 111*, e203–e207.

Lattal, K. A., & Perone, M. (1998). The experimental analysis of human operant behavior. In K. A. Lattal & M. Perone (Eds.), *Handbook of Research Methods in Human Operant Behavior* (pp. 3–14). New York, NY: Plenum.

Lawton, C., France, K. G., & Blampied, N. M. (1991). Treatment of infant sleep disturbance by graduated extinction. *Child & Family Behavior Therapy, 13*, 39–56.

Lawton, C., Blampied, N. M., & France, K. G. (1995). Help them make it through the night: The behavioural treatment of infant sleep disturbance. *Children Australia, 20*, 30–34.

Lerman, D. C. (2003). From the laboratory to community application: Translational research in behavior analysis. *Journal of Applied Behavior Analysis, 36*, 415–419.

Lerman D. C., & Iwata, B. A. (1995). Prevalence of the extinction burst and its attenuation during treatment. *Journal of Applied Behavior Analysis, 28*, 93–94.

Lerman D. C., & Iwata, B. A. (1996). Developing a technology for the use of operant extinction in clinical settings: An examination of basic and applied research. *Journal of Applied Behavior Analysis, 29*, 345–382.

Lewandowski, A. S., Toliver-Sokol, M., & Palermo, T. M. (2011). Evidence-based review of subjective pediatric sleep measures. *Journal of Pediatric Psychology, 36*, 780–793.

MacCorquodale, K. (1970). On Chomsky's review of Skinner's *Verbal Behavior. Journal of the Experimental Analysis of Behavior, 13*, 83–99.

Madden, G. (Editor-in-Chief). (2013). *Handbook of Behavior Analysis, Vol 1., Methods and Principles and Vol. 2, Translating Principles into Practice.* Washington, DC: American Psychological Association.

Mash, E. J., & Lee, C. M. (1993). Behavioral assessment with children. In R. T. Ammerman & M. Hersen (Eds.), *Handbook of Behavior Therapy with Children and Adults* (pp. 13–31). Boston, MA: Allyn & Bacon.

McGarr, R. J., & Hovell, M. F. (1980). In search of the sandman: Shaping an infant to sleep. *Education & Treatment of Children, 3*, 173–182.

McNair, D., Lorr, M., Droppleman, L. (1971). *Manual for the Profile of Mood States.* San Diego, CA: Educational and Industrial Testing Service.

McReynolds, P. (1997). *Lightner Witmer: His Life and Times.* Washington, DC: American Psychological Association.

Michael, J. (2000). Implications and refinement of the establishing operations concept. *Journal of Applied Behavior Analysis, 33*, 401–410.

Minde, K., Faucon, A., & Falkner, S. (1994). Sleep problems in toddlers: Effects of treatment on their daytime behavior. *Journal of the American Academy of Child & Adolescent Psychiatry, 33*, 1114–1121.

Mindell, J. A., & Durand, V. M. (1993). Treatment of childhood sleep disorders: Generalization across disorders and effects on family members. *Journal of Pediatric Psychology, 18*, 731–750.

Mindell, J. A. (1999). Empirically supported treatments in pediatric psychology: Bedtime refusal and night waking in young children. *Journal of Pediatric Psychology, 24*, 464–481.

Mindell, J. A., Telofski, L. S., Weigand, B., & Kurtz, E. S. (2009). A nightly bedtime routine: Impact on sleep in young children and maternal mood. *Sleep, 32*, 599–606.

Mitchel, R. B., & Kelly, J. (2008). Sleep and quality of life in children. In J. C. Verster, S. E. Pandi-Perumel, & D. C. Streiner (Eds), *Sleep and Quality of Life in Clinical Medicine* (pp. 139–145). Totowa, NJ: Humana.

Morell, J. M. (1999). The Infant Sleep Questionnaire: A new tool to assess infant sleep problems for research and clinical purposes. *Child Psychology & Psychiatry Review, 4*, 20–26.

Moore, B. A., Friman, P. C., Fruzetti, A. E., & MacAleese, K. (2007). Brief Report: Evaluating the bedtime pass program for child resistance to bedtime—a randomized controlled trial. *Journal of Pediatric Psychology, 32*, 283–287.

Moore, J. (1984). Privacy, causes, and contingencies. *The Behavior Analyst, 7*, 3–16.

Moore, J., & Cooper, J. O. (2003). Some proposed relations among domains of behavior analysis. *The Behavior Analyst, 26*, 69–84.

Moore, J., & Shook, G. L. (2001). Certification, accreditation, and quality control in behavior analysis. *The Behavior Analyst, 24*, 45–55.

Morris, E. K. (1988). Contextualism: The world view of behavior analysis. *Journal of Experimental Child Psychology, 46*, 289–323.

Morris, E. K. (1992). The aim, progress, and evolution of behavior analysis. *The Behavior Analyst, 15*, 3–29.

Moxley, R. A. (1992). From mechanistic to functional behaviorism. *American Psychologist, 47*, 1300–1311.

Moxley, R. A. (2005). Ernst Mach and B.F. Skinner: Their similarities with two traditions for verbal behavior. *The Behavior Analyst, 28*, 29–48.

O'Brien, W. H., Mcgrath, J. J., & Haynes, S. N. (2003). Assessment of psychopathology with behavioral approaches. In J.R. Graham & J.A. Naglieri (Eds.), *Handbook of Psychology, Vol. 10, Assessment Psychology* (pp. 509–529). Hoboken, NJ: Wiley.

O'Brien, W. H., & Carhart, V. (2011). Functional analysis in behavioral medicine. *European Journal of Psychological Assessment, 27*, 4–16.

O'Donohue, W., & Krasner, L. (1995). Theories in behavior therapy: Philosophical and historical contexts. In W. O'Donohue & L. Krasner (Eds.), *Theories of Behavior Therapy: Exploring Behavior Change* (pp. 1–22). Washington, DC: American Psychological Association.

Ollendick, T. H., Alvarez, H. K., & Greene, R. W. (2004). Behavioral assessment: History of underlying concepts and methods. In S. N. Haynes & E. M. Heiby (Eds.), *Comprehensive Handbook of Psychological Assessment, Vol. 3, Behavioral Assessment* (pp. 19–34). Hoboken, NJ: Wiley.

O'Reilly, M. F. (1995). Functional analysis and treatment of escape-maintained aggression correlated with sleep deprivation. *Journal of Applied Behavior Analysis, 28*, 225–226.

Owens, J. A., & Mindell, J. A. (2005). *Take Charge of Your Child's Sleep*. New York, NY: Marlowe & Co.

Owens, J. A, Palermo, T. M., & Rosen, C. L. (2002). Overview of current management of sleep disturbances in children: II – Behavioral interventions. *Current Therapeutic Research, 63*, B38–B52.

Page, L. O., & Golden, J. A. (2009). Review: Functional behavioral assessment as a model for multidisciplinary assessment and treatment. *Journal of Health Care, 13*, 347–360.

Palmer, D. C. (1998). On Skinner's rejection of S-R psychology. *The Behavior Analyst, 21*, 93–96.

Parker, R. I., & Hagen-Burke, S. (2007). Useful effect sizes for single case research. *Behavior Therapy, 38*, 95–105.

Patterson, G. R., & Reid, J. B. (1973). Reciprocity and coercion: Two facets of social systems. In C. Neuringer & J.L. Michael (Eds.). *Behavior Modification in Clinical Psychology* (pp. 133–177). New York, NY: Appleton-Century-Crofts.

Patterson, G. R. (1982). *Coercive Family Processes*. Eugene, OR: Castilia.

Piazza, C. C., & Fisher, W. (1991). A faded bedtime with response cost protocol for treatment of multiple sleep problems in children. *Journal of Applied Behavior Analysis, 24*, 129–140.

Pincus, D. B., Weiner, C. L., & Friedman, A. G. (2012). Differential efficacy of home monitoring and cognitive-behavioral treatment for decreasing children's maladaptive nighttime fears. *Child & Family Behavior Therapy, 34*, 1–19.

Price, A. M. H., Wake, M., Ukoumunne, O. C., & Hiscock, H. (2012). Five-year follow-up of harms and benefits for behavioral infant sleep intervention: Randomized trial. *Pediatrics, 130*, 643–651.

Reid, J. B., Patterson, G. R., & Snyder, J. (Eds.). (2002). *Antisocial Behavior in Children and Adolescents: A Developmental Analysis and Model for Intervention*. Washington, DC: American Psychological Association.

Reid, M. J., Walter, A. L., & O'Leary, S. G. (1999). Treatment of young children's bedtime refusal and nighttime waking: A comparison of "standard" and graduated ignoring procedures. *Journal of Abnormal Child Psychology, 27*, 5–16.

Richman, N. (1985). A double-blind drug trial of sleep problems in young children. *Journal of Child Psychology & Psychiatry, 26*, 59 1–598.

Richman, N., Douglas, J., Hunt, H., Lansdown, R, & Levere, R. (1985). Behavioural methods in the treatment of sleep disorders–A pilot study. *Journal of Child Psychology & Psychiatry, 26*, 581–590.

Rolider, A., & Van Houten, R. (1984). Training parents to use extinction to eliminate nighttime crying by gradually increasing the criteria for ignoring crying. *Education & Treatment of Children, 7*, 119–124.

Ronen, T. (1991). Intervention package for treating sleep disorders in a four-year old girl. *Journal of Behavior Therapy & Experimental Psychiatry, 22*, 141–148.

Rucci, A. J., & Tweney, R. D. (1980). Analysis of variance and the "second discipline" of scientific psychology: A historical account. *Psychological Bulletin, 87*, 166–184.

Sadeh, A. (1994). Assessment of intervention for infant night waking: Parent reports and activity-based home monitoring. *Journal of Consulting & Clinical Psychology, 62*, 63–68.

Sadeh, A. (2004). A brief screening questionnaire for infant sleep problems: Validation and findings from an Internet sample. *Pediatrics, 113*, e570–e577.

Sadeh, A., Mindell, J., Luedtke, K., & Wiegand, B. (2009). Sleep and sleep ecology in the first three years: A web-based study. *Journal of Sleep Research, 18*, 60–73.

Sadeh, A., Tikotzky, L., & Scher, A. (2010). Parenting and infant sleep. *Sleep Medicine Reviews, 14*, 89–96.

Sanders, M. R. (1992). *Every Parent: A Positive Approach to Children's Behavior*. Sydney: Addison-Wesley.

Sanders, M. R., & Dadds, M. R. (1993). *Behavioral Family Intervention*. Boston, MA: Allyn & Bacon.

Sanders, M. R., & Lawton, J. M. (1993). Discussing assessment findings with families: A guided participation model of information transfer. *Child & Family Behavior Therapy, 15*, 5–35.

Sarsour, K., van Brunt, D. L., Johnston, J. A., Foley, K. A., Morin, C. M., & Walsh, J. K. (2010). Associations of nonrestorative sleep with insomnia, depression, and daytime function. *Sleep Medicine Reviews, 11*, 965–972.

Schlinger, H. D. (1992). Theory in behavior analysis: An application to child development. *American Psychologist, 47*, 1396–1410.

Schmidt, S. (2009). Shall we really do it again? The powerful concept of replication is neglected in the social sciences. *Review of General Psychology, 13*, 90–100.

Schneider, S. M., & Morris, E. K. (1987). A history of the term *radical behaviorism*: From Watson to Skinner. *The Behavior Analyst, 10*, 27–39.

Scott, G., & Richards, M. P. M. (1989). Night waking in infants: Effects of providing advice and support for parents. *Journal of Child Psychology & Psychiatry, 31*, 551–567.

Selim, C. A., France, K. G., Blampied, N. M., & Liberty, K. A. (2006). Treating treatment-resistant infant sleep disturbance with combination pharmacotherapy and behavioural family interventions. *Australian Psychologist, 41*, 193–204.

Sidman, M. (1960). *Tactics of Scientific Research*. New York, NY: Basic Books.

Siegel, J. M. (2005). Clues to the functions of mammalian sleep. *Nature, 437*, 1264–1271.

Skinner, B. F. (1937). Two types of conditioned reflex: A reply to Kornski and Miller. *Journal of General Psychology, 16*, 272–279.

Skinner, B. F. (1938). *The Behavior of Organisms*. New York, NY: Appleton-Century-Croft.

Skinner, B. F. (1953). *Science and Human Behavior*. New York, NY: Macmillan.

Skinner, B. F. (1966). The phylogeny and ontogeny of behavior. *Science, 153*, 1205–1213.

Skinner, B. F. (1969). *Contingencies of Reinforcement: A Theoretical Analysis*. New York, NY: Appleton-Century-Crofts.

Skinner, B. F. (1974). *About Behaviorism*. New York, NY: Knopf.

Skinner, B. F. (1979). *The Shaping of a Behaviorist. Part two of an Autobiography*. New York, NY: Knopf.

Spanier, G. B. (1976). Measuring dyadic adjustment: New scales for measuring the quality of marriage and similar dyads. *Journal of Marriage & Family, 38*, 15–28.

Speilberger, C. D., (1983). *Manual for the State-Trait Anxiety Inventory*. Palo Alto, CA: Consulting Press.

Spruyt, K., & Gozal, D. (2011a). Development of pediatric sleep questionnaires as diagnostic or epidemiological tools: A brief review of Dos and Don'ts. *Sleep Medicine Reviews, 15*, 7–17.

Spruyt, K., Gozal, D. (2011b). Pediatric sleep questionnaires as diagnostic or epidemiological tools: A review of currently available instruments. *Sleep Medicine Reviews, 15*, 19–32.

Stepanski, E. J., & Wyatt, J. K. (2003). Use of sleep hygiene in the treatment of insomnia. *Sleep Medicine Reviews, 7,* 215–225.

Teng, A., Bartle, A., Sadeh, A., & Mindell, J. (2012). Infant and toddler sleep in Australia and New Zealand. *Journal of Pediatrics & Child Health, 48,* 268–273.

Thoman, E. B. (1990). Sleeping and waking states in infants: A functional perspective. *Neuroscience & Biobehavioral Reviews, 14,* 93–107.

Thompson, T. (2007). Relations among functional systems in behavior analysis. *Journal of the Experimental Analysis of Behavior, 87,* 423–440.

Thorndike, E. L. (1911). *Animal Intelligence.* New York, NY: Macmillan.

Thyer, B. A. (1999). Clinical behavior analysis and clinical social work: A mutually reinforcing relationship. *The Behavior Analyst, 22,* 17–29.

Van den Bulck, J. (2007). Adolescent use of mobile phones for calling and for sending text messages after lights-out. Results from a prospective cohort study with a one year follow-up. *Sleep, 30,* 1220–1223.

Varni, J. W., Seid, M., & Kurtin, P. S. (2001). PedsQL 4.0: Reliability, and validity of the Pediatric Quality of Life Inventory, version 4.0 generic cores scales in healthy and patient populations. *Medical Care, 39,* 800–812.

Verster, J. C., Pandi-Perumel, S. R., & Streiner, D. C. (Eds.), (2008). *Sleep and Quality of Life in Clinical Medicine.* Totowa, NJ: Humana

Ward, T. M., Gay, C., Anders, T. F., Alkon, A., & Lee, K. A. (2007). Sleep and napping patterns in 3-to 5-year old children attending full-day childcare centers. *Journal of Pediatric Psychology, 32,* 1–7.

Weiner, I. B. (2003). The assessment process. In J. R. Graham & J. A. Naglieri (Eds.), *Handbook of Psychology, Vol. 10, Assessment Psychology* (3–25). Hoboken, NJ: Wiley.

Williams, B. A. (1994). Conditioned reinforcement: Experimental and theoretical issues. *The Behavior Analyst, 17,* 261–285.

Williams, C. D. (1959). The elimination of tantrum behavior by extinction procedures. *Journal of Abnormal & Social Psychology, 59,* 269.

Wilson, S. (2013). *Effects on sleep-state organization of a behavioral intervention for infant sleep disturbance.* Unpublished Masters thesis, University of Canterbury, Christchurch, New Zealand.

Witmer, L. (1996). Clinical psychology. *American Psychologist, 51,* 248–251. (Original work published 1907)

Wolf, M. M. (1978). Social validity: The case for subjective measurement, or how applied behavior analysis is finding its heart. *Journal of Applied Behavior Analysis, 11,* 203–214.

Wolfson, A., Lacks, P., & Futterman, A. (1992). Effects of parent training on infant sleeping patterns, parents' stress and perceived parental competence. *Journal of Consulting & Clinical Psychology, 60,* 41–48.

Zeifman, D. M. (2001). An ethological analysis of human infant crying: Answering Tinbergen's four questions. *Developmental Psychobiology, 39,* 265–285.

Zeskind, P. S., & Lester, B. M. (2001). Analysis of infant crying. In L.T. Singer & P. S. Zeskind (Eds.), *Biobehavioral Assessment of the Infant* (pp. 149–166). London, UK: Guilford.

CHAPTER

16 Actigraphy and Sleep/Wake Diaries

Rosemary S. C. Horne *and* Sarah N. Biggs

Abstract

Although polysomnography is the gold standard for recording sleep, the use of actigraphy in conjunction with a sleep diary is now common in the study of sleep/wake patterns in infants, children, and adolescents. Actigraphy has the advantage of being able to record data over long periods of time while the subject carries out his or her normal routine. The devices are small, lightweight, and can be worn on the wrist in a similar manner to a wristwatch, or on the ankle as is often used in infant studies. A number of studies have validated actigraphy against polysomnography for determining sleep and found good agreements; however, the specificity for determining wake is low across all ages of children. In conjunction with a sleep diary, the accuracy of actigraphy is significantly improved. Conversely, accuracy of parental reporting of sleep and wake using a sleep diary can be significantly improved when used in conjunction with actigraphy. The use of actigraphy in clinical medicine is expanding as it provides important supplementary information to clinicians regarding a variety of sleep disorders.

Key Words: actigraphy, sleep diary, sleep/wake patterns, infant, child, adolescent

Introduction

The gold standard for the assessment of sleep is overnight polysomnography (PSG), which involves attachment of a number of sensors for neurophysiological recording, and is usually carried out in a specialist sleep laboratory. However, the nature of this environment may alter a subject's normal sleep (Iber et al., 2004). Other limitations of PSG are that it is typically only tolerated for one or two nights; it is costly, time-consuming, labor intensive, and may be difficult to use in infants and young children (Thoman & Acebo, 1995). An alternative to PSG for assessing sleep is actigraphy, which has gained increasing popularity over the last 20 years (Tryon, 2004). Actigraphy uses an accelerometer to measure the presence or absence of movement which provides an estimate of sleep and wake. Unlike PSG, however, actigraphy does not provide physiological measures of sleep, but rather sleep/wake patterns that in turn are used to estimate sleep time and quality. Acebo et al. (1999) determined that a minimum of 7 nights of recording, which is likely to yield over 90% of 5 usable nights of data, is required to produce reliable results. In 1972, Kupfer and colleagues (Kupfer, Detre, Foster, Tucker, & Delgado, 1972) reported a significant correlation between wrist activity and encephalogram-measured movement and wakefulness in adults. In 1995, the Standards of Practice Committee of the American Sleep Disorders Association found enough evidence to support the use of actigraphy in evaluating some aspects of sleep disorders; for example, as an adjunct to a detailed history, examination, and subjective sleep diary for the diagnosis and treatment of insomnia, circadian rhythm disorders, and excessive sleepiness (AASD, 1995). In 2002, they found further evidence that actigraphy was reliable for detecting normal sleep in adult populations and could also be useful for characterizing and monitoring circadian rhythm patterns or disturbances in newborns, infants, children, and adolescents (Littner et al., 2003). The use of actigraphy was further expanded in recommendations made in 2007 (Morgenthaler et al., 2007). In addition to changes to recommendations for the use of actigraphy in adults, the Standards of Practice Committee of the American Academy of Sleep Medicine stated that "Actigraphy is indicated for delineating sleep patterns, and to document treatment responses in normal infants and children (in whom traditional sleep monitoring by polysomnography can be difficult to perform and/or interpret), and in special pediatric populations." (Morgenthaler et al., 2007; p. 525). The growth in popularity in the use of actigraphy over the past 20 years is evidenced by the number of publications which report using this method of sleep pattern assessment, which has risen exponentially from 10 in 1991 to 125 in 2009 (Sadeh, 2011). This growth in the use of actigraphy is particularly evident in pediatric research, where the number of studies published in 2010 (n = 41) is similar to the combined total of studies published between 1991–2001 (n = 38) (Meltzer, Montgomery-Downs, Insana, & Walsh, 2012). Despite this growth in the use of actigraphy there are, however, no pediatric practice standards for recording and scoring of actigraphy (Meltzer, Montgomery-Downs et al., 2012). This lack of standardized methods has made it difficult to compare between studies.

Sleep logs or sleep diaries have been used extensively to assess sleep in adults, infants, and children. Sleep diaries have the advantage of being an inexpensive method of collecting sleep/wake information from large numbers of subjects over long periods of time. However, they are dependent on the accuracy and reliability of the person completing them, and thus have a number of limitations. It is standard practice for sleep diaries to be used in conjunction with actigraphy for greater reliability in reporting of sleep/wake patterns.

This chapter will review the literature pertaining to the use of actigraphy and sleep diaries in infants, children, and adolescents and their usefulness for assessing normal sleep patterns, along with their use in clinical situations.

Actigraphy

The fundamental principal behind actigraphy is that the presence of movements indicates wakefulness and the absence of movements indicates sleep. Actigraphs are small wristwatch-like movement detectors (accelerometers) that are generally placed on the nondominant wrist, but can also be placed on the leg or trunk as illustrated in Figure 16.1.

Actigraphy distinguishes sleep from wake using algorithms to quantify the reduced movement associated with sleep. The actigraph continuously records the occurrence of limb movements and then sums the number and amplitude for a given epoch length. Each epoch is then given a classification of sleep or wake dependent on the activity count of that epoch compared to those around it. If the activity count of the epoch in question is less than or equal to the predetermined wake threshold, then the epoch will be scored as sleep. Actigraphs commonly have a number of sensitivity threshold settings that can be altered to adjust for different movement intensities. These thresholds can be low, medium, high, or automatic. A low threshold will identify sleep at a lower level of movement than a high threshold. They usually also have an inbuilt event marker which can be activated to indicate

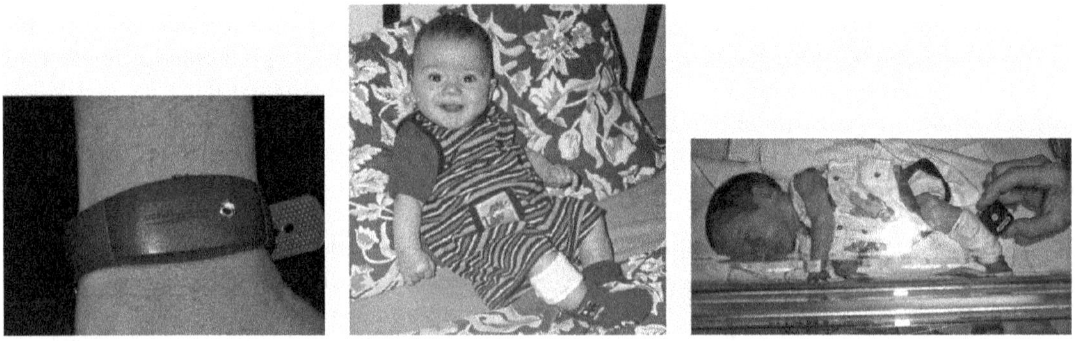

Figure 16.1 Actigraphs are usually worn on the wrist. However, in infants they are commonly placed on the leg and can be held securely with a soft bandage. In this manner they can be concealed under clothing. This method of attachment can also be used in preterm infants. (Used with permission)

when the watch is put on and removed. More recent models have light detection capabilities. This complicated analysis is conducted automatically within most actigraphy software; however, it is important to note that each device uses a slightly different algorithm that makes comparison between devices difficult. Additionally, researchers may also elect to manually score sleep and wake rather than rely on the inbuilt algorithms (Sadeh, Lavie, Scher, Tirosh, & Epstein, 1991) which negates direct comparison between studies.

Once epochs of sleep and wake are identified, the outcome variables provided through actigraphy include sleep onset, sleep latency, sleep period time (time available for sleep), wake after sleep onset, actual sleep time, sleep offset, sleep efficiency, number and length of sleep and wake bouts, and a sleep fragmentation index. One algorithm reportedly is able to distinguish between REM and non-REM sleep (Sadeh et al., 1991); however, all others only distinguish sleep and wake. An example of the output of actigraphy is illustrated in Figure 16.2.

A number of studies have been carried out in normal healthy adults, adolescents, children, and infants to assess the validity of actigraphy for assessing sleep and wake against the gold standard of PSG. In adults, good agreement (97%) has been found for total sleep time (Jean-Louis et al., 1996) with a sleep/wake determination agreement level of 91%–93% (Jean-Louis, Kripke, Cole, Assmus, & Langer, 2001; Sadeh, Sharkey, & Carskadon, 1994). Overall agreement rates of 89%–94% between actigraphy and PSG were found in a cohort of infants aged 2–4 weeks, 2–4 months, and 5–6 months (So, Buckley, Adamson, & Horne, 2005). This study showed a predictive value for determining sleep of 97% and sensitivity for sleep between 91%–96%. A recent study comparing two different actigraphy devices against PSG in children aged 3–18 years demonstrated that actigraphy was a valid measure of detecting sleep (level of agreement 89%–97%) and overall accuracy across total sleep period (level of agreement 87%–90%) when compared with PSG; however, actigraphy was limited in its ability to detect wake (overall agreement 54%–77%; see Meltzer, Walsh, Traylor, & Westin, 2012). In adolescents, comparison of three different actigraphic data modes to PSG revealed an underestimation of total sleep time in every case (Johnson et al., 2007); however, when examining time above threshold (or wake after sleep onset), the mean difference was 11 minutes. This suggests that although there is a tendency for actigraphy to underestimate sleep and overestimate wake, this can be minimized by the choice of analysis.

Sleep Diaries

Typically, pediatric sleep diaries rely on parents to record bedtime, the time the child went to sleep, the number and duration of nocturnal awakenings, the time the child awoke in the morning, and any daytime napping. This is then used to estimate both time in bed and total sleep time. As sleep diaries are an inexpensive method of collecting sleep/wake information from large numbers of subjects over long periods of time, they are the assessment tool of choice for large epidemiological studies.

For example, Seo et al. (2010) used sleep diaries to examine the sleep patterns in 3639 school-aged children in Korea. In that study, parents of children aged 7–12 years were asked to keep a sleep diary over two consecutive days, recording bedtime, wake-up time, sleep latency, number and duration of night awakenings, and any daytime napping. While this assessment method is adequate for providing a "snapshot" of sleep/wake patterns in large cohorts, it is not without its limitations. As with any parental or self-report measure, there is inherent bias in this reporting method (see Spruyt, pp. XX, this volume). Bedtimes, wake times, and particularly nocturnal awakenings may be over- or underestimated due to lack of knowledge or imprecise recordings. In the case of parent report, this becomes particularly problematic as children get older and begin to manage their own bedtimes. As such, self-report sleep diaries are often used when assessing sleep/wake patterns in adolescents. Wolfson et al. (2003) compared self-report sleep diary, retrospective survey, and actigraphy in a cohort of adolescents aged 13–19 years and found that reports of sleep/wake patterns were comparable across the three measures for weekdays, although less so for weekends. The above limitations do not suggest, however, that sleep diaries should not be utilized. Validation of sleep diaries against PSG or actigraphy have shown that while there is often an overestimation of sleep time and underestimation of night awakenings, sleep diaries are adequate for determining differences in sleep patterns across ages (Canet, 2010; Seo et al., 2010) and clinical groups (Corkum, Tannock, Moldofsky, Hogg-Johnson, & Humphries, 2001; Kieckhefer, Ward, Tsai, & Lentz, 2008). Examples of sleep diaries used for clinical and research purposes are presented in Figures 16.3, 16.4, and 16.5 respectively.

(a)

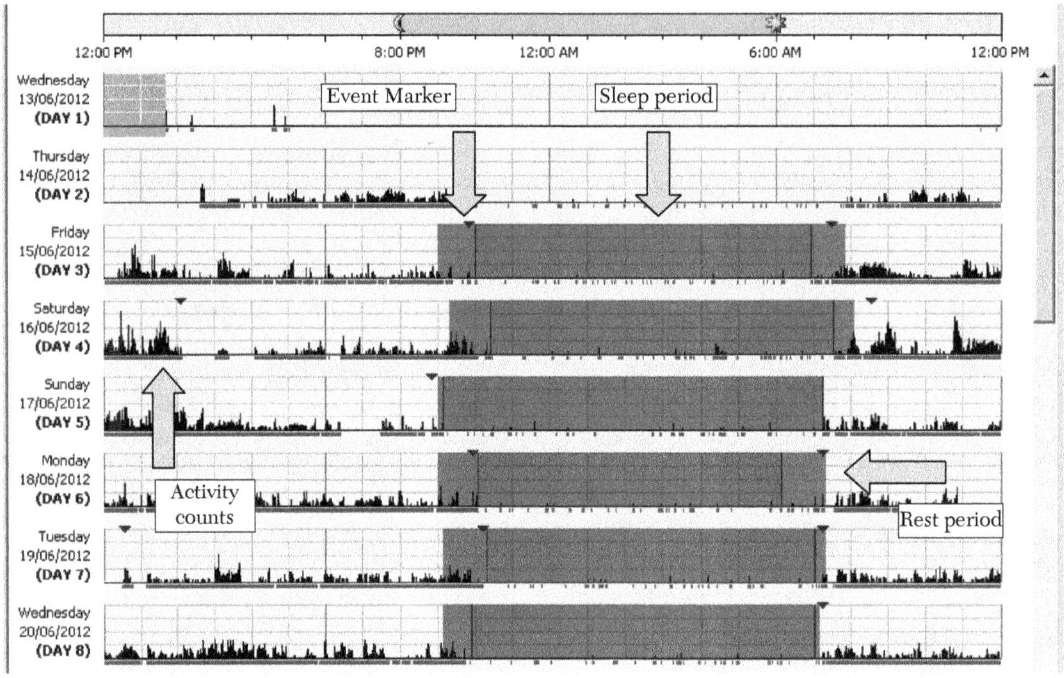

(b)

59	---------------------- Statistics ----------------------												
60													
61	Interval Ty	Interval#	Start Date	Start Time	End Date	End Time	Duration	%Invalid S	Efficiency	Wake Tim	%Wake	Sleep Tim	%Sleep
62							(minutes)	(%)	(%)	(minutes)	(%)	(minutes)	(%)
63													
64	SLEEP	1	15/06/2012	10:02:00 PM	16/06/2012	6:56:00 AM	534	0	74.62	49	9.18	485	90.82
65	SLEEP	2	16/06/2012	10:27:00 PM	17/06/2012	7:32:00 AM	545	0	70.39	91	16.7	454	83.3
66	SLEEP	3	17/06/2012	9:08:00 PM	18/06/2012	7:14:00 AM	606	0	86.5	74	12.21	532	87.79
67	SLEEP	4	18/06/2012	10:05:00 PM	19/06/2012	6:08:00 AM	483	0	69.35	53	10.97	430	89.03
68	SLEEP	5	19/06/2012	10:21:00 PM	20/06/2012	7:03:00 AM	522	0	76.07	58	11.11	464	88.89
69	SLEEP	6	20/06/2012	9:55:00 PM	21/06/2012	7:04:00 AM	549	0	82.33	55	10.02	494	89.98
70	SLEEP	7	21/06/2012	9:36:00 PM	22/06/2012	6:56:00 AM	560	0	81.9	85	15.18	475	84.82
71	SLEEP	8	22/06/2012	10:43:00 PM	23/06/2012	7:48:00 AM	545	0	77.94	54	9.91	491	90.09
72	SLEEP	9	23/06/2012	10:32:00 PM	24/06/2012	7:43:00 AM	551	0	78.37	69	12.52	482	87.48
73	Sleep Sum	n	NaN	NaN	NaN	NaN	9	9	9	9	9	9	9
74	Sleep Sum	Minimum	NaN	NaN	NaN	NaN	483	0	69.35	49	9.18	430	83.3
75	Sleep Sum	Maximum	NaN	NaN	NaN	NaN	606	0	86.5	91	16.7	532	90.82
76	Sleep Sum	Average(r	NaN	NaN	NaN	NaN	543.89	0	77.5	65.33	11.98	478.56	88.02
77	Sleep Sum	Std Dev(n	NaN	NaN	NaN	NaN	32.56	0	5.61	15.17	2.52	28.48	2.52

Figure 16.2 A. An example of an actigram. The actigram displays the sleep and wake periods over 24 hours. The black lines indicate the activity count for each epoch. The dark blue areas are sleep and the light blue is determined as a rest period. A rest period indicates a period of low movement prior to sleep onset or after sleep offset, scored as wake but within the sleep interval. The sleep/rest periods can be automatically allocated by the software or manually defined in accordance with the sleep diary. In this diagram, sleep/rest periods have been manually allocated. **B.** The associated sleep statistics output for the actigram. Depending on the software program, the user can request a number of statistics that are then exported. In this case, the output displays the sleep periods for each 24-hour period and includes duration of sleep period, whether there were any invalid epochs, sleep efficiency, the amount of time awake after sleep onset both in minutes and as a percentage of sleep time, and total sleep in minutes and as a percentage. Again depending on the software, a summary of the whole recording period is often available.

Validation Studies of Actigraphy

When validating actigraphy against the gold standard measurement of sleep and wake measured using PSG, a number of parameters are frequently calculated. Agreement rate (AR) is defined as the proportion of observations for which PSG ratings accord with actiwatch ratings for both sleep and awake; predictive value for sleep (PVS) is calculated as the probability that the actiwatch prediction is correct by PSG criteria for sleep; and predictive value for wake (PVW) is calculated as the probability that the actiwatch prediction is

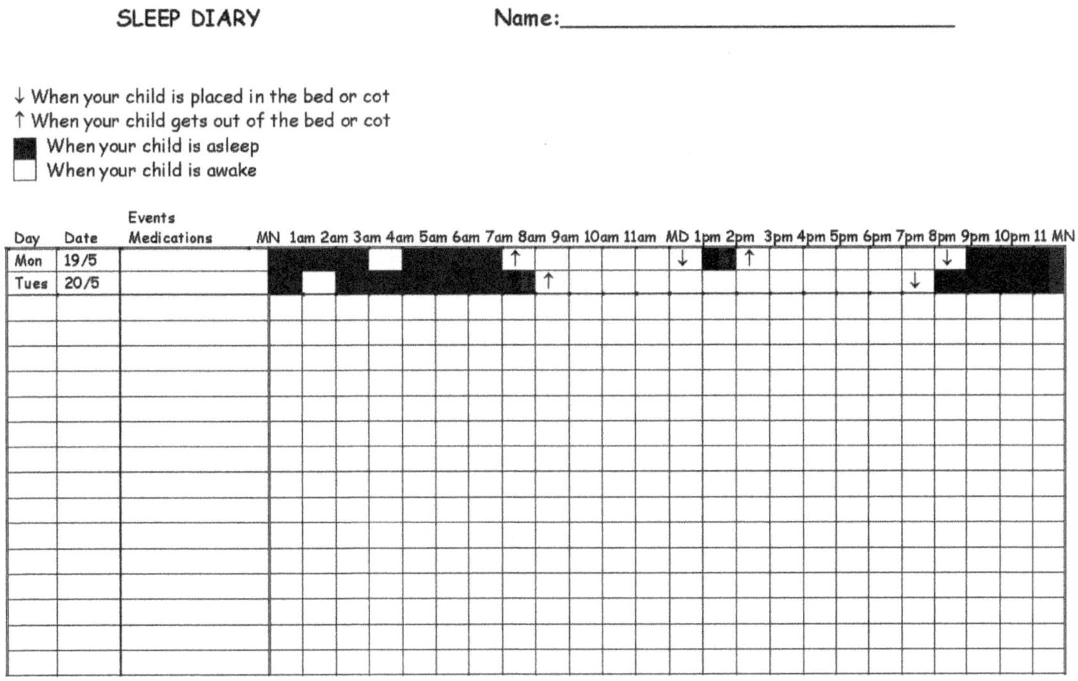

Figure 16.3 Example of a sleep diary used for clinical purposes. Parents are asked to shade the areas when the child is asleep and indicate with arrows when they are put to bed and get up.

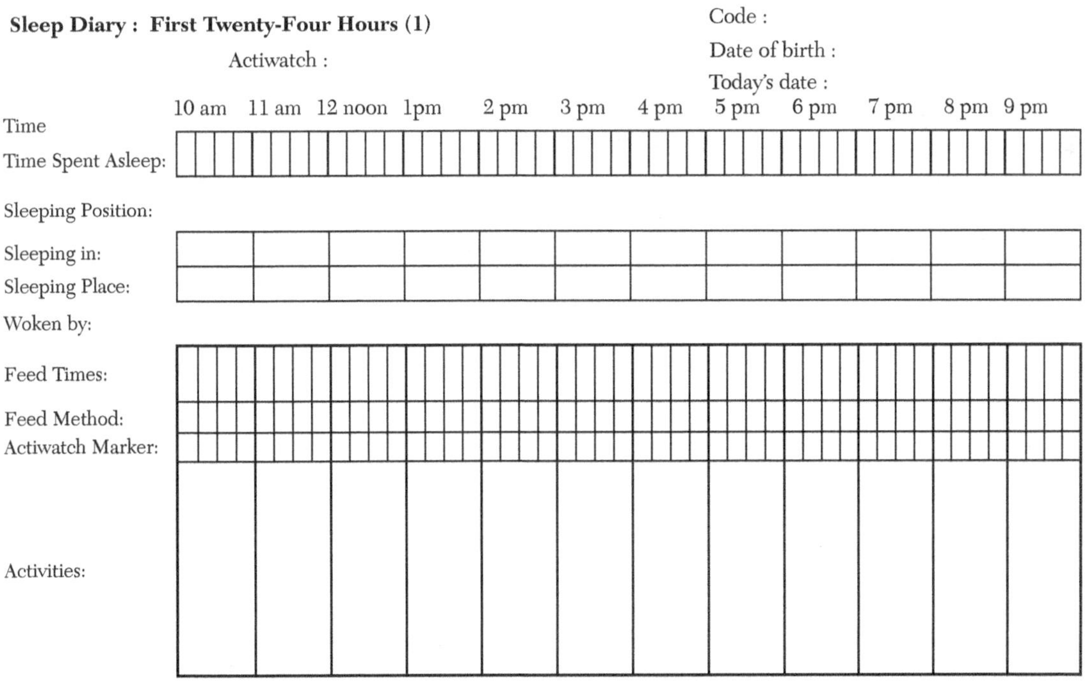

Figure 16.4 An example of an infant sleep research diary as used in studies by So and colleagues (So, Adamson, & Horne, 2007). Parents were asked to complete the diary over 72 hours, recording infant sleep/wake every 15 minutes. They were also asked to note when their infant was fed and other activities such as external movements associated with traveling in a car, being held, or being rocked.

SELF REPORT SLEEP DIARY

Your Full Name:	Office use only Study ID:

Do you share a room? Yes / No *(please circle)*

Do you share a bed with anyone for the whole night? Yes / No *(please circle)*

Did you consume caffeine (e.g. coke, coffee) in the hour before bed? Yes / No *(please circle)* If yes, how often? Every night / 3-4 nights per week / 1-2 nights per week *(please circle)*

Date	Day	Number of daytime naps	Total time of all daytime naps (mins)	Time went to bed in evening	After going to your bedroom, what did you do? (*Tick all that apply*)	Time went to sleep	Number of awakenings during night	Total time awake during night (mins)	Did you move to another bed during the night (Y/N)	Time woke up next morning	Who or what woke you up in the morning? *(Please tick)*	Time got out of bed
2/7/12	*Mon*	*1*	*30 min*	*10:15pm*	Went straight to sleep ☐ Watched TV ☑ Read a book ☐ Played on the computer ☐ Listened to music ☐ Talked/text on phone ☐ Other: ________	*10:50pm*	2	*20 min*	*Yes*	*7:15am*	Woke myself ☐ A family member ☐ Alarm clock ☑ Other: ________	*7:20am*
					Went straight to sleep ☐ Watched TV ☐ Read a book ☐ Played on the computer ☐ Listened to music ☐ Talked/text on phone ☐ Other: ________						Woke myself ☐ A family member ☐ Alarm clock ☐ Other: ________	
					Went straight to sleep ☐ Watched TV ☐ Read a book ☐ Played on the computer ☐ Listened to music ☐ Talked/text on phone ☐ Other: ________						Woke myself ☐ A family member ☐ Alarm clock ☐ Other: ________	
					Went straight to sleep ☐ Watched TV ☐ Read a book ☐ Played on the computer ☐ Listened to music ☐ Talked/text on phone ☐ Other: ________						Woke myself ☐ A family member ☐ Alarm clock ☐ Other: ________	

Page 1

Figure 16.5 An example of a self-report sleep diary for use in adolescents. In addition to the standard documentation of sleep and wake, subjects are asked to record events that may influence sleep, such as caffeine use and bedtime activities. This provides an indication of sleep hygiene—pre-sleep behaviors that affect sleep schedules, duration and quality—which can be useful in assessing sleep patterns and problems in teenagers.

correct by PSG criteria for wake. Sensitivity, the ability of the actiwatch to predict true sleep, and specificity, the ability of the actiwatch to predict true wake, are also frequently reported. In addition Bland-Altman plots are used to compare the two methods.

Validation Studies in Preterm Infants

In adults, adolescents, children, and older infants, PSG is the standard method of assessing sleep/wake; however, in preterm infants in a neonatal unit environment the attachment of leads necessary for PSG is frequently not possible due to the size of the infant and fragility of the infant's skin. A study using actigraphy in preterm infants in the neonatal intensive care setting found it to be a valid method for determining sleep before term-equivalent age when compared against behavioral observations (Sung, Adamson, & Horne, 2009). Overall, on the low activity threshold they found agreement rates of 84.5%–88.9% between actigraphy and behavioral scoring with the predictive value for determining sleep being between 91.3%–95.6% and sensitivity between 88.2%–96.8%. However, the actiwatch was not reliable for determining wakefulness, with low predictive values (31.1%–53.7%) and specificity (31.5–33.6%). Previous studies have shown that actigraphy is less reliable in younger infants, with agreement rates of 88.9% (So et al., 2005) and 88.7% (Gnidovec, Neubauer, & Zidar, 2002) and have also reported no difference in agreement rates across age between 2–4 weeks and 5–6 months at the low and auto activity threshold settings (So et al., 2005). The Sung et al. (2009) actigraphic study did, however, find that the predictive value for sleep increased significantly between 30–33 weeks and 37–40 weeks post-natal age. The low predictive value for wake and the lower overall agreement rates in this age group could be due to the relatively high number of body movements, especially during active sleep (see Lushington, Pamula, Martin, and Kennedy, Chapters 5 and 6). Previous reports have shown that the amount of movement during sleep decreases with age (Hayes & Mitchell, 1998). Since actigraphy uses activity levels to determine sleep and wakefulness, and there is a high level of activity during the sleep of preterm infants, it is not surprising that actigraphy scores a high percentage of sleep as wakefulness. Despite this limitation actigraphy provides a useful noninvasive method for determining sleep patterns in preterm infants.

Validation Studies in Infants

The first validation studies of actigraphy in infants were conducted comparing actigraphy with behavioral observations of infant sleep/wake. The first study by Sadeh et al. (1995) assessed sleep–wake patterns in 41 infants (10 newborns, 11 at 3 months, 10 at 6 months and 10 at 12 months) who were studied using actigraphy over a 2–2.5 hour period with behavioral assessments (Thoman, 1990). The aim of that study was to develop an algorithm for automatic scoring in infants and then to test the validity of this algorithm. Minute-by-minute agreement rates with behavioral scoring reached 95.3%; however, distinction between active and quiet sleep states was less accurate and ranged between 54%–87% at the different ages. The study concluded that actigraphy provided a valid measurement of sleep/wake over the first year of life. A later study by Gnidovec et al. (Gnidovec, 2002) also compared actigraphy data with behaviorally scored sleep and wakefulness in 10 healthy term infants at 1, 3, and 6 months of age over 3 hours. Overall agreement rates were between 87%–95% at 3 and 6 months; however, at 1 month these did not exceed 72%. The actiwatch did not, however, allow active sleep and quiet sleep to be distinguished. A study by Sazonov et al. (Sazonov, Sazonova, Schuckers, & Neuman, 2004) used an actigraph positioned over the sacral region on the infant's diaper, which determined not only sleep/wake states but also the position of the infant in the cot. The study used logistic regression and nonlinear mapping as predictors, rather than the more broadly used discriminant analysis techniques, and results were compared to PSG. The study reported similar accuracies of 77%–92% and prediction rates of 85%–95% to those previously reported with actigraphs on the infant ankle (Sadeh, Acebo, Seifer, Aytur, & Carskadon, 1995).

There have been a small number of studies in infants comparing actigraphy to PSG. A study which compared actigraphy to daytime PSG in 13 term and 9 preterm infants at three different matched postconceptional ages: 2–4 weeks (n = 8, mean 21 ± 2d), 2–4 months (n = 13, mean 84 ± 4d) and 5–6 months (n = 11, mean 171 ± 3d) found overall agreement rates of 89%–94% between actigraphy and PSG, with the predictive value for determining sleep being 97% and sensitivity between 91%–96% (So et al., 2005). However, the actiwatch was not reliable for determining wakefulness, with low values for predictive value for wake and specificity. This could have been because a relatively low number of epochs of wake were recorded during the study (460 minutes wake compared with 6546 minutes sleep). A recent study of 22 healthy infants aged 13–15 months, using the same actiwatch reported above, used Bland Altman analysis rather than minute-by-minute agreement rates and showed that although there was a strong statistically significant correlation between total sleep time recorded by both devices, the actiwatch underestimated total sleep time and overestimated wake after sleep onset time (Insana, Gozal, & Montgomery-Downs, 2010). Unlike standard correlational analysis, which can show a relationship even if one does not exist, a Bland Altman determines the 95% confidence intervals by plotting the difference between the measures against the mean of both. This allows the determination of the level of agreement between the measures within a 5% error margin. If the Bland Altman plot shows the difference in the means falls within this 95% confidence interval, then one measure can be confidently substituted for the other (Bland & Altman, 1995). Insana et al. (2010), concluded that improved software device and/or software development was needed before the device could be considered a valid method of identifying infant sleep–wake patterns.

A study which utilized a large dataset of infant sleep recorded during the Collaborative Home Infant Monitoring Evaluation (CHIME) study compared PSG and actigraphy to develop new methods of utilizing artificial neural networks and decision trees, which capture nonlinear classification characteristics, rather than the traditional linear methods (Tilmanne, Urbain, Kothare, Wouwer, & Kothare, 2009). The study reported improved tradeoffs between sensitivity and specificity in groups of healthy term and preterm infants, those with apnea of prematurity, and siblings of SIDS infants. Accuracy rates across the groups was 79.3%–86.9%, with the highest accuracy in the term infants and lowest in the preterm infants (Tilmanne et al., 2009). The researchers recommend that these new techniques be added to newer actigraphic models as they are produced.

One of the limitations of actigraphy is that external movement can have a significant impact on measurements, particularly in infants. In a study where actigraphs were placed on dolls, external movement from being placed in normal situations that an infant would experience, such as a stroller, shopping cart, being held and rocked, or travelling in a car, all influenced activity counts (Tsai & Thomas, 2010). In a previous report the same group studied infants over 4–7 days and identified that 40% of recording time involved external motion as reported by parents (Tsai, Burr, & Thomas, 2009). Approximately 75% of the external motion involved the caregiver holding the infant, and the remainder included infants being placed in an infant bouncer, car seat, infant stroller, or shopping trolley. When external motion was excluded from analysis, the correlation between actigraphy and sleep diary improved. It is therefore important that the type and extent of external movement, and also the sensitivity threshold of the actigraph, is accounted for. In some studies, external movement has been excluded before analysis (Acebo et al., 2005; So et al., 2005); in others, external movement has been included (Jenni, Deboer, & Achermann, 2006; So et al., 2007); however, in the majority of studies how the data were analyzed in relation to external movement has not been specified.

Overall, validation studies in infants have found good agreement between actigraphy and PSG-measured sleep but less specificity for determining wake. As can be seen by the above studies reporting a high prevalence of movement artifact, limitations of the technology exist in naturalistic settings. In the absence of a complementary measure, such as a sleep diary, the likelihood of underestimation of sleep in infants is high. Thus, while actigraphy is currently the best method for objectively estimating sleep/wake patterns in infants in the naturalistic setting, the limitations of the technology must be acknowledged.

Validation Studies in Children

In a study comparing the agreement between actigraphy and PSG in a cohort of clinically referred children aged 1–12 years (N = 45), Hyde and colleagues (2007) determined the validity of the tool to accurately determine sleep and wake over four different thresholds: low, medium, high, and automatic. A high threshold allows for a greater amplitude of movement before deeming it as wake, a low threshold determines wake at a small amplitude of movement, and an automatic threshold determines the average movement amplitude for that subject and uses an algorithm based on that average to determine what wake would be for that particular person. That study determined that actigraphy was most accurate in determining total sleep time and sleep efficiency when at the low and automatic thresholds, but did not accurately estimate nocturnal waking. That is, actigraphy cannot differentiate between a period of quiet wakefulness (e.g., lying still in bed) and sleep. Actigraphy best predicted wake when set at the high or medium threshold; however, there were still some discrepancies with actigraphy confusing gross body movements (e.g., rolling over) as wake. In a later study by the same group, 130 children and adolescents aged 2–18 years referred for assessment of sleep disordered breathing wore an actigraph while undergoing clinical PSG (O'Driscoll, Foster, Davey, Nixon, & Horne, 2010). The arousal index scored from the PSG study was compared to the actigraphically derived sleep fragmentation index. The ability of actigraphic measures to correctly classify a child as having an arousal index >10 events/h was rated as fair for the fragmentation index and poor for wake bouts/h (area under the receiver operator characteristic curve, 0.73 and 0.67, respectively). The authors concluded that actigraphy had significant limitations for being used as a diagnostic tool for children with sleep disordered breathing (O'Driscoll et al., 2010).

In a recent study comparing two different actigraphy devices against PSG in a group (N = 115) of clinically referred children aged 3–18 years, Meltzer and colleagues (Meltzer, Walsh et al., 2012) also demonstrated that actigraphy was a valid measure of detecting sleep (level of agreement 89%–97%) and overall accuracy across total sleep period (level of agreement 87%–90%) when compared with PSG but was limited in its ability to detect wake (overall agreement 54%–77%). The range of agreement level altered depending on the device, scoring algorithm, and sensitivity threshold, highlighting the difficulty of comparison across studies and the need for standardization of actigraphy analysis. In a study of 58 preschool children with a variety of disorders including autism, autism without developmental delay, and typically developing children, nocturnal sleep and wake was recorded with both actigraphy and videosomnography (Sitnick, Goodlin-Jones, & Anders, 2008). When compared, there was overall 94% agreement epoch-by-epoch with a sensitivity of 97% and a specificity of only 24%, indicating that actigraphy had poor agreement for detecting night awakenings in this age group and should be used in conjunction with other recording methods (Sitnick et al., 2008).

There are also discrepancies in regard to how sleep variables are defined from actigraphy data, as there are currently no standard rules for scoring the sleep parameters. For example, sleep onset has been defined as 3, 5, 15, or even 20 minutes of immobility (Meltzer & Westin, 2011). These differences can have an effect on sleep latency, total sleep time, and wake after sleep onset. Meltzer and Westin (2011) conducted a study comparing outcome variables of two commonly reported non-automated actigraphy scoring methods in a cohort of children aged 8–12 years (N = 38). In the first analysis, sleep onset was defined as the first minute of 15 minutes of consecutive sleep following the time indicated on the sleep diary that sleep was attempted. Sleep offset was the last minute of 15 minutes of consecutive sleep prior to diary-reported awakening. The second analysis defined sleep onset as the first minute of 3 consecutive minutes of sleep, and sleep offset as the last minute of 5 consecutive minutes of sleep, both following diary-report attempted sleep and awakening as outlined above. A third condition, where the sleep diary was not available, was also included. Significantly different results were found between the scoring methods for sleep offset, sleep period, wake after sleep onset, and sleep efficiency. Overall, the 15-minute condition resulted in shorter sleep duration but higher sleep efficiency. However, while these were statistically significant differences, actual discrepancies between sleep outcomes were minimal. Differences in sleep offset were 8 and 11 minutes between the 15-minute condition and 3/5-minute and no diary condition, respectively. Differences in sleep efficiency were approximately 1%. Thus, the authors concluded that while differences did exist between scoring methods, they are unlikely to be of any clinical significance. Despite this, standard scoring rules are required if one wishes to make comparisons across studies.

Validation Studies in Adolescents

Johnson et al. (2007) examined the accuracy of actigraphically measured total sleep time against PSG in 181 adolescents aged 12–16 years, with and without sleep disordered breathing. In this study, the authors compared three different data modes within actigraphy: time above threshold (TAT), zero crossing mode (ZCM), and proportional integration mode (PIM). TAT describes the amount of time the activity count exceeds the threshold. ZCM is the number of times the activity count crosses the threshold (set close to zero) and PIM is the area under the curve for each epoch. Results of that study revealed that when compared to PSG, actigraphy underestimated total sleep time irrespective of which data mode was used. TAT, however, showed the greatest accuracy, with a mean difference of 11 minutes. The discrepancy between PSG and actigraphic total sleep time increased in the sleep disordered breathing group. From this, the authors concluded that actigraphy was a good estimate in healthy sleeping adolescents but was less accurate for adolescents with sleep disordered breathing.

Meltzer and colleagues (Meltzer, Walsh et al., 2012) also found reduced sensitivity—ability to determine true sleep—and increased specificity—ability to determine true wake—of actigraphy in adolescents with sleep disordered breathing compared to healthy controls. In that study, depending on the algorithm used, sensitivity decreased by approximately 10% in adolescents with moderate to severe obstructive sleep apnea (OSA:85%) compared to non-snoring adolescents (92%). Specificity increased by approximately 5% (59% in non-snoring adolescents; 63% in moderate to severe OSA). Due to the inherent problem with the technology—that is, the inability to distinguish movement from wake—it is likely that the increased arousal associated with sleep disordered breathing led to this result.

Thus, while actigraphy is an adequate estimate of sleep in healthy adolescents, its accuracy reduces in the presence of sleep disorders. As such, the choice of activity thresholds and scoring algorithms are of utmost importance when using actigraphy to examine sleep and wake in healthy versus clinical populations of children and adolescents.

Comparison of Sleep Diaries and Actigraphy

Parental sleep diaries have been used extensively over many years to record infant and child sleep/wake patterns (Coons & Guilleminault, 1984). This method has the advantage of being economical and not requiring any specialized equipment. Actigraphy is more expensive, particularly the initial cost of purchasing the equipment, and requires some technical expertise to interpret the results.

Sleep Diaries and Actigraphy in Infants

Usually sleep diaries are recorded on paper, but recently electronic versions of the same diary have been developed and compared in conjunction with actigraphy (Muller, Hemmi, Wilhelm, Barr, & Schneider, 2011). Overall, a good correlation was found between both types of diaries and actigraphy over 24 hours and when the study was separated into day and night. However, both types of diaries recorded more sleep over 24 hours and during the day than actigraphy (Muller et al., 2011). Interestingly, although parents reported that they preferred the electronic diary they were less adherent in completing it, and 16% of records were lost due to technical difficulties (Muller et al., 2011). When choosing electronic versus paper diaries the cost of recording needs to be weighed against the increased acceptability and ease of use of the electronic versions.

Studies have reported overall a good agreement between parental logs of sleep and actigraphy in infants (Sadeh, 1994, 1996; So et al., 2007). Two studies that compared sleep patterns of infants referred for assessment of sleep disturbances using parental sleep diaries and actigraphy, showed that parents accurately reported sleep onset and sleep duration but overestimated the time their infant spent asleep and underestimated the number of night awakenings (Sadeh, 1994, 1996). Importantly, the parental records became less reliable as the study progressed, suggesting that parents became either less motivated or exhausted in completing the sleep diaries (Sadeh, 1994). These findings have also been reported in longitudinal studies of healthy term infants where there was a good agreement between parental report and actigraphy during the day, but at night parents underreported time spent awake (So et al., 2007; Spruyt et al., 2008). It has been suggested that these discrepancies could have been due to the infants waking during the night but not crying and alerting parents, or that parents were not as conscientious about reporting night awakenings due to tiredness (So et al., 2007).

Studies that have compared parental reports with actigraphy or a home-based limited sleep recording system have found that there was significant variability in the reliability of mothers' reports of their infants' sleep patterns (Sadeh, 1994, 1996; Whitney & Thoman, 1993). This may arise because mothers cannot always know what their baby is doing—for example, some babies are able to self-soothe back to sleep without crying; thus, their mothers are unaware that their babies have awoken and report that they were asleep the whole time. Thus, it is important to validate each method of recording, and a combination of actigraphy and sleep diary is recommended.

A recent study compared parental sleep diaries against actigraphy to determine whether they could be reliably used clinically without the cost or expertise required for actigraphy. That study of 52 infants at around 1 year of age, studied for 7 days, found that sleep diaries scored in 30-minute epochs provided accurate reporting of sleep onset and offset time, nocturnal sleep duration, and number of night awakenings (Asaka & Takada, 2011). However, wake after sleep onset was significantly underreported on the diaries compared to actigraphy. The study also found that the reliability of the diaries varied considerably across the week of the study, with lower correlations in the middle of the study period. The results add to the argument of the validity of sleep diaries, as in this study the majority (50/52) of infants slept in the same room as the parents, indicating that sleep quality determination by diary is not just dependent on parents not hearing their infant awake.

Sleep Diaries and Actigraphy in Children

Acebo et al. (2005) conducted a study, using both actigraphy and sleep diary data, to profile sleep/wake patterns in the home in a cohort of healthy children aged 1 to 5 years. In that study, 169 children wore an actigraph for approximately 7 days while their parents completed a sleep/wake diary, reporting all nocturnal and daytime sleep over the same period. On average, sleep diary reports revealed that children were in bed approximately 11 hours 20 minutes per night at 1 year of age and 10 hours 20 minutes at 5 years of age. Actigraphy also reported this decline with age, but sleep period time was estimated at 10 hours 50 minutes at age 1 to 9 hours 40 minutes at age 5. Therefore, while there may be a tendency for overestimation of sleep duration using sleep diaries, this assessment method can provide valuable information regarding the profile of sleep/wake patterns in infants and children. Werner et al. (Werner, Molinari, Guyer, & Jenni, 2008) conducted a study that examined the agreement rates between questionnaire, sleep diary, and actigraphy data in a sample of kindergarten children (N = 50, 4–7 years). Actigraphy monitoring was conducted for a period of 6–8 consecutive nights, and parents completed a sleep diary for their child for the same period. A questionnaire describing normal sleep patterns was also completed. A standardized interview was used to determine behavioral sleep problems. The degree of agreement between the sleep assessment measures was analyzed using a Bland Altman plot. Comparison between actigraphy and sleep diary showed adequate agreement for sleep start (±28 minutes), sleep end (±24 minutes), and assumed sleep (±32 minutes). Actual sleep time (±72 minutes) and nocturnal wake time (±55 minutes) failed to reach agreement. Comparison between actigraphy and the questionnaire failed to reach acceptable agreement on any sleep parameter. In a similar study of 59 kindergarten children aged 3–6 years, monitored for 4–5 consecutive nights, correlation between actigraphy measures and parental reports for sleep schedule measures were 66%–79%, indicating the patterns of sleep/wake were similar between the two measures. However, parents had a tendency to significantly underestimate night wakings and overestimate sleep quality when compared to actigraphy (Tikotzky & Sadeh, 2001). These studies suggest that actigraphy and sleep diaries are complementary when measuring sleep start, sleep end, and assumed sleep time; however, they cannot be used interchangeably for actual sleep time or nocturnal wakings.

Sleep Diaries and Actigraphy in Adolescents

Short and colleagues (Short, Gradisar, Lack, Wright, & Carskadon, 2012) examined the discrepancies between sleep and wake after sleep onset in a cohort of adolescents (N = 290, 13–18 years) and showed that there were large differences between self-reported sleep diary and actigraphic recorded sleep time and wake after sleep onset. In that study, actigraphy overestimated wake after sleep onset and underestimated total sleep time as compared to sleep diaries. Additionally, an increase in wake after sleep onset as measured on actigraphy did not predict adolescent's reports of excessive nocturnal restlessness, problems with nocturnal awakenings, or sleep problems. However, the activity threshold of this analysis was not reported. Interestingly, the discrepancy between actigraphy and self-reported sleep diary was greater in boys than girls in this study. The authors suggested that this may be due to a higher amount of nocturnal movement in the boys than the girls, or it may be that the girls were more diligent in the accuracy of their diary reporting. Overall, a combination of sleep diaries and actigraphy is being widely used to determine sleep patterns in children and it appears that despite some limitations they provide accurate measures over sustained periods of time.

Summary

Actigraphy and sleep diaries provide a cost-effective way of gathering sleep and wake information from large cohorts over extended periods of time; however, they are not without their limitations. In regard to the sleep diary, parents may not be aware of how often their child awakens if the child does not disturb the parent. In addition, as the child ages and begins to manage his/her own bedtime routines, parents may be unaware of when the child actually goes to bed and attempts to fall asleep. This would lead to an overestimation of bedtime and underestimation of night time arousals, resulting in an overestimation of total sleep time. Actigraphy is, however, unable to distinguish between *(1)* two categories of wakefulness, crying and non-crying in infants, or *(2)* periods of quiet wakefulness and sleep. Actigraphy is prone to movement artifacts, often recording nocturnal movements such as rolling over or twitching, as wake. This then leads to an overestimation of wake after sleep onset, underestimating total sleep time. It appears that when it comes to gathering the most accurate information regarding sleep/wake patterns in infants, children, and adolescents, outside of the gold standard PSG, a combination of actigraphy and sleep diary measures are required.

Clinical Use of Actigraphy and Sleep Diaries

Infant and child sleep problems are of great concern to parents and can have important clinical consequences. The exact prevalence of sleep disorders in children is unknown; however, questionnaire-based estimates suggest that up to 40% of children and adolescents report sleep problems that either disrupt or restrict sleep (Blunden et al., 2004; Mindell & Durand, 1993). Excessive daytime sleepiness has been reported in 17%–21% of children and adolescents, and this may be as high as 68% in high school students (Gibson et al., 2006). Difficulties in initiating and maintaining sleep and the total amount of daily sleep have considerable implications for infant and child development, behavior, and overall health. Parents with children who exhibit developmental, affective, or executive disorders often report sleep disturbances, especially sleep disruption and shortened sleep duration. In addition, sleep deprivation may indicate an underlying medical disorder such as sleep disordered breathing or restless leg syndrome. Interpreting a parent's report of their child's sleep patterns is often challenging for clinicians. Frequently parents are asked to keep a sleep diary for this, but more commonly actigraphy is now being used in conjunction with sleep diaries.

In 1995, Sadeh et al. conducted an extensive literature review examining the usefulness of actigraphy in evaluating sleep disorders. These authors concluded that while actigraphy was adequate in assessing the natural patterns of sleep and wake, it was not suitable as a diagnostic tool. More recently, however, actigraphy has been recommended as a valid tool for assessing sleep disorders such as circadian phase disorders, sleep disturbances associated with insomnia and hypersomnia, sleep duration in patients with obstructive sleep apnea, sleep problems in older adults, and in children with behavioral concerns such as attention deficit hyperactivity disorder (ADHD) (Morgenthaler et al., 2007). Thus, actigraphy is useful in determining differences in sleep/wake patterns in different clinical populations, potentially identifying a comorbid behavioral sleep problem that may be amenable to treatment or intervention.

For example, actigraphy has been used in children with learning disabilities and autism spectrum disorders to determine sleep disruption in these populations, and correlated with parental sleep diary report (Wiggs & Stores, 2004). Interestingly, the actigraphic reports of those children whose parents reported daytime sleepiness in their children did not differ from those who did not, although both groups of children had disturbed sleep (took longer to fall asleep, spent more time awake at night, had reduced sleep efficiency and more extreme sleep times) compared to normal values (Wiggs & Stores, 2004). In a study which compared actigraphic and both parental report and self-report of sleep in children with ADHD and control children, it was found that all three measures suggested that the children with ADHD had reduced sleep quality and more disturbed sleep than controls (Owens et al., 2009; see Corkum and Coulombe, Chapter 34). In contrast, another study of children with ADHD demonstrated a very poor correlation between parental report of sleep and actigraphy (Wiggs, Montgomery, & Stores, 2005). In this study the majority of children also had an underlying sleep disorder, such as restless leg syndrome or sleep disordered breathing, highlighting the importance of clinicians also screening for these disorders (Wiggs et al., 2005). In a study of preschool children aged 2–5 years, although it was found that parental reports of ADHD symptoms were associated with parental reports of sleep problems, no significant differences in actigraphic sleep patterns or night-to-night sleep/wake variability were found (Goodlin-Jones, Waters, & Anders, 2009). Thus, there is still controversy regarding the relationship between sleep patterns and ADHD, but using both subjective and objective measures of sleep provides better clinical evidence than the use of parental report alone.

In a study of infants born to depressed and non-depressed mothers over the first 6 months of life, which used both actigraphy and sleep diaries, it was found that the infants of depressed mothers took longer to fall asleep, had lower sleep efficiencies, and had more sleep bouts at nighttime than did the control infants (Armitage et al., 2009). Actigraphy has also been proposed as a novel method to detect infantile colic in 3-month-old infants (Martin-Martinez et al., 2010).

In summary, actigraphy is becoming more widely used in pediatric clinical practice, but does have the limitation of not being able to distinguish between sleep states. In addition there are problems of providing an accurate measure of sleep and wake if the patient has a concurrent movement disorder or if they lie quietly awake and do not move.

Conclusions

Sleep in infants, children, and adolescents is of major clinical importance and most frequently has been assessed using parental sleep diaries. However, the use of diaries is subjective and they are only as reliable as the extent to which the parents are able to observe the child sleeping. If the child spends time during the night awake without alerting parents then these diaries can be inaccurate. It has also been shown that when parents are required to keep diaries over extended periods of time their reporting becomes less accurate. Over the past two decades there has been a dramatic growth in the use of actigraphy for estimating sleep/wake patterns in infants and children, in both research studies and in clinical settings. In comparison with polysomnography, actigraphy is low cost and can be used for prolonged periods of time in the individual's usual environment. Actigraphy is thus an important tool for estimating sleep patterns in pediatric populations. Actigraphy has been validated for determining sleep and wake against polysomnography and, in most studies, has good agreement for determining sleep but is very limited for detecting wakefulness during sleep periods. Actigraphy also has good agreement in most instances with self-reports and parental diary reports of sleep/wake patterns when reporting sleep onset time and duration; however, there is poorer agreement for sleep quality variables such as night waking. Another limitation of the use of actigraphy, particularly in infants, is that of external movement, which is very common during infancy, and this significantly influences results. Thus the use of actigraphy in conjunction with sleep diaries, which identify these periods, is recommended.

Currently there are many actigraph models available and that number is steadily increasing. Each device uses a different algorithm, making it difficult to compare between devices. New algorithms are being developed that will provide greater accuracy, particularly for determining wake periods during sleep, and these will be of great benefit both to researchers and clinicians.

In conclusion, both sleep diaries and actigraphy have limitations and strengths. When used in conjunction these two methods enhance each other and can provide important insights into sleep/wake patterns in infants, children, and adolescents.

Future Directions

- Development of standardized rules for recording, scoring, and reporting actigraphy in infants children and adolescents.
- Development and refinement of current algorithms needs to continue, particularly to allow more specific assessment of wake periods that occur during sleep.
- More sensitive detection of when devices have been removed will also allow more accurate assessment of sleep/wake patterns.
- The further development of algorithms to distinguish active sleep (REM sleep) from quiet sleep (NREM sleep) would be beneficial, particularly in the study of the development of infant sleep/wake patterns.
- As models of actigraphs become cheaper they will become more widely used in clinical research.
- The use of electronic sleep diaries has some benefits over the use of traditional paper diaries; however, more research is needed into these new devices.

References

American Sleep Disorders Association. (1995). Practice parameters for the use of actigraphy in the clinical assessment of sleep disorders. *Sleep, 18*(4), 283–287.

Acebo, C., Sadeh, A., Seifer, R., Tzischinsky, O., Wolfson, A. R., Hafer, A., et al. (1999). Estimating sleep patterns with activity monitoring in children and adolescents: How many nights are necessary for reliable measures? *Sleep, 22*(1), 95–103.

Acebo, C., Sadeh, A., Seifer, R., Tzischinsky, O., Hafer, A., & Carskadon, M. A. (2005). Sleep/wake patterns derived from activity monitoring and maternal report for healthy 1- to 5-year-old children. *Sleep, 28*(12), 1568–1577.

Armitage, R., Flynn, H., Hoffmann, R., Vazquez, D., Lopez, J., & Marcus, S. (2009). Early developmental changes in sleep in infants: The impact of maternal depression. *Sleep, 32*(5), 693–696.

Asaka, Y., & Takada, S. (2011). Comparing sleep measures of infants derived from parental reports in sleep diaries and acceleration sensors. *Acta Paediatrica, 100*(8), 1158–1163.

Bland, J. M., & Altman, D. G. (1995). Comparing methods of measurement: Why plotting difference against standard method is misleading. *Lancet, 346*, 1085–1087.

Blunden, S., Lushington, K., Lorenzen, B., Ooi, T., Fung, F., & Kennedy, D. (2004). Are sleep problems under-recognised in general practice? *Archives of Disease in Childhood, 89*(8), 708–712.

Canet, T. (2010). Sleep-wake habits in Spanish primary school children. *Sleep Medicine, 11*(9), 917–921.

Coons, S., & Guilleminault, C. (1984). Development of consolidated sleep and wakeful periods in relation to the day/night cycle in infancy. *Developmental Medicine and Child Neurology, 26*(2), 169–176.

Corkum, P., Tannock, R., Moldofsky, H., Hogg-Johnson, S., & Humphries, T. (2001). Actigraphy and parental ratings of sleep in children with attention-deficit/hyperactivity disorder (ADHD). *Sleep, 24*(3), 303–312.

Gibson, E. S., Powles, A. C., Thabane, L., O'Brien, S., Molnar, D. S., Trajanovic, N., et al. (2006). "Sleepiness" is serious in adolescence: two surveys of 3235 Canadian students. *BMC Public Health, 6*, 116.

Gnidovec, B., Neubauer, D., & Zidar, J. (2002). Actigraphic assessment of sleep-wake rhythm during the first 6 months of life. *Clinical Neurophysiology, 113*(11), 1815–1821.

Goodlin-Jones, B. L., Waters, S., & Anders, T. F. (2009). Objective sleep measurement in typically and atypically developing preschool children with ADHD-like profiles. *Child Psychiatry & Human Development, 40*(2), 257–268.

Hayes, M. J., & Mitchell, D. (1998). Spontaneous movements during sleep in children: Temporal organization and changes with age. *Developmental Psychobiology, 32*(1), 13–21.

Hyde, M., O'Driscoll, D. M., Binette, S., Galang, C., Tan, S. K., Verginis, N., et al. (2007). Validation of actigraphy for determining sleep and wake in children with sleep disordered breathing. *Journal of Sleep Research, 16*, 213–216.

Iber, C., Redline, S., Kaplan Gilpin, A. M., Quan, S. F., Zhang, L., Gottlieb, D. J., et al. (2004). Polysomnography performed in the unattended home versus the attended laboratory setting—Sleep Heart Health Study methodology. *Sleep, 27*(3), 536–540.

Insana, S. P., Gozal, D., & Montgomery-Downs, H. E. (2010). Invalidity of one actigraphy brand for identifying sleep and wake among infants. *Sleep Medicine, 11*(2), 191–196.

Jean-Louis, G., von Gizycki, H., Zizi, F., Fookson, J., Spielman, A., Nunes, J., et al. (1996). Determination of sleep and wakefulness with the actigraph data analysis software (ADAS). *Sleep, 19*(9), 739–743.

Jean-Louis, G., Kripke, D. F., Cole, R. J., Assmus, J. D., & Langer, R. D. (2001). Sleep detection with an accelerometer actigraph: Comparisons with polysomnography. *Physiology & Behavior, 72*(1–2), 21–28.

Jenni, O. G., Deboer, T., & Achermann, P. (2006). Development of the 24-h rest-activity pattern in human infants. *Infant Behavior and Development, 29*(2), 143–152.

Johnson, N. L., Kirchner, H. L., Rosen, C. L., Storfer-Isser, A., Cartar, L. N., Ancoli-Israel, S., et al. (2007). Sleep estimation using wrist actigraphy in adolescents with and without sleep disordered breathing: A comparison of three data modes. *Sleep, 30*(7), 899–905.

Kieckhefer, G. M., Ward, T. M., Tsai, S. Y., & Lentz, M. J. (2008). Nighttime sleep and daytime nap patterns in school age children with and without asthma. *Journal of Developmental & Behavioral Pediatrics, 29*(5), 338–344.

Kupfer, D. J., Detre, T. P., Foster, G., Tucker, G. J., & Delgado, J. (1972). The application of Delgado's telemetric mobility recorder for human studies. *Behavioral Biology, 7*(4), 585–590.

Littner, M., Kushida, C. A., Anderson, W. M., Bailey, D., Berry, R. B., Davila, D. G., et al. (2003). Practice parameters for the role of actigraphy in the study of sleep and circadian rhythms: An update for 2002. *Sleep 26*(3), 337–341.

Martin-Martinez, D., Casaseca-de-la-Higuera, P., Vegas-Sanchez-Ferrero, G., Cordero-Grande, L., Andres-de-Llano, J. M., Garmendia-Leiza, J. R., et al. (2010). Characterization of activity epochs in actimetric registries for infantile colic diagnosis: Identification and feature extraction based on wavelets and symbolic dynamics. *Conference Proceedings of the IEEE Engineering in Medicine & Biology Society, 2010*, 2383–2386.

Meltzer, L. J., & Westin, A. M. (2011). A comparison of actigraphy scoring rules used in pediatric research. *Sleep Medicine, 12*(8), 793–796.

Meltzer, L. J., Montgomery-Downs, H. E., Insana, S. P., & Walsh, C. M. (2012). Use of actigraphy for assessment in pediatric sleep research. *Sleep Medicine Reviews, 16*(5), 463–475.

Meltzer, L. J., Walsh, C. M., Traylor, J., & Westin, A. M. (2012). Direct comparison of two new actigraphs and polysomnography in children and adolescents. *Sleep, 35*(1), 159–166.

Mindell, J. A., & Durand, V. M. (1993). Treatment of childhood sleep disorders: Generalization across disorders and effects on family members. *Journal of Pediatric Psychology, 18*(6), 731–750.

Morgenthaler, T., Alessi, C., Friedman, L., Owens, J., Kapur, V., Boehlecke, B., et al. (2007). Practice parameters for the use of actigraphy in the assessment of sleep and sleep disorders: An update for 2007. *Sleep, 30*(4), 519–529.

Muller, S., Hemmi, M. H., Wilhelm, F. H., Barr, R. G., & Schneider, S. (2011). Parental report of infant sleep behavior by electronic versus paper-and-pencil diaries, and their relationship to actigraphic sleep measurement. *Journal of Sleep Research, 20*(4), 598–605.

O'Driscoll, D. M., Foster, A. M., Davey, M. J., Nixon, G. M., & Horne, R. S. (2010). Can actigraphy measure sleep fragmentation in children? *Archives of Disease in Childhood, 95*(12), 1031–1033.

Owens, J., Sangal, R. B., Sutton, V. K., Bakken, R., Allen, A. J., & Kelsey, D. (2009). Subjective and objective measures of sleep in children with attention-deficit/hyperactivity disorder. *Sleep Medicine, 10*(4), 446–456.

Sadeh, A., Lavie, P., Scher, A., Tirosh, E., & Epstein, R. (1991). Actigraphic home-monitoring sleep-disturbed and control infants and young children: A new method for pediatric assessment of sleep-wake patterns. *Pediatrics, 87*(4), 494–499.

Sadeh, A. (1994). Assessment of intervention for infant night waking: Parental reports and activity-based home monitoring. *Journal of Consulting and Clinical Psychology, 62*(1), 63–68.

Sadeh, A., Sharkey, K. M., & Carskadon, M. A. (1994). Activity-based sleep-wake identification: An empirical test of methodological issues. *Sleep, 17*(3), 201–207.

Sadeh, A., Acebo, C., Seifer, R., Aytur, S., & Carskadon, M. A. (1995). Activity-based assessment of sleep-wake patterns during the 1st year of life. *Infant Behaviour and Development, 18*, 329–337.

Sadeh, A., Hauri, P. J., Kripke, D. F., & Lavie, P. (1995). The role of actigraphy in the evaluation of sleep disorders. *Sleep, 18*(4), 288–302.

Sadeh, A. (1996). Evaluating night wakings in sleep-disturbed infants: A methodological study of parental reports and actigraphy. *Sleep, 19*(10), 757–762.

Sadeh, A. (2011). The role and validity of actigraphy in sleep medicine: An update. *Sleep Medicine Reviews, 15*(4), 259–267.

Sazonov, E., Sazonova, N., Schuckers, S., & Neuman, M. (2004). Activity-based sleep-wake identification in infants. *Physiological Measurement, 25*(5), 1291–1304.

Seo, W. S., Sung, H. M., Lee, J. H., Koo, B. H., Kim, M. J., Kim, S. Y., et al. (2010). Sleep patterns and their age-related changes in elementary-school children. *Sleep Medicine, 11*(6), 569–575.

Short, M. A., Gradisar, M., Lack, L. C., Wright, H., & Carskadon, M. A. (2012). The discrepancy between actigraphic and sleep diary measures of sleep in adolescents. *Sleep Medicine, 13*(4), 378–384.

Sitnick, S. L., Goodlin-Jones, B. L., & Anders, T. F. (2008). The use of actigraphy to study sleep disorders in preschoolers: Some concerns about detection of nighttime awakenings. *Sleep, 31*(3), 395–401.

So, K., Buckley, P., Adamson, T. M., & Horne, R. S. (2005). Actigraphy correctly predicts sleep behavior in infants who are younger than six months, when compared with polysomnography. *Pediatric Research, 58*(4), 761–765.

So, K., Adamson, T. M., & Horne, R. S. C. (2007). The use of actigraphy for assessment of the development of sleep/wake patterns in infants during the first 12 months of life. *Journal of Sleep Research, 16*, 181–187.

Spruyt, K., Aitken, R. J., So, K., Charlton, M., Adamson, T. M., & Horne, R. S. (2008). Relationship between sleep/wake patterns, temperament and overall development in term infants over the first year of life. *Early Human Development, 84*(5), 289–296.

Sung, M., Adamson, T. M., & Horne, R. S. (2009). Validation of actigraphy for determining sleep and wake in preterm infants. *Acta Paediatrica, 98*(1), 52–57.

Thoman, E. B. (1990). Sleeping and waking states in infants: A functional perspective. *Neuroscience & Biobehavioral Reviews, 14*(1), 93–107.

Thoman, E. B., & Acebo, C. (1995). *Monitoring of Sleep in Neonates and Young Children*. Philadelphia: W. B. Saunders.

Tikotzky, L., & Sadeh, A. (2001). Sleep patterns and sleep disruptions in kindergarten children. *Journal of Clinical Child Psychology, 30*(4), 581–591.

Tilmanne, J., Urbain, J., Kothare, M. V., Wouwer, A. V., & Kothare, S. V. (2009). Algorithms for sleep-wake identification using actigraphy: a comparative study and new results. *Journal of Sleep Research, 18*(1), 85–98.

Tryon, W. W. (2004). Issues of validity in actigraphic sleep assessment. *Sleep, 27*(1), 158–165.

Tsai, S. Y., Burr, R. L., & Thomas, K. A. (2009). Effect of external motion on correspondence between infant actigraphy and maternal diary. *Infant Behavioral Development, 32*(3), 340–343.

Tsai, S. Y., & Thomas, K. A. (2010). Actigraphy as a measure of activity and sleep for infants: a methodological study. *Archives of Pediatrics & Adolescent Medicine, 164*(11), 1071–1072.

Werner, H., Molinari, L., Guyer, C., & Jenni, O. G. (2008). Agreement rates between actigraphy, diary, and questionnaire for children's sleep patterns. *Archives of Pediatrics & Adolescent Medicine, 162*(4), 350–358.

Whitney, M. P., & Thoman, E. B. (1993). Early sleep patterns of premature infants are differentially related to later developmental disabilities. *Developmental and Behavioral Pediatrics, 14*(2), 71–80.

Wiggs, L., & Stores, G. (2004). Sleep patterns and sleep disorders in children with autistic spectrum disorders: Insights using parent report and actigraphy. *Developmental Medicine & Child Neurology, 46*(6), 372–380.

Wiggs, L., Montgomery, P., & Stores, G. (2005). Actigraphic and parent reports of sleep patterns and sleep disorders in children with subtypes of attention-deficit hyperactivity disorder. *Sleep, 28*(11), 1437–1445.

Wolfson, A. R., Carskadon, M. A., Acebo, C., Seifer, R., Fallone, G., Labyak, S. E., et al. (2003). Evidence for the validity of a sleep habits survey for adolescents. *Sleep, 26*(2), 213–216.

CHAPTER

17

Assessment of Circadian Rhythms

Stephanie J. Crowley

Abstract

This chapter will focus on methods used to measure the endogenous circadian timing system in a pediatric population. To provide a basic understanding of the system that is being measured, the chapter begins by reviewing basic circadian terms and physiology. Then, behavioral measures, which are often associated with daily rhythms and can be used as global estimates of the circadian system, are reviewed. The focus will subsequently shift to physiological measures of the circadian system, with a specific focus on the endogenous rhythm of melatonin because currently it is the most commonly used physiological measure in human circadian research. The chapter will conclude with a brief description of how these physiological measures are used to make inferences about the central circadian clock. These circadian measures may complement and inform research studies relevant to health and behavior during development.

Key Words: melatonin, dim light melatonin onset (DLMO), core body temperature, chronotype, morningness/eveningness

The circadian timing system is one of two processes that regulate the timing of sleep and wake (Borbély, 1982). Ideally, the homeostatic sleep system and the circadian timing system interact in such a way to promote wake during the "biological day" and promote sleep during the "biological night" (Dijk & Czeisler, 1995; Edgar, Dement, & Fuller, 1993). This interaction likely changes across development (Carskadon & Acebo, 2002; Jenni & LeBourgeois, 2006), and when the systems are misaligned, problems with mood, cognition, and physical health may develop. This chapter focuses on measurement of the circadian timing system in a pediatric population. Utilizing these circadian measures can complement research studies relevant to health and behavior during development, and can inform our understanding of circadian-based sleep disorders that commonly emerge during development, such as Delayed Sleep Phase Disorder (see Chapter 23).

To begin, the human circadian timing system is reviewed to provide a basic understanding of the system that is being measured. Then, behavioral measures that are often associated with the daily rhythmicity of the circadian system are reviewed. The focus subsequently shifts to physiological measures of the circadian system, with a specific emphasis on the endogenous rhythm of melatonin because it is the most commonly used physiological measure in current human circadian research. The chapter will conclude with a brief description of how these physiological measures are used to make inferences about the central circadian clock.

The Circadian Timing System

The circadian timing system is an endogenous, genetically regulated, self-sustaining system that provides organization to daily variation in physiology and a number of adaptive behaviors, including the drives to be asleep and be awake (Moore, 1992; see Auger and Crowley, Chapter 23). The "master clock" that organizes these rhythms in mammals has been localized to a small paired nucleus in the hypothalamus, the suprachiasmatic nucleus (SCN; Moore, 1997). In mammals, the SCN begins to develop in utero or shortly after birth (Davis & Reppert, 2001).

Circadian literally translates to "about" (*circa*) "one day" (*diem*); thus rhythms regulated by the circadian system oscillate with an endogenous period (*tau*) close to, but slightly different from, 24 hours. For the majority of humans, tau is longer than 24 hours (Duffy & Wright, 2005). Tau of healthy human adults ranges from 23.5 to 24.9 hours (Burgess & Eastman, 2008; Czeisler et al., 1999; Duffy et al., 2011; Smith, Burgess, Fogg, & Eastman, 2009; Wright, Hughes, Kronauer, Dijk, & Czeisler, 2001; Wyatt, Ritz-DeCecco, Czeisler, & Dijk, 1999). Carskadon and colleagues reported a range of 24.08 to 24.60 hours in 10 young adolescents aged 10.9 to 15.2 years (Carskadon, Labyak, Acebo, & Seifer, 1999). A similar range in tau (23.86 to 24.59 h) is emerging in a preliminary study of older adolescents (aged 14.2–17.9 years, n = 11) from our laboratory (Crowley, unpublished data). When external cues or "zeitgebers" are present, the circadian system is able to synchronize—or "entrain"—to a 24-hour day. The primary entraining stimulus to the circadian system is light and dark (Aschoff, Hoffmann, Pohl, & Wever, 1975; Czeisler, Richardson, Zimmerman, Moore-Ede, & Weitzman, 1981). Light/dark (LD) cues come from the daily cycles of daylight and darkness, but can also be artificially imposed in modern environments by switching an electric light on and off or by drawing a window shade.

According to one theory, entrainment is a daily adjustment of the circadian clock to make tau equal to 24 hours. This process is predicted by a phase response curve (PRC) to light. A light PRC describes how light shifts circadian rhythms earlier or later in time. In general, light exposure during the beginning of the habitual sleep time shifts circadian rhythms later (phase delay), while light exposure at the end of habitual sleep shifts circadian rhythms earlier (phase advance) (Eastman, Molina, Burgess, & Revell, 2010; Khalsa, Jewett, Cajochen, & Czeisler, 2003; Kripke, Elliott, Youngstedt, & Rex, 2007; Minors, Waterhouse, & Wirz-Justice, 1991; Revell & Eastman, 2005; St. Hilaire et al., 2012). A preliminary PRC to light for older adolescents aged 14–17 years shows a similar pattern (Crowley & Eastman, 2012); however, more data are needed to fully characterize the adolescent PRC to light to understand whether the adult and adolescent PRCs are similar. No PRCs to light are available for younger children. Morning exposure to a light source facilitates entrainment in humans with tau greater than 24 hours, whereas evening light exposure entrains individuals with tau shorter than 24 hours. The majority of humans entrain by a small phase advance, while a small proportion entrains by a small phase delay (Duffy & Wright, 2005). When zeitgebers—like the light/dark cycle—are removed, then the clock continues to keep time, though at its own pace according to its endogenous circadian period (tau), and is said to "free-run."

As shown in Figure 17.1, light/dark signals are interpreted by retinal photoreceptors in the eye. A small subset of intrinsically photosensitive retinal ganglion cells (ipRGCs) contain melanopsin and project to the SCN (Berson, Dunn, & Takao, 2002; Gooley, Lu, Chou, Scammell, & Saper, 2001; Hannibal, Hindersson, Knudsen, Georg, & Fahrenkrug, 2002; Provencio et al., 2000). These ipRGCs are necessary for circadian entrainment by light (Güler et al., 2008), but are modulated by synaptic input from rods and cones (Wong, Dunn, Graham, & Berson, 2007). The transduced light/dark signals from the retina reach the SCN primarily through the retinohypothalamic tract (Gooley et al., 2001).

The SCN regulates many systems and is often likened to a conductor of an orchestra; it controls the tempo of many individual parts (the instruments) to make a cohesive, harmonious system (a pleasant-sounding symphony). When studying the circadian timing system in humans, researchers measure physiological or behavioral outputs of these systems regulated by the SCN (see Figure 17.1). When measured over extended periods of time (hours to days), events associated with a rhythm (e.g., when a hormone "turns on" and "turns off") can be marked, and these markers are used experimentally or clinically to infer circadian time, or "phase." This chapter will focus on "central-clock" (SCN)-driven rhythms. For more information about peripheral clocks see the review of Cermakian and Boivin (2009).

Behavioral Measures

Chronotype

Often referred to as morningness/eveningness or M/E, chronotype is a self-assessed (or parent-assessed in the case of younger children) construct that reflects the individual difference of when someone feels "at their peak" or "at their best." Morningess/eveningess questionnaires typically ask what time of day one would choose to engage in different

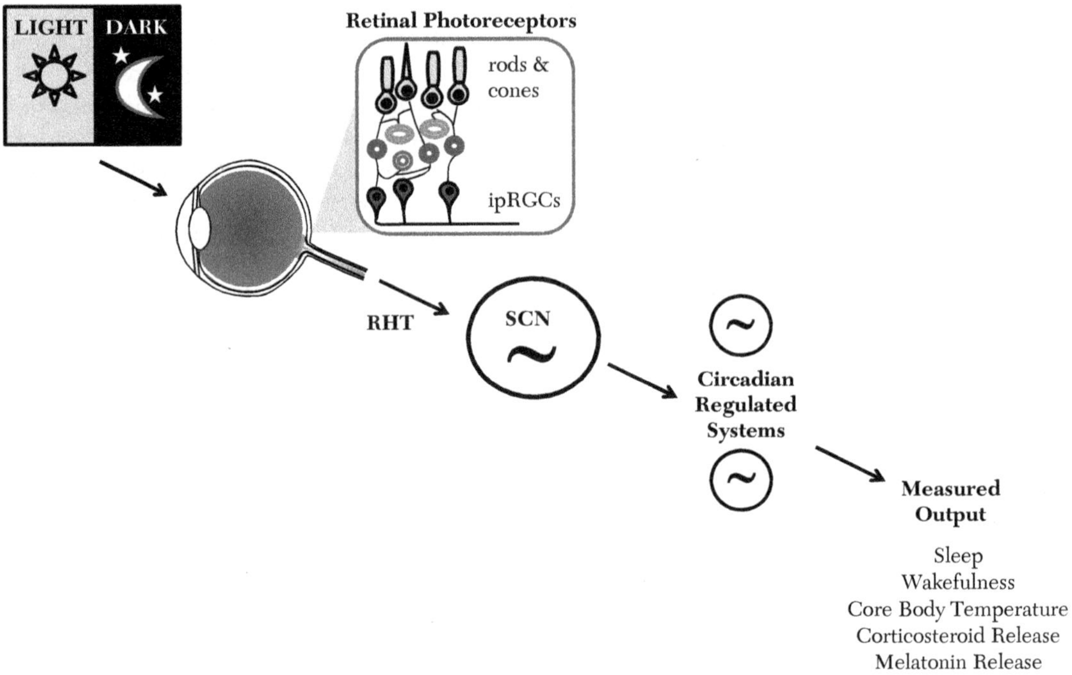

Figure 17.1 A simplified schematic illustration to summarize the main components of the circadian timing system. The primary stimulus (*zeitgeber*) to the system is light and dark exposure to the eye. In humans, intrinsically photosensitive retinal ganglion cells (ipRGCs), with input from rods and cones, transduce light/dark signals, which reach the suprachiasmatic nucleus (SCN) via the retinohypothalamic tract (RHT). The SCN—or "master clock"—regulates many systems, such as those related to sleep and arousal, thermoregulation, feeding and metabolism, and endocrine function. The output of these systems can be measured over the course of hours or days to make inferences about the human circadian system. These outputs can also feedback to modulate the system. Environmental conditions, behavior, and substances during measurement must be controlled to avoid masking of the endogenous circadian signal (see text for details).

activities, such as when they prefer to wake up, go to bed, take a test, exercise, and so forth. Chronotype is conventionally split into three groups: morning ("lark"), evening ("owl"), and intermediate ("neither") types. Morningness/eveningness usually has a normal distribution, with owls and larks sitting at either end of the continuum and most individuals rating themselves as intermediate types. Of note, however, is that morning/evening tendency changes across the life span. Carskadon and colleagues were the first to demonstrate an association between morningness/eveningness and self-assessed pubertal development and age; more mature and older participants endorse more evening tendencies (Carskadon, Vieira, & Acebo, 1993). Others have since confirmed this finding (Giannotti, Cortesi, Sebastiani, & Ottaviano, 2002; Kim, Dueker, Hasher, & Goldstein, 2002; Randler & Bilger, 2009; Roenneberg et al., 2007; Roenneberg et al., 2004). This evening tendency typically reverses in the third decade of life, and aging is associated with a change toward morningness (Carrier, Monk, Buysse, & Kupfer, 1997; Duffy & Czeisler, 2002; Roenneberg et al., 2004). Sex and cultural factors may also contribute to differences in distributions; therefore, adapting questionnaires to fit the appropriate demographic is advised (Adan & Natale, 2002; Caci et al., 2005; Kerkhof, 1985; Smith, Tisak, Bauman, & Green, 1991).

Studies of adults have demonstrated that evening types have a later circadian phase measured from physiological outputs (core body temperature and the onset of melatonin) and later sleep times compared to intermediate and morning types (Baehr, Revelle, & Eastman, 2000; Foret, Touron, Benoit, & Bouard, 1985; Goulet, Mongrain, Desrosiers, Paquet, & Dumont, 2007; Ostberg & Nicholl, 1973; Taillard, Philip, Coste, Sagaspe, & Bioulac, 2003). Similar results emerge in children and adolescents (Crowley, Bushnell, Acebo, & Carskadon, 2006; Laberge et al., 2000; Tzischinsky & Shochat, 2011; Werner, Lebourgeois, Geiger, & Jenni, 2009). Data from adults also suggest that the temporal alignment between the circadian system and sleep behavior differs between morning and evening types; evening types sleep at an *earlier* circadian phase compared to morning types (Baehr et al., 2000; Duffy, Dijk, Hall, & Czeisler, 1999). Conceptualized another way, evening types wake at an earlier part of their circadian cycle compared to the morning types. More recent evidence suggests, however, that when individuals are allowed to sleep on a schedule unconstrained by environmental factors (e.g., school or work), this is only the case for individuals with extremely early or extremely late phases (Goulet et al., 2007; Mongrain, Lavoie, Selmaoui, Paquet, & Dumont, 2004). Variation in several core "clock genes," including *CLOCK, PER1/2/3,* and *CK1ε/δ*, has also been associated with morningness/eveningness (Archer et al., 2003; Carpen, Archer, Skene, Smits, & von Schantz, 2005; Carpen, von Schantz, Smits, Skene, & Archer, 2006; Jones et al., 2007; Katzenberg et al., 1998; Mishima, Tozawa, Satoh, Saitoh, & Mishima, 2005; Pereira et al., 2005). Differences in circadian phase, how the circadian system temporally aligns with sleep/wake behavior, and genetic variation between morning and evening types suggests that this construct of morningness/eveningness likely has a physiological basis and is not only a product of self-selected sleep/wake (and LD) patterns.

Horne and Östberg (1976) developed the first questionnaire in English to assess the construct of morningness/eveningness. This 19-item, mixed-format questionnaire is the most widely used, and it has been translated into several languages including French (Goulet et al., 2007; Taillard, Philip, Chastang, & Bioulac, 2004), Dutch (Kerkhof, 1985), Italian (Mecacci & Zani, 1983), Spanish (Adan & Almirall, 1990), Japanese (Ishihara, Saitoh, Inoue, & Miyata, 1984), and Chinese (Li et al., 2011). The morningness/eveningness questionnaire (MEQ) was originally tested in a group of British young adults (18–32 years), and 5 categories were created based on cutoff scores: Definite Morning Type (70–86), Moderate Morning Type (59–69), Neither Type (42–58), Moderate Evening Type (31–41), and Definite Evening Type (16–30). The rationale for these cutoff scores was not described. It has been argued that since this questionnaire was developed based on mostly college-age, nonworking students, these cutoffs need to be adjusted for age and to account for working status, as these change the natural preference of an individual (Paine, Gander, & Travier, 2006; Taillard et al., 2004). The MEQ has also been criticized for its length; thus, Adan and Almirall (1991) developed a version with only 5 items (rMEQ). Both questionnaires may be difficult for younger children to comprehend, though they have been used with adolescents (~15–16 years) (Laberge et al., 2000; Urban, Magyarodi, & Rigo, 2011). Internal consistency from adult samples is good for the MEQ (Cronbach alpha > .80) (Adan & Natale, 2002; Paine et al., 2006; Smith, Reilly, & Midkiff, 1989).

Based on a comprehensive assessment of the psychometric properties of three different morningness/eveningness scales (Folkard, Monk, & Lobban, 1979; Horne & Östberg, 1976; Torsvall & Akerstedt, 1980), Smith and colleagues (1989) developed a Composite Morningness Scale (CMS) by taking the best items from the MEQ of Horne and Östberg (1976) and the scale of Torsvall & Akerstedt (1980). This 13-item scale was tested on college-age students, but has been used with children and adolescents (Crowley, Bushnell, et al., 2006; Randler, 2008; Randler & Bilger, 2009). In contrast to the MEQ's 5 categories, the Composite Scale of Morningness categorizes individuals into 3 different groups based on a 10–90 percentile split: Evening Type (22 and less), Intermediate Type (23–43), and Morning Type (44 and above). This scale has been translated to other languages, including German (Randler & Bilger, 2009), French (Caci, Nadalet, Staccini, Myquel, & Boyer, 1999, 2000), Italian (Natale & Alzani, 2001), Spanish (Adan, Caci, & Prat, 2005), and Thai (Pornpitakpan, 1998); however, cross-cultural differences need to be considered (Caci et al., 2005; Smith et al., 1991).

Carskadon and colleagues (1993) developed a new scale specifically for children largely based on the above-mentioned Composite Morningness Scale of Smith and colleagues (1989). This 10-item scale questions the youngster about preferred bedtime, wake-up time, and the optimal time to take a test, but phrases questions using language easily understood by the child and also puts questions in the context of typical events or behaviors of younger children like school and gym class. In a group of fourth- and fifth-grade American students (aged ~10–13 years), this scale shows a good internal consistency (Cronbach's alpha = .76) and moderate construct validity when compared to sleep times (Crowley, Bushnell, et al., 2006). Similarly, in a group of Italian high school students aged 14.1 to 18.6 years, internal consistency is also good (Cronbach's alpha = .73) and morningess/eveningness scores are predictive of differences in sleep patterns (Giannotti et al., 2002). This scale has also been translated to other languages, such as Spanish (Escribano, Diaz-Morales, Delgado, & Collado,

2012), Hebrew (Tzischinsky & Shochat, 2011) and Italian (Giannotti et al., 2002).

The questions in the scales described thus far are subjective, asking individuals to choose preferred sleep times based on their own "feeling best rhythm," and are also contextualized within hypothetical situations or circumstances (e.g., "...at what time would you get up if you were entirely free to plan your day?"). Roenneberg and colleagues (2003) argue that inquiring about actual behavior—not what you "would" do, but rather what you actually do—may be a better way to assess the construct of chronotype. Therefore, they developed the Munich ChonoType Questionnaire (MCTQ), which asks individuals to record clock times of their sleep behavior (e.g., go to bed time, try to fall asleep time, wake up time, get out of bed time, etc.), as well as record the number of minutes it takes to fall asleep. Individuals record this information separately for work/school days and nonwork/nonschool days ("free days"), since sleep timing usually differs between these day types in most individuals across the life span (Crowley, Acebo, & Carskadon, 2007; Roenneberg et al., 2007; Werner et al., 2009). Mid-sleep time on free days is used to quantify chronotype because it is argued that sleep is less constrained by work or school schedules and would therefore more accurately reflect the individual's true chronotype. Mid-sleep time on free days is the midpoint between sleep onset time (try to fall asleep time + number of minutes to fall asleep) and wake time. Also, because sleep duration is often restricted during the school/work week, many sleep longer on weekends or on vacation to "recover" from the accumulated sleep debt. Roenneberg and colleagues (2007) argue that this potential confounding factor of sleep debt needs to be accounted for in their chronotype metric, and they correct the mid-sleep time on free days by subtracting the individual's "sleep need" (weighted average of sleep duration on school/work days and nonschool/nonwork days) from their estimated mid-sleep time of free days. This metric of chronotype shows a normal distribution (Roenneberg et al., 2007; Roenneberg et al., 2004; Roenneberg, Wirz-Justice, & Merrow, 2003), and large range (~12 hours) (Roenneberg et al., 2007). This research group continues to update the MCTQ and has amassed an extremely large dataset (~65,000). Using this large dataset, Roenneberg and colleagues observed a gradual delay of chronotype in the second decade of life and then an abrupt advance at around the age of 20 years; this abrupt change is thought to be a "biological marker of the end of adolescence" (Roenneberg et al., 2004).

Finally, Werner and colleagues (2009) recently developed the Children's Chronotype Questionnaire, which is an adaptation of the MCTQ (Roenneberg et al., 2003), and the Morningness/Eveningness Scale for Children (Carskadon et al., 1993). This parent-report, 27-item scale was originally tested in a group of 4- to 11-year-old Swiss children and shows high test–retest reliability and validity against parent-reported sleep times (Werner et al., 2009). In a more recent analysis of children aged 30–36 months (n = 19), parents who rated their children as evening types had later melatonin rhythms and slept at an earlier circadian phase (Simpkin, Akacem, Garlo, Jenni, & Lebourgeois, 2012), which mimics findings in adults. Thus, this individual difference of chronotype is apparent in early childhood and can serve as a good global estimate of circadian timing in young children.

Sleep/Wake Patterns

Sleep/wake patterns assessed by field measures, such as actigraphy and daily sleep/wake diaries (see Horne and Biggs, Chapter 16) may provide a way to estimate circadian timing in entrained individuals when phase cannot be measured more directly. The timing of sleep and wake is partly controlled by the circadian timing system; however, the sleep/wake pattern in a human is not a circadian measure per se, because the behavior is voluntary or parent-imposed (i.e., can override the endogenous system). Nevertheless, an individual's sleep/wake schedule is the primary behavioral modulator of the 24-hour light/dark pattern, which in turn signals the central clock. Thus, timing of sleep and wake is usually coupled with the timing of the circadian system.

Three previous studies of adults (aged 18 to 43 years) demonstrated that the average timing of the sleep/wake schedule is correlated with physiological measures of circadian phase and can predict measured phase within 1 to 2 hours (Burgess & Eastman, 2005; Burgess et al., 2003; Martin & Eastman, 2002). A similar analysis of youngsters aged 9 to 17 years, either during the school year or while on summer vacation, showed similar results (Crowley, Acebo, Fallone, & Carskadon, 2006). Average mid-sleep time (over the proximal 5 days), in particular, predicted the onset of the melatonin rhythm during both the school year and during summer vacation. Linear regression equations using mid-sleep time estimated melatonin onset phase within ± 1 hour of actual phase for 82% and 86%

of participants during the school year and during summer, respectively.

Using sleep/wake behavior to provide a gross estimate of endogenous circadian phase can be quite practical. Estimated phase from sleep/wake schedules can guide timing of the data collection window to sample physiological measures of the circadian timing system, such as salivary melatonin (see below). An estimate of circadian phase could also provide context when interpreting neurobehavioral data or other outcome measures that vary over the course of 24 hours. Collecting physiological measures of phase in the clinic is often hindered by the expense and labor-intensive nature of collecting such measures. Using habitual sleep times as a gross estimate of phase could help guide treatment strategies (e.g., bright light or exogenous melatonin) for circadian-based sleep disorders.

Physiological Measures

Core Body Temperature

Core body temperature (CBT) is a circadian output that can be measured in humans and is the classic measure of circadian phase and amplitude that was used in older studies of human circadian timing (Czeisler et al., 1985; Kleitman, 1939; Mills, Minors, & Waterhouse, 1978a, 1978b). The CBT minimum, a common phase marker, usually occurs during the second half of the habitual sleep period. Measurement of CBT requires participants to wear a rectal thermistor over at least 24 hours. The thermistor is placed 10 cm into the rectum and is only removed for bowel movements and showers. Some participants find the procedure invasive; however, most participants become unaware of the thermistor once in place and even adolescents have completed the procedure successfully (Carskadon et al., 1999; Labyak, Acebo, & Carskadon, 1998). The thermistor can move from the desired position, which can result in data loss; taping the thermistor to the lower back may reduce this risk. An alternative to the rectal thermistor is an ingestible capsule that travels through the gastrointestinal tract and transmits core temperature to a monitor close to the body via a radio frequency transmission. Studies in the field and in the laboratory that have measured CBT using the rectal thermistor and the ingestible pill simultaneously show similar results between the two methods; however, the pill reads slightly higher temperature than the rectal thermistor (Darwent, Zhou, van den Heuvel, Sargent, & Roach, 2011; Edwards, Waterhouse, Reilly, & Atkinson, 2002). Some drawbacks to the ingestible pill are that the rate at which the pill moves through the body varies widely among individuals and temperature varies depending on what part of the gastrointestinal tract the pill is traveling through (Darwent et al., 2011).

The CBT rhythm can be hidden or "masked" by behavior. CBT changes with body posture (Minors & Waterhouse, 1989), is elevated by physical activity, and is lower during the sleeping state compared to the waking state (Minors, Waterhouse, & Akerstedt, 1994; Waterhouse et al., 2000). Therefore, participants must stay awake in a constant posture throughout the night to accurately measure the endogenous CBT rhythm (Czeisler et al., 1985; Duffy, 1995; Duffy & Dijk, 2002; Mills et al., 1978a). Alternatively, a complex mathematical estimate (Eastman, 1992; Eastman, Liu, & Fogg, 1995) or other "purification" methods (Waterhouse et al., 2000) can be used to account for masking effects on CBT while participants are in their natural environment. Some caution with these correction factors must taken, however, since the amount of change in the rhythm in response to these masking factors differs among individuals and by the time of day (Duffy & Dijk, 2002). Masking effects and the somewhat invasive procedures that CBT measurement requires have prompted many laboratories to switch to using the secretory pattern of melatonin to determine circadian phase. Circadian markers using the melatonin rhythm are also more reliable than CBT markers (Klerman, Gershengorn, Duffy, & Kronauer, 2002; Klerman et al., 2012).

Endogenous Melatonin

Melatonin is a neurohormone that is secreted by the pineal gland and has a distinct circadian pattern: circulating melatonin concentration is low during the day, abruptly increases close to habitual bedtime, remains high throughout the night, and decreases close to habitual wake-up time. This rhythmic pattern of melatonin release is driven by activity of the enzyme arylalkylamine N-acetyltransferase (AANAT), which is a critical enzyme in melatonin synthesis from serotonin. The activity of AANAT in the pinealocyte, and thus the release of melatonin, is regulated by the SCN (see Ganguly, Coon, & Klein, 2002 for a review). Melatonin is released immediately into the bloodstream; thus, what is measured in circulation is temporally very close to the production of the hormone. Melatonin can be sampled from blood or saliva, and the melatonin metabolite 6-sulfatoxymelatonin can be sampled from urine.

SAMPLING

Plasma melatonin samples are collected from blood drawn through an indwelling catheter inserted into a forearm vein. It is suggested to insert the catheter at least 2 hours before sampling begins to ensure that any increase in adrenergic levels in response to catheter insertion does not affect melatonin levels (Benloucif et al., 2008). Blood is sampled at frequent intervals (every 20 to 30 minutes), and often sampling occurs over 24 hours. Samples can be taken without disturbing a sleeping individual by attaching a long tube that runs from the bedroom to an outside control room. The precise time of each sample must be recorded. Serial plasma melatonin samples have been collected in young people (Attanasio, Borrelli, & Gupta, 1985; Cavallo, 1992; Ehrenkranz et al., 1982; Salti et al., 2000); however, this procedure can be frightening or painful. Moreover, a trained phlebotomist or someone with medical training (e.g., a nurse) is needed to start and maintain the indwelling intravenous catheter. This procedure is best carried out in an inpatient facility, making this method impractical for field studies.

Salivary melatonin is typically collected using a swab (absorbent) method. Saliva collection systems, like the one shown in Figure 17.2 (Salivette®, Sarstedt AG & Co.), typically consist of a large plastic collection tube (A) in which another smaller tube is nested (B). This nested tube holds the absorbent untreated cotton roll (C). The untreated cotton is placed into the mouth by the individual and saliva is absorbed into the cotton. In the case of an infant or very small child, an adult inserts the cotton into the child's mouth while holding onto an attached string or a stick so that the child does not choke. In most cases, saliva saturates the cotton in fewer than 5 minutes. The sample needs to be centrifuged and then frozen for later analysis. The nested tube (B) has a small hole on the bottom, which allows saliva to collect at the bottom of the large tube when it is centrifuged. A typical assay requires about 0.5 mL per sample and a minimum of 1 mL is needed to assay samples in duplicate. Our laboratory aims to collect 2 mL of saliva in every sample. The nested tube and cotton can be discarded after enough saliva is pulled to the bottom of the collection tube. Serial saliva samples are typically taken at 30- to 60- minute intervals. Food and drink (including water) should not be consumed in the 5 to 10 minutes before saliva collection. If food is consumed in the time between samples, then participants need to brush their teeth with water (no toothpaste) so as not to contaminate the sample with food particles. Similarly, if participants drink anything besides water they must rinse with water (no mouthwash). Participants should be advised not to brush their teeth too hard because their gums may bleed, and blood would inflate the amount of detected melatonin in the sample. Our laboratory uses ultra-soft toothbrushes to reduce the risk of this problem. As with plasma melatonin sampling, the precise time of each sample must be recorded. Serial salivary melatonin samples are routinely collected from children and adolescents (Carskadon, Acebo, Richardson, Tate, & Seifer, 1997; Carskadon, Wolfson, Acebo, Tzischinsky, & Seifer, 1998; Crowley, Acebo, & Carskadon, 2012; Crowley, Acebo, et al., 2006; Crowley & Carskadon, 2010), and have been collected from children as young as 30 to 36 months (Garlo, Crossin, Carskadon, & LeBourgeois, 2008; LeBourgeois, Wright, LeBourgeois, & Jenni). Sampling saliva may also be a valid, noninvasive, and practical way to measure melatonin in infants (Bagci et al., 2009, 2010), though the melatonin rhythm does not seem to emerge until about 9–12 weeks in normally developing infants (Kennaway, Stamp, & Goble, 1992). Collecting melatonin from saliva is less invasive than blood sampling, and does not require professional medical training. Sampling melatonin via saliva, however, requires that the individual remain awake, which makes 24-hour sampling difficult. Many groups time saliva sampling to coincide with the onset phase of the melatonin rhythm, though overnight sampling is possible and has been done in adults (Burgess & Eastman, 2004, 2006) and adolescents (Carskadon et al., 1997; Carskadon et al., 1999; Crowley et al., 2012; (see Figure 17.3). To catch the evening onset of melatonin, sampling should begin about 5 to 7 hours before and end about 1 to 2 hours after habitual bedtime. Salivary melatonin is typically collected in the laboratory, though a new procedure to collect these data in the home is currently being validated in adults (Burgess, 2012).

In our laboratory, we collect salivary melatonin samples from adolescent research participants in a dimly lit room (< 5 lux) with a sink for staff to wash their hands. Participants remain seated in comfortable recliners throughout the sampling session (sometimes up to 18 hours), except when they need to use the attached restroom (also < 5 lux). They can watch age-appropriate television shows or movies (approved by their parents) or play board games. The participants are supervised continuously by research staff, who prepare them food and noncaffeinated, nonalcoholic drinks in between

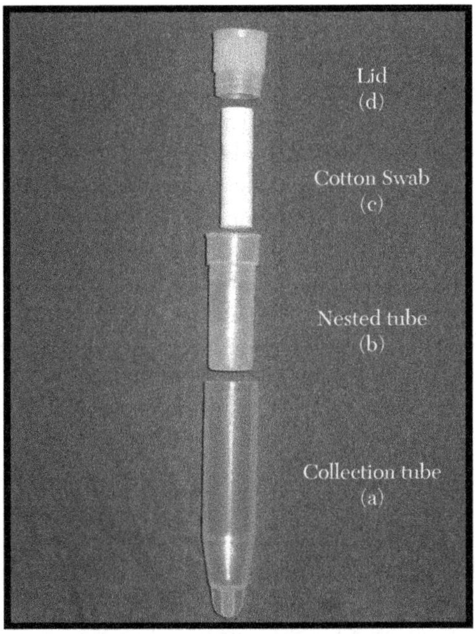

Figure 17.2 A picture of a Salivette® (Sarstedt AG & Co.) used to collect saliva and later assay for hormones, such as melatonin (see text).

samples. Frequent light readings with a light meter at the level of the eye ensure that light levels remain dim (see *Factors that Affect Endogenous Melatonin*, below). Many adolescents have successfully completed this salivary melatonin sampling procedure in our laboratory.

The primary metabolite of melatonin, 6-sulfatoxymelatonin (aMT6s), can be measured in urine. All urine voids are collected for at least 48 hours in 4-hour intervals during waking, plus an 8-hour overnight collection interval. Sample times and the total urine volume must be documented. A summary of the typical collection procedure in adults is described by Wright, Drake, and Lockley (2008). Briefly, participants collect all of their urine for 48 hours. After waking on day 1, participants void their bladder but do not collect this first urine. All other voids thereafter are collected in sex-appropriate containers or a toilet hat throughout consecutive 4-hour intervals. As an example, if wake-up time on day 1 (Monday) is at 6:00am, the participant should void her bladder, but not collect it. Then, all of the urine from 6:00am to 10:00am is collected in the same container. At 10:00am, the total volume is measured and the collection interval time (6:00am–10:00am) is recorded. Using a small plastic disposable pipette, a 5mL sample of the urine collected between 6:00am and 10:00am is then transferred to a small (5–10 mL) labeled urine vial. This urine sample should be double-bagged and frozen. The remaining urine from the large container can be discarded, and the container should be rinsed with warm water. The same procedure is repeated for each 4-hour time interval (10:00 am–2:00 pm, 2:00 pm–6:00 pm, and 6:00 pm–10:00 pm). The final collection interval of the first day will be the 8-hour overnight collection, in which any urine excreted throughout the night and the first void the next morning (e.g., Tuesday) is collected in the same container. This procedure is repeated again on the second day and sampling concludes with the last overnight collection on day 3 (e.g., Wednesday morning). This method of urinary aMT6s collection has been used with children as young as about 4 years old (Gebru & LeBourgeois, 2009) and with adolescents (Laberge et al., 2000). Urinary aMT6s can also be extracted from diapers of infants (Kennaway et al., 1992; Tauman, Zisapel, Laudon, Nehama, & Sivan, 2002). Parents are asked to save all diapers over the course of 24 to 48 hours and to record the time of each diaper change. The volume of urine is often measured by weighing the diaper. Measuring the urinary aMT6s is practical for field studies or when working with a special population (e.g., infants) to estimate the global timing and amount of melatonin secretion. This method, however, is less precise than sampling plasma or salivary melatonin because of its infrequent sampling rate, which is limited by the need to urinate. If small changes in circadian timing are expected, then the higher resolution of salivary or plasma melatonin is more informative. Also, the urinary aMT6s rhythm peak typically occurs about 2 hours after the peak in plasma, suggesting that the metabolite is not as temporally close to SCN activity. This lag should be considered when using the melatonin metabolite to infer phase of the circadian system (see review by Wright and colleagues,2008). Finally, this method may not reflect the endogenous melatonin rhythm since masking factors in the field (e.g., ambient light levels) are difficult to control.

FACTORS THAT AFFECT ENDOGENOUS MELATONIN

Melatonin synthesis is suppressed by light (Lewy, Wehr, Goodwin, Newsome, & Markey, 1980), and studies show that room light levels (< 200 lux) suppress endogenous melatonin synthesis (Boivin & James, 2002; Gooley et al., 2011; Santhi et al., 2012; Zeitzer, Dijk, Kronauer, Brown, & Czeisler, 2000); thus, sampling must be completed in dim light conditions. A consensus workgroup (Benloucif et al.,

2008) recommends that light levels should remain lower than 30 lux, though many researchers sample melatonin in light < 5 or 10 lux. Recent data also suggests that light from an LED computer screen can suppress endogenous melatonin (Cajochen et al., 2011), which suggests that devices with back lights that are typically used close to the eye (electronic tablets, laptop computers, and so forth) should be prohibited during sampling.

Posture can also affect melatonin levels. Measured melatonin levels are higher when the individual is seated compared to when lying down (Deacon, Arendt, & English, 1993; Nathan, Jeyaseelan, Burrows, & Norman, 1998) but are highest when standing (Cajochen, Jewett, & Dijk, 2003; Deacon & Arendt, 1994a; Nathan et al., 1998). Changes in melatonin levels as a result of standing can typically be reversed within about 10 minutes (Deacon & Arendt, 1994a). Therefore, individuals should remain seated or reclined for at least 5 to 10 minutes before a sample is taken. One study shows little effect of posture on phase of the melatonin rhythm (Voultsios, Kennaway, & Dawson, 1997); however, if the amplitude of the curve is used to derive melatonin phase markers (see below), then posture needs to be controlled.

Finally, some substances must be controlled when sampling melatonin as they alter the timing and/or the amount of melatonin secretion (see Table 1 of Arendt, 2005). Beta-blockers (Arendt, Bojkowski, Franey, Wright, & Marks, 1985; Cowen, Bevan, Gosden, & Elliott, 1985; Rommel & Demisch, 1994; Stoschitzky et al., 1999), alpha-blockers (Palazidou, Franey, Arendt, Stahl, & Checkley, 1989; Palazidou, Papadopoulos, Sitsen, Stahl, & Checkley, 1989; Stankov et al., 1990), antidepressants (Carvalho, Gorenstein, Moreno, Pariante, & Markus, 2009; Miller, Ekstrom, Mason, Lydiard, & Golden, 2001; Palazidou, Papadopoulos, Ratcliff, Dawling, & Checkley, 1992; Palazidou, Skene, Arendt, Everitt, & Checkley, 1992; Thompson et al., 1985), benzodiazepines (Mann et al., 1996; Monteleone, Forziati, Orazzo, & Maj, 1989), nonsteroidal anti-inflammatory drugs (NSAIDs) (Murphy, Myers, & Badia, 1996), and oral contraceptives (Wright & Badia, 1999) can alter the timing and/or the amount of detected melatonin. Alcohol suppresses melatonin (Ekman, Leppaluoto, Huttunen, Aranko, & Vakkuri, 1993; Rupp, Acebo, & Carskadon, 2007), while caffeine (Wright, Badia, Myers, Plenzler, & Hakel, 1997) and marijuana (Lissoni et al., 1986) increase melatonin; therefore, prohibiting these substances a few days before and on the day of sampling is necessary. Exogenous melatonin pills should also be avoided on the day of sampling, as this will increase detected melatonin levels to supraphysiological levels. Some laboratories prohibit specific foods during saliva collection, such as those with artificial coloring and bananas; however, there is no published literature to support that these items affect salivary melatonin or its analysis. Use of diuretics, and any liver or kidney disorders that may affect metabolism or excretion of melatonin, should be noted when sampling urinary aMT6s (Wright et al., 2008).

MELATONIN ASSAY

Once samples have been collected, a hormone assay is used to determine the melatonin concentrations at each time point. Direct radioimmunoassay (RIA) is the typical assay used for melatonin, though enzyme-linked immunosorbent assay (ELISA) has also been used for this purpose. Immunoassays are based on the interaction between an antibody and its antigen (the hormone), such that when the antigen comes in contact with its antibody, an antigen-antibody complex is formed. The salivary melatonin RIA is a competitive-binding assay. Radioactive melatonin (^{125} I melatonin) and unlabeled melatonin compete for the binding sites on an antibody (anti-melatonin).

The salivary melatonin RIA procedure takes two days to complete. Participant samples and "standard" samples are treated with radioactive melatonin and antibody on day 1. After a 16- to 24-hour incubation period there should be proportional binding (unlabeled vs. labeled) to the antibody. A second antibody separates the bound complex (unlabeled and labeled complex) as a solid white substance ("pellet"). Radioactivity is counted in the pellet using a gamma counter. If the counter detects a lot radioactivity, then unlabeled melatonin (from the saliva sample) is low. Conversely, if the counter detects little radioactivity then unlabeled melatonin (from saliva samples) is high. Standard samples with a known amount of melatonin provide a calibration curve that allows for estimation of the amount of melatonin in the unknown (participant) samples.

If specimens are shipped to another laboratory to be assayed, the samples are packed in insulated boxes with dry ice according to the International Air Transport Association (IATA) packing instruction 650 UN3373. The US Centers for Disease Control and Prevention (CDC) guidelines for transporting biological specimens within the United States (USPS 18 USC 1716) should also be followed.

PLASMA AND SALIVARY MELATONIN PHASE MARKERS

Abrupt changes in the melatonin secretory pattern provide distinct points on the curve that can be marked. The abrupt-onset phase of melatonin secretion is called the *dim light melatonin onset* (DLMO; Lewy, Cutler, & Sack, 1999; Lewy & Sack, 1989). The DLMO is the most reliable phase marker (Benloucif et al., 2005; Klerman et al., 2002; Klerman et al., 2012), and therefore is most often used to estimate circadian timing. The decline of melatonin, also called the *dim light melatonin offset* (DLMOff) phase, and the midpoint between DLMO and DLMOff are also phase markers of the circadian timing system derived from the melatonin rhythm.

The DLMO is defined as the clock time at which endogenous melatonin surpasses and stays above a predetermined threshold for several hours. The DLMOff is the time at which melatonin falls below the threshold again and does not rise above the threshold for several hours. A standard threshold procedure is not established for determining the DLMO or DLMOff. Four common methods include: *(1)* an absolute value threshold in the range of 3 to 10 pg/mL; *(2)* a relative threshold based on a percentage of a maximum value; *(3)* a threshold that is 2 standard deviations above mean daytime levels or the limit of detection of the assay; and *(4)* a 24-hour mean threshold. Another method is to visually estimate the change from baseline levels to a clear rising (or declining) of melatonin concentrations to estimate the DLMO (or DLMOff); consensus of these visual estimates is needed. The best method to estimate DLMO or DLMOff will depend on the research or clinical question under investigation, how melatonin is sampled (e.g., salivary versus plasma), and the time frame of sampling (e.g., overnight versus evening collection).

Figure 17.3 illustrates an example of a salivary melatonin profile collected overnight from a 13-year-old female. Saliva was sampled every 30 minutes while the youngster remained awake in a constant posture in dim light (< 40 lux). This female kept a sleep schedule of 22:00 to 08:00 for about 10 days before these data were collected. Three different thresholds are illustrated with horizontal dashed lines to compute the DLMO and DLMOff. One is an absolute threshold of 4 pg/mL. The absolute threshold most often used for plasma melatonin is 10 pg/mL based on the original work of Lewy and colleagues (Lewy et al., 1999). Because salivary melatonin levels are approximately 30% (Voultsios et al., 1997) to 40% (Deacon & Arendt, 1994b) of

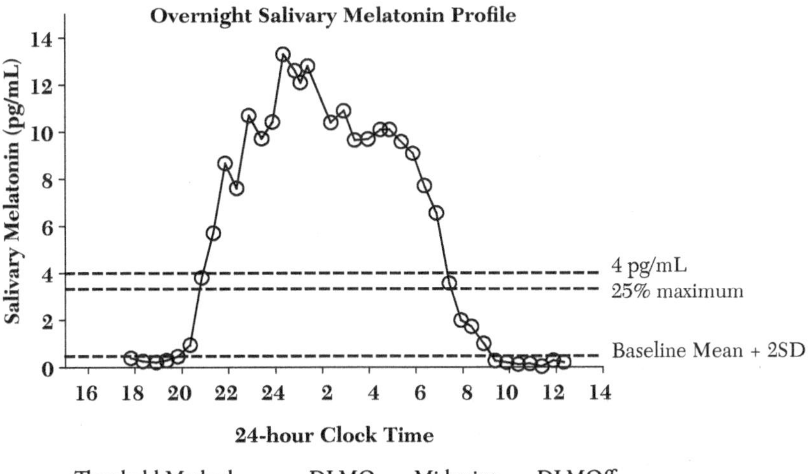

Threshold Method	DLMO	Midpoint	DLMOff
4 pg/mL	20:54	2:07	7:20
25% maximum	20:46	2:07	7:30
Baseline Mean + 2 SD	19:50	2:33	9:15

Figure 17.3 Salivary melatonin data collected over the course of one night (17:50 to 12:20 the next day) from a 13-year-old girl (data from the laboratory of Mary A. Carskadon, PhD, with permission). Melatonin values derived from radioimmunoassay (RIA) at each time point are illustrated by an open circle. The hashed lines illustrate three different thresholds that are commonly used to determine the dim light melatonin onset (DLMO) and dim light melatonin offset (DLMOff) (see text for more detail). The table shows the time of the DLMO, DLMOff, and the midpoint between these two markers for each threshold.

plasma levels, absolute thresholds for salivary melatonin are typically 3 or 4 pg/mL. A second threshold is computed as 25% of the maximum melatonin concentration. This method is considered a relative threshold because the threshold is tailored to the individual to account for large individual differences in melatonin amplitude (Burgess & Fogg, 2008). Some caution, however, must be taken when applying a relative threshold in developmental research, especially in a longitudinal study over a number of years, because melatonin amplitude changes across the life span (Iguchi, Kato, & Ibayashi, 1982; Sack, Lewy, Erb, Vollmer, & Singer, 1986; Waldhauser & Steger, 1986; Waldhauser et al., 1988; Zhao, Xie, Fu, Bogdan, & Touitou, 2002), particularly during puberty (Attanasio et al., 1985; Crowley et al., 2012; Salti et al., 2000; Waldhauser et al., 1984; Wilson & Gordon, 1989). Changes in amplitude would also change this relative threshold across repeated assessments. A relative threshold based on a percentage of the maximum or the 24-hour mean can only be used when overnight or 24 hours of data are available. The third method uses daytime or baseline values to derive a threshold. The example threshold here is based on the work of Voultsios, Kennaway, and Dawson (1997), in which the threshold is computed as the mean plus 2 standard deviations of the first three low daytime samples. This threshold is typically lower than the others shown, which may better estimate the physiological onset or offset of melatonin secretion (the start or end of the biological night) (Molina & Burgess, 2011).

The time at which melatonin rises above a threshold (DLMO) or falls below a threshold (DLMOff) will differ depending on the threshold method used. Figure 17.3 shows the calculated DLMO and DLMOff for each of the three thresholds. The highest threshold in this case (4 pg/mL) marks the DLMO later and the DLMOff earlier than the lower thresholds (25% maximum and Baseline + 2 SD). The melatonin midpoint phase is calculated as the midpoint between the DLMO and DLMOff, and may be less impacted by the threshold method. To compute all three of these phase markers, overnight data collection is necessary.

Although overnight saliva collection is possible in young people, its feasibility is limited by the need to remain awake all night. Plasma melatonin collection allows the participants to sleep; however, this procedure requires medical staff and an inpatient facility. Therefore, many research laboratories and clinicians use evening salivary melatonin collection to measure the onset of melatonin (DLMO) only. Figure 17.4 illustrates a typical evening melatonin profile from a 15-year-old male. This research participant kept a fixed sleep schedule for 7 nights during the school year before saliva collection in the laboratory. Sampling started 5 hours before and ended 1 hour after his fixed bedtime of 22:30. Saliva was sampled every 30 minutes in dim light (< 20 lux), and the participant was seated for at least 5 minutes before each sample was taken. The raw data for this participant are in the table on the bottom of Figure 17.4. The sample clock time for each of the 13 samples is listed in column A. In column B, sample time is converted to decimal hours to make DLMO computations easier (note: if sample time is midnight use 24.00 h, and if later than midnight, add 24 h to the clock time (e.g., 1:00am = 25.00 h)). Salivary melatonin concentration measured using RIA is listed in column C. In this example, the mean plus 2 SD of samples 1, 2, and 3 is 0.69 pg/mL. This threshold value falls between the melatonin values of samples 7 and 8, which are bracketed in column C, and the DLMO will therefore fall between the sample times bracketed in column B. Linear interpolation is used to estimate the time at which melatonin values equal the threshold value. Using the column letters (B and C) and sample numbers (7 and 8) in Figure 17.4, the following formula is used:

$$\text{DLMO} = \text{B7} + \frac{(\text{threshold} - \text{C7})*(\text{B8} - \text{B7})}{(\text{C8} - \text{C7})}$$

$$\text{DLMO} = 20.50\text{ h} + \frac{(0.69\text{ pg/mL} - 0.25\text{ pg/mL})*\ (21.00\text{ h} - 20.50\text{ h})}{(1.29\text{ pg/mL} - 0.25\text{ pg/mL})}$$

$$\text{DLMO} = 20.71\text{ h}$$

The TREND function in Microsoft Excel will automate this formula: "=TREND (sample time immediately before the threshold: sample time immediately after the threshold, melatonin value immediately below the threshold: melatonin value immediately above the threshold, threshold)." The result will be expressed in decimal hours. To convert back to 24-hour clock time (hh:mm), simply multiply the fraction of the hour (e.g., 0.71) by 60 minutes. The DLMO in 24-hour clock time in the above example is 20:43.

URINARY AMT6S PHASE MARKERS

Urinary data are analyzed with different procedures compared to saliva and plasma. The aMT6s assay results (in ng/mL) are converted into hourly rates for each collection interval using this formula:

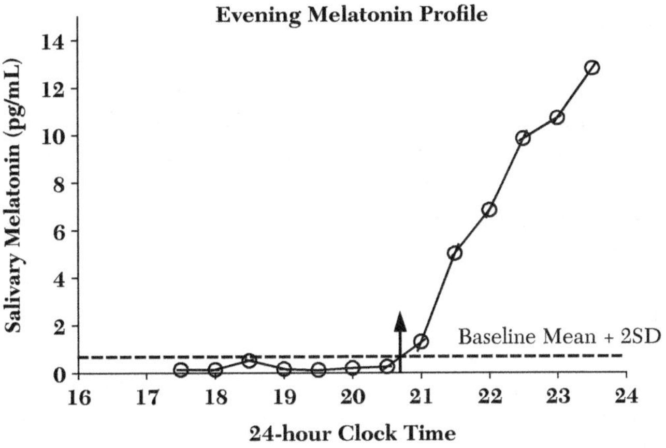

Sample #	A Sample Time (24-h clock time)	B Sample Time (decimal h)	C Salivary Melatonin (pg/mL)
1	17:30:00	17.50	0.14
2	18:00:00	18.00	0.14
3	18:30:00	18.50	0.51
4	19:00:00	19.00	0.17
5	19:30:00	19.50	0.12
6	20:00:00	20.00	0.2
7	20:30:00	(20.50	(0.25
8	21:00:00	21.00)	1.29)
9	21:30:00	21.50	5.01
10	22:00:00	22.00	6.83
11	22:30:00	22.50	9.84
12	23:00:00	23.00	10.7
13	23:30:00	23.50	12.8

Figure 17.4 Salivary melatonin data collected during the evening from a 15-year-old male participant to measure the dim light melatonin onset (DLMO). *Top*: Melatonin values derived from radioimmunoassay (RIA) at each time point are illustrated by an open circle. The hashed horizontal line illustrates the threshold, which equals the mean plus 2 standard deviations of the first 3 points (Voultsios et al., 1997). The DLMO is the clock time that melatonin concentrations rise above this threshold, and is noted by the upward facing arrow. *Bottom*: A table of the raw data is listed to illustrate an example DLMO calculation (see text).

(ng/mL x total volume)/total sample hours. The hourly rate (in ng/h) for each collection interval is plotted on the y-axis, and the midpoint time of the collection interval is plotted on the x-axis. The peak of the curve is used as the phase marker of the rhythm. The peak can be derived from the raw data, or from a fitted cosine curve.

Measuring Circadian Phase Shifts

In some cases, phase changes—or phase shifts—of the circadian system may be of interest; for example, to objectively assess effectiveness of circadian-based interventions or treatments to shift the clock earlier (phase advance) or later (phase delay) in time. Phase after the clinical or experimental intervention is subtracted from phase before the intervention so that negative numbers indicate a phase delay shift, and positive numbers indicate a phase advance shift as per standard circadian nomenclature.

Measuring Intrinsic Circadian Period (tau)

Tau is measured in controlled conditions in the laboratory using a light/dark (wake/sleep) cycle over several days that is too far from 24 hours, such that the SCN cannot capture the light/dark cues and therefore cannot entrain to a 24-hour day. The protocol's light/dark cycle is said to be *outside of the range of entrainment* and, as a result, the clock runs at its own pace, or "free-runs." The classic method to measure the free-running intrinsic period (tau) is a "forced desynchrony" (FD) protocol, which was first described by Kleitman (1939) and later refined by Czeisler and colleagues (Czeisler, Dijk, & Duffy, 1994; Czeisler et al., 1999; Dijk & Czeisler, 1994). Before the FD protocol begins, participants keep a stable sleep schedule for at least 3 baseline days. Physiological markers of the circadian clock are subsequently measured in a 36- to 40-hour constant routine (Duffy & Dijk, 2002; Minors & Waterhouse, 1984), in which participants remain awake in a constant posture and are restricted to very low activity levels and isocaloric snacks or meals distributed throughout the duration of the constant routine. The FD protocol then begins and lasts for about 2 to 3 weeks. A common FD "day" is 28 hours, in which participants have a sleep opportunity in the dark for approximately one-third of the 28 hours (9h 20 mins) and are awake in dim light for the remainder of the "day" (18 h and 40 mins). The sleep opportunity times are shifted 4 clock hours later each cycle compared to the previous cycle. A 20-hour day is another FD day length that has been used (Wyatt et al., 1999) with the same proportion of sleep to wake (6 h and 40 mins sleep/dark:13 h and 20 mins wake/light). Physiological rhythms, such as core body temperature and melatonin, are measured repeatedly over several cycles of the FD protocol. A second constant routine begins after wake-up of the last cycle. A regression line can be fit to the computed phase markers (CBT minimum, DLMO, and DLMOff) measured during the constant routines and throughout several cycles of the FD protocol to estimate tau. This protocol has been successfully carried out in children as young as 10 years, though the sleep/wake durations were slightly modified (11 h and 40 min sleep opportunity in the dark: 16 h and 20 mins awake in dim light) (Carskadon et al., 1999). In addition to measuring tau, the FD protocol is the only protocol that can disentangle the relative contributions of the tightly coupled circadian and homeostatic sleep systems. Many use the FD protocol to understand the independent contributions of the sleep homeostat and the circadian timing system on several outcomes, including cardiac and metabolic health (Scheer, Hilton, Mantzoros, & Shea, 2009), cognitive performance, and sleepiness (Dijk, Duffy, & Czeisler, 1992; Johnson et al., 1992; Wright, Hull, & Czeisler, 2002; Wyatt et al., 1999).

If tau is the only outcome of interest, however, then the FD protocol may not be as feasible given how long and labor-intensive it is, the participant burden of being isolated for 2 to 3 weeks continuously, and the expense. In recent years, an ultradian light/dark protocol has been used to estimate tau (Burgess & Eastman, 2008; Kripke et al., 2005; Lack, Micic, De Bruyn, Wright, & Lovato, 2012; Smith et al., 2009). This protocol is similar to a FD protocol in that the light/dark (wake/sleep) schedule is out of the range of entrainment. In these protocols, participants are kept on a short "day." Kripke and colleagues (2005) used a 1.5-hour day in which adult participants were awake for 60 minutes and asleep for 30 minutes across about 72 hours. Eastman and colleagues (Burgess & Eastman, 2008; Smith et al., 2009) adapted this ultradian LD cycle such that participants were exposed to a 4-hour day (2.5 h awake:1.5 h sleep opportunity in the dark) over the course of about 4 days. An ongoing study of adolescents aged 14 to 17 years in our laboratory utilizes a similar 4-hour ultradian LD protocol, except sleep and wake are both 2 hours to provide more sleep opportunity to this younger group (Crowley & Eastman, 2012). Melatonin or its metabolite is sampled throughout the ultradian protocol (Kripke et al., 2005; Lack et al., 2012) or can be measured before and after the ultradian light/dark cycle, from which a change in phase is computed (Burgess & Eastman, 2008; Smith et al., 2009). The phase shift is interpreted as the drift over the ultradian light/dark protocol that could be attributed to free-running.

Conclusion

In summary, the circadian system can be assessed with varying amounts of precision. Behavioral measures serve as a global estimate of circadian timing, whereas physiological measures, especially plasma and salivary melatonin, provide a more precise and unmasked estimate of circadian phase. The research or clinical question under investigation and the age of the child will largely drive which method to use. Core body temperature and melatonin collection protocols are labor-intensive, restrict the individual's behavior, and usually require laboratory or clinical space. These factors may limit the feasibility of collecting these measures, especially in vulnerable populations like young children. The circadian timing system is a powerful modulator of behavior. Using the tools described in this chapter, developmental psychologists are urged to consider the circadian system's impact on physical, emotional, and social development, which may in turn inform social policy.

Future Directions

- Validating melatonin collection in the home is currently underway with adults (Burgess, 2012); however, future studies are needed to determine feasibility and validity of such a procedure with young children and their caregiver(s).
- Computations of the DLMO—the most commonly measured circadian marker in humans—are not standardized in the field. While some efforts have been made to standardize this procedure in adults (Benloucif et al., 2008), a similar effort is needed for the younger pediatric population.

Acknowledgments

The author would like to thank Helen J. Burgess, PhD, for her helpful comments on this chapter. Some of the data described here were collected as part of NIH grants (F31MH078662 and R01HL105395) awarded to S. Crowley. The content is solely the responsibility of the author and does not necessarily represent the official views of the National Institutes of Health.

References

Adan, A., & Almirall, H. (1990). Adaptation and standardization of a Spanish version of the morningness-eveningness questionnaire: Individual differences. *Personality and Individual Differences, 11*(11), 1123–1130.

Adan, A., & Almirall, H. (1991). Horne & Ostberg morningness-eveningness questionnaire: A reduced scale. *Personality and Individual Differences, 12*(3), 241–253.

Adan, A., & Natale, V. (2002). Gender differences in morningness-eveningness preference. *Chronobiology International, 19*(4), 709–720.

Adan, A., Caci, H., & Prat, G. (2005). Reliability of the Spanish version of the Composite Scale of Morningness. *European Psychiatry, 20*(7), 503–509.

Archer, S. N., Robilliard, D. L., Skene, D. J., Smits, M., Williams, A., Arendt, J., et al. (2003). A length polymorphism in the circadian clock gene per3 is linked to delayed sleep phase syndrome and extreme diurnal preference. *Sleep, 26*, 413–415.

Arendt, J., Bojkowski, C., Franey, C., Wright, J., & Marks, V. (1985). Immunoassay of 6-hydroxymelatonin sulfate in human plasma and urine: Abolition of the urinary 24-hour rhythm with atenolol. *Journal of Clinical Endocrinology and Metabolism, 60*(6), 1166–1173.

Arendt, J. (2005). Melatonin: Characteristics, concerns, and prospects. *Journal of Biological Rhythms, 20*(4), 291–303.

Aschoff, J., Hoffmann, K., Pohl, H., & Wever, R. (1975). Re-entrainment of circadian rhythms after phase shifts of the zeitgeber. *Chronobiologia, 2*, 23–78.

Attanasio, A., Borrelli, P., & Gupta, D. (1985). Circadian rhythms in serum melatonin from infancy to adolescence. *Journal of Clinical Endocrinology and Metabolism, 61*(2), 388–390.

Baehr, E. K., Revelle, W., & Eastman, C. I. (2000). Individual differences in the phase and amplitude of the human circadian temperature rhythm: with an emphasis on morningness-eveningness. *Journal of Sleep Research, 9*, 117–127.

Bagci, S., Mueller, A., Reinsberg, J., Heep, A., Bartmann, P., & Franz, A. R. (2009). Saliva as a valid alternative in monitoring melatonin concentrations in newborn infants. *Early Human Development, 85*(9), 595–598.

Bagci, S., Mueller, A., Reinsberg, J., Heep, A., Bartmann, P., & Franz, A. R. (2010). Utility of salivary melatonin measurements in the assessment of the pineal physiology in newborn infants. *Clinical Biochemistry, 43*(10–11), 868–872.

Benloucif, S., Guico, M. J., Reid, K. J., Wolfe, L. F., L'Hermite-Baleriaux, M., & Zee, P. C. (2005). Stability of melatonin and temperature as circadian phase markers and their relation to sleep times in humans. *Journal of Biological Rhythms, 20*(2), 178–188.

Benloucif, S., Burgess, H. J., Klerman, E. B., Lewy, A. J., Middleton, B., Murphy, P. J., et al. (2008). Measuring melatonin in humans. *Journal of Clinical Sleep Medicine, 4*(1), 66–69.

Berson, D. M., Dunn, F. A., & Takao, M. (2002). Phototransduction by retinal ganglion cells that set the circadian clock. *Science, 295*(5557), 1070–1073.

Boivin, D. B., & James, F. O. (2002). Phase-dependent effect of room light exposure in a 5-h advance of the sleep-wake cycle: Implications for jet lag. *Journal of Biological Rhythms, 17*(3), 266–276.

Borbely, A. A. (1982). A two process model of sleep regulation. *Human Neurobiology, 1*, 195–204.

Burgess, H. (2012). A new method for the valid measurement of the dim light melatoin onset at home. *Sleep, 35*(Supplement), A205.

Burgess, H. J., Savic, N., Sletten, T., Roach, G., Gilbert, S. S., & Dawson, D. (2003). The relationship between the dim light melatonin onset and sleep on a regular schedule in young healthy adults. *Behavioral Sleep Medicine, 1*, 102–114.

Burgess, H. J., & Eastman, C. I. (2004). Early versus late bedtimes phase shift the human dim light melatonin rhythm despite a fixed morning lights on time. *Neuroscience Letters, 356*, 115–118.

Burgess, H. J., & Eastman, C. I. (2005). The dim light melatonin onset following fixed and free sleep schedules. *Journal of Sleep Research, 14*, 229–237.

Burgess, H. J., & Eastman, C. I. (2006). A late wake time phase delays the human dim light melatonin rhythm. *Neuroscience Letters, 395*, 191–195.

Burgess, H. J., & Eastman, C. I. (2008). Human tau in an ultradian light-dark cycle. *Journal of Biological Rhythms, 23*(4), 374–376.

Burgess, H. J., & Fogg, L. F. (2008). Individual differences in the amount and timing of salivary melatonin secretion. *PLoS One, 3*(8), e3055.

Caci, H., Nadalet, L., Staccini, P., Myquel, M., & Boyer, P. (1999). Psychometric properties of the French version of the composite scale of morningness in adults. *European Psychiatry, 14*(5), 284–290.

Caci, H., Nadalet, L., Staccini, P., Myquel, M., & Boyer, P. (2000). The composite scale of morningness: Further psychometric properties and temporal stability. *European Psychiatry, 15*(4), 278–281.

Caci, H., Adan, A., Bohle, P., Natale, V., Pornpitakpan, C., & Tilley, A. (2005). Transcultural properties of the composite scale of morningness: The relevance of the "morning affect" factor. *Chronobiology International, 22*(3), 523–540.

Cajochen, C., Jewett, M. E., & Dijk, D. J. (2003). Human circadian melatonin rhythm phase delay during a fixed sleep-wake schedule interspersed with nights of sleep deprivation. *Journal of Pineal Research, 35*, 149–157.

Cajochen, C., Frey, S., Anders, D., Spati, J., Bues, M., Pross, A., et al. (2011). Evening exposure to a light-emitting diodes (LED)-backlit computer screen affects circadian physiology and cognitive performance. *Journal of Applied Physiology, 110*(5), 1432–1438.

Carpen, J. D., Archer, S. N., Skene, D. J., Smits, M., & von Schantz, M. (2005). A single-nucleotide polymorphism in the 5'-untranslated region of the hPER2 gene is associated with diurnal preference. *Journal of Sleep Research, 14*(3), 293–297.

Carpen, J. D., von Schantz, M., Smits, M., Skene, D. J., & Archer, S. N. (2006). A silent polymorphism in the PER1 gene associates with extreme diurnal preference in humans. *Journal of Human Genetics, 51*(12), 1122–1125.

Carrier, J., Monk, T. H., Buysse, D. J., & Kupfer, D. J. (1997). Sleep and morningness-eveningness in the "middle" years of life (20–59 y). *Journal of Sleep Research, 6*(4), 230–237.

Carskadon, M. A., Vieira, C., & Acebo, C. (1993). Association between puberty and delayed phase preference. *Sleep, 16*(3), 258–262.

Carskadon, M. A., Acebo, C., Richardson, G. S., Tate, B. A., & Seifer, R. (1997). An approach to studying circadian rhythms of adolescent humans. *Journal of Biological Rhythms, 12*(3), 278–289.

Carskadon, M. A., Wolfson, A. R., Acebo, C., Tzischinsky, O., & Seifer, R. (1998). Adolescent sleep patterns, circadian timing, and sleepiness at a transition to early school days. *Sleep, 21*(8), 871–881.

Carskadon, M. A., Labyak, S. E., Acebo, C., & Seifer, R. (1999). Intrinsic circadian period of adolescent humans measured in conditions of forced desynchrony. *Neuroscience Letters, 260*, 129–132.

Carskadon, M. A., & Acebo, C. (2002). Regulation of sleepiness in adolescents: Update, insights, and speculation. *Sleep, 25*(6), 606–614.

Carvalho, L. A., Gorenstein, C., Moreno, R., Pariante, C., & Markus, R. P. (2009). Effect of antidepressants on melatonin metabolite in depressed patients. *Journal of Psychopharmacology, 23*(3), 315–321.

Cavallo, A. (1992). Plasma melatonin rhythm in normal puberty: Interactions of age and pubertal stages. *Neuroendocrinology, 55*(4), 372–379.

Cermakian, N., & Boivin, D. B. (2009). The regulation of central and peripheral circadian clocks in humans. *Obesity Reviews, 10*(Suppl 2), 25–36.

Cowen, P. J., Bevan, J. S., Gosden, B., & Elliott, S. A. (1985). Treatment with B-adrenoceptor blockers reduces plasma melatonin concentration. *British Journal of Clinical Pharmacology, 19*(2), 258–260.

Crowley, S. J., Acebo, C., Fallone, G., & Carskadon, M. A. (2006). Estimating dim light melatonin onset (DLMO) phase in adolescents using summer or school-year sleep/wake schedules. *Sleep, 29*(12), 1632–1641.

Crowley, S. J., Bushnell, D. L., Acebo, C., & Carskadon, M. A. (2006). Internal consistency and construct validity of two morningness/eveningness questionnaires in children. *Sleep, 29*(Supplement), A66.

Crowley, S. J., Acebo, C., & Carskadon, M. A. (2007). Sleep, circadian rhythms, and delayed phase in adolescence. *Sleep Medicine, 8*(6), 602–612.

Crowley, S. J., & Carskadon, M. A. (2010). Modifications to weekend recovery sleep delay circadian phase in older adolescents. *Chronobiology International, 27*(7), 1469–1492.

Crowley, S. J., Acebo, C., & Carskadon, M. A. (2012). Human puberty: Salivary melatonin profiles in constant conditions. *Developmental Psychobiology, 54*(4), 468–473.

Crowley, S. J., & Eastman, C. I. (2012). Shedding light on the adolescent phase response curve (PRC). *Sleep, 35*(Supplement), A64.

Czeisler, C. A., Richardson, G. S., Zimmerman, J. C., Moore-Ede, M. C., & Weitzman, E. D. (1981). Entrainment of human circadian rhythms by light-dark cycles: A reassessment. *Photochemistry and Photobiology, 34*, 239–247.

Czeisler, C. A., Brown, E. N., Ronda, J. M., Kronauer, R. E., Richardson, G. S., & Freitag, W. O. (1985). A clinical method to assess the endogenous circadian phase (ECP) of the deep circadian oscillator in man. *Sleep Research, 14*, 295.

Czeisler, C. A., Dijk, D. J., & Duffy, J. F. (1994). Entrained phase of the circadian pacemaker serves to stabilize alertness and performance throughout the habitual waking day. In R. D. Ogilvie & J. R. Harsh (Eds.), *Sleep Onset: Normal and Abnormal Processes* (pp. 89–110). Washington, DC: American Psychological Association.

Czeisler, C. A., Duffy, J. F., Shanahan, T. L., Brown, E. N., Mitchell, J. F., Rimmer, D. W., et al. (1999). Stability, precision, and near-24-hour period of the human circadian pacemaker. *Science, 284*, 2177–2181.

Darwent, D., Zhou, X., van den Heuvel, C., Sargent, C., & Roach, G. D. (2011). The validity of temperature-sensitive ingestible capsules for measuring core body temperature in laboratory protocols. *Chronobiology International, 28*(8), 719–726.

Davis, F. C., & Reppert, S. M. (2001). Development of mammalian circadian rhythms. In J. S. Takahashi, F. W. Turek, & R. Y. Moore (Eds.), *Handbook of Behavioral Neurobiology: Circadian Clocks* (Vol. 12, pp. 247–290). New York: Kluwer Academic / Plenum Publishers.

Deacon, S., & Arendt, J. (1994a). Posture influences melatonin concentrations in plasma and saliva in humans. *Neuroscience Letters, 167*, 191–194.

Deacon, S. J., Arendt, J., & English, J. (1993). Posture: A possible masking factor of the melatonin circadian rhythm. In Y. Touitou, J. Arendt, & P. Pevet (Eds.), *Melatonin and the Pineal Gland—From Basic Science to Clinical Application* (pp. 387–390). New York: Excerpta Medica.

Deacon, S. J., & Arendt, J. (1994b). Phase-shifts in melatonin, 6-sulphatoxymelatonin and alertness rhythms after treatment with moderately bright light at night. *Clinical Endocrinology, 40*, 413–420.

Dijk, D. J., Duffy, J. F., & Czeisler, C. A. (1992). Circadian and sleep/wake dependent aspects of subjective alertness and cognitive performance. *Journal of Sleep Research, 1*(2), 112–117.

Dijk, D. J., & Czeisler, C. A. (1994). Paradoxical timing of the circadian rhythm of sleep propensity serves to consolidate sleep and wakefulness in humans. *Neuroscience Letters, 166*, 63–68.

Dijk, D. J., & Czeisler, C. A. (1995). Contribution of the circadian pacemaker and the sleep homeostat to sleep propensity, sleep structure, electroencephalographic slow waves, and sleep spindle activity in humans. *Journal of Neuroscience, 15*(5 Pt 1), 3526–3538.

Duffy, J. F. (1995). Constant Routine. In M. A. Carskadon, A. Rechtschaffen, G. Richardson, T. Roth, & J. Siegel (Eds.), *Encyclopedia of Sleep and Dreaming* (pp. 134–136). Philadelphia: Simon & Schuster Macmillan.

Duffy, J. F., Dijk, D. J., Hall, E. F., & Czeisler, C. A. (1999). Relationship of endogenous circadian melatonin and temperature rhythms to self-reported preference for morning or evening activity in young and older people. *Journal of Investigative Medicine, 47,* 141–150.

Duffy, J. F., & Czeisler, C. A. (2002). Age-related change in the relationship between circadian period, circadian phase, and diurnal preference in humans. *Neuroscience Letters, 318*(3), 117–120.

Duffy, J. F., & Dijk, D. J. (2002). Getting through to circadian oscillators: Why use constant routines? *Journal of Biological Rhythms, 17*(1), 4–13.

Duffy, J. F., & Wright, K. P. (2005). Entrainment of the human circadian system by light. *Journal of Biological Rhythms, 20*(4), 326–338.

Duffy, J. F., Cain, S. W., Chang, A., Phillips, A. J. K., Munch, M. Y., Gronfier, C., et al. (2011). Sex difference in the near-24-hour intrinsic period of the human circadian timing system. *Proceedings of the National Academy of Sciences of the United States of America, 108*(Supplement 3), 15602–15608.

Eastman, C. I. (1992). High intensity light for circadian adaptation to a 12-h shift of the sleep schedule. *American Journal of Physiology, 263*(32), R428–R436.

Eastman, C. I., Liu, L., & Fogg, L. F. (1995). Circadian rhythm adaptation to simulated night shift work: Effect of nocturnal bright-light duration. *Sleep, 18*(6), 399–407.

Eastman, C. I., Molina, T. A., Burgess, H. J., & Revell, V. L. (2010). Ongoing goLITE (blue light) phase response curve in humans. *Sleep, 33*(Supplement), A64.

Edgar, D. M., Dement, W. C., & Fuller, C. A. (1993). Effect of SCN lesions on sleep in squirrel monkeys: Evidence for opponent processes in sleep-wake regulation. *Journal of Neuroscience, 13*(3), 1065–1079.

Edwards, B., Waterhouse, J., Reilly, T., & Atkinson, G. (2002). A comparison of the suitabilities of rectal, gut, and insulated axilla temperatures for measurement of the circadian rhythm of core temperature in field studies. *Chronobiology International, 19*(3), 579–597.

Ehrenkranz, J. R., Tamarkin, L., Comite, F., Johnsonbaugh, R. E., Bybee, D. E., Loriaux, D. L., et al. (1982). Daily rhythm of plasma melatonin in normal and precocious puberty. *Journal of Clinical Endocrinology and Metabolism, 55*(2), 307–310.

Ekman, A. C., Leppaluoto, J., Huttunen, P., Aranko, K., & Vakkuri, O. (1993). Ethanol inhibits melatonin secretion in healthy volunteers in a dose-dependent randomized double blind cross-over study. *Journal of Clinical Endocrinology and Metabolism, 77*(3), 780–783.

Escribano, C., Diaz-Morales, J. F., Delgado, P., & Collado, M. J. (2012). Morningness/eveningness and school performance among Spanish adolescents: Further evidence. *Learning and Individual Differences, 22*(3), 409–413.

Folkard, S., Monk, T. H., & Lobban, M. C. (1979). Towards a predictive test of adjustment to shift work. *Ergonomics, 22*(1), 79–91.

Foret, J., Touron, N., Benoit, O., & Bouard, G. (1985). Sleep and body temperature in "morning" and "evening" people. *Sleep, 8*(4), 311–318.

Ganguly, S., Coon, S. L., & Klein, D. C. (2002). Control of melatonin synthesis in the mammalian pineal gland: The critical role of serotonin acetylation. *Cell and Tissue Research, 309*(1), 127–137.

Garlo, K. G., Crossin, R. A., Carskadon, M. A., & LeBourgeois, M. K. (2008). Assessment of salivary dim light melatonin onset (DLMO) and reported sleep in preschool children. *Sleep, 31*(Supplement), A48.

Gebru, H., & LeBourgeois, M. K. (2009). Circadian assessment with urinary 6-sulfatoxymelatonin (aMT6s) secretion in healthy preschool children. *Sleep 32*(Supplement), A91.

Giannotti, F., Cortesi, F., Sebastiani, T., & Ottaviano, S. (2002). Circadian preference, sleep and daytime behaviour in adolescence. *Journal of Sleep Research, 11*(3), 191–199.

Gooley, J. J., Lu, J., Chou, T. C., Scammell, T. E., & Saper, C. B. (2001). Melanopsin in cells of origin of the retinohypothalamic tract. *Nature Neuroscience, 4*(12), 1165.

Gooley, J. J., Chamberlain, K., Smith, K. A., Khalsa, S. B., Rajaratnam, S. M., Van Reen, E., et al. (2011). Exposure to room light before bedtime suppresses melatonin onset and shortens melatonin duration in humans. *Journal of Clinical Endocrinology and Metabolism, 96*(3), E463-E472.

Goulet, G., Mongrain, V., Desrosiers, C., Paquet, J., & Dumont, M. (2007). Daily light exposure in morning-type and evening-type individuals. *Journal of Biological Rhythms, 22*(2), 151–158.

Guler, A. D., Ecker, J. L., Lall, G. S., Haq, S., Altimus, C. M., Liao, H. W., et al. (2008). Melanopsin cells are the principal conduits for rod-cone input to non-image-forming vision. *Nature, 453*(7191), 102–105.

Hannibal, J., Hindersson, P., Knudsen, S. M., Georg, B., & Fahrenkrug, J. (2002). The photopigment melanopsin is exclusively present in pituitary adenylate cyclase-activating polypeptide-containing retinal ganglion cells of the retinohypothalamic tract. *Journal of Neuroscience, 22,* RC191

Horne, J. A., & Östberg, O. (1976). A self-assessment questionnaire to determine morningness-eveningness in human circadian rhythms. *International Journal of Chronobiology, 4,* 97–110.

Iguchi, H., Kato, K., & Ibayashi, H. (1982). Age-dependent reduction in serum melatonin concentrations in healthy human subjects. *Journal of Clinical Endocrinology and Metabolism, 55*(1), 27–29.

Ishihara, K., Saitoh, T., Inoue, Y., & Miyata, Y. (1984). Validity of the Japanese version of the morningness-eveningness questionnaire. *Perceptual and Motor Skills, 59,* 863–866.

Jenni, O. G., & LeBourgeois, M. K. (2006). Understanding sleep-wake behavior and sleep disorders in children: The value of a model. *Current Opinion in Psychiatry, 19*(3), 282–287.

Johnson, M. P., Duffy, J. F., Dijk, D. J., Ronda, J. M., Dyal, C. M., & Czeisler, C. A. (1992). Short-term memory, alertness and performance: A reappraisal of their relationship to body temperature. *Journal of Sleep Research, 1,* 24–29.

Jones, K. H. S., Ellis, J., Von Schantz, M., Skene, D. J., Dijk, D. J., & Archer, S. N. (2007). Age-related change in the association between a polymorphism in the PER3 gene and preferred timing of sleep and waking activities. *Journal of Sleep Research, 16,* 12–16.

Katzenberg, D., Young, T., Finn, L., Lin, L., King, D. P., Takahashi, J. S., et al. (1998). A CLOCK polymorphism associated with human diurnal preference. *Sleep, 21*(6), 569–576.

Kennaway, D. J., Stamp, G. E., & Goble, F. C. (1992). Development of melatonin production in infants and the impact of prematurity. *Journal of Clinical Endocrinology and Metabolism, 75*(2), 367–369.

Kerkhof, G. A. (1985). Inter-individual differences in the human circadian system: A review. *Biological Psychology, 20,* 83–112.

Khalsa, S. B. S., Jewett, M. E., Cajochen, C., & Czeisler, C. A. (2003). A phase response curve to single bright light pulses in human subjects. *Journal of Physiology, 549.3*, 945–952.

Kim, S., Dueker, G. L., Hasher, L., & Goldstein, D. (2002). Children's time of day preference: age, gender and ethnic differences. *Personality and Individual Differences, 33*(7), 1083–1090.

Kleitman, N. (1939). *Sleep and Wakefulness.* Chicago: The University of Chicago Press.

Klerman, E. B., Gershengorn, H. B., Duffy, J. F., & Kronauer, R. E. (2002). Comparisons of the variability of three markers of the human circadian pacemaker. *Journal of Biological Rhythms, 17*(2), 181–193.

Klerman, H., St. Hilaire, M. A., Kronauer, R. E., Gooley, J. J., Gronfier, C., Hull, J. T., et al. (2012). Analysis method and experimental conditions affect computed circadian phase from melatonin data. *PLoS One, 7*(4), e33836.

Kripke, D. F., Youngstedt, S. D., Elliott, J. A., Tuunainen, A., Rex, K. M., Hauger, R. L., et al. (2005). Circadian phase in adults of contrasting ages. *Chronobiology International, 22*(4), 695–709.

Kripke, D. F., Elliott, J. A., Youngstedt, S. D., & Rex, K. M. (2007). Circadian phase response curves to light in older and young women and men. *Journal of Circadian Rhythms, 5*(1), 4.

Laberge, L., Carrier, J., Lesperance, P., Lambert, C., Vitaro, F., Tremblay, R. E., et al. (2000). Sleep and circadian phase characteristics of adolescent and young adult males in a naturalistic summertime condition. *Chronobiology International, 17*(4), 489–501.

Labyak, S. E., Acebo, C., & Carskadon, M. A. (1998). Circadian phase of core body temperature minimum in adolescents. *Sleep, 21* (Supplement), 203.

Lack, L. C., Micic, G., De Bruyn, A., Wright, H., & Lovato, N. (2012). Circadian rhythm period length in delayed sleep phase disorder. *Sleep, 35*(Supplement), A203.

LeBourgeois, M. K., Wright, K. P., LeBourgeois, H. B., & Jenni, O. G. (in press). Dissonance between parent-selected bedtimes and young children's circadian physiology influences nighttime settling difficulties. *Mind, Brain, and Education.*

Lewy, A. J., Wehr, T. A., Goodwin, F. K., Newsome, D. A., & Markey, S. P. (1980). Light suppresses melatonin secretion in humans. *Science, 210*(4475), 1267–1269.

Lewy, A. J., & Sack, R. L. (1989). The dim light melatonin onset as a marker for circadian phase position. *Chronobiology International, 6*(1), 93–102.

Lewy, A. J., Cutler, N. L., & Sack, R. L. (1999). The endogenous melatonin profile as a marker of circadian phase position. *Journal of Biological Rhythms, 14*(3), 227–236.

Li, S.-X., Li, Q.-Q., Wang, X.-F., Liu, L.-J., Liu, Y., Zhang, L.-X., et al. (2011). Preliminary test for the Chinese version of the morningness-eveningness questionnaire. *Sleep and Biological Rhythms, 9*, 19–23.

Lissoni, P., Resentini, M., Mauri, R., Esposti, D., Esposti, G., Rossi, D., et al. (1986). Effects of tetrahydrocannabinol on melatonin secretion in man. *Hormone and Metabolic Research, 18*, 77–78.

Mann, K., Bauer, H., Hiemke, C., Roschke, J., Wetzel, H., & Benkert, O. (1996). Acute, subchronic and discontinuation effects of zopiclone on sleep EEG and nocturnal melatonin secretion. *European Neuropsychopharmacology, 6*(3), 163–168.

Martin, S. K., & Eastman, C. I. (2002). Sleep logs of young adults with self-selected sleep times predict the dim light melatonin onset. *Chronobiology International, 19*(4), 695–707.

Mecacci, L., & Zani, A. (1983). Morningness-eveningness preferences and sleep-waking diary data of morning and evening types in student and worker samples. *Ergonomics, 26*(12), 1147–1153.

Miller, H. L., Ekstrom, R. D., Mason, G. A., Lydiard, R. B., & Golden, R. N. (2001). Noradrenergic function and clinical outcome in antidepressant pharmacotherapy. *Neuropsychopharmacology, 24*(6), 617–623.

Mills, J. N., Minors, D. S., & Waterhouse, J. M. (1978a). Adaptation to abrupt time shifts of the oscillator(s) controlling human circadian rhythms. *Journal of Physiology, 285*, 455–470.

Mills, J. N., Minors, D. S., & Waterhouse, J. M. (1978b). Endogenous rhythms after living on 21 hr "days." *Journal of Physiology, 281*, 22p–23p.

Minors, D. S., & Waterhouse, J. M. (1984). The use of constant routines in unmasking the endogenous component of human circadian rhythms. *Chronobiology International, 1*(3), 205–216.

Minors, D. S., & Waterhouse, J. M. (1989). Masking in humans: The problem and some attempts to solve it. *Chronobiology International, 6*(1), 29–53.

Minors, D. S., Waterhouse, J. M., & Wirz-Justice, A. (1991). A human phase-response curve to light. *Neuroscience Letters, 133*, 36–40.

Minors, D. S., Waterhouse, J. M., & Akerstedt, T. (1994). The effect of the timing, quality and quantity of sleep upon the depression (masking) of body temperature on an irregular sleep/wake schedule. *Journal of Sleep Research, 3*, 45–51.

Mishima, K., Tozawa, T., Satoh, K., Saitoh, H., & Mishima, Y. (2005). The 3111T/C polymorphism of hClock is associated with evening preference and delayed sleep timing in a Japanese population sample. *American Journal of Medical Genetics. Part B, Neuropsychiatric Genetics, 133B*(1), 101–104.

Molina, T. A., & Burgess, H. J. (2011). Calculating the dim light melatonin onset: The impact of threshold and sampling rate. *Chronobiology International, 28*(8), 714–718.

Mongrain, V., Lavoie, S., Selmaoui, B., Paquet, J., & Dumont, M. (2004). Phase relationships between sleep-wake cycle and underlying circadian rhythms in morningness-eveningness. *Journal of Biological Rhythms, 19*(3), 248–257.

Monteleone, P., Forziati, D., Orazzo, C., & Maj, M. (1989). Preliminary observations on the suppression of nocturnal plasma melatonin levels by short-term administration of diazepam in humans. *Journal of Pineal Research, 6*(3), 253–258.

Moore, R. Y. (1992). The organization of the human circadian timing system. *Progress in Brain Research, 93*, 101–117.

Moore, R. Y. (1997). Circadian rhythms: Basic neurobiology and clinical applications. *Annual Review of Medicine, 48*, 253–266.

Murphy, P. J., Myers, B. L., & Badia, P. (1996). Nonsteroidal anti-inflammatory drugs alter body temperature and suppress melatonin in humans. *Physiology & Behavior, 59*, 133–139.

Natale, V., & Alzani, A. (2001). Additional validity evidence for the Composite Scale of Morningness. *Personality and Individual Differences, 30*(2), 293–301.

Nathan, P. J., Jeyaseelan, A. S., Burrows, G. D., & Norman, T. R. (1998). Modulation of plasma melatonin concentrations by changes in posture. *Journal of Pineal Research, 24*, 219–223.

Ostberg, O., & Nicholl, A. G. M. (1973). The preferred thermal conditions for "morning" and "evening" types of subjects during day and night–preliminary results. *Build International, 6*, 147–157.

Paine, S. J., Gander, P. H., & Travier, N. (2006). The epidemiology of morningness/eveningness: Influence of age, gender, ethnicity, and socioeconomic factors in adults (30–49 years). *Journal of Biological Rhythms, 21*(1), 68–76.

Palazidou, E., Franey, C., Arendt, J., Stahl, S., & Checkley, S. (1989). Evidence for a functional role of alpha-1 adrenoceptors in the regulation of melatonin secretion in man. *Psychoneuroendocrinology, 14*(1–2), 131–135.

Palazidou, E., Papadopoulos, A., Sitsen, A., Stahl, S., & Checkley, S. (1989). An alpha 2 adrenoceptor antagonist, Org 3770, enhances nocturnal melatonin secretion in man. *Psychopharmacology (Berlin), 97*(1), 115–117.

Palazidou, E., Papadopoulos, A., Ratcliff, H., Dawling, S., & Checkley, S. A. (1992). Noradrenaline uptake inhibition increases melatonin secretion, a measure of noradrenergic neurotransmission, in depressed patients. *Psychological Medicine, 22*(2), 309–315.

Palazidou, E., Skene, D., Arendt, J., Everitt, B., & Checkley, S. A. (1992). The acute and chronic effects of (+) and (-) oxaprotiline upon melatonin secretion in normal subjects. *Psychological Medicine, 22*(1), 61–67.

Pereira, D. S., Tufik, S., Louzada, F. M., Benedito-Silva, A. A., Lopez, A. R., Lemos, N. A., et al. (2005). Association of the length polymorphism in the human Per3 gene with the delayed sleep-phase syndrome: Does latitude have an influence upon it? *Sleep, 28*(1), 29–32.

Pornpitakpan, C. (1998). Psychometric properties of the composite scale of morningness: A shortened version. *Personality and Individual Differences, 25*(4), 699–709.

Provencio, I., Rodriguez, I. R., Jiang, G., Hayes, W. P., Moreira, E. F., & Rollag, M. D. (2000). A novel human opsin in the inner retina. *Journal of Neuroscience, 20*(2), 600–605.

Randler, C. (2008). Differences in sleep and circadian preference between Eastern and Western German adolescents. *Chronobiology International, 25*(4), 565–575.

Randler, C., & Bilger, S. (2009). Associations among sleep, chronotype, parental monitoring, and pubertal development among German adolescents. *Journal of Psychology, 143*(5), 509–520.

Revell, V. L., & Eastman, C. I. (2005). How to trick Mother Nature into letting you fly around or stay up all night. *Journal of Biological Rhythms, 20*(4), 353–365.

Roenneberg, T., Wirz-Justice, A., & Merrow, M. (2003). Life between clocks: Daily temporal patterns of humans chronotypes. *Journal of Biological Rhythms, 18*(1), 80–90.

Roenneberg, T., Kuehnle, T., Pramstaller, P. P., Ricken, J., Havel, M., Guth, A., et al. (2004). A marker for the end of adolescence. *Current Biology, 14*(24), R1038–1039.

Roenneberg, T., Kuehnle, T., Juda, M., Kantermann, T., Allebrandt, K., Gordijn, M., et al. (2007). Epidemiology of the human circadian clock. *Sleep Medicine Reviews, 11*(6), 429–438.

Rommel, T., & Demisch, L. (1994). Influence of chronic beta-adrenoreceptor blocker treatment on melatonin secretion and sleep quality in patients with essential hypertension. *Journal of Neural Transmission, 95*, 39–48.

Rupp, T. L., Acebo, C., & Carskadon, M. A. (2007). Evening alcohol suppresses salivary melatonin in young adults. *Chronobiology International, 24*(3), 463–470.

Sack, R. L., Lewy, A. J., Erb, D. L., Vollmer, W. M., & Singer, C. M. (1986). Human melatonin production decreases with age. *Journal of Pineal Research, 3*, 379–388.

Salti, R., Galluzzi, F., Bindi, G., Perfetto, F., Tarquini, R., Halberg, F., et al. (2000). Nocturnal melatonin patterns in children. *Journal of Clinical Endocrinology and Metabolism, 85*(6), 2137–2144.

Santhi, N., Thorne, H. C., van der Veen, D. R., Johnsen, S., Mills, S. L., Hommes, V., et al. (2012). The spectral composition of evening light and individual differences in the suppression of melatonin and delay of sleep in humans. *Journal of Pineal Research, 53*(1), 47–59.

Scheer, F. A., Hilton, M. F., Mantzoros, C. S., & Shea, S. A. (2009). Adverse metabolic and cardiovascular consequences of circadian misalignment. *Proceedings of the National Academy of Sciences of the United States of America, 106*(11), 4453–4458.

Simpkin, C. T., Akacem, L. D., Garlo, K. G., Jenni, O. G., & Lebourgeois, M. K. (2012). Chronotype in early childhood: Associations with dim light melatonin onset (DLMO), phase angle of entrainment, and parent reports of sleep. *Sleep, 35*(Supplement), A20.

Smith, C. S., Reilly, C., & Midkiff, K. (1989). Evaluation of three circadian rhythm questionnaires with suggestions for an improved measure of morningness. *Journal of Applied Psychology, 74*(5), 728–738.

Smith, C. S., Tisak, J., Bauman, T., & Green, E. (1991). Psychometric equivalence of a translated circadian rhythm questionnaire: Implications for between- and within-population assessments. *Journal of Applied Psychology, 76*(5), 628–636.

Smith, M. R., Burgess, H. J., Fogg, L. F., & Eastman, C. I. (2009). Racial differences in the human endogenous circadian period. *PLoS One, 4*(6), e6014.

St. Hilaire, M. A., Gooley, J. J., Khalsa, S. B., Kronauer, R. E., Czeisler, C. A., & Lockley, S. W. (2012). Human phase response curve (PRC) to a 1-hour pulse of bright white light. *Journal of Physiology, 590*(Pt 13), 3035–3045.

Stankov, B., Lucini, V., Mariani, M., Scaglione, F., Demartini, G., & Fraschini, F. (1990). Alpha-1 adrenoceptor involvement in the control of melatonin secretion in the golden hamster. *Journal of Pineal Research, 9*(1), 21–28.

Stoschitzky, K., Sakotnik, A., Lercher, P., Zweiker, R., Maier, R., Liebmann, P., et al. (1999). Influence of beta-blockers on melatonin release. *European Journal of Clinical Pharmacology, 55*(2), 111–115.

Taillard, J., Philip, P., Coste, O., Sagaspe, P., & Bioulac, B. (2003). The circadian and homeostatic modulation of sleep pressure during wafefulness differs between morning and evening chronotypes. *Journal of Sleep Research, 12*, 275–282.

Taillard, J., Philip, P., Chastang, J. F., & Bioulac, B. (2004). Validation of Horne and Ostberg morningness-eveningness questionnaire in a middle-aged population of French workers. *Journal of Biological Rhythms, 19*(1), 76–86.

Tauman, R., Zisapel, N., Laudon, M., Nehama, H., & Sivan, Y. (2002). Melatonin production in infants. *Pediatric Neurology, 26*(5), 379–382.

Thompson, C., Mezey, G., Corn, T., Franey, C., English, J., Arendt, J., et al. (1985). The effect of desipramine upon melatonin and cortisol secretion in depressed and normal subjects. *British Journal of Psychiatry, 147*, 389–393.

Torsvall, L., & Akerstedt, T. (1980). A diurnal type scale: Construction, consistency and validation in shift work. *Scandinavian Journal of Work, Environment and Health, 6*, 283–290.

Tzischinsky, O., & Shochat, T. (2011). Eveningness, sleep patterns, daytime functioning, and quality of life in Israeli adolescents. *Chronobiology International, 28*(4), 338–343.

Urban, R., Magyarodi, T., & Rigo, A. (2011). Morningness-eveningness, chronotypes and health-impairing behaviors in adolescents. *Chronobiology International, 28*(3), 238–247.

Voultsios, A., Kennaway, D. J., & Dawson, D. (1997). Salivary melatonin as a circadian phase marker: Validation and comparison to plasma melatonin. *Journal of Biological Rhythms, 12*(5), 457–466.

Waldhauser, F., Weiszenbacher, G., Frisch, H., Zeitlhuber, U., Waldhauser, M., & Wurtman, R. J. (1984). Fall in nocturnal serum melatonin during prepuberty and pubescence. *Lancet, 1*(8373), 362–365.

Waldhauser, F., & Steger, H. (1986). Changes in melatonin secretion with age and pubescence. *Journal of Neural Transmission, 21*(Suppl), 183–197.

Waldhauser, F., Weiszenbacher, G., Tatzer, E., Gisinger, B., Waldhauser, M., Schemper, M., et al. (1988). Alterations in nocturnal serum melatonin levels in humans with growth and aging. *Journal of Clinical Endocrinology and Metabolism, 66*(3), 648–652.

Waterhouse, J., Weinert, D., Minors, D., Folkard, S., Owens, D., Atkinson, G., et al. (2000). A comparison of some different methods for purifying core temperature data from humans. *Chronobiology International, 17*(4), 539–566.

Werner, H., Lebourgeois, M. K., Geiger, A., & Jenni, O. G. (2009). Assessment of chronotype in four- to eleven-year-old children: Reliability and validity of the Children's Chronotype Questionnaire (CCTQ). *Chronobiology International, 26*(5), 992–1014.

Wilson, M. E., & Gordon, T. P. (1989). Nocturnal changes in serum melatonin during female puberty in rhesus monkeys: A longitudinal study. *Journal of Endocrinology, 121*(3), 553–562.

Wong, K. Y., Dunn, F. A., Graham, D. M., & Berson, D. M. (2007). Synaptic influences on rat ganglion-cell photoreceptors. *Journal of Physiology, 582*(Pt 1), 279–296.

Wright, K. P., Badia, P., Myers, B. L., Plenzler, S. C., & Hakel, M. (1997). Caffeine and light effects on nighttime melatonin and temperature levels in sleep-deprived humans. *Brain Research, 747,* 78–84.

Wright, K. P., & Badia, P. (1999). Effects of menstrual cycle phase and oral contraceptives on alertness, cognitive performance, and circadian rhythms during sleep deprivation. *Behavioural Brain Research, 103*(2), 185–194.

Wright, K. P., Hughes, R. J., Kronauer, R. E., Dijk, D. J., & Czeisler, C. A. (2001). Intrinsic near-24-h pacemaker period determines limits of circadian entrainment to a weak synchronizer in humans. *Proceedings of the National Academy of Sciences of the United States of America, 98*(24), 14027–14032.

Wright, K. P., Hull, J. T., & Czeisler, C. A. (2002). Relationship between alertness, performance, and body temperature in humans. *American Journal of Physiology. Regulatory, Integrative, and Comparative Physiology, 283,* R1370–R1377.

Wright, K. P., Drake, C. L., & Lockley, S. W. (2008). Diagnostic tools for circadian rhythm sleep disorders. In C.A. Kushida (Ed.), *Handbook of Sleep Disorders* (pp. 147–175). New York: Taylor & Francis Group.

Wyatt, J. K., Ritz-DeCecco, A., Czeisler, C. A., & Dijk, D. J. (1999). Circadian temperature and melatonin rhythms, sleep, and neurobehavioral function in humans living on a 20-h day. *American Journal of Physiology, 277*(4 Pt 2), R1152–R1163.

Zeitzer, J. M., Dijk, D. J., Kronauer, R. E., Brown, E. N., & Czeisler, C. A. (2000). Sensitivity of the human circadian pacemaker to nocturnal light: Melatonin phase resetting and suppression. *Journal of Physiology, 526.3,* 695–702.

Zhao, Z. Y., Xie, Y., Fu, Y. R., Bogdan, A., & Touitou, Y. (2002). Aging and the circadian rhythm of melatonin: A cross-sectional study of Chinese subjects 30–110 yr of age. *Chronobiology International, 19*(6), 1171–1182.

CHAPTER

18 Sleep Surveys and Screening: To Measure Is to Know

Karen Spruyt

Abstract

There is a pervasive lack of awareness of the relatively frequent presence of sleep problems in children, which in turn can manifest in a myriad of clinical presentations that may be easily misconstrued as other pediatric conditions and mistreated accordingly. To measure is to know! Here, we touch upon the theoretical and pragmatic processes required for instrument design and evaluation in the rapidly developing scientific world of pediatric sleep. There are too many tools being used that have not undergone careful and methodical psychometric evaluation and, as such, may be fraught with biased or invalid findings. The field of pediatric sleep can only continue to grow and exert its impact on other fields if researchers and clinicians thoroughly investigate and report the psychometric properties of the tool(s) they develop and use.

Key Words: reliability, validity, equivalence, item-analysis, standardization, Likert scale, questionnaire, diary, log

Introduction

"When you can measure what you are speaking about, and can express it in numbers, you know something about it; but when you cannot measure it, when you cannot express it in numbers, then your knowledge is of a meager and unsatisfactory kind" – Lord Kelvin, 1883 (quoted in Stellman, 1998)

A systematic screening for sleep issues might assist in early identification of academic, behavioral, health, and quality of life problems, which if treated will result in a better learning, happier, and healthier child. In the field of pediatric sleep research, a trend toward implementation of large-scale sleep surveys has surfaced. Unfortunately, only a fraction of the manuscripts seem to report on the psychometric criteria of the applied tool and rarely, if at all, describe endorsement rates of items.

Previously, (Spruyt & Gozal, 2011a) we described in detail 11 methodological steps needed to develop and evaluate a sleep assessment tool (See Figure 18.1): *(1)* Purpose, or *the use of a tool*; (2) Research Question, or *the tool's intended application*; (3) Response Format, or *how to question*; (4) Generation of Items, or *what to question*; (5) Pilot, or *trials to perfect the tool*; (6) Item-analyses and non-response analyses, or *the preciseness and representativeness of the tool*; (7) Structure, or *the identification of underlying concepts*; (8) Reliability, or *the consistency of measurement*; (9) Validity, or *the representation of the attribute under investigation*; (10) Confirmatory analyses, or *verifying the stability of aforementioned steps*; and (11) Standardization and *norm development*, or *the large-scale usage*. (For more details see (Spruyt & Gozal, 2011a). Additionally, translating tools to other languages requires a process that will fulfill conceptual equivalence (e.g., how sleep is conceptualized) and item/content equivalence (i.e., validity or relevance of items), but also semantic equivalence, operational equivalence

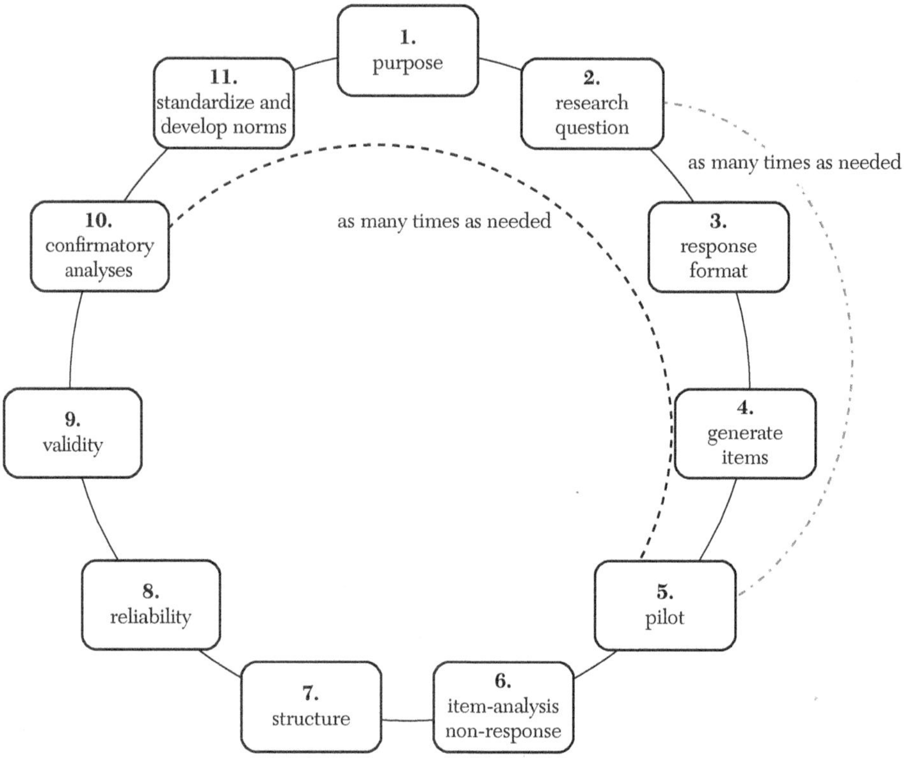

Figure 18.1 Steps in Tool Development or Evaluation (Spruyt & Gozal, 2011a)

(i.e., the way data were collected), measurement (i.e., psychometric properties), and functional (i.e., equivalence throughout the development steps) equivalence need to be evaluated (Sagheri, Wiater, Steffen, & Owens, 2010; Spruyt & Gozal, 2011a). These psychometric approaches should be implemented using appropriate manuals and scholarly manuscripts on this topic, because inappropriate tools and lack of rigor inevitably lead to poor quality data, misleading conclusions, and inaccurate recommendations.

Indeed, similar to daytime diagnostic tools, the core principles on which development of tools aiming to obtain valid information on nighttime behaviors are heavily dependent on the psychometric quality of the "subjective tool" (i.e., instrument, test, interview, measure, scale, diary, log, and questionnaire, hereafter referred to as "tool"). It is still somewhat disconcerting how undervalued "nighttime" behavior is when reflecting upon the abundance of standardized "daytime" behavior assessment tools and the relative scarcity of such tools for the "dark hours" in infants, children and adolescents. As a result, it is imperative that researchers, clinicians, and publishers should be as transparent as possible regarding the subjective tool(s) utilized and reported. It is the only way through which our field will continue to grow, as per Lord Kelvin: (continued) *"it may be the beginning of knowledge, but you have scarcely in your thoughts advanced to the state of Science, whatever the matter may be."* A tool forms the bridge between the researcher or clinician and the respondent, and thus it is of utmost importance that their "perception" of a sleep behavior is nearly identical. Therefore, we want precise questions that measure what we want to measure, time after time, regardless of the sociodemographics of the respondents.

Questionnaires

"Ask and ye shall be answered"— is it really that simple? Questionnaires are a useful and extensively used tool in clinical sleep medicine and in sleep research (Krieger & Vitiello, 2011; Moul, 2011; Spruyt & Gozal, 2011b). The number of sleep questionnaires targeting the pediatric age range has tremendously increased in recent years (i.e., five-fold after 2000), and with such explosion in the number of instruments, their heterogeneity has become all the more apparent.

Fifty-seven tools were found to have been psychometrically evaluated to some extent (Spruyt & Gozal, 2011b). On average, 5.4 steps were performed and 38% fulfilled 7 out of the 11 psychometric steps. Of these were specifically the Steps 1–4 among the more popular steps, yet reliability of the instrument used was assessed in 93% of the tools (Figure 18.2). Unfortunately, reliability does not imply validity, although a tool cannot be considered valid if it is not reliable. Validity is only questioned in about 63% of the questionnaires reviewed. Hence, what are we questioning? In clear contrast to general (non-sleep) assessment tools, only 8.8% of the sleep questionnaires have some form of norms. Furthermore, questionnaires have been primarily used or developed for a school-age population, and in 63.2% of these tools the caregiver was the key respondent. During infancy, tools tend to focus on sleep environment and settling, whereas for school-age children, sleep–wake patterns as well as a diversity of sleep behaviors (e.g., snoring, insomnia) are mostly assessed. Toward adolescence, more questions surfaced regarding sleepiness or circadian typology and emotional well-being, as well as scholastic achievement. The time to complete the questionnaire was reported only for 21% of the tools. Overall, the number of items ranged from about 6 to 140, of which few are of descriptive or demographic nature. About 66% of the questionnaires used solely closed-ended questions, with the frequency or Likert-type scale being the most common answer format. In contrast, the psychometric characteristics of open-ended questions or interviews have seldom been assessed. Also, few tools created through a dissertation study will be peer reviewed and eventually published in journals.

Only two tools fulfilled all methodological steps: The Sleep Disturbance Scale for Children (SDSC) and Sleep Disorders Inventory for Student-Children and Adolescent form (SDIS-C, SDIS-A). More specifically, they assess sleep–wake patterns and sleep behaviors, and both have been applied in community and clinical settings. Each of these tools provides T-scores, a type of standardized score that can be mathematically transformed into other types of standardized scores, and has an average range of 40–60 and thus, more importantly, about 68% of the sample would score within that range (i.e., normal, bell-shaped curve).

The Sleep Disorders Inventory for Student-Children and Adolescent form (SDIS-C, SDIS-A) (Luginbuehl, Bradley-Klug, Ferron, Anderson, & Benbadis, 2008; Luginbuehl, 2003) is commercially available (see Pearson website), largely designed for school psychologists, and is the result of a doctoral dissertation in collaboration with an expert panel and seven pediatric sleep centers in four regions of the country. Its subscales are: obstructive sleep apnea syndrome, excessive daytime sleepiness, periodic limb movement disorder, delayed sleep phase syndrome, and narcolepsy disorders. Their combined age range goes from 2 to 18 year old children, and demographics of the population are as reflected by the 2000 US Census. This parental rating tool is also available in Spanish. Items are scored on a 7-point Likert scale questioning the past 6–12 months, and

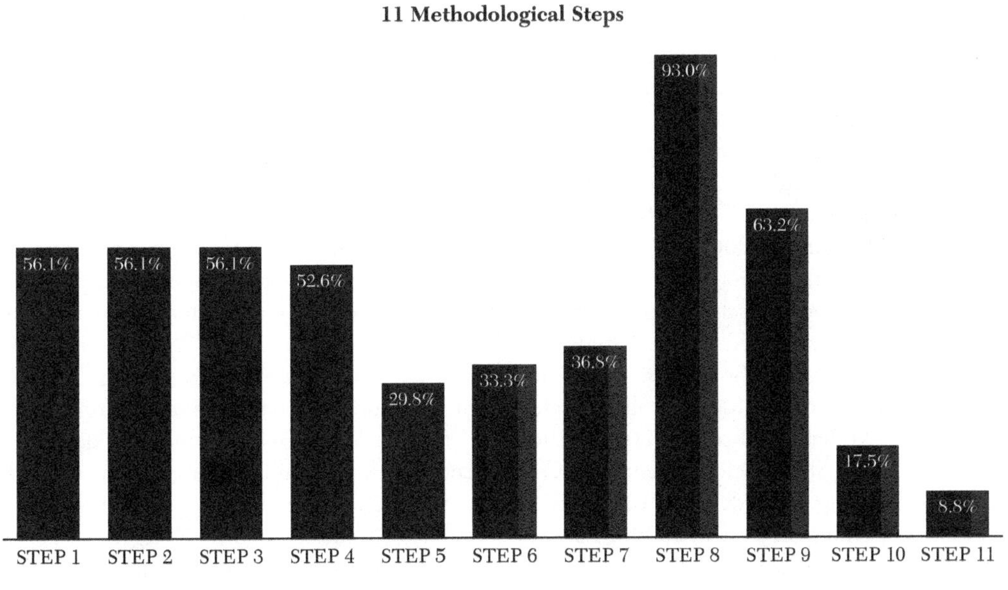

Figure 18.2 The 11 Methodological Steps for 57 Tools Reviewed.

they each take about 10 minutes to complete. The author strongly advocates its screening purpose, and therefore has developed a clinician-friendly format of the tool that includes computer scoring and the generation of graphs and reports. Luginbuehl et al. (2008) further advocate the need for additional studies in clinical populations and Hispanic population.

The Sleep Disturbance Scale for Children (SDSC) is freely available through its publications in the *Journal of Sleep Research* (Bruni et al., 1996), and comprises six subscales fitting into the categories of Association of Sleep Disorders Centers and the Association for the Psychophysiological Study of Sleep diagnostic classification of sleep and arousal disorders. It assesses disorders of initiating and maintaining sleep, sleep disordered breathing disorders, disorders of arousal, sleep–wake transition disorders, disorders of excessive somnolence, and sleep hyperhydrosis. Although no American norms are available, this instrument has been widely translated and used, maintaining its psychometric soundness. The scoring format is a 5-point Likert scale comprising the past 6 months. Time to complete is about 10 minutes. It was developed for 6.5–15.3-year-old children, yet translations have been applied to other age ranges. Norms of the original tool have only been generated for an Italian sample.

For the following tools not all steps of tool development have been discussed extensively, but the tools are generally satisfactory to adequate (see Spruyt & Gozal, 2011b for more details, and Tables 18.1–18.3). Sleep problems of infancy can be assessed by use of the Sleep and Settle Questionnaire (SSQ; Matthey, 2001), Parental Interactive Bedtime Behavior Scale (PIBBS; Morell & Cortina-Borja, 2002), Maternal Cognitions about Infant Sleep Questionnaire (MCISQ; Morrell, 1999) or, for older children, Bedtime Routines Questionnaire (BRQ; Henderson & Jordan, 2009) or Tayside Children's Sleep Questionnaire (TCSQ; McGreavey, Donnan, Pagliari, & Sullivan, 2005), which mainly focus on sleep–wake patterns, routines, or hygiene. For preschoolers and young school-age children, these problems can be surveyed by the Children's Sleep Wake Scale (CSWS; LeBourgeois, 2003) or Behavioral Evaluation of Disorders of Sleep Scale (BEDS; Schreck, Mulick, & Rojahn, 2003). The well-known Pediatric Sleep Questionnaire (PSQ) sleep-related breathing disorder (SRBD) scale (Chervin, Hedger, Dillon, & Pituch, 2000; Chervin et al., 2007) has been extensively studied and shows adequate psychometric properties. Conversely, the Dream Content Questionnaire for Children (ChDCQ; Bruni, Lo Reto, Recine, Ottaviano, & Guidetti, 1999) and Cleveland Adolescent Sleepiness Questionnaire (CASQ; Spilsbury, Drotar, Rosen, & Redline, 2007) are the only self-report tools in this list and have been somewhat overlooked despite their relatively high psychometric qualities. In fact, the CASQ offers a visual alternative to the verbal sleepiness questionnaires. Nearly all of these tools use a 5-point Likert scale, although the time frame questioned varies (i.e., recent to past 6 months) depending on the purpose or targeted population.

As a final note, nearly all instruments focus on frequency of sleep problems but few have an eye for severity or change. A trend toward emergence of diagnostic tools is noticeable. To date, each of the instruments remains largely a screening tool and, strikingly, tools for specific clinical populations are lacking (e.g., developmental disabilities). Tables 18.1–18.3 report more detail on their use of the 11 methodological steps.

When developing, using, or reviewing sleep tools, we advocate considering the following points:

- Most instruments are generic in content, such that few study in detail specific sleep behaviors.
- Most instruments query the frequency of sleep behaviors, while their severity or change also may be pertinent.
- Most instruments are parental reports; therefore, more tools for other informants (e.g., self-report, teacher report) should be developed.
- Generation of items, piloting, and item analysis should be (more) extensively reported.
- The 11 steps need to be implemented and reported in instrument development.
- Sleep surveys are primarily used to (retrospectively) study sleep behaviors or habits, while few focus on sleep patterns or sleep environment.
- Most instruments focus on nighttime sleep, yet few tools incorporate napping.
- Tools sensitive to changes in sleep characteristics throughout development should be developed.
- Discuss administration, scoring, interpretation and handling of missing data.
- Differentiation between school days, non-school days, and holidays might be advocated.
- Bedtime, wake-up time, sleep onset latency, and sleep duration are often categorical; boundaries of categories differ or overlap, hampering potential statistical analysis.

Table 18.1 Tools in which Nearly All Psychometric Properties were Evaluated: Basic Information

	Tool acronym	Place of origin	Age	Respondent	Steps fulfilled (see Figure 18.1)
1	**Sleep and Settle Questionnaire** **SSQ** (Matthey, 2001)	Australia	6-week-old infants	Parent	All steps; step 3 and step 10 are not reported in detail
2	**Parental Interactive Bedtime Behavior Scale** **PIBBS** (Morell & Cortina-Borja, 2002)	UK	12–19 months	Parent	All steps except 5, 10, and 11
3	**Maternal Cognitions about Infant Sleep Questionnaire** **MCISQ** (Morrell, 1999)	UK	12.9–16.8 months	Parent	All steps except 10 and 11
4	**Tayside Children's Sleep Questionnaire** **TCSQ** (McGreavey et al., 2005)	UK	1–5 yrs	Parent	All steps except 10 and 11; step 9 is not reported in detail
5	**Bedtime Routines Questionnaire** **BRQ** (Henderson & Jordan, 2009)	USA	2–8 yrs	Parent	All steps except 5, 10, and 11
6	**Children's Sleep Wake Scale** **CSWS** (LeBourgeois, 2003) abstract Sleep 2001 360G 370G	USA	2–8 yrs	Parent	All steps except 5, 7, and 11
7	**Sleep Disorders Inventory for Students—Children** **SDIS-C** (Luginbuehl et al., 2008; Luginbuehl, 2003)	USA	2–10 yrs	Parent	All steps (in step 11 a T-score was applied for ROC analyses)
8	**Pediatric Sleep Questionnaire** **PSQ** (Chervin et al., 2000)	USA	2–18 yrs	Parent	For the 22 items: all except step 11
9	**Behavioral Evaluation of Disorders of Sleep Scale** **BEDS** (Schreck et al., 2003)	USA	5–12 yrs	Parent	All steps except 11; step 5 was not reported

(*continued*)

Table 18.1 (Continued)

	Tool acronym	Place of origin	Age	Respondent	Steps fulfilled (see Figure 18.1)
10	**Sleep-Related Breathing Disorders scale** **SRBD** (Chervin et al., 2002; 2007)	USA	5–12.9 yrs	Parent	9 *See PSQ*
11	**Sleep Disturbance Scale for Children** **SDSC** (Bruni et al., 1996)	Italy	6.5–15.3 yrs	Parent	All steps
12	**Dream Content Questionnaire for Children** **ChDCQ** (Bruni et al., 1999)	Italy	9–13 yrs	Self	All steps except 11
13	**Cleveland Adolescent Sleepiness Questionnaire** **CASQ** (Spilsbury et al., 2007)	USA	11–17 yrs	Self	All steps except 11
14	**Sleep Disorders Inventory for Students—Adolescents** **SDIS-A** (Luginbuehl et al., 2008; Luginbuehl, 2003)	USA	11–18 yrs	Parent	All steps (in step 11 a T-score was applied for ROC analyses)

Table 18.2 Tools in which Psychometric Properties were Evaluated: The how, the which, the type, and the number.

	Tool	Time to complete	Number of questions	Concept details	Time frame/period evaluated	Response format
1	**Sleep and Settle Questionnaire** **SSQ** (Matthey, 2001)	Not specified	34	Baby sleep patterns Time it takes to settle the baby to sleep The duration of crying The temperament of the baby when awake The confidence of the parent at the time of getting the baby to sleep The attributions of the parent to unsettled infant behavior Extent to which the baby's sleep patterns as temperament bother the parent	Last week	5-point Likert scale
2	**Parental Interactive Bedtime Behavior Scale** **PIBBS** (Morell & Cortina-Borja, 2002)	Not specified	22 →19 (but 2 are not incorporated in total score)	Active physical comforting Encouraging infant autonomy Movement Passive physical comforting Social comforting	Not specified	5-point Likert scale
3	**Maternal Cognitions about Infant Sleep Questionnaire** **MCISQ** (Morrell, 1999)	Not specified	27 → 20	Limit setting Anger Doubt Feeding Safety	How you feel with your 13-month old	6-point Likert scale
4	**Tayside Children's Sleep Questionnaire** **TCSQ** (McGreavey et al., 2005)	Not specified	10	Core sleeping problems Parental interventions	Previous 3 months	5-point Likert scale

(continued)

Table 18.2 (Continued)

	Tool	Time to complete	Number of questions	Concept details	Time frame/period evaluated	Response format
5	**Bedtime Routines Questionnaire** **BRQ** (Henderson & Jordan, 2009)	Not specified	35 → 31	Consistency (routine behavior and routine environment: 10 items) Reactivity (to changes in routines: 5 items) Activities (a 2-factor scale comprising adaptive and maladaptive activities: 16 items)	Past month	5-point Likert
6	**Children's Sleep Wake Scale** **CSWS** (LeBourgeois, 2003)	10 min.	77 → 39 (43?)	Going to bed (10 items) Falling asleep (7 items) Awakening/arousing (8 items) Reinitiating sleep (6 items) Returning to wakefulness (8 items)	Past month	3-point Likert scale
7	**Sleep Disorders Inventory for Students—Children** **SDIS-C** (Luginbuehl et al., 2008; Luginbuehl, 2003)	~10min.	25	OSAS: obstructive sleep apnea syndrome EDS: excessive daytime sleepiness PLMD: periodic limb movement disorder DSPS: delayed sleep phase syndrome	Past 6 to 12 months	7-point Likert scale
8	**Pediatric Sleep Questionnaire** **PSQ** (Chervin et al., 2000)	20–30 min.	~70 (Archbold, Pituch, Panahi, & Chervin, 2002)→ 49 (Chervin et al., 2000)→ 22 Being reported in several papers	SRBD: sleep-related breathing disorder (4 items) S: snoring (4 items) SS: sleepiness (4 items) B: inattentive/hyperactive behavior (behavioral problems) (6 items) Other	In general the past month	For sleep items: 3 categories—Yes, No, Do not know Dichotomous Open

9	**Behavioral Evaluation of Disorders of Sleep Scale** **BEDS** (Schreck et al., 2003)	Not specified	107 → 40 → 28	Expressive sleep disturbances (10 items) Sensitivity to the environment (8 items) Disoriented awakening (4 items) *Sleep facilitators (3 items) is dropped in the confirmatory analyses* Apnea/bruxism (3 items)	Past six months	5-point Likert scale
10	**Sleep-Related Breathing Disorders scale** **SRBD or also SDB** (Chervin et al., 2002, 2007)	Not specified	14 (16 or10)	Snoring (4 items) Sleepiness (4 items) Inattention/hyperactivity (6 items)	In general the past month	3 categories
11	**Sleep Disturbance Scale for Children** **SDSC** (Bruni et al., 1996)	10 min (5 min data-entry)	27 → 26	DIMS: disorders of initiating and maintaining sleep (7 items) SBD: sleep breathing disorders (3 items) DA: disorders of arousal (3 items) SWTD: sleep wake transition disorders (6 items) DOES: disorders of excessive somnolence (6 items) SHY: sleep hyperhydrosis (2 items)	Past 6 months	5-point Likert scale

(*continued*)

Table 18.2 (Continued)

	Tool	Time to complete	Number of questions	Concept details	Time frame/period evaluated	Response format
12	**Dream Content Questionnaire for Children** **ChDCQ** (Bruni et al., 1999)	Not specified	63 →44	Action of aggressiveness (8 items) Friendly interactions (7 items) Inhibition of aggressiveness (10 items) Characters and sexual interactions (5 items) Negative emotions (4 items) Positive emotions (3 items) Bizarreness/archetypal (7 items)	Recent dreams or any other remembered	4-point Likert scale and 3 items on frequency of dream recall, nightmare, and look forward to dreams
13	**Cleveland Adolescent Sleepiness Questionnaire** **CASQ** (Spilsbury et al., 2007)	Not specified	46 →40 →35 →16	Sleep in school Alert in school Sleep in evening Sleep in transport	Usual week	5-point Likert scale
14	**Sleep Disorders Inventory for Students—Adolescents** **SDIS-A** Luginbuehl et al., 2008; Luginbuehl, 2003)	~10min	30	OSAS: obstructive sleep apnea syndrome EDS: excessive daytime sleepiness PLMD: periodic limb movement disorder DSPS: delayed sleep phase syndrome NARC: narcolepsy	Past 6 to 12 months	7-point Likert scale

Table 18.3 Tools in which Psychometric Properties were Evaluated: Norms, Validity and Reliability

	Tool	Norms	Validity type	Validity results		Reliability type	Reliability results
1	**Sleep and Settle Questionnaire SSQ** (Matthey, 2001)	Yes		Derived from reports of experiences of women, and men from previous study sample, and piloted with new parents		Test-retest item correlations for "bothersome" items 7–14 days N = 20	0.01 to 0.99
			Concurrent validity	Semistructured interview at 6-weeks postpartum: range 0.18 to 0.43			
			Criterion validity	Comparing SSQ data of the mothers from the class: range 0.46 to 0.64			
			Discriminant validity	Comparison of scores of those reporting no problems versus those that went to class: significant			
			Construct validity of the both-ersome score	Factor analysis of the 9 bother items			
			Sensitivity to change	Filled out by mothers following a treatment program, conducted separately Comparison reports at 6 weeks and 6 months postpartum			
2	**Parental Interactive Bedtime Behavior Scale PIBBS** (Morell & Cortina-Borja, 2002)	No	Convergent validity (Pearson Correlation) with Richman's sleep diary	Active physical comforting:	0.501	Cronbach Alpha of Total (17 items)	0.721
				Encouraging autonomy:	−0.265		
				Settle by movement:	0.103		
				Passive physical comforting:	0.413		
				Social comforting:	0.1		
				Diary derived average weekly hours in parental bed and "settle in parents bed":	0.727		

(continued)

Table 18.3 (Continued)

	Tool	Norms	Validity type	Validity results		Reliability type	Reliability results
			Construct validity (Mann-Whitney U test) control to clinical	Significant at $p < 0.000$ for total percentage scores: active physical comforting minus encourage autonomy plus settle by movement, passive physical comforting and social comforting		Alpha for those fulfilling Richman's criteria of a sleep problem (n = 54)	0.626
				Significant differences for active physical comforting and encourage autonomy subscales			
			Developmental change by Linear Mixed Effects modeling	1-year follow-up show developmental trend (n = 259) (note: effect of temperament was separately modeled)		Alpha for those not fulfilling Richman's criteria of a sleep problem (n = 234)	0.721
				1-year follow-up of 4 sub-groups according to the Richman criteria (presence/absence at time 1 and 2) indicating change			
3	**Maternal Cognitions about Infant Sleep Questionnaire MCISQ** (Morrell, 1999)	No	Construct validity by extreme groups method (Mann-Whitney U test) based on research criteria and based on maternal criteria	Limit setting:	significant	Test-retest reliability (Pearson correlation) N = 34 6 weeks	0.81
				Anger:	significant		
				Doubt:	significant		
				Feeding:	non-significant		
				Safety:	non-significant		
				Total:	significant		
			Convergent validity with composite sleep diary score (n = 59)	Limit setting:	0.52	Cronbach Alpha on remaining items after discarding items with item-total Pearson correlation <0.15, i.e., 20 items	0.82

				Anger:	0.39		
				Doubt:	0.37		
				Feeding:	0.26		
				Safety:	−0.009		Sleep problem group (n = 22): 0.80
				Total:	0.48		
			Convergent validity with Richman's diary when controlling for General Health Questionnaire (GHQ-28)	Limit setting:	0.39		
				Anger:	0.31		
				Doubt:	0.31		Control group (n = 37): 0.84
				Feeding:	n.s.		
				Safety:	n.s.		
				Total:	0.36		
4	**Tayside Children's Sleep Questionnaire TCSQ** (McGreavey et al., 2005)	No		A pilot study in 1–10 years old		Cronbach Alpha	0.85
				Interview mothers of children with and without sleep problems, asses corroboration with test results		Item-total correlations	Range: 0.30–0.72
				Expert consultation			
5	**Bedtime Routines Questionnaire BRQ** (Henderson & Jordan, 2009)	No	Content validation	Theoretically relevant aspects of bedtime routines and review of sleep literature Expert panel for the activity subscale items		Item-total correlation for Consistency factor	0.50–0.73
			Construct validity	Correlations between BRQ and child routines questionnaire, children's sleep hygiene scale, children's sleep wake scale, BASC-2 externalizing score		Item-total correlation for Reactivity factor	0.5–0.61
				Total consistency	0.85–0.88	Item-total correlation	0.26–0.56
				Routine behaviors	0.04–0.56	Cronbach Alpha Total Consistency	0.88

(continued)

Table 18.3 (Continued)

	Tool	Norms	Validity type	Validity results		Reliability type	Reliability results
				Routine environment	−0.03–0.42	Routine behaviors	0.90
				Reactivity	−0.25–0.17	Routine environment	0.83
				Adaptive activities	−0.03–0.70	Reactivity	0.76
				Maladaptive activities	−0.39–0.07	Adaptive activities	0.74
						Maladaptive Activities	0.69
6	**Children's Sleep Wake Scale** **CSWS** (LeBourgeois, 2003)	No	Content validity	Existing literature search and expert consultation		Internal consistency total	0.89
			Structural Equation modeling	AGFI: 0.77 RMSEA: 0.64		Cronbach Alpha	
			Construct validity	6 items were selected as potential indicators of problem severity and correlated to subscale scores: range: 0.018–0.576		Going to bed	0.83
						Falling asleep	0.71
						Arousing/awakening	0.73
						Reinitiating sleep	0.78
						Returning to wakefulness	0.89
7	**Sleep Disorders Inventory for Students—Children** **SDIS-C** (Luginbuehl et al., 2008; Luginbuehl, 2003)	Yes	Content validity	Expert Test Review Panel		Cronbach Alpha	
			Concurrent validity (Pearson correlation) with NPSG	RDI: 0.33 (n = 106) Snore loudly at night: 0.43 (n = 98) N too small for other subscales		total	0.91
						OSAS	0.84

			Sensitivity(Se), specificity(Sp), positive predictive power (PPP), negative predictive power (NPP) (ROC) in hospital diagnosed sample	scale	Se	PPP	Sp	NPP	EDS	0.85	
				DSPS	1	0.71	0.98	1	PLMD	0.85	
				NARC	0.80	0.67	0.98	0.99			
				OSAS	0.91	0.75	0.62	0.84			
				PLMD/RLS	0.50	0.54	0.93	0.91			
					0.83	0.71	0.91	0.95			
			Overall Se	0.83					DSPS	0.76	
			Overall Sp	0.91					Test-retest reliability N = 30 2–6 months	0.97	
8	**Pediatric Sleep Questionnaire PSQ** (Chervin et al., 2000)	No	Logistic regression analyses on SRBD# presence or absence in both groups (controlled for age and gender)	OR: range 3.6–52.4 # = SRBD based on NPSG					Cronbach Alpha	Group A	Group B
			ROC towards SRBD# diagnosis (presence/absence)	AUC			Group A	Group B	S:	0.86	0.86
				S:			0.85	0.85	SS:	0.66	0.77
				SS:			0.8	0.77	B:	0.84	0.83
				B:			0.84	0.79	SRBD:	0.89	0.88
				SRBD:			0.95	0.92	Test-retest (spearman correlation) N = 21 19–67 days		
									S:	0.92	
									SS:	0.66	
									B:	0.83	
									SRDB:	0.75	

(continued)

Table 18.3 (Continued)

	Tool	Norms	Validity type	Validity results		Reliability type	Reliability results	
9	**Behavioral Evaluation of Disorders of Sleep Scale** **BEDS** (Schreck et al., 2003)		Construct face validity	Review of ICSD diagnostic criteria 107 items		Test-retest reliability N = 102 2–3 weeks		
			Parental report of yes/no sleep problem	Spearman correlation 0.14		Internal consistency	Factor 1	0.80 [0.85]
							Factor 2	0.60 [0.65]
							Factor 3	0.78 [0.79]
							Factor 4	*0.69*
							Factor 5	0.25 [0.60]
						total	0.77	
10	**Sleep-Related Breathing Disorders scale** **SRBD** (Chervin et al., 2002, 2007)	No	Spearman correlation between normalized SRBD-score and NPSG parameters	Baseline: –0.30 to 0.52	Follow-up: –0.02 to 0.22 (all n.s.)			
			Logistic regression (adjusted for age)	Baseline: OR: 2.8	Follow-up: OR:1.89			
11	**Sleep Disturbance Scale for Children** **SDSC** (Bruni et al., 1996)	Yes T-score of 70	Comparison between controls and clinical of factors scores	Significant for all		Cronbach Alpha	control	clinical
							0.79	0.71
						Item-total correlation	0.46 – 0.17	0.48 – 0.08
			Factor-total correlation matrix	Control Range: 0.11–0.77 Clinical Range: 0.01–0.69		Test-retest reliability (spearman rank) N = 100 28–46 days	Total: 0.71 Items:0.66 to 0.21	

12	**Dream Content Questionnaire for Children** **ChDCQ** (Bruni et al., 1999)	No	Correlations with Student Sleep Habits Questionnaire (SSHS)	Range: – 0.01 to 0.43		Cronbach Alpha	0.81
						Item-total correlation	0.17–0.47
						Test-retest reliability N = 30 15 days	0.13–0.84
13	**Cleveland Adolescent Sleepiness Questionnaire** **CASQ** (Spilsbury et al., 2007)	No		Expert panel and pre-test in 23 children		Cronbach Alpha	0.89
			Pearson correlation	Control (n = 411)	Clinical (n = 62)		
			with PDSS	0.75	0.70		
			with sleepiness subscale of SSHS	0.72	0.66		
			Sleep-wake patterns	Non-school night: –0.05 – School-night: –0.40 Sleep debt: 0.24	Nonschool night: –0.02 – School-night: –0.34 Sleep debt: 0.20		
			NPSG	With AHI: 0.16—With SEI: –0.15			
14	**Sleep Disorders Inventory for Students—Adolescents** **SDIS-A** (Luginbuehl et al., 2008; Luginbuehl, 2003)	Yes	Content validity	Expert Test Review Panel		Cronbach Alpha	
			Concurrent validity (Pearson correlation) with NPSG	RDI: 0.57 (n = 48) Snore loudly at night: 0.64 (n = 43) N too small for other subscales		total	0.92
						OSAS	0.88
			sensitivity(Se), specificity(Sp), positive predictive power (PPP), negative predictive power (NPP) (ROC)	scale DSPS NARC OSAS PLMD/RLS	se PPP sp NPP 1 0.78 0.95 1 0.88 0.70 0.92 0.97 0.86 0.86 0.88 0.88 0.55 0.75 0.94 0.87 0.81 0.79 0.93 0.94	NARC	0.92
						PLMD/RLS	0.83
						DSPS	0.71
			Overall Se	0.81		EDS	0.83
			Overall Sp	0.93		Test-retest reliability N = 24 2–6 months	0.86

Diaries and Logs

The literature search revealed that these terms are used interchangeably and that a clear distinction was not made between these and the often concomitantly applied actigraphy and its parameter report. Even in these tools, heterogeneity is remarkably apparent in the wording, the order, the layout, the number of questions and when to complete, and in the time-frame or even calculations based on the tool. In addition, a plethora of interpretations are derived from diaries and logs—but the most striking aspect is the lack of any psychometric evaluation.

The proposed 11 methodological steps should be implemented in the development and evaluation of diaries and logs. For example, the Sleep Habits Survey (Wolfson & Carskadon, 1998), developed by one of the editors, is a self-report survey querying students about usual sleeping and waking behaviors over the past 2 weeks. First, besides the sleep time, bedtime, and rise time, the authors investigated weekend delay (i.e., the difference between weekend bedtime and school-night bedtime) and weekend oversleep (i.e., the difference between weekend total sleep time and school-night total sleep time). Second, it questioned whether the respondent had struggled to stay awake or had fallen asleep in 10 different situations in the last 2 weeks. Third, indicators of erratic sleep/wake behaviors over the course of the last 2 weeks (e.g., being late due to oversleeping) were included. More specifically, Wolfson and colleagues (Wolfson & Carskadon, 1998; Wolfson et al., 2003) successfully compared self-reported survey estimates of sleep patterns in adolescents with retrospective survey descriptions of usual school-night and weekend-night sleep habits, diary-reported sleep patterns, and actigraphically estimated sleep behaviors over a subsequent week.

Nonetheless, in logs and diaries researchers and clinicians all too often implicitly expect to have fulfilled these 11 psychometric criteria even though, for example, question order or format potentially has an impact on response and so will additional questions that increase awareness of nighttime behavior or patterns. Therefore, delivery of instructions, training, or try-out has to be considered as well as the feasibility of using the tool within the home environment, family schedules, and so forth. It might be advisable to have the respondent repeat what is expected, how important the gathered information is, and the need for precision. For instance, a confusing layout might affect compliance or completeness. Finally, we advocate that a clear distinction should be made between diary (i.e., a record of what has happened over the course of the recording period, potentially also including person's experiences, thoughts, feelings) and log (i.e., a record as of the performance of equipment or the progress of an undertaking). In the current e-world, 24-hour interfaces with respondents might be enabled as a twenty-first century approach to diaries or logs.

With respect to diaries and logs, the following considerations are noteworthy:

- No psychometric evaluation could be found in the sleep literature
- Diaries and logs are primarily used for (prospectively) studying sleep patterns
- Tremendous heterogeneity rules, hampering comparability
- Differentiation from actigraphic logs should be made, such that the diary or other type of log is seen as an adjunct to manually scoring the actigraphic recording
- Layout is crucial

Sleep Items in Standardized Tools

The first potentially "diagnostic" sleep questions, historically and not surprisingly, were embedded in daytime psychopathology tools, such as Achenbach's Child Behavior Checklist (CBCL; Achenbach, 2011; Gregory et al., 2011) and Sines' Missouri Children's Picture Series (MCPS; Sines, Pauker, Sines, & Owen, 1969), Conners Rating Scales (Conners, 2011), and the Louisville Behavior Checklist (Miller, Hampe, Barrett, & Noble, 1971; Miller & Roid, 1988), all of which were developed in the 1970s. However, only a handful of sleep items appear in each of the 21 instruments we reviewed (Spruyt & Gozal, 2011b), and their psychometric properties are diluted within the realm of daytime indicators with content that is often generic. Such lack of pediatric sleep tools or items within standardized tools available through test publishers underscores the low level of importance given to sleep within a screening process or overall health care approach. Nonetheless, high scores on such sleep items might be a signal for the clinician to discuss sleep in greater depth.

A recent review (Bonuck et al., 2011) on 47 existing tools used for children in the Individuals with Disabilities and Education Act (IDEA) and Early Childhood Special Education (ECSE) programs assessing *(1)* their social-emotional or adaptive functioning, behavior, or temperament; *(2)* employed caregiver direct report; or *(3)* children in the 0–60 month age range indicated that on average, 1.5 items were sleep-related. Indeed, in children whose cognitive impairment or expressive difficulties prevent them from being able to articulate their complaints, sleep problems are often not recognized or are mistaken as part of the challenging behavior or developmental delay/intellectual disability. Overall, 38% of total existing instruments reviewed (n = 67) had no sleep-related items. None of the tools contained a sleep-related breathing item. Similar to an existing tool for a typically developing child, the top questions were about resistance to bedtime, night waking, and parental concern about the child's sleep. Often these were the only items. In Box 18.1 the five most commonly used tools by IDEA are reprinted (Bonuck et al., 2011). In any case these findings are particularly troubling given that in clinical populations there is an increased risk for problematic sleep, and furthermore that 84% of those with sleep problems are reported to have at least two types of sleep disturbances (Kronk et al., 2010).

Even though the above list of standardized tools is not exhaustive, the standardized tools should be considered in light of the following:

- No sleep expertise was mentioned in the manuals, potentially resulting, for example, in generic and few items.
- No sleep validation of items exists, for example, in comparison to other tools.

Unpublished Tools

All the above is likely just the tip of the iceberg, and the vast amount of tools used remain unpublished.

Box 18.1 The 5 most commonly used tools by IDEA

1.	Battelle Developmental Inventory	0–7 years 11 months
2.	Bayley Scales of Infant and Toddler Development	1 to 42 months
3.	Hawaii Early Learning Profile	0–3 years and 3–6 years
4.	Early Learning Accomplishment Profile-revised	0–36 months
5.	Developmental Assessment of Young Children	0–5 years

Through the willingness of colleagues to share their tools we were able to review about 28 instruments. (Spruyt & Gozal, 2011b) In these we discovered that instruments in practice tend toward a history-taking format with descriptive or demographic questions and health status of the child, and sometimes of the child's relatives, in addition to sleep–wake patterns and sleep behaviors. Unfortunately little of such collected data are being entered into a database, which would be an incredibly valuable pool for item analyses and data mining. Of interest might be the newer perspectives; namely, an RLS/PLMD (Restless Legs Syndrome/Periodic Limb Movement Disorder) pediatric screening questionnaire, dream habits, hospitalized children's sleep, and others suggestive of a diversification of the field.

Unpublished tools are to be considered in light of the following:

- Most tools are highly generic.
- Lack of psychometric validation or discussion of the tool tends to be a rule rather than the exception.
- Most focus on nighttime sleep; few include napping.
- Most focus on frequency (hence not severity or changes).
- Tools should be screened for adherence to 11 steps prior to use.

Conclusion

It is clear that much remains to be done, even if in recent years the psychometric evaluation of tools created and applied within the field of pediatric sleep has been growing. Sleep-related breathing and sleepiness disorder questionnaires are probably leading this trend. The majority of sleep questionnaires assess frequency or occurrence, whereas questioning the severity of sleep complaints is seldom performed. It is possible that other response formats (e.g., severity) might be more suitable for certain sleep problems, and this should be explored in the future. Another trend is the application of sleep questionnaires and especially diaries or logs in children with developmental disabilities. With the aid of computers or other e-devices, the field might expand; for example, parents recording behavior through smart phones or a sleep applet in the iPhone, and so forth. Though infrequently reported, endorsement rates could help us toward conducting meta-analyses of sleep items and would further allow visualization of cultural boundaries.

Since 2000 the number of subjective sleep tools has increased substantially (Spruyt & Gozal, 2011b).

However, quantity does not guarantee quality and several important questions need to be addressed: *(1)* What is the conceptual domain of sleep? *(2)* Is the construct "sleep" limited to only objective measures, for example, overnight polysomnography? *(3)* Does the subjective measure need to include all facets of sleep? *(4)* How well do subjective measures correlate or discriminate? *(5)* What are the underlying dimensions of sleep? While acknowledging that a perfect instrument does not exist, a tool still needs to be evaluated by weighing its pros and cons.

In conclusion, very few tools fulfill all the necessary psychometric properties, and few standardized tools exist thus far. None of the tools has any diagnostic power, in other words an independently confirmed adequate sensitivity and specificity to diagnose. It is worthy of note that alpha (reliability) is not a panacea and needs to be interpreted in terms of the number of items, item intercorrelations, and dimensionality. Also, the influence of response format needs to be considered. We welcome studies that compare the psychometric properties and screening performance of subjective sleep tools.

Future Directions

- Studies applying questionnaires or other subjective sleep tools should assess and report their psychometric criteria.
- More subjective tools that measure change or treatment outcome with respect to sleep problems should be developed.
- A clear need is present for tools that incorporate the bidirectional relationship between sleep and medical disorders, neurodevelopmental, and mental health disorders, since these children are at significantly increased risk for sleep problems and may experience exacerbation of emotional and cognitive disturbances because of poor sleep.

Author Note

The author certifies that there is no conflict of interest regarding the material discussed in this chapter.

References

Achenbach, T. M. (2011). Child Behavior Checklist, from http://www.aseba.org. Accessed April 11, 2013.

Archbold, K. H., Pituch, K. J., Panahi, P., & Chervin, R. D. (2002). Symptoms of sleep disturbances among children at two general pediatric clinics. *Journal of Pediatrics, 140*(1), 97–102.

Bonuck, K. A., Hyden, C., Ury, G., Barnett, J., Ashkinaze, H., & Briggs, R. D. (2011). Screening for sleep problems in early intervention and early childhood special education: A systematic review of screening and assessment instruments. *Infants and Young Children, 24*(4), 295–308.

Bruni, O., Ottaviano, S., Guidetti, V., Romoli, M., Innocenzi, M., Cortesi, F., et al. (1996). The Sleep Disturbance Scale for Children (SDSC). Construction and validation of an instrument to evaluate sleep disturbances in childhood and adolescence. *Journal of Sleep Research, 5*(4), 251–261.

Bruni, O., Lo Reto, F., Recine, A., Ottaviano, S., & Guidetti, V. (1999). Development and validation of a dream content questionnaire for school age children. *Sleep and Hypnosis, 1*(1), 41–46.

Chervin, R. D., Hedger, K., Dillon, J. E., & Pituch, K. J. (2000). Pediatric Sleep Questionnaire (PSQ): Validity and reliability of scales for sleep-disordered breathing, snoring, sleepiness, and behavioral problems. *Sleep Medicine, 1*, 21–32.

Chervin, R. D., Archbold, K. H., Dillon, J. E., Panahi, P., Pituch, K. J., Dahl, R. E., et al. (2002). Inattention, hyperactivity, and symptoms of sleep-disordered breathing. *Pediatrics, 109*(3), 449–456.

Chervin, R. D., Weatherly, R. A., Garetz, S. L., Ruzicka, D. L., Giordani, B. J., Hodges, E. K., et al. (2007). Pediatric Sleep Questionnaire: Prediction of sleep apnea and outcomes. *Archives of Otolaryngology—Head & Neck Surgery, 133*(3), 216–222.

Conners, C. K. (2011). Conners Rating Scales, from http://psychcorp.pearsonassessments.com/HAIWEB/Cultures/en-us/Productdetail.htm?Pid=Conners_3. Accessed April 11, 2013.

Gregory, A. M., Cousins, J. C., Forbes, E. E., Trubnick, L., Ryan, N. D., Axelson, D. A., et al. (2011). Sleep items in the child behavior checklist: A comparison with sleep diaries, actigraphy, and polysomnography. *Journal of the American Academy of Child & Adolescent Psychiatry, 50*(5), 499–507.

Henderson, J. A., & Jordan, S. S. (2009). Development and preliminary evaluation of the Bedtime Routines Questionnaire. *Journal of Psychopathology and Behavioral Assessment, 32*, 271–80.

Krieger, J., & Vitiello, M. V. (2011). Another milestone. *Sleep Medicine Reviews, 15*(1), 1.

Kronk, R., Bishop, E. E., Raspa, M., Bickel, J. O., Mandel, D. A., & Bailey, D. B., Jr. (2010). Prevalence, nature, and correlates of sleep problems among children with fragile X syndrome based on a large scale parent survey. *Sleep, 33*(5), 679–687.

LeBourgeois, M. K. (2003). *Validation of the Children's Sleep-Wake Scale.* Unpublished PhD dissertation, The University of Southern Mississippi, United States—Mississippi.

Luginbuehl, M., Bradley-Klug, K. L., Ferron, J., Anderson, W. M., & Benbadis, S. R. (2008). Pediatric sleep disorders: Validation of the Sleep Disorders Inventory for students. *School Psychology Review, 37*(3), 409–431.

Luginbuehl, M. L. (2003). *The initial development and validation study of the Sleep Disorders Inventory for Students.* Unpublished PhD dissertation, University of South Florida, United States—Florida.

Matthey, S. (2001). The Sleep and Settle Questionnaire for parents of infants: Psychometric properties. *Journal of Paediatrics & Child Health, 37*(5), 470–470.

McGreavey, J. A., Donnan, P. T., Pagliari, H. C., & Sullivan, F. M. (2005). The Tayside children's sleep questionnaire: A simple tool to evaluate sleep problems in young children. *Child: Care, Health and Development, 31*(5), 539–544.

Miller, L. C., Hampe, E., Barrett, C. L., & Noble, H. (1971). Children's deviant behavior within the general population. *Journal of Consulting and Clinical Psychology, 37*(1), 16–22.

Miller, L. C., & Roid, G. H. (1988). Factor-analytically derived scales for the Louisville Behavior Checklist. *Journal of Consulting and Clinical Psychology, 56*(2), 302–304.

Morell, J., & Cortina-Borja, M. (2002). The developmental change in strategies parents employ to settle young children to sleep, and their relationship to infant sleeping problems, as assessed by a new questionnaire: The Parental Interactive Bedtime Behaviour Scale. *Infant and Child Development, 11*(1), 17–41.

Morrell, J. M. B. (1999). The role of maternal cognitions in infant sleep problems as assessed by a new instrument, the Maternal Cognitions about Infant Sleep Questionnaire. *Journal of Child Psychology and Psychiatry and Allied Disciplines, 40*(2), 247–258.

Moul, D. E. (2011). The house of questionnaires now has a bedroom, but what is the house's floorplan? *Sleep Medicine Reviews, 15*(1), 3–5.

Sagheri, D., Wiater, A., Steffen, P., & Owens, J. A. (2010). Applying principles of good practice for translation and cross-cultural adaptation of sleep-screening instruments in children. *Behavioral Sleep Medicine, 8*(3), 151–156.

Schreck, K. A., Mulick, J. A., & Rojahn, J. (2003). Development of the Behavioral Evaluation of Disorders of Sleep Scale. *Journal of Child and Family Studies, 12*(3), 349–359.

Sines, J. O., Pauker, J. D., Sines, L. K., & Owen, D. R. (1969). Identification of clinically relevant dimensions of children's behavior. *Journal of Consulting and Clinical Psychology, 33*(6), 728–734.

Spilsbury, J. C., Drotar, D., Rosen, C. L., & Redline, S. (2007). The Cleveland Adolescent Sleepiness Questionnaire: A new measure to assess excessive daytime sleepiness in adolescents. *Journal of Clinical Sleep Medicine, 3*(6), 603–612.

Spruyt, K., & Gozal, D. (2011a). Development of pediatric sleep questionnaires as diagnostic or epidemiological tools: A brief review of dos and don'ts. *Sleep Medicine Reviews, 15*(1), 7–17.

Spruyt, K., & Gozal, D. (2011b). Pediatric sleep questionnaires as diagnostic or epidemiological tools: A review of currently available instruments. *Sleep Med Rev, 15*(1), 19–32.

Stellman, J. M. (Ed.). (1998). *Encyclopaedia of Occupational Health and Safety.*

Wolfson, A. R., & Carskadon, M. A. (1998). Sleep schedules and daytime functioning in adolescents. *Child Development, 69*(4), 875–887.

Wolfson, A. R., Carskadon, M. A., Acebo, C., Seifer, R., Fallone, G., Labyak, S. E., et al. (2003). Evidence for the validity of a sleep habits survey for adolescents. *Sleep, 26*(2), 213–216.

CHAPTER

19 Role of Behavioral Sleep Medicine in Health Care

Valerie McLaughlin Crabtree, Amanda M. Rach, *and* Heather L. Gamble

Abstract

Because many childhood sleep disturbances can be effectively treated by behavioral sleep medicine providers, understanding when and how to refer children for such services is essential to assist families in obtaining the right treatment. A stepped care model of service delivery is an appropriate model, particularly given the high prevalence of behavioral sleep disturbance in childhood and the limited number of trained pediatric behavioral sleep medicine providers. Securing appropriate referrals requires understanding physicians' educational needs with regard to assessment for sleep disturbances and referrals to behavioral sleep medicine providers. The goal of the field of pediatric behavioral sleep medicine, then, is to determine which patients are in greatest need of referrals, match interventions accordingly, and effectively communicate this to physician referral sources.

Key Words: patient referrals, manualized interventions, stepped care, physician education, tailored interventions

Behavioral sleep disturbances are common in infancy, childhood, and adolescence and are identified by hallmark features of difficulty initiating and/or maintaining sleep. In comparison to primary sleep disturbances with a clear medical etiology, behavioral sleep disturbances are precipitated and/or perpetuated by cognitive and behavioral factors that lend themselves to behavioral sleep interventions. As such, many behavioral sleep disturbances can be effectively treated by behavioral sleep medicine providers. Of course, for treatment to be effective, the child or adolescent must first access the provider. The goal of this chapter is to outline empirical support for behavioral sleep medicine interventions, identify referral flow for behavioral sleep medicine providers including appropriate referrals for sleep intervention to and from mental health providers, and propose a model of stepped care delivery in pediatric behavioral sleep medicine.

For psychologists and other behavioral health providers, determining sources and flow of patient referrals is crucial to maintaining a thriving practice and providing the highest quality care to patients with the greatest need for services. For infants, children, and adolescents with sleep disturbances, parents most often seek initial information and treatment from pediatricians and other primary care providers. Unfortunately, few studies have examined the thought process underlying physicians' decisions to refer patients with sleep complaints to behavioral sleep medicine providers. Much of what is known regarding referrals from physicians is more specific to specialty medical care providers, including sleep clinics, rather than specific to behavioral sleep medicine providers.

Support for Behavioral Sleep Interventions

Several sleep disruptions can be effectively treated with behavioral and cognitive-behavioral sleep interventions. Empirical support exists for the treatment of difficulty initiating and maintaining sleep (see Roane and Taylor, Chapter 22), nocturnal enuresis (see Caldwell and Waters, Chapter 26), sleep terrors, recurrent nightmares, somnambulism, and circadian rhythm disturbances, as well as improving adherence to continuous positive airway pressure (CPAP) and bilevel positive airway pressure (BiPAP) used to treat obstructive sleep apnea (OSA) (Hasler & Germain, 2009; Pigeon, Crabtree, & Scherer, 2007; also see Archbold, Chapter 25). Adjunctive nonpharmacologic management of narcolepsy and restless legs syndrome can also be effectively utilized by behavioral sleep medicine providers.

Parasomnias are estimated to affect between 1% and 27% of children, with the least common parasomnia (night terrors) affecting 1%–7% and the most common (sleep talking) affecting 5%–27% (Arruda, Guidetti, Galli, Albuquerque, & Bigal, 2010; Avidan & Kaplish, 2010; Goodwin et al., 2004; Liu et al., 2005; Simola et al., 2010). Parasomnias, such as somnambulism (sleepwalking) in particular, which between 3% and 17% of children experience, can be triggered and/or exacerbated by insufficient sleep in children (Arruda et al., 2010; Avidan & Kaplish, 2010; Goodwin et al., 2004). Behavioral sleep medicine providers can provide nonpharmacologic management of parasomnias through the use of appropriate and adequate sleep scheduling as well as scheduled awakenings. Delayed sleep phase is the most commonly seen circadian rhythm sleep disturbance in adolescents, with a prevalence rate of 0.1% to 3% in the general population (Crowley, Acebo, & Carskadon, 2007), and can often result in truancy and mood disturbance. This circadian rhythm disturbance can be effectively treated through the use of sleep scheduling, light therapy, and appropriate use of melatonin, with secondary improvements in mood and school attendance.

Obstructive sleep apnea is estimated to occur in 1%–4% of children (Lumeng & Chervin, 2008; Praud & Dorion, 2008), and despite adenotonsillectomy (A/T) being the treatment of choice for most cases of pediatric OSA, it is associated with a cure rate of only 80% (Lipton & Gozal, 2003). Thus, a substantial proportion of children still require CPAP/BiPAP treatment for management of their OSA following A/T. Adherence rates in children prescribed CPAP/BiPAP vary widely between 50% and 100% (Marcus et al., 1995; Massa, Gonsalez, Laverty, Wallis, & Lane, 2002; Uong, Epperson, Bathon, & Jeffe, 2007), with adolescents having the lowest rates of adherence (Uong et al., 2007). Behavioral interventions can improve acceptance and use of CPAP/BiPAP mask and equipment. As adherence to CPAP/BiPAP in children and adolescents can be a complex process, psychologists can play an important role in improving adherence to, and therefore benefit from, the intervention. (Koontz, Slifer, Cataldo, & Marcus, 2003; O'Donnell, Bjornson, Bohn, & Kirk, 2006; Rains, 1995).

Behavioral and cognitive-behavioral interventions have also proven useful as adjunctive interventions for treatment of narcolepsy and restless legs syndrome. Although less empirical support exists, many behavioral sleep medicine specialists also have training to assist in the treatment of bruxism, REM sleep behavior disorder, and sleep disturbances comorbid with many psychiatric and medical disorders, such as depression, anxiety, and chronic pain disorders (Pigeon et al., 2007).

Evidence certainly exists to support the role of behavioral sleep interventions in improving sleep in patients. To provide these services, behavioral sleep medicine providers must determine the most appropriate and effective routes for seeking referrals. Little is known regarding the circumstances under which primary care physicians request consultation and what physicians are seeking specifically from a consultation with a behavioral sleep medicine provider. Consultation may involve no transfer of patient care responsibility, transfer of patient care to the specialist, or shared management of a patient's health care (Forrest, Glade, Baker, Bocian, Kang, & Starfield, 1999). Knowing the model of consultation preferred by the referral source a priori will assist behavioral sleep medicine providers in maintaining collaborative relationships with referring physicians to provide the most beneficial patient care.

Who Refers Patients?

Primary Care Physicians' Knowledge of Sleep Disorders Management

Although medical schools and residency programs are placing a greater emphasis on educating students and interns in sleep medicine, in comparison to other specialty areas physicians receive little or no formal training in the assessment and treatment of sleep disorders (Ball et al., 1997; Kramer, Cook, Carlisle, Corwin, & Millman, 1999; Namen et al., 2002). A United Kingdom study of medical students found that the median time formally allocated to sleep and its disorders was 5 minutes (Stores & Wiggs, 1998), with students in the United States reporting an average of 2 hours of training in sleep (Kramer et al., 1999). Unfortunately, the paucity of sleep disorder education is not unique to physicians and also exists within psychology training programs. Meltzer and colleagues found that only 6% of psychology graduate programs and pre-doctoral internship sites offered formal didactic courses in sleep (Meltzer, Phillips, & Mindell, 2009). The insufficient quantity of sleep education for front-line professionals (see Thomas, Avis, and Lichstein Chapter 41) should be considered partially responsible for the low rates of referrals to sleep disorder clinics, which are lower than expected when compared to sleep disorder prevalence rates in adult populations (Bailes et al., 2008; Ball et al., 1997; Kramer et al., 1999; Namen et al., 2002).

Referral from Primary Care in Adult Patients

Because a larger literature base exists to explain referral practices in adult medicine, it is important to first understand how adult primary care physicians make specialty referral decisions before discussing the role of pediatricians in referring to behavioral sleep medicine specialists. Insufficient sleep education and training may underlie the lower than expected referral rates of adult patients to sleep specialists, as health care providers may be unable to recognize the symptoms of sleep disorders that would benefit from specialized treatment. However, physician characteristics also appear to contribute to referral practices. A study examining a group of 55 primary care physicians caring for over 54,000 patients found only 68 (0.13%) patients were referred for polysomnography to rule out OSA over a 1-year period (Kramer et al., 1999). Distribution of referrals across physicians, though, was not even, as 72% of physicians ordered one or no studies, 5% ordered 31% of the studies, and 11% ordered almost half (49%) of all studies (Kramer et al., 1999).

Ten years later, Thornton and colleagues compared rates of physician referral for polysomnography (Thornton et al., 2010). Using the Berlin, a self-report screen for sleep apnea inquiring about OSA risk factors (e.g., snoring, wake-time sleepiness or fatigue, and the presence of obesity or hypertension) (Netzer, Stoohs, Netzer, Clark, & Strohl, 1999), patients scoring within the high-risk range on the Berlin were more likely to receive a polysomnography referral; however, the rate for the entire sample was low, as only 11% of patients were referred (Thornton et al., 2010). Although the authors describe the 11% as disappointing and significantly lower than the rates for mammograms and colonoscopies (63% and 80% respectively), this is substantially higher than the results of Kramer and colleagues (1999) 10 years prior.

It is encouraging that a self-report measure highlighting the potential presence of a problem may increase referral rates for those most in need. As such, behavioral sleep medicine providers should consider providing primary care providers with tools that assist in the identification of patients who are at increased risk for sleep disorders that a qualified behavioral sleep medicine provider could effectively treat. Additional measures that have proven beneficial in increasing rates of referral to sleep specialists have included providing education to and ongoing consultation with primary care physicians (Ball et al., 1997). Thus, behavioral medicine providers with specialized training in the treatment of sleep disorders may further impact referral practices by educating primary care providers and the general community as to the symptoms and treatment options for sleep disorders. Playing the role of informal consultant and support for physicians is an excellent opportunity for behavioral sleep medicine specialists to influence referral practices.

Physicians' opinions regarding treatment approaches for insomnia indicated a preference for modification of lifestyle factors (e.g., caffeine intake, exercise, and daytime napping) as front-line treatment of insomnia (Dollman, LeBlanc, & Roughead, 2003). Second to modifying lifestyle factors, physicians reported that prescriptions, specifically benzodiazepines, followed by referrals to other health care professionals were the most appropriate targets of intervention. Although physicians reported preferring nonpharmacologic interventions, they described patients' strong desires for medication as a barrier to suggesting nondrug alternatives but reported being willing to discuss nondrug treatments if the patient initiated the conversation (Dollman et al., 2003). This suggests that physicians consider both their own preferences and those of the patient when making referral decisions. Thus, psychologists can influence referral practices by educating parents to initiate conversations with their child's health care provider regarding nonpharmacological treatment options for their behavioral sleep disturbances.

Pediatricians' Knowledge of Sleep Disorders Management

Sleep disturbances in children and adolescents are a common concern among behavioral problems presented to pediatricians, with approximately 25% to 40% of all children and adolescents experiencing a behavioral sleep disturbance of some kind (Mindell & Owens, 2003; Owens, 2005). Mindell and colleagues (1994) sought to better understand pediatricians' training and knowledge of sleep and sleep disorders in children as well as their actual treatment practices for sleep problems. Findings revealed a staggering lack of training in sleep and sleep disorders across pediatric residency programs, despite the fact that sleep problems in children is a major concern for parents. Despite practicing pediatricians being well informed about developmental sleep needs and sleep hygiene, they lacked crucial knowledge for diagnosis and managing specific sleep disorders in children (Mindell, Moline, Zendell, Brown, & Fry, 1994). Finally, the majority of surveyed pediatricians reported recommending appropriate behavioral interventions for sleep problems; however, 15% endorsed prescribing often contraindicated pharmacotherapy or misinforming parents that their child would outgrow his or her sleep difficulty (Mindell et al., 1994). The authors did not assess whether or how often the participating pediatricians made referrals for children with sleep difficulties to sleep specialists; however, 65% reported "usually" or "always" successfully treating children's sleep problems (Mindell et al., 1994).

More than 15 years later, in a study designed to evaluate the prevalence of International Classification of Disease, 9th Revision (ICD-9) sleep disorders diagnosed by pediatric medical providers, 3.7% of youth received an ICD-9 sleep diagnosis, which is significantly lower than prevalence rates previously reported in epidemiological studies (Meltzer, Johnson, Crosette, Ramos, & Mindell, 2010). The authors suggested that primary care providers may be underdiagnosing sleep disorders in children and adolescents, and they suggested additional education and support for pediatric primary care providers to assist in the diagnosis and treatment of pediatric sleep problems (Meltzer et al., 2010).

Two separate studies examining basic sleep disorders knowledge in primary care pediatricians have revealed deficits in basic knowledge of pediatric sleep and sleep disorders, as well as low perceived ability to accurately identify and successfully treat such disorders (Owens, 2001; Tamay et al., 2006). Pediatricians were most knowledgeable in developmental and behavioral aspects of children's sleep but less knowledgeable with regard to specific sleep disorders such as sleep disordered breathing, disorders of excessive daytime sleepiness, and sleep-related movement disorders. Furthermore, although the majority of pediatricians reported routinely inquiring about sleep issues during well-child examinations, many failed to ask more than a single sleep question, suggesting that an inadequate assessment may fail to accurately identify patients with sleep problems. More concerning was the finding that the percentage of pediatricians who did not screen for sleep disturbances or asked only one sleep question ranged from 42% in infants, to 52% in school-age children, to 74% in adolescents (Owens, 2001). Findings also highlighted that 53% of respondents never or rarely suggested overnight polysomnographies to evaluate and subsequently treat pediatric sleep problems such as obstructive sleep apnea (Owens, 2001). Of note, those with subspecialty training, such as pediatric pulmonologists, exhibited better knowledge of sleep disordered breathing, suggesting the need for improved training in sleep disorders in general pediatrics residency programs (Tamay et al., 2006).

Referrals from Pediatricians to Subspecialists

Because pediatric behavioral sleep medicine providers most often seek referrals from pediatricians and pediatric subspecialists, understanding the referral process taken most often by pediatric specialists is important. Unfortunately, very little information regarding pediatricians' referrals to behavioral providers is available. When investigating referrals to other pediatric specialists, in a prospective study utilizing a national primary care practice–based research network, pediatricians referred patients to specialists during approximately 2% of office visits. Seeking advice on patient diagnosis or treatment accounted for the majority of reasons for referral (74%), and referral to mental health specialists typically resulted in shared management of patient care (Forrest et al., 1999). Most physicians referring for dental care provide parents with the name of the dentist, though slightly over half will also have their staff call the dental office to schedule an appointment for the child (de la Cruz, Rozier, & Slade, 2004). Important conclusions can be drawn and applied to referrals to behavioral sleep medicine specialists. Behavioral providers must develop working partnerships with primary care physicians in their local community so that physicians are aware of appropriate referral services.

Which Patients Should Be Referred?

Understanding and evaluating a child's sleep needs according to developmental stage is key to physicians making appropriate decisions regarding referral for sleep problems. Babcock (2011) argues that sleep assessment should be a standard component of children's routine medical exams, with referrals outside of the primary care office dependent upon the child's developmental level, comorbid medical conditions, and specific sleep disturbances reported by parents. For example, infant sleep problems may not require referral to a sleep physician. Instead, a behavioral sleep medicine provider or primary care provider may be more appropriate, as many infant sleep problems can be addressed through behavioral intervention and modified parenting strategies (Babcock, 2011).

During the school-age years, common sleep complaints include snoring and other symptoms of sleep disordered breathing, including neuropsychological and neurocognitive deficits such as symptoms of attention-deficit/hyperactivity disorder, learning disabilities, and psychological disorders. For such concerns, a referral may be necessary for psychoeducational assessment and/or nocturnal polysomnography (Babcock, 2011). Certainly, school-age children also may exhibit specific behavioral sleep disturbances including difficulty initiating and maintaining sleep, undesired co-sleeping, nocturnal enuresis, and recurrent nightmares, all of which would likely benefit from referral to a behavioral sleep medicine provider.

During adolescence, fatigue and daytime sleepiness may become a more specific complaint and thorough assessment by the primary care physician should include medical (e.g., acute and chronic illness, medication reactions, snoring or respiratory problems, diabetes), psychological (e.g., depression, anxiety, substance use, family or personal stress), and sleep-related (e.g., sleep phase delay, late bedtime, use of electronics at sleep onset, caffeine consumption) factors. For many adolescent sleep concerns related to sleep hygiene factors, providing adolescents and their families with information regarding appropriate sleep hygiene may suffice (Babcock, 2011); however, adolescents whose sleep does not improve relatively quickly following provision of information and those with psychological etiologies of their sleep disturbance should be referred to a behavioral sleep medicine provider.

Not all infants, children, and adolescents with sleep disturbances will require the specialized intervention services of a behavioral sleep specialist. Use of a "stepped care" model ensures that children and adolescents most in need of services reach the providers with the most specialized training, which is especially important given the limited resource of trained behavioral sleep medicine specialists. Espie (2009) proposed a stepped care model of cognitive-behavioral therapy for insomnia (CBT-I) that could be applied to infant and child behavioral sleep disturbances as well. As is the case in stepped care models, thorough assessment of the problem is necessary to determine the appropriate entry pathway for the patient. Some children with less severe sleep disturbances may see significant improvement with proper parent/child education, sleep hygiene instruction, bibliotherapy, or web-based intervention. For example, with the assistance of Jodi Mindell, PhD, Johnson & Johnson Co. developed an online tool for parents to assist with their children's sleep disturbances that demonstrated significant improvement in children's parent-reported sleep difficulties, as well as improvement in maternal mood and sleep (Mindell et al., 2011). An online sleep assessment tool may be a particularly salient method to provide parents with educational material regarding minimal intervention techniques such as calming routines at bedtime and sleep hygiene practices.

Children with only moderate sleep problems may be well served by their primary care provider and/or by providers trained in delivering manualized interventions. Currently, manualized CBT-I interventions have been empirically validated for use in adults (see Figure 19.1; Espie, 2009), and certainly the need exists for empirically supported manualized behavioral sleep interventions for infants and children that could be administered by providers trained in manual administration. Promising interventions have been trialed in adolescents (Bootzin & Stevens, 2005; Schlarb, Liddle, & Hautzinger, 2011) and can provide the basis for manualized interventions that can be conducted with the full range of pediatric patients. At the time of this writing, a team of researchers led by Greg Clarke and Allison Harvey are funded by the National Institute of Mental Health to empirically evaluate a behavioral sleep medicine intervention in youth with depression, lending further support to the use of manualized interventions. When empirically supported manualized interventions are appropriately disseminated, only a small fraction of patients, then, would require specific behavioral sleep intervention.

The Need for a Stepped Care Model in Children's Behavioral Sleep Disturbances

A large number of children with sleep disorders are seen outside of sleep specialty centers by pediatricians, general practitioners, and child psychiatrists; however, it is likely that many children (and adults) do not receive specialized services by sleep specialists and perhaps when they do, the care

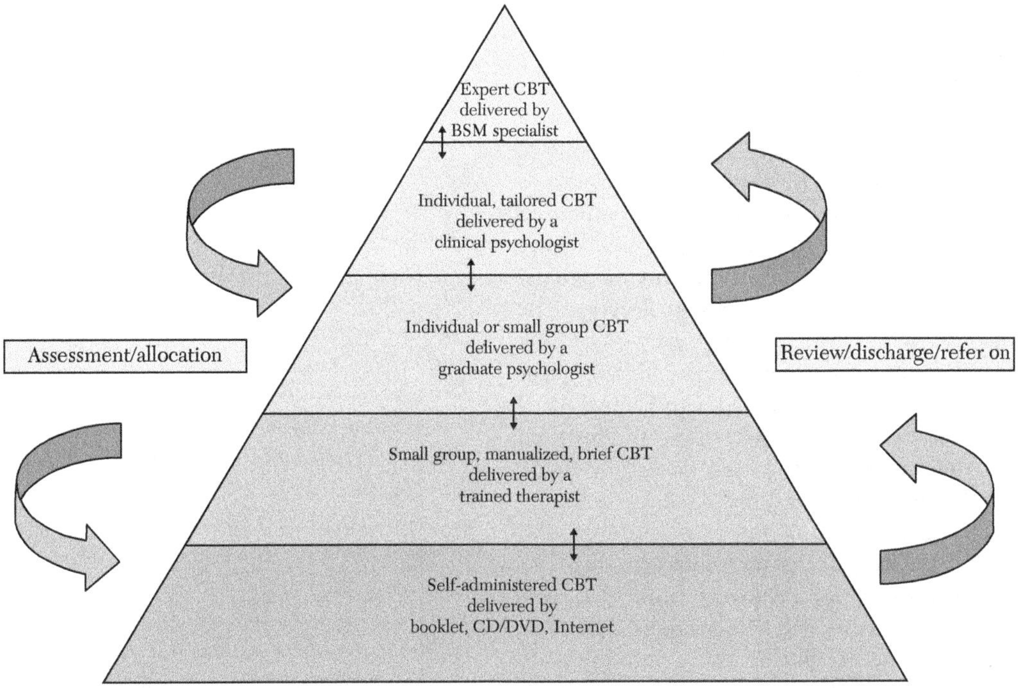

Figure 19.1 Espie's (2009) Model of Stepped Care Delivery of Insomnia Interventions.

is inadequate (Stores & Wiggs, 1998). Stores and Wiggs (1998) suggested that postgraduate medical training in the United Kingdom, United States, and Europe provides minimal instruction in pediatric sleep and sleep disorders, and that services, when provided, tend to be restricted to general night wakings or nocturnal enuresis rather than the broad range of sleep difficulties that exist. Similar to Espie's pyramid model of referral, Stores and Wiggs (1998) proposed a three-tiered system of provision of treatment for children's medical and behavioral sleep disorders. First, it was recommended that a majority of sleep problems could be assessed and adequately treated within the primary care setting. For more severe disorders and those requiring more intensive treatment, referrals may be made to other pediatric services such as pediatric neurologists, psychologists, and child psychiatrists, who may work collaboratively to provide services. Finally, when such attempts have limited effects or the sleep disorder requires more specialized diagnostic, assessment, and treatment options, the authors recommended that referrals be made to regional tertiary services, such as a comprehensive pediatric medical center (see Table 19.1).

For mental health professionals needing to make a referral to a regional tertiary care service, resources are available to assist in finding the most appropriate referral. For a child who requires evaluation and/or treatment at a regional sleep medicine center, the American Academy of Sleep Medicine maintains a website with a list of accredited sleep centers that can be found at www.sleepcenters.org. Board-certified sleep medicine physicians can be identified through the American Board of Medical Specialties at www.abms.org. All board-certified sleep medicine physicians will have completed a residency in a primary care specialty, anesthesiology, otolaryngology, neurology, or psychiatry, followed by specialty training in sleep medicine. Board-certified sleep medicine physicians may provide diagnosis and management of children and adults. As a result, it is in the best interest of a mental health professional making a referral to ensure that the physician has experience

Table 19.1 Indicators of Need for Referral to a Sleep Medicine Provider

Excessive daytime sleepiness
Restless sleep
Significant daytime fatigue
Sleep maintenance difficulties
Snoring/breathing pauses in sleep
Sweating in sleep
Persistent sleep disturbance following appropriate implementation of intervention

in treating children and adolescents either by confirming with the sleep medicine clinic, locating a clinic affiliated with a children's hospital, or identifying board-certified sleep medicine physicians who have completed a residency in a pediatric specialty.

To assist this referral process, we propose a model whereby children with more commonly seen and transient sleep disruptions could have recommendations made for alterations of parenting behaviors, environmental cues, or sleep hygiene instructions within the primary care physician's office. Sleep disturbances appropriate for this entry point would include undesired co-sleeping, bedtime refusal, nocturnal awakenings, pre-bedtime anxiety, and transient nightmares (See Table 19.2). Those children who continue to have difficulty sleeping after provision of advice, or children who require more specific behavioral interventions (i.e., nocturnal enuresis), would then be provided with resources for parents including books, websites, and sleep hygiene pamphlets. These would provide more detailed instructions to parents regarding how to implement behavioral modification packages to address commonly seen childhood sleep disturbances. For those children whose sleep disturbances persist, or for children who present to their primary care provider with long-standing sleep disruption, manualized interventions are most appropriate. As mentioned, manualized interventions for childhood sleep disturbances do not yet have the overwhelming support that currently exists for adult CBT-I manuals. Thus, it is necessary for behavioral sleep medicine researchers to empirically validate manuals for childhood behavioral sleep disorders that can be implemented by advanced practice nurses, licensed clinical social workers, and other behavioral sleep medicine providers interested in and trained to deliver such interventions on a broader scope and in small group formats.

Table 19.2 Pediatricians' Decision Tree for Behavioral Sleep Medicine Referrals

Treat
Undesired co-sleeping
Bedtime resistance
Common nightmares
Primary nocturnal enuresis
Refer
Persistent nocturnal enuresis
Frequent night wakings
Circadian rhythm sleep disturbances
Sleep disruption comorbid with a psychiatric disorder
Primary sleep disorder
Recurrent nightmares
Any sleep disturbance that is not readily ameliorated with advice and reassurance

Clinical Case Example

A 3-year-old girl presents to her pediatrician for a well-child visit. Her parents report that she has been sleeping in their bed since infancy. Her mother is pregnant and wishes to have her daughter sleep in her own room to prepare for the arrival of the new baby. The pediatrician provides advice in the form of suggesting that the parents place the child in her room, sit with her until she falls asleep, and then leave the room. She then suggests that the parents move their chair to the hallway until the child falls asleep, eventually allowing her to fall asleep independently. The parents return to the pediatrician one month later to report that she has been getting out of bed repeatedly throughout the night, crying for her parents, and refusing to fall asleep such that they are now allowing her into their bed at the beginning of the night. The pediatrician then provides the parents with a brochure targeting undesired co-sleeping and suggests that if following a more specific plan described in the brochure is unhelpful, they should enroll in a group parenting session at the local children's hospital provided by a nurse practitioner trained in behavioral sleep interventions. The parents enroll in the course after repeated failed attempts at encouraging their daughter to fall asleep in her room. They are guided through a manualized intervention targeted at bedtime resistance and undesired co-sleeping in young children. After four weeks, their daughter is falling asleep independently in her bed and sleeping through the night.

Children whose sleep problems continue to persist following manualized interventions would then be "stepped up" to treatment by a licensed psychologist. Furthermore, a licensed mental health provider would be the entry point for children with comorbid mood difficulties or other psychiatric disorders such as attention-deficit/hyperactivity disorder (ADHD), significant behavioral disturbances, and/or recurrent nightmares. A further step up would be treatment by a licensed psychologist with specific behavioral sleep medicine training and expertise. A pediatric psychologist certified in behavioral sleep medicine is the referral of choice for children whose sleep disturbances persist after treatment by general licensed psychologists and the entry point for children with specific sleep disorders, such as circadian rhythm sleep disturbances, narcolepsy, or

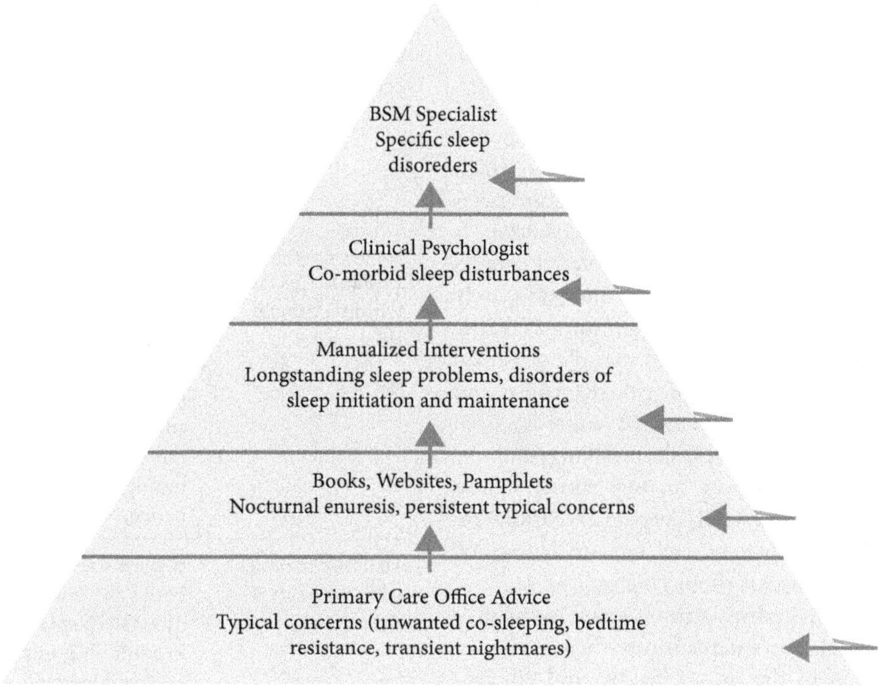

Figure 19.2 Proposed Stepped Care Model of Pediatric BSM Delivery.

obstructive sleep apnea who require CPAP/BiPAP adherence interventions. In this way, treatment approaches and referrals can be tailored specifically to the individual child's needs while ensuring that a limited resource (licensed psychologists with behavioral sleep medicine expertise) is providing service to those patients with greatest need. Ideally, this referral practice would be disseminated to providers who are the primary source of patient referrals (see Figure 19.2).

Clinical Case Example

A 9-year-old boy presents to his pediatrician for routine medication management of his ADHD. His mother reports that he is having significant difficulty initiating sleep more often than not, has very restless sleep, and is extremely difficult to awaken in the morning. He has recently had more behavioral problems at school, is making increasingly poor grades, and is at risk of failing the 3rd grade. His pediatrician refers him to a clinical child psychologist in the community. The psychologist coordinates with the school to institute a behavior modification package to address the classroom disruptions and works with the mother to normalize the child's pre-bedtime routine, bedtime/waketime schedule, and provide incentives for following all aspects of the behavioral intervention package. His behavioral difficulties at school improve to some degree, though he continues to struggle academically. His mother reports that she has been able to normalize his bedtime/waketime schedule but that he still has significant difficulty initiating and maintaining sleep on many nights. The psychologist refers him to a pediatric psychologist certified in behavioral sleep medicine. The behavioral sleep medicine specialist then refers the child to a pediatric sleep physician in his group. A nocturnal polysomnography reveals restless legs syndrome, and laboratory studies indicate low serum ferritin. Iron supplementation is recommended by the physician, and the behavioral sleep medicine specialist continues to work with the mother on improving the child's pre-bedtime routine and sleep/wake schedule. The psychologist also addresses nonpharmacologic adjunctive management of his restless legs syndrome. After 3 months, the child is initiating and maintaining sleep well and performing significantly better, both academically and behaviorally, in the classroom.

How Is the Need for Referrals Communicated?

Behavioral sleep medicine providers need to communicate to referral sources both how to identify children and adolescents most in need of specialized intervention and how to make the referral.

Of significant importance in each of these decisions is the knowledge base of the referring provider.

Educating Pediatric Specialists

Behavioral sleep medicine providers have a significant role in educating referring providers as to which patients fall in the top tier of the stepped care pyramid and how to refer for behavioral intervention. It is crucial to provide information to referral sources as to the sleep disturbances that are most effectively ameliorated with behavioral interventions. Pediatric specialists must be educated as to the role of behavioral sleep interventions in improving sleep onset and maintenance difficulties, nocturnal enuresis, sleep terrors, recurrent nightmares, sleepwalking, and circadian rhythm disturbances. As they gain awareness of the impact of behavioral sleep interventions on sleep disturbances, their referral rates to behavioral sleep medicine providers should increase.

As pediatric specialists become aware of the utility of behavioral sleep interventions, they then must be educated as to the most effective and efficient ways to provide patients and families with referrals. The model of practice of both the sleep clinic and the behavioral sleep medicine provider dictates how referrals will be made.

Models of Pediatric Sleep Practice

Pediatric sleep medicine emphasizes the developmental aspects of sleep and includes a number of clinical sleep disorders that are unique to children and adolescents (Owens & Mindell, 2002). Due to the biopsychosocial nature of sleep problems, the high prevalence of dual and triple diagnoses, especially comorbid behavioral issues in children, the underlying medical conditions, and the neuropsychological and social functioning of patients and their families, pediatric sleep specialists and sleep centers need to be prepared to assess and treat a wide range of disorders across a range of ages and developmental levels (Owens & Mindell, 2002; Wiggs, 2003). This multidisciplinary nature means that in addition to physicians, a number of other disciplines (behavioral pediatricians, child psychiatrists, pediatric psychologists, pediatric and family nurse practitioners, psychiatric social workers, and other behavioral sleep medicine providers) should be involved in the development and delivery of these services (Owens & Mindell, 2002). To accomplish this goal, a number of practice models have been identified for the provision of children's sleep services with significant diversity in the conceptualization of these services (see Table 19.3; Owens & Mindell, 2002).

Table 19.3 Practice Models for Pediatric Sleep Treatment

Pediatric sleep center	• Freestanding sleep practice exclusively dedicated to pediatric patients • Some will have their own pediatric laboratory, while others refer patients to an affiliated adult sleep laboratory
Pediatric specialist within a general sleep center	• Incorporating a pediatric sleep medicine specialist within the context of general sleep center • One individual maintains a practice devoted exclusively to children and adolescents, with the affiliated sleep laboratory testing both adults and pediatric patients
Pediatric patients within a general sleep center	• A general sleep specialist sees both adult and pediatric patients • These sleep specialists are trained in adult sleep medicine but also treat children and adolescents
Pediatric sleep practice within a general practice	• Incorporation of a pediatric sleep service within a general setting • This appears to be more common of psychologists working within a psychology setting (department of psychology or pediatric center)

Note: Adapted with permission from Owens & Mindell (2002).

Due to the multiple models for pediatric sleep interventions, practitioners who provide behavioral sleep medicine services may have different roles within each practice. While some behavioral sleep medicine providers may be embedded within the practice, others may maintain a separate practice. For providers embedded within the sleep medicine clinic, referrals will often come from within the sleep medicine practice. In this context, children and adolescents are often first evaluated by the sleep medicine physician and, as behavioral sleep medicine disturbances are discovered, referrals are made for behavioral intervention within the clinic. In other cases, children and adolescents are referred directly to the behavioral sleep medicine provider when the clear reason for referral is a behavioral sleep disturbance. For behavioral sleep medicine providers who are located in practices outside of a sleep center, referrals may come from sleep centers or from primary care physicians. For this reason, education of physicians regarding when behavioral sleep disturbances require referrals and how to best make those referrals is essential. Although most sleep medicine physicians are acutely aware of the role of behavioral sleep specialists in improving insomnia and other behavioral sleep disturbances, it is imperative for behavioral sleep medicine providers to ensure that sleep medicine physicians are educated as to the adjunctive role that can be provided in managing narcolepsy, restless legs syndrome, bruxism, sleep disturbances with comorbid medical and psychiatric disorders, and CPAP/BiPAP adherence.

Just as pediatric sleep providers have multiple models of intervention, so do behavioral sleep providers. The distinction primarily is drawn between integrated versus outside services (see Table 19.4).

Interdisciplinary Treatment

In an ideal setting, a team treatment approach best addresses the multifaceted nature of sleep disorders. The two primary approaches (multidisciplinary and interdisciplinary) share certain characteristics but differ in important ways. A traditional multidisciplinary team includes members from different disciplines who have independent roles and meet to share patient information. Although team members may meet regularly, there is not necessarily an attempt to create a common plan. Interdisciplinary teams, on the other hand, include members from different disciplines; however, the team works collaboratively with interdependent roles. The team makes assessment and decisions about treatment together.

Table 19.4 Models of Behavioral Sleep Medicine Practice

Integrated Center	BSM integrated within sleep center
Medical Center Referral	Referral outside sleep center but within medical center
Psychology/Psychiatry Department	Referral to outside large psychology/psychiatry department
Outside Referral	Referral to outside psychotherapy practice with behavioral sleep expertise
Contract	Referral to contracted behavioral sleep provider with specific follow-up provided.

Note: Adapted with permission from Pigeon et al. (2007).

Benefits of interdisciplinary care in the treatment of pediatric behavioral sleep disturbances involve the ability to approach each presenting problem from a number of angles, resulting in comprehensive and immediate feedback (Meltzer, Moore, & Mindell, 2008) and integrating information across disciplines to reduce the likelihood parents will receive contradictory recommendations from different providers (Sheehan, Robertson, & Ormond, 2007). This latter benefit is important, as a review of pediatric sleep clinics in the United Kingdom found that poor outcomes at follow-up were not related to the nature or complexity of the sleep disorder or the type of treatment recommended, but rather to poor communication between health professionals involved in the child's care (Wiggs, 2003).

As awareness regarding sleep disorders and treatment options grows, multidisciplinary and interdisciplinary teams will become increasingly important in the delivery of behavioral interventions for sleep disorders. Currently, most behavioral interventions are delivered in mental health or sleep disorder clinics, which means only a small fraction of those who could benefit are actually provided with the service (Goodie, Isler, Hunter, & Peterson, 2009). By incorporating psychologists and other behavioral health specialists into the provision of primary care, the barriers to treatment implementation such as limited training in behavioral approaches (Richardson, 2000), limited appointment time (Goodie et al., 2009), and patient expectations regarding medication (Dollman et al., 2003) will no longer be applicable. Further, using a psychologist or other health care provider trained to deliver behavioral interventions may also enable a small-group approach, which is highly cost-efficient, (Espie, Inglis, Tessier, & Harvey, 2001).

Future Directions

Certainly, pediatric behavioral sleep medicine providers are a limited resource with a large number of infants, children, and adolescents presenting to their primary care physicians with identified sleep problems. Because of this limited resource, a stepped care model is an appropriate framework for identifying those children and adolescents at greatest need of the most specialized intervention services. It should be the mission of the field of behavioral sleep medicine, then, to *(1)* identify which patients should receive which level of specialized care; *(2)* develop and empirically evaluate manualized interventions for the most common childhood behavioral sleep disturbances; *(3)* train care providers to implement empirically supported manualized interventions; and *(4)* educate the referral sources as to which patients to refer to which level of care.

References

Arruda, M. A., Guidetti, V., Galli, F., Albuquerque, R. C. A. P., & Bigal, M. E. (2010). Childhood periodic syndromes: a population-based study. *Pediatric Neurology, 43*(6), 420–424.

Avidan, A. Y., & Kaplish, N. (2010). The parasomnias: Epidemiology, clinical features, and diagnostic approach. *Clinics in Chest Medicine, 31*(2), 353–370.

Babcock, D. A. (2011). Evaluating sleep and sleep disorders in the pediatric primary care setting. *Pediatric Clinics of North America, 58*(3), 543–554.

Bailes, S., Baltzan, M., Rizzo, D., Fichten, C. S., Amsel, R., & Libman, E. (2008). A diagnostic symptom profile for sleep disorder in primary care patients. *Journal of Psychosomatic Research, 64*(4), 427–433.

Ball, E. M., Simon, R. D., Jr, Tall, A. A., Banks, M. B., Nino-Murcia, G., & Dement, W. C. (1997). Diagnosis and treatment of sleep apnea within the community. The Walla Walla Project. *Archives of Internal Medicine, 157*(4), 419–424.

Bootzin, R.R., & Stevens, S.J. (2005). Adolescents, substance abuse, and the treatment of insomnia and daytime sleepiness. *Clinical Psychology Review, 25(5),* 629–644.

Crowley, S. J., Acebo, C., & Carskadon, M. A. (2007). Sleep, circadian rhythms, and delayed phase in adolescence. *Sleep Medicine, 8*(6), 602–612.

de la Cruz, G. G., Rozier, R. G., & Slade, G. (2004). Dental screening and referral of young children by pediatric primary care providers. *Pediatrics, 114*(5), e642-e652.

Dollman, W. B., LeBlanc, V. T., & Roughead, E. E. (2003). Managing insomnia in the elderly—what prevents us using non-drug options? *Journal of Clinical Pharmacy and Therapeutics, 28*(6), 485–491.

Espie, C. A., Inglis, S. J., Tessier, S., & Harvey, L. (2001). The clinical effectiveness of cognitive behaviour therapy for chronic insomnia: Implementation and evaluation of a sleep clinic in general medical practice. *Behaviour Research and Therapy, 39*(1), 45–60.

Espie, C.A. (2009). "Stepped care": A health technology solution for delivering cognitive behavioral therapy as a first line insomnia treatment. *Sleep, 32(12),* 1549–1558.

Forrest, C. B., Glade, G. B., Baker, A. E., Bocian, A. B., Kang, M., & Starfield, B. (1999). The pediatric primary-specialty care interface: How pediatricians refer children and adolescents to specialty care. *Archives of Pediatrics & Adolescent Medicine, 153*(7), 705–714.

Goodie, J. L., Isler, W. C., Hunter, C., & Peterson, A. L. (2009). Using behavioral health consultants to treat insomnia in primary care: A clinical case series. *Journal of Clinical Psychology, 65*(3), 294–304.

Goodwin, J., Kaemingk, K., Fregosi, R., Rosen, G., Morgan, W., Smith, T., & Quan, S. (2004). Parasomnias and sleep disordered breathing in Caucasian and Hispanic children—the Tucson children's assessment of sleep apnea study. *BMC Medicine, 2*(1), 14.

Hasler, B., & Germain, A. (2009). Correlates and treatments of nightmares in adults. *Sleep Medicine Clinics, 4*(4), 507–517.

Koontz, K. L., Slifer, K. J., Cataldo, M. D., & Marcus, C. L. (2003). Improving pediatric compliance with positive airway pressure therapy: The impact of behavioral intervention. *Sleep, 15*(26), 1010–1015.

Kramer, N. R., Cook, T. E., Carlisle, C. C., Corwin, R. W., & Millman, R. P. (1999). The role of the primary care physician in recognizing obstructive sleep apnea. *Archives of Internal Medicine, 159*(9), 965–968.

Lipton, A. J., & Gozal, D. (2003). Treatment of obstructive sleep apnea in children: Do we really know how? *Sleep Medicine Reviews, 7*(1), 61–80.

Liu, X., Ma, Y., Wang, Y., Jiang, Q., Rao, X., Lu, X., & Teng, H. (2005). Brief report: An epidemiologic survey of the prevalence of sleep disorders among children 2 to 12 years old in Beijing, China. *Pediatrics, 115*(Supplement 1), 266–268.

Lumeng, J. C., & Chervin, R. D. (2008). Epidemiology of pediatric obstructive sleep apnea. *Proceedings of the American Thoracic Society, 5*(2), 242–252. d

Marcus, C. L., Ward, S. L. D., Mallory, G. B., Rosen, C. L., Beckerman, R. C., Weese-Mayer, D. E., et al. (1995). Use of nasal continuous positive airway pressure as treatment of childhood obstructive sleep apnea. *The Journal of Pediatrics, 127*(1), 88–94.

Massa, F., Gonsalez, S., Laverty, A., Wallis, C., & Lane, R. (2002). The use of nasal continuous positive airway pressure to treat obstructive sleep apnoea. *Archives of Disease in Childhood, 87*(5), 438–443.

Meltzer, L. J., Moore, M., & Mindell, J. A. (2008). The need for interdisciplinary pediatric sleep clinics. *Behavioral Sleep Medicine, 6*(4), 268–282.

Meltzer, L. J., Phillips, C., & Mindell, J. A. (2009). Clinical psychology training in sleep and sleep disorders. *Journal of Clinical Psychology, 65*(3), 305–318.

Meltzer, L. J., Johnson, C., Crosette, J., Ramos, M., & Mindell, J. A. (2010). Prevalence of diagnosed sleep disorders in pediatric primary care practices. [Research Support, N.I.H., Extramural]. *Pediatrics, 125*(6), e1410–1418.

Mindell, J. A., Moline, M. L., Zendell, S. M., Brown, L. W., & Fry, J. M. (1994). Pediatricians and sleep disorders: Training and practice. *Pediatrics, 94*(2), 194–200.

Mindell, J. A., & Owens, J. (2003). *A Clinical Guide to Pediatric Sleep: Diagnosis and Management of Sleep Problems.* Philadelphia: Lippincott Williams Wilkins.

Mindell, J. A., Du Mond, C. E., Sadeh, A., Telofski, L. S., Kulkarni, N., & Gunn, E. (2011). Efficacy of an internet-based intervention for infant and toddler sleep disturbances. [Randomized Controlled Trial Research Support, Non-U.S. Gov't]. *Sleep, 34*(4), 451–458.

Namen, A. M., Dunagan, D. P., Fleischer, A., Tillett, J., Barnett, M., McCall, W. V., & Haponik, E. F. (2002). Increased physician-reported sleep apnea: The National Ambulatory Medical Care Survey. *Chest, 121*(6), 1741–1747.

Netzer, N. C., Stoohs, R. A., Netzer, C. M., Clark, K., & Strohl, K. P. (1999). Using the Berlin questionnaire to identify patients at risk for the sleep apnea syndrome. *Annals of Internal Medicine, 131*(7), 485–491.

O'Donnell, A. R., Bjornson, C. L., Bohn, S. G., & Kirk, V. G. (2006). Compliance rates in children using noninvasive continuous positive airway pressure. *Sleep, 29*(5), 651–658.

Owens, J. A. (2001). The practice of pediatric sleep medicine: Results of a community survey. *Pediatrics, 108*(3), e51.

Owens, J. A., & Mindell, J. A. (2002). Clinical sleep services for children: Clinical and administrative considerations. *Sleep Medicine, 3*(3), 291–294.

Owens, J. A. (2005). Epidemiology of sleep disorders during childhood. In S. H. Sheldon, R. Ferber & M. H. Kryger

(Eds.), *Principles and Practices of Pediatric Sleep Medicine* (pp. 27–33). Philadelphia: Elsevier Saunders.

Pigeon, W., Crabtree, V., & Scherer, M. (2007). The future of behavioral sleep medicine. *Journal of Clinical Sleep Medicine, 15*(3), 73–79.

Praud, J.-P., & Dorion, D. (2008). Obstructive sleep disordered breathing in children: Beyond adenotonsillectomy. *Pediatric Pulmonology, 43*(9), 837–843.

Rains, J. C. (1995). Treatment of obstructive sleep apnea in pediatric patients. Behavioral intervention for compliance with nasal continuous positive airway pressure. *Clinical Pediatrics, 34*(10), 535–541.

Richardson, G. S. (2000). Managing insomnia in the primary care setting: Raising the issues. *Sleep, 23* (Suppl 1), S9.

Schlarb, A.A., Liddle, C.C., & Hautzinger, M. (2011). JuST—A multimodal program for treatment of insomnia in adolescents: A pilot study. *Nature and Science of Sleep, 3,* 13–20.

Sheehan, D., Robertson, L., & Ormond, T. (2007). Comparison of language used and patterns of communication in interprofessional and multidisciplinary teams. *Journal of Interprofessional Care, 21*(1), 17–30.

Simola, P., Niskakangas, M., Liukkonen, K., Virkkula, P., Pitkäranta, A., Kirjavainen, T., & Aronen, E. T. (2010). Sleep problems and daytime tiredness in Finnish preschool-aged children-a community survey. *Child: Care, Health and Development, 36*(6), 805–811.

Stores, G., & Wiggs, L. (1998). Clinical services for sleep disorders. *Archives of Disease in Childhood, 79*(6), 495–497.

Tamay, Z., Akcay, A., Kilic, G., Suleyman, A., Ones, U., & Guler, N. (2006). Are physicians aware of obstructive sleep apnea in children? *Sleep Med, 7*(7), 580–584.

Thornton, D. J., Chandriani, K., Thornton, J. G., Farooq, S., Moallem, M., Krishnan, V., & Auckley, D. (2010). Assessing the prioritization of primary care referrals for polysomnograms. *Sleep 33*(9), 1255–1260.

Uong, E. C., Epperson, M., Bathon, S. A., & Jeffe, D. B. (2007). Adherence to nasal positive airway pressure therapy among school-aged children and adolescents with obstructive sleep apnea syndrome. *Pediatrics, 120*(5), e1203-e1211.

Wiggs, L. D. (2003). Paediatric sleep disorders: The need for multidisciplinary sleep clinics *International Journal of Pediatric Otorhinolaryngology, 67*(Suppl 1), S115.

CHAPTER

20 Helping Children and Parents Manage their Sleep Study Experience

Lissy Zaremba

Abstract

With the increasing recognition of pediatric sleep disorders, there is a growing demand for pediatric sleep medicine services, including polysomnography (PSG). Treating a child's and parent's emotional, developmental, and psychosocial needs simultaneously with their medical needs has a significant positive and lasting impact on them, improving their future health care experiences and overall family satisfaction. This chapter will present the Rainbow Comfort Measures© (RCM©) model of care and how the model's guiding principles can be effectively integrated in a pediatric sleep center's operations and clinical practices. Practical interventions and coping strategies, integral to RCM©, will also be discussed. By incorporating these foundational principles into a pediatric sleep center's standard of care, a parent and child's anxiety will decrease and their understanding, cooperation, achievement, self-control, and self-esteem will be enhanced. Additionally, the sleep center staff's knowledge base and confidence will be strengthened, the ability to gather high quality PSG data will improve, and overall patient satisfaction scores will increase.

Key Words: pediatrics, polysomnography, medical procedures, rainbow comfort measures, rainbow comfort positioning, procedural distress, psychological preparation, parental participation, child participation, coping skills

Introduction

There is a growing demand for pediatric sleep medicine services, including polysomnography (PSG), with the increasing recognition of pediatric sleep disorders and sleep disordered breathing (Sinha & Guilleminault, 2010). Sleep disordered breathing peaks in children between the ages of 2 and 8 years (Hoban, 2010). Additionally, children with certain medical conditions and/or developmental disabilities are at a greater risk for sleep disordered breathing (Sinha & Guilleminault, 2010; Richdale & Schreck, 2009; see Richdale, Chapter 33). Children with the greatest need for diagnostic services in sleep medicine fall within these two groups. Even though a sleep study is considered by adults to be a noninvasive, relatively painless test, it still may raise many concerns for parents and children. The anticipation of sleeping with medical sensors and wires while in an unfamiliar environment, experiencing new sensations, and having limited mobility can be quite anxiety-provoking for children and parents despite reassurance from sleep center staff. Parents may find the PSG sensors and wires a physical barrier to comforting their child. Furthermore, younger children with busy fingers and children with developmental disabilities and/or sensory integration issues may have an even more challenging time tolerating the sleep study experience due to their tactile sensitivities, the need to restrict their movement, and their overall decreased ability to understand, manage, and cooperate. Perhaps the sleep center's staff most helpful interventions for a child and parent are listening to *and hearing* their concerns, preparing them for what to expect, problem-solving creative solutions to possible challenges along with them, and encouraging to them to be an active part of their experience. With a sleep center's respectful and team-based approach, a child and parent will have an increased opportunity to *own* their sleep study experience and feel positive about how they handled any challenges.

The RCM© model of care helps children and families manage their health care experiences by promoting their comfort, achievement, and sense of control. The guiding principles of the RCM© model can be adapted to any medical experience and/or environment and involve: *(1)* preparing the child and family for what to expect; *(2)* providing a role for everyone involved; *(3)* positioning the child and parent comfortably (sitting upright whenever possible); *(4)* encouraging the child to choose his or her coping strategies; and *(5)* creating a calm and supportive environment (Stephens, Barkey, & Hall, 1999). This chapter will help the reader understand and assess the child's and parent's needs before, during, and after their sleep center experiences. Strategies will be discussed which incorporate the emotional, developmental, and psychological needs of a child and parent. Sleep center staff can integrate these concepts and strategies into their clinical practice, enhancing their child-friendly interactions while gathering high-quality PSG data and, in turn, increasing family satisfaction outcomes.

Understanding Child and Parent Needs

Essential concerns of children and parents in the health care setting are pain, separation, lack of information, and the uncertainty of the environment or experience (Salmela, Aronen, & Salantera, 2010; Gaynard et al., 1990). Children and parents may have a variety of feelings as they wait for their scheduled sleep study. A child and/or parent may be anxious about what to expect, whether they can manage the experience, or what the results of the sleep study may conclude. They may envision the worst possible scenario or fear possible painful events. These thoughts and feelings may stem from their own imaginations or memories from past medical experiences. On the other hand, a child and/or parent may not be worried about their upcoming experience or may be eager to find answers and possible solutions to their medical concerns. Whether during interactions with the sleep medicine specialist at the clinic visit, the sleep center coordinator during their scheduling process, or with the sleep study technologist on the study night, there are multiple needs that a child and parent have beyond completing the task at hand (i.e., ordering the sleep study, scheduling the sleep study, conducting the sleep study). When providing care for a child and parent, consider this question: "Are we (the sleep center staff, parent, and child) on the same page, working together to achieve the same goals?" Identical to any health care professional's goals for children and families, the sleep center staff's goals should be: *(1)* to assist the overall procedural experience to be safe and satisfying with productive, high-quality data; *(2)* to minimize the trauma and distress for the child, parent, and the sleep center staff; and *(3)* to maintain the integrity of the whole child during a potentially stressful procedure (Stephens et al., 1999; Cavender et al., 2004; Leahy et al., 2008).

Consider the possible perspectives and/or needs of everyone involved in the sleep center experiences. A sleep center staff member may be thinking, "I need to remain calm, confident, and competent so I can successfully interact and perform the task or procedure with care, speed, and skill. I need the parent to trust that I have the best interest of their child in mind. I need the parent to remain calm and supportive and not overprotective of the child so that he or she resists or pressures me. I need the child to be cooperative, calm, and still. I need to not cause any added distress for the child or the parent." Then, a parent may be thinking, "I need my child to receive expert care from the sleep center staff that I trust has the best interest of my child in mind. I need for my child to remain comfortable and without pain or distress. I need to be able to advocate for my child, to be heard and respected. I need to be with my child and know *how **I** can help*." Finally, a child may be thinking, "I need to understand what is happening to me. I need to have choices and not be forced to do something that I don't want or understand. I need for everyone to stay calm. I need to feel safe, protected, and not feel pain. I want to trust what people are telling me is the truth and that they *want* to help me. I need to be able to speak my mind, be heard, and have my thoughts respected. I need to know *what **I*** can do to help." Be mindful that there may be discrepancies between what *health care professionals* ***think*** *the needs of the child or parent might be* and what the *child and parent* ***feel*** *are their needs.* The question becomes... "How do we, as sleep center staff, figure out the true needs of the child and parent?" A very good question; read on.

When a task presents itself, sometimes health care professionals may be quick to set their agenda with their familiar routines. Tasks that may seem very simple may become quite complex. Examples may include: scheduling a young child for a sleep study; greeting an active child and his or her overtired parent on the study night; applying the PSG sensors on an extremely anxious and possibly defensive child; optimizing the child's and parent's sleep onset; or maintaining sensor integrity on an easily awakened child throughout the night. However, if we slow down our actions, pause in the moment, and expand our viewpoint to consider the child's and parent's variety of needs from *their* perspectives, we may find ourselves challenged to accomplish our basic and familiar tasks. The tasks as we know them are suddenly not so easy. We realize that our agenda, what we planned to do, does not necessarily take into account the child's and parent's palpable needs—the needs for safety, security, trust, comfort from pain, predictability, and control. We realize that we need to expand our goals to align with those of the child and parent (Zaremba & Mitchell, 2011). But, how is this done? Another good question; read on.

Marcel Proust, a famous French novelist (1871–1922), was quoted as saying, "The real voyage of discovery consists not in seeking new landscapes but in having new eyes" (retrieved from: http//www.quotationspage.com, July 22, 2012). A simple interpretation, we must look at our given situation from a different angle; new and improved possibilities or solutions can be discovered. As a health care professional, begin to think and see the potentially stressful PSG experience as a child or parent may view it. What do the child and parent want and need on an emotional and developmental level? What actions can we take that will help a child and parent feel cared for and informed? Just as important as the concrete *act* of imparting information may be the *feeling* we are giving them when we listen, attend and respond to their cues, take our time with them, ask for their thoughts, or help them understand information through an approach which connects best with their learning style and needs. This requires our true *willingness to listen* to a child and parent and our *ability to hear* what they are saying. By incorporating into our practice developmentally appropriate knowledge and strategies that take into account a child's and parent's needs, their medical experiences can become positive and psychologically growth-producing. We are investing in the child, investing in the child's future. A child's and parent's interactions with caring and trusted professionals during their sleep center experiences will have far-reaching effects for them. Our investment now helps to pave their path for future successful medical and nonmedical experiences and possibly their life course.

The Rainbow Comfort Measures© Model of Care

RCM© is a model of care pioneered at University Hospitals Rainbow Babies and Children's Hospital in Cleveland, Ohio, by Mary Barkey, MA, CCLS and Barbara Stephens, MAN, CRRN, CNS in the early 1990s. The model uses a family-centered and relationship-based care framework of evidence-based clinical practices that meet the psychosocial, emotional and developmental needs of children and their families during potentially stressful health care experiences. RCM© promotes the parent and child's capacity for the highest level of participation in their care. Honoring the family unit, health care professionals partner with the parent's and child to create strategies that empower them to cope with their health care experiences (Stephens et al., 1999). The RCM© model of care's Mission Statement, Foundational Cornerstones and Guiding Principles are outlined in Table 20.1. The model's guiding principles which are directly applicable to and influence a child and family care experiences in a pediatric sleep center environment include the following:

- Create a calm, positive, child-friendly and supportive environment.
- Assess a child's and parent's understanding of the current experience and the impact of their past experiences and coping abilities.
- Assess a child's and parent's developmental level, learning style and verbal/nonverbal actions and reactions.
- Prepare a child and parent for the experience individualizing developmentally appropriate explanations using child-friendlier wording and active participation with hands-on demonstration and/or role rehearsal.
- Develop and support a child's and parent's active participation including specific roles and realistic choices.
- Guide and support a child's pre-existing or newly learned coping and relaxation strategies.
- Use the Rainbow Comfort Positioning© model maintaining a child's and parent's physical and emotional connection while maximizing their comfort and minimizing the child's movement.
- Provide positive guidance, coaching and specific praise to reinforce a child's and parent's efforts and accomplishments.
- Listen, hear and support a child's and parent's verbal and/or emotional processing and integrate improvements into current and future experiences.

Table 20.1 Rainbow Comfort Measures© Model of Care

Rainbow Comfort Measures© Model of Care*
Mission Statement
Helping children and families manage health care experiences by addressing their psychosocial, emotional and developmental needs while promoting their comfort, participation, sense of control and achievement.
4 Foundational Cornerstones of RCM©
1. Parent Participation 2. Preparation 3. Positioning 4. Processing
Guiding Principles of RCM©
• Develop and implement an integrated **pain management plan** with the parent/caregiver (and the child) for optimal physical and emotional pain prevention and relief.
• Create **a calm, positive, child-friendly and supportive environment** by minimizing unnecessary stimuli.
• Perform stressful experiences in the **treatment room** (in areas where a treatment room exists).
• Assess the child's and parent/caregiver's **understanding of the current health care experience** and the **impact of their past experiences and coping abilities.**
• Assess and consider the child's and parent/caregiver's **developmental level**, learning style and verbal/nonverbal actions and reactions.
• **Prepare** the child and parent/caregiver for the health care experience. Individualize and integrate developmentally appropriate explanations using child-friendlier wording and active participation with hands-on demonstration and/or role rehearsal.
• Develop, integrate and support a **coping plan** with the child's and/or parent/caregiver's input and active participation. Include realistic choices, the child's and parent/caregiver's specific roles, and their pre-existing and/or newly learned coping and relaxation strategies.
• Use the **Rainbow Comfort Positioining© Model**. Preserve the child's and parent/caregiver's physical and emotional connection with each other while maximizing their comfort and security, minimizing the child's movement and maintaining easy access to the site.
• Provide the child and parent/caregiver with **positive guidance and coaching** while offering **specific praise** to reinforce their efforts and accomplishments.
• Before, during and after the health care encounter, provide time with the child and parent/caregiver for **verbal and/or emotional processing** of their experience. Listen, hear and provide support to the child and/or parent/caregiver and integrate improvements into the child's and parent/caregiver's current and future health care experiences.

*Adapted with permission from: Family and Child Life Services. (2010). *Comfort Measures: Helping children and families manage their stressful health care experiences – Comfort Measures principles.* [in Rainbow Comfort Measures© educational handout series]. University Hospitals Rainbow Babies and Children's Hospital, Cleveland, OH.

As health care professionals expand their knowledge and skill base, to incorporate the emotional and developmental needs of the child and parent as well as the RCM© guiding principles into their practice, they are better able to effectively teach, model, and coach a child and parent through their medical experience. The child and parent can take what they have learned during their current experience, build upon and refine the strategies that worked well, and then apply those strategies and skills they have learned as they encounter future medical or challenging life experiences. For a child and parent, the skills, confidence, and positive self-esteem that develop from their medical experience(s) can be carried with them throughout their lifetime. The RCM© model of care can be easily integrated to any sleep center's culture and standard of practice.

Addressing the Child's and Parent's Needs

When assessing and addressing children's and parents' needs to create child-friendlier health care experiences, the RCM© guiding principles should be incorporated into the sleep center's standard of care and philosophy of practice. The guiding principles of RCM© will be further discussed, including: redefining the medical team; inviting the child's and/or parent's participation while supporting their involvement; providing psychological preparation for the experience; establishing positive and defined roles for the child and parent while integrating coping strategies; and creating a calm and supportive environment.

Redefine the Medical Team

The Comfort Measures model begins with defining, or redefining, the medical team (Stephens et al., 1999). The American Academy of Pediatrics (2006) strongly supports incorporating the parent and the child as vital, active, and respected members of the medical team. Parents are knowledgeable about their child's medical history, temperament, what comforts them, how they have managed past medical experiences, and the best approaches to gain their child's cooperation during stressful experiences. Much insight can also be gained from actively listening, reading nonverbal cues, and involving the child. Altogether, *everyone* has a hand in contributing to the success of the experience.

In a team approach, there are no "good guys" or "bad guys." The parent is not the "rescuer" or the "good guy" after the PSG setup is complete, just as the sleep study technologist is not the "bad guy" because he/she needs to put PSG sensors on the protesting child. A parent's active and supportive involvement with their child during the PSG setup and overall experience communicates to the child that this test is needed and important to his/her health and well-being. Essentially, the parent agrees with the doctor's plan and we are all on the same team together. In the long run, the parent's active involvement in his or her child's current experience fosters the child's trust that the parent is supporting him or her now and will continue to support him or her during any future challenging times (Stephens et al., 1999).

As members of the medical team, the parent and child should be engaged as active participants in the medical procedure and plan of care, rather than being passive recipients. Children want to feel in control, respected, and successful. Involving the child in his or her experience provides just that—a greater sense of accomplishment, self-worth, and self-confidence. Additionally, parents want to be involved with their child's care, offering comfort and help to manage challenging experiences whether the child is in the hospital, at home, or elsewhere (Bauchner, Vinci, Bak, Pearson, & Corwin, 1996). Everyone—the child, parent and sleep center staff—has an important and helpful role to play on the team.

Invite the Child's and Parent's Participation and Support their Involvement

Life is filled with ups and downs, challenges and successes. The parent's role is to be the continuous support throughout his or her child's life, helping the child to navigate turbulent times and celebrate successes. This role should not change during medical experiences. Research supports that children want their parents to be with them during procedures (Ross & Ross, 1984) and parents want to be with their children (Bauchner et al., 1991; Bauchner et al., 1996). Parental anxiety has been shown to decrease when a parent is with his or her child, which in turn reduces the child's anxiety (Bauchner et al., 1996). By actively encouraging the parent and child's participation, we are communicating our genuine respect for the family unit and our sincere desire for parent and child involvement rather than merely just being present. It communicates that we are doing things *for* and *with* the child rather than *to them*. The parent's and child's medical experience should be viewed as more than just something they need to "tolerate" or "get through." A parent's and child's involvement and participation in their experience can help them to *own* their experience, making it *meaningful* to them. They are able to internalize their feelings of accomplishment and success, thereby building their self-confidence and self-esteem.

Parents have much to offer to the success of their child's medical experience, to the comfort of their child, and to the strengthening of their parent–child bond. However, within the unfamiliar and stressful medical environment, sometimes parents may feel overwhelmed, anxious, or inadequate in their parental role. Studies have shown that parents' behaviors are significantly related to their child's distress (Cohen, Manimala, Blount,

2000; Dahlquist & Pendley, 2005). A parent may not know *how* to effectively support and comfort his or her child, especially as he or she learns the number of PSG sensors that need to be placed. As sleep center professionals, we can teach, guide, and coach the parents in their roles.

Just as the parent has an integral role, the child does as well. Attempting to gain his/her compliance is key. Be attuned to the child's emotional and nonverbal cues, and respond appropriately. Addressing the child's concerns, and then inviting and encouraging his/her participation in the PSG set-up will be helpful (for example, holding the "stickers," helping to buckle the "stretchy bands" like a belt, etc.). Giving a child a job with realistic choices will foster a sense of inclusion, that his/her help is meaningful and important. The knowledge gained, skills learned and self-confidence developed from one experience can be built upon and integrated into a child's and parent's future medical and life experiences.

Provide Psychological Preparation for the Experience

Psychological preparation refers to the interactive process of helping children and parents know and understand in advance what to expect and possible strategies to manage the experience. It reduces the uncertainty, which might otherwise lead to increased misconceptions, anxiety, and fear (Wolfer & Visintainer, 1979). Preparation involves verbal explanation, familiarization and desensitization with medical equipment and the environment, as well as hands-on demonstration of what will be happening, all delivered in a developmentally appropriate, sensitive, and timely manner. Within the preparation process, coping strategies are discussed that allow the child and parent to constructively participate in their care (Melamed & Ridley-Johnson, 1988). Table 20.2 outlines a summary of essential preparation components. The time spent preparing a child and parent can vary depending on the child's individual needs and time available; preparation could occur 15 minutes prior to beginning the PSG setup, or even in the moment as each step occurs. Providing preparation significantly decreases a child's and parent's anxiety and misconceptions and enhances their ability to manage what is asked of them, thereby increasing their cooperation and positive experiences (Kain, Mayes, & Caramico, 1996; Wolfer & Visintainer, 1979). The Child Life Council's (http://www.childlife.org, March 13, 2012) evidenced-based practice statement discusses preparing children and adolescents for medical procedures and offers a comprehensive summary of psychological preparation for health care experiences. (Koller, 2007).

CONSIDER THE CHILD'S AND PARENT'S INDIVIDUAL NEEDS

Every child and family unit carries with it its own unique styles and past experiences that shape how the child and family respond to future events, stressful or not. Developmental age, previous experience with medical procedures, illness, hospitalization or separation, innate or acquired coping skills, seriousness of the diagnosis, and available support systems will all influence how a child and parent respond to upcoming stressors (Brewer et al., 2006; Melamed, Dearborn & Hermecz, 1983). To help create a supportive environment for the child and parent, it is important to understand the parent's and child's perspective on such things as how the child has managed past challenging experiences or transitions to new environments, how the child processes information, the child's temperament, and the child's comfort level with strangers (for example, shy and quiet, slow to warm up, or eager to make new friends). Asking about the parent's expectations of his or her child's ability to cooperate and eliciting helpful suggestions he or she may have is also crucial for a thorough assessment.

Successful interactions with children and their parents occur when a health care professional demonstrates a clear understanding of child growth and development. However, it is important to keep in mind that children process information in different ways. Additionally, a child and parent may regress in their understanding and coping abilities as their stress increases (Heard, 2008; Salmela, Salantera, & Aronen, 2010). Key developmental issues and needs for infants, toddlers, and preschool-age children include parental presence and involvement, active involvement for learning, and less developed language abilities. Key developmental issues and needs for school-age children and adolescents include increasing language skills but difficulty with new words and abstract ideas, self-esteem that is influenced by performance, and growing independence and decision-making skills (Family and Child Life Services, 2010; Heard, 2008). To further facilitate a general understanding of child development and the impact the medical environment may have on a child, Appendix A offers a condensed overview of each developmental stage (infancy through adolescence) highlighting possible stressors at each stage, subsequent cognitive impact and coping

Table 20.2 Preparation Considerations for Health Care Professionals

Preparing Children and Parents/Caregivers for Medical Procedures *

• **Create a calm, positive, child-friendly and supportive environment.**
  • Provide a welcoming atmosphere.
  • Minimize unnecessary stimuli.

• **Gather and assess pertinent information from the child and parent/caregiver in order to individualize their preparation and coping plans.**   • Determine the child's and parent/caregiver's current understanding, the impact of their past experiences, and strategies for improved coping.

• **Prepare the child and parent/caregiver for what to expect.**
  • Help the child and parent/caregiver know what to expect using developmentally appropriate explanations, hands-on demonstration, active participation and/or role rehearsal.
  • Use developmentally appropriate, child-friendlier wording.
  • Be honest and only make promises that can be kept.
  • Encourage questions.
  • Continually assess the child's and parent/caregiver's understanding, nonverbal behaviors, and emotional reactions; then modify the approach as needed.

• **Develop a plan with the child and parent/caregiver to manage their experience using pre-existing and/or newly learned coping and relaxation strategies.**
  • Use the Rainbow Comfort Positioning© model.
  • Offer realistic choices, specific roles, and provide diversional items or strategies.

• **Continually assess the child's and parent/caregiver's understanding and reactions throughout the procedure and modify the approach as needed.**   • Continue to provide explanations and positive guidance, adjust comfort positioning, and/or redirect the child's and parent/caregiver's role as needed.
• **Offer specific praise to reinforce the child's and parent/caregiver's accomplishments to help them know what was done well.**

* Adapted with permission from: Family and Child Life Services. (2010). *Comfort Measures: Helping children and families manage their stressful health care experiences – Preparing children for medical procedures.* [in Rainbow Comfort Measures© educational handout series]. University Hospitals Rainbow Babies and Children's Hospital, Cleveland, OH.

behaviors, and possible interventions and support. Understanding the needs and strengths specific to each child can help the sleep study staff, in partnership with the parent and child, to prepare and plan developmentally appropriate interventions that will assist them in managing the demands of the sleep study.

WHAT TO SAY, HOW TO SAY IT AND WHAT TO DO

Effective preparation is more than providing just information. It is a way of integrating positive messages into what is said, to inspire confidence and to empower and reassure children and parents that we will work with them to have the most successful outcome possible. An effective preparation contains several essential elements: *(1)* why the procedure is important ("Why do I need to have a sleep study?"); *(2)* what to expect during the procedure ("What is going to happen to me?"); and *(3)* how we will manage the procedure together ("What do I need to do and how can I help?") (Breiner, 2009; Stephens et al., 1999). In order to be emotionally invested in the experience, a parent needs to understand why the procedure is important to his or her child's health. If cognitively able, it is helpful when a child recognizes the importance of the procedure as well. For a child, clarifying the purpose of the sleep study can also diminish misconceptions or guilty feelings about the reason for the procedure (for example, a punishment for an imagined wrongdoing; Breiner, 2009). To assess the child and parent's knowledge about their sleep study experience, ask, "Tell me what you know about your sleepover tonight." A simple explanation for the child may be, "This test will help your doctor know how your body works when you are sleeping. It will help your doctor know (… or make decisions about) how to help you sleep better at night." To quell uncertainties, the child and parent need to understand what they will experience (i.e., what they may feel, see, hear, and smell), as well as their individual roles (Stephens et al., 1999). For example, "I will show and tell you everything that I am doing so there will be no surprises. My job will be to put these small stickers on different parts of your body, like your legs, chest, and head. Your job will be to sit on the bed, and you can even help me with the stickers. Mom's job will be sit next to you on your bed, and she can even help, too." Explore the parent's and child's thoughts and expectations by saying, "Let's figure out how we can be helpful to each other. Would you like to help me with the stickers?"

Honest, concrete, and simple words are most effective when helping children and families understand an upcoming procedure or event. Using accurate medical terminology with clarification is also helpful (Breiner, 2009; Gaynard et al., 1990). For example, "I need to put this little disc on your head. Some kids think it looks like a little cup. It has a long string on it. The real name for it is an electrode (… or a lead). It helps the doctor understand what your brain is telling your body to do, like if you are sleeping or if you are dreaming. But I won't be able to know what you are thinking or dreaming about." Since every child's language skills, understanding, and past medical experiences will be different, be attuned to the child's cues and/or situation to modify word choices or provide further explanation.

Word choices and phrasing can be tricky in regard to honesty, connotations, and interpretation. Words can help shift a person's mindset from a negative to a positive frame of thinking (Breiner, 2009; Gaynard et al., 1990). For example, use a softer word such as "bother" or "uncomfortable" instead of the stronger word, "hurt." Provide positive guidance and comments that boost rather than weaken a child's self-esteem and confidence (Stephens et al., 1999). Positive alternatives to the harsh, "don't cry," "that doesn't hurt," or "be a big boy/girl" can be, "You may feel more comfortable when you … (hug your mom, snuggle with your blankie, etc.)" or "The look on your face tells me you might feel worried. Some kids find it helpful to look in the mirror and watch as we put the stickers on your chin." Direct a child's attention to acceptable behaviors such as, "Hold yourself very still" or "Put your hands on your book," rather than "Don't move" or "Don't touch." Try to include sensory information in an explanation (Breiner, 2009; Gaynard et al., 1990; Stephens et al., 1999; Wolfer & Visintainer, 1979). However, many adults offer their own assessment of how something will likely feel. Since feelings and sensations may be experienced or perceived differently by each individual, whether adult or child, it is helpful to first *ask a child how he or she thinks something may feel* instead of *telling them* too specifically what he/she will feel or experience. For example, instead of saying "This skin prep lotion feels scratchy," an alternative may be, "I need to clean this spot on your skin with some cleaning lotion and a Q-Tip. Then I will put a sticker where I cleaned. Some kids say they can feel little bumps in the lotion (offer to let them feel the lotion between their fingers). Those tiny little bumps help to clean your skin. You can tell me what you notice as I clean this spot on your skin."

Language and word choice has the potential to affect how a person feels or what he or she perceives during an experience (Gaynard et al., 1990). Many children often ask, "Will this hurt?" Since pain is a subjective feeling, it is difficult to promise that something won't hurt. In fact, it is best if this promise is never made. You may try saying, "You may notice … " or "You might be surprised at … (how relaxed you feel, how easy this may be, etc.)." Describing a realistic range of feelings may also help, such as, "You may notice some bumps in the lotion as I rub it on your skin. Some kids say the lotion feels a bit like toothpaste, or like it has sand or crumbs in it. You can let me know how it feels to you." If a child says, "Ouch, that hurts!" a response may be, "I'm sorry. Lets figure out a way to make this more comfortable." By offering acceptable choices, a child is more likely to feel in control and not forced to do something (Heard, 2008). For example, instead of saying "Can I … ?" an alternative might be, "I need to put two stickers on each of your legs, (point to where). These stickers will show how much your legs wiggle while you sleep. Which leg should we put the stickers on first? Would you like to help by taking the back off the sticker?" Additionally, make statements that are true and only make promises that can be kept. For example, "I'm just looking (... at your leg, tummy, etc.)" is commonly said when actually "I'm gently touching (... your leg, tummy, etc.)" is a more accurate statement. Finally, always encourage and be open to a child's and parent's questions before, during, and after an experience (Breiner, 2009; Heard, 2008; Zaremba et al., 2005). Appendix B offers a guide to suggested child-friendlier word choices and lead-in statements when talking with children about their sleep study experience.

Although literal thinking is developmentally appropriate for younger children and school-age children, when children and parents are in an unfamiliar situation or environment they become a bit more serious and literal in their interpretations, or they may possibly misinterpret well-meaning actions. A child and parent may not readily catch on to casual humor or jokes. Consequently, an adult who makes a comment in a joking manner may unintentionally misrepresent him or herself as lacking understanding, empathy, and compassion (Ross & Ross, 1982). Additionally, tickling a child crosses a personal boundary and adds an element of surprise to the predicable environment the sleep technologist is trying to create. Although sometimes PSG sensors may need to be placed where a child is ticklish, the sleep technologist's conscious act of tickling a child in an attempt to build rapport or gain a smile or laughter should always be avoided. These approaches by the sleep technologist may be done with the goal of lightening a child and parent's mood and with no conscious harm intended. However, the sleep technologist should consistently and carefully read the child and parent's behavioral cues for their appropriateness and their possible need for clarification of their actions.

Preparation using hands-on demonstration and visual aids (for example, photographs of a cooperative child during each stage of the PSG setup) contribute to a child's ease in understanding the procedure and also becoming more interested in his or her body functions (Tanaka et al., 2011). Since toddlers, preschool, and school-age children learn best through interaction with their environment, combining verbal explanations with opportunities to handle, explore, and role-play using the medical supplies appropriate to the procedure is helpful. Demonstrating what will happen, as well as providing the opportunity for the child to handle the PSG sensors and stickers, creates a hands-on, kinesthetic experience which helps a child internalize the procedural steps, making the experience more manageable, predictable, and understandable. Allowing the child to actively touch and play with the various sensors will help the child become increasingly more desensitized to the equipment on their own terms and in their own time frame (Breiner, 2009; Zaremba et al., 2005). This approach is often helpful when introducing and gaining a child's compliance with the thermister and nasal cannula, since these sensors are frequently the most challenging for a child to tolerate. A thermister or nasal cannula can be introduced to a child in a positive and encouraging approach. For example, a sleep technologist may introduce the thermister to a child by saying, "some kids say the next sticker reminds them of a mustache...something like this (then place a small piece of tape or fun-type sticker under your nose and/or parent's nose). You can hold and touch this sticker that will rest under your nose. It is called a *thermister* and this is what it looks like (allow the child to hold the thermister). Some kids like to choose a fun sticker to decorate it. Some kids like to hold a mirror so they can watch while I gently place the sticker under their nose. Would you like to choose a fun sticker to decorate it? Here is a mirror if you'd like to watch."

Additionally, a doll (i.e., inexpensive plain muslin cloth dolls, which a child can use to draw a face and/or decorate with markers) or stuffed animal is ideal to demonstrate the PSG setup (Figure 20.1). Provide the child with a preparation doll or a stuffed animal to practice and role-play with the PSG sensors. If the child brought his or her own doll or stuffed animal from home, it is important to still

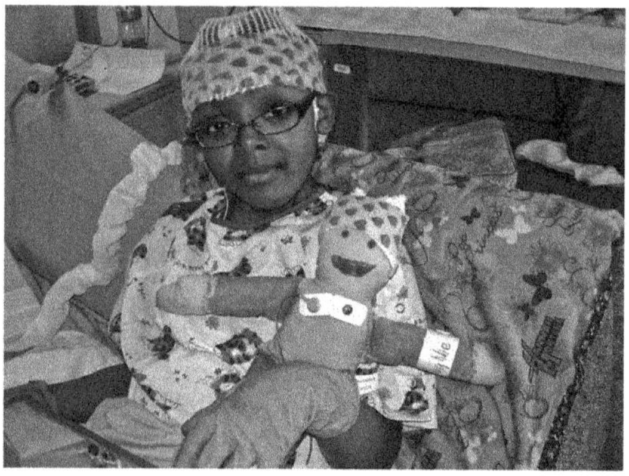

Figure 20.1 Hands-on preparation increases understanding, control, and sense of accomplishment. A school-age patient proudly displays her "patient." She learned about her own PSG set-up as she placed the PSG sensors on her doll.

offer a choice of using their doll/stuffed animal or one that they are not attached to. Some children are very protective of their cherished comfort items and will not want to use them in this manner (Zaremba et al, 2005). To introduce this preparation strategy to the child, the sleep technologist might say, "I have a doll/stuffed animal for you to keep and take home. Some kids like to put the same stickers on the doll/stuffed animal that they will have on their body for their sleepover. We can do this for you and your doll/stuffed animal." Show the child on the doll/stuffed animal where and how each sticker and sensor will be placed. This can be done step-by-step, prior to placement of each sticker and sensor on the child. Explain to the child and encourage their involvement by saying, "First, we need to clean the little spot on your doll's chest with a Q-Tip like this (demonstrate on doll) before we put a sticker there. While you are cleaning the spot on your doll's chest, I'll clean this spot on your chest (touch the spot with your finger first). Great job cleaning, and great job holding your body still." The child is encouraged to take the doll/stuffed animal home with them in the morning. Broken EEG leads and other sensors can be saved and disinfected to create a reusable preparation kit. Table 20.3 provides a suggested list of preparation supplies. For the child who is apprehensive with the PSG sensors and setup process, sometime the parent can be a role model to demonstrate what the PSG sensors look and may feel like on the parent before it is the child's turn. After discussing this strategy with the parent, the sleep technologist may say, "Mom, I have a sticker for your chin (place the sticker on mom's chin). Thank you Mom, nice job holding so still while I put the sticker under your chin. It's Johnny's turn. Johnny, thank you for holding so still, too. Your turn again, mom. I have a sticker that rests by your eye."

Establish Positive and Defined Roles for the Child and Parent while Integrating Coping Strategies

Assess a child's and parent's ability, interest, and readiness to participate with the experience. Some children are able to manage new experiences quite well with very little prior preparation, and some children become more comfortable, relaxed, and cooperative when given ample time and opportunity to touch, explore, and play with the PSG sensors prior to their own setup beginning. Anxious parents may be overly protective and restrict their child's opportunity to interact with the environment (Dahlquist & Pendley, 2005). Parents may doubt their own ability to help their child manage a possibly challenging experience. They may withdraw completely from actively supporting their child and allow the sleep technologist to assume their parenting role. This disengagement may be interpreted by the sleep center staff as not caring. However, parents whose behavior is anxious, withdrawn, and/or disengaged should signal to the technologist that further assessment and an increased emphasis on helping the parent feel comfortable in his or her role during the sleep study experience is needed. On the other hand, some parents may intuitively know how to comfort and support their child in feeling confident to continue their coping strategies in new and possibly challenging

Table 20.3 Suggested Preparation Supplies and Diversional Items for Sleep Studies *

Preparation Supplies	Diversional Items
• Small stuffed animals and/or plain muslin cloth dolls • Markers to draw face/clothes on plain muslin cloth dolls • Small fun-type stickers • Broken PSG sensors and EEG leads • PSG stickers, sensors and other PSG supplies used in the setup • Unbreakable mirror	• Books (ex. lift-the-flap books, push button music/sounds books, "I Spy" books, etc.) • Push button water toys • Cause and effect toys (ex. pop-up, lights, music) • "Meteor Storms" (ie. hand-held lighted spinning globes) • "Find-It" game (ie. objects hidden within a bead-filled cylinder) • Bubbles (ie. no-spill mini-bubble tumbler) • Portable DVD player • Commonly viewed child-appropriate DVDs (ex. Elmo, SpongeBob, etc) • Ipod; iTouch; iPad

* Adapted with permission from: Family and Child Life Services. (2010). *Comfort Measures: Helping children and families manage their stressful health care experiences – Diversional Tools* [in Rainbow Comfort Measures© educational handout series]. University Hospitals Rainbow Babies and Children's Hospital, Cleveland, OH.

situations. When given the opportunity to express their concerns or fears, when prepared for the procedure and their role, and when receiving guidance, support, and encouragement from the health care professionals, parents and children are often more willing to participate and become involved in their medical experience (Breiner, 2009; Stephens et al., 1999). Subsequently, parents are frequently able to comfort and support their child effectively and children are more likely to successfully manage the more challenging unfamiliar and/or uncomfortable experiences (Stephens et al., 1999).

INVOLVE AND SUPPORT THE CHILD AND PARENT IN HIS/HER "JOB"

Establishing positive, integrated roles (or "jobs") for the child, parent, and health care professional is essential within the RCM© model of care philosophy (Stephens et al., 1999). During a PSG setup, the parent's main role/job is to be with his or her child and to support and comfort him or her; the child's main role/job is to hold their body (or leg, face, head, and hand) as still as he/she can while the sleep technologist places the PSG sensors on his or her body; the sleep technologist's main role/job is to place the PSG sensors on the child as accurately as possible and to gather the best quality PSG data possible. Everyone's roles/jobs can be expanded upon or adapted depending on the child's interests and individual needs during the changing circumstances of the PSG setup and study. Consider an example of a busy toddler who is pulling off his PSG sensors. This is a developmentally appropriate behavior, considering toddlers are focused on themselves and the environment around them. A curious toddler uses his or her senses to learn about the environment by mouthing, touching, or pulling at objects. The child knows the PSG sensors feel different and do not belong on his or her body. The colorful wires are tempting to explore and pull, and the wires are also making it difficult for him to move around on the bed and reach the toys. However, for the sleep study to proceed the toddler needs help to keep his or her hands busy and remain still while the sleep technologist replaces her leg stickers and some of the EEG leads. If the parent does not intuitively notice and respond to the technologist's and child's challenges, the technologist may need to refocus the parent back to his or her role/job and coach him or her on helpful strategies that will assist the technologist's and child's role/job. The sleep technologist may guide the parent on how to securely hold their child on their lap while also providing coping strategies such as redirection to an appropriate activity, distraction such as singing a song that may require hand movements (for example, The Itsy Bitsy Spider, The Wheels on the Bus, Peek-a-Boo, etc.) or playing with a cause-and-effect toy, encouraging the parent's hand-over-hand assistance with his or her child.

Anxiety is reduced when everyone's job is known and everyone's task at hand can be their focus. Having a specific role helps to refocus a parent's and child's energy and anxiety in a more positive and productive direction. When the parent and child are focused on their role during a procedure, such as decorating their PSG sensors with fun stickers, giving big hugs, holding a mirror, and blowing bubbles, their attention is redirected away from the sleep technologist's performance (Cavender et al., 2004; Stephens et al., 1999). In turn, this decreases a technologist's preoccupation and worry over the child resisting and fighting, which allows for a stronger level of confidence in procedural performance. This ultimately allows the technologist to focus on the task and increases the speed and likelihood of success in accomplishing the procedure (Bauchner et al., 1996).

USE THE RAINBOW COMFORT POSITIONING© MODEL

Once a child has achieved the developmental milestone of sitting unassisted at approximately 6 months of age, being forced to lie down creates a sense of vulnerability, stress, and an increased struggle to sit up (Stephens et al., 1999). Rainbow Comfort Positioning© (RCP©) is a fundamental component of the RCM© model of care and addresses this developmental issue during medical procedures by having a child sit upright, whenever possible, enhancing his or her sense of control. Additionally, a parent's active involvement of securely holding and comforting his or her child supports the need for a parent and child's close physical, visual, and emotional contact with each other. Furthermore, the parent and child's secure hugging hold limits the child's movements, providing a parent's positive assistance to the procedure (i.e., a hugging hold, a *bigger* hugging hold to further minimize movement) rather than negative restraint (i.e., holding down). Using RCP©, the parent can adjust the strength of his or her hold to the needs of his or her child from minimal holding (for example, parent and child sitting next to each other with the need for the parent's occasional hand placement on the child's cheek for a reminder to hold still) to more secure holding (for example, parent and child are coached to hug each other, giving each other a bigger hug when needed). In general, hugging is a positive action that comforts children and adults and is beneficial for many people, especially during stressful times. Also, the act of hugging requires a person's arms/body to stiffen and ultimately lessens their movements. Coincidentally, these results are equally beneficial for medical procedures (Stephens et al., 1999). Encouraging the child to hug his or her parent assists in their comfort and their success in their only "job" which is to hold still... "Your hugs with mom help your body hold so still. I am able to put these little stickers on your head so quickly." This also reinforces the parent's and child's teamwork and accomplishments by helping them know what they are doing well (Cavender et al., 2004; Lacey et al., 2008; Sparks et al., 2007; Stephens et al., 1999).

Integrating RCP© model into a child's sleep study experience will set a positive tone for a calm, child-friendly PSG setup. Encourage the parent and child to sit together on the bed with each other or, if more comfortable, encourage the parent to sit the child on his or her lap. For the child who is a bit more anxious or apprehensive, in need of more parental reassurance, or having a difficult time holding still, the parent should be encouraged to sit on the bed (or in a chair bedside the bed) while the child comfortably sits on his or her lap. The sleep technologist can then begin or continue the PSG setup. Also, plenty of space should be on the child's bed for a few diversional toys that can be readily accessible for redirection of busy hands. RCP© Positions should be creatively adapted for a child's age and individual needs. For example, a chair or rocking chair can be provided for the parent of an infant so the parent can hold the child during the setup. An added benefit to this individualized accommodation: the parent who usually rocks his or her child as part of their bedtime routine at home is able to continue this comforting ritual during their sleep study experience.

While a child's minimal movement is helpful to the sleep technologist when applying the PSG sensors, this fortunately is not an absolute requirement. The technologist should be flexible in his or her approach and adapt to and accommodate some of the child's movements within reason. If a child's movements increase too much and prevent any PSG sensor placement, a parent can be coached to a Comfort Position's more secure hugging hold. Particularly for younger children (infants, toddlers, and some preschool-age children), the child sits upright on the parent's lap, with the child's back to the parent's chest (Figure 20.2, "Back-to-Chest"); the child's chest to the parent's chest (Figure 20.3, "Chest-to-Chest"); or the child sitting sideways on the parent's lap (Figure 20.4, "Sideways Sitting"). The parent and child are coached to hug one another, or to give each other a bigger hug (i.e. more firm and secure hug), when the child needs increasing restraint. However, if a child becomes frantic the technologist should stop and reassess the situation and approach together with the parent, to determine how to proceed in the best interest of the child.

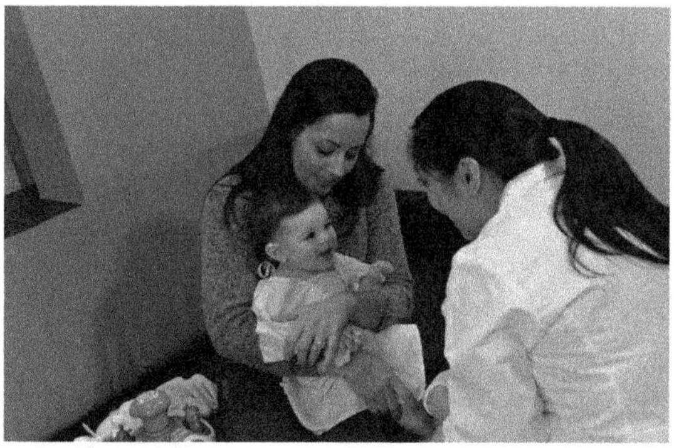

Figure 20.2 Comfort Positioning—"Back-to-Chest" on a Parent's Lap. A "hugging hold" with the child's back against the parent's chest. The parent's arm is around and securing the child's body. A more secure hug is given when the child needs more help to hold his or her body still. Provide diversional items or strategies to help manage the set-up.

Using the treatment room is central to RCM© model of care, particularly in an inpatient hospital setting. During stressful medical experiences, Stephens et al. (1999) emphasize the importance of moving the child and parent to the treatment room for stressful events in order to maintain the child's bed as a space to relax, sleep, and heal. In a hospital setting, often staff enter a patient's room unannounced and at unexpected times. In some cases stressful procedures may be performed in a child's bed. Consequently, a child has difficulty differentiating if a health care professional is coming into their room for something stressful or not. Unfortunately, a child may become fearful and distrustful of any staff entering their room, worrying that something uncomfortable may happen without notice. A child's insecurity and anxious feelings may continue at home after their hospitalization. Sleep study centers might be located in a hospital or hotel setting, and treatment rooms are not usually an option to use for the PSG setup. Generally, placement of the PSG sensors on a child will take place in his or her bed. Therefore, it is essential to create a positive experience that is rich in preparation, parent and child interaction, and support (Figure 20.5).

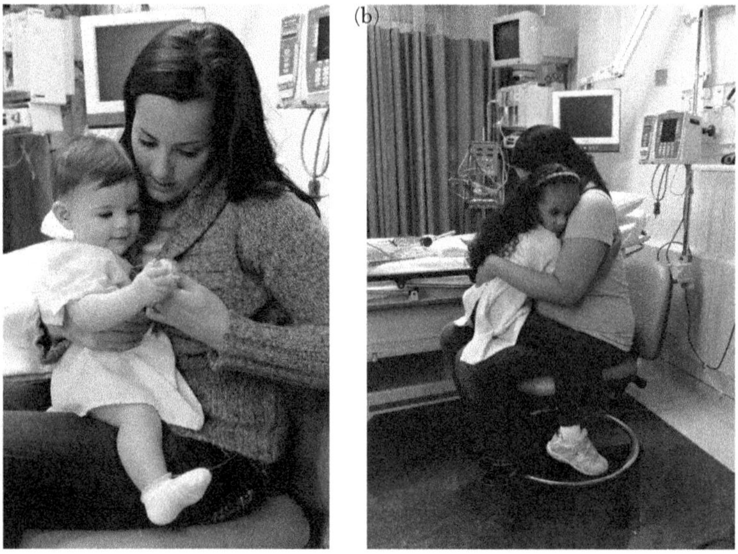
(a) (b)

Figure 20.3 Comfort Positioning—"Chest-to-Chest" on a Parent's Lap. A chest-to-chest "hugging hold" with the parent's arms around the child's body. A secure hug is given when the child needs more help to hold his or her body still. Provide diversional items or strategies to help manage the set-up.

Paramount for the successful use of RCP© is the continued assessment, guidance, and adjustment of a parent's and child's positioning throughout the procedure in order to maximize the child's cooperation, minimize his or her movement, and maintain the child's and parent's emotional connection. Whether sitting independently, sitting on a parent's lap, or sitting in a parent's hugging hold, the sitting position enhances a child's sense of security, sense of control, comfort, and cooperation (Cavender et al., 2004; Lacey et al., 2008; Sparks et al., 2007; Stephens et al., 1999).

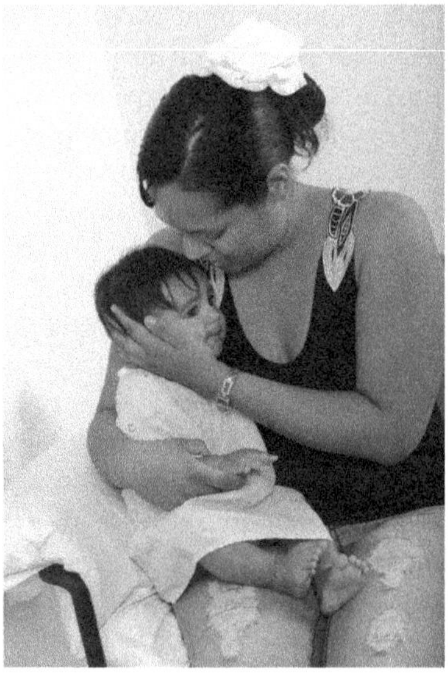

Figure 20.4. Comfort Positioning—"Sideways Sitting on a Parent's Lap". A "hugging hold" with the child sitting sideways on the parent's lap. The parent's arm cradles around and holds the child's body. The parent's free hand can be placed on the child's cheek, head, legs or body to minimize the child's movements as needed. Provide diversional items or strategies to help manage the set-up.

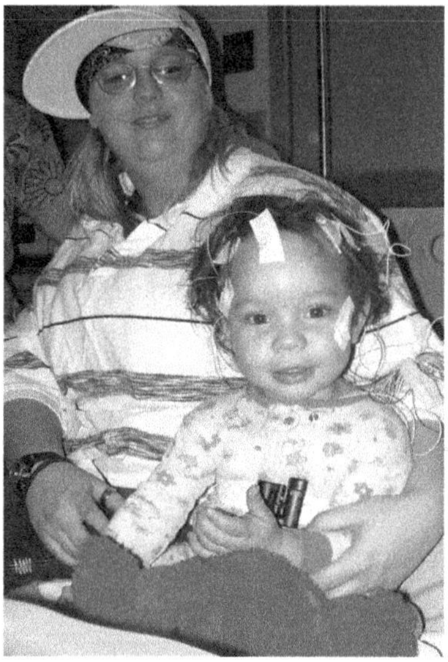

Figure 20.5 A content toddler and mom during her PSG set-up. This active 16-month-old feels safe with her mom by her side. Her mom was able to easily redirect her attention away from the sensors and wires with cause-and-effect toys, which helped the sleep technologist's successful placement of PSG sensors. Consent for image reproduction provided.

GUIDE AND SUPPORT THE CHILD'S AND PARENT'S COPING STRATEGIES

Coping strategies help children participate in constructive ways in their care and during their procedures. This in turn enhances the child's sense of mastery and appropriate control over a potentially stressful experience (Salmela, Salantera & Aronen, 2010). Using coping strategies can decrease a child's anxiety and pain while improving his/her cooperation and ability to manage stressful experiences. Additionally, active forms of coping result in less pain and less behavioral distress (Cavender et al., 2004). For example, offer the child a mirror to hold with both hands as he or she watches the leads, stickers and sensors being placed on the chest, face, and head. This coping strategy increases the child's sense of control by being able to watch the sleep technologist apply the PSG stickers rather than just feeling the unfamiliar sensations on his or her body. Additionally, the child's hands are occupied, resulting in less likelihood for tugging at the sensors. Another challenge might be a child who is very sensitive to textures and finds the skin preparation (i.e., Nuprep, Lemon Prep, etc.) uncomfortable and possibly intolerable. In this case, provide the child a bit more control and involvement in the experience by encouraging the child to help clean his or her skin with you. Offer the child a Q-Tip with a small amount of "cleaning lotion," then guide his or her participation in helping you clean his or her skin. Follow the child's cues with either more encouragement if the child's interest is piqued by his or her involvement, or a different approach if the child still seems overwhelmed or is not responding. Additionally, using the medical equipment in fun but accurate ways is often helpful. For example, have an assortment of small-size fun stickers with different pictures and interests available (for example, cars, animals, princesses, cartoon characters, etc.) for the child to decorate the PSG sensors. When ready to apply the PSG sensors to the child, encourage the child to select each sensor that he or she decorated for placement.

Diversional items are another effective coping strategy to use during a child's sleep study experience. Diversional items and toys can enhance a child's cooperation, coping, and sense of control (Breiner, 2009; Heard, 2008; Salmela, Salantera & Aronen, 2010). Table 20.3 suggests a variety of diversional items that can be helpful to children during PSG experiences. The use of diversional items does not eliminate the need to explain to a child and parent the sequence of events as they happen during the PSG setup. Preparation helps to eliminate any surprises for a child and is essential, even if it is as simple as, "while you are watching the movie, I'm going to put these blue stickers on your chest right here, here, and here (as you point the areas on the child's chest)." Diversional items also offer a bridge for a heath care professional to establish rapport, trust, and cooperation with a child. For safety and infection control, all diversional items must be easily disinfected with an approved hospital cleaner/disinfectant after each child's use.

Engaging a parent and child in creating a coping plan for managing their sleep study experience cannot be overemphasized (Salmela, Salentera & Aronen, 2010). Appendix C offers suggestions on a variety of developmentally appropriate coping strategies that can be used during a child's sleep study. Essential is remembering to ask a parent for their ideas on how he or she can be most supportive to their child, as well as how *you* can be most supportive to both of them (Figure 20.6). This same question can also be asked of a child. For example, "I'm having a hard time putting the sticker on your leg. You are wiggling your legs away from me. What will be helpful so you are able to keep your leg relaxed?" Try to incorporate the child's and parent's ideas or, if needed, provide a few acceptable options to them. This may involve considering, or adapting to, an approach that might be new or different from your typical routine. In the event that their suggestions cannot be accommodated or adapted, it is important

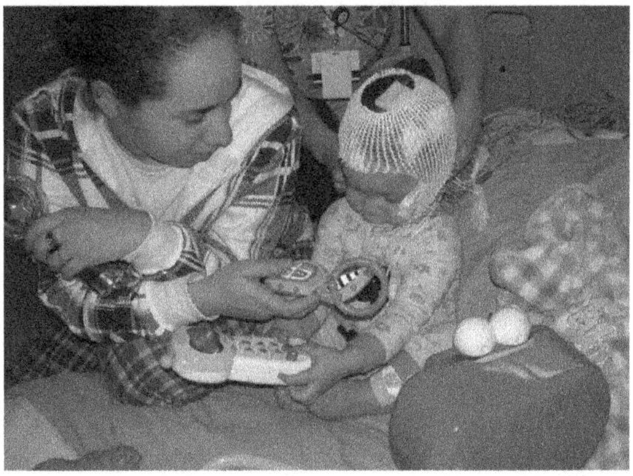

Figure 20.6 A content toddler and mom at the end of her PSG set-up. All PSG sensors, except the nasal cannula and thermister, were able to be placed on the toddler prior to her falling asleep. She remained happy and cooperative during the entire PSG set-up with no attempt to pull at the PSG sensors and wires. The sleep technologist and parents decided to place the nasal cannula and thermister after the toddler was in a deeper stage of sleep. All sensors were successfully placed and sensor integrity was easily maintained throughout the night. Consent for image reproduction provided.

to validate the child's and parent's thoughts, feelings, or input, then discuss the reason their suggestion cannot be realistically implemented.

Having an open mind, patience, flexibility, and a positive, calm attitude are prerequisites for working with children. Even with the best preparation and coping strategies, children may become overwhelmed by the sleep study experience. A child's uncooperativeness is most likely an attempt to communicate his or her needs. A child may exhibit increased anxiety (for example, self-stimulating behaviors, disengaging, screaming, etc.), uncooperative or aggressive behaviors to protect his or her body, even to the extent of panic when a child's fight or flight response is triggered (for example, blocking placement of sensors, pulling off sensors, hitting, biting, screaming, etc.). Could a child's reactions be due to limited understanding, overstimulation, discomfort, hunger, sensory overload, unfamiliar environment and people, inability to follow established routines and rituals, or could it be something else (Salmela, Aronen & Salantera, 2010; Salmela, Salantera, Aronen, 2010)? It is crucial for a sleep technologist to be attentive to a child's and parent's cues, talk with a parent about the child's anxiety triggers, recognize a need to adapt to a new approach that is less threatening, or discuss other strategies with a parent. One helpful approach may be placing the least intrusive sensors on the child first, such as the leg sensors, then progressively working up to placing the sensors on the torso, neck, head, and then face. The sleep technologist may prefer to begin a child's PSG setup with the EEG electrodes and face sensors because it is easier for the technologist and part of his or her established routine. However, the placement of the sensors should correspond with what is easiest, most comfortable, and less threatening for the child and not necessarily the simplest for the sleep technician. For example, the sleep technician begins the PSG setup with the sensors farthest away from the child's head and face (i.e., the leg, then chest sensors) while leaving the more sensitive head and face sensors until last. This allows the child to feel more in control by being able to watch and easily participate with the initial sensors. Once the child is familiar with the process, he or she can watch in a mirror as the head and face sensors are placed. Another suggestion, and less bothersome for the child, may be placing the pulse-oximeter on the child's toe instead of the finger, especially if the child is a thumb-sucker or uses his or her hands for self-soothing sleep onset activities (for example, rubbing their ear, hair, blanket, or stuffed animal).

Many children manage their sleep study experience and tolerate the PSG sensors better than their parents or staff would have otherwise predicted. Much success may be due to the positive, calm, and child-friendly RCM© practices of the sleep center's staff. However, some children with sensory issues, anxiety issues, or children with a limited ability to cooperate are still not able to tolerate a full PSG setup at the beginning of or throughout the night, despite the sleep technician's caring efforts and despite exhausting all RCM© coping strategies. While achieving a full polysomnography study is the ideal goal, for some children with sensory issues, anxiety issues, or limited ability to cooperate, this may not be a reality. Some children still are not able to tolerate all the PSG sensors even when all RCM© and coping strategies have been exhausted. Research has shown that excessive restraint during procedures increases a child's distress (Sparks, Setlik, & Luhman, 2007). Therefore, the sleep technologist and parents will need to discuss options for a less traumatic approach to applying the sensors while still being able to gather quality data for a clinical diagnosis. By minimizing a child's distress during the PSG setup through alternate approaches, a child is more apt to tolerate and maintain the crucial PSG sensors that can be placed, and his or her typical sleep onset will most likely occur. One consideration may be placing the most needed sensors on the child prior to sleep onset; then, when the child achieves a deeper sleep stage, place the challenging or remaining PSG sensors (Zaremba et al., 2005). Ultimately, while not ideal, a limited channel study may become the only viable option for the extremely anxious or uncooperative child. The number of sensors needed for the child depends on the clinical question being asked. When sleep disordered breathing is in question, the more severe the breathing problem, the fewer sensors are needed. When moderate to severe sleep apnea is in question, the problem will not be missed by simple oximetry and good technician observation of snoring and difficulty breathing. The fewer the number of signals available for review, the more experienced the interpreting physician needs to be in terms of lab–clinical correlations (C. Rosen, personal communication, May 16, 2012). Useful and quality data can still be gained while ultimately supporting the emotional integrity of the whole child. The entire sleep center staff's creative thinking and concern for the child's overall well-being, in addition to the collaboration with the parents on the child's individual needs, make alternate approaches to the sleep study experience possible while still leading to quality data collection.

Create an Inviting, Calm and Supportive Environment

Creating an inviting, calm, and relaxing child-friendly atmosphere (Stephens et al.,1999) will set the tone for a child's and parent's sleep center experience (Zaremba et al, 2005). Pay attention to each area of the sleep center that a child and parent will encounter, such as the waiting room and exam rooms in the sleep clinic and the reception area and "bedrooms" on the sleep unit. Look at the areas or rooms from a child's point of view, and at a child's eye level. What would a child see first as he or she walks into the area or room? A medical assistant in the sleep clinic might write an individualized greeting for the child on the exam table's paper (for example, "Hi Anna!"). Have a variety of books available in the exam room for the child to look at or read as the parents talk with the sleep medicine specialist. For a child-friendlier welcome on the sleep unit, place a few developmentally appropriate, interactive toys and books on the bed in the child's "bedroom." The parent's bed or cot can be made up in advance as well, so the child can be reassured that his or her parent is staying for the "sleepover," too (Figure 20.7). These approaches, along with the caring and child-friendly staff, instantly welcome a child and parent and help them to relax and feel more comfortable.

BUILD RAPPORT WITH THE CHILD AND PARENT

Making a concentrated effort to establish a trusting and supportive relationship with a child and parent has been shown to significantly increase patient/family satisfaction with the experience (Salmela, Aronen, & Salantera, 2010; Salmela, Salantera, & Aronen, 2010; Wolfer & Visintainer, 1979). As the child and parent arrive at the sleep clinic or to the sleep unit/laboratory, the importance of establishing rapport and a trusting relationship begins immediately. If the child is very quiet or reluctant to walk with his or her parent to the exam room at the sleep clinic or the "bedroom" in the sleep unit/laboratory, it may be an indication that he or she is nervous or worried. Parental involvement will be crucial in order to gain a child's cooperation, and a bit more time may need to be spent with the child in relationship-building and step-by-step preparation. Using toys and bubbles are helpful strategies to ease transitions and build rapport. For example, create a bubble parade by blowing bubbles as everyone walks down the hallway to the exam room or "bedroom." The child and parent can pop the bubbles as they walk to their "bedroom." With proper preparation, the child should have no surprises from the sleep study technologist, which in turn will foster an increasingly trusting relationship.

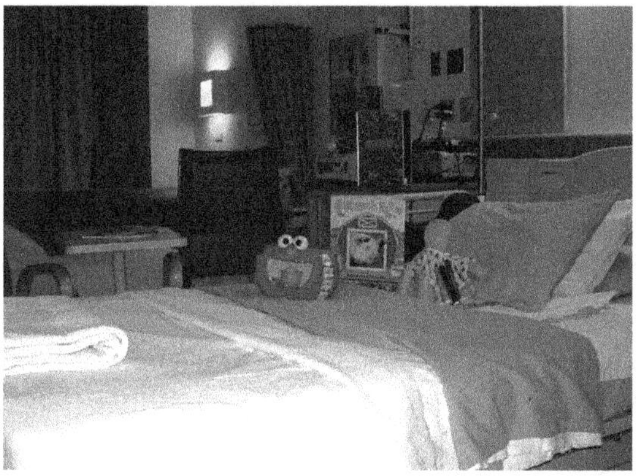

Figure 20.7 A child-friendly "bedroom" with toys to welcome a child and a comfortable parent sleep space. (University Hospitals Rainbow Babies and Children's Hospital, Cleveland, OH).

Additionally beneficial to gaining a child's trust and cooperation is the health care professional's ability to adapt his or her demeanor to match a child's emotions (Stephens et al., 1999). For example, a typically outgoing and exuberant sleep technologist tones down those behaviors when caring for an introverted and timid child. The technologist's approach becomes softer, gentle and quiet. As the evening progresses, and if the child becomes more relaxed and comfortable, the technologist may slowly incorporate a bit more of his or her outgoing personality, keeping in mind to continually assess the child's behavioral cues for further adjustment. On the other hand, a child with attention deficit disorder may find the new and stimulating environment too much, making it near impossible for the child to calm down, sit still, and focus, let alone fall asleep. In this case, a sleep technologist will need to create a quiet atmosphere with very little stimulation. During the child's setup suggestions may include using quieter voices, lowering the lights in the bedroom, turning off the TV, limiting the amount of choices, and choosing appropriate and calming diversional items. Additionally, when building rapport with parents conversations can be easily sidetracked to unrelated topics apart from the child's interests, needs, or experiences, or to the parent's pertinent needs and questions. Help maintain a child-focused experience with conversations focused on the child's interests, comfort, preparation, questions, and coping strategies.

PROVIDE POSITIVE GUIDANCE AND PRAISE

Stress affects a person's ability to successfully manage an experience. Demonstrating confidence in children's and parents' ability to succeed will help to decrease their stress and positively impact their experience (Breiner, 2009; Dahlquist & Pendley, 2005). The sleep technologist can role-model, coach, and gently guide a parent and child through the experience, adapting approaches to meet the parent's and child's specific emotional, developmental, and psychological needs. To redirect the busy child back to a book and gently coach the parent to become more involved, a technologist might say, "Dad, I wonder what picture is under the flap with the picture of a train? Johnny, can you guess?" or "Which flap are you and dad going to open next?"

Praise helps to reinforce a person's accomplishments. Even during the most challenging situations, something positive can be found. For example, "Your crying tells me you don't like this... but I noticed you and Dad gave each other big hugs while you watched in the mirror. I was able to put these stickers on very quickly." By acknowledging a child's and parent's teamwork and specific efforts such as trying, listening, holding still, helping, or even "being done," they will feel more confident in their own abilities and be more apt to apply the strategies they learned to future experiences (Breiner, 2009; Stephens et al., 1999; Zaremba et al., 2005). For example, "Great teamwork! Thank you for handing me the stickers, you and Dad decorated with the animal stickers. We've got quite a zoo here! I need to put the next sticker beside your eye. Which sticker would you like to hand me next?... Cool! It is a sticker with a turtle on it!" (Refer to Table 20.4 for suggested positive guidance and positive phrasing).

Practical Interventions Prior to the Child's Sleep Study Night

Many practical coping strategies and interventions have been discussed to facilitate a child's and parent's psychological preparation process and coping skill development during a sleep study. In addition, organizational and environmental considerations, as well as preadmission interventions, may be helpful to consider prior to a child's study night. Implementing these interventions can enhance a child's and parent's experience as well as the overall sleep study quality.

Organizational and Environmental Considerations

When working with a pediatric population, organizational and environmental considerations may be overlooked, such as in the scheduling process, in accommodations for the parent and child, and in safety concerns in the sleep unit/laboratory. When scheduling a child's sleep study, or when the technologist is determining the start time for the PSG setup on the sleep study night, the child's typical sleep/wake cycles should be taken into consideration. For convenience, all studies in the sleep unit/laboratory may need to be consistently scheduled for the same patient arrival time (for example, 7:30pm). As a child and parent arrive, allow a bit of time for them to relax and become comfortable

Table 20.4 Suggested Phrases for Positive Guidance and Praise*

Positive Guidance	Praise
• "Mom, you can hold Matt on your lap. This will help Matt be more still. You both can continue to play with the toy while I put the EEG leads on Matt's head." • "Hug each other a little tighter." • "Dad, what will you and Anna look for next in the 'I-Spy' book?" • "I notice it is hard for you to keep your head still Alan. Mom, can you put your hand on Alan's cheek. This may help remind him to keep his head still." • "You can hold this mirror with both hands. Now you can watch as I put the stickers on your chin."	• "You did it Abby! You held your head very still so I could gently put the sticker mustache under your nose. That was so helpful!" • "You and Dad make a great team!" • "Eliza, you are holding your head so still. That is so helpful. We are really working together." • "Your crying tells me you don't like this Emma, but I notice you are holding your body very still. I'm able to put these stickers on your legs much quicker. Your mom's hugs seem very comforting." • "Wow Becky! You kept your body so still for me while you and mom were looking at the book together. That was great teamwork!" • "What a big hug you are giving each other!"

* Adapted with permission from: Family and Child Life Services. (2010). *Comfort Measures: Helping children and families manage their stressful health care experiences – Positive Guidance and Praise* [in Rainbow Comfort Measures© educational handout series]. University Hospitals Rainbow Babies and Children's Hospital, Cleveland, OH.

in their "bedroom." For a cooperative child, the setup may take approximately an hour to complete. However, anticipate and plan for additional time when younger children, anxious children, or children with special needs are scheduled, as well as when extended montages or CPAP studies have been ordered by the sleep medicine specialist. If the child has a late bedtime at home, consider waiting to begin the child's PSG setup until closer to his/her actual bedtime. By shortening the length of time between the child's completed setup (i.e., all the tolerable sensors are applied prior to sleep onset) and when he or she falls asleep, there is less opportunity for the child to fidget, become increasingly frustrated with the sensors being on them, or possibly pull off the sensors.

As a health care professional, consider that you are inviting a child and parent into your own "home"—the sleep clinic or in the sleep unit. What should this feel like for a child and parent? Take into account what a child and parent see and experience upon entering the waiting room, the exam room, the sleep unit or the "bedroom." These areas all need to be child-friendly, comfortable, safe, and quiet. This first impression helps to pave the path for the child's and parent's visit. In the waiting areas, seeing unfamiliar and/or ill-appearing adult patients may heighten a child's anxiety and potentially begin their visit with more apprehension. A separate, child-friendly area for meeting and greeting pediatric patients may be helpful to consider. Additionally, common safety considerations in a sleep unit include beds with optional safety rails, access to extra linens and padding, safety plugs for wall outlets, limited medical equipment within the child's view and reach, bedside emergency equipment, staff training for emergency situations, medical-alert procedures, and medical backup appropriate for children (Zaremba et al., 2005).

During a sleep study it is essential to keep in mind sleeping arrangements for a child and parent (Dahlquist & Pendley, 2005). There must be comfortable sleeping accommodations for the parent in the same room as the child, like a cot or pullout couch with pillows and linens provided. The sleep/laboratory unit will need to anticipate and be flexible to sometimes accommodate two parents rooming-in due to a variety of reasons, such as families traveling long distances or when having the presence of both parents may feel more normal, familiar, and supportive to the child. Parents can then support each other, as well, capitalizing on each other's strengths in helping the child to cooperate.

Co-sleeping should also be an option for a parent and child during their sleep study. The parent and child may routinely sleep together at home. Requiring the parent and child to sleep in different beds on the study night may be a disruption to their normal routine at home, potentially leading to the child's uncooperative behaviors and adding to the child's distress. Even when co-sleeping is not a typical pattern at home, it still may need to be considered during the study night for a busy, anxious, or upset child. Co-sleeping may provide the child additional closeness, security, and reassurance needed from the parent in order to cooperate. While the parent and child are lying together, the parent can continue to comfort his or her child while redirecting unwanted behaviors such as pulling at the sensors or getting out of bed. Depending on the child's need, co-sleeping may be needed until the child falls asleep or perhaps for the entire night. While the parent remains in his or her child's bed, the technologist's detailed notes during the night will provide helpful information for study interpretation (for example, documenting the parent's snoring, movement, etc.).

People understand and assimilate information differently. Some people respond well to written information, some to verbal information, some to hands-on experiences, and some to a combination of the above. Parents should receive a confirmation letter via email or postal mail confirming their child's appointment, as well as a confirmation phone call a day or two prior to their child's visit. The sleep study confirmation letter should include the study's date, arrival time, type of test, parking logistics, directions to the sleep unit/laboratory, and any registration information needed. Also helpful is adding a brief explanation of what to expect during the study night, such as the routine of the night and an overview of the PSG sensors. Provide a reminder to bring anything that would enhance the child's comfort sleeping away from home, facilitate their typical bedtime routine, or help with diversion during the setup (for example, pajamas, comfort items, pillow, bedtime stories, favorite toy or DVD, etc.). Additionally, provide a reminder of what not to do or use prior to the study night (for example, no caffeine, limited naps, no skin or scalp lotions, etc.). Finally, include contact information to a designated resource person (further described below) in the sleep center and encourage a parent to call with any questions or if they feel their child may have difficulty with the experience.

As mentioned above, pediatric sleep centers should consider incorporating a designated resource person on their staff, such as a child life specialist or a sleep technician specifically trained in providing developmental preparations and guiding and teaching coping skill strategies to parents and children. A resource person is able to provide the additional time needed for families prior to their study night by supporting their emotional and psychological needs, helping them to manage their sleep study experience, and providing essential communication and support to the sleep center staff (Zaremba et al., 2005).

Pre-Procedural Assessment and Preparation Strategies

Ideally, preparation for a child and parent's sleep study starts in advance of the sleep study night. Preparation and information interchange can be accomplished in many different ways, including telephone, mail, Internet or pre-study visits. Pre-study assessment helps to determine the emotional readiness and coping abilities of the child and parent for their experience (Heard, 2008). Many children who are referred to the sleep clinic for a consultation or to the sleep unit for a sleep study are children with higher-acuity disorders such as certain medical, genetic, behavioral, or neurodevelopmental or neuromuscular comorbidities (for example, Trisomy 21, Prader Willi syndrome, autism spectrum disorder, sensory integration disorders, anxiety disorders, ADD/ADHD, etc.; Sinha & Guilleminault, 2010; Richdale & Schreck, 2009). These comorbidities may make managing the sleep study experience especially challenging for the child (Reynolds & Malow, 2011). Pre-study preparation is extremely helpful for children with developmental disabilities (Slifer & Frutchey, 2008).

The assessment process should begin during the initial contact with the family, either upon their first visit to the sleep clinic with the sleep medicine specialist and/or during their sleep study scheduling process with the sleep coordinator. When a child and parent are seen in the sleep clinic prior to scheduling their sleep study, a sleep medicine specialist can gain an appreciation for how a child and parent may tolerate the study night by personally observing and interacting with a child, observing parent–child dynamics, and gathering a parent's perceptions of how his or her child may manage the upcoming sleep study (for example, a child's cooperation with past sleep study or similar testing experiences or in unfamiliar and/or stressful situations). Additionally, reviewing a referring physician's notes can shed light on a child's developmental, social, and medical history, as well as past medical experiences.

Another key assessment period is during the scheduling process with a parent for the sleep study. The sleep coordinator gathers the child's demographic, general sleep, and health information needed for scheduling. The sleep coordinator can also take this opportunity with the parent to gain additional information about the child, which may signal the need for further interventions prior to his or her sleep study. For example, the coordinator may ask, "Does your child have any medical conditions (any disabilities or genetic conditions), behavioral problems, or accommodations needs that we should be aware of?" Then list a few possibilities, such as Down's Syndrome, Prader Willi syndrome, developmental delays, mental or learning disabilities, severe behavior problems, visual or hearing impairments, autism, sensory issues, seizures, cerebral palsy, craniofacial diagnosis, ADHD/ADD. Children with higher-acuity disorders may be at an increased risk for poor coping during medical procedures (Slifer & Frutchey, 2008). To gather further helpful information about the child, the coordinator may ask, "Is there anything you know about your child that might make it hard for him or her to do or cooperate for a sleep test?" Some parents can only answer this question honestly if they have an understanding of what the sleep study entails and what will be required of their child. A brief overview of the PSG sensors may need to be repeated. Additionally, it may be helpful to ask about the child's cooperation, coping skills, and possible challenges with transitions; then briefly discuss possible interventions and coping strategies (Zaremba et al., 2005). A referral to the sleep center's resource person for further support and preparation should be made when the sleep coordinator feels the parent would benefit from more time or expertise beyond what he or she is able to give during the scheduling process.

During the above key information-gathering opportunities, decisions can be made on the acuity and staffing level of the sleep study and the communication process can begin with the sleep center staff (Zaremba et al., 2005). For those children who are identified as high risk for anxiety and uncooperative behaviors, a designated child life specialist or sleep study resource person can provide a more detailed follow-up with a parent and child prior to their sleep night. This person can provide a pre-procedural preparation telephone call to a parent, as well as conducting a pre-procedural daytime visit to the sleep unit with a parent and child. Both are successful strategies that are beneficial to meeting children's and parents' pre-procedural emotional, psychological, developmental, and preparation needs.

PRE-PROCEDURAL PREPARATION TELEPHONE CALL WITH THE PARENT

A pre-procedural preparation phone call to a parent is made by a sleep center's designated resource person when a parent and/or child has been identified by the sleep medicine staff as needing more emotional and preparation support prior to the study night. Due to the detailed nature of most pre-procedural telephone calls, more time will be spent on the telephone with a parent than during the sleep study scheduling phone call. Every phone conversation is individualized to the parent's needs. Depending on those needs, a telephone call may last 30 minutes or more. Parents of children with higher-acuity disorders have been found to benefit most from these telephone calls, since their children may be more easily overwhelmed by the sleep study experience and PSG sensor setup (Zaremba et al., 2005).

The pre-procedural preparation telephone call offers the opportunity to gain additional insight into a child's personality, temperament, and past coping with challenging experiences or medical events. It is an opportunity for a parent to sort out worries and concerns and to ask further questions (Heard, 2008). The resource person making the call is able to share with the parent a more detailed explanation of the study night, including the various PSG sensors and how they are applied. Even though the sleep medicine specialist or referring physician may have described a sleep study experience and PSG sensors to the parent, it is not uncommon for a parent to hear and retain only a small portion of the explanation. Hearing explanations again may prompt further questions that were not previously considered. Additional dialogue can then take place, discussing different preparation and coping strategies that may enhance the child's coping with and tolerance of a sleep study experience. Parents' questions or concerns regarding their child's medicines, diagnosis, or future treatment plans should be directed to the sleep medicine specialist.

Parents also can be encouraged to begin the preparation process at home. It may be helpful to discuss with parents the importance of appropriate timing and approaches, as well as to suggest developmentally appropriate word choices to use with the child. Parents can begin talking about the sleep study with the child by introducing it as a "sleepover," then continue with a preparation plan that corresponds to the child's developmental level and need for information. Simple wording for a child developmentally functioning at a preschool level may be, "Matt, you and I are going to have a sleepover at Rainbow tomorrow. Your sleep doctor and I want to know why you are so tired during the day and what we can do to help you. At our sleepover we will meet a few people that will help us. They will put a few stickers on your legs, chest, face, and head... maybe you can even help them. These stickers will help your sleep doctor know how your body is working while you are sleeping. You will need to sleep all night with the stickers on you. I will sleep in a bed next to you. The next morning you can help take the stickers off your body and we will come home."

Parents can also role-play a PSG setup at home with the child by placing fun-type stickers (which can be purchased at many stores) in the appropriate places on a doll, stuffed animal, themselves and/or the child. in a playful but educational manner. Long strings to simulate the PSG sensor wires can be added to each "sensor" if the parent feels this would be helpful. The child may benefit greatly from this approach to preparation, since the process begins in the comfort of home. The parent also has the ability to offer a number of short preparation sessions, which can increase in length and content according to the child's needs. To further facilitate the child's preparation process and the transition from home to the sleep study unit/laboratory, the parents can encourage their child to help pack a suitcase for the sleepover. The child can help decide what to bring (for example, favorite pajamas, comfort items, pillow, favorite items or toys that may facilitate distraction during the setup, etc.), along with any items involved with their typical bedtime routine (bedtime stories, non-caffeinated bedtime drinks and snacks, soft bedtime music, etc.)

The information gathered during a pre-procedure preparation telephone call should be communicated with the sleep center staff through documentation in the child's medical records. The sleep center's medical director, manager, and/or lead technician should review this information so that any additional concerns that may impact the study are anticipated and proactively managed.

OPTIONAL PRE-PROCEDURAL DAYTIME VISIT

Pre-procedural and presurgical preparation programs for children have been found to decrease both a child's and parent's anxiety and increase their comfort level and cooperation with upcoming experiences. Tours and preparation sessions prior to a procedure or surgical experience improve a child's understanding of what to expect on the procedure or surgery day and offers opportunities to become familiar with the environment and begin building a rapport with the medical staff (Ellerton & Merriam, 1994; Slifer & Frutchey, 2008; DeMore, Cataldo, Tierney, & Slifer, 2009). Given the tremendous benefits that pre-procedural preparation visits can offer to children, parents, and staff, sleep centers should consider providing optional pre-procedural daytime visits for children and parents and encourage their participation, especially when children have poor coping abilities.

Supporting the benefits of pre-procedural preparation visits are two studies conducted with children with developmental and behavioral disabilities. Slifer & Frutchey (2008) and DeMore et al. (2009) determined helpful strategies for children who have neurodevelopmental disabilities, such as autism, to help them successfully manage and complete standard electroencephalographic (EEG) procedures (Slifer & Frutchey 2008) and overnight EEG procedures (DeMore et al., 2009). In both studies, children were involved with pre-procedural mock EEG sessions in which each child had a systematic and gradual exposure to the procedural steps, helping them form increasingly positive associations, tolerance, and success with the EEG routine while also using additional behavioral intervention strategies to increase compliance (i.e., differential reinforcement, escape extinction, counterconditioning, shaping procedures). The researchers found that with incremental preparation, desensitization, and behavioral training provided during the children's pre-visit(s), children's cooperation, tolerance of sensory stimulation, and coping abilities increased. In addition, their uncooperative behaviors (i.e., aggression, blocking placement of or removing EEG leads, crying, screaming, attempting to run away) decreased during the actual procedure, providing successful completion of the children's EEG studies. Since the successful completion of both an EEG procedure and a sleep study test involves similar behavioral requirements for a child (i.e., the ability to tolerate sensory stimulation, transitions, unfamiliar environment and equipment, and limited mobility for an extended period of time), these interventions and positive results from Slifer & Frutchey and DeMore et al. studies can be generalized to benefit children undergoing sleep studies.

Providing multiple pre-procedural training sessions using incremental desensitization paired with other behavioral training strategies may not be feasible for sleep centers to offer due to time constraints. However, a sleep center program should offer parents and children an option of at least a single pre-procedural daytime visit. The visit to the sleep unit/laboratory should include a tour of the sleep unit/laboratory and bedroom. In the bedroom, encourage the child to safely explore the room. Sitting or lying on the bed, working the TV remote control, and so forth may help the child feel more comfortable in the space. Then offer opportunities for the child's familiarization with the PSG sensors and hands-on preparation for the actual PSG setup. A doll or stuffed animal can be used to help the child and parent learn more about the PSG sensors and setup. Demonstrate on the doll or stuffed animal (which can be taken home) where and how the PSG sensors will be placed, and encourage the child's help. Being able to touch the PSG sensors and participate in the demonstration and role-playing will continue to increase the child's familiarity, understanding, and comfort level with the PSG equipment and experience. During a pre-visit, a plan for managing the PSG experience also needs to be discussed and possibly role-played with the parent and child. Strategies may include hands-on demonstration, participation, RCP©, relaxation, and distraction.

Similar to a preparation approach during a child's sleep study night, preparation during the pre-visit involves a parent but should progress at the child's pace and observed level of anxiety, but never to the extent of overly distressing the child. Continual assessment of the child's understanding, nonverbal cues, and emotional reactions are important when adapting an approach to meet the child's individual needs. For example, if the child seems distracted, not listening or unable to focus, attempts should be made to redirect the child's attention back to the preparation. If the child still is not responding or inattentive, continue the preparation process with just the parent. Even though the child may seem inattentive, he or she may still be listening and taking in all overheard information. The preparation experience may have become too overwhelming for the child, and a slower or different approach may be needed. It may be helpful to encourage the parent to review with his or her child the sleep study information and sensors shared at the pre-visit once in the familiar and nonthreatening environment of their home.

Additional ideas to facilitate further preparation at home after the pre-visit include: taking a photograph of the child during the pre-visit preparation session (for example, sitting on the bed with the doll that he/she helped place the PSG sensors), which can be referred at home and help continue discussion, preparation, and transition back to the sleep unit/laboratory for the child's study night; or providing the child and parent with a few extra sensors to take home (for example, EKG sensors, EEG electrode with a shortened wire nasal cannula, etc.), which may add to further hands-on practice and desensitization opportunities.

Conclusion

Health care experiences typically elicit some stress, if not a great amount of stress from individuals enduring them. Positively speaking, when stress is anticipated it can be seen as an opportunity for growth, to learn how to cope, manage adversity, and develop resiliency. Stress is also more tolerable when coupled with support from trusted individuals. A person's stress level may rise as his or her physician discusses a plan of care, as they receive preparation for an upcoming medical procedure, or as they talk about different strategies to manage an experience. However, discussion, preparation, and the implementation of coping strategies will contribute to a person's development of resiliency. As preparation unfolds, it is combined with support from knowledgeable and caring staff committed to helping a child and parent manage their challenging hurdles ahead. On the other hand, unexpected stress—stress from the unknown, unpredictable, or threatening event—creates a loss of control and increases anxiety. We as health care professionals need to understand *how* to promote resiliency within children and not inhibit, obstruct, or send mixed messages. We can help a child and parent not only to cope in the moment during a procedure or situation, but also to gain the confidence and skills to cope better in the future. Ultimately, the child's resiliency will help him or her overcome the many adversities they will face in life (Bernard vanLeer Foundation, 1995).

A child's and parent's involvement in their medical experience must be seen as a process that evolves over time according to their needs, circumstances, and motivation. The RCM© model of care's foundations rooted in child development and uses evidence-based strategies to enhance a child's and parent's understanding of their experiences and builds their coping skills. The model promotes a child's and parent's increased participation, comfort, achievement, self-control, self-esteem, and resilience. The benefits of incorporating the RCM© model of care into a sleep center's philosophy, policies and practice guidelines are summarized in Table 20.5.

What a child experiences during a medical experience and how he/she remembers that event has significant implications for how that child will manage future medical experiences (Salmon et al., 2006; Chen et al., 2000). A child and parent should not be required to totally conform to all of our needs and practices when this may create negative experiences for them. Instead, a child's and parent's needs should guide, influence, and change how we practice. Intentionally take note: *how* do your actions and words translate to the child and parent?...what *words* do you choose?...how are your messages delivered and how are they received?...are you doing things *for* and *with* a child instead of just *to* them? These questions may seem inconsequential in the overall goal of completing a task or medical procedure. However, these questions and considerations are not inconsequential to the child and family. These questions, considerations, and responsive actions are crucial to the respectful humanization of the child's and family's experience. ***This*** is the art of caring. In order to empower the child and parent in the medical experience, ask yourself these questions, am I open to examining my own approach?...am I willing to integrate the RCM© model of care components—this family centered, relationship-based approach—into my clinical perspective and practice? Additionally, for the sleep technician and the sleep center's benefit, this reflective mindset and approach will make the difference between a successful sleep study and diagnostic outcome versus possibly not being able to complete the sleep study at all. During the child's and parent's health care experiences, we have the ideal opportunity as sleep medicine professionals to help strengthen the child and parent in their spirit, in their relationship, in their view of healthcare professionals and medical experiences, and in their confidence in being able to cope positively with future medical and life experiences.

Future Directions

There is an abundance of research that supports a child's and parent's emotional, psychological, and developmental growth when pre-procedural preparation, parent–child involvement, RCP©, and coping strategies are integrated into their care plans. Unfortunately, there is only limited literature and

Table 20.5 Benefits of Rainbow Comfort Measures© Model of Care*

For the Parent and the Child ...	For the Health Care Professional ...
• **Decreased Anxiety and Emotional Stress** RCM© promotes physical and emotional contact between the child and parent. Anxiety and fear is reduced and lower levels of fear correlate to a decreased perception of pain.	• **Decreased Number of Staff Needed for Immobilization** RCM© upholds the importance of parental involvement and preparation which leads to the child's enhanced cooperation. Fewer staff members are needed due to the child's increased cooperation and decreased movement.
• **Increased Self-esteem, Mastery and Resiliency** RCM© facilitates and promotes the child's feeling of control and therefore his/her ability to cooperate. The child's self confidence, mastery over an experience, self esteem, and resiliency are all increased.	• **Decreased Time for Procedural Success** RCM© promotes a collaborative working relationship between the child, parent and staff members. There is a focus on individual roles while also working toward the overall combined goal of a successful outcome, both physically and emotionally.
• **Maintained and Strengthened Parent-Child Bond** Parents want to help their child get through challenging experiences but sometimes they don't know how. RCM© involves and coaches a parent's active role to positively support their child leading to a strengthened and trusted parent-child bond.	• **Decreased Stress and Pressure on Procedural Performance** Since RCM© assumes the child and parent are prepared for their experience and their role during the procedure, an environment is created for staff to have a better frame of mind for accuracy. There is a decreased preoccupation and worry over the child resisting and fighting which allows for a strong level of confidence in procedural performance. Ultimately, the likelihood of success in accomplishing the task at hand is increased.
• **Increased Satisfaction with Immediate and Future Health Care Experiences** RCM© promotes positive experiences and memories that will have a far reaching impact on the child's and family's perception and response to their current and future health care experiences.	• **Increased Trust and Confidence Toward Health Care Professionals** RCM© empowers a sense of trust, confidence, and camaraderie among the parent, child, and staff members which will extend to future health care experiences.

* Adapted with permission from: Zaremba & Mitchell (2011).

research documenting effective approaches and strategies to help children and families manage the emotional, psychological, and procedural challenges of sleep studies. Future research investigations are needed with children and parents who undergo sleep studies to determine successful interventions and coping strategies that increase cooperation, decrease anxiety, and provide a child and parent with positive growth-producing experiences. Areas of investigational research within pediatric sleep medicine may include a focus on the benefits and outcomes of providing pre-procedural preparation visits for a child and family, providing pre-procedural preparation phone calls to parents, and integrating the RCM© guiding principles into a child's care plan on the study night.

Another area in need of further investigation is that of children requiring continuous positive airway pressure (CPAP) titration and CPAP titration studies (see Archbold, Chapter 25). With the national obesity epidemic, sleep centers are seeing more obese children with obstructive sleep apnea that cannot be medically managed with adenotonsillectomy alone. Many of these children are looking at long-term therapies like CPAP to manage their sleep apnea (Sinha & Guilleminault, 2010). CPAP therapy involves wearing a cushioned mask over the nose and sometime nose and mouth. These masks deliver humidified airflow and pressure to open up the child's collapsed airway at night so that the child can achieve good quality, safe sleep. Sleep units are increasingly involved in providing CPAP titration studies and CPAP treatment in children. Tasks on the study night include fitting the child for the CPAP mask and wearing the medical device all night for sleep. This adds a new level of complexity to the sleep study procedure. However, the principles of the RCM© model of care can be effectively applied to the initiation of CPAP therapy. Creating a positive first CPAP experience for a child and parent may result in greater likelihood of cooperation and compliance compared to a CPAP titration study performed without incorporating the guiding principles of the RCM©. Future research investigations would be helpful to determine successful strategies that increase a child's and parent's understanding, adjustment, and adherence to their CPAP procedures and treatment (C. Rosen, personal communication, March 13, 2012).

In order to provide the support necessary to integrate the RCM© model of care into a sleep center's policies and procedures, formalized educational opportunities need to be provided to all sleep medicine professionals. RCM© education should be built into a new employee's orientation process. For continued professional growth, frequent didactic in-service programs on the RCM© guiding principles should be provided by a child life specialist or other health care professional who has training in the emotional, psychological, and developmental needs of children and families. Additionally, providing and encouraging ongoing mentoring and discussion among staff is crucial to successfully integrate the RCM© components into practice. As colleagues are able to debrief with and positively support one another on their successes and challenges with children and families, new perspectives can be gained, problem-solving can begin, and motivation to provide outstanding child-friendly and child-focused care can flourish. This support in staff development and personal growth positively impacts and upgrades pediatric sleep study services and improves both sleep study quality and child and parent satisfaction.

Future Directions for Pediatric Sleep Medicine

- Research investigations on the benefits and outcomes of:
    - Providing pre-procedural phone calls to parents.
    - Providing pre-procedural preparation visits for children and parents
    - Integrating the RCM© model of care's guiding principles into sleep study procedural practices.
- Research investigation to determine successful strategies that increase children's and parents' understanding, adjustment, and adherence to CPAP procedures and treatment
- Incorporate the RCM© model of care into the education and training of all sleep center health care professionals through new employee orientations and ongoing didactic in-services and clinical mentoring.

References

American Academy of Pediatrics. (2006). Child life council and committee on hospital care. Child Life services. *Pediatrics, 118*(4), 1757–1763.

Bauchner, H., Waring, C., & Vinci, R. (1991). Parental presence during procedure in an emergency room: Results from 50 observations. *Pediatrics, 87*(4), 544–548.

Bauchner, H., Vinci, R., Bak, S., Pearson, C., & Corwin, M. J. (1996). Parents and procedures: A randomized controlled trial. *Pediatrics, 98*(5), 861–867.

The Bernard vanLeer Foundation. (1995) *A guide to promoting resilience in children: Strengthening the human spirit.* The International Resilience Project from the Early Childhood Development: Practice and Reflections Series. ISSN 1382–4813.

Breiner, S. M. (2009). Preparation of the pediatric patient for invasive procedures. *Journal of Infusion Nursing, 32*(5), 252–256.

Brewer, S., Gleditsch, S.L., Syblik, D., Tietjens, M. E., Vacik, H.W. (2006). Pediatric anxiety: Child life intervention in day surgery. *Journal of Pediatric Nursing, 21*(1), 13–22.

Cavender, K., Goff, M. D., Hollon, E. C., & Guzzetta, C. E. (2004). Parents' positioning and distracting children during venipuncture: Effects on children's pain, fear, and distress. *Journal of Holistic Nursing, 22*(1), 32–56.

Chen, E., Zeltzer, L.K., Craske, M. G., & Katz, E. (2000). Children's memories for painful cancer treatment procedures: Implications for distress. *Child Development, 71*, 933–947.

Cohen, L. L., Manimala, R., & Blount, R. L. (2000). Easier said than done: What parents say they do and what they do during children's immunizations. *Children's Health Care, 29*(2), 79–86.

Dahlquist, L. M., & Pendley, J. S. (2005). When distraction fails: Parental anxiety and children's responses to distraction during cancer procedures. *Journal of Pediatric Psychology, 30*(7), 623–628.

DeMore, M., Cataldo, M., Tierney, E., & Slifer, K. (2009). Behavioral approaches to training developmentally disabled children for an overnight EEG procedure. *Journal of Developmental and Physical Disabilities, 21*, 245–251.

Ellerton, M. L., & Merriam, C. (1994). Preparing children and families psychologically for day surgery: An evaluation. *Journal of Advanced Nursing, 19*(6), 1057–1062.

Family and Child Life Services. (2010). *Comfort measures: Helping children and families manage their stressful health care experiences.* [in Rainbow Comfort Measures educational handout series]. Cleveland, OH: University Hospitals/Rainbow Babies and Children's Hospital.

Gaynard, L., Wolfer, J., Goldberger, J., Thompson, R., Redbum, L., & Laidley, L. (1990). *Psychosocial care of children in hospitals: A clinical practice manual from the ACCH child life research project.* Bethesda, MD: The Association for the Care of Children's Health.

Heard, L. (2008). Taking care of the little things: Preparation of the pediatric endoscopy patient. *Gastroenterology Nursing, 31*(2), 108–112.

Hoban, T. F. (2010). Sleep disorders in children. *Annals of the New York Academy of Sciences, 1184*, 1–14.

Kain, Z. N., Mayes, L. C., & Caramico, L. A. (1996). Preoperative preparation in children: a cross-sectional study. *Journal of Clinical Anesthesia, 8*, 508–514.

Koller, D. (2007). Preparing children and adolescents for medical procedures. [Child Life Council evidence-based practice statement]. Retrieved from http://www.childlife.org.

Lacey, C. M., Finklestein, M., & Thygeson, M. V. (2008). The impact of positioning on fear during immunization: Supine versus sitting up. *Journal of Pediatric Nursing, 23*(3), 32–56.

Leahy, S., Kennedy, R. M., Hesselgrave, J., Gurwitch, K., Barkey, M., & Millar, T. (2008). On the front lines: Lessons learned in implementing multidisciplinary peripheral venous access pain-management programs in pediatric hospitals. *Pediatrics, 122*(3), S161–S167.

Melamed, B. G., Dearborn, M., & Hermecz, D. A. (1983). Necessary considerations for surgery preparation: Age and previous experience. *Psychosomatic Medicine. 45*(6), 517–525.

Melamed, B. G., Ridley-Johnson, R. (1988). Psychological preparation of families for hospitalization. *Journal of Developmental & Behavioral Pediatrics, 9*(2), 96–102.

Richdale, A. L. & Schreck, A. A. (2009). Sleep problems in autism spectrum disorders: prevalence, nature and possible biopsychosocial actiologies. *Sleep Medicine Reviews, 13*, 403–411.

Reynolds, A. M., & Malow, B. A. (2011). Sleep and autism spectrum disorders. *Pediatric Clinics of North America, 58*, 685–698.

Ross, D. M., & Ross, S. A. (1982). A study of the pain experiences in children. Final report Ref No. 1 ROIDH 13672–01. Bethesda, MD: National Institute of Child Health and Human Development.

Ross, D. M., & Ross, S. A. (1984). Childhood pain: The school-aged child's viewpoint. *Pain, 20*, 179–191.

Salmela, M., Aronen, E. T., & Salantera, S. (2010). The experience of hospital-related fears of 4- to 6-year-old children. *Child: Care, Health and Development, 37*(5), 719–726.

Salmela, M., Salantera, S., & Aronen, E. T. (2010). Coping with hospital-related fears: Experiences of pre-school-aged children. *Journal of Advanced Nursing, 66*(6), 1222–1231.

Salmon, D., McGuigan, F., & Pereira, J. K. (2006). Brief report. Optimizing children's memory and management of an invasive medical procedure: The influence of procedural narration and distraction. *Journal of Pediatric Psychology, 31*(5), 522–527.

Sinha, D. & Guilleminault, C. (2010). Sleep disordered breathing. *Indian Journal of Medical Research, 131*, 311–320.

Slifer, K., & Frutchey, R. A. (2008). Behavioral interventions to increase compliance with electroencephalographic procedures in children with developmental disabilities. *Epilepsy & Behavior, 13*, 189–195.

Sparks, L. A., Setlik, J., & Luhman, J. (2007). Parental holding and positioning to decrease IV distress in young children: A randomized control trial. *Journal of Pediatric Nursing, 22*(6), 440–447.

Stephens, B. K., Barkey, M. E., & Hall, H. R. (1999). Techniques to comfort children during stressful procedures. *Advances in Mind-Body Medicine, 15*, 49–60.

Tanaka, K., Oikawa, N., Terao, R., Negishi, Y., Fujii, T., Kudo, T., & Shimizu, T. (2011). Psychological preparation for children undergoing endoscopy. *Journal of Pediatric Gastroenterology andNutrition, 52*(2), 227–229.

Wolfer, J. A., & Visintainer, M. A. (1979). Prehospital psychological preparation for tonsillectomy patients: Effects on children's and parent's adjustment. *Pediatrics, 64*, 646–655.

Zaremba, E. K., Barkey, M. E., Mesa, C., Sanniti, K., & Rosen, C. (2005). Making polysomnography more "child-friendly": A family-centered care approach. *Journal of Clinical Sleep Medicine, 1*(2), 189–198.

Zaremba, L. & Mitchell, D. (May, 2011). "Hold Me... PLEASE!": Parental participation during stressful procedures. [Conference presentation] 3a Journada Humanization of Children's Hospitals. Hospital Sant Joan de Deu Universitat de Barcelona, Barcelona, Spain.

Appendix A

Developmental Considerations for Infants through Adolescents

Infants (birth to 12 months)*

Developmental Considerations	Possible Stressors	Cognitive Impact and Coping Behaviors	Interventions and Support
• Attachment and bonding to parent • Developing trust • Meeting basic physical needs are of primary importance	• Separation from parents • Stranger anxiety • Senses parent's stress • Change in routines	• Intense anxiety when separated from familiar caregiver (begins at 6mos) • Generalized anxiety (crying, fussing, clinging behaviors, etc.) • Hyper-alertness • Expects basic physical needs to be met	• Support parent participation in care and procedures including Rainbow Comfort Positioning© • Prepare parent for procedure and enable comforting role • Minimize number of medical caregivers • Meet physical needs and avoid hunger • Incorporate familiar routines
• Learns through senses and repetition	• Overstimulation (lights, noises, people, etc.) • Restrained for procedures • Painful touch • Loss of normal stimulation	• Hand-mouth activity	• Talk quietly before touching • Decrease unnecessary stimuli • Provide opportunities for sucking (breastfeeding, bottle, pacifier, etc.) • Provide tactile stimulation for comfort
• Developing purposeful communication • Minimal language abilities	• Unresponsiveness to nonverbal cues/stress signals	• Increased agitation in movements • Crying • Tantrums	• Respond to nonverbal cues • Mimic child's sounds, rhythms or words

* Adapted with permission from: Family and Child Life Services. (2010). *Comfort Measures: Helping children and families manage their stressful health care experiences – Developmental considerations for infant, toddlers and preschool Age children.* [in Rainbow Comfort Measures© educational handout series]. University Hospitals Rainbow Babies and Children's Hospital, Cleveland, OH.

Toddlers (1 to 2 years)*

Developmental Considerations	Possible Stressors	Cognitive Impact and Coping Behaviors	Interventions and Support
• Attachment to parent • Learns through active participation and play • Focuses on one thing at a time • Imitates routine tasks • Short attention span	• Separation from parent and familiar environment • Fear of abandonment • Stranger anxiety • Overstimulation (lights, noise, people, many events at once, etc.) • Unfamiliar environment • Anything touching the body can be seen as a threat	• Generalized anxiety (crying, clinging, fussing behaviors, etc.) • Regression • Expects to participate in routine tasks	• Support parents participation in care and procedures including Rainbow Comfort Positioning© • Provide brief details of sensory information • Demonstrate just prior to action (using doll/stuffed animal, etc.) • Encourage manipulation of equipment and imitation of procedural steps • Allow expression of feelings through play
• Developing language skills • Receptive language more advanced than expressive language • No concept of time	• Overwhelmed by directions	• Difficulty understanding directions when overwhelmed	• Provide simple, concrete description for each medical step with visual and tactile support
• Learning new skills (walking, potty training, etc.) • Beginning to make choices • Wants to do things "all by myself" • Acts on impulse and has assertive will • Loves rituals • Expects basic physical needs to be met	• Loss of autonomy • Restriction of movement • Loss of control (physical and emotional) • Change in routine	• Intense dislike of being retrained • May resist treatment • Tantrums • Pain may be seen as a punishment for a prior misbehavior	• Actively involve in procedures and treatment • Offer choices when possible • Minimize excessive restraint and allow for some means of movement if possible (legs, hands, etc.) • Maintain daily schedule and bedtime routine • Meet basic physical needs and avoid hunger

* Adapted with permission from: Family and Child Life Services. (2010). *Comfort Measures: Helping children and families manage their stressful health care experiences – Developmental considerations for infant, toddlers and preschool Age children.* [in Rainbow Comfort Measures© educational handout series]. University Hospitals Rainbow Babies and Children's Hospital, Cleveland, OH.

Preschool Age Children (3 to 5 years)*

Developmental Considerations	Possible Stressors	Cognitive Impact and Coping Behaviors	Interventions and Support
• Parent is a secure base • Learns through active participation and play • Imitates through play • Uses play to understand and master experiences • Understands the "here" and "now" • Focuses on one thing at a time • Limited concept of time • Little understanding of body functions	• Separation from parent • Loss of appropriate sensory and motor stimulation • Overstimulation (too many experiences happening at once, etc.) • Fear of unknown events	• Misconceptions develop from lack of understanding • Concepts about "inside the body" may be too abstract • Understands the "job" of medical equipment	• Support parent participation in care and procedures including Rainbow Comfort Positioning© • Demonstrate prior to the procedure (using doll/ stuffed animal, etc.) • Encourage manipulation of equipment and imitation of procedural steps • Use concrete markers for time ("same amount of time as a SpongeBob show") • Allow expression of feelings through play
• Increasing language skills but still limited • Literal interpretation of language • Increasing development of fears and fantasies • Mixes fears with reality	• Fears are intensified in a medical setting • Worried about being hurt • Anything touching the body can be seen as a threat • Inability to distinguish reality from fantasy • Fear of body mutilation • Fear of death and monsters • Use of humor or playful teasing	• Fantasy and misconceptions • Medical experiences may be seen as a punishment for a prior misbehavior	• Provide simple, concrete, and truthful descriptions for each medical step with visual and tactile support • Use words and phrases that are familiar • Avoid words with multiple meanings • Encourage use of familiar soothing items
• Egocentric • Increasing autonomy and becoming more self-sufficiency	• Loss of control and choices • Loss of competence and initiative in newly acquired skills	• Guilt • Regression • Anger and aggression • Temper tantrums • Oppositional behavior	• Allow participation in procedures and care • Focus on immediate event and offer concrete, realistic choices • Teach and support coping skills • Offer specific praise, even for small helpful behaviors

* Adapted with permission from: Family and Child Life Services. (2010). *Comfort Measures: Helping children and families manage their stressful health care experiences – Developmental considerations for infant, toddlers and preschool Age children.* [in Rainbow Comfort Measures© educational handout series]. University Hospitals Rainbow Babies and Children's Hospital, Cleveland, OH.

School Age Children (6 to 12 years)*

Developmental Considerations	Possible Stressors	Cognitive Impact and Coping Behaviors	Interventions and Support
• Active learner and curious about how things work • Understands cause/effect and sequential relationships • Concrete thinking (something is either good or bad) • Rules and "doing things the right way" are important • Able to reason and compromise • Increasing concept of time • Increasing understanding of body functions and structure	• Separation from parents • Fear of the unknown • Fear of pain • Fear of disability and/or death • Fear of bodily harm and/or change	• Learning styles are established (verbal, hands-on, demonstration) • Understand more about the "inside of the body" concepts • Often has expectations of medical events • Connects expectations with previous experiences	• Support parent participation including Rainbow Comfort Positioning© • Describe steps involved in procedure using appropriate individual learning style • Encourage active involvement in procedures and own care • Realistically reassure about progress (procedure, course of treatment, etc.)
• Self-esteem influenced by performance • Increasing participation in self-care • Concern for body integrity • Increasing modesty	• Fear of failure • Lack of privacy • Loss of independence and enforced dependence • Loss of bodily control • Fear of altered body image and/or functions	• Strives to accomplish tasks • Understands limits • Acting out • Regression	• Observe and respond to cues and behaviors • Respect thoughts and feelings • Provide activities that foster sense of accomplishment • Offer choices when possible • Teach and support coping strategies • Give "jobs" to help during procedures • Recognize and praise aspects of effective coping • Respect modesty
• Increasing autonomy and becoming more self-sufficient • Peers and peer approval are important	• Loss of control and choices • Loss of competence and initiative in newly acquired skills • Conscious of being different • Loss of status in school or peer group	• Guilt • Anger and aggression • Oppositional behavior • Hesitant to ask questions or talk about concerns directly • Withdrawal from peer group or socialization opportunities	• Encourage participation in procedures and care • Offer concrete, realistic choices • Teach and support coping skills • Offer specific praise, even for small helpful behaviors • Facilitate continued and new peer connections

* Adapted with permission from: Family and Child Life Services. (2010). *Comfort Measures: Helping children and families manage their stressful health care experiences – Developmental considerations for school age children and adolescents.* [in Rainbow Comfort Measures© educational handout series]. University Hospitals Rainbow Babies and Children's Hospital, Cleveland, OH.

Adolescents (13 to 18 years)*

Developmental Considerations	Possible Stressors	Cognitive Impact and Coping Behaviors	Interventions and Support
• Uses deductive reasoning and abstract thought • Thinks about the future • Struggles with more advanced concepts related to mortality	• Impact on current and/or future plans • Fear of the unknown • Fear of pain • Fear of disability and/or death	• Intellectualization • Knowledgeable about body functions	• Honest explanations and procedures and diagnosis • Ask about preferred learning mode • Describe steps involved in procedures and ask if more detailed explanations would be helpful • Encourage active role in procedures and decision-making • Use Rainbow Comfort Positioning©
• Struggles to develop self-identity • Growing sense of personal values • Increasing independence and responsibility • Increasing decision-making skills • Self-determination	• Increased restrictions (lifestyle, diet, medications, treatments, etc.) • Threat to future competence • Loss of independence and enforced dependence • Loss of control • Medical diagnosis is concerning	• Defense mechanisms • Conformity • Reluctant to see rationale to medical interventions • Uncooperative behavior and noncompliance • Feels invincible • Risk-taking behaviors • Mood swings	• Observe and respond to cues and behavior • Communicate honestly • Involve in care and decisions • Teach and support coping strategies • Allow choices and control • Respect autonomy • Respond by linking concerns with ways to help self • Discuss potential psychological and physical changes • Provide opportunities for follow-up discussion and guidance
• Need for physical and emotional privacy • Rapidly changing body image • Body image relates to self- esteem • Need for socialization and peer relations • Strong peer influence • Interest in sexuality beginning	• Lack of privacy and control • Fear of altered body image and/or function • Concern about other's perceptions • Social isolation • Loss of peer acceptance or fear of rejection • Fear of failure in school	• Secrecy • Embarrassment or avoidance • Withdrawal from peer group or socialization opportunities	• Respect and maintain privacy • Minimize unnecessary touch • May prefer discussing upcoming events or issues in private environment • Facilitate continued and new peer connections

* Adapted with permission from: Family and Child Life Services. (2010). *Comfort Measures: Helping children and families manage their stressful health care experiences – Developmental considerations for schoolage children and adolescents.* [in Rainbow Comfort Measures© educational handout series]. University Hospitals Rainbow Babies and Children's Hospital, Cleveland, OH.

Appendix B

Child-Friendlier Wording Alternatives: Sleep Study Environment

Child-Friendlier Wording Alternatives: Sleep Study Environment*

Word or Phrase	Potential Perception or Reaction	Alternatives
Sleep study; Test	Unknown word; Confusion – "I'm not in school, I can't have a test!"	"Sleep over"; "Your doctor wants to understand how your body is working while you are sleeping."
Is it ok if I . . . ?; Can I . . . ?	Avoid offering a choice when there is not a choice	"I need to . . . (put 3 stickers on your chest)." *Then offer real choices,* "Would you like to decorate the stickers first?"; "You can take the back off the sticker and help me place it on your leg."
Take your vitals	Unknown word; Confusion – "Take away from me?"	"Check your temperature (. . . how warm your body is)."; "Check your blood pressure (. . . a hug around your arm)."; "Listen to your heart beat (. . . how strong your heart is beating)."
You will feel . . . ; It feels like . . .	Avoid stating a certain feeling or sensation since feelings may be perceived differently for each child	*Describe a realistic range of feelings,* "You may notice . . . "; "Some kids say it feels . . . (bumpy, smooth). You can tell me how it feels for you."
Pressure	Unknown word	"A push"; "A touch"
Hurt; This part will hurt	Words can have a hard or soft connotation	"Bother"; "Uncomfortable"; "You may notice . . ."; "Some kids say it feels . . . (bumpy, like toothpaste or crumbs). You can tell me how it feels for you."; "You may feel more comfortable when . . . (you hug your mom)." *Pair statement with positive suggestions,* "Some kids like to help clean their skin with a Q-Tip. Would you like to help?"
Special; Funny	Words may have different meanings for each individual – "It doesn't look special to me."; "That isn't funny"	"Different"; "Unusual"
Don't touch; Don't move	Attention directed to unwanted behavior; Avoid phrasing with a negative connotation	"You want . . . (the stickers off your face), so you are . . . (pulling them off). The stickers stay on . . . (your face)." *Then, redirect to an appropriate action,* "You can put this green string into the box", "Which button on the book makes the cow noise?"; *Or state the desired behavior,* "Hold yourself very still and quiet"; "Please keep your hands down. You can hold the mirror to watch."

Word or Phrase	Potential Perception or Reaction	Alternatives
If you . . . (don't sit still), then you can't . . . (play with the toy); If you . . . (keep the stickers on), I'll give you/let you . . . (a prize/ watch TV)	Avoid bribery to achieve a goal; Diminishes self-esteem and opportunity to learn self-control; Potential for power struggle	*Set limits respectfully,* "You may . . . (help me put the sticker under your nose) or . . . (watch in the mirror, hold mom's hands). What is your choice?"; "After I . . . (put the sticker under your nose), you may . . . (drink your milk)"
Be a big boy/girl; That doesn't hurt; Don't cry	Diminishes self-esteem; May cause guilty feelings; Avoid phrasing with a negative connotation	*Provide coping strategies,* "Let's have you sit on mom's lap."; "When I count to three blow that feeling away."
You are . . . (angry, scared, worried); That was hard for you	Avoid telling a child what he/she feels without first asking him/her	"Your body is hunched over and you seem sad. Something must . . . (have happened, be bothering you). You're safe. You can talk to me when you are ready."; "How was that for you?"; "Was it the way you thought it would be?"; "Was it harder or easier than you thought?"; "Is there something else we should tell other kids about this . . . (test) that might help them?"
We're all done; The hard part is over	Anger or mistrust if more events are added; The "hard part" may be different for each child	"Almost done"; "We are done with this part. Next we need to . . . "
Will you still be my friend?; Will you smile for me?	May cause guilty feelings; Attention is directed toward medical caregiver's feelings	"You did a great job . . . (holding your body still, keeping the plastic mustache under your nose)."
Sensor; Electrodes; Leads; EKG leads; Leg movement sensors	Unknown word; Confusion – "electricity?"; "leash?"; "lead me where?"	"Stickers for your . . . (chest, chin, face, head)"; "The stickers have a little wet spot that will rest against your skin. The sticker also has a long string attached to it. While you sleep, the sticker will show . . . (how fast or slow your heart beats, how relaxed your muscles are)."
Belts; Respiratory effort belts	Unknown word; Confusion – "belt for my pants?"; "belt for spanking?"	"Stretchy bands"; "One stretchy band will go around your tummy, the other around your chest. The stretchy bands rest on top of your pajamas. They will show how you breathe while you sleep."
Pulse oximeter; pulse-ox;	Unknown word	"A night light (. . . little flashlight) for your . . . (finger, toe)."; "Some kids say it reminds them of a Band-Aid with a little red light. It will show . . . (your breathing while you sleep, how much oxygen is in your body)."
EEG leads; EEG electrodes	Unknown word; Confusion – "electricity?"; "a leash?"; "lead me where?"	"Tiny gold cups (. . . stickers, discs, hair jewelry)"; "They are about the size of an eraser on a pencil with a skinny string on it. Nine of them will rest on your head. A little bit of paste with a tiny blanket (. . . little piece of gauze) on top will help hold it in place. The gold cups will show when you are sleeping."

Word or Phrase	Potential Perception or Reaction	Alternatives
Snore sensor	Unknown word	"Little microphone"; "It is a small sticker that rests on your neck. A soft piece of tape will help hold it in place. It will show when you make noises or snore while you are sleeping."
Thermister	Unknown word	"Sticker moustache"; "The sticker will rest under your nose. It will tell if your air comes out of your nose or mouth while you are sleeping."
Cannula	Unknown word; Confusion – "Can I . . . what?"	"Plastic moustache"; "It is a skinny, soft plastic tube that will rest under your nose. It will tell how much air you breathe out of your nose while you are sleeping."
Video Camera	Lack of privacy; Tendency to become self-conscious	"You are a movie star tonight"; "The doctor is able to see a movie of you sleeping. Both the movie and the stickers on your body will help the doctor understand how you sleep. The doctor wants to find way to help you . . . (sleep better at night, not be so tired during the day)."
Hook you up; Set you up; Plug you in	Unknown phrase; Confusion – "Where are you going to put me?"; "Plug me into a wall?"	"I need to put a few stickers . . . (on your leg, on your chest)."; "Now that all the different stickers are on your body, you and mom can lie down, relax and read your books together. When you are sleepy, it is ok to fall asleep. Your mom will . . . (sleep next to you all night, move to her bed next to you once you fall asleep)."
Take you down	Unknown phrase; Confusion – "You are going to take me down to where?"; "Are you going to beat me up?"	"Your sleepover is all done. Would you like to help me take the stickers off your body? When the stickers are all off, you can get dressed, eat some breakfast then you can go home."

* Adapted with permission from: Family and Child Life Services. (2010). *Comfort Measures: Helping children and families manage their stressful health care experiences – Child-friendlier wording alternatives.* [in Rainbow Comfort Measures© educational handout series]. University Hospitals Rainbow Babies and Children's Hospital, Cleveland, OH.; Zaremba et al. (2005).

Appendix C

Coping Strategies for Infants through Adolescents

Infants (birth to 12 months)*

FAMILIAR=COMFORT *Provide familiar people, objects, stimulation*	**ACTIVE ENGAGEMENT** *Give the child something they CAN do*	**BUILD RAPPORT** *Let the child and parent know you are here to help*	**REALISTIC CHOICES** *Promote a sense of control and participation*
• Parent holding • Swaddling • Soothing touch • Eye contact • Calm, rhythmic voice • Favorite comfort items • Familiar, calm music	• Opportunities for sucking (breast feeding, bottle, sucking) • Cause & effect toys for diversion (lights, music, lift-the-flap books, etc)	• Sing or talk quietly • Guide and support parent's involvement through procedures • Use Rainbow Comfort Positioning©	• Involve parent's suggestions (preferred cuddling position, routines, etc.)

Toddlers (1 year to 2 years)*

FAMILIAR=COMFORT *Provide familiar people, objects, stimulation*	**ACTIVE ENGAGEMENT** *Give the child something they CAN do*	**BUILD RAPPORT** *Let the child and parent know you are here to help*	**REALISTIC CHOICES** *Promote a sense of control and participation*
• Parent holding • Soothing touch • Eye contact • Calm voice • Clothes from home • Favorite comfort items • Familiar, calm music	• Elicit "help" with the procedure (decorate the medical sticker with fun sticker, hold the mirror, etc.) • Cause & effect toys for diversion (toys with lights, buttons & music, lift-the-flap books, etc) • Sing familiar songs • Bubbles, pinwheels	• Play together for a few minutes • Demonstrate just prior to the action (using a doll/stuffed animal, etc.) • Give brief details of sensory information just prior to experience ("lotion may feel bumpy") • Use Rainbow Comfort Positioning©	• Involve parent's suggestions (preferred cuddling positions, routines, etc.) • Books (push button music or lift-the-flap books, etc.) • Favorite DVD

Preschool Age Children (3 to 5 years)*

FAMILIAR=COMFORT *Provide familiar people, objects, stimulation*	ACTIVE ENGAGEMENT *Give the child something they CAN do*	BUILD RAPPORT *Let the child and parent know you are here to help*	REALISTIC CHOICES *Promote a sense of control and participation*
• Parent holding • Soothing touch • Eye contact • Calm voice • Clothes from home • Favorite toy or comfort items • Familiar, calm music	• Elicit "help" with the procedure • Slow, deep breathing ("blow the feeling away") • Count, say alphabet • Talk about favorite tings (pets, movies, favorite places, cartoon characters or super heros, etc.)	• Talk or play together for a few minutes • Use developmentally appropriate words to describe actions ("hold your body very still and quiet") • Demonstrate prior to procedure (using doll/ stuffed animal, etc.) • Provide brief details of sensory information ("the stretch bands hug your tummy") • Use Rainbow Comfort Positioning©	• Involve parent's suggestions (preferred cuddling position, routines, etc.) • Books (push button music or lift-the-flap books simple 'I-Spy', etc.) • Favorite DVD • iPad; iTouch • Cause & effect toys for diversion (toys with lights, buttons & music, lift-the-flap books, etc) • Interactive games ('Find-It', push button water toys, etc.)

School Age Children (6 to 12 years)*

FAMILIAR=COMFORT *Provide familiar people, objects, stimulation*	ACTIVE ENGAGEMENT *Give the child something they CAN do*	BUILD RAPPORT *Let the child and parent know you are here to help*	REALISTIC CHOICES *Promote a sense of control and participation*
• Parent's presence, possible parent holding • Soothing touch • Eye contact • Calm voice • Clothes from home • Favorite toy or comfort items • Favorite music	• Elicit "help" with the procedure • Slow, deep breathing ("blow the feeling away") • Counting • Squeezing a ball • Talk about favorite things (pets, movies, favorite place, hobbies, etc.)	• Talk or play together for a few minutes • Explain/demonstrate steps involved in the procedure using developmentally appropriate words to describe actions ("a sticker that helps me how fast or slow your heart is beating) • Provide details of sensory information ("it may feel like a push or a touch") • Be honest when answering questions, then plan coping strategies together	• Books ('I-Spy', etc.) • Interactive games (Find it, push button water toys, etc) • Hand-held games or game systems (20 Questions, etc) • Favorite DVD • iPad, iTouch • Guided imagery (child's script of their pleasurable real/pretend experiences including sensory elements; "see the colors", "hear the soft hum"

Adolescents (13 to 18 years)*

FAMILIAR=COMFORT *Provide familiar people, objects, stimulation*	ACTIVE ENGAGEMENT *Give the child something they CAN do*	BUILD RAPPORT *Let the child and parent know you are here to help*	REALISTIC CHOICES *Promote a sense of control and participation*
• Parent's presence • Soothing touch • Eye contact • Calm voice • Clothes from home • Favorite toy or comfort items • Favorite music	• Elicit "help" with the procedure • Slow, deep breathing ("blow the feeling away") • Counting • Squeezing a ball • Talk about favorite things (pets, movies, favorite place, hobbies, school, etc.)	• Talk together for a few minutes • Describe steps involved in the procedure and ask if more detailed explanation would be helpful ("soft, skinny tubing that rests under your nose and measures how much carbon dioxide your breathing out") • Be hones when answering questions, then plan coping strategies together	• Books ('I-Spy", etc.) • Hand-held games/ game systems ('20 Questions', etc.) • Favorite DVD • iPod, iTouch • Guided imagery (child's script of their pleasurable real/pretend experiences including sensory elements; "feel the warm breeze", "smell the salty air")

* Adapted with permission from: Family and Child Life Services. (2010). *Comfort Measures: Helping children and families manage their stressful health care experiences – Coping strategies.* [in Rainbow Comfort Measures© educational handout series]. University Hospitals Rainbow Babies and Children's Hospital, Cleveland, OH.

CHAPTER

21 The Role of Schools in Identification, Treatment, and Prevention of Children's Sleep Problems

Joseph A. Buckhalt

Abstract

Increasing academic achievement and promoting behavioral adjustment of children and adolescents are primary missions of schools. Considerable research shows that cognitive functioning and emotion regulation are compromised by insufficient sleep, with deleterious effects for school achievement and behavior. In response to concerns about low achievement, maladaptive behavior, and inadequate sleep, a number of actions are described that schools can take toward improving the sufficiency of sleep in children. For example, observing sleepiness at school may help identify children with sleep disorders; primary and secondary school curricula can be expanded to include the relations of sleep to health and performance; and system-wide policies that facilitate adequate sleep may be considered for change.

Key Words: sleep, school achievement, school behavior, role of schools

Sleep Problems and the Role of Schools

What does children's sleep have to do with the mission of schools? It is a fair question to ask, "Is this the business of schools?" If sleep were not related to school academic performance or social behavior, it might not be the school's business. Further, if sleep disorders at a clinical level were the only problem then even if performance at school were affected, sleep might be considered more the business of health care professionals. Finally, if there were no actions school personnel could take to influence sleep, it might not be a domain of child functioning that should be a responsibility of schools. In this chapter, I will argue that none of those three assumptions are valid. A case will be made that sleep does affect children's learning and social behavior at school. Evidence will be provided that sleep problems that do not rise to the level of a clinical disorder have become pervasive in children and often do not come to the attention of health care providers. Most importantly, many actions to facilitate children's sleep with the potential to improve school performance at school will be outlined. In short, it will be argued that sleep definitely is the school's business.

Primary and secondary schools constitute a significant component of the sociocultural infrastructure of American society. The majority of children (~87%; IES, National Center for Educational Statistics, US Department of Education) attend government-funded public schools, a substantial percent attend private and parochial schools (~10%: IES), and an increasing number are schooled at home (~3%; IES). But whatever the type of school, law demands that all children attend schools for many years. It was not always so in the United States, as compulsory education laws were enacted only during the latter nineteenth to early twentieth century. But for many decades, children from the ages of 5 or 6 up to around 16 have been required to attend school. Because attendance is mandatory, school is arguably the only societal institution where all children are required to be present. It is the one place where all children come into regular and frequent contact with professionals who are trained and motivated to look after their broad interests.

The mission of schools has evolved over the years from their inception to the present. Instruction in so-called "academic" subjects is universally agreed to be the number one mission of schools. Basic knowledge and skill in mathematics, language arts (especially reading), science, and history (and a few others) are considered essential to prepare children for jobs and participation as citizens in essential societal activities including voting and serving on a jury. Secondary to the academic mission, it has been acknowledged that school serves a socializing mission. At school, children learn to inhibit their impulses ("Raise your hand"), get along with others ("Wait for your turn"), and interact with children who are alike and different from them in many ways. School is also a place where "extracurricular" activities such as music, art, and athletics are taught.

But while those missions would likely get broad agreement among the American public, many other missions have been questioned. Whether or not school is an appropriate venue to teach character, moral development, and religious values has been a matter of intense debate. Are schools responsible for children's nutrition? Beginning with the National School Lunch Act in 1946, lunch has been provided (for a charge) in schools (School Nutrition Association, 2011). Free or reduced-cost breakfast and lunch are newer programs that have been enacted with some controversy. In the minds of some, feeding poor children at school has been an extension of an already too large social welfare program (Currie, 1979; McDonnell, 2004). But congress has repeatedly reauthorized the programs that served 31.7 million school children in 2010 (U.S. Department of Agriculture, 2011).

Are schools responsible for children's health? Nursing care is provided and mandated by many state boards of education in the United States, but standards vary widely from state to state. At least one state requires that a school nurse be present in every school, but only around a third of states have a mandated nurse-to-student ratio, and those range from 1–500 up to 1–5000 with a median of 1–750 (National Association of State School Boards, NASBE). Even preventive measures such as vaccinations, once routinely administered at schools, are rarely seen in today's schools. Health education in schools has generally been seen as important but, as in the case of nursing care, standards vary widely. Requirements vary from state to state, with some states requiring instruction in health education but not specifying grade levels or amounts of instruction required. The majority of states require health education to be taught in elementary, middle, and junior high grades, but in some states there is no minimum number of hours set. At the high school level, requirements vary from state to state, ranging from no requirement to a half-credit (one semester) to one or more credits (full year). Many states mandate instruction in particular health education topics (e.g., reproductive health and pregnancy prevention; alcohol, tobacco, and drugs). Physical education has often been viewed as a component of health education and promotion, but emphasis has waxed and waned over past decades. A call for renewal of focus on health in schools has been made in a policy report, *A Broader, Bolder Approach to Education*: "Health and nutrition supports ensure that children come to school immunized, well fed, and without toothaches or acute asthma attacks that prevent them from focusing and learning." (Economic Policy Institute, 2011). To meet that objective, the report recommends that health care clinics be located in US schools, consistent with a similar initiative by the National Assembly on School Based Health Care (2011).

In the early history of American schools, the school was a place where health topics were addressed. Surprisingly, sleep was one of those concerns. For example, J. Mace Andress of the State Normal School in Worcester, Massachusetts, writing in the *Journal of Educational Psychology* (1911) states in the opening sentence,

> "Sleep is so vitally related to the mental and physical health and
> efficiency of human beings that I decided to investigate the sleep
> of my own pupils." (p. 153)

Andress goes on to report that following "... some instruction in the physiology and hygiene of sleep..." (p. 153) a questionnaire was answered by 23 seniors (20–21 years old) and 26 juniors (17–19 years old), and they kept daily records of their sleep. The average durations of sleep are remarkable compared with the much lower numbers adolescents and young adults report today. Juniors averaged 8 hours, 54 minutes, with no individual reporting fewer than 8 hours. The average for seniors was 8 hours, 34 minutes with only one person reporting fewer than 8 hours.

Andress closes with,

> "The principal value of this investigation was the arousal of enthusiasm in the students for the study of psychology and hygiene and for the practice of the laws of health. Many pupils have told the writer since this investigation that they were getting more sleep. Similar information should be of value to every administrator of schools because it throws light on the mental and physical condition of students. Sleep is the great prophylactic and is comparable in its influence to fresh air, pure water, nutritious food and healthful exercise." (p. 156)

The question of whether sleep is the business of schools must be considered in the context of the many important responsibilities society has assigned to schools. We should expect parents and school professionals to be skeptical of adding a new role, and their questions deserve close attention. Over 60 years ago the realization that that hungry children did not learn well led to schools assuming more responsibility for children's nutrition. We need to consider the proposition that sleepy children are not optimally receptive learners and do not regulate their emotions well, and it is appropriate to consider what can and should be done by school personnel.

The Scope and Extent of Children's School Problems

Concerns about underachievement of American schoolchildren have been expressed frequently over the years, but perhaps never more so than recently. Reports from The National Assessment of Educational Progress (NAEP) annually state that the United States continues to fall further behind other countries in crucial academic subjects, including science and mathematics. Many federal and state initiatives over a very long time (e.g., the No Child Left Behind Act of 2001) have been directed at improving academic performance, but results have been largely disappointing. Particularly troubling have been low scores of children from lower socioeconomic status and minority ethnicity families, whom many programs have been designated to help (NAEP, 2011; ETS, 2009; 2010). Also pertinent are the reports of increases in the numbers of children with disorders that impair learning, including autism, learning disability (LD), and attention-deficit/hyperactivity disorder (ADHD). The percentage of children who are LD has doubled since its origination as a special education category in 1975 (Pierangelo & Giuliani, 2006) to 5% of all public school students children in 2009 (Cortiella, 2011). ADHD prevalence has also increased to 6.69% of all children, a 33% increase over 10 years (CDC 2010b). Autism prevalence has increased as well, to 0.47%, up an astounding 289.5% in the last decade (CDC, 2010a).

While most of the attention has been directed to problems of academic achievement, some evidence also suggests that behavior problems of schoolchildren have been increasing in frequency and severity. Examining results from a restandardization of the Behavior Assessment System for Children (BASC-II, Reynolds & Kamphaus, 2004), Distefano, Kamphaus, and Mindrilă (2010) reported differences from the original standardization sample published in 1996. In 8 years, teacher-reported disruptive behavior had increased from 8% to 12% of the 2338 children in the stratified national sample. Children with elevated clinical scales of both externalizing (e.g., serious behavior problems) and internalizing (e.g., anxiety, depression) had risen from 4% in 1996 to 15% in 2004. Among all children in US schools, prevalence figures for those who have serious emotional or behavioral problems are estimated by the CDC at 5.1% of all children ages 4–17. And for poor children aged 11–14, that figure is 9.3% compared with 3.5% of children from affluent families (CDC, 2011; Boyle et al., 2011). It is clear that problematic behavior at school constitutes a growing challenge for educators.

How Sleep Relates to School Problems

All available evidence suggests that children, adolescents, and adults are getting less sleep than in previous times and less than they need (Olds, Blunden, Petkov, & Forchino, 2010; Smaldone, Honig, & Byrne, 2007). The National Sleep Foundation has conducted a nationwide survey every year since 2002, with each year's topic addressing a different aspect of sleep. In the 2004 poll (Children and Sleep) and the 2006 poll (Teens and Sleep), respondents indicated that sleep duration and sleep quality is suboptimal. In the 2011 poll (Technology Use and Sleep), children 13–18 years old reported an average of 7 hours 26 minutes sleep on school nights, and 18% of them reported being awakened a few nights a week by a text message, phone call, or e-mail. Although it is difficult to determine exact figures for many reasons, estimates have ranged from 20% of children and adolescents with a sleep problem at the present to 40% who experience a sleep problem at some point for some duration in childhood and adolescence (Mindell & Owens, 2010). Using the smaller of those two figures and an estimated 55 million children in Grades K–12 as of Fall, 2011 (U.S. Census Bureau, 2011), around 11 million children have an ongoing chronic sleep problem or an acute sleep problem that is manifesting now or occurred at some point during the school years. It is important to remember that the vast majority of children are not likely to have their sleep problems come to the attention of primary health care providers. Some evidence shows that in most cases, parents do not report sleep problems to their physicians (Blunden et al. 2004). In a survey of around 150,000 children seen by primary care physicians during 2007, only 3.7% had a sleep disorder diagnosis compared with a much higher prevalence rate estimated in epidemiological studies (Meltzer, Johnson, Crosette, Ramos, & Mindell, 2010). Thus, school is the only place where the preponderance of those children with problems have a chance of being discovered. Among these 11 million children at school are:

1. Children with diagnosed clinical sleep disorders.
2. Children who have serious sleep problems that have not come to the attention of health care providers or who have subclinical levels of problems.
3. Children who have diagnosed learning and behavior problems in school, but have sleep problems that have not been recognized as related to their disorder (e.g., autism, ADHD, LD, intellectual disability, other health impairments).
4. Children whose long-term maintenance medication (for conditions such as ADHD and asthma) or short-term medication (e.g., for colds) have a disruptive influence on sleep.
5. Children who have psychological problems such as depression and anxiety, for which sleep problems is one of an array of symptoms.
6. Children whose families live in poverty and have both poor sleep environments (beds, bedding, air quality) and poor parent-monitored habits that are associated with sleep (e.g., irregular and late bedtimes, access to caffeinated beverages).
7. Children with insufficient sleep that is not chronic, but is related to a transitory situation in the family (e.g., recent move, economic stress, serious illness or death in the family, family conflict).
8. Children whose sleep is chronically insufficient in duration or quality but is unrecognized as related to academic underachievement and behavior problems at school.

The learning, behavior, and emotional problems that are the consequences of sleep disorders have been amply documented (Mindell & Owens, 2010; O'Brien, 2011). Children with sleep disordered breathing, to take one example, have been shown to have impaired cognitive functioning (e.g., Bourke et al., 2011). Similarly, the sleep problems of children with a wide range of disabilities have been documented. For example, 40%–60% of children with autism are estimated to have sleep problems (Richdale & Schreck, 2009), and rates of problems for children with intellectual disabilities and ADHD are also high (Doran, Harvey, & Horner, 2006; Konofal, Lecendreux, & Cortese, 2010). Further, children with a number of prevalent health problems, notably asthma and obesity, have been found to have concomitant sleep problems (Desager, Nelen, Weyler, & De Backer, 2004; Hart, Cairns, & Jelalian, 2011).

While the groups of children mentioned above deserve special attention, the consequences of insufficient sleep for the majority of children who have no clinical disorder of sleep, learning, or health are also becoming clearer. Researchers have only recently begun to explore sleep in these children, and some of the findings are alarming. In the cognitive domain, shorter sleep duration, poorer sleep quality, and higher levels of daytime sleepiness have all been associated with poor performance on cognitive and academic measures of many types, including grades, standardized test scores, and teacher ratings (Dewald, Meijer, Oort, Kerkhof, & Bogels, 2010). While most of these studies have been cross-sectional, measuring sleep and cognitive outcomes concurrently, recent evidence suggests that the relations endure over years. For example, Bub, Buckhalt, and El-Sheikh (2011) followed children over 3 years and discovered that children whose sleepiness increased over that time had scores on cognitive tests as much as a standard deviation below those of children whose sleepiness had not increased. Studies of experimental sleep deprivation in adults indicate that impairments in attention and vigilance are most sensitive to sleep insufficiency, while higher-order cognitive functions are less affected (Lim & Dinges, 2010). But in children, poor sleep has been linked to a wide array of cognitive functioning not only in attention and processing speed, comparable to adults, but also in memory and verbal comprehension (Bub et al., 2011; Kopasz et al., 2010).

Turning to the behavioral domain, children with more sleep problems and higher levels of sleepiness are more likely to have school conduct problems (O'Brien et al. 2011). These results are consistent with those of other studies that have linked higher levels of internalizing problems (i.e., depression, anxiety) and externalizing problems (i.e., aggression, impulsivity) to poor sleep (e.g., El-Sheikh, Kelly, Buckhalt, & Hinnant, 2010; Gregory et al., 2005; Paavonen et al., 2002). Children who have problems with sleep, emotion regulation, and behavior are likely also to have difficulties in academic achievement.

School achievement and behavior of children from families of low socioeconomic status (SES) and those who are ethnic minorities are particularly problematic. Considerable effort has been expended to understand and ameliorate the achievement gap between these children and others. Only recently have SES and ethnicity been the primary focus of investigation in sleep of typically developing children, and the results are informative. Poorer sleep has been found in persons of African-American and Hispanic ethnicity (e.g., Ruiter, DeCoster, Jacobs, & Lichstein, 2010) and in children from poorer families. For example, Marco, Wolfson, Sparling, and Azuaje (2012) reported that lower SES adolescents went to bed later, had more variability in bedtime, and slept less on school nights. Moreover, SES and ethnicity have been found to moderate the relations between sleep and outcomes. Specifically, children from lower class and minority ethnicity families have been shown to have larger correlations between poor sleep and poor cognitive performance (Buckhalt, El-Sheikh, & Keller, 2007; Buckhalt, El-Sheikh, Keller, & Kelly, 2009) and between poor sleep and problematic behavior (El-Sheikh et al., 2010). These findings have led to the hypothesis that sleep insufficiency may be of central importance in the persistent academic gap that has defied reduction by many proposed remedies for over 40 years (Buckhalt, 2011; Buckhalt & Staton, 2011).

What Can Schools Do?

School personnel are very familiar with the learning and behavior problems of their students. They are also very knowledgeable about students with disabilities. At present, though, they lack knowledge about the relations of sleep to these children's problems. Sleep has not been a topic that is covered in the education of school teachers, school counselors, school psychologists, or school administrators. To take one example, in the first three editions of *The Handbook of School Psychology* (Gutkin & Reynolds, 1999; Reynolds & Gutkin 1982; 1990), each a 1100 + page comprehensive volume, sleep is not an index term and sleep problems are not addressed. In the 4th edition (Gutkin & Reynolds, 2009), one paragraph on sleep disorders is found in a chapter on neuropsychological assessment. A few articles describing the relations of sleep to school performance and behavior have been published in journals that school professionals read (i.e., Bergin & Bergin, 2009; Buckhalt & El-Sheikh, 2010; Buckhalt, Wolfson, El-Sheikh, 2007; 2009; Carskadon, 1999; Wolfson & Carskadon, 2005), but sleep has not made its way into the primary topics of educational curricula for any professionals who work in schools.

School personnel are well situated to implement aspects of recently formulated broad health policy initiatives. The Institute of Medicine, a unit of the National Academy of Sciences (2011), included several recommendations related to sleep improvement in a recent policy report:

> Recommendation 5-2: Healthcare providers should counsel parents and children's caregivers not to permit televisions, computers, or other digital media devices in children's bedrooms or other sleeping spaces.
>
> Recommendation 6-1: Child care regulatory agencies should require child care providers to adopt practices that promote age-appropriate sleep durations.
>
> Recommendation 6-2: Health and education professionals should be trained in how to counsel parents about their children's age-appropriate sleep durations.

In Healthy People 2020 (NIH, 2011), an initiative of the National Institutes of Health, several objectives are related to improving sleep, including one specifically related to adolescents:

> **SH–3:** Increase the proportion of students in grades 9 through 12 who get sufficient sleep.

The preceding discussion provides a compelling rationale that sleep is the appropriate business of the schools. But what can be done by school professionals about insufficient sleep and consequent sleepiness at school? The following are among many possible potential courses of action

1. School professionals can learn about nighttime sleep, daytime sleepiness, and their relations to attention, learning, memory, emotion regulation, and behavioral adjustment. This goal should not be difficult to attain. Teachers are very motivated to discover information that will improve student performance and behavior. Sleep science and practice should become an integral part of training curricula for teachers and other school professionals, particularly administrators, counselors, and psychologists.

2. Teachers and other school professionals should learn to recognize and screen for serious sleep disorders and, through the parents, refer children to pediatric sleep specialists for diagnosis and treatment. If children are sleepy at school, in many cases the signs are obvious if we choose to notice them. The model for this action is already in place for other disorders that are considered the domain of health care. For example, schools monitor immunization for children and identify children with numerous health conditions who need referral for treatment.

3. For children with identified learning disabilities that have been associated with high prevalence of sleep problems, their individual education plans can be modified to include sleep improvement among other objectives. Many of the specific measures will require the cooperation of parents and, while engaging parents is challenging, teachers and others at school are better positioned to consult with parents than anyone else.

4. School professionals can be informed about relations of sleep to conditions such as obesity and overweight, asthma, and allergies. All of these conditions have increased significantly in recent years and are related to insufficient sleep. When children with these and other health conditions have learning and behavior problems at school, it should be recognized that poor sleep needs to be considered as a possible contributing factor beyond any other direct effects of the conditions on school learning and behavior.

5. When a child is referred for assessment of cognitive and academic functioning due to underachievement, school professionals should routinely rule out the presence of sleep problems before assuming that a disability is present. Ruling out vision and hearing problems that interfere with learning are already part of the assessment process, and sleep problems should be treated similarly.

6. When high stakes testing is scheduled, such as group administered achievement tests or individually administered tests to determine eligibility for special services, a concerted effort can be made to optimize the sleep of children in days and weeks leading up to the tests. Many schools now provide extra snacks on testing days, and some suggest in materials sent home to parents that children should come to school well rested. They also provide focused classroom time devoted to test preparation. All of these actions imply that schools realize children need to have energy and mental preparation to perform their best, so trying to maximize the duration and quality of sleep is consistent with other ongoing efforts.

7. Especially for younger children, school administrators and policymakers need to take a hard look at the practice of having children take naps at school. It was not uncommon in past years for the youngest children to have a nap time at school. But napping is rare now in kindergarten. Many educators believe that the curriculum is too full of academic demands to consider having children spend time napping that would otherwise be devoted to instruction. Beyond kindergarten, it is very common for children and adolescents to be discouraged or even punished for sleeping at school. A child who falls asleep at school is responding to a basic need and should be referred for evaluation of the factors causing excessive sleepiness.

8. Schools begin early, and while attempts to move start times later in the morning have been met with resistance in some places (Appleman, and Stavitsky, Chapter 38), more school districts are adopting later start times for high schools. In some rural areas where bus rides are long, children board buses before 7:00 am, which means rise times of 6:30 am at the latest and in many cases much earlier. Particularly for adolescents who are experiencing sleep phase delay and who have heavy homework demands along with afterschool sports or other activities, getting to bed early enough to have sufficient sleep is all but impossible. In many schools, "zero period" has been initiated for honors courses, tutoring and remedial classes, or art and music instruction, and begins as early as 7:00 am. School administrators must weigh the evidence for and against later start times and make wise decisions in the best interest of students.

9. School administrators and policymakers need to take a close look at how school and community

activities in athletics and other domains have encroached upon school nights with the effect of delaying bedtimes. To take one example, since high school football games are scheduled on Friday nights in most communities, middle and junior high games are increasingly being scheduled on school nights. In many communities, it is not unusual for a 12-year-old to get home as late as 9 or 10 pm after an away game. For some community sports such as soccer, games and practices are held on school nights. After vigorous physical activity and emotional arousal, players, and in many cases their siblings, travel with their families from the fields to home, then take care of baths, often have an evening meal and engage in other activities, all of which delay bedtime and make it impossible to have sufficient sleep.

10. Education about sleep needs and good sleep practices should be infused into the health and science education curriculum beginning in kindergarten and continuing through high school. A few sets of materials suitable for lesson plans and activities have been developed by national organizations, but many more resources will need to be developed.

Conclusion

All available evidence suggests that children's sleep is as vital for their optimal performance as good nutrition and regular exercise. When children's sleep is insufficient, there are deleterious consequences for cognitive processing, learning, memory, and emotion regulation. These problems in turn lead to poor academic achievement and behavior problems, both of which have posed increasing challenges for schools. School professionals could help prevent sleep problems, recognize them when they are present, and intervene in a number of different ways. Before assuming that learning or behavior disorders are the cause of low achievement and problem behavior, chronic or acute sleep disorders or inadequate sleep at the subclinical level should be ruled out. Screening for sleep disorders and sleep insufficiency can be accomplished as easily as screening for vision and hearing problems. By administering brief screening instruments recognizing overt behavioral signs of sleepiness, children who might have sleep disorders may be identified early and referred for further assessment and treatment. Teachers already reach out to parents to help them structure and monitor home activities that foster school success. Homework is the most obvious example, but teachers also work with parents when health or nutrition problems are interfering with school performance. Consulting with parents about good sleep habits can be incorporated into the existing teacher–parent alliance. Current health education curricula can be expanded to include the relations of sleep to numerous health and performance outcomes. Finally, system-wide policies that facilitate adequate sleep, such as discontinuing very early school start times and school night sports, need to be considered.

Future Directions

- Much of the evidence leading to the conclusion that sleep insufficiency affects school performance comes from studies that use correlational designs. We may also logically infer that if experimental studies of voluntary sleep deprivation in adults show that cognitive functioning is impaired, the same holds true for children and adolescents. Still, more experimental studies are needed, including those that take advantage of naturally occurring sleep deprivation in groups of children such as sleepovers. Further, more studies need to be done to determine sources of individual differences in the response to sleep loss. The optimal amount of sleep no doubt varies from child to child, as does their response to sleeping poorly.
- A few well-designed intervention studies have demonstrated that when children's sleep is improved, there is a concomitant improvement in school performance. More such studies with individual children and with groups of children are needed that provide information about the strategies that work.
- Further research is always needed, but sufficient evidence suggests that prevention and intervention programs should be implemented in schools. Model programs need to be developed and field-tested in schools. These programs need to be built upon existing frameworks of screening for problems that inhibit learning and adaptive behavior, upon existing methods of teacher–parent consultation and education, and infused into already existing health education curricula. Changes at the system-wide level, such as delaying school start times, need to be considered within existing ways schoolwide policies are formulated and implemented.

Resources for Educators

Tools for School Assessment of Sleep Problems and Sleepiness

BEARS—A screening interview for sleep problems (Owens & Dalzell, 2005)

Pediatric Sleep Questionnaire (Chervin, Hedger, Dillon, & Pituch, 2000)

Children's Sleep Habits Questionnaire (Owens, Spirito, & McGuinn, 2000)

School Sleep Habits Survey (Wolfson et al., 2003)

Sleep Disorders Inventory for Students (Luginbuehl, 2003; 2008)

Pediatric Daytime Sleepiness Scale (Drake et al., 2003)

Children's Report of Sleep Patterns-Sleepiness (Meltzer et al. 2012)

For a review of these and other available instruments, see Spruyt, K. & Gozal, D. (2011). Pediatric sleep questionnaires as diagnostic or epidemiological tools: A review of currently available instruments. *Sleep Medicine Reviews, 15*, 19–32.

Materials for Sleep Education

National Institutes of Health (NIH). Sleep, sleep disorders, and biological

rhythms: NIH curriculum supplement series—Grades 9–12. Retrieved 11–4-2011

from http://science.education.nih.gov/supplements/nih3/sleep/default.htm.

American Academy of Sleep Medicine. Lesson Plans for K-12 Teachers. Retrieved 11-4-2011 from http://www.sleepeducation.com/.

Books for Professionals

Carskadon, M. A. (2002). *Adolescent Sleep Patterns: Biological, Social, and Psychological Influences*. New York: Cambridge University Press.

El-Sheikh, M. (Ed.). (2011). *Sleep and Development: Familial and Socio-Cultural Considerations*. New York: Oxford University Press.

Ivanenko, A. (Ed.). (2008). *Sleep and Psychiatric Disorders in Children and Adolescents*. New York: Informa Healthcare.

Mindell, J. A., & Owens, J. A. (2010). *A Clinical Guide to Pediatric Sleep*. Philadelphia: Lippincott, Williams & Wilkins.

Books for Parents

Ferber, R. (2006). *Solve Your Child's Sleep Problems*. New York: Fireside.

Owens, J. A. & Mindell, J. A. (2005). *Take Charge of Your Child's Sleep: The All-in-One Resource for Solving Sleep Problems in Kids and Teens*. New York: Marlowe.

Weissbluth, M. (2003). *Healthy Sleep Habits, Happy Child*. New York: Ballantine.

Websites

National Sleep Foundation: http://www.sleepfoundation.org/

(NSF also sponsors Sleep for Kids: http://www.sleepforkids.org/)

American Academy of Sleep Medicine: http://www.aasmnet.org/

(Includes www.sleepcenters.org to locate a sleep diagnosis and treatment center in the United States)

Child Uplift, Inc.: *Wake Up America! Eliminate Sleep Problems and Improve Children's Performance*. http://70.38.93.194/index.cfm?ID=1

Acknowledgments

Research discussed in this paper was supported by grants from the National Science Foundation (0339115, 0623936, & 0843185) and the National Institutes of Health (R01HL093246 & R01HD046795). I also wish to acknowledge the support of Dr. Mona El-Sheikh, other colleagues who have been collaborators, graduate students, laboratory employees, school district personnel, parents, and the children who participated in our studies.

References

Andress, J. M. (1911). An investigation of the sleep of normal school students. *Journal of Educational Psychology, 2*, 153–156.

Bergin, C. S., & Bergin, D. A. (2009). Sleep: The E-ZZZ intervention. *Educational Leadership, 67*, 44–47.

Blunden, S., Lushington, K., Lorenzen, B., Ooi, T., Fung, F., & Kennedy, D. (2004). Are sleep problems under-recognized in general practice? *Archives of Diseases in Childhood, 89*, 708–712.

Bourke, R., Anderson, V., Yang., Jackman, A. R., Killedar, A., Nixon, G. M., Davey, M. J., et al. (2011). Cognitive and academic functions are impaired in children with all severities of sleep-disordered breathing. *Sleep Medicine, 12*, 489–496.

Bub, K. L., Buckhalt, J. A., & El-Sheikh, M. (2011). Children's sleep and cognitive performance: A cross-domain analysis of change over time. *Developmental Psychology, 47*, 1504–1514.

Buckhalt, J. A., El-Sheikh, M., & Keller, P. (2007) Children's sleep and cognitive functioning: Race and socioeconomic status as moderators of effects. *Child Development, 78*, 213–231.

Buckhalt, J. A., Wolfson, A., & El-Sheikh, M. (2007). Children's sleep, academic performance, and school behavior. *NASP Communique, 35*, 40–43.

Buckhalt, J. A., El-Sheikh, M., Keller, P., & Kelly, R. (2009). Concurrent and longitudinal relations between children's sleep and cognitive functioning. *Child Development, 80*, 875–892.

Buckhalt, J. A. & Wolfson, A., & El-Sheikh, M. (2009). Children's sleep and school psychology practice. *School Psychology Quarterly, 24*, 60–69.

Buckhalt, J. A., & El-Sheikh, M. (2010). Assessment and intervention for sleep problems. In P. McCabe & S. Shaw

(Eds.), *Pediatric Disorders: Current Topics and Interventions for Educators* (pp. 52–60). Thousand Oaks, CA: National Association of School Psychologists & Corwin Press.

Buckhalt, J. A. (2011). Insufficient sleep and the socioeconomic status achievement gap. *Child Development Perspectives, 5,* 59–65.

Buckhalt, J. A., & Staton, L. (2011). Children's sleep, cognition, and academic performance in the context of socioeconomic status and ethnicity. In M. El-Sheikh (Ed.). *Sleep and Development: Familial and Socio-Cultural Considerations* (pp. 219–244). New York: Oxford University Press.

Carskadon, M. A. (1999). When worlds collide: Adolescent needs for sleep and societal demands. *Phi Delta Kappan, 80,* 348–353.

Centers for Disease Control (2010a). Increasing prevalence of parent-reported attention-deficit/hyperactivity disorder among children: United States, 2003–2007. *Morbidity and Mortality Weekly Report (MMWR), 59,* 1439–1443 http://www.cdc.gov/mmwr/preview/mmwrhtml/mm5944a3.htm. Retrieved April 11, 2013.

Centers for Disease Control (2010b). Key Findings: Trends in the Prevalence of Developmental Disabilities in U. S. Children, 1997–2008. http://www.cdc.gov/ncbddd/features/birthdefects-dd-keyfindings.html. Retrieved April 11, 2013. Also published as Boyle, C. A., Boulet, S., Schieve, L., Cohen, R. A., Blumberg, S. J., Yeargin-Allsopp, M., et al. (2011). Trends in the prevalence of developmental disabilities in US children, 1997–2008. *Pediatrics, 127,*1034–1042.

Centers for Disease Control (2011). QuickStats: Percentage of children with serious emotional or behavioral difficulties, by age group and family income group. National Health Interview Survey, United States, 2004—2009. *Morbidity and Mortality Weekly Report (MMWR), 60,* 555 (May 6, 2011). http://www.cdc.gov/mmwr/preview/mmwrhtml/mm6017a10.htm. Retrieved April 11, 2013.

Chervin, R. D., Hedger, K., Dillon, J. E., & Pituch, K. J. (2000). Pediatric sleep questionnaire (PSQ): Validity and reliability of scales for sleep-disordered breathing, snoring, sleepiness, and behavioral problems. *Sleep Medicine, 1,* 21–32.

Cortiella, C. (2011). *The State of Learning Disabilities.* New York: National Center for Learning Disabilities. http://issuu.com/ncld/docs/state_of_ld?mode=embed&layout=http%3A%2F%2Fskin.issuu.com%2Fv%2Flight%2Flayout.xml. Retrieved April 11, 2013.

Currie, J. (1979). Health care: School breakfast in the South—Federal funds available compared with funds used 1978. *Southern Changes, 1,* 22–23. http://beck.library.emory.edu/southernchanges/article.php?id=sc01-8_009. Retrieved April 11, 2013.

Desager, K. N., Nelen, V., Weyler, J. J., & De Backer, W. A. (2004). Sleep disturbance and daytime symptoms in wheezing school- aged children. *Journal of Sleep Research, 14,* 77–82.

Dewald, J. F., Meijer, A. M., Oort, F. J., Kerkhof, G. A., & Bogels, S. M. (2010). The influence of sleep quality, sleep duration, and sleepiness on school performance in children and adolescents: A meta-analytic review. *Sleep Medicine Reviews, 14,* 179–189.

DiStefano, C. A., Kamphaus, R. W., & Mindrilă, D. L. (2010). A typology of teacher-rated child behavior: Revisiting subgroups over 10 years later. *School Psychology Quarterly, 25,* 152–163.

Doran, S. M., Harvey, M. T., & Horner, R. H. (2006). Sleep and developmental disabilities: Assessment, treatment, and outcome measures. *Mental Retardation, 44,* 13–27.

Drake, C., Nickel, C., Burduvali, E., Roth, T., Jefferson, C., & Pietro, B. (2003). The Pediatric Daytime Sleepiness Scale (PDSS): Sleep habits and school outcomes in middle-school children. *Sleep, 26,* 455–458.

Economic Policy Institute (2011). A broader, bolder approach to education. http://www.boldapproach.org/index.php?id=01. Retrieved April 11, 2013.

Educational Testing Service. (2009). *Parsing the achievement gap II.* Princeton, NJ: ETS. Retrieved from http://www.ets.org/Media/Research/pdf/PICPARSINGII.pdf. Retrieved April 11, 2013.

Educational Testing Service. (2010). *The black-white achievement gap: When progress stopped.* http://www.ets.org/research/policy_research_reports/pic-bwgap. Retrieved April 11, 2013.

El-Sheikh, M., Kelly, R., Buckhalt, J. A., & Hinnant, J. (2010). Children's sleep and adjustment over time: The role of the socio-economic context. *Child Development, 81,* 870–883.

Gregory, A. M., Caspi, A., Eley, T. C., Moffitt, T. E., O'Conner, T. G., & Pouton, R. (2005). Prospective longitudinal associations between persistent sleep problems in childhood and anxiety and depression disorders in adults. *Journal of Abnormal Child Psychology, 33,* 157–163.

Gutkin, T. B., & Reynolds, C. R. (1999). *The Handbook of School Psychology,* (3rd Ed.). NY: Wiley.

Gutkin, T. B., & Reynolds, C. R. (2009). *The Handbook of School Psychology* (4th Ed.). NY: Wiley.

Hart, C. N., Cairns, A., & Jelalian, E. (2011) Sleep and obesity in children and adolescents. *Pediatric Clinics of North America, 58,* 715–733.

IES National Center for Educational Statistics, U.S. Department of Education (2011). *Participation in Education.* http://nces.ed.gov/programs/coe/introduction1.asp. Retrieved April 11, 2013.

Konofal, E., Lecendreux, M., & Cortese, S. (2010). Sleep and ADHD. *Sleep Medicine, 11,* 652–658.

Kopasz, M., Loessl, B., Hornyak, M., Riemann, D., Nissen, C., Pioczyk, H., & Voderholzer, U. (2010). Sleep and memory in healthy children and adolescents. *Sleep Medicine Reviews, 14,* 167–177.

Lim, J., & Dinges, D. F. (2010). A meta-analysis of the impact of short-term sleep deprivation on cognitive variables. *Psychological Bulletin, 136,* 375–389.

Luginbuehl, M. (2003). *Sleep Disorders Inventory for Students.* Fairview, WY: Child Uplift, Inc.

Luginbuehl, M., Bradley-Klug, K. L., Ferron, J., Anderson, W. M., & Benbadis, S. R. (2008). Pediatric sleep disorders: Validation of the sleep disorders inventory for students. *School Psychology Review, 37,* 409–431.

McDonnell, E. (2004). School breakfast programs: Perceptions and barriers. *The Journal of Child Nutrition and Management, 2,* http://docs.schoolnutrition.org/newsroom/jcnm/04fall/mcdonnell/index.asp (Retrieved April 11, 2013 from online journal with no page numbers).

Marco, C. A., Wolfson, A. R., Sparling, M., & Azuaje, A. (2012). Family socioeconomic status and sleep patterns of young adolescents. *Behavioral Sleep Medicine, 10,* 70–80.

Meltzer, L. J., Johnson, C., Crosette, J., Ramos, M., & Mindell, J. A. (2010). Prevalence of diagnosed sleep disorders in pediatric primary care practices. *Pediatrics, 125,* e1410–1418.

Meltzer, L. J., Biggs, S., Reynolds, A., Avis, K. T., Mclaughlin-Crabtree, V., & Bevans, K. B. (2012). Children's report of sleep patterns-sleepiness: A self-report measure for school age children. *Sleep Medicine, 13*(4), 385–389.

Mindell, J. A. & Owens, J. A. (2010). *A Clinical Guide to Pediatric Sleep*. Philadelphia: Lippincott, Williams & Wilkins.

National Assessment of Educational Progress (2011). http://nces.ed.gov/nationsreportcard/National Association of State School Boards (NASBE, 2012). http://nasbe.org/healthy_schools/hs/index.php. Retrieved April 11, 2013.

National Assembly on School Based Health Care. (2011). http://www.nasbhc.org/site/pp.aspx?c=ckLQKbOVLkK6E&b=7453519. Retrieved April 11, 2013.

National Institutes of Health. (2011). *Healthy People* 2020. http://www.healthypeople.gov/2020/topicsobjectives2020/overview.aspx?topicid=38. Retrieved April 11, 2013.

National Sleep Foundation. (NSF, 2004). *Sleep in America Poll: Children and Sleep*. http://www.sleepfoundation.org/category/article-type/sleep-america-polls. Retrieved April 11, 2013.

National Sleep Foundation. (NSF, 2006). *Sleep in America Poll: Teens and Sleep* http://www.sleepfoundation.org/category/article-type/sleep-america-polls. Retrieved April 11, 2013.

National Sleep Foundation. (NSF, 2011). *Sleep in America Poll: Technology Use and Sleep*. http://www.sleepfoundation.org/category/article-type/sleep-america-polls. Retrieved April 11, 2013.

No Child Left Behind (NCLB) Act of 2001, Pub. L. No. 107–110, § 115, Stat. 1425. (2002).

O'Brien, L. M. (2011). The neurocognitive effects of sleep disruption in children and adolescents. *Sleep Medicine Clinics, 6*, 109–116.

O'Brien, L. M., Lucas, N. H., Felt, B. T., Hoban, T. F., Ruzicka, D. L., Jordan, R., et al. (2011). Aggressive behavior, bullying, snoring, and sleepiness in schoolchildren. *Sleep Medicine, 12*, 652–658.

Olds, T., Blunden, S., Petkov, J., & Forchino, F. (2010). The relationships between age, sex, geography and time in bed in adolescents: A meta-analysis of data from 23 countries. *Sleep Medicine Reviews, 14*, 371–378.

Owens, J. A., Spirito, A., & McGuinn, M. (2000). The Children's Sleep Habits Questionnaire (CSHQ): Psychometric properties of a survey instrument for school-aged children. *Sleep, 23*, 1043–1051.

Owens, J. A. & Dalzell, V. (2005). Use of the "BEARS" sleep screening tool in a pediatric residents' continuity clinic: A pilot study. *Sleep, 6*, 63–69.

Paavonen, E. J., Almqvist, F., Tamminen, T., Moilanen, J., Piha, J., Rasenen, E., et al. (2002). Poor sleep and psychiatric symptoms at school: An epidemiological study. *European Child and Adolescent Psychiatry, 11*, 10–17.

Pierangelo, R. & Giuliani, G. (2006). *Learning Disabilities: A practical approach to foundations, assessment, diagnosis, and teaching*. NY: Allyn-Bacon.

Reynolds, C. R. & Gutkin, T. B. (1982). *The Handbook of School Psychology*. NY: Wiley.

Reynolds, C. R. & Gutkin, T. B. (1990). *The Handbook of School Psychology* (2nd Ed.). New York: Wiley.

Reynolds, C. R. & Kamphaus, R. W. (2004). *Behavior Assessment System for Children* (2nd Ed.) *(BASC-2)*. San Antonio: Pearson Assessments.

Richdale, A. L. & Schreck, K. A. (2009). Sleep problems in autism spectrum disorders: Prevalence, nature, and possible biopsychosocial aetiologies. *Sleep Medicine Reviews, 13*, 403–411.

Ruiter, M. E., DeCoster, J., Jacobs, L., & Lichstein, K. L. (2010). Normal sleep in African-Americans: A meta-analysis. *Sleep Medicine, 12*, 209–214.

School Nutrition Association. (2011). http://www.schoolnutrition.org/Content.aspx?id=2374. Retrieved April 11, 2013.

Smaldone, A., Honig, J. C., & Byrne, M. W. (2007). Sleepless in America: Inadequate sleep and relationships to health and well-being of our nation's children. *Pediatrics, 119*, (Supplement 1), S29–S37

Spruyt, K., & Gozal, D. (2011). Pediatric sleep questionnaires as diagnostic or epidemiological tools: A review of currently available instruments. *Sleep Medicine Reviews, 15*, 19–32.

U.S. Census Bureau. (2011). School Enrollment in the United States. http://www.census.gov/compendia/statab/2012/tables/12s0219.pdf. Retrieved April 11, 2013.

U.S. Department of Agriculture. (2011). National school lunch program. http://www.fns.usda.gov/cnd/lunch/. Retrieved April 11, 2013.

Wolfson, A. R., Carskadon, M. A., Acebo, C., Seifer, R., Fallone, G., Labyak, S. E., & Martin, J. L. (2003). Evidence for the validity of a sleep habits survey for adolescents. *Sleep, 26*, 213–216.

Wolfson, A. R. & Carskadon, M. A. (2005). A survey of factors influencing high school start times. *NASSP Bulletin, 89*, 47–66.

PART 4

Sleep Challenges, Problems, and Disorders

CHAPTER

22 Pediatric Insomnia

Brandy M. Roane *and* Daniel J. Taylor

Abstract

Across the life span the presentation of disordered sleep varies greatly, but probably never more so than the changes that occur from infancy to adolescence. A major factor in this distinction is who reports the complaint. For infants and young children, parents are more likely to initiate contact with a professional with reports of insomnia that resembles limit setting, sleep onset association, or a combination of these two types. Conversely, older children and adolescents more often self-report difficulties, and their presentations typically consist of difficulties falling asleep and staying asleep. Children and their families experience adverse effects such as daytime sleepiness, depressed mood, and attention/concentration difficulties as a result of the child's sleep disturbance. Across the ages, behavioral interventions are the treatment of choice with the addition of cognitive therapy for adolescents. The current chapter highlights the distinctions in presentation of pediatric insomnia from early childhood to adolescence and discusses the empirically validated treatments in each age group.

Key Words: pediatric, adolescent, insomnia, behavioral insomnia of childhood, pediatric insomnia treatment, adolescent insomnia treatment

Introduction

While the basic physiology of sleep changes little after the first year of life, presentation of disordered sleep varies greatly across the life span. Insomnia is no exception. Numerous changes are observed in the presentation of insomnia coinciding with maturation in pediatric populations. No matter the age, insomnia refers to difficulties falling asleep, staying asleep, awakening too early, or sleep that is nonrestorative for at least a month, and these symptoms result in daytime impairment (American Academy of Sleep Medicine, 2005; American Psychiatric Association, 2000). The *Diagnostic and Statistical Manual of Mental Disorders* (DSM; American Psychiatric Association, 2000) distinguishes between primary insomnia and insomnia due to an Axis I or II disorder, while the *International Classification of Sleep Disorders* (ICSD-2; American Academy of Sleep Medicine, 2005) identifies seven types of insomnia determined by the presentation. For instance, behavioral insomnia of childhood (BIC) and psychophysiological insomnia would fall under primary insomnia in the DSM, but each would have their own type in the ICSD-2. The ICSD-2 determines types based on their presentation so, for instance, insomnia caused by an immediate stressor would be classified as *adjustment insomnia.* The ICSD-2 also considers inadequate sleep hygiene to be a type of insomnia. Clinically, insomnia is often discussed in terms of the time period when sleep is being disrupted, which results in three "types": sleep onset—difficulties initiating sleep at the beginning of the sleep period; maintenance—difficulties maintaining sleep during the night; and terminal—awaking prematurely before the desired wake time.

One theory used to explain the etiology of insomnia is the *behavioral model of insomnia* (Spielman, Caruso, & Glovinsky, 1987). This model conceptualizes physiological, psychological, and behavioral factors as predisposing, precipitating, and perpetuating events. Predisposing factors are typically the underlying pathophysiological mechanisms that place individuals at risk for insomnia. The exact etiology of insomnia is unclear, but recent lines of research suggest predisposing factors are likely genetics (Gehrman et al., 2011; Moore, Slane, Mindell, Burt, & Klump, 2011) and hyperactivity of corticotropin-releasing factor neurons (Richardson & Roth, 2001).

While little is known about the etiology of insomnia, similar predisposing factors likely affect predisposition across the age groups; however, precipitating and perpetuating factors change with age. At the core of these differences is the normal developmental shift in the central role parents have in the child's functioning. Infants require constant attention that progressively lessens as children mature. For younger children, the learned behaviors of both parents and children initiate and maintain insomnia, while for older children and adolescents, the learned behaviors they independently adopt often maintain insomnia.

What constitutes disturbed sleep varies greatly across the life span based on family and individual definition of "disturbed"(Jenni & O'Connor, 2005; Mindell, Sadeh, Wiegand, How, & Goh, 2010; Sadeh, Flint-Ofir, Tirosh, & Tikotzky, 2007; *Sleep in America Poll*, 2006). What one family may consider "disturbed" another may consider "normal." Numerous factors contribute to this determination, including cultural practices, parental expectations, and the child's developmental stage (Goodlin-Jones, Tang, Liu, & Anders, 2009; Jenni & O'Connor, 2005; Mindell, Kuhn, Lewin, Meltzer, & Sadeh, 2006; Mindell, Sadeh, Wiegand, et al., 2010). Maturation brings about an awareness of the sleep disturbance and the associated daytime consequences (Bibace & Walsh, 1980). Thus as children mature, their own experiences along with their family's perspectives influence how they define disturbed sleep and subsequently self-report sleep disturbances.

The progressive independence of children as they mature also affects the presentation of insomnia. Younger children are at the mercy of their parents in the determination of bedtime, whereas older children and adolescents begin to develop more autonomy surrounding bedtime. Thus, younger children may attempt to impose control over their bedtime by resisting falling asleep or insisting that specific circumstances always be present to fall asleep. Alternatively, the resulting sleep disturbance may not be children attempting to impose control, but more a misalignment between children's internal timing systems and their imposed bedtime. As a result, children are not sleepy when bedtime comes to pass. The latter is more often true for older children and adolescents, who experience a natural delaying of their internal timing system (Carskadon, 2008; Carskadon, Labyak, Acebo, & Seifer, 1999; Carskadon, Vieira, & Acebo, 1993). Unlike younger children, adolescents and older children do not resist sleep but instead present more like adults with insomnia who, despite their best efforts to fall asleep, are unable to.

Parents of younger children are more involved in the bedtime routine, bedtime, and, by proxy, more aware of sleep disturbances. They also are more likely to experience secondary sleep difficulties and daytime consequences as a result of their child's sleep disturbance (e.g., secondary sleep loss, missed work days, bed sharing with the child; Martin, Hiscock, Hardy, Davey, & Wake, 2007; Meltzer & Mindell, 2007). Conversely, parents of older children and adolescents may not be aware of the problem because they are not witnessing the difficulty (e.g., the parent is not present to "tuck" the child in bed) or contributing to the disturbance (e.g., child requires mom to lie down with her in order to fall asleep). As a result, older children and adolescents are more likely to self-report the sleep disturbance because parents are less likely to know what is going on at bedtime and throughout the night. For instance, the National Sleep Foundation found that 7% of caregivers polled reported their adolescents experienced a sleep disorder, whereas over twice as many (16%) of the adolescents self-reported a sleep disorder (*Sleep in America Poll*, 2006). Yet, these reports were not always congruent. For instance, 12% of the caregivers reported their adolescent had no sleep problems, but the adolescent self-reported a possible or definite problem. Conversely, 3% of the caregivers who reported their adolescents had a sleep disorder, which the adolescent denied.

Schreck and Richdale (2011) looked beyond parental reports of sleep disorders to explore factors that influenced their observations. They found parents' knowledge of sleep and sleep disorders was poor in general, but significantly worse in older children and adolescents compared to younger children. For instance, almost one-third of parents were unsure if adolescents snored on a nightly basis or if adolescents slept more on school nights or non-school nights.

Both closeness to the problem (i.e., being the individual reporting the problem versus observer of the reported sleep disturbance) and definition of disturbance influence these discrepancies. Parents' knowledge about "normal" sleep and their observations provide the point of reference when determining if their children's sleep is poor. Thus, a dearth of knowledge and no observed sleep disturbances enable parents to think their older child or teen is sleeping just fine.

The distinctions in presentation of insomnia and treatment by the various age groups will be elucidated further in the sections below. Please note, the following sections focus on insomnia and treatments for children and adolescents ages 1 to 18 from a Western cultural perspective. In addition, the authors use the term *parents*, but recognize that family situations arise such that two parents are not always present or involved in treatment.

Preschoolers (Ages 1 to 5)

Sleep disturbances, in general, are one of the most common complaints in pediatrician and child psychotherapy offices with reports as high as approximately 20%–30% (Armstrong, Quinn, & Dadds, 1994; Burnham, Goodlin-Jones, Gaylor, & Anders, 2002; Goodlin-Jones, Burnham, Gaylor, & Anders, 2001; Lozoff, Wolf, & Davis, 1985; Mindell, 1999). Topping the list of sleep problems in young children is behavioral insomnia of childhood (BIC), characterized by parent-reported bedtime struggles and frequent night awakenings. BIC includes two subtypes: sleep-onset association type (BIC-SOA) and limit-setting type (BIC-LST), which frequently coexist and have symptom overlap. While some children may display only one difficulty or the other, many display features of both, or combined type (BIC-C). The function of the behavior drives the determination of the sub-type.

Sleep-Onset Association Type. Children who seek parental intervention or assistance to create or recreate a specific situation (e.g., feeding, rocking, parental presence) required for sleep onset to occur present with BIC-SOA (American Academy of Sleep Medicine, 2005; Mindell, Kuhn, et al., 2006). These children are unable to self-soothe, and seek out parental attention by either signaling or leaving their rooms. They have learned a non-adaptive sleep-onset association through repeated pairings of the situation with sleep (Goodlin-Jones et al., 2001; Van Tassel, 1985). The repeated pairings of the learned cue with sleep occur not just from night to night at bedtime, but also throughout the night each time the child awakes and requests the situation to be recreated in order to return to sleep. Children, like adolescents and adults, experience nocturnal arousals and awakenings throughout the night as they cycle through the sleep stages (Anders, Halpern, & Hua, 1992). Children who have learned to independently initiate sleep will use this skill to return to sleep; however, children with insomnia will respond by seeking out the situation (e.g., feeding, rocking, parental presence) they used to fall asleep initially.

Limit-Setting Type. Children who present with BIC-LST engage in a host of noncompliant behaviors as bedtime or naptime approaches, such as stalling or complete refusal to go to bed, verbal protests, tantrums, crying, and repeated demands (e.g., hugs, kisses, glass of water; American Academy of Sleep Medicine, 2005; Mindell, Kuhn, et al., 2006). Children most often engage in these behaviors at bedtime, but they can reappear during the night if the child awakens and is expected to return to bed. This pattern of behavior results from an established learning history in which parents impose bedtime, children engage in the noncompliant behaviors, and parents do not impose limits. When parents do impose limits, children will often escalate their behaviors (i.e., "extinction burst"). As a result, parents back down from the limit they imposed and children are reinforced for engaging in this new, more escalated behavior. By the time the family arrives for an office visit, the interplay between parents and children has frequently exacerbated the severity of this subtype. A frequent adverse consequence of BIC-LST is that children truncate their total sleep time, leading to an increase in daytime behavior problems.

BIC adversely influences the child, the parents, and the family. Children frequently exhibit daytime impairments expressed as mood disturbances, performance impairments, and daytime sleepiness (Beebe, 2011; Fallone, Owens, & Deane, 2002). The disruptive behaviors that surround bedtime are often a reflection of what is occurring throughout the day, only now all parties involved are sleepier. Increased sleepiness impairs judgment and decision making ultimately increasing the likelihood that conflict may occur between the child and parents and a less desirable outcome may result (e.g., child sleeping in the parents' bed, parent sleeping in the child's room). Similarly, children under 5 who are still within napping age often exhibit these disruptive bedtime behaviors during naptime. The sleep disturbances adversely impact the family both during the night and daytime. For instance, parents may be reactively co-sleeping (i.e., sleeping with the child in an attempt to address the sleep problem), consequently disrupting their own sleeping arrangements, or the child's behavior may be disturbing other siblings who share the room (Kataria, Swanson, & Trevathan, 1987). The subsequent daytime impairments experienced by the child and parents also take a toll the next day on all family members.

Younger children often exhibit "paradoxical" behaviors in the aftermath of sleep loss such as hyperactivity, impulsivity, or risk-taking behaviors, unlike their parents who experience daytime sleepiness (Boergers, Hart, Owens, Streisand, & Spirito, 2007; Meltzer & Mindell, 2007). Parent-reported daytime impairments include increased mood disturbances, fatigue, daytime sleepiness, stress, marital conflict, negative parent–child interactions, and decreased level of effective parenting (Boergers et al., 2007; Mindell, Kuhn, et al., 2006; Owens, 2008). In addition, studies have documented that infant sleep disturbances persist into young childhood (Kataria et al., 1987; Stein, Mendelsohn, Obermeyer, Amromin, & Benca, 2001; Zuckerman, Stevenson, & Bailey, 1987). Thus, the detrimental effects on the child, parents, and family can become pervasive as these behavioral patterns become engrained if problems persist for years.

Several intrinsic and extrinsic factors contribute to the likelihood that young children will develop BIC (Burnham et al., 2002; Hiscock, 2010; Mindell, Sadeh, Kohyama, & How, 2010; Sadeh, Mindell, Luedtke, & Wiegand, 2009; Sadeh, Tikotzky, & Scher, 2010). These factors can be clustered into parental, individual, and environmental variables, but should always be considered within a cultural context. Parental variables include how parents manage bedtime and night awakenings (strongest predictor), parenting style, family stress (Bates, Viken, Alexander, Beyers, & Stockton, 2002), parental temperament (Sadeh et al., 2010), differences in parental perceptions of their child's sleep (Boergers et al., 2007; Sadeh et al., 2007), mental health concerns such as maternal depression (Bayer, Hiscock, Hampton, & Wake, 2007; Boergers et al., 2007; Sadeh et al., 2010), parent education, and knowledge about childhood sleep (Schreck & Richdale, 2011) and typical development (Reich, 2005). Child variables that influence sleep include temperament, developmental age, cognitive and emotional development, and medical conditions (Owens, 2008; Owens & Mindell, 2011). Environmental factors very widely, encompassing areas like the sleeping environment (light, noise, room sharing, bed sharing, sleeping space, sleeping surface, perceived safety, electronics), family composition (family roles, family size, ages, medical and mental health status), family lifestyle (parental work status, family schedules, household rules), and socioeconomic status.

Cultural factors impact a family's and individual's perception of normal sleep, thereby influencing what they perceive as disordered (see Chapters 9, 10, and 11). Mindell and colleagues (2010) examined sleep patterns and problems of infants and toddlers ages birth to 36 months in predominately Asian (P-A) and predominantly Caucasian (P-C) countries by assessing 29,287 parents. Significant cross-cultural differences resulted, with parents in P-A countries reporting higher perceptions of sleep disorders and that their children had later bedtimes, shorter total sleep times, and increased room sharing compared to parents in P-C countries. Thus, the cultural and racial/ethnic makeup of the family are important considerations when evaluating and treating children's sleep disturbances (Jenni & O'Connor, 2005; Mindell, Sadeh, Wiegand, et al., 2010).

Behavioral Treatments for Children Ages 1 Through 5

A host of strategies have been used to address pediatric sleep disturbances, but behaviorally based therapies in children ages 1 through 5 are by far the strongest (Kuhn & Elliott, 2003; Mindell, Kuhn, et al., 2006; Morgenthaler, Owens, et al., 2006). The primary treatments used generalize to both symptoms and subtypes. The generalization of the treatment is important and likely due to the very nature of the sleep cycle. Children, like adults, experience repeated brief nighttime awakenings following initial sleep onset. Each of these brief periods of wakefulness often turn into prolonged awakenings for children with BIC and represent an opportunity for the child—and for the parent to allow the child—to practice independent sleep initiation.

A task force appointed by the American Academy of Sleep Medicine convened and reviewed 52 studies using modified Sackett criteria (Sackett,1993) and a clinical grading system (i.e., standard, guideline, or option; Eddy, 1992). They established the first pediatric practice parameters for the clinical management of BIC (Mindell, Kuhn, et al., 2006). Their findings were consistent with two prior clinical reviews (Kuhn & Elliott, 2003; Mindell, 1999). They reported a 94% efficacy rate for behaviorally based treatments, with over 80% of the children maintaining improvements at 3 or 6 months. The evidence provides the most support for younger children, but the few studies in children closer to age 5 also support the use of behavioral interventions.

This task force identified unmodified extinction and preventive parent education as *Standard Treatments*, supported by a plethora of well-designed randomized trials. *Guideline Treatments*, with support from randomized trials or nonrandomized concurrently controlled studies, included graduated extinction, positive routines/faded bedtime, and scheduled awakenings. Insufficient evidence was available to recommend bedtime routines and positive reinforcement as stand-alone treatments.

Research clearly supports behavioral interventions for the treatment of BIC. The daunting task for clinicians becomes choosing which treatment intervention to use and appropriately tailoring it to meet the needs of the child and family. Behaviorally based therapies apply the principles of learning to bring about change in sleep-related behaviors. Predictability and consistency enable learning to occur (Kazdin, 2000). The child learns to anticipate sleep at the end when parents implement a bedtime routine. In addition, the outcome becomes a predictable consequence when the child experiences the same consequence each time a specific behavior occurs. The judicious use of reinforcement, another component of behavioral therapies, aids in the child learning by establishing a contrast in experience. For instance, parents can use differential attention to create this contrast by attending to (reinforcement) a wanted behavior (e.g., praise the child for getting ready for bed) and not attending to (extinguish) unwanted behaviors (e.g., actively ignore the child crying once in bed).

The parent is the active agent of change in these therapies (Mindell, 1999; Owens, 2006; Sadeh, 2005), but an important and often underappreciated component of these therapies is the fact that the caregivers and children are both changing their behaviors. This latter point is likely the primary reason these treatments are so effective. Behavioral therapies produce a family level of change (i.e., both parents and children are changing behaviors) versus an individual level of change (i.e., expecting just the child to change). The benefit of parents learning effective tools for handling bedtime struggles and night awakenings is that if, and more realistically when, these sleep problems reappear following unexpected events in the child's life (e.g., transition to a bed from the crib, vacation, illness), parents are prepared.

PARENT EDUCATION AND PREVENTION

Preventive measures are the most effective, economical, and time-efficient of any behaviorally based pediatric sleep medicine intervention (Mindell, Kuhn, et al., 2006). During the prenatal period through 6 months postnatal, proactive educational approaches are used with parents that aim to avert sleep disorders by helping them to establish positive sleep habits for their children. Caregivers learn appropriate expectations about sleep in infants and how to establish limits. Parent management of bedtime is the strongest predictor of future BIC for younger children (Hiscock, 2010; Mindell, Sadeh, Kohyama, et al., 2010; Sadeh et al., 2010). The primary take-home message with preventative education is that babies should be placed in bed "drowsy but awake," enabling them to develop independent sleep initiation skills (Mindell, Kuhn, et al., 2006). In a large randomized control trial of 268 parents and their 2- to 3-week-old infants, nurses delivered one 45-minute consultation with written materials. Infants in the intervention group slept on average 1 hour 20 minutes more than the control group per day at 6 weeks, and gains were maintained at 3-month follow-up (Symon, Marley, Martin, & Norman, 2005).

The primary advantages are the use of skill-building and the focus on prevention. Unfortunately, the limited availability of these programs and their limited utility once sleep difficulties develop in children results in other intervention methods being necessary.

UNMODIFIED EXTINCTION

Unmodified extinction, or "systematic ignoring," is the most effective behavioral intervention for BIC (Kuhn & Elliott, 2003; Mindell, Kuhn, et al., 2006). Parents often refer to this intervention as the "cry-it-out approach." Yet, extinction in its true form does not equate to "crying it out" but instead involves removing the reinforcing consequence that maintains an unwanted behavior in order to reduce the frequency of this behavior over time (Lerman & Iwata, 1996).

In the treatment of BIC, unmodified extinction involves having parents place the child in bed and not attend to him or her until the next morning (Chadez & Nurius, 1987; France & Hudson, 1990; Rapoff, Christophersen, & Rapoff, 1982; Rickert & Johnson, 1988; Sanders, Bor, & Dadds, 1984).

Possible exceptions to this last instruction include legitimate illness, danger of self-harm, or property destruction. Most often these basic instructions are modified to include other behavioral strategies that can make the treatment plan more successful (Lerman, Iwata, & Wallace, 1999). These strategies include establishing a regular bedtime and bedtime routine (Rapoff et al., 1982; Seymour, Bayfield, Brock, & During, 1983), handling refusals to stay in bed (Reid, Walter, & O'Leary, 1999), and preparing the parents for the potential extinction burst (Wade, Ortiz, & Gorman, 2007).

Two potential concerns with any behavioral treatment is the occurrence of an extinction burst, a temporary escalation (increase in frequency, duration, and/or magnitude) in the unwanted behavior, or an extinction-induced emotional outburst and a spontaneous reappearance of the unwanted behavior (Kazdin, 2000). Children are likely to exhibit this spontaneous reappearance in response to changes in their environment (bed, bedroom routine, or caregivers) or schedule. While the extinction burst can be too adverse for some parents to endure, especially when the burst can last 2 to 3 days (Rickert & Johnson, 1988), the major advantage of unmodified extinction is the rapid response if done correctly. Most children go to bed with little to no protest by the third day (France, Henderson, & Hudson, 1996).

GRADUATED EXTINCTION

An alternative to unmodified extinction is graduated extinction. Numerous interventions fit under the umbrella term *graduated extinction*, but all integrate into the unmodified extinction intervention parent "check-ins" that are faded over time (Adams & Rickert, 1989; Ferber, 1985; Kuhn & Weidinger, 2000; Lawton, France, & Blampied, 1991; Meltzer & Mindell, 2010; Mindell, Kuhn, et al., 2006). Check-ins are brief, planned visits (e.g., 15 to 60 seconds) into the child's room until the child falls asleep. The schedule and length of time between checks varies. A fixed time schedule establishes a set interval between checks (e.g., 5 minutes) that remains constant between checks, whereas a graduated time schedule, more commonly called "incremental" graduated extinction, progressively increases the length of time between each check (e.g., 5-minutes, 10-minutes, 15-minutes). During the check-ins, parents are instructed to minimize social interactions and attention (i.e., no excessive talking, touching, or looking at the child). The goal of check-ins is to reassure the parent that the child is safe and to provide assurance to the child that the parents are close.

Graduated extinction has the benefits of maintaining the regular bedtime and parents returning to the room for quick checks. Reid and colleagues (1999) found both extinction and graduated extinction produced similar improvements in bedtime refusal and night awakenings when compared to a waitlist control group. Analysis of maternal stress about treatment showed no significant difference between groups, but within-group comparisons found that mothers using graduated extinction reported significantly lower treatment-related stress by weeks 2 and 3. Regarding potential additive benefits of treatments, extinction was associated with reductions in distress about parenting and in verbose discipline strategies (e.g., excessive talking about the behavior, scolding) following treatment, while graduated extinction was associated with improved parent–child interactions compared to no intervention. Thus, these findings suggest that the extinction techniques provide parents with helpful tools that are generalizable to their parenting skills.

The main note of caution with this procedure is the risk of inadvertently reinforcing inappropriate behavior with the noncontingent parental presence provided by the checks. In essence, parents are reentering the room whether the child is behaving appropriately or not. In some instances, parents may unwittingly shape longer and longer bouts of crying through the incremental check procedure.

EXTINCTION WITH PARENTAL PRESENCE

Another variant, called *extinction with parental presence*, requires parents to remain in the bedroom feigning sleep in a separate bed or cot while actively ignoring inappropriate behaviors (France, 2010; France & Blampied, 2005; Mindell, Kuhn, et al., 2006). The only exceptions to ignoring are if the child is ill or in danger (Mindell, Kuhn, et al., 2006; Wolfson, 1998). Parents remain in the room for up to one week or until the child is independently initiating and maintaining sleep, whichever occurs first. Once parents are out of the child's bedroom and back in their own bed, they employ unmodified extinction for crying out and other inappropriate behaviors.

This modification of extinction, like graduated extinction, can ease parents' concerns about safety because they can "see" their child throughout the process. Evidence shows this approach produces less crying than extinction and graduated extinction (France & Blampied, 2005). France (2010) proposes the parent's presence reduces the child's separation anxiety. Some concerns that need further empirical evaluation are the stress on the parent who remains in the room pretending to not know the child is crying and upset, and adherence with the request that parents temporarily alter their sleeping arrangements.

THE BEDTIME PASS

The bedtime pass is a more recent modification of extinction for children at least 3 years of age with bedtime refusal. The bedtime pass is intended for children who have shown mastery of independent sleep initiation but are calling out, coming out of the room, or engaging in other bedtime struggles (Freeman, 2006; Friman et al., 1999; Moore, Friman, Fruzzetti, & MacAleese, 2007). Prior to initiating this intervention, parents need to assist the child in choosing or creating an object to serve as the bedtime pass. Objects that typically work well are decorated index cards, stuffed animals, or other small toys. Items to avoid include the child's transitional object or strings with beads (for safety reasons). After making or selecting an item to be the bedtime pass, the child is told the ground rules of the bedtime pass. The bedtime pass can be exchanged for one, and only one, trip or small request (e.g., drink of water, extra hug or kiss) that takes less than 3 minutes. When the child uses the pass, parents respond immediately by readily fulfilling the request and collecting the bedtime pass from the child. The child is also told that once the bedtime pass is used, additional trips or calling out are not allowed. Parents use systematic ignoring (extinction) for any subsequent problematic bedtime behaviors once the child hands over the bedtime pass. In the morning, parents are encouraged not to discuss the use or nonuse of the bedtime pass. Each night at bedtime, the child is reminded of the bedtime pass rules. Once the child consistently goes to bed without struggles, the bedtime pass is gradually faded out.

Evidence indicates the bedtime pass is effective in reducing bedtime struggles in typically developing toddlers and school-age children (Freeman, 2006; Moore et al., 2007). In addition, the bedtime pass appears to minimize the post-extinction response bursts, and parents respond well to the treatment.

POSITIVE ROUTINES

While extinction and its various modifications focus on removing inappropriate behaviors, positive routines shift the focus to increasing appropriate pre-sleep behaviors. The use of positive routines combines two components: establishing a pre-bedtime routine, and temporarily delaying the bedtime to more closely match when the child is naturally falling asleep pre-treatment (Milan, Mitchell, Berger, & Pierson, 1981; Mindell, Kuhn, et al., 2006). Similar to sleep restriction therapy described later, this instruction helps to build intrinsic sleep pressure through the homeostatic sleep drive. The homeostatic sleep drive is a sleep–wake dependent system that regulates sleep propensity. Prolonged wakefulness increases the need for sleep and sleeping decreases this need.

The delayed bedtime also serves to simultaneously reduce bedtime struggles by increasing the likeliness the child will be sleepy closer to their bedtime. In addition, a pre-bedtime routine is established that should simultaneously lead up to the child's bedtime and bedroom, which lasts up to 20 minutes and consists of four to seven activities. Parents provide positive reinforcement, often in the form of verbal praise, with successful completion of each activity. Activities may include going to the bathroom, brushing teeth, putting on pajamas, and reading a story. In essence, parents establish a behavior "chain" with these activities that in turn serve as cues for sleep. If the child begins to tantrum or engage in other bedtime refusal behaviors during the routine, parents leave the child alone for 15 minutes. Upon returning, parents pick up the chain where they left off. Parents are instructed to engage in systematic ignoring when the child is in bed. Once the behavioral chain is established and the child is falling asleep quickly without resistance, the pre-bedtime routine gradually advances earlier in the evening until reaching a preestablished bedtime goal (Adams & Rickert, 1989; Milan et al., 1981).

The focus on establishing cues for sleep and teaching the child what to do versus what not to do are benefits of this approach. In a 6-week comparison of graduated extinction, positive routines, and no treatment group, positive routines showed similar improvements in frequency of tantrums compared to graduated extinction, but by week 4 the children in the positive routines group were tantruming for less time compared to the graduated extinction and control groups (Adams & Rickert, 1989). Post-treatment outcomes indicated the positive routines and graduated extinction groups meet treatment goals in terms of reduced bedtime struggles; however, the parents in the positive routines group reported the greatest improvements in marital satisfaction. Adam and Rickert also noted that parents in the positive routines group asked fewer questions about the protocol. While this intervention includes extinction, the context is differential reinforcement (i.e., attending to the desired behaviors and systematically ignoring the undesired behaviors), and the combination of reinforcement with extinction appears to cushion the use of the latter.

BEDTIME FADING AND BEDTIME FADING WITH RESPONSE COST

Bedtime fading, like positive routines, temporarily delays the child's bedtime to facilitate more rapid sleep onset. The distinction in the two bedtime delay procedures is that the use of positive routines delays the initial treatment bedtime to match the typical pretreatment sleep onset time, whereas bedtime fading establishes the initial treatment bedtime by adding an additional 30 minutes to the typical pretreatment sleep onset time (Kodak & Piazza, 2010; Piazza & Fisher, 1991a, 1991b). In addition to delaying bedtime, bedtime fading establishes a scheduled wake-up time each morning. Parents continue to interact with the child at bedtime and during night awakenings as they did pre-treatment. The key shift is the management of times. Parents are instructed to rigorously manage the child's sleep/wake schedule to insure no sleep is occurring outside of the prescribed sleep times. Exceptions can be made for children 4 years and under who are still napping (Kodak & Piazza, 2010). Fading the bedtime involves advancing the bedtime by 30 minutes each night the child fell asleep within 15 minutes the night before, or delaying the bedtime 30 minutes if the child took longer than 15 minutes to fall asleep the night before. In many ways, bedtime fading is similar to sleep restriction therapy used for the treatment of insomnia in older children, adolescents, and adults.

The addition of response cost requires parents to remove the child from bed for 1 hour if sleep onset does not occur within 15 minutes of the prescribed bedtime (Piazza & Fisher, 1991a, 1991b). The focus is on increasing the reinforcement value of sleep. The rationale is that the reinforcement value of sleep will outweigh that of parental attention through the cumulative effect of increasing the homeostatic sleep drive via stringent management of the sleep/wake schedule and removing the child from bed when sleep onset does not occur swiftly. Bedtime fading with response cost parallels stimulus control therapy used for the treatment of insomnia in older children, adolescents, and adults (Piazza & Fisher, 1991a). By removing the individual from bed, sleep becomes the dominant association with bed versus the established wake associations. Sleep becoming the strongest association with bed increases the likelihood that sleep onset will occur at bedtime. The pairing of response cost with faded bedtime further increases this likelihood, because delaying the bedtime results in greater homeostatic sleep pressure.

While this treatment shows promise, more research is needed to determine how effective it is in populations aside from children ages 3 and older and children with special needs residing in institutionalized settings, and to explore the active treatment mechanisms to know the necessity of response cost in the protocol. In addition, adherence to the full bedtime fading with response cost protocol needs to be evaluated, as the majority of studies have assessed treatment implemented by trained professionals. The benefit of this treatment is that parents are not required to alter their management of bedtime and nighttime awakenings; however, they must be willing to stringently manage the child's sleep/wake schedule and accept night-to-night fluctuations in their child's bedtime during treatment.

SCHEDULED AWAKENINGS

The scheduled awakenings protocol breaks the association between middle of the night awakenings and parental attention by establishing a noncontingent reinforcement with schedule thinning in children up to age 5 (Adams & Rickert, 1989; Mindell, Kuhn, et al., 2006). Parents closely monitor their child's sleep to establish a baseline pattern of nocturnal awakening times (e.g., 11:30 AM, 1:30 AM, and 3:30 AM). Parents are instructed to preemptively wake their child up 15 to 30 minutes prior to these night awakenings and engage in the usual caregiving activities (e.g., rocking, feeding) until sleep is reinitiated. The time of each awakening is gradually delayed to facilitate the child sleeping uninterrupted for longer periods of time (Rickert & Johnson, 1988).

While scheduled awakenings are an effective treatment, the procedure has several drawbacks that make it less likely to be the treatment of choice for most BIC cases. Scheduled awakenings address only night awakening difficulties, which limits the treatment's utility. The procedure is complex, disruptive, and gradual. These three characteristics are not always preferable to parents. Parents must anticipate every night awakening, causing disruption to their own sleep schedule. In addition, treatment course is often several weeks (e.g., 8 weeks) versus swifter periods shown with extinction-based protocols (e.g., 1–3 weeks).

Despite these drawbacks, scheduled awakenings are a good alternative for children who are resistant to extinction-based procedures or who engage in self-harming behaviors (Kuhn & Weidinger, 2000). If parents prematurely end extinction-based procedures (e.g., attend to the child at the peak of an extinction burst), they may inadvertently teach their child more severe behaviors or establish a learning history in which the child escalates rapidly because the parents will "give in." Repeated exposure to situations such as this can result in the child becoming resistant to extinction-based procedures. These children escalate more quickly and engage in more severe behaviors than their peers when an extinction-based procedure is introduced. In addition, children who engage in self-harming behaviors (e.g., scratching themselves, severe head banging) should not be left unattended under normal circumstances and, as such, should not be left unattended during the peak of an extinction burst. Parents of these children need to be able to observe the child, which contradicts systematic ignoring.

Comorbid Conditions and Considerations

Comorbid and occult sleep disorders should be a consideration when evaluating for and treating BIC. Children presenting with night awakenings may also have obstructive sleep apnea, sleep terrors, or, in some cases, both. Any child presenting with middle of the night awakenings, especially if this is the primary complaint, should also be assessed for obstructive sleep apnea (OSA). In these cases, a referral for a polysomnography study (PSG) is necessary for determining if OSA should be ruled in or out (see McLaughlin Crabtree, Rach, and Gamble, Chapter 19). In these cases, treating the OSA may be effective in eliminating the night awakenings even though additional treatment using behavioral interventions may be necessary to treat residual bedtime struggles and night awakenings.

The second comorbid disorder, sleep terrors, is a common consequence as a result of the sleep loss experienced by children with BIC. Sleep terrors are a partial-arousal parasomnia in which the autonomic nervous system becomes activated during delta sleep (stages 3 and 4). As a result, the child may scream out or cry as though he or she is scared or in pain despite remaining asleep. Parents are often the most alarmed by these events because they are unsure if their child is hurt or has been hurt and is now recalling that past event. The good news for these children is that treatment for BIC will reduce the occurrence of sleep terrors, but parents must also be educated. In some instances a child who is predisposed to sleep terrors will also present with both BIC and OSA. These children are likely suffering sleep loss from both the OSA and BIC and that triggers the sleep terrors. The BIC may have arisen independently of the OSA or may be a by-product of the OSA-induced night awakenings. In most cases, treating the OSA and BIC will result in a cessation of the sleep terrors.

Middle Childhood (Ages 6 to 10)

School-age children have usually mastered independent sleep initiation. They are less inclined to need parental presence in order to fall asleep. If children are unable to fall asleep immediately upon going to bed, instead of signaling they are more likely to occupy themselves quietly (e.g., reading a book, lying quietly) until sleep onset occurs (Owens, Spirito, McGuinn, & Nobile, 2000). School enables this transition to independence. School provides opportunities for children to expand their social circles to include peer relationships, and their interests to include academics and extracurricular activities. All of which introduces new reinforcers that are as reinforcing if not more so than parental attention.

Parents allow children more independence of their bedtime and bedtime routines as the children show mastery of skills both at bedtime and during the day. Simultaneously, children become more aware and accepting of their need for sleep with maturation (Dement, 1999). With less interference around bedtime pushing sleep onset later, the strong opposing forces of clock-dependent alertness and homeostatic sleep drive work in harmony such that school-age children often fall asleep and awaken with ease.

Despite these maturational changes, parent-reported rates of bedtime problems (~15%–30%) remain as high during middle childhood (Blader, Koplewicz, Abikoff, & Foley, 1997; Owens et al., 2000; Stein et al., 2001) as those reported during early childhood. As children hit middle childhood, the presentation of insomnia begins to change. Although most of these children continue to present with bedtime refusal (~15%–27%), a small portion develop insomnia that more closely resembles the presentation seen in adolescents and adults (Mindell, Emslie, et al., 2006; Stein et al., 2001; described in the next section).

Comorbid Conditions and Considerations

The majority of evidence-based treatment of pediatric insomnia literature targets infants and preschool children, with less focus on school-age children (Owens et al., 2000; Tikotzky & Sadeh, 2010). Unfortunately, clinicians working with school-age children and adolescents must rely on the scant literature to date and make inferences from the literature available in other age groups. The few BIC studies that have included school-age children support the use of positive routines, faded bedtime with response cost, and the bedtime pass, all described previously. Developing a treatment plan for a school-age child presenting with insomnia like that seen in adolescents and adults requires clinicians to borrow from the adult treatment literature (described in the next section). No matter the treatment of choice for a school-age child, the family unit should continue to be the mechanism of treatment delivery and monitoring adherence.

School-age children who present with insomnia are frequently more complex cases than infants or toddlers. Often etiology is multifactorial including environmental, psychiatric, medical, and psychosocial factors (Sadeh, Raviv, & Gruber, 2000), making the list of rule-ins and rule-outs longer. Insomnia in school-age children can be comorbid with other medical, neurodevelopmental, and psychiatric disorders. Common conditions frequently associated with insomnia are attention-deficit/hyperactivity disorder (ADHD), pervasive developmental disorder, autism, anxiety, depression, and oppositional defiant disorder (Stein et al., 2001). Insomnia due to medication is also a consideration if the child is taking psychostimulants or selective serotonin reuptake inhibitors (SSRIs). Obstructive sleep apnea is still a necessary rule-out when evaluating insomnia in school-age children. Rates of sleep terrors decrease with age, so this is less likely to be a comorbid disorder but may still be present in some children who are predisposed and experiencing stress or restricting their sleep. Occurring at the opposite end of the night (latter third versus first third) are nightmares, which occur most frequently in school-age children. These events can easily escalate and result in a comorbid case of BIC-SOA if the child seeks out parental assistance to initiate or reinitiate sleep. Circadian disorders, particularly delayed sleep phase disorder, may begin to emerge in children closer to puberty.

Adolescence (Ages 10 to 18)

Adolescence is a developmental period that encompasses numerous neuroendocrine and structural brain changes and the reactivation of the hypothalamus-pituitary-gonadal axis, triggering the onset of puberty (see Carskadon and Tarokh, Chapter 8). Structural reorganization of the brain occurs throughout the second decade of life, the most prominent being cortical synaptic pruning (Huttenlocher, 1979). These changes influence physiological correlates of sleep, as shown by the sharp decrease in the amount of slow wave and high-amplitude sleep experienced by adolescents.

Adolescents also experience changes in both processes that regulate the timing of sleep, Process S (the homeostatic sleep pressure) and Process C (intrinsic circadian timing system). Older adolescents experience a slower accumulation of Process S during wake compare to pre- and early pubertal adolescents following sleep deprivation (Jenni, Achermann, & Carskadon, 2005). A slower accumulation of sleep pressure means older adolescents are able to stay awake for longer periods of time (Taylor, Jenni, Acebo, & Carskadon, 2005). Simultaneously, pubertal development is associated with a delayed phase preference (Carskadon et al., 1993). Interestingly, despite a notable delay in bedtimes and the emergence of a delayed preference, sleep need of approximately 8 hours 54 minutes to 9 hours 12 minutes (SD 16–33 min) does not change across the adolescent age range (Carskadon et al., 1980).

Adolescents' intrinsic forces work against them falling asleep earlier as they mature; yet, their intrinsic sleep need continues to be the same. Simultaneously, society-imposed school start times do not compensate for these factors but instead push against them by shifting school starts to the earliest times of all school-age children and adolescents (see Au, Appleman, and Stavitsky, Chapter 38). As a result, many adolescents adopt irregular schedules that become worse with age. These schedules often reflect a pattern of shorter school-day sleep periods with extended "catch-up" sleep periods on non-school nights. For instance, younger adolescents average 30 minutes to 1 hour more sleep on non-school nights, while this average increases to 1 hour 30 minutes to 2 hours for older adolescents (Carskadon, Wolfson, Acebo, Tzischinsky, & Seifer, 1998; Strauch & Meier, 1988; Wolfson, Acebo, Fallone, & Carskadon, 2003). Some adolescents are able to maintain a fairly stable schedule and do not rack up a high sleep debt. Unfortunately, not all adolescents fare as well. For those adolescents who instead maintain a highly irregular schedule, the extended sleep times on the non-school nights do not make up for the sleep loss they incurred on school nights, so they fare worse. Their poorer outcomes are reflected in the higher reports of behavior and academic problems, daytime sleepiness, and depressed mood in this group (Wolfson & Carskadon, 1998).

Adolescence is a critical point in development due to the numerous physiological, psychosocial, and environmental changes occurring. These simultaneous changes occurring put adolescents at an increased risk for development of psychopathology, including insomnia, compared to preadolescents and younger children. Rates of adolescent insomnia range from 4%–39% for prevalence, 5%–23% for new onset, and 2%–20% for chronic (Johnson, Roth, Schultz, & Breslau, 2006; Ohayon, Roberts, Zulley, Smirne, & Priest, 2000; Patten, Choi, Gillin, & Pierce, 2000; Roberts, Lewinsohn, & Seeley, 1995; Roberts, Roberts, & Chan, 2008). Differences in criteria for insomnia play a large role in the variable rates from study to study. Roberts and colleagues used DSM-IV criteria and found a prevalence rate of 7.03% and incidence rate of 5.5% with a chronicity rate of 34.71% and remission rate of 65.29% at follow-up (Roberts et al., 2008). Using similar DSM-IV criteria plus a frequency requirement of at least four times per week, Johnson and colleagues reported 9.4% of adolescents met criteria for insomnia (Johnson, Roth, Schultz, et al., 2006).

As indicated previously, the behavioral model of insomnia (Spielman, Caruso, et al., 1987) uses a three-factor model (predisposing, precipitating, and perpetuating events) to explain insomnia. Older children and adolescents likely experience predisposing events, genetics (Gehrman et al., 2011; Moore et al., 2011), and hyperactivity of corticotropin-releasing factor neurons (Richardson & Roth, 2001) similar to those of younger children and adults, but precipitating and perpetuating events differ.

Psychological precipitating events, or events that "trigger" the onset of insomnia, include psychological disorders such as mood disorders and anxiety disorder. Almost 73% adolescents with major depression reported sleep problems, with insomnia as the most prominent complaint (Liu et al., 2007). Depression and insomnia are frequently comorbid (see Harvey, Alfano, and Clarke, Chapter 35), and insomnia symptoms during adolescence predict future depression (Johnson, Roth, & Breslau, 2006; Roane & Taylor, 2008; Roberts, Roberts, & Chen, 2002). Similarly, adolescents with bipolar disorder (Harvey, 2008) and anxiety disorders frequently report insomnia (Alfano, Pina, Zerr, & Villalta, 2010). For instance, 54% of children and adolescents with anxiety disorders report trouble sleeping (Alfano et al., 2010).

Underlying sleep disorders such as obstructive sleep apnea or restless legs syndrome can act as physiological precipitants. Other physiological triggers include caffeine, medication, alcohol or drug use or abuse, and medical conditions such as chronic pain (Palermo, Wilson, Lewandowski, Toliver-Sokol, & Murray, 2011). Another important physiological consideration for adolescents are the changes in sleep–wake bioregulatory processes that result in circadian phase delays (Carskadon, Acebo, Richardson, Tate, & Seifer, 1997; Carskadon et al., 1993; Carskadon, Acebo, & Jenni, 2004; Feinberg, 1982; Huttenlocher, 1979; Jenni et al., 2005). For some adolescents the delay and subsequent extended wakefulness may trigger acute insomnia onset. For instance, the extended wakefulness experienced while trying to adjust to an early school-day schedule following a delayed sleep schedule creates a potential for compensatory behaviors and unhelpful beliefs to develop. Initially the adolescent may just lie awake exerting effort to sleep. After repeat episodes, the time awake could allow for other compensatory behaviors to creep in, such as watching TV, playing video games, or texting. Before long, the acute case of insomnia becomes chronic. The extra time in bed also provides opportunities for anxiety about not falling asleep and rumination over the inability to sleep to occur, with both facilitating the development of unhelpful beliefs about insomnia (Gregory et al., 2009). In turn, these compensatory behaviors are reinforced by the detriments to daytime functioning such as daytime sleepiness, inattention, and mood disturbances (Roth & Ancoli-Israel, 1999; Ustinov et al., 2010) that are associated with an insomnia sleep pattern and delays in the circadian system.

Associations between insomnia, phase preference, and circadian systems exist in the literature. For instance, evening types report more daytime sleepiness (Carrier, Monk, Buysse, & Kupfer, 1997; National Sleep Foundation, 2005) and unhelpful beliefs about sleep (Adan, Fabbri, Natale, & Prat, 2006) compared to morning types. Delays in circadian core body temperature rhythm occur with sleep onset insomnia (Morris, Lack, & Dawson, 1990), whereas advances in the circadian core body temperature rhythm occur in early morning awakening insomnia (Lack & Wright, 1993) and are associated with shorter and more restless sleep (Kerkhof & van Vianen, 1999). In adults with insomnia, those who were identified as evening types reported longer time in bed, greater variability in their sleep/wake schedules, higher rates of unhelpful beliefs about sleep, and higher depression scores than morning or intermediate types (Ong, Huang, Kuo, & Manber, 2007). Fewer studies exist in the adolescent literature; however, evidence does support similar findings to those in adults. Specifically, adolescents with self-reported sleep difficulties exhibited later dim light melatonin onset (DLMO), or onset of melatonin secretion and a marker of the circadian timing system, than their peers without self-reported sleep difficulties, and later DLMOs were associated with longer sleep onset latencies (Hasler, Bootzin, Cousins, Fridel, & Wenk, 2008).

At times, the close connections between insomnia and circadian dysregulation can complicate the diagnosis. While adolescents with insomnia and those with delayed sleep phase disorder (DSPD) each experience symptoms of the other, there are a few ways to distinguish the two. For instance, adolescents who present with sleep-onset insomnia and difficulties waking in the morning, but the complaint is schedule-specific, most likely have DSPD (Wyatt, 2004). What this means is that when these adolescents are free to pick their schedule (e.g., vacation, summer), they experience no difficulties initiating and are able to sleep for a full sleep period (Crowley, Acebo, & Carskadon, 2007; Wyatt, 2004); yet, when constrained by a society-imposed "normal" schedule, these adolescents experience difficulties.

Many of the neuroendocrine and structural brain changes adolescents experience result in a differentiation of the sexes (Buchanan, Eccles, & Becker, 1992; Giedd et al., 2006). This divergence of their physiology manifests in observable gender differences in their sleep patterns (Laberge et al., 2001; Lee, McEnany, & Weekes, 1999), sleep hygiene practices (Eggermont & Van den Bulck, 2006), and rates of insomnia (Johnson, Roth, Schultz, et al., 2006). Following menarche, gender differences in insomnia are the most striking. Prior to menses onset, boys and girls show no difference in insomnia rates; however, menarche marks a well-documented 2.75-increased risk for insomnia in girls (Johnson, Roth, Schultz, et al., 2006). Studies in adults indicate this gender differentiation in rates remains until post-menopause (Foley, Ancoli-Israel, Britz, & Walsh, 2004).

Researchers have explored the menstrual cycle to better elucidate what could be driving this increased risk. Despite the point of divergence occurring at or around puberty, these studies have been conducted in young and middle-aged adult women. A primary reason for this is likely due to the irregularity present in an adolescent female's cycle, but this very factor may also be an important catalyst to study. A few studies have looked at objective measures of sleep disturbance. Shibui and colleagues (2000) found decreased amplitude of the core body temperature rhythm, increased occurrence of slow wave sleep during the daytime, and increased reports of daytime sleepiness during the luteal phase compared to the follicular phase. The reported daytime sleepiness was thought to be a result of the occurrence of slow wave sleep during the daytime. Schechter and colleagues (Shechter, Varin, & Boivin, 2010) found increased progesterone concentrations were correlated with a blunted decline in core body temperature and decreased amplitude. Subjectively, women reported longer sleep onset latencies and more sleepiness upon awakening during the mid-luteal phase compared to the mid-follicular phase. Objective PSG findings indicated a decrease in REM time. Manber and Bootzin found increased subjective reports of disturbed sleep during the late luteal phase (1997). Baker and Driver (2004) triangulated the specific time window when women were most likely to experience subjective sleep disturbances by confirming the ovulatory cycle and found that the last 3–6 days of the late luteal phase and the first 4 days of menstruation was the specific timeframe of increased reports. Unfortunately, no studies could be found evaluating this phenomenon in adolescent females.

While healthy adult women experience changes in their subjective sleep and markers for sleep across the menstrual cycle (Baker et al., 2001; Baker & Driver, 2004; Manber & Bootzin, 1997; Shechter et al., 2010; Shibui et al., 2000), these associations are complex. A large source of this complexity resides with the menstrual cycle. Age of menses onset varies among females and regularity in the cycle takes several years to be established, making the menstrual cycle an extremely diverse event despite its occurring in nearly every female.

In context of the behavioral model of insomnia (Spielman, Caruso, et al., 1987), the menstrual cycle is a perfect storm for encouraging insomnia to manifest and maintain in adolescent females. First, adolescent girls experiencing sleep disturbances coinciding with their menstrual cycle will do so frequently and repeatedly given the menstrual cycle's length of 21–45 days during the first 3 years (Treloar, Boynton, Behn, & Brown, 1967; Vollman, 1977). Second, the innate variability in length of the menstrual cycle during the first 3 years (American Academy of Pediatrics, Committee on

Adolescence, American College of Obstetricians and Gynecologists, & Committee on Adolescent Health Care, 2006; Treloar et al., 1967; Vollman, 1977) results in a frequent but unpredictable event that does not allow their sleep disturbance to be easily tied to it. The result is recurring, irregular bouts of sleep disturbance with an instigating factor. Third, post-pubescent adolescent females are prone to experience a delayed circadian phase, increasing sleep onset difficulties (Carskadon et al., 1993). Last, many of the medications used to treat menstrual symptoms include caffeine, which further exacerbates sleep disturbances.

Finally, numerous behavioral and environmental factors contribute to the maintenance or perpetuation of insomnia. Irregular schedules, particularly those kept by adolescents, contribute to a phase delay on the non-school nights, which in turn leads to delayed sleep onsets at the beginning of the school week (Crowley & Carskadon, 2010). In addition, unhelpful beliefs about insomnia (Morin, Vallières, & Ivers, 2007) and poor sleep hygiene practices contribute to the maintenance of insomnia.

Behavioral Treatments for Insomnia in Older Children and Adolescents

Very few treatment outcome studies exist in the literature for older children and adolescents. The scant literature available and the larger treatment outcome research base in adults provide data that supports the use of cognitive and behavioral treatments for insomnia in adolescents (Barowsky, Moskowitz, & Zweig, 1990; Bootzin & Stevens, 2005; Weil & Goldfried, 1973). One case study with an 11-year-old showed self-relaxation training improved insomnia (Weil & Goldfried, 1973). Another case study with three adolescents showed improvements in onset and maintenance insomnia with biofeedback (Barowsky et al., 1990). Two recent studies provide the most solid evidence to date that some of the empirically validated approaches used in adults could be used with adolescents (Bootzin & Stevens, 2005; Gradisar et al., 2011). Bootzin and Stevens (2005) evaluated insomnia treatment outcomes in adolescents with a history of a substance abuse disorders and self-reported sleep problems or daytime sleepiness. They used a polytherapeutic treatment approach consisting of stimulus control therapy, bright light therapy, cognitive therapy, mindfulness-based stress reduction, and sleep hygiene education. Adolescents reported significant improvements following treatment, but drawing treatment outcome conclusions from this study was difficult due to a few limitations including ambiguity about whether the driving factor in changes in sleep was the treatment itself or to improvements in their comorbid condition (i.e., participants were substance abuse patients); the control group was not well selected; and the simultaneous inclusion of bright light into the treatment intervention makes it difficult to parse the effects of the light versus behavioral interventions. A more recent study by Gradisar and colleagues (2011) treated adolescents with DSPD using a similar polytherapeutic treatment including sleep education, sleep hygiene, bright light therapy, and stimulus control therapy. Their sample included a significant number with comorbid insomnia symptoms. Like Bootzin and colleagues, the effects were high, but the use of bright light confounds the interpretation of treatment effects.

Analogies from the adult literature and preliminary evidence from studies currently underway also support the use of behavioral and cognitive interventions, which are discussed in the next sections. The behavioral and cognitive interventions for the treatment of insomnia are typically used as monotherapies or combined into the polytherapeutic intervention called *cognitive-behavioral therapy for insomnia* (CBTi). CBTi may look different depending on who is delivering the therapy, but generally uses some combination of the monotherapies of stimulus control therapy, sleep restriction therapy, and cognitive therapy with a relaxation technique and sleep hygiene education. The rationale behind this multimodal approach is that the combination of both behavioral and cognitive therapies better addresses the multifaceted nature of insomnia. To date, no studies have dismantled CBTi to determine if all components typically included are necessary (Morin et al., 2006).

Some of the monotherapies that comprise CBTi have solid empirical evidence while others do not (Morgenthaler, Kramer, et al., 2006). Similar to the behavioral interventions for BIC, a task force appointed by the American Academy of Sleep Medicine convened to determine effective treatments for insomnia in adults using the Sackett criteria to review 37 articles (Morgenthaler, Kramer, et al., 2006; Morin et al., 2006). Currently, there has been no task force that specifically addresses empirical treatment of insomnia in adolescents. In place of such a review, clinicians rely on the empirical treatments recommended for adults and may modify these interventions to address the needs of adolescents participating in treatment (e.g., circadian delay in addition to insomnia, living space consists of their bedroom). Stimulus control therapy (SCT), relaxation training, and CBTi were identified as *Standard Treatments* (same criteria as indicated previously). *Guideline Treatments* were sleep restriction therapy (SRT), multicomponent therapy (without cognitive therapy), and biofeedback. Despite effect sizes similar to SCT, SRT is frequently used in conjunction with SCT, limiting the studies that evaluated it as a monotherapy. Insufficient evidence was available to recommend sleep hygiene education as a monotherapy or to know the additive value of it included with other therapeutic treatments. Currently, bright light therapy is an empirically supported treatment for DSPD but is not on the list of supported treatments for insomnia.

Cognitive and Behavioral Therapies for Insomnia (CBTi)

STIMULUS CONTROL THERAPY

Stimulus control therapy (SCT) is the most effective single treatment method for insomnia. The goal of this behavioral intervention is to strengthen the association between the bedroom and sleep by removing competing sleep-incompatible associations (e.g., eating, watching TV, worrying; Bootzin, 1972). At the core of these sleep-incompatible associations is wakefulness. Thus when these become the dominant associations with the bedroom, the bedroom no longer promotes sleepiness. In fact, the exact opposite happens. The bedroom becomes associated with wakefulness, which in turn activates the arousal system and reduces the likelihood of sleep onset. Continued wakefulness in bed results in the individual becoming more aroused, either out of frustration or worry, and the likelihood of sleep onset is reduced. The result is a negative cycle that can spiral out of control for the individual.

In order to break the wake-promoting associations and strengthen the sleep and bed association, access to the bed is made contingent on being sleepy. The 5 key instructions of SCT are: *(1)* use the bed for sleep only, *(2)* go to bed only when sleepy, *(3)* get out of bed within 15 to 20 minutes when unable to sleep, *(4)* wake up at the same time each morning, and *(5)* no daily naps. The first step of SCT is to remove electronics out of the room and to establish it as a sleep-only zone. For adolescents this may be more difficult, since adolescents often spend much more time in their rooms and engage in many more nonsleep behaviors in their rooms than adults do (see Gradisar and Short, Chapter 11). Thus, educating the adolescent and family is a crucial step for this intervention to be effective. In addition, working with the adolescent and family on the implementation of these instructions given their life situation is important in order to increase adherence when beginning the intervention. This might mean for some families sitting down with a floor plan, identifying sanctioned areas in the room where schoolwork can be done, and establishing a clearly defined boundary (e.g., sheet, shoji screen) that partitions the room so the bed is clearly distinct from the area where sleep-incompatible behaviors are allowed to occur. For other families, discussing alternative areas for activities to occur will be important.

Once the room is ready, adolescents are instructed to only get into bed if they are sleepy; however, they cannot engage in just any activity when they are not sleepy. You do not want adolescents increasing their alertness by texting, playing video games, or engaging in the numerous other recreational (i.e., "fun") activities that would decrease the likelihood of sleepiness occurring. Instead, adolescents are instructed to engage in a mundane activity (e.g., reading a dictionary, reading a school book, writing sentences) in dim light to reduce stimulation and the impact of light on the circadian timing system. Once they feel sleepy, they get into bed. If they cannot fall asleep in what *feels like* 15–20 minutes they can get out of bed, engage in a mundane activity, and return to bed only when sleepy. Adolescents are instructed not to clock-watch but instead to get out of bed if they have to ask, "Has it been 15–20 minutes?" Two advantages of SCT are reestablishing the association of sleep with the bedroom through repeated experiences of falling asleep quickly in bed. and helping adolescents begin to better determine what signs (e.g., yawning, tired eyes, nodding off) occur when they are actually "sleepy" rather than fatigued.

SLEEP RESTRICTION THERAPY

Sleep restriction therapy (SRT) prompts the body's natural drive to sleep while re-entraining the circadian timing system, which can become dysregulated as a result of the irregular sleep schedules common to people with insomnia. These schedules can be even more dysregulated in an adolescent already prone to a delayed circadian phase. In order to accomplish these feats, the sleep/wake schedule is regulated so that the time spent in bed matches the individual's true sleep needs (Spielman, Caruso, et al., 1987). Access to bed is initially restricted to increase sleep pressure, thereby increasing the likelihood that sleep onset occurs quickly and continues uninterrupted throughout the night. Starting with a restricted schedule also allows you to extend the hours for sleep until the individual's true sleep need is determined.

Prior to starting SRT, adolescents should keep a sleep diary for 2 to 3 weeks to determine their average total sleep time (TST). In collaboration with the adolescent and parents, an allowable time in bed (TIB) for the next week is determined. A good rule of thumb is TIB equals the average TST. Some therapists will allow an additional 30 minutes. For adults, the recommendation is TIB is no less than 5 hours to 5 hours 30 minutes (Spielman, Saskin, & Thorpy, 1987). For school-age children and adolescents, the TIB is typically more conservative due to the unknown effects of restricting sleep at this critical developmental time or period, and to the known effects of mood dysregulation resulting from restricted sleep in children and adolescents. To establish the "prescribed schedule" for the week, first establish the earliest time the adolescent must get up for the week. This time becomes the wake time for the week and the bedtime is determined by TIB (e.g., TIB = 7 hr 30 min; earliest wake time = 7 am; bedtime = 11:30 pm). The adolescent's TIB progressively lengthens by 15 minutes weekly if the average sleep efficiency ([total sleep time/total time in bed] x 100) is greater than 87% for that week. If the sleep efficiency falls below 85%, the adolescent's TIB is decreased by 15–30 minutes. Incremental increases occur each week until the optimal time in bed is achieved (i.e., TIB cannot be extended without sleep efficiency dropping below 87%).

The advantage of SRT is the rapid consolidation of the sleep period; however, adolescents and parents may not initially agree with the restricted sleep schedule. Thus, education about why the schedule is being restricted and the long-term plans of sleep extension are important. In addition, discuss with adolescents and parents the side effects of both SCT and SRT. They will likely experience daytime sleepiness and potentially other side effects of decreased total sleep times. Discussing with parents and adolescents what to expect beforehand will reduce premature treatment termination and inability or unwillingness to follow the intervention.

SLEEP COMPRESSION THERAPY

One alternative to sleep restriction, sleep compression, has also shown effectiveness in treating insomnia (Lichstein, Riedel, Wilson, Lester, & Aguillard, 2001). The goal of sleep compression is to gradually reduce time in bed until the patient's optimal time in bed has been established. This intervention may be more acceptable to some parents and teens who find the sleep restriction technique too drastic. As in SRT, prior to starting adolescents should keep a sleep diary for 2–3 weeks to determine their average TST and TIB. They should then reduce their TIB by 30 minutes each night per week until their sleep efficiency increases to greater than 87%.

RELAXATION THERAPY

Various relaxation techniques exist, including progressive muscle relaxation (PMR), diaphragmatic breathing, visual imagery, meditation, and yoga. PMR has historically shown the most support in the treatment for insomnia (Morgenthaler, Kramer, et al., 2006; Morin et al., 2006). In more recent years the combination of mindfulness meditation with CBTi has shown promising results (Ong, Shapiro, & Manber, 2008, 2009; Ong & Sholtes, 2010). For any relaxation technique, the overarching goal is to induce relaxation through diverting focus. For instance, adolescents learn to focus on tensing and relaxing muscle groups in PMR, while they learn to be aware of their thoughts and actions in the present with mindfulness meditation. Through sustained focus, the body is allowed time to relax. Adolescents are reminded that relaxation techniques are a skill that requires daily practice. Once they learn the skill with the therapist, they are instructed to practice daily. Usually, practice initially occurs before bed and not when they require it to fall asleep or return to sleep. Once they master the skill, they can begin to use it when they are unable to sleep.

COGNITIVE THERAPY

Cognitive therapy (CT) for insomnia targets the unhelpful beliefs that interfere with sleep and replaces them with more adaptive substitutes (Harvey, Sharpley, Ree, Stinson, & Clark, 2007; Sloan et al., 1993). More adaptive thoughts should reduce arousal, therefore reducing the likelihood of extended wakefulness. These unhelpful beliefs are often identified through the initial interview and standardized assessments such as the Dysfunctional Beliefs and Attitudes about Sleep Scale (Morin et al., 2007). Once unhelpful beliefs are identified, work begins with the adolescent to challenge and replace these through education and behavioral experiments. Advantages to CT are the replacement of unhelpful beliefs about sleep. Preliminary data suggests CT is effective at altering unhelpful beliefs about sleep as a standalone treatment in adults, but effects on sleep outcomes are not as clear and no research has been conducted to test the efficacy in children and adolescents (Harvey et al., 2007).

SLEEP HYGIENE EDUCATION

If evidence from your assessment indicates the adolescent engages in poor sleep hygiene behaviors, then a diagnosis of inadequate sleep hygiene should be given (see Gruber, Constantin, Cassoff, and Michaelson, Chapter 39). In these cases, sleep hygiene education would be included in treatment (Mindell, 2003; Owens & Witmans, 2004) focusing on the specific areas where the adolescent endorsed difficulties. In general, sleep hygiene education covers several topics like insuring your sleep environment is conducive to sleep, avoiding stimulating activities the hour before bedtime, and avoiding naps. Sleep hygiene education as a monotherapy is ineffective (Taylor, Schmidt-Nowara, Jessop, & Ahearn, 2010); Yet, non–sleep specialists often offer it as the first and only line of treatment to their patients. As a result, adolescents and families may feel like behavioral therapies are ineffective because sleep hygiene did not work.

Bright Light Therapy

Bright light therapy (BLT) is not a typical component of insomnia treatment, but it is an empirically supported treatment for delayed sleep phase disorder (DSPD; Morgenthaler et al., 2007; Sack et al., 2007). Bright light therapy may also be beneficial with adolescents due to their predisposed tendency to phase delay. The scant literature in adolescents that has used BLT to treatment insomnia symptoms, alone or in the context of DPSD, suggests it is effective (Bootzin & Stevens, 2005; Gradisar et al., 2011). BLT targets the circadian timing system and aims to phase advance or phase delay the system. For adolescents, most often treatment will focus on phase advancing (i.e., shifting the intrinsic timing system earlier).

Bright light therapy is derived from experimental research that has demonstrated light to be the most effective mechanism to entrain the circadian system. The effect light has on the circadian timing system depends on several factors including timing, light intensity, duration, and wavelength. For treatment purposes, bright light therapy relies on the Phase Response Curve (PRC) literature that identified the shifting effects of light based on the timing of administration. Bright light administered after the core body temperature minimum will phase advance the circadian system (i.e., move it to an earlier clock time) while bright light administered before the core body temperature minimum will phase delay the circadian timing system (i.e., move it to a later clock time). In order to phase advance for adolescents, BLT is typically used in the mornings upon waking up. Currently there is no general agreement on optimal timing, duration, and dosing of morning light for DPSD or insomnia. Often, adolescents are recommended to obtain 30–45 minutes of bright light either via natural light or a bright light box. The use of bright light therapy is quite a complicated procedure and should not be attempted without the help of a board certified sleep medicine specialist, preferably one who is certified in behavioral sleep medicine.

Comorbid Conditions and Considerations

Differential diagnoses to consider when evaluating for insomnia are DSPD, inadequate sleep hygiene, and behavioral sleep restriction. The previously mentioned study by Johnson and colleagues (2006) evaluated the role DSPD plays in diagnosing insomnia. They found DSPD did not significantly account for the insomnia cases (4/95) studied. While adolescents may not be experiencing DSPD that accounts for their insomnia symptoms, they may be experiencing a dysregulated circadian system, which does need to be a consideration in treatment. Similarly, if adolescents engage in poor sleep hygiene behaviors, then a diagnosis of inadequate sleep hygiene should be given. This diagnosis does not preclude them from a comorbid diagnosis of insomnia, circadian rhythm disorder, or behavioral sleep restriction.

As with younger children, underlying sleep and medical disorders can trigger insomnia and should be considered in the evaluation. OSA often presents as frequent night awakenings, but is accompanied by other symptoms such as loud snoring, gasping for air, pauses in breathing, night sweats, and enuresis. Another sleep disorder that can present with nocturnal awakenings is periodic limb movement disorder (PLMD), whereas restless legs syndrome (RLS) appears more like sleep onset insomnia. OSA and PLMD require further evaluation via a PSG, while RLS is based on subjective reports. As indicated previously, insomnia is frequently comorbid with Axis I disorders. Recent research supports the treatment of insomnia in the context of a comorbid disorder, and doing so can help to reduce the severity of the comorbid condition (Manber et al., 2008; Taylor, Lichstein, Weinstock, Sanford, & Temple, 2007). Any time a comorbid condition is present, treatment consideration should be made. Considerations may include waiting to treat until after the insomnia is improving, co-treating, or treating the comorbid condition first.

Pharmacological Treatment for Pediatric Insomnia

Currently, evidence supports behavioral and cognitive therapies for the treatment of pediatric insomnia. Despite the evidence, pharmacological treatments have been proposed on numerous occasions as possible alternatives. In order to evaluate the potential use of pharmacological treatments, the National Sleep Foundation collaborated with Best Practice Project Management, Inc., to establish a panel of experts who could convene and evaluate the evidence (Mindell, Emslie, et al., 2006). These experts drew two primary conclusions: *(1)* scant evidence supports the use of pharmacological interventions in pediatric insomnia, and *(2)* effectiveness and safety studies are needed to empirically evaluate hypnotic use in pediatric populations.

Despite the first conclusion, evidence suggests 77% of pediatricians have recommended over-the-counter remedies and 58% have prescribed medication for BIC in a 6-month period (Owens, Rosen, & Mindell, 2003). A more recent study evaluating prescription practices by psychiatrists noted insomnia was a concern of a third of the patients seen and nearly one-fourth of these children and adolescents were receiving pharmacological treatment for insomnia (Owens, Rosen, Mindell, & Kirchner, 2010). On average each month, 96% of psychiatrists in study recommended a prescription medication and 88% recommended an over-the-counter medication. This and other evidence brought about the panels' second recommendation that empirical evidence is needed to guide prescription practices in treating pediatric insomnia. To date, the Food and Drug Administration has not approved the use of hypnotics in pediatric populations, which means these medications are being used off-label. Prescription practices often vary by clinician, as limited evidence supports the use of these medications in pediatric populations. A review panel of experts in the pediatric sleep field convened recently in an attempt to provide physicians and psychiatrists guidelines for prescribing, but again these guidelines are based on the scant evidence available and clinical experience (Owens & Moturi, 2009). As such, behavioral and cognitive therapies are still recommended as the treatment of choice for pediatric insomnia.

Conclusions

Pediatric insomnia encompasses a large range of clinical manifestations. Understanding of insomnia in pediatric populations requires clinicians to appreciate numerous factors such as developmental age, family context, cultural and social factors, biological factors, and comorbid conditions. The majority of research has been conducted in infants and young children, and supports the use of behavioral interventions in the treatment of BIC. Less research guides clinicians in the treatment of insomnia present in older children and adolescents. Fortunately, more studies are underway and hopefully soon the bounty of these studies will be reaped for the children and adolescents who experience difficulties sleeping. Until then, the literature offers guidance and supports the use of behavioral and cognitive therapies for the treatment of insomnia in older children and adolescents. One major limitation is the lack of qualified professionals to treat these individuals (see Thomas, Avis, and Lichstein, Chapter 41). Future studies also need to focus on dissemination of those interventions that have been shown to work in these populations. For more information on curricula, systematic strategies, strategies for working with adolescents, clinical sleep training, and the impact of behavioral interventions see Chapters 37–41 that focus on prevention and intervention.

Future Directions

- Despite evidence that shows prevention is effective, current rates of pediatric insomnia in infants and toddlers are still extremely high. What needs to be done to improve the utilization of preventive education?
- Evidence shows that older children and adolescents often do not come forward indicating a problem. What can be done to reach these age groups and increase their access to treatment?
- Research indicates that young children with insomnia are more likely to experience insomnia as older children, adolescents, and adults. What influence does treatment at an early age have on outcomes when these children are older, with regard to insomnia and other disorders?
- Despite the noted prevalence rates of insomnia in school-age children and adolescents, treatment studies are lacking in these populations. What treatments are most effective for these populations? Are there adjuvant treatments that may increase the effectiveness and/or adherence to already established treatments?

• Research shows a sex difference emerges with adolescents in rates of insomnia. What protective factors may be present for males that are not for females? If there are protective factors, aside from the lack of a menstrual cycle, can these factors be introduced to females to reduce their risk? Along these lines, can preventive interventions be used to reduce the rate of insomnia in females?

• Few trained pediatric behavioral sleep medicine specialists are available to handle patient needs. More training programs need to be developed to educate clinicians in pediatric behavioral sleep medicine.

References

Adams, L. A., & Rickert, V. I. (1989). Reducing bedtime tantrums: Comparison between positive routines and graduated extinction. *Pediatrics, 84*(5), 756–761.

Adan, A., Fabbri, M., Natale, V., & Prat, G. (2006). Sleep Beliefs Scale (SBS) and circadian typology. *Journal of Sleep Research, 15*(2), 125–132.

Alfano, C. A., Pina, A. A., Zerr, A. A., & Villalta, I. K. (2010). Pre-sleep arousal and sleep problems of anxiety-disordered youth. *Child Psychiatry and Human Development, 41*(2), 156–167.

American Academy of Pediatrics, Committee on Adolescence, American College of Obstetricians and Gynecologists, & Committee on Adolescent Health Care. (2006). Menstruation in girls and adolescents: Using the menstrual cycle as a vital sign. *Pediatrics, 118*(5), 2245–2250.

American Academy of Sleep Medicine. (2005). *International Classification of Sleep Disorders: Diagnostic and Coding Manual* (2nd ed.). Westchester, IL: American Academy of Sleep Medicine.

American Psychiatric Association. (2000). *Diagnostic and Statistical Manual of Mental Disorders* (4th ed., text rev.). Washington, DC: American Psychiatric Association.

Anders, T. F., Halpern, L. F., & Hua, J. (1992). Sleeping through the night: A developmental perspective. *Pediatrics, 90*(4), 554–560.

Armstrong, K. L., Quinn, R. A., & Dadds, M. R. (1994). The sleep patterns of normal children. *The Medical Journal of Australia, 161*(3), 202–206.

Baker, F. C., Waner, J. I., Vieira, E. F., Taylor, S. R., Driver, H. S., & Mitchell, D. (2001). Sleep and 24 hour body temperatures: A comparison in young men, naturally cycling women and women taking hormonal contraceptives. *The Journal of Physiology, 530*(Pt 3), 565–574.

Baker, F. C., & Driver, H. S. (2004). Self-reported sleep across the menstrual cycle in young, healthy women. *Journal of Psychosomatic Research, 56*(2), 239–243.

Barowsky, E. I., Moskowitz, J., & Zweig, J. B. (1990). Biofeedback for disorders of initiating and maintaining sleep. *Annals of the New York Academy of Sciences, 602*, 97–103.

Bates, J. E., Viken, R. J., Alexander, D. B., Beyers, J., & Stockton, L. (2002). Sleep and adjustment in preschool children: Sleep diary reports by mothers relate to behavior reports by teachers. *Child Development, 73*(1), 62–74.

Bayer, J. K., Hiscock, H., Hampton, A., & Wake, M. (2007). Sleep problems in young infants and maternal mental and physical health. *Journal of Paediatrics and Child Health, 43*(1–2), 66–73.

Beebe, D. W. (2011). Cognitive, behavioral, and functional consequences of inadequate sleep in children and adolescents. *Pediatric Clinics of North America, 58*(3), 649–665.

Bibace, R., & Walsh, M. E. (1980). Development of children's concepts of illness. *Pediatrics, 66*(6), 912–917.

Blader, J. C., Koplewicz, H. S., Abikoff, H., & Foley, C. (1997). Sleep problems of elementary school children. A community survey. *Archives of Pediatrics & Adolescent Medicine, 151*(5), 473–480.

Boergers, J., Hart, C., Owens, J. A., Streisand, R., & Spirito, A. (2007). Child sleep disorders: Associations with parental sleep duration and daytime sleepiness. *Journal of Family Psychology: JFP: Journal of the Division of Family Psychology of the American Psychological Association (Division 43), 21*(1), 88–94.

Bootzin, R. R. (1972). A stimulus control treatment for insomnia (Vol. 7). Presented at the American Psychological Association 80th Annual Convention Proceedings.

Bootzin, R. R., & Stevens, S. J. (2005). Adolescents, substance abuse, and the treatment of insomnia and daytime sleepiness. *Clinical Psychology Review, 25*(5), 629–644.

Buchanan, C. M., Eccles, J. S., & Becker, J. B. (1992). Are adolescents the victims of raging hormones: Evidence for activational effects of hormones on moods and behavior at adolescence. *Psychological Bulletin, 111*(1), 62–107.

Burnham, M. M., Goodlin-Jones, B. L., Gaylor, E. E., & Anders, T. F. (2002). Nighttime sleep-wake patterns and self-soothing from birth to one year of age: A longitudinal intervention study. *Journal of Child Psychology and Psychiatry, and Allied Disciplines, 43*(6), 713–725.

Carrier, J., Monk, T. H., Buysse, D. J., & Kupfer, D. J. (1997). Sleep and morningness-eveningness in the "middle" years of life (20–59 y). *Journal of Sleep Research, 6*(4), 230–237.

Carskadon, M. A., Harvey, K., Duke, P., Anders, T. F., Litt, I. F., & Dement, W. C. (1980). Pubertal changes in daytime sleepiness. *Sleep, 2*(4), 453–460.

Carskadon, M. A., Vieira, C., & Acebo, C. (1993). Association between puberty and delayed phase preference. *Sleep, 16*(3), 258–262.

Carskadon, M. A., Acebo, C., Richardson, G. S., Tate, B. A., & Seifer, R. (1997). An approach to studying circadian rhythms of adolescent humans. *Journal of Biological Rhythms, 12*(3), 278–289.

Carskadon, M. A., Wolfson, A. R., Acebo, C., Tzischinsky, O., & Seifer, R. (1998). Adolescent sleep patterns, circadian timing, and sleepiness at a transition to early school days. *Sleep, 21*(8), 871–881.

Carskadon, M. A., Labyak, S. E., Acebo, C., & Seifer, R. (1999). Intrinsic circadian period of adolescent humans measured in conditions of forced desynchrony. *Neuroscience Letters, 260*(2), 129–132.

Carskadon, M. A., Acebo, C., & Jenni, O. G. (2004). Regulation of adolescent sleep: Implications for behavior. *Annals of the New York Academy of Sciences*, 1021, 276–291.

Carskadon, M. A. (2008). Maturation of processes regulating sleep in adolescents. In L. Marcus, J. L. Caroll, D. F. Donnelly, & G. M. Loughlin (Eds.), *Sleep in Children: Developmental Changes in Sleep Patterns* (2nd ed., pp. 95–114). New York, NY: Informa Healthcare USA, Inc.

Chadez, L. H., & Nurius, P. S. (1987). Stopping bedtime crying: Treating the child and the parents. *Journal of Clinical Child Psychology, 16*(3), 212–217.

Crowley, S. J., Acebo, C., & Carskadon, M. A. (2007). Sleep, circadian rhythms, and delayed phase in adolescence. *Sleep Medicine*, *8*(6), 602–612.

Crowley, S. J., & Carskadon, M. A. (2010). Modifications to weekend recovery sleep delay circadian phase in older adolescents. *Chronobiology International*, *27*(7), 1469–1492.

Dement, W. C. (1999). *The Promise of Sleep*. New York: Dell.

Eddy, D. M. (1992). *A manual for assessing health practices and designing practice policies: The explicit approach*. Philadelphia, PA: American College of Physicians.

Eggermont, S., & Van den Bulck, J. (2006). Nodding off or switching off? The use of popular media as a sleep aid in secondary-school children. *Journal of Paediatrics and Child Health*, *42*(7–8), 428–433.

Fallone, G., Owens, J. A., & Deane, J. (2002). Sleepiness in children and adolescents: clinical implications. *Sleep Medicine Reviews*, *6*(4), 287–306.

Feinberg, I. (1982). Schizophrenia: caused by a fault in programmed synaptic elimination during adolescence? *Journal of Psychiatric Research*, *17*(4), 319–334.

Ferber, R. (1985). *Solve Your Child's Sleep Problems*. New York: Simon & Schuster.

Foley, D., Ancoli-Israel, S., Britz, P., & Walsh, J. (2004). Sleep disturbances and chronic disease in older adults: Results of the 2003 National Sleep Foundation Sleep in America Survey. *Journal of Psychosomatic Research*, *56*(5), 497–502.

France, K. G., & Hudson, S. M. (1990). Behavior management of infant sleep disturbance. *Journal of Applied Behavior Analysis*, *23*(1), 91–98.

France, K. G., Henderson, J. M., & Hudson, S. M. (1996). Fact, act, and tact: A three-stage approach to treating the sleep problems of infants and young children. *Child and Adolescent Psychiatric Clinics of North America*, *5*(3), 581–599.

France, K. G., & Blampied, N. M. (2005). Modifications of Systematic ignoring in the management of infant sleep disturbance: Efficacy and infant distress. *Child & Family Behavior Therapy*, *27*(1), 1–16.

France, K. G. (2010). Extinction with parental presence. In M. Perlis, M. Aloia, & B. R. Kuhn (Eds.), *Behavioral Treatments for Sleep Disorders: A Comprehensive Primer of Behavioral Sleep Medicine Interventions* (pp. 275–284). Boston: Elsevier/Academic Press.

Freeman, K. A. (2006). Treating bed time resistance with the bed time pass: A systematic replication and component analysis with 3-year-olds. *Journal of Applied Behavior Analysis*, *39*(4), 423–428.

Friman, P. C., Hoff, K. E., Schnoes, C., Freeman, K. A., Woods, D. W., & Blum, N. (1999). The bedtime pass: An approach to bedtime crying and leaving the room. *Archives of Pediatrics & Adolescent Medicine*, *153*(10), 1027–1029.

Gehrman, P. R., Meltzer, L. J., Moore, M., Pack, A. I., Perlis, M. L., Eaves, L. J., & Silberg, J. L. (2011). Heritability of insomnia symptoms in youth and their relationship to depression and anxiety. *Sleep*, *34*(12), 1641–1646.

Giedd, J. N., Clasen, L. S., Lenroot, R., Greenstein, D., Wallace, G. L., Ordaz, S., Molloy, E. A., et al. (2006). Puberty-related influences on brain development. *Molecular and Cellular Endocrinology*, 254–255, 154–162.

Goodlin-Jones, B. L., Burnham, M. M., Gaylor, E. E., & Anders, T. F. (2001). Night waking, sleep-wake organization, and self-soothing in the first year of life. *Journal of Developmental and Behavioral Pediatrics*, *22*(4), 226–233.

Goodlin-Jones, B., Tang, K., Liu, J., & Anders, T. F. (2009). Sleep problems, sleepiness and daytime behavior in preschool-age children. *Journal of Child Psychology and Psychiatry and Allied Disciplines*, *50*(12), 1532–1540.

Gradisar, M., Dohnt, H., Gardner, G., Paine, S., Starkey, K., Menne, A., Slater, A., et al. (2011). A randomized controlled trial of cognitive-behavior therapy plus bright light therapy for adolescent delayed sleep phase disorder. *Sleep*, *34*(12), 1671–1680.

Gregory, A. M., Cox, J., Crawford, M. R., Holland, J., Harvey, A. G., & The Steps Team. (2009). Dysfunctional beliefs and attitudes about sleep in children. *Journal of Sleep Research*, *18*(4), 422–426.

Harvey, A., Sharpley, A., Ree, M., Stinson, K., & Clark, D. (2007). An open trial of cognitive therapy for chronic insomnia. *Behaviour Research and Therapy*, *45*(10), 2491–2501.

Harvey, A. G. (2008). Sleep and circadian rhythms in bipolar disorder: Seeking synchrony, harmony, and regulation. *The American Journal of Psychiatry*, *165*(7), 820–829.

Hasler, B. P., Bootzin, R. R., Cousins, J. C., Fridel, K., & Wenk, G. L. (2008). Circadian phase in sleep-disturbed adolescents with a history of substance abuse: A pilot study. *Behavioral Sleep Medicine*, *6*(1), 55–73.

Hiscock, H. (2010). Rock-a-bye baby? Parenting and infant sleep. *Sleep Medicine Reviews*, *14*(2), 85–87.

Huttenlocher, P. R. (1979). Synaptic density in human frontal cortex—developmental changes and effects of aging. *Brain Research*, *163*(2), 195–205.

Jenni, O. G., Achermann, P., & Carskadon, M. A. (2005). Homeostatic sleep regulation in adolescents. *Sleep*, *28*(11), 1446–1454.

Jenni, O. G., & O'Connor, B. B. (2005). Children's sleep: An interplay between culture and biology. *Pediatrics*, *115*(1 Suppl), 204–216.

Johnson, E. O., Roth, T., & Breslau, N. (2006). The association of insomnia with anxiety disorders and depression: Exploration of the direction of risk. *Journal of Psychiatric Research*, *40*(8), 700–708.

Johnson, E. O., Roth, T., Schultz, L., & Breslau, N. (2006). Epidemiology of DSM-IV insomnia in adolescence: Lifetime prevalence, chronicity, and an emergent gender difference. *Pediatrics*, *117*(2), e247–256.

Kataria, S., Swanson, M. S., & Trevathan, G. E. (1987). Persistence of sleep disturbances in preschool children. *The Journal of Pediatrics*, *110*(4), 642–646.

Kazdin, A. E. (2000). *Behavior Modification in Applied Settings* (6th ed., pp. 33–66, Principles of operant conditioning). Independence, KY: Wadsworth Publishing.

Kerkhof, G., & van Vianen, B. (1999). Circadian phase estimation of chronic insomniacs relates to their sleep characteristics. *Archives of Physiology and Biochemistry*, *107*(5), 383–392.

Kodak, T., & Piazza, C. C. (2010). Bedtime fading with response cost for children with multiple sleep problems. In M. Perlis, M. Aloia, & B. R. Kuhn (Eds.), *Behavioral Treatments for Sleep Disorders: A Comprehensive Primer of Behavioral Sleep Medicine Interventions* (pp. 285–292). Boston: Elsevier/Academic Press.

Kuhn, B. R., & Weidinger, D. (2000). Interventions for infant and toddler sleep disturbance: A review. *Child & Family Behavior Therapy*, *22*(2), 33–50.

Kuhn, B. R., & Elliott, A. J. (2003). Treatment efficacy in behavioral pediatric sleep medicine. *Journal of Psychosomatic Research*, *54*(6), 587–597.

Laberge, L., Petit, D., Simard, C., Vitaro, F., Tremblay, R. E., & Montplaisir, J. (2001). Development of sleep patterns in early adolescence. *Journal of Sleep Research, 10*(1), 59–67.

Lack, L., & Wright, H. (1993). The effect of evening bright light in delaying the circadian rhythms and lengthening the sleep of early morning awakening insomniacs. *Sleep, 16*(5), 436–443.

Lawton, C., France, K. G., & Blampied, N. M. (1991). Treatment of infant sleep disturbance by graduated extinction. *Child & Family Behavior Therapy, 13*(1), 39–56.

Lee, K. A., McEnany, G., & Weekes, D. (1999). Gender differences in sleep patterns for early adolescents. *The Journal of Adolescent Health, 24*(1), 16–20.

Lerman, D. C., & Iwata, B. A. (1996). Developing a technology for the use of operant extinction in clinical settings: An examination of basic and applied research. *Journal of Applied Behavior Analysis, 29*(3), 345–382; discussion 383–385.

Lerman, D. C., Iwata, B. A., & Wallace, M. D. (1999). Side effects of extinction: Prevalence of bursting and aggression during the treatment of self-injurious behavior. *Journal of Applied Behavior Analysis, 32*(1), 1–8.

Lichstein, K. L., Riedel, B. W., Wilson, N. M., Lester, K. W., & Aguillard, R. N. (2001). Relaxation and sleep compression for late-life insomnia: A placebo-controlled trial. *Journal of Consulting and Clinical Psychology, 69*(2), 227–239.

Liu, X., Buysse, D. J., Gentzler, A. L., Kiss, E., Mayer, L., Kapornai, K., Vetró, A., et al. (2007). Insomnia and hypersomnia associated with depressive phenomenology and comorbidity in childhood depression. *Sleep, 30*(1), 83–90.

Lozoff, B., Wolf, A. W., & Davis, N. S. (1985). Sleep problems seen in pediatric practice. *Pediatrics, 75*(3), 477–483.

Manber, R., & Bootzin, R. R. (1997). Sleep and the menstrual cycle. *Health Psychology: Official Journal of the Division of Health Psychology, American Psychological Association, 16*(3), 209–214.

Manber, R., Edinger, J. D., Gress, J. L., San Pedro-Salcedo, M., Kuo, T. F., & Kalista, T. (2008). Cognitive behavioral therapy for insomnia enhances depression outcome in patients with comorbid major depressive disorder and insomnia. *Sleep, 31*(4), 489–495.

Martin, J., Hiscock, H., Hardy, P., Davey, B., & Wake, M. (2007). Adverse associations of infant and child sleep problems and parent health: An Australian population study. *Pediatrics, 119*(5), 947–955.

Meltzer, L. J., & Mindell, J. A. (2007). Relationship between child sleep disturbances and maternal sleep, mood, and parenting stress: A pilot study. *Journal of Family Psychology: Journal of the Division of Family Psychology of the American Psychological Association (Division 43), 21*(1), 67–73.

Meltzer, L. J., & Mindell, J. A. (2010). Graduated extinction: Behavioral treatment for bedtime problems and night wakings in young children. In M. Perlis, M. Aloia, & B. R. Kuhn (Eds.), *Behavioral Treatments for Sleep Disorders: A Comprehensive Primer of Behavioral Sleep Medicine Interventions* (pp. 275–284). Boston: Elsevier/Academic Press.

Milan, M. A., Mitchell, Z. P., Berger, M. I., & Pierson, D. F. (1981). Positive routines: A rapid alternative to extinction for elimination of bedtime tantrum behavior. *Child Behavior Therapy, 3*(1), 13–25.

Mindell, J. A. (1999). Empirically supported treatments in pediatric psychology: Bedtime refusal and night wakings in young children. *Journal of Pediatric Psychology, 24*(6), 465–481.

Mindell, J. A. (2003). Insomnia in children and adolescents. In M. P. Szuba, J. D. Kloss, & D. F. Dinges (Eds.), *Insomnia Principles and Management* (pp. 125–135). New York: Cambridge University Press.

Mindell, J. A., Emslie, G., Blumer, J., Genel, M., Glaze, D., Ivanenko, A., Johnson, K., et al. (2006). Pharmacologic management of insomnia in children and adolescents: Consensus statement. *Pediatrics, 117*(6), e1223–1232.

Mindell, J. A., Kuhn, B., Lewin, D. S., Meltzer, L. J., & Sadeh, A. (2006). Behavioral treatment of bedtime problems and night wakings in infants and young children. *Sleep, 29*(10), 1263–1276.

Mindell, J. A., Sadeh, A., Kohyama, J., & How, T. H. (2010). Parental behaviors and sleep outcomes in infants and toddlers: A cross-cultural comparison. *Sleep Medicine, 11*(4), 393–399.

Mindell, J. A., Sadeh, A., Wiegand, B., How, T. H., & Goh, D. Y. T. (2010). Cross-cultural differences in infant and toddler sleep. *Sleep Medicine, 11*(3), 274–280.

Moore, B. A., Friman, P. C., Fruzzetti, A. E., & MacAleese, K. (2007). Brief report: Evaluating the Bedtime Pass Program for child resistance to bedtime—a randomized, controlled trial. *Journal of Pediatric Psychology, 32*(3), 283–287.

Moore, M., Slane, J., Mindell, J. A., Burt, S. A., & Klump, K. L. (2011). Genetic and environmental influences on sleep problems: A study of preadolescent and adolescent twins. *Child: Care, Health and Development.*

Morgenthaler, T., Kramer, M., Alessi, C., Friedman, L., Boehlecke, B., Brown, T., Coleman, J., et al. (2006). Practice parameters for the psychological and behavioral treatment of insomnia: an update. An American Academy Of Sleep Medicine report. *Sleep, 29*(11), 1415–1419.

Morgenthaler, T., Owens, J., Alessi, C., Boehlecke, B., Brown, T. M., Coleman, J., Jr., Friedman, L., et al. (2006). Practice parameters for behavioral treatment of bedtime problems and night wakings in infants and young children. *Sleep, 29*(10), 1277–1281.

Morgenthaler, T., Lee-Chiong, T., Alessi, C., Friedman, L., Aurora, R. N., Boehlecke, B., et al. (2007). Practice parameters for the clinical evaluation and treatment of circadian rhythm sleep disorders. An American Academy of Sleep Medicine report. *Sleep, 30*(11), 1445–1459.

Morin, C., Vallières, A., & Ivers, H. (2007). Dysfunctional beliefs and attitudes about sleep (DBAS): Validation of a brief version (DBAS-16). *Sleep, 30*(11), 1547–1554.

Morin, C. M., Bootzin, R. R., Buysse, D. J., Edinger, J. D., Espie, C. A., & Lichstein, K. L. (2006). Psychological and behavioral treatment of insomnia: Update of the recent evidence (1998–2004). *Sleep, 29*(11), 1398–1414.

Morris, M., Lack, L., & Dawson, D. (1990). Sleep-onset insomniacs have delayed temperature rhythms. *Sleep, 13*(1), 1–14.

National Sleep Foundation. (2005). *Sleep in America Poll.* Washington, D.C. Retrieved from http://www.sleep-foundation.org/. Accessed August 13, 2010.

National Sleep Foundation. (2006). *Sleep in America Poll.* Washington, D.C. Retrieved from http://www.sleepfoundation.org/. Accessed August 13, 2010.

Ohayon, M. M., Roberts, R. E., Zulley, J., Smirne, S., & Priest, R. G. (2000). Prevalence and patterns of problematic sleep among older adolescents. *Journal of the American Academy of Child and Adolescent Psychiatry, 39*(12), 1549–1556.

Ong, J., & Sholtes, D. (2010). A mindfulness-based approach to the treatment of insomnia. *Journal of Clinical Psychology, 66*(11), 1175–1184.

Ong, J. C., Huang, J. S., Kuo, T. F., & Manber, R. (2007). Characteristics of insomniacs with self-reported morning and evening chronotypes. *Journal of Clinical Sleep Medicine, 3*(3), 289–294.

Ong, J. C., Shapiro, S. L., & Manber, R. (2008). Combining mindfulness meditation with cognitive-behavior therapy for insomnia: A treatment-development study. *Behavior Therapy, 39*(2), 171–182.

Ong, J. C., Shapiro, S. L., & Manber, R. (2009). Mindfulness meditation and cognitive behavioral therapy for insomnia: A naturalistic 12-month follow-up. *Explore (New York, N.Y.), 5*(1), 30–36.

Owens, J. (2008). Classification and epidemiology of childhood sleep disorders. *Primary Care, 35*(3), 533–546, vii.

Owens, J. A., Spirito, A., McGuinn, M., & Nobile, C. (2000). Sleep habits and sleep disturbance in elementary school-aged children. *Journal of Developmental and Behavioral Pediatrics, 21*(1), 27–36.

Owens, J. A., Rosen, C. L., & Mindell, J. A. (2003). Medication use in the treatment of pediatric insomnia: results of a survey of community-based pediatricians. *Pediatrics, 111*(5 Pt 1), e628–635.

Owens, J. A., & Witmans, M. (2004). Sleep problems. *Current Problems in Pediatric and Adolescent Health Care, 34*(4), 154–179.

Owens, J. A. (2006). When a child can't sleep, start by treating the parents. *The Journal of Family Practice, 5*(21–22), 27–30.

Owens, J. A., & Moturi, S. (2009). Pharmacologic treatment of pediatric insomnia. *Child and Adolescent Psychiatric Clinics of North America, 18*(4), 1001–1016.

Owens, J. A., Rosen, C. L., Mindell, J. A., & Kirchner, H. L. (2010). Use of pharmacotherapy for insomnia in child psychiatry practice: A national survey. *Sleep Medicine, 11*(7), 692–700.

Owens, J. A., & Mindell, J. A. (2011). Pediatric insomnia. *Pediatric Clinics of North America, 58*(3), 555–569.

Palermo, T. M., Wilson, A. C., Lewandowski, A. S., Toliver-Sokol, M., & Murray, C. B. (2011). Behavioral and psychosocial factors associated with insomnia in adolescents with chronic pain. *Pain, 152*(1), 89–94.

Patten, C. A., Choi, W. S., Gillin, J. C., & Pierce, J. P. (2000). Depressive symptoms and cigarette smoking predict development and persistence of sleep problems in US adolescents. *Pediatrics, 106*(2), E23.

Piazza, C. C., & Fisher, W. (1991a). A faded bedtime with response cost protocol for treatment of multiple sleep problems in children. *Journal of Applied Behavior Analysis, 24*(1), 129–140.

Piazza, C. C., & Fisher, W. W. (1991b). Bedtime fading in the treatment of pediatric insomnia. *Journal of Behavior Therapy and Experimental Psychiatry, 22*(1), 53–56.

Rapoff, M. A., Christophersen, E. R., & Rapoff, K. E. (1982). The management of common childhood bedtime problems by pediatric nurse practitioners. *Journal of Pediatric Psychology, 7*(2), 179–196.

Reich, S. (2005). What do mothers know? Maternal knowledge of child development. *Infant Mental Health Journal, 26*, 143–156.

Reid, M. J., Walter, A. L., & O'Leary, S. G. (1999). Treatment of young children's bedtime refusal and nighttime wakings: A comparison of "standard" and graduated ignoring procedures. *Journal of Abnormal Child Psychology, 27*(1), 5–16.

Richardson, G. S., & Roth, T. (2001). Future directions in the management of insomnia. *The Journal of Clinical Psychiatry, 62*(Suppl 10), 39–45.

Rickert, V. I., & Johnson, C. M. (1988). Reducing nocturnal awakening and crying episodes in infants and young children: A comparison between scheduled awakenings and systematic ignoring. *Pediatrics, 81*(2), 203–212.

Roane, B. M., & Taylor, D. J. (2008). Adolescent insomnia as a risk factor for early adult depression and substance abuse. *Sleep, 31*(10), 1351–1356.

Roberts, R. E., Lewinsohn, P. M., & Seeley, J. R. (1995). Symptoms of DSM-III-R major depression in adolescence: Evidence from an epidemiological survey. *Journal of the American Academy of Child and Adolescent Psychiatry, 34*(12), 1608–1617.

Roberts, R. E., Roberts, C. R., & Chen, I. G. (2002). Impact of insomnia on future functioning of adolescents. *Journal of Psychosomatic Research, 53*(1), 561–569.

Roberts, R. E., Roberts, C. R., & Chan, W. (2008). Persistence and change in symptoms of insomnia among adolescents. *Sleep, 31*(2), 177–184.

Roth, T., & Ancoli-Israel, S. (1999). Daytime consequences and correlates of insomnia in the United States: Results of the 1991 National Sleep Foundation Survey. II. *Sleep, 22*(Suppl 2), S354–358.

Sack, R. L., Auckley, D., Auger, R. R., Carskadon, M. A., Wright, K. P., Jr., Vitiello, M. V., & Zhdanova, I. V. (2007). Circadian rhythm sleep disorders: Part II, advanced sleep phase disorder, delayed sleep phase disorder, free-running disorder, and irregular sleep-wake rhythm. An American Academy of Sleep Medicine review. *Sleep, 30*(11), 1484–1501.

Sackett, D. L. (1993). Rules of evidence and clinical recommendations for the management of patients. *Canadian Journal of Cardiology, 9*, 487–489.

Sadeh, A., Raviv, A., & Gruber, R. (2000). Sleep patterns and sleep disruptions in school-age children. *Developmental Psychology, 36*(3), 291–301.

Sadeh, A. (2005). Cognitive-behavioral treatment for childhood sleep disorders. *Clinical Psychology Review, 25*(5), 612–628.

Sadeh, A., Flint-Ofir, E., Tirosh, T., & Tikotzky, L. (2007). Infant sleep and parental sleep-related cognitions. *Journal of Family Psychology: Journal of the Division of Family Psychology of the American Psychological Association (Division 43), 21*(1), 74–87.

Sadeh, A., Mindell, J. A., Luedtke, K., & Wiegand, B. (2009). Sleep and sleep ecology in the first 3 years: A web-based study. *Journal of Sleep Research, 18*(1), 60–73.

Sadeh, A., Tikotzky, L., & Scher, A. (2010). Parenting and infant sleep. *Sleep Medicine Reviews, 14*(2), 89–96.

Sanders, M. R., Bor, B., & Dadds, M. (1984). Modifying bedtime disruptions in children using stimulus control and contingency management techniques. *Behavioural & Cognitive Psychotherapy, 12*(02), 130–141.

Schreck, K. A., & Richdale, A. L. (2011). Knowledge of childhood sleep: A possible variable in under or misdiagnosis of childhood sleep problems. *Journal of Sleep Research, 20*(4), 589–597.

Seymour, F. W., Bayfield, G., Brock, P., & During, M. (1983). Management of night-waking in young children. *Australian Journal of Family Therapy, 4*(4), 217–223.

Shechter, A., Varin, F., & Boivin, D. B. (2010). Circadian variation of sleep during the follicular and luteal phases of the menstrual cycle. *Sleep, 33*(5), 647–656.

Shibui, K., Uchiyama, M., Okawa, M., Kudo, Y., Kim, K., Liu, X., et al. (2000). Diurnal fluctuation of sleep propensity and hormonal secretion across the menstrual cycle. *Biological Psychiatry, 48*(11), 1062–1068.

Sloan, E. P., Hauri, P., Bootzin, R., Morin, C., Stevenson, M., & Shapiro, C. M. (1993). The nuts and bolts of behavioral therapy for insomnia. *Journal of Psychosomatic Research, 37*(Suppl 1), 19–37.

Spielman, A. J., Caruso, L. S., & Glovinsky, P. B. (1987). A behavioral perspective on insomnia treatment. *The Psychiatric Clinics of North America, 10*(4), 541–553.

Spielman, A. J., Saskin, P., & Thorpy, M. J. (1987). Treatment of chronic insomnia by restriction of time in bed. *Sleep, 10*(1), 45–56.

Stein, M. A., Mendelsohn, J., Obermeyer, W. H., Amromin, J., & Benca, R. (2001). Sleep and behavior problems in school-aged children. *Pediatrics, 107*(4), E60.

Strauch, I., & Meier, B. (1988). Sleep need in adolescents: A longitudinal approach. *Sleep, 11*(4), 378–386.

Symon, B. G., Marley, J. E., Martin, A. J., & Norman, E. R. (2005). Effect of a consultation teaching behaviour modification on sleep performance in infants: A randomised controlled trial. *The Medical Journal of Australia, 182*(5), 215–218.

Taylor, D. J., Jenni, O. G., Acebo, C., & Carskadon, M. A. (2005). Sleep tendency during extended wakefulness: Insights into adolescent sleep regulation and behavior. *Journal of Sleep Research, 14*(3), 239–244.

Taylor, D. J., Lichstein, K. L., Weinstock, J., Sanford, S., & Temple, J. R. (2007). A pilot study of cognitive-behavioral therapy of insomnia in people with mild depression. *Behavior Therapy, 38*(1), 49–57.

Taylor, D. J., Schmidt-Nowara, W., Jessop, C. A., & Ahearn, J. (2010). Sleep restriction therapy and hypnotic withdrawal versus sleep hygiene education in hypnotic using patients with insomnia. *Journal of Clinical Sleep Medicine, 6*(2), 169–175.

Tikotzky, L., & Sadeh, A. (2010). The role of cognitive-behavioral therapy in behavioral childhood insomnia. *Sleep Medicine, 11*(7), 686–691.

Treloar, A. E., Boynton, R. E., Behn, B. G., & Brown, B. W. (1967). Variation of the human menstrual cycle through reproductive life. *International Journal of Fertility, 12* (1 Pt 2), 77–126.

Ustinov, Y., Lichstein, K. L., Wal, G. S. V., Taylor, D. J., Riedel, B. W., & Bush, A. J. (2010). Association between report of insomnia and daytime functioning. *Sleep Medicine, 11*(1), 65–68.

Van Tassel, E. B. (1985). The relative influence of child and environmental characteristics on sleep disturbances in the first and second years of life. *Journal of Developmental and Behavioral Pediatrics, 6*(2), 81–86.

Vollman, R. F. (1977). The menstrual cycle. *Major Problems in Obstetrics and Gynecology, 7*, 1–193.

Wade, C. M., Ortiz, C., & Gorman, B. S. (2007). Two-session group parent training for bedtime noncompliance in head start preschoolers. *Child & Family Behavior Therapy, 29*(3), 23–55.

Weil, G., & Goldfried, M. (1973). Treatment of insomnia in an eleven-year-old child through self-relaxation. *Behavior Therapy, 4*(2), 282–284.

Wolfson, A. (1998). Working with parents on developing efficacious sleep/wake habits for infants and young children. In C. E. Schaefer & J. M. Briesmeister (Eds.), *Handbook of Parent Training: Parents as co-therapists for children's behavior problems* (2nd ed., pp. 166–188). New York: Wiley.

Wolfson, A. R., & Carskadon, M. A. (1998). Sleep schedules and daytime functioning in adolescents. *Child Development, 69*(4), 875–887.

Wolfson, A. R., Acebo, C., Fallone, G., & Carskadon, M. A. (2003). Actigraphically-estimated sleep patterns of middle school students. *Sleep, 26*(Suppl), 313.

Wyatt, J. K. (2004). Delayed sleep phase syndrome: Pathophysiology and treatment options. *Sleep, 27*(6), 1195–1203.

Zuckerman, B., Stevenson, J., & Bailey, V. (1987). Sleep problems in early childhood: Continuities, predictive factors, and behavioral correlates. *Pediatrics, 80*(5), 664–671.

CHAPTER

23 Circadian Timing: Delayed Sleep Phase Disorder

R. Robert Auger *and* Stephanie J. Crowley

Abstract

Delayed sleep phase disorder (DSPD), common among adolescents, is characterized by an extreme "eveningness" circadian preference. Various etiologies have been proposed for this presumably multifactorial condition. As those afflicted frequently present during a time of transition to earlier school start times, sleep restriction can be profound, which may mediate described associated emotional and mental health difficulties, poor academic performance, and increased risk of unintentional injuries or death. A thorough assessment is required for accurate diagnosis and appropriate treatment. More studies are needed to establish evidence-based clinical guidelines for this young population, particularly as implementation of adult-based therapies are met with numerous barriers.

Key Words: circadian, delayed sleep phase disorder, adolescents, light, melatonin, sleep

Introduction

This chapter aims to educate the reader about adolescent delayed sleep phase disorder (DSPD). Background information is provided regarding the normal developmental delay in the sleep/wake schedule in association with puberty, as DSPD is widely viewed as an extreme expression of this phenomenon. The observed frequency of DSPD is then reviewed, which is contingent upon varying diagnostic criteria and differences in school start times. Predominant biological etiological hypotheses are discussed, with acknowledgment that the condition has multifactorial origins. This detailed preface segues into a review of clinical presentation, comorbidities, and treatment options. We begin with a primer of human circadian biology and terminology (see Chapters 8 and 17).

Circadian Rhythms and Light

Sleep and wakefulness are conceptually governed by two processes, "Process S" and "Process C" (Borbely & Achermann, 1992). The homeostatic drive to sleep (Process S) is proportional to the duration of wakefulness and, among young adults, becomes maximal at about 40 hours (Carskadon & Dement, 1979). In contrast, Process C creates a drive for wakefulness that variably opposes Process S and is dependent upon circadian ("approximately daily") rhythms intrinsic to the organism. Master coordination of this sleep/wake rhythm (and numerous other behavioral and physiological variables) is provided by the neurons of the suprachiasmatic nuclei located within the hypothalamus (Moore & Eichler, 1972; Stephan & Zucker, 1972; Ralph, Foster et al., 1990; Welsh, Logothetis et al., 1995), whose rhythmic output results from an autoregulatory feedback loop within which oscillating gene products regulate their own transcription and translation (reviewed in Piggins, 2002). As this intrinsic period (termed τ) is typically slightly longer than 24 hours (Czeisler, Duffy et al., 1999), synchronization to the 24-hour day (entrainment) is accomplished by various environmental inputs, the most important of which is light and dark exposure (Waterhouse & DeCoursey, 2004).

The relationship between the timing of a stimulus and the magnitude and direction of a phase shift is described by a phase response curve (PRC; see Figure 23.1; Carskadon and Tarokh, Chapter 8). The time at which the stimulus response shifts from phase delay to phase advance is known as the *crossover point.* In the adult human light PRC, this occurs near the time of the minimum core body temperature (MCBT; inverted triangle in Figure 23.1), which typically manifests a few hours prior to habitual sleep offset and corresponds with maximal sleepiness (Cagnacci, Elliott et al., 1992). The transition from low daytime melatonin (a "darkness" hormone) secretion to robust nocturnal secretion can be assessed serially (e.g., with salivary samples) during a window that precedes and overlaps the typical time of sleep onset (Pandi-Perumal, Smits et al., 2007). As this procedure is performed under dim light conditions (to avoid light-induced melatonin suppression), the time at which the transition occurs is termed the *dim light melatonin onset* (DLMO; see Figure 23.1; Crowley, Chapter 17; also (Sack, Auckley et al., 2007a) The DLMO serves as a rough crossover point for the melatonin PRC (see Figure 23.1).

In an individual normally entrained to the light/dark cycle, evening light exposure (i.e., exposure prior to the MCBT) delays circadian rhythms, and morning light exposure (i.e., exposure after the MCBT) advances rhythms (see Figure 23.1; (Eastman & Burgess, 2009). These opposing effects allow the majority of the population to be properly attuned to the light/dark cycle such that sleep and wakefulness occur at a conventional schedule (Duffy & Wright, 2005). Failure to synchronize can alter the phase relationships between internal rhythms and the light/dark cycle, which may manifest in the form of circadian rhythm sleep disturbances such as irregular sleep–wake and free-running types, advanced sleep phase disorder and, most pertinent to this chapter, delayed sleep phase disorder (American Academy of Sleep Medicine, 2005).

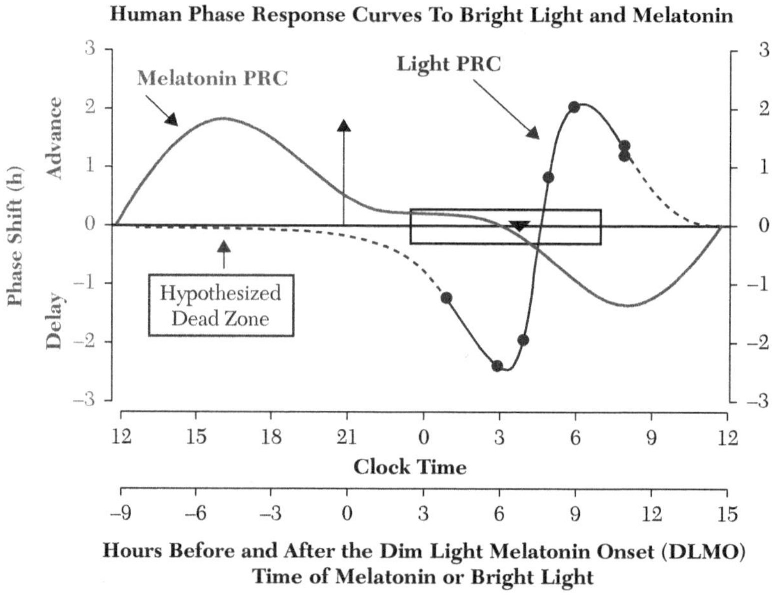

Figure 23.1 Phase response curves (PRCs) generated from subjects free-running through an ultradian light–dark cycle (2.5 hours: 1.5 hours) for three 24-hour days. Melatonin pills (3.0 mg; Burgess, Revell, et al., 2008) or bright light pulses (2 hours of ~3500 lux; Revell, 2005) were given each day, with different subjects receiving the stimulus at different times of day. Phase shifts were derived from circadian phase assessments conducted before and after the 3 days of the protocol. The X axis shows the time the pill was given or the time the bright light pulse began relative to each subject's dim light melatonin onset (DLMO), represented by zero on the bottom time line and the upward arrow. The clock time axis allows for depiction of a subject with a DLMO at approximately 21:00, sleep from about 23:30 until 07:00 (rectangle), and a core body temperature minimum (MCBT) at about 04:00 (inverted triangle). These represent typical times and phase relationships among these rhythms when the circadian clock is entrained to a 24-hour day (Burgess & Eastman, 2005; Lee, Smith et al., 2006; Burgess & Fogg, 2008).

Source: Eastman & Burgess, 2009.

Delayed Sleep/Wake Timing in Association with Developmental Changes

A delay in the preferred timing of sleep and wakefulness in association with adolescence has been demonstrated within numerous societies worldwide (Andrade, Benedito-Silva et al., 1993; Wolfson & Carskadon, 1998; National Sleep Foundation, 2000; Laberge, Petit et al., 2001; Carskadon & Acebo, 2002; Giannotti, Cortesi et al., 2002; Gau & Soong, 2003; National Sleep Foundation, 2006; Ouyang, Lu et al., 2009; Sadeh, Dahl et al., 2009), and coincides with a variety of physiologic pubertal changes, as well as nonphysiologic changes (see Chapters 8 and 11) in the social milieu (reviewed in Crowley, Acebo et al., 2007). A systematic assessment of circadian preference involving over 20,000 participants demonstrated a crescendo pattern of increasing "eveningness" until the age of approximately 20 with a subsequent gradual decline, proposed to be a marker for the "end of adolescence"(Roenneberg, Kuehnle et al., 2004). Commonly observed adolescent DSPD appears to represent an extreme expression of this scheduling preference. (Pelayo, Thorpy et al., 1988; Dagan, Stein et al., 1998; Thorpy, Korman et al., 1998; American Academy of Sleep Medicine, 2005; Carskadon, Vieira et al., 1993; Carskadon, Acebo et al., 1997; Jenni, Achermann et al., 2005).

DSPD Clinical Presentation

DSPD can be construed as a pronounced "night owl" circadian preference, such that those affected habitually retire and arise significantly later than conventional or desired clock times (see Table 23.1). As the condition is felt to relate primarily to an aberration in timing (but not quality) of sleep, the characterization of a disorder is invoked only if the schedule interferes significantly with social or occupational functioning. Adolescents with DSPD live at a circadian phase that is incompatible with personal and academic obligations.

Primary considerations within the differential diagnosis include depression and anxiety, which often manifest with sleep complaints (Ohayon, 1997), as well as inadequate sleep hygiene and numerous other conditions associated with sleep initiation complaints. One must encourage elaboration among those presenting with "insomnia," as approximately 10% of such patients within sleep medicine clinics ultimately prove to have DSPD (American Academy of Sleep Medicine, 2005). Psychophysiological insomnia can be differentiated from DSPD with the patient's endorsement of readily initiating sleep when allowed to sleep according to his/her desired sleep/wake schedule. The simultaneous presence of more than one condition seems to be the norm rather than the exception (Gradisar, Dohnt et al., 2011), however, and each needs to be treated accordingly.

Table 23.1 International Classification of Sleep Disorders, Second Edition, Diagnostic Criteria for Delayed Sleep Phase Disorder*

A. There is a delay in the phase of the major sleep period in relation to the desired sleep time and wake-up time, as evidenced by a chronic or recurrent complaint of inability to fall asleep at a desired conventional clock time together with the inability to awaken at a desired and socially acceptable time.

B. When allowed to choose their preferred schedule, patients will exhibit normal sleep quality and duration for age and maintain a delayed but stable phase of entrainment to the 24-hour sleep-wake pattern.

C. Sleep log or actigraphy monitoring (including sleep diary) for at least seven days demonstrates a stable delay in the timing of the habitual sleep period.

D. The sleep disturbance is not better explained by another current sleep disorder, medical or neurological disorder, medication use, or substance use disorder.

*Source: American Academy of Sleep Medicine, 2005.

Diagnosis and Assessment

As there are no discrete clock times associated with the International Classification of Sleep Disorders 2nd Edition diagnostic criteria for DSPD (American Academy of Sleep Medicine, 2005), and only sparse normative data regarding adolescent sleep–wake times in general, a simplistic approach is to elicit a typical weekday bedtime of 00:00 or later for those >14 years of age, and a threshold clock time of 23:00 h for those ≤14 years (Auger, Burgess et al., 2011) These timings cutoffs are based, in part, upon the average bedtimes reported by 6th- through 8th–graders in the 2006 Sleep in America Poll (National Sleep Foundation, 2006). As wake times are typically enforced due to school attendance 5 days of the week, they do not accurately represent internal preferences. Both sleep onset and offset times are likely to be later on weekends, but sole attention to this schedule is less likely to identify those with an obligate delayed circadian preference.

Various assessment tools can complement the clinical history in establishing a diagnosis of DSPD (see Crowley, Chapter 17). Either sleep logs or actigraphy are required to demonstrate stability of the complaint (and to rule out extraneous influences), but the latter typically generates more reliable data (Bradshaw, Yanagi et al., 2007). Actigraphs are compact "motion detectors" (which may or may not contain photosensors) used commonly in clinical and research settings, the output of which allows longitudinal assessment of various sleep/wake parameters (Morgenthaler, Alessi et al., 2007). Eveningness tendencies of presumptive DSPD patients can be further verified with morningness/eveningness questionnaires (Horne & Ostberg, 1976). Lower score values are associated with evening types, which are felt to correspond to the endogenous circadian period or phase, and can therefore be helpful in narrowing the differential diagnosis for sleep-initiation complaints (reviewed in Sack, Auckley et al., 2007). See Spruyt, Chapter 18 Crowley (Chapter 17) also describes ME questionnaires, for a full description of morningness/eveningness questionnaires.

Physiological assessments for diagnosis show promise. Although studied almost exclusively among adult patients, DSPD has been associated with delayed circadian rhythms of melatonin, cortisol, thyroid-stimulating hormone, and body temperature (Ozaki, Uchiyama et al., 1996; Shibui, Uchiyama et al., 1999; Shibui et al., 2003) As a result, such tests (particularly salivary melatonin immunoassays) appear to have potential clinical utility but are not yet routinely used (see Crowley, Chapter 17; reviewed in Sack, Auckley et al., 2007a) To preface, the DLMO typically begins 14 hours after natural sleep offset (about 2 hours before sleep onset; Burgess & Eastman, 2005), and the MCBT occurs approximately 7 hours thereafter (reviewed in Lee, Smith et al., 2006) or, as discussed above, a few hours prior to natural awakening (Cagnacci, Elliott et al., 1992). Rahman and colleagues (2009) contend that DLMO values can be used to distinguish between those with DSPD and those with prolonged sleep latency due to non-circadian-based entities. As the distinction between their comparison groups was based solely upon greater polysomnographically measured sleep onset latency within the DSPD group, however, these results should not be considered definitive, as those with insomnia do not reliably exhibit reduced sleep latency subsequent to a 1-night laboratory adaptation.

The development of comprehensive normative values represent another hurdle to the use of DLMO in the clinical setting, as exemplified by comparing phase markers obtained from familial advanced sleep phase disorder (FASPD) to nonfamilial ASPD and/or patients with maintenance or terminal insomnia attributed primarily to circadian phase advances. A case-control comparison of FASPD patients (representative of the extreme phenotype) demonstrated markedly advanced DLMO (17:31 ± 1:49 vs. 21:21 ± 0:28, $p < 0.0005$) and MCBT (23:22 ± 2:55 vs. 03:35 ± 1:33, $p = 0.002$) clock times (Jones, Campbell et al., 1999) A review of MCBT values obtained from nonfamilial ASPD patients (DLMO values not available for comparison) and those with advance-related complaints reveals a wider range of values (ranging from approximately 01:30–04:00; Campbell, Dawson et al., 1993; Lack & Wright, 1993; Lack, Wright et al., 2005), however, with the latter range approaching those expected in unaffected populations. Taking into account that changes in circadian rhythms can be produced by voluntary manipulation of the sleep/wake schedule alone (Wyatt, 2004), a physiological assay will be useful in clinical practice only if extremes in values can be readily identified, prompting providers to search for further clinical correlation if results fall into a "gray zone." Such an approach is familiar to those who interpret multiple sleep latency testing values on a regular basis (Arand, Bonnet et al., 2005). Phase assessments may have greater potential to guide the timing of melatonin and/or light therapy.

Delayed Sleep Phase Disorder Epidemiology

Prevalence estimates of DSPD range widely. Reports based on questionnaires, telephone surveys, or mixed subjective and objective measures estimate a general population prevalence between 0.13–3.1% (Schrader, Bovim et al., 1993; Ando, Kripke et al., 1995; Yazaki, Shirakawa et al., 1999; Wyatt, 2004). Adolescent prevalence in particular varies with the country of origin, but predominance in comparison to adults appears uniform (Pelayo, Thorpy et al., 1988; Ando, Kripke et al., 1995; Yazaki, Shirakawa et al., 1999; Hazama, Inoue et al., 2008; Saxvig, Pallesen et al., 2012). Both US and Norwegian estimates exceed 7% in select studies (Pelayo, Thorpy et al., 1988; American Academy of Sleep Medicine, 2005; Saxvig, Pallesen et al., 2012), although the latter applied less rigid diagnostic criteria than the former. A Japanese survey that queried students from "junior high to university age" (precise ages unspecified) described a strikingly different prevalence rate of 0.48%, with an increase in association with advanced age (1.7% among 4th-year university students; (Hazama, Inoue et al., 2008). A systematic

Table 23.2 Diagnostic and Statistical Manual of Mental Disorders, Fourth Edition, Text Revision Criteria for Circadian Rhythm Sleep Disorder*

A. A persistent or recurring pattern of sleep disruption leading to excessive sleepiness or insomnia that is due to a mismatch between the sleep–wake schedule required by a person's environment and his or her circadian sleep–wake pattern.
B. The sleep disturbance causes clinically significant distress or impairment in social, occupational, or other important areas of functioning.
C. The disturbance does not occur exclusively during the course of another Sleep Disorder or other mental disorder.
D. The disturbance is not due to the direct physiological effects of a substance (e.g., a drug of abuse, a medication) or a general medical condition.

*Source: American Psychiatric Association, 2000

study involving over 1000 Western European adolescents aged 15–18 years structured interview questions in relation to discrete Diagnostic and Statistical Manual of Mental Disorders 4th Edition criteria (American Psychiatric Association, 2000; see Table 23.2) and reported a similarly low rate (0.4%) of circadian disorders of any type (Ohayon, Roberts et al., 2000). As the authors reported later school start times than in many areas of the United States, marked discrepancies in regional prevalence may be due in part to this variable, particularly as a large number in the European group were excluded from estimates solely due to an absence of reported negative daytime consequences. With respect to gender differences, a pronounced male predominance (10:1) was reported in a UK-based study (Alvarez, Dahlitz et al., 1992) but was not described in a subsequent Japanese report (Hazama, Inoue et al., 2008).

Findings and Proposed Etiologies

Although DSPD is undoubtedly heterogeneous in nature and comprises varying amounts of endogenous and exogenous contributors, current diagnostic schemas emphasize biological underpinnings. Proposed etiologies are concordant with this emphasis.

Molecular Genetics

The identification of DSPD pedigrees (Ancoli-Israel, Schnierow et al., 2001) has led to attempts to correlate polymorphisms or mutations of clock genes with the observed phenotype, but the research is in its early stages (reviewed by Sack and colleagues, 2007b) and has been generated primarily from adult subjects. Several studies have focused on the *hPer3* gene. Among five polymorphisms (occurring within four haplotypes) reported by a Japanese group, one haplotype occurred at a higher frequency among adult DSPD subjects, but associations with specific polymorphisms were not explored (Ebisawa, Uchiyama et al., 2001). Taking a different approach, a British group focused on a length-polymorphic repeat region of *hPer3* (composed of either 4 or 5 units), and found a higher frequency of the 4-repeat allele among a DSPD patient group aged 16–27 years (88%; (Archer, Robilliard et al., 2003). In contrast, the 5-repeat allele was associated with a morningness phenotype. Complicating the picture (and perhaps pertinent to the regional differences in DSPD prevalence described above), a Brazilian group found homozygosity for the 5-repeat allele among nearly 30% of adult DSPD patients (Pereira, Tufik et al., 2005) and suggested that discrepancies may be due to differences in patients' ethnic origins or other environmental factors (e.g., latitude). The British group subsequently expanded their search to the promoter region of the gene (Archer, Carpen et al., 2010). Among 3 single nucleotide polymorphisms identified, 2 alleles (G-320T and C-319A) occurred more frequently in the adult DSPD cohort than among comparison groups of morning and evening types. A particular allele combination (TA2G) was also more prevalent among these subjects.

A separate Japanese group identified two more genes associated with DSPD: arylalkylamine N-acetyltransferase (AA-NAT) and human leukocyte antigen (HLA) DR1 (Hohjoh, Takahashi et al., 1999; Hohjoh, Takasu et al., 2003). Intriguingly, AA-NAT is the rate-limiting enzyme in melatonin synthesis. The frequency of a single nucleotide polymorphism (amino acid substitution from alanine to threonine at position 129) was significantly higher among those with DSPD (16%) versus controls (3.1%; the age of the studied population is unspecified) (Hohjoh, Takasu et al., 2003). The positivities of the DR1 antigen were 26.2% and 9.4% among cases (14–45 years of age) and controls, respectively, although the corrected p value failed to reach statistical significance (Hohjoh, Takahashi et al., 1999) Finally, Takano and colleagues (Takano, Uchiyama et al., 2004) identified a polymorphism in a specific human caseine kinase gene (CKIε; S408N) that may be protective in the development of DSPD, as it occurred significantly less frequently among both adult Japanese DSPD and free-running subjects than in controls. The presence of the same polymorphism was documented as extremely rare among the adult Brazilian population, however, indicating that its presence exerts no impact on the expression of the condition (Castro, Barbosa et al., 2008).

A number of additional studies have endeavored to correlate circadian propensity (i.e., morningness versus eveningness, rather than a circadian rhythm sleep disorder per se) with clock gene variations. An early investigation involved over 400 middle-aged American adults, among whom phase preferences were measured with the morningness/eveningness questionnaire (MEQ; (Katzenberg, Young et al., 1998) A single nucleotide polymorphism was identified, with a cytosine for threonine (C for T) substitution at the immediate 3′ region of the human CLOCK gene (*hClock*; 3111C versus 3111T). Participants homozygous for the T allele were less "evening type" than heterozygotes or all C carriers. Similarly, C allele homozygotes exhibited lower but statistically insignificant MEQ values (greater eveningness) when compared to T homozygotes, a result perhaps influenced by the small sample size of the former group. A Japanese group demonstrated similar findings among adult subjects (Mishima, Tozawa et al., 2005) but a separate British group failed to identify an association with either circadian preference or DSPD (Robilliard, Archer et al., 2002). Iwase and colleagues noted an infrequent overall presence of *hClock* polymorphisms within an adult Japanese DSPD cohort, and without differences versus controls (Iwase, Kajimura et al., 2002). Further studies are needed to clarify these and other findings, with acknowledgment that multiple genes could underlie circadian rhythm disorders and with alterations in different genes potentially resulting in a similar circadian phenotype or a mutation in a different site of the same gene producing an opposite effect on the circadian system. In support of the latter notion, a murine study showed that, depending upon the site of *Per2* phosphorylation, the expression, degradation, and/or nuclear entry and retention of the protein can change, resulting in a different degree of advance or delay in the circadian period (Xu, Padiath et al., 2005).

Lengthening of the Intrinsic Period of the Circadian Clock

It has long been suggested that the intrinsic circadian period (τ) of DSPD subjects is abnormally long, which would require greater adjustment to entrain to the 24-hour solar day (Weitzman, Czeisler et al., 1981). This was definitively described in temporal isolation with only one adult subject, however, who demonstrated a τ >25 hours (Campbell & Murphy, 2007). A very recent study (published in abstract form) compared the τ of six DSPD adults to that of seven normal controls and described a significantly greater length in the former (25.2 ± 0.47 hours) versus the latter group (24.6 ± 0.27 hours; Lack, 2012). In the context of development, Carskadon and colleagues (2005) measured τ in 27 healthy adolescents aged 9–15 years and showed an average length of 24.27 hours. Although the sample size was too small to determine whether period lengthens across pubertal development, τ was longer than that measured from an adult sample (mean = 24.12 hours; ages 21–41 years) in a separate laboratory (Czeisler, Duffy et al., 1999). With respect to animal studies, a longer τ has been reported in the pubertal degu (Hummer, 2007) and Long-Evans rat (McGinnis, Lumia et al., 2007) in comparison to healthy adult counterparts. These cumulative findings form the basis of an intriguing etiological hypothesis for adolescent DSPD. Longitudinal studies with a larger number of participants at various stages of pubertal development are required for confirmation.

Alterations of Response to Light

Although a light PRC for adolescent humans has not yet been developed, an investigation by Aoki and colleagues (involving predominantly adults) supports the possibility of hypersensitivity to nocturnal photic stimulation among select DSPD patients as compared to unaffected counterparts, as assessed by the degree of melatonin suppression with 2000 lux-hours of light exposure (Aoki, Ozeki et al., 2001), resulting in excessive stimulation of the phase delay portion of the PRC (see Figure 23.1). Such heightened sensitivity was not supported with indirect assessments within a separate study that examined evening light exposure in association with various sleep parameters, however (Auger, Burgess et al., 2011), nor within a separate study that assessed differences in sensitivity among (non-DSPD) adolescents at various stages of pubertal development (Carskadon, 2002). The latter two studies may have been confounded by differences in daytime light exposure, which can alter melatonin suppression to subsequent exposure and phase-shifting responses (reviewed in Crowley, Acebo et al., 2007). More work is needed to definitively explore the prospect of augmented responses to light among DSPD patients.

The notion of a blunted phase advance response among pubertal humans has also been proposed

(Hagenauer, Perryman et al., 2009). Potentially supporting this contention, two multifaceted interventional studies (involving non-DSPD adolescents aged 15–16 years and delayed young adults aged 18–30 years) failed to phase-advance subjects receiving 1 hour of blue light exposure during two weekend mornings (Crowley & Carskadon, 2010) or six consecutive days (Sharkey, Carskadon et al., 2011) of post-awakening treatments. These results are unexpected based on the PRC to short-wavelength light among adults, which was determined with light delivered by the same commercially available devices used for those protocols (but for a total treatment duration of 1.5 hours, administered intermittently), with descriptions of 30–60 minute advances of the circadian system in response to post-awakening exposure (Revell, 2012). Since the intervention studies delivered treatments in participants' homes (without strict control by laboratory staff), observed differences might be due to discrepancies in light delivery protocols (e.g., varying participant distance from the light source, differing angles of gaze, etc.). Studies to understand normal developmental differences in circadian phase-shifting responses to light are ongoing.

Changes in Light Exposure Patterns

Independent of issues regarding sensitivity to light, an increase in evening light exposure and/or a decrease in morning exposure could theoretically contribute to the DSPD phenotype (see Figure 23.1). A study of non-DSPD adolescents demonstrated delayed circadian phase and sleep onset times during spring as compared to winter months, related to extended daylight hours (seasonal differences were not observed with respect to electrical light usage subsequent to sunset; Figueiro & Rea, 2010a). An investigation by Harada and colleagues (2002) demonstrated a negative correlation between high school students' propensity to seek outdoor light and delayed circadian preference. Nevertheless, a recently published prospective cohort study that investigated light exposure patterns among adolescents with rigorously defined DSPD demonstrated comparatively *less* pre-sleep light exposure (i.e., during a period of time expected to impact the phase delay portion of the PRC) and equivalent amounts of post-sleep exposure (i.e., during a period of time expected to impact the phase advance portion of the PRC; see Figure 23.1; (Auger, Burgess et al., 2011) The negation of receipt of higher light intensity (lux) among these patients does not detract from the possibility of higher exposure to blue wavelengths as contributory, however. In a recent proof-of-concept study involving adult insomnia patients, participants who wore "blue-blocker" glasses during the 3 hours prior to habitual bedtime demonstrated improved subjective sleep quality compared with the placebo intervention (Burkhart & Phelps, 2009). Taking into account circadian sensitivity of the human eye to this shorter wavelength light (Brainard, Hanifin et al., 2001), this finding is of considerable interest. Further investigations are required to clarify the relative contribution of varying light intensities and wavelengths to the sleep complaints associated with DSPD.

Alterations in Phase Relationships

Alterations in phase relationships between the circadian timing system and sleep behavior could impact the ability of light to exert circadian-based changes in a manner predicted by the PRC (see Figure 23.1). Longer intervals from various melatonin parameters (Shibui, Uchiyama et al., 1999) and MCBT (Ozaki, Uchiyama et al., 1996; Uchiyama, Okawa et al., 2000a; Watanabe, Kajimura et al., 2003) to sleep offset have been frequently described among adult DSPD patients as compared to controls. These data lend support to a role of decreased exposure to the phase-advance portion of the PRC as an etiological factor. However, this finding has not been demonstrated among protocols in which subjects are forced to maintain a more conventional sleep/wake schedule (Mundey, Benloucif et al., 2005; Chang, Reid et al., 2009), similar to the scenario of adolescents suffering from this condition whose wake times are inflexible on school days, suggesting that this observation may simply be a consequence of longer habitual sleep times.

Other Potential Etiological Contributors

Uchiyama and colleagues contend that homeostatic sleep processes are impaired among (predominantly adult) DSPD patients, as their investigation demonstrated a lesser ability to initiate sleep following sleep loss compared with controls. (Uchiyama, Okawa et al., 2000b) Isolated case reports describe the emergence of DSPD subsequent to traumatic brain injury, including among adolescents (Patten & Lauderdale, 1992; Nagtegaal, Kerkhof et al., 1997; Quinto, Gellido et al., 2000; Ayalon, Borodkin et al., 2007). Numerous exogenous factors, such as increased autonomy with respect to sleep time, employment, and involvement in extracurricular activities, have been identified as factors contributing to the general changes in the sleep patterns of adolescents (Crowley, Acebo et al., 2007) but have not been studied specifically among adolescent DSPD cohorts (Carskadon, 1990; Wyatt, 2004).

Consequences and Comorbidities of Adolescent Delayed Sleep Phase and DSPD

Sleep Impairments

Observed delays in the preferred timing of sleep and wakefulness in association with pubertal development significantly contributes to the reductions in total sleep time associated with adolescence (Andrade, Benedito-Silva et al., 1993; Wolfson & Carskadon, 1998; National Sleep Foundation, 2000, 2006; Laberge, Petit et al., 2001; Carskadon & Acebo, 2002; Giannotti, Cortesi et al., 2002; Gau & Soong, 2003; Crowley, Acebo et al., 2007; Ouyang, Lu et al., 2009; Sadeh, Dahl et al., 2009). Data from the Centers for Disease Control and Prevention Youth Risk Behavior Survey describe insufficient school night sleep (<8 hours nightly) among nearly 69% of respondents and optimal sleep (≥9 hours nightly) among less than 8% (Eaton, McKnight-Eily et al., 2010). An alarming 26% of adolescents from a separate survey study reported typically sleeping 6.5 hours or less (Wolfson & Carskadon, 1998) One group demonstrated an objective degree of sleepiness (during the early periods of school) equivalent to that of narcoleptics (Carskadon, Wolfson et al., 1998).

The numerous adverse consequences associated with chronic sleep restriction have led to adolescents' characterization as a high-risk group for problematic sleepiness by the US National Institutes of Health (National Sleep Foundation, 2000). High school students with average or below average grades report less sleep, later bedtimes, and more irregular sleep schedules than students reporting higher grades (Wolfson & Carskadon, 1998; Saxvig, Pallesen et al., 2012). Such sleep complaints have also been associated with increased use of stimulants and alcohol, symptoms of depression and anxiety, and a higher frequency of behavioral problems than those without complaints (Carskadon, 1990; Wolfson, Tzischinsky et al., 1995; Wolfson & Carskadon, 1998; Noland, Price et al., 2009; Negriff, Dorn et al., 2011; Urban, Magyarodi et al., 2011; Saxvig, Pallesen et al., 2012). Perhaps most sobering, one study reported that drivers age 25 or younger caused 55% of all crashes attributed to sleepiness (Pack, Pack et al., 1995).

DSPD further increases students' susceptibility to chronic sleep restriction and associated deleterious outcomes (Alvarez, Dahlitz et al., 1992; Ohta, Iwata et al., 1992; Thorpy, Korman et al., 1998; Nagtegaal, Laurant et al., 2000; Fernandez-Mendoza, 2010). In a large survey of high school students, of the 63% who felt they needed more sleep on school nights there was a significant "eveningness" preference as compared to the cohort that described sufficient sleep, suggesting that some of those complaining suffered from DSPD (Mercer, Merritt et al., 1998). In a series investigating 22 adolescents with DSPD, 59% demonstrated poor scholastic performance, and 45% displayed a variety of behavioral problems (Thorpy, Korman et al., 1998).

Reflecting the ongoing struggles associated with this chronic condition, a study investigating quality of life impairments among DSPD adults demonstrated significantly worse scores as compared to age and gender adjusted norms, and worse performance on two scales (social functioning and role disability due to physical problems) in comparison to patients suffering from sleep apnea, clinical depression, migraine headaches, and osteoarthritis (Nagtegaal, Laurant et al., 2000). Data regarding the long-term course of this condition among adolescents is sparse. In a prospective study involving 14 patients (5 adolescents) with DSPD, followed over a period of 5 years in a clinical setting, subjects reported severe disability as a result of failure of morning arousal, with considerable educational, work, and social problems (Alvarez, Dahlitz et al. 1992). All had made attempts to adopt a conventional sleep onset time, successfully achieved by only one patient. A Japanese adolescent case series (Ando, 1994) involving seven participants (mean age at study entry 16.9 years) collected responses to a questionnaire pertaining to ongoing sleep disturbances and social adaptation (both deemed impaired at the time of initial contact) subsequent to completion of initial treatment (mean follow-up duration 3.9 years). Apart from noting that three participants (43%) no longer required treatment at the time of follow-up (presumably due in large part to the fact that they no longer needed to arise at a specified time in the morning), the authors provided no treatment details regarding the remaining patients. Nevertheless, only two participants (29%) endorsed continuing DSPD severity, one of whom remained in school as a university student and was therefore presumably confined to a relatively rigid rise time. The same individual continued to endorse poor social adaptation at follow-up, as did one additional individual (who actually described a diminution of severity with respect to sleep onset and offset times). In the sole adolescent case control study (published in abstract form) to investigate long-term outcomes, questionnaires were obtained from 71 DSPD subjects (median age of onset 13–14 years) and compared to controls (Krahn, Kubas et al., 2003). During a follow-up duration ranging from 2 to 8 years, those afflicted exhibited psychosocial impairment (e.g., truancy, social functioning) similar to psychiatrically ill controls.

Daytime complaints related to DSPD may not be entirely related to chronic sleep restriction. In a prospective study involving adolescents (10–18 years of age), there were no group differences in total sleep time as compared to controls, as afflicted subjects routinely arose later (Auger, Burgess et al., 2011). Group differences in sleep quality and/or circadian desynchronization ("social jet lag") may therefore be implicated. An adult case control DSPD study demonstrated objective decrements in sleep quality measured polysomnographically (Campbell and Murphy 2007).

Affective Instability

Comorbid affective disorder was noted in the initial description of DSPD (Weitzman, Czeisler et al., 1981) and has subsequently been described among other adult cohorts (Regestein & Monk, 1995; Takahashi, Hohjoh et al., 2000; Shirayama, Shirayama et al., 2003; Kripke, Rex et al., 2008) and, to a lesser extent, adolescent cohorts (Dagan, Stein et al., 1998; Thorpy, Korman et al., 1998; Krahn, Kubas et al., 2003). A US-based prospective case control study involving adults demonstrated higher current depression ratings as well as a greater lifetime history of unipolar depression, depression treatment, and antidepressant use than controls (Kripke, Rex et al., 2008). A separate Japanese study systematically investigated the association of depressive symptoms among predominantly adult patients and found that 64% endorsed symptoms of at least moderate severity (Abe, Inoue et al., 2011). Other adult groups have reported a significantly higher prevalence of seasonal affective disorder (as assessed by a standardized questionnaire) in comparison to controls (approximately threefold higher) (Lee, Rex et al., 2011).

Rahman and colleagues (2010) demonstrated a marked delay in the melatonin excretion rhythm among depressed DSPD patients as compared to euthymic DSPD controls, suggesting a direct relationship between the degree of circadian misalignment and mood severity, although their sample size was small. At least two groups have described correlations with respect to chronotype (an innate trait), but not in relation to self-reported sleep onset and offset times, suggesting that the findings are independent of sleep complaints per se (Kitamura, Hida et al., 2010; Abe, Inoue et al., 2011). Of significant relevance in the clinical arena, the simultaneous occurrence of both conditions has been reported to result in an antidepressant-refractory depressive state, necessitating the introduction of circadian-based interventions (Okawa & Uchiyama, 2007).

Emerging adult research has supported a specific association between delayed circadian preference and bipolar I disorder (in comparison to a control group with schizophrenia) even after controlling for age, with assertions that this chronotype may represent a trait characteristic of affectively ill patients even during periods of remission (Ahn, Chang et al., 2008) This association has been limited to a singular case report in the pediatric literature (Faedda and Teicher 2005). Interestingly, in addition to the associations with increased eveningness described above, bipolar adults carrying the C allele of the previously specified *hclock* gene polymorphism demonstrate higher illness recurrence rates, in addition to a higher incidence of comorbid insomnia, suggesting the possibility of a shared pathophysiology (reviewed in Staton, 2008). Future studies need to examine the directionality of these affective-circadian relationships on a large scale, with rigorous control for confounding variables.

Other Psychiatric Comorbidities

Van der Heijden and colleagues compared attention deficit hyperactivity disorder (ADHD) pediatric patients (ages 6–12) with and without sleep onset insomnia and demonstrated phase delays in salivary melatonin secretion in the former group, suggestive of comorbid DSPD (Van der Heijden, Smits et al., 2005). Various case reports similarly describe the occurrence of both conditions, with select demonstration of improvement in behavioral symptoms with the introduction of circadian-based interventions (Dahl, Pelham et al., 1991; Gruber, Grizenko et al., 2007; Khurshid & Khan, 2009). A study by Kissling and colleagues (2008) demonstrated an association with a specific *hClock* polymorphism (rs1801260) among adults with ADHD.

An uncontrolled study of adults with obsessive-compulsive disorder revealed a high frequency of comorbid DSPD, which correlated with increased severity of disability (Turner, Drummond et al., 2007) A separate retrospective study examining this comorbid relationship reported an earlier age of psychiatric symptom onset (Mukhopadhyay, Fineberg et al., 2008). Monteleone and colleagues (1994) found that nocturnal peak melatonin levels were significantly lower in adult OCD patients than in healthy controls (and delayed by approximately two hours), but a separate case control study failed to demonstrate any phase differences among both physiologic and other parameters (Millet, Touitou et al., 1998) Such studies have not yet been performed within pediatric/adolescent populations.

Circadian dysrhythmias may occasionally be medication-related. Among adult schizophrenic patients, receipt of typical neuroleptics (haloperidol and flupenthixol) was associated with circadian dyssynchrony (including delayed and free-running patterns), while receipt of clozapine was associated with a highly regular rest–activity cycle (Wirz-Justice, Haug et al., 2001). Hermesh and colleagues (2001) described 10 cases of DSPD associated with initiation of fluvoxamine (the age of only one adult participant was specified). There are no data that bear upon this association within younger patient populations.

Finally, Dagan and colleagues (1966) found a particularly high rate of personality disorders among (predominantly adult) DSPD patients in comparison to controls. No characteristic personality pattern was identified. The authors suggest that these disorders arise as a result of early-onset developmental difficulties whereby the differing schedules of the child and the caretaker impair the attachment process.

DSPD Treatments

DSPD treatments consist primarily of post-awakening bright light therapy and exogenous melatonin, in an effort to advance the internal clock (reviewed in Sack, Auckley et al., 2007). Despite its prevalence among adolescents, relatively few treatment studies solely involving this population have been published, with identification of only four randomized placebo-controlled trials of melatonin (Smits, Nagtegaal et al., 2001; Smits, van Stel et al., 2003; Weiss, Wasdell et al., 2006; Van der Heijden, Smits et al., 2007) and one multi-interventional trial that employed light therapy (Gradisar, Dohnt et al., 2011). Additional pediatric studies are retrospective in nature or presented as case series (Dahl, Pelham et al., 1991; Okawa, Uchiyama et al., 1998a; Szeinberg, Borodkin et al., 2006; Gruber, Grizenko et al., 2007; Iwamitsu, 2007). Remaining controlled studies (Rosenthal, Joseph-Vanderpool et al., 1990; Dahlitz, Alvarez et al., 1991; Nagtegaal, Kerkhof et al., 1998; Kayumov, Brown et al., 2001; Cole, Smith et al., 2002; Mundey, Benloucif et al., 2005; Lack, Bramwell, Wright, & Kemp, 2007) and case reports/uncontrolled studies (Czeisler, Weitzman et al., 1981; Uruha, 1987; Mizuma, 1991; Oren & Wehr, 1992; Ito, Ando et al., 1993; Oldani, Ferini-Strambi et al., 1994; Regestein & Pavlova, 1995; Weyerbrock, Timmer et al., 1996; Dagan, Yovel et al., 1998; Okawa, Uchiyama et al., 1998b; Watanabe, Kajimura et al., 1999; Kamei, Hayakawa et al., 2000) either consist entirely of adult populations (Czeisler, Weitzman et al., 1981; Uruha, 1987; Oren & Wehr, 1992; Ito, Ando et al., 1993; Weyerbrock, Timmer et al., 1996; Nagtegaal, Kerkhof et al., 1998; Watanabe, Kajimura et al., 1999; Mundey, Benloucif et al., 2005; Lack et al., 2007), include a significant minority of pediatric subjects (Dahlitz, Alvarez et al., 1991; Mizuma, 1991; Oldani, Ferini-Strambi et al., 1994; Regestein & Pavlova, 1995; Dagan, Yovel et al., 1998; Okawa, Uchiyama et al., 1998b; Kamei, Hayakawa et al., 2000; Kayumov, Brown et al., 2001; Cole, Smith et al., 2002), or do not specify the demographics of participants (Rosenthal, Joseph-Vanderpool et al., 1990).

Light Therapy

In a controlled treatment study (ages of participants unspecified), Rosenthal and colleagues (1990) demonstrated that properly timed post-awakening bright light therapy (≥ 2500 lux) can exert physiologically measured phase advances, objective improvements in daytime alertness, and earlier reported bedtimes as compared to controls. The minimum duration of treatment has not been determined (the Rosenthal study administered therapy for 2 hours), but most begin with 30 minutes exposure, which has been deemed effective for the treatment of seasonal affective disorder (Wirz-Justice, Benedetti et al., 2009). Clinical experience suggests that longer treatment lengths are impractical among adolescents. Despite claims by industry, there is currently no evidence to support devices that solely deliver blue light. A recent study of healthy adults demonstrated no benefit with blue-enriched polychromatic light in comparison to standard polychromatic light (Smith, Revell et al., 2009).

Physiologic determinations of phase are not routinely performed in the clinical setting but can be estimated based upon the individual's sleep timing using published algorithms for adults (Burgess & Eastman, 2005) or adolescents (Crowley, Acebo et al., 2006). Light therapy should be timed to occur after the estimated MCBT (~7 hours subsequent to estimated DLMO; Lee, Smith et al., 2006; see Figure 23.1). Although the timing of light treatment is based upon healthy adult subjects, alternate methods for children/adolescents cannot be recommended, as affiliated data are not yet available. As mentioned above, select studies have demonstrated alterations in phase relationships among those with DSPD (Ozaki, Uchiyama et al., 1996; Uchiyama, Okawa et al., 2000a; Watanabe, Kajimura et al., 2003), potentially altering strategic timing of circadian-based interventions—but comparison studies involving young adults have demonstrated equivalent and persistent phase relationships in settings where sleep times are not inordinately prolonged (Wyatt, Stepanski et al., 2006; Chang, Reid et al., 2009).

Bearing in mind that documented MCBTs of (primarily adult) DSPD patients occur between approximately 07:30–08:00 (Ozaki, Uchiyama et al., 1996; Mundey, Benloucif et al., 2005; Chang, Reid et al., 2009) and that the typical occurrence is between 04:00–06:00 (Cagnacci, Elliott et al., 1992), the possibility exists to further provoke phase delays if treatments occur before MCBT (Cagnacci, Elliott et al., 1992; Czeisler, 1999; see Figure 23.1). As the initial timing of light therapy (based on the estimates described above) may be too late to occur prior to school start times, it is sometimes necessary to commence treatment during extended breaks from school. A schedule that slowly advances morning light exposure each or every other morning is recommended to accommodate gradual advances until the target time of awakening is reached (Lack & Wright, 2007). There are no specific guidelines to dictate maintenance treatment, but Lack and Wright (2007) recommend a minimum of seven additional treatment days. Subsequent strict adherence to a specified sleep/wake schedule is required, in addition to accompanying aspects of sleep hygiene, with resumption of light therapy if phase delays reemerge.

Although knowledge of the effect of light therapy on adolescent DSPD is limited, sparse data regarding compliance with the intervention paints a bleak picture (Krahn, Kubas et al., 2003; Bjorvatn & Pallesen, 2009), perhaps because it requires yet an earlier wake time among those already arising near the physiologic nadir of sleepiness to attend school (Ozaki, Uchiyama et al., 1996; Mundey, Benloucif et al., 2005; Chang, Reid et al., 2009). Recognizing this and other barriers, the sole randomized controlled adolescent trial (mean age approximately 15 years) implemented the treatment in combination with multicomponent behavioral therapy (six 45–60 minute sessions, 8 weeks total treatment duration) and demonstrated a respectable 12% dropout rate, with 26% dropout from the waitlist control group (Gradisar, Dohnt et al., 2011). Light exposure was obtained either from the outdoors or from a broad-spectrum lamp (~1000 lux) for a duration of 0.5–2.0 hours. Each participant initially began treatment at his/her natural time of awakening, with advances of 30 minutes daily until a target time of 06:00 was reached or the 8-week protocol terminated. If the target time was reached prior to study termination, multicomponent behavioral interventions ensued with a specific emphasis on stimulus control measures (Morgenthaler, Kramer et al., 2006). Relative to the control group, active participants demonstrated improved sleep latency, total sleep time, and earlier sleep onset and offset times (all subjectively determined). Concomitant benefits in fatigue and sleepiness were also observed. At 6-month follow-up, a select group who received active treatment demonstrated continual improvements in sleep latency and sleep onset time on weekend days, as compared to baseline. Significantly fewer participants in the active group met criteria for DSPD post-treatment (13% vs. 82% for cases and controls, respectively). Since physiologic phase assessments were not employed (and because these interventions were multi-armed), however, it is not possible to definitively attribute these benefits to circadian advances.

Important for implementation in the clinical realm, school nonattendance, unrestricted sleep during vacation periods, and lack of motivation have all been noted to be barriers to successful outcomes with light therapy (Gradisar, Dohnt et al., 2011). Relief from accompanying behavioral problems may provide a treatment incentive for patients and caregivers. A recent case report described a misdiagnosis of ADHD in an adolescent with DSPD (Gruber, Grizenko et al., 2007). Behavioral symptoms resolved with morning light therapy and a concomitant advance in the sleep phase. Similar benefits have been noted in adult studies (Rybak, McNeely et al., 2006).

Others have attempted to surmount the compliance barrier by eliminating the need for active participation. Cole and colleagues (2002) used a light mask that exposed participants to 2700 lux of white light on closed eyelids (about 57 lux at the cornea) and, compared with placebo (0.1 lux of red light), demonstrated significant melatonin phase shifts among select adults (18–40 years) with DSPD. The use of dawn simulators for this condition also shows promise, but have not been studied specifically as a treatment for DSPD (Terman & Jiuan Su, 2010).

Melatonin

Published *American Academy of Sleep Medicine Practice Parameters* (based primarily upon adult data) support the role of properly timed melatonin to achieve phase advances among participants with DSPD (Morgenthaler, Lee-Chiong et al., 2007). Pediatric/adolescent data are not abundant. In a study with participants aged 6–12 years (some with comorbid ADHD), 1-month treatment with 5 milligrams melatonin between 18:00–19:00 significantly improved phase and sleep disturbances (advanced sleep and melatonin onsets, sleep latency, and sleep offset) in comparison to placebo (Smits, Nagtegaal et al., 2001; Smits, van Stel et al., 2003). A separate randomized controlled trial containing solely stimulant-treated children with ADHD + DSPD (mean age = 10.3 years) described decreased sleep latency (subjectively and objectively assessed) with administration of 5 milligrams melatonin (taken 20 minutes before bedtime for a duration of 30 days) and implementation of sleep hygiene recommendations (Weiss, Wasdell et al., 2006). Mixed results have been reported regarding isolated non-sleep-related behavioral effects of melatonin among ADHD + DSPD patients abstaining from stimulant treatment. A study utilizing doses of 3 or 6 milligrams (depending upon body weight) failed to demonstrate singular benefits with respect to emotional and behavioral problems, cognitive performance, or quality of life with a treatment duration of 4 weeks (Van der Heijden, Smits et al., 2007). When these same participants were followed longitudinally (mean of approximately 4 years), however, improvement of mood and behavior was reported in 71% and 61%, respectively. Although not possible to directly attribute these improvements to the effect of melatonin and/or improved sleep, 65% continued to use the medication daily and 88% described the medication as persistently effective for sleep-related difficulties (Hoebert, van der Heijden et al., 2009). A retrospective study of adolescents with DSPD (nearly 50% of whom had comorbid ADHD) undergoing long-term treatment with 3 to 6 milligrams melatonin (1–16 months), taken at a mean of nearly 2 hours prior to desired sleep onset, demonstrated decreases in behaviors detrimental to school performance (Szeinberg, Borodkin et al., 2006) Finally, among adult DSPD patients, an open trial of 5 milligrams melatonin (given 5 hours prior to calculated DLMO) lasting 2 to 9 months demonstrated significantly improved health-related quality of life scores on a standardized questionnaire in all but one of the evaluated domains as compared to the pretreatment period (Nagtegaal, Laurant et al., 2000).

Select additional data describe melatonin treatment among DSPD patients with comorbidities other than ADHD. Wasdell and colleagues (2008) performed a randomized, placebo-controlled crossover trial of 5 milligrams controlled-release melatonin in the treatment of DSPD (10 days per treatment arm) among approximately 50 children (ages 2–18, mean 7.4 years) with neurodevelopmental disabilities (Wasdell, Jan et al., 2008). Participants were recruited in part based upon sleep latency ≥ 30 minutes in relation to the desired time of sleep onset, and melatonin was administered 20–30 minutes prior to this caregiver-determined time. Significant improvements were observed in subjectively and actigraphically recorded total sleep time, sleep latency, and clinician- and caregiver-assessed overall sleep disorder severity and other functional and health dimensions. Decreases in family stress were also observed, as determined by the Family Stress Scale. During the 3-month open-label phase of the trial, 58% escalated the melatonin dosage to 10–15 milligrams. Additive subjective improvements were noted only with respect to longest sleep episode and sleep efficiency, and no changes were observed with respect to actigraphically derived parameters. A follow-up open-label prospective study (duration up to 3.8 years) demonstrated continued caregiver-reported benefits on sleep, overall health, behavior, education, and learning (Carr, Wasdell et al., 2007). Finally, despite the documentation of depression in frequent coexistence with DSPD, only one randomized placebo-controlled trial has been published (involving adults). Five milligrams melatonin (administered between 19:00–21:00) taken for 4 weeks was described as beneficial within both affective and sleep realms as determined by structured clinical assessments and polysomnographic measures, respectively (Rahman, Kayumov et al., 2010).

As for light therapy, estimates of phase are required to optimize the timing of oral melatonin (to affect a maximal phase advance) in the absence of physiologic circadian assessments. Best evidence (as extrapolated from the adult literature) would appear to support dosing approximately 8 hours after an individual's natural (i.e., preferred) wake time (Burgess & Eastman, 2005; Mundey, Benloucif et al., 2005). Doses of 0.5 milligrams or less appear optimal with respect to achievement of maximal chronobiotic effects among adults (Lewy, Emens et al., 2005). Although rather nonspecific in its recommendations, a recent meta analysis (including both children and adults with DSPD) vaguely endorsed both recommendations, as it concluded that "low dose" melatonin administered "as early as tolerable" was most effective (van Geijlswijk, Korzilius et al., 2010).

Among healthy adults, a synergistic effect can be obtained when melatonin is used in combination with light therapy (Revell, Burgess et al., 2006) Although physiologic phase assessments were not employed, a recent case series (n = 28) described success with this treatment combination among DSPD patients in the field (age range 15–60 years, median = 22 years). Three milligrams melatonin was taken 2 hours prior to desired bedtime in conjunction with either outdoor or 5000 lux light exposure for a minimum of 30 minutes between 06:00–08:00. During a median follow-up period of 6.4 weeks, 82% reported improvements in sleep patterns, with a mean sleep phase advance of approximately 2 hours (Samaranayake, Fernando et al., 2010).

Pediatric/adolescent patients and/or their caregivers are frequently wary of melatonin use due to concerns related to adverse effects on reproductive function and the regulation of growth hormone (Valcavi, Zini et al., 1993; Luboshitzky, Shen-Orr et al., 2002; Committee on the Framework for Evaluating the Safety of Dietary Supplements, 2005; Szeinberg, Borodkin et al., 2006). A randomized placebo-controlled trial that investigated the toxicology of "long-term" treatment (28 days) with 10 milligrams melatonin (solely comprising male adult participants) revealed no group differences with respect to adverse effects on polysomnographically recorded sleep, subjective sleepiness, numerous clinical laboratory examinations, or other subjectively recorded events (Seabra, Bignotto et al., 2000). Data are more limited within the pediatric population and do not specifically address concerns related to reproductive organs. A long-term follow-up study of patients with DSPD + ADHD utilizing melatonin doses up to 10 milligrams (mean follow-up time of approximately 4 years, mean age at follow-up 12.4 years) detected no serious adverse events as a result of serial interviews with the children's parents, and 65% of participants continued to use the medication daily (Hoebert, van der Heijden et al., 2009). A follow-up open-label prospective study of subjects with neurodevelopmental disabilities comorbid with DSPD receiving controlled-release melatonin (max dosage 15 mg, duration up to 3.8 years) similarly described no adverse events (Wasdell, Jan et al., 2008; Carr, Wasdell et al., 2007).

Prescribed Sleep/Wake Scheduling

Chronotherapy is a treatment whereby patients are prescribed a sleep schedule that is delayed several hours incrementally until sleep is aligned to a target bedtime. After this goal is reached, the individual is advised to rigorously maintain a regular sleep/wake schedule, repeating the process as necessary. Although there are positive case reports describing the use of this treatment for DSPD (Czeisler, Weitzman et al., 1981; Dahl, Pelham et al., 1991), there have been no controlled trials of its efficacy or safety. One study reported that relapse was common when adult patients were followed long-term (Ito, Ando et al., 1993). In addition, there is one report of an adult patient who developed free-running circadian rhythms after engaging in this treatment (Oren & Wehr, 1992). In the sole pediatric case report, Dahl et al. (1991) described a 10-year-old girl with ADD and a 5-year history of sleep disturbance. A trial of chronotherapy and accompanying behavioral modifications resulted in significant improvement in the ADD symptomatology.

For the sufficiently motivated adolescent, strict adherence to a fixed advanced sleep/wake may be sufficient. Sharkey and colleagues (2011) studied a cohort that included older adolescents (age range 18–30 years, mean 21.8) with subthreshold DSPD (the social/occupational impairment criterion was not applied). Participants advanced sleep schedules by 1–2.5 hours earlier than the average bedtime prior to study entry, and continued this schedule for 6 days (actigraphically and subjectively monitored). Amber filters covered backlit screens after sunset, to minimize competing delaying photic stimuli. An average phase advance of 1.4 hours was observed with DLMO. As would be expected in an intervention of this duration, however, the majority of participants exhibited decreased sleep time. Pointing to the challenges inherent to those with the more extreme phenotype, Iwamitsu and colleagues (2007) demonstrated uniform sleep-related improvements with sleep/wake scheduling interventions among DSPD patients in the inpatient setting, but only 57% showed persistent improvement subsequent to discharge, such that they resumed school attendance. Finally, recognizing that some DSPD cases are refractory to treatment, Dagan and Abadi (2001) recommend implementation of rehabilitation and accommodation to the delayed sleep schedule in select instances, including support for disability from duties that require strict sleep/wake schedules, and encouragement to pursue endeavors with more flexible scheduling.

Hypnotics

There is limited evidence to support the use of hypnotics in DSPD (Uruha, 1987; Ohta, Iwata et al., 1992; Ito, Ando et al., 1993), and patients may exhibit resistance to their effects (Mizuma, 1991; Yamadera, Takahashi et al., 1996; Auger, 2008). Nevertheless, in individuals with a concomitant conditioned insomnia, they can serve in some instances to heighten confidence with respect to the ability to initiate sleep. No hypnotics are approved by the US Food and Drug Administration for use within the pediatric population.

Other Behavioral Approaches

A later school start time may be sought if practical and available within the district (see Au, Appleman, and Stavitsky, Chapter 38). This intervention alone can significantly increase total sleep time and mitigate associated impairments (National Sleep Foundation, 2000; Wahlstrom, 2002; Owens, Belon et al., 2010). A recent study reported an approximately 17% drop in the average crash rate for adolescents 2 years subsequent to a 1-hour delay in school start times, in conjunction with increased mean hours of nightly sleep (Danner & Phillips, 2008). Unfortunately, the implementation of this policy change frequently encounters staunch political resistance (Wahlstrom, 1999), and is presently available in select regions only.

In all instances, external contributors to DSPD complaints should be pursued and addressed, including poor sleep hygiene practices and/or substance misuse. As can occur in anyone with chronic sleep initiation complaints, DSPD patients may have a concomitant conditioned insomnia, which is often responsive to evidence-based behavioral treatments (reviewed in Morgenthaler, Kramer et al., 2006)). Implementation of non-extreme wake times on weekends should be emphasized (perhaps varying no more than 30 minutes from the weekday time), as later rise times can themselves cause phase delays (Burgess & Eastman, 2006; Taylor, 2008; Crowley & Carskadon, 2010). If one can convince the adolescent to maintain regular rise times, he/she might be better served by taking a midday nap to relieve sleep deprivation. Naps taken during a window of 6 hours centered 12 hours from the midpoint of the unrestricted weekend sleep bout have been shown to have nil effects on circadian rhythms (Eastman, Gazda et al., 2005).

Conclusion

DSPD is common among adolescents (particularly in the United States), and may in part represent an exaggeration of normal developmental tendencies. Its characterization as a disorder hinges predominantly upon the degree to which the desired sleep/wake schedule conflicts with what is externally required, and its severity therefore varies with the flexibility of the imposed schedule. A multifactorial etiology is apparent, with contributions from numerous endogenous and exogenous factors. The eventual elucidation of various DSPD subtypes will enable the development of more sophisticated multicomponent interventions. The identification of successful treatments is an essential "first step" in establishing whether resolution of complaints can directly address other comorbidities and may serve to further characterize directional relationships, potentially in conjunction with emerging clock gene research. The most commonly utilized treatments consist of post-awakening light therapy and oral melatonin. Integration of physiologic circadian assessments into the clinical arena could assist with optimal timing of these therapies and potentially also assist with diagnosis. Devices that deliver light stimuli during sleep and/or post-awakening protocols with a more flexible schedule need to be further developed to address compliance barriers and to accommodate adolescents' academic and social schedules. Equally relevant, school lighting environments should be optimized for maximal circadian benefits to account for the proportion of time adolescents spend within this setting (Figueiro & Rea, 2010b). Although serious adverse events have not been associated with melatonin to date, definitive pediatric/adolescent data are lacking, particularly with respect to long-term effects on reproductive organs. In many respects, clinical circadian research remains in its early infancy in comparison to the relative adulthood of bench research. Increasing recognition of DSPD and related funding will hopefully allow for increased evidence-based data for the oft-neglected pediatric/adolescent population.

Future Directions

• Examine, assess, and develop the most effective treatments for adolescent DSPD, recognizing the current lack of evidence-based data.

• Studies need to investigate and understand the predominant exogenous and exogenous contributors to the development and perpetuation of adolescent DSPD, so that different DSPD subtypes may be identified.

• Examine whether successful treatment of DSPD decreases the deleterious outcomes associated with affective and other comorbidities.

References

Abe, T., Inoue, Y., Komada, Y., Nakamura, M., Asaoka, S., Kanno, M.,, et al. (2011). Relation between morningness-eveningness score and depressive symptoms among patients with delayed sleep phase syndrome. *Sleep Medicine, 12*(7), 680–684.

Ahn, Y. M., J. Chang, et al. (2008). Chronotype distribution in bipolar I disorder and schizophrenia in a Korean sample. *Bipolar Disorders, 10*(2), 271–275.

Alvarez, B., M. J. Dahlitz, et al. (1992). The delayed sleep phase syndrome, clinical and investigative findings in 14 subjects. *Journal of Neurology, Neurosurgery & Psychiatry, 55*(8), 665–670.

American Academy of Sleep Medicine (2005). *International Classification of Sleep Disorders. Diagnostic and Coding Manual.* Westchester, IL: American Academy of Sleep Medicine.

American Psychiatric Association (2000). *Diagnostic and Statistical Manual of Mental Disorders, Fourth Edition, Text Revision.* Washington, DC: American Psychiatric Association.

Ancoli-Israel, S., B. Schnierow, et al. (2001). A pedigree of one family with delayed sleep phase syndrome. *Chronobiology International, 18*(5), 831–840.

Ando, K., Hayakawa, T., Ohta, T., Kayukawa, Y., Ito, A., Iwata, T., Okada, T. (1994). Long-term follow up of study of 10 adolescent patients with sleep-wake schedule disorders. *The Japanese Journal of Psychiatry and Neurology, 48*(1), 37–41.

Ando, K., D. F. Kripke, et al. (1995). Estimated prevalence of delayed and advanced sleep phase syndromes [abstract]. *Sleep Research, 24*, 509.

Andrade, M. M., A. A. Benedito-Silva, et al. (1993). Sleep characteristics of adolescents: a longitudinal study. *Journal of Adolescent Health, 14*(5), 401–406.

Aoki, H., Y. Ozeki, et al. (2001). Hypersensitivity of melatonin suppression in response to light in patients with delayed sleep phase syndrome. *Chronobiology International, 18*(2), 263–271.

Arand, D., M. Bonnet, et al. (2005). The clinical use of the MSLT and MWT. *Sleep, 28*(1), 123–144.

Archer, S. N., J. D. Carpen, et al. (2010). Polymorphism in the PER3 promoter associates with diurnal preference and delayed sleep phase disorder. *Sleep, 33*(5), 695–701.

Archer, S. N., D. L. Robilliard, et al. (2003). A length polymorphism in the circadian clock gene Per3 is linked to delayed sleep phase syndrome and extreme diurnal preference. *Sleep, 26*(4), 413–415.

Auger, R. R. (2008). *Circadian Rhythm Sleep Disorder, Delayed Sleep Phase Type (Pediatric Case)* (pp. 195–199). Westchester, IL: American Academy of Sleep Medicine.

Auger, R. R., H. J. Burgess, et al. (2011). Light exposure among adolescents with delayed sleep phase disorder: A prospective cohort study. *Chronobiology International, 28*(10), 911–920.

Ayalon, L., K. Borodkin, et al. (2007). Circadian rhythm sleep disorders following mild traumatic brain injury. *Neurology, 68*(14), 1136–1140.

Bjorvatn, B., & S. Pallesen (2009). A practical approach to circadian rhythm sleep disorders. *Sleep Medicine Reviews, 13*(1), 47–60.

Borbely, A. A., & P. Achermann (1992). Concepts and models of sleep regulation: An overview. *Journal of Sleep Research 1*(2), 63–79.

Bradshaw, D. A., M. A. Yanagi, et al. (2007). Nightly sleep duration in the 2-week period preceding multiple sleep latency testing. *Journal of Clinical Sleep Medicine 3*(6), 613–619.

Brainard, G., J. Hanifin, et al. (2001). Action spectrum for melatonin regulation in humans: Evidence for a novel circadian photoreceptor. *Journal of Neuroscience, 21*(16), 6405–6412.

Burgess, H. J., & C. I. Eastman (2005). The dim light melatonin onset following fixed and free sleep schedules. *Journal of Sleep Research, 14*(3), 229–237.

Burgess, H. J., & C. I. Eastman (2006). A late wake time phase delays the human dim light melatonin rhythm. *Neurosci Lett 395*(3), 191–195.

Burgess, H. J., & L. F. Fogg (2008). Individual differences in the amount and timing of salivary melatonin secretion. *PLoS ONE, 3*(8), e3055.

Burgess, H. J., V. L. Revell, et al. (2008). A three pulse phase response curve to three milligrams of melatonin in humans. *Journal of Physiology, 586*(2), 639–647.

Burkhart, K., & J. R. Phelps (2009). Amber lenses to block blue light and improve sleep: a randomized trial. *Chronobiology International, 26*(8), 1602–1612.

Cagnacci, A., J. A. Elliott, et al. (1992). Melatonin: a major regulator of the circadian rhythm of core temperature in humans. *Journal of Clinical Endocrinology & Metabolism, 75*(2), 447–452.

Campbell, S. S., D. Dawson, et al. (1993). Alleviation of sleep maintenance insomnia with timed exposure to bright light. *Journal of the American Geriatric Society, 41*(8), 829–836.

Campbell, S. S., & P. J. Murphy (2007). Delayed sleep phase disorder in temporal isolation. *Sleep, 30*(9), 1225–1228.

Carr, R., M. B. Wasdell, et al. (2007). Long-term effectiveness outcome of melatonin therapy in children with treatment-resistant circadian rhythm sleep disorders. *Journal of Pineal Research, 43*(4), 351–359.

Carskadon, M. A., & W. C. Dement (1979). Effects of total sleep loss on sleep tendency. *Perceptual and Motor Skills, 48*(2), 495–506.

Carskadon, M. A. (1990). Patterns of sleep and sleepiness in adolescents. *Pediatrician, 17*(1), 5–12.

Carskadon, M. A., C. Vieira, et al. (1993). Association between puberty and delayed phase preference. *Sleep, 16*(3), 258–262.

Carskadon, M. A., C. Acebo, et al. (1997). An approach to studying circadian rhythms of adolescent humans. *Journal of Biological Rhythms, 12*(3), 278–289.

Carskadon, M. A., A. R. Wolfson, et al. (1998). Adolescent sleep patterns, circadian timing, and sleepiness at a transition to early school days. *Sleep, 21*(8), 871–881.

Carskadon, M. A., & C. Acebo (2002). Regulation of sleepiness in adolescents: update, insights, and speculation. *Sleep, 25*(6), 606–614.

Carskadon, M. A., Acebo, C., Arendt, J. (2002). Failure to identify pubertally-mediated melatonin sensitivity to light in adolescents [abstract]. *Sleep, 25*(Abstract Supplement), A191.

Carskadon, M. A., Acebo, C. (2005). Intrinsic circadian period in adolescents versus adults from forced desynchrony [abstract]. *Sleep, 28*(Abstract Supplement), A71.

Castro, R. M., A. A. Barbosa, et al. (2008). Casein kinase I epsilon (CKIvarepsilon) N408 allele is very rare in the Brazilian population and is not involved in susceptibility to circadian rhythm sleep disorders. *Behavioural Brain Research, 193*(1), 156–157.

Chang, A. M., K. J. Reid, et al. (2009). Sleep timing and circadian phase in delayed sleep phase syndrome. *Journal of Biological Rhythms, 24*(4), 313–321.

Cole, R., J. Smith, et al. (2002). Bright-light mask treatment of delayed sleep phase syndrome. *Journal of Biological Rhythms, 17*(1), 89–101.

Committee on the Framework for Evaluating the Safety of Dietary Supplements, F. a. N. B., Board on Life Sciences, Institute of Medicine and National Research Council of the National Academies. (2005). *Dietary Supplements: A Framework for Evaluating Safety.* Washington, DC: The National Academies Press.

Crowley, S. J., C. Acebo, et al. (2006). Estimating dim light melatonin onset (DLMO) phase in adolescents using summer or school-year sleep/wake schedules. *Sleep, 29*(12), 1632–1641.

Crowley, S. J., C. Acebo, et al. (2007). Sleep, circadian rhythms, and delayed phase in adolescence. *Sleep Medicine, 8*(6), 602–612.

Crowley, S. J., & Carskadon, M. A. (2010). Modifications to weekend recovery sleep delay circadian phase in older adolescents. *Chronobiology International, 27*(7), 1469–1492.

Czeisler, C., J. Duffy, et al. (1999). Stability, precision, and near-24-hour period of the human circadian pacemaker. *Science, 284*(5423), 2177–2181.

Czeisler, C., & Wright Jr., K. (1999). *Influence of Light on Circadian Rhythmicity in Humans.* New York: Marcel Dekker, Inc.

Czeisler, C., E. Weitzman, et al. (1981). Chronotherapy: Resetting the circadian clocks of patients with delayed sleep phase insomnia. *Sleep, 4,* 1–21.

Dagan, Y., H. Sela, et al. (1996). High prevalence of personality disorders among circadian rhythm sleep disorders (CRSD) patients. *Journal of Psychosomatic Research, 41*(4), 357–363.

Dagan, Y., D. Stein, et al. (1998). Frequency of delayed sleep phase syndrome among hospitalized adolescent psychiatric patients. *Journal of Psychosomatic Research, 45*(1 Spec No), 15–20.

Dagan, Y., I. Yovel, et al. (1998). Evaluating the role of melatonin in the long-term treatment of delayed sleep phase syndrome (DSPS). *Chronobiology International, 15*(2), 181–190.

Dagan, Y., & Abadi, J. (2001). Sleep-wake schedule disorder disability: A lifelong untreatable pathology of the circadian time structure. *Chronobiology International, 18*(6), 1019–1027.

Dahl, R. E., W. E. Pelham, et al. (1991). The role of sleep disturbances in attention deficit disorder symptoms: A case study. *Journal of Pediatric Psychology, 16*(2), 229–239.

Dahlitz, M., B. Alvarez, et al. (1991). Delayed sleep phase syndrome response to melatonin. *Lancet, 337*(8750), 1121–1124.

Danner, F., & B. Phillips (2008). Adolescent sleep, school start times, and teen motor vehicle crashes. *Journal of Clinical Sleep Medicine, 4*(6), 533–535.

Duffy, J. F., & K. P. Wright, Jr. (2005). Entrainment of the human circadian system by light. *Journal of Biological Rhythms, 20*(4), 326–338.

Eastman, C. I., C. J. Gazda, et al. (2005). Advancing circadian rhythms before eastward flight: A strategy to prevent or reduce jet lag. *Sleep, 28*(1), 33–44.

Eastman, C. I., & H. J. Burgess (2009). How to travel the world without jet lag. *Sleep Medicine Clinics, 4*(2), 241–255.

Eaton, D. K., McKnight-Eily, L. R, Lowry, R., Perry, G. S., Presley-Cantrell, L., Croft, J. B. (2010). Prevalence of insufficient, borderline, and optimal hours of sleep among high school students—United States, 2007. *Journal of Adolescent Health, 46*(4), 399–401.

Ebisawa, T., M. Uchiyama, et al. (2001). Association of structural polymorphisms in the human period3 gene with delayed sleep phase syndrome. *EMBO Reports, 2*(4), 342–346.

Faedda, G. L., & M. H. Teicher (2005). Objective measures of activity and attention in the differential diagnosis of psychiatric disorders of childhood. *Essential Psychopharmacology, 6*(5), 239–249.

Fernandez-Mendoza, J., Iliuodi, C., Montes, M.I., Olavarrieta-Bernardino, S., Aguirre-Berrocal, A., De La Cruz-Troca, J.J., Vela-Bueno, A. (2010). Circadian preference, nighttime sleep and daytime functioning in young adulthood. *Sleep and Biological Rhythms, 8,* 52–62.

Figueiro, M. G., & M. S. Rea (2010a). Evening daylight may cause adolescents to sleep less in spring than in winter. *Chronobiology International, 27*(6), 1242–1258.

Figueiro, M. G., & M. S. Rea (2010b). Lack of short-wavelength light during the school day delays dim light melatonin onset (DLMO) in middle school students. *Neuroendocrinology Letters, 31*(1), 92–96.

Gau, S. F., & W. T. Soong (2003). The transition of sleep-wake patterns in early adolescence. *Sleep,* 26(4), 449–454.

Giannotti, F., F. Cortesi, et al. (2002). Circadian preference, sleep and daytime behaviour in adolescence. *Journal of Sleep Research, 11*(3), 191–199.

Gradisar, M., H. Dohnt, et al. (2011). A randomized controlled trial of cognitive-behavior therapy plus bright light therapy for adolescent delayed sleep phase disorder. *Sleep, 34*(12), 1671–1680.

Gruber, R., N. Grizenko, et al. (2007). Delayed sleep phase syndrome, ADHD, and bright light therapy. *Journal of Clinical Psychiatry, 68*(2), 337–338.

Hagenauer, M. H., J. I. Perryman, et al. (2009). Adolescent changes in the homeostatic and circadian regulation of sleep. *Developmental Neuroscience, 31*(4), 276–284.

Harada, T., H. Morisane, et al. (2002). Effect of daytime light conditions on sleep habits and morningness-eveningness preference of Japanese students aged 12–15 years. *Psychiatry and Clinical Neurosciences,Psychiatry and Clinical Neurosciences 56*(3), 225–226.

Hazama, G. I., Y. Inoue, et al. (2008). The prevalence of probable delayed-sleep-phase syndrome in students from junior high school to university in Tottori, Japan. *Tohoku Journal of Experimental Medicine, 216*(1), 95–98.

Hermesh, H., H. Lemberg, et al. (2001). Circadian rhythm sleep disorders as a possible side effect of fluvoxamine. *CNS Spectrums, 6*(6), 511–513.

Hoebert, M., K. B. van der Heijden, et al. (2009). Long-term follow-up of melatonin treatment in children with ADHD and chronic sleep onset insomnia. *Journal of Pineal Research, 47*(1), 1–7.

Hohjoh, H., Y. Takahashi, et al. (1999). Possible association of human leucocyte antigen DR1 with delayed sleep phase syndrome. *Psychiatry and Clinical Neurosciences, 53*(4), 527–529.

Hohjoh, H., M. Takasu, et al. (2003). Significant association of the arylalkylamine N-acetyltransferase (AA-NAT) gene with delayed sleep phase syndrome. *Neurogenetics, 4*(3), 151–153.

Horne, J. A., & O. Ostberg (1976). A self-assessment questionnaire to determine morningness-eveningness in human circadian rhythms. *International Journal of Chronobiology, 4*(2), 97–110.

Hummer, D. L., Jechura, T. J., Mahoney, M. M., & Lee, T. M. (2007). Gonadal hormone effects on entrained and free-running circadian activity rhythms in the developing diurnal rodent Octodon degus. *American Journal of Physiology – Regulatory, Integrative and Comparative Physiology, 292*(1), R586–597.

Ito, A., K., &o, et al. (1993). Long-term course of adult patients with delayed sleep phase syndrome. *Japanese Journal of Psychiatry and Neurology, 47*(3), 563–567.

Iwamitsu Y., Ozeki, Y., Konishi M., Murakami J., Kimura, S., & Okawa M. (2007). Psychological characteristics and the efficacy of hospitalization treatment on delayed sleep phase syndrome patients with school refusal. *Sleep and Biological Rhythms, 5*, 15–22.

Iwase, T., N. Kajimura, et al. (2002). Mutation screening of the human Clock gene in circadian rhythm sleep disorders. *Psychiatry Research, 109*(2), 121–128.

Jenni, O. G., P. Achermann, et al. (2005). Homeostatic sleep regulation in adolescents. *Sleep, 28*(11), 1446–1454.

Jones, C., S. Campbell, et al. (1999). Familial advanced sleep phase syndrome, A short-period circadian rhythm variant in humans. *Nature Medicine, 5*(9), 1062–1065.

Kamei, Y., T. Hayakawa, et al. (2000). Melatonin treatment for circadian rhythm sleep disorders. *Psychiatry and Clinical Neurosciences, 54*(3), 381–382.

Katzenberg, D., T. Young, et al. (1998). A CLOCK polymorphism associated with human diurnal preference. *Sleep, 21*(6), 569–576.

Kayumov, L., G. Brown, et al. (2001). A randomized, double-blind, placebo-controlled crossover study of the effect of exogenous melatonin on delayed sleep phase syndrome. *Psychosomatic Medicine, 63*(1), 40–48.

Khurshid, K. A., & Khan, A. A. (2009). Delayed sleep phase disorder and attention deficit and hyperactivity symptoms in a teenager. *Attention Deficit and Hyperactactivity Disorders, 1*(2), 211–213.

Kissling, C., W. Retz, et al. (2008). A polymorphism at the 3'-untranslated region of the CLOCK gene is associated with adult attention-deficit hyperactivity disorder. *American Journal of Medical Genetics Part B: Neuropsychiatric Genetics, 147*(3), 333–338.

Kitamura, S., A. Hida, et al. (2010). Evening preference is related to the incidence of depressive states independent of sleep-wake conditions. *Chronobiology International, 27*(9–10), 1797–1812.

Krahn, L. E., S. M. Kubas, et al. (2003). Long-term outcome of adolescents with delayed sleep phase disorder [abstract]. *Sleep, 26*, A115.

Kripke, D. F., K. M. Rex, et al. (2008). Delayed sleep phase cases and controls. *Journal of Circadian Rhythms, 6*, 6.

Laberge, L., D. Petit, et al. (2001). Development of sleep patterns in early adolescence. *Journal of Sleep Research, 10*(1), 59–67.

Lack, L., & Wright, H. (1993). The effect of evening bright light in delaying the circadian rhythms and lengthening the sleep of early morning awakening insomniacs. *Sleep, 16*(5), 436–443.

Lack, L., H. Wright, et al. (2005). The treatment of early-morning awakening insomnia with 2 evenings of bright light. *Sleep, 28*(5), 616–623.

Lack, L., Bramwell, T., Wright, H., & Kemp, K. (2007). Morning blue light can advance the melatonin rhythm in mild delayed sleep phase syndrome. *Sleep and Biological Rhythms, 5*, 78–80.

Lack, L. C., & Wright, H. R. (2007). Clinical management of delayed sleep phase disorder. *Behavioral Sleep Medicine, 5*(1), 57–76.

Lack, L. C., Micic, G., De Bruyn, A., Wright, H., & Lovato, N. (2012). Circadian rhythm period length in delayed sleep phase disorder [abstract]. *Sleep, 35*(Abstract Supplement), A203.

Lee, C., M. R. Smith, et al. (2006). A compromise phase position for permanent night shift workers: Circadian phase after two night shifts with scheduled sleep and light/dark exposure. *Chronobiology International, 23*(4), 859–875.

Lee, H. J., K. M. Rex, et al. (2011). Delayed sleep phase syndrome is related to seasonal affective disorder. *Journal of Affective Disorders, 133*(3), 573–579.

Lewy, A. J., J. S. Emens, et al. (2005). Melatonin entrains free-running blind people according to a physiological dose-response curve. *Chronobiology International, 22*(6), 1093–1106.

Luboshitzky, R., Z. Shen-Orr, et al. (2002). Melatonin administration alters semen quality in healthy men. *Journal of Andrology, 23*(4), 572–578.

McGinnis, M. Y., A. R. Lumia, et al. (2007). Effects of anabolic androgenic steroids on the development and expression of running wheel activity and circadian rhythms in male rats. *Physiology & Behavior, 92*(5), 1010–1018.

Mercer, P. W., S. L. Merritt, et al. (1998). Differences in reported sleep need among adolescents. *Journal of Adolescent Health, 23*(5), 259–263.

Millet, B., Y. Touitou, et al. (1998). Plasma melatonin and cortisol in patients with obsessive-compulsive disorder: Relationship with axillary temperature, physical activity, and clinical symptoms. *Biological Psychiatry, 44*(9), 874–881.

Mishima, K., T. Tozawa, et al. (2005). The 3111T/C polymorphism of hClock is associated with evening preference and delayed sleep timing in a Japanese population sample. *American Journal of Medical Genetics Part B: Neuropsychiatric Genetics, 133B*(1), 101–104.

Mizuma H., Miyahara, Y., Sakamoto, T., Kotorii, T., & Nakazawa, Y. (1991). Two cases of delayed sleep phase syndrome (DSPS). *Japanese Journal of Psychiatry and Neurology, 45*(1), 163–164.

Monteleone, P., F. Catapano, et al. (1994). Circadian rhythms of melatonin, cortisol and prolactin in patients with obsessive-compulsive disorder. *Acta Psychiatrica Scandinavia, 89*(6), 411–415.

Moore, R. Y., & Eichler, V. B. (1972). Loss of a circadian adrenal corticosterone rhythm following suprachiasmatic lesions in the rat. *Brain Research, 42*(1), 201–206.

Morgenthaler, T., M. Kramer, et al. (2006). Practice parameters for the psychological and behavioral treatment of insomnia: An update. An American Academy of Sleep Medicine report. *Sleep, 29*(11), 1415–1419.

Morgenthaler, T. I., C. Alessi, et al. (2007). Practice parameters for the use of actigraphy in the assessment of sleep and sleep disorders, An update for 2007. *Sleep, 30*(4), 519–529.

Morgenthaler, T. I., T. Lee-Chiong, et al. (2007). Practice parameters for the clinical evaluation and treatment of circadian rhythm sleep disorders. An American Academy of Sleep Medicine report. *Sleep, 30*(11), 1445–1459.

Mukhopadhyay, S., N. A. Fineberg, et al. (2008). Delayed sleep phase in severe obsessive-compulsive disorder: A systematic case-report survey. *CNS Spectrums, 13*(5), 406–413.

Mundey, K., S. Benloucif, et al. (2005). Phase-dependent treatment of delayed sleep phase syndrome with melatonin. *Sleep. 28*(10), 1271–1278.

Nagtegaal, J. E., G. A. Kerkhof, et al. (1997). Traumatic brain injury-associated delayed sleep phase syndrome. *Functional Neurology, 12*(6), 345–348.

Nagtegaal, J. E., G. A. Kerkhof, et al. (1998). Delayed sleep phase syndrome: A placebo-controlled cross-over study on the effects of melatonin administered five hours before the individual dim light melatonin onset. *Journal of Sleep Research, 7*(2), 135–143.

Nagtegaal, J. E., M. W. Laurant, et al. (2000). Effects of melatonin on the quality of life in patients with delayed sleep phase syndrome. *Journal of Psychosomatic Research, 48*(1), 45–50.

National Sleep Foundation. (2000). *Adolescent Sleep Needs and Patterns: Research Report and Resource Guide.* Washington, DC: National Sleep Foundation.

National Sleep Foundation. (2006). *2006 Sleep In America Poll Summary Findings.* Accessed July 3, 2008 at http,//www.sleepfoundation.org/sites/default/files/2006_summary_of_findings.pdf, 2008.

Negriff, S., L. D. Dorn, et al. (2011). Morningness/eveningness, pubertal timing, and substance use in adolescent girls. *Psychiatry Research, 185*(3), 408–413.

Noland, H., J. H. Price, et al. (2009). Adolescents' sleep behaviors and perceptions of sleep. *Journal of School Health, 79*(5), 224–230.

Ohayon, M. (1997). Prevalence of DSM-IV diagnostic criteria of insomnia: Distinguishing insomnia related to mental disorders from sleep disorders. *Journal of Psychiatric Research, 31*(3), 333–346.

Ohayon, M. M., R. E. Roberts, et al. (2000). Prevalence and patterns of problematic sleep among older adolescents. *Journal of the American Academy of Child and Adolescent Psychiatry, 39*(12), 1549–1556.

Ohta, T., T. Iwata, et al. (1992). Daily activity and persistent sleep-wake schedule disorders. *Progress in Neuro-Psychopharmacology & Biological Psychiatry, 16*(4), 529–537.

Okawa, M., M. Uchiyama, et al. (1998a). Circadian rhythm sleep disorders in adolescents: Clinical trials of combined treatments based on chronobiology. *Psychiatry and Clinical Neurosciences, 52*(5), 483–490.

Okawa, M., M. Uchiyama, et al. (1998b). Melatonin treatment for circadian rhythm sleep disorders. *Psychiatry and Clinical Neurosciences, 52*(2), 259–260.

Okawa, M., & Uchiyama, M. (2007). Circadian rhythm sleep disorders: Characteristics and entrainment pathology in delayed sleep phase and non-24-h sleep-wake syndrome. *Sleep Medicine Reviews, 11*(6), 485–496.

Oldani, A., L. Ferini-Strambi, et al. (1994). Melatonin and delayed sleep phase syndrome: Ambulatory polygraphic evaluation. *Neuroreport, 6*(1), 132–134.

Oren, D. A., & Wehr, T. A. (1992). Hypernyctohemeral syndrome after chronotherapy for delayed sleep phase syndrome. *New England Journal of Medicine, 327*(24), 1762.

Ouyang, F., B. S. Lu, et al. (2009). Sleep patterns among rural Chinese twin adolescents. *Sleep Medicine, 10*(4), 479–489.

Owens, J. A., K. Belon, et al. (2010). Impact of delaying school start time on adolescent sleep, mood, and behavior. *Archives of Pediatrics & Adolescent Medicine, 164*(7), 608–614.

Ozaki, S., M. Uchiyama, et al. (1996). Prolonged interval from body temperature nadir to sleep offset in patients with delayed sleep phase syndrome. *Sleep, 19*(1), 36–40.

Pack, A. I., A. M. Pack, et al. (1995). Characteristics of crashes attributed to the driver having fallen asleep. *Accident Analysis & Prevention, 27*(6), 769–775.

Pandi-Perumal, S. R., M. Smits, et al. (2007). Dim light melatonin onset (DLMO): A tool for the analysis of circadian phase in human sleep and chronobiological disorders. *Progress in Neuro-Psychopharmacology & Biological Psychiatry, 31*(1), 1–11.

Patten, S. B., & W. M. Lauderdale (1992). Delayed sleep phase disorder after traumatic brain injury. *Journal of the American Academy of Child and Adolescent Psychiatry, 31*(1), 100–102.

Pelayo, R., M. Thorpy, et al. (1988). Prevalence of delayed sleep phase disorder among adolescents. *Sleep, 17*, 392.

Pereira, D. S., S. Tufik, et al. (2005). Association of the length polymorphism in the human Per3 gene with the delayed sleep-phase syndrome: Does latitude have an influence upon it? Sleep, 28(1), 29–32.

Piggins, H. D. (2002). Human clock genes. *Annals of Medicine, 34*(5), 394–400.

Quinto, C., C. Gellido, et al. (2000). Posttraumatic delayed sleep phase syndrome. *Neurology, 54*(1), 250–252.

Rahman, S. A., L. Kayumov, et al. (2009). Clinical efficacy of dim light melatonin onset testing in diagnosing delayed sleep phase syndrome. *Sleep Medicine, 10*(5), 549–555.

Rahman, S. A., L. Kayumov, et al. (2010). Antidepressant action of melatonin in the treatment of Delayed Sleep Phase Syndrome. *Sleep Medicine, 11*(2), 131–136.

Ralph, M. R., R. G. Foster, et al. (1990). Transplanted suprachiasmatic nucleus determines circadian period. *Science, 247*(4945), 975–978.

Regestein, Q., & Monk, T. H. (1995). Delayed sleep phase syndrome: A review of its clinical aspects. *American Journal of Psychiatry, 152*(4), 602–608.

Regestein, Q. R., & Pavlova, M. (1995). Treatment of delayed sleep phase syndrome. *General Hospital Psychiatry, 17*(5), 335–345.

Revell, V. L., & Eastman, C. I. (2005). How to trick mother nature into letting you fly around or stay up all night. *Journal of Biological Rhythms, 20*(4), 353–365.

Revell, V. L., H. J. Burgess, et al. (2006). Advancing human circadian rhythms with afternoon melatonin and morning intermittent bright light. *Journal of Clinical Endocrinology & Metabolism, 91*(1), 54–59.

Revell, V. L., Molina, T. A., & Eastman, C.I. (2012). Human phase response curve to intermittent blue light using a commercially available device (in press). *Journal of Physiology, 590*(Pt 19), 4859–4868.

Robilliard, D. L., S. N. Archer, et al. (2002). The 3111 Clock gene polymorphism is not associated with sleep and circadian rhythmicity in phenotypically characterized human subjects. *Journal of Sleep Research, 11*(4), 305–312.

Roenneberg, T., T. Kuehnle, et al. (2004). A marker for the end of adolescence. *Current Biology, 14*(24), R1038–1039.

Rosenthal, N. E., J. R. Joseph-Vanderpool, et al. (1990). Phase-shifting effects of bright morning light as treatment for delayed sleep phase syndrome. *Sleep, 13*(4), 354–361.

Rybak, Y. E., H. E. McNeely, et al. (2006). An open trial of light therapy in adult attention-deficit/hyperactivity disorder. *Journal of Clinical Psychiatry, 67*(10), 1527–1535.

Sack, R. L., D. Auckley, et al. (2007a). Circadian rhythm sleep disorders: Part I, basic principles, shift work and jet lag disorders. An American Academy of Sleep Medicine review. *Sleep, 30*(11), 1460–1483.

Sack, R. L., D. Auckley, et al. (2007b). Circadian rhythm sleep disorders: Part II, advanced sleep phase disorder, delayed sleep phase disorder, free-running disorder, and irregular sleep-wake rhythm. An American Academy of Sleep Medicine review. *Sleep, 30*(11), 1484–1501.

Sadeh, A., R. E. Dahl, et al. (2009). Sleep and the transition to adolescence: A longitudinal study. *Sleep, 32*(12), 1602–1609.

Samaranayake, C. B., A. Fernando, et al. (2010). Outcome of combined melatonin and bright light treatments for delayed sleep phase disorder. *Australian and New Zealand Journal of Psychiatry, 44*(7), 676.

Saxvig, I. W., S. Pallesen, et al. (2012). Prevalence and correlates of delayed sleep phase in high school students. *Sleep Medicine, 13*(2), 193–199.

Schrader, H., G. Bovim, et al. (1993). The prevalence of delayed and advanced sleep phase syndromes. *Journal of Sleep Research, 2*(1), 51–55.

Seabra, M. L., M. Bignotto, et al. (2000). Randomized, double-blind clinical trial, controlled with placebo, of the toxicology of chronic melatonin treatment. *Journal of Pineal Research, 29*(4), 193–200.

Sharkey, K. M., M. A. Carskadon, et al. (2011). Effects of an advanced sleep schedule and morning short wavelength light exposure on circadian phase in young adults with late sleep schedules. *Sleep Medicine, 12*(7), 685–692.

Shibui, K., M. Uchiyama, et al. (1999). Melatonin rhythms in delayed sleep phase syndrome. *Journal of Biological Rhythms, 14*(1), 72–76.

Shibui, K., Uchiyama, M., Kim, K., Tagaya, H., Kuriyama, K., Suzukim H., et al. (2003). Melatonin, cortisol and thyroid-stimulating hormone rhythms are delayed in patients with delayed sleep phase syndrome. *Sleep and Biological Rhythms, 1*, 209–214.

Shirayama, M., Y. Shirayama, et al. (2003). The psychological aspects of patients with delayed sleep phase syndrome (DSPS). *Sleep Medicine, 4*(5), 427–433.

Smith, M. R., V. L. Revell, et al. (2009). Phase advancing the human circadian clock with blue-enriched polychromatic light. *Sleep Medicine, 10*(3), 287–294.

Smits, M. G., E. E. Nagtegaal, et al. (2001). Melatonin for chronic sleep onset insomnia in children: A randomized placebo-controlled trial. *Journal of Child Neurology, 16*(2), 86–92.

Smits, M. G., H. F. van Stel, et al. (2003). Melatonin improves health status and sleep in children with idiopathic chronic sleep-onset insomnia: A randomized placebo-controlled trial. *Journal of the American Academy of Child and Adolescent Psychiatry, 42*(11), 1286–1293.

Staton, D. (2008). The impairment of pediatric bipolar sleep: Hypotheses regarding a core defect and phenotype-specific sleep disturbances. *Journal of Affective Disorders, 108*(3), 199–206.

Stephan, F. K., & Zucker, I. (1972). Circadian rhythms in drinking behavior and locomotor activity of rats are eliminated by hypothalamic lesions. *Proceedings of the National Academy of Sciences USA, 69*(6), 1583–1586.

Szeinberg, A., K. Borodkin, et al. (2006). Melatonin treatment in adolescents with delayed sleep phase syndrome. *Clinical Pediatrics (Philadelphia), 45*(9), 809–818.

Takahashi, Y., H. Hohjoh, et al. (2000). Predisposing factors in delayed sleep phase syndrome. *Psychiatry & Clinical Neurosciences, 54*(3), 356–358.

Takano, A., M. Uchiyama, et al. (2004). A missense variation in human casein kinase I epsilon gene that induces functional alteration and shows an inverse association with circadian rhythm sleep disorders. *Neuropsychopharmacology, 29*(10), 1901–1909.

Taylor, A., Wright, H. R., & Lack, L. C. (2008). Sleeping-in on the weekend delays circadian phase and increases sleepiness the following week. *Sleep and Biological Rhythms, 6*, 172–179.

Terman, M., & Jiuan Su, T. (2010). Circadian rhythm phase advance with dawn simulation treatment for winter depression. *Journal of Biological Rhythms, 25*(4), 297–301.

Thorpy, M. J., E. Korman, et al. (1998). Delayed sleep phase syndrome in adolescents. *Journal of Adolescent Health Care, 9*(1), 22–27.

Turner, J., L. M. Drummond, et al. (2007). A prospective study of delayed sleep phase syndrome in patients with severe resistant obsessive-compulsive disorder. *World Psychiatry, 6*(2), 108–111.

Uchiyama, M., M. Okawa, et al. (2000a). Altered phase relation between sleep timing and core body temperature rhythm in delayed sleep phase syndrome and non-24-hour sleep-wake syndrome in humans. *Neuroscience Letters, 294*(2), 101–104.

Uchiyama, M., M. Okawa, et al. (2000b). Poor compensatory function for sleep loss as a pathogenic factor in patients with delayed sleep phase syndrome. *Sleep, 23*(4), 553–558.

Urban, R., T. Magyarodi, et al. (2011). Morningness-eveningness, chronotypes and health-impairing behaviors in adolescents. *Chronobiology International, 28*(3), 238–247.

Uruha, S., Mikami, A. Teshima, Y. Sugita, Y. Honda, H. Inatani, K., et al. (1987). Effect of triazolam for delayed sleep phase syndrome [abstract]. *Sleep Research, 16*, 650.

Valcavi, R., M. Zini, et al. (1993). Melatonin stimulates growth hormone secretion through pathways other than the growth hormone-releasing hormone. *Clinical Endocrinology (Oxford), 39*(2), 193–199.

Van der Heijden, K. B., M. G. Smits, et al. (2005). Idiopathic chronic sleep onset insomnia in attention-deficit/hyperactivity disorder: A circadian rhythm sleep disorder. *Chronobiology International, 22*(3), 559–570.

Van der Heijden, K. B., M. G. Smits, et al. (2007). Effect of melatonin on sleep, behavior, and cognition in ADHD and chronic sleep-onset insomnia. *Journal of the American Academy of Child and Adolescent Psychiatry, 46*(2), 233–241.

van Geijlswijk, I. M., H. P. Korzilius, et al. (2010). The use of exogenous melatonin in delayed sleep phase disorder: A meta-analysis. *Sleep, 33*(12), 1605–1614.

Wahlstrom, K. (1999). The prickly politics of school starting times. *Phi Delta Kappan, 80*(5), 344–347.

Wahlstrom, K. (2002). Changing times: Findings from the first longitudinal study of later high school start times. *NASSP Bulletin 86*(633), 3–21.

Wasdell, M. B., J. E. Jan, et al. (2008). A randomized, placebo-controlled trial of controlled release melatonin treatment of delayed sleep phase syndrome and impaired sleep maintenance in children with neurodevelopmental disabilities. *Journal of Pineal Research, 44*(1), 57–64.

Watanabe, T., N. Kajimura, et al. (1999). Effects of phototherapy in patients with delayed sleep phase syndrome. *Psychiatry and Clinical Neurosciences, 53*(2), 231–233.

Watanabe, T., N. Kajimura, et al. (2003). Sleep and circadian rhythm disturbances in patients with delayed sleep phase syndrome. *Sleep, 26*(6), 657–661.

Waterhouse, J., & DeCoursey, P. J. (2004). *Chronobiology: Biological Timekeeping.* Sunderland, MA: Sinauer Associates, Inc.

Weiss, M. D., M. B. Wasdell, et al. (2006). Sleep hygiene and melatonin treatment for children and adolescents with ADHD and initial insomnia. *Journal of the American Academy of Child and Adolescent Psychiatry, 45*(5), 512–519.

Weitzman, E. D., C. A. Czeisler, et al. (1981). Delayed sleep phase syndrome. A chronobiological disorder with sleep-onset insomnia. *Archives of General Psychiatry, 38*(7), 737–746.

Welsh, D. K., D. E. Logothetis, et al. (1995). Individual neurons dissociated from rat suprachiasmatic nucleus express independently phased circadian firing rhythms. *Neuron, 14*(4), 697–706.

Weyerbrock, A., J. Timmer, et al. (1996). Effects of light and chronotherapy on human circadian rhythms in delayed sleep phase syndrome, cytokines, cortisol, growth hormone, and the sleep-wake cycle. *Biological Psychiatry, 40*(8), 794–797.

Wirz-Justice, A., H. J. Haug, et al. (2001). Disturbed circadian rest-activity cycles in schizophrenia patients, an effect of drugs? *Schizophrenia Bulletin, 27*(3), 497–502.

Wirz-Justice, A., F. Benedetti, et al. (2009). *Chronotherapeutics for Affective Disorders, A Clinician's Manual for Light and Wake Therapy.* Basel, Switzerland: S. Karger AG.

Wolfson, A. R., O. Tzischinsky, et al. (1995). Sleep, behavior, and stress at the transition to senior high school [abstract]. *Sleep Research, 24.*

Wolfson, A. R., & Carskadon, M. A. (1998). Sleep schedules and daytime functioning in adolescents. *Child Development, 69*(4), 875–887.

Wyatt, J. K. (2004). Delayed sleep phase syndrome: Pathophysiology and treatment options. *Sleep, 27*(6), 1195–1203.

Wyatt, J. K., E. J. Stepanski, et al. (2006). Circadian phase in delayed sleep phase syndrome: Predictors and temporal stability across multiple assessments. *Sleep, 29*(8), 1075–1080.

Xu, Y., Q. S. Padiath, et al. (2005). Functional consequences of a CKIdelta mutation causing familial advanced sleep phase syndrome. *Nature, 434*(7033), 640–644.

Yamadera, H., K. Takahashi, et al. (1996). A multicenter study of sleep-wake rhythm disorders: Clinical features of sleep-wake rhythm disorders. *Psychiatry and Clinical Neurosciences, 50*(4), 195–201.

Yazaki, M., S. Shirakawa, et al. (1999). Demography of sleep disturbances associated with circadian rhythm disorders in Japan. *Psychiatry and Clinical Neurosciences, 53*(2), 267–268.

CHAPTER

24 Nighttime Distractions: Fears, Nightmares, and Parasomnias

Anna Ivanenko *and* Kymberly Larson

Abstract

This chapter encompasses a discussion of nighttime fears, nightmares, and parasomnias in healthy, normally developing children and among children with anxiety disorders. Prevalence, presentation, differential diagnosis, and treatment are discussed from a developmental perspective. The relationship between anxiety disorders and sleep is discussed, highlighting the anxiety disorders most commonly associated with nighttime fears and nightmares: generalized anxiety disorder (GAD), separation anxiety, and post-traumatic stress disorder (PTSD).

Key Words: nighttime fears, nightmares, anxiety disorders, parasomnias, sleep disorders, bedtime resistance

Introduction

Sleep disorders are common across the life span and affect healthy individuals as well as those with compromised health. In children, sleep disorders manifest in myriad ways, from fearfulness to the inability to sleep or the propensity to sleep too much, to autonomic, neuromuscular, respiratory, behavioral, social, and academic dysfunction. Two of the most prevalent yet benign sleep disturbances in the pediatric population are the experience of nighttime fears and nightmares. Nighttime fears are a heterogeneous group of fears that children experience before sleep onset and during nocturnal awakenings. Nighttime fears are normal and typically short-lived. The specific content of a child's nocturnal fear(s) is typically related to their neurocognitive development. Nightmares are dream sequences of distressful content that occur during REM sleep and frequently result in waking in an unpleasant emotional state. Often children have difficulty falling back to sleep after a nightmare, for fear the nightmare will continue. Parasomnias are sleep disorders that present with behavioral or physiological events associated with both REM and NREM sleep, as well as transitions from one sleep state to another. Although for the most part parasomnias have a benign clinical course, they can present with dramatic behavioral manifestations that can be potentially dangerous to the child or his environment and require thorough assessment and treatment. Nocturnal fears, nightmares, and parasomnias are more prevalent among children with psychiatric disorders and should be addressed as part of a comprehensive evaluation and treatment plan for those children who suffer from both sleep and psychiatric comorbidities.

This chapter will provide an overview of prevalence, clinical characteristics, evaluation, and treatment of nocturnal fears and parasomnias in children and adolescents across different stages of their development. Interaction between nighttime fears, parasomnias, and common psychiatric disorders will be discussed.

Nighttime Fears

In normally developing children, the experience of nighttime fears is quite prevalent. Muris et al.

(2001) conducted a study of nighttime fears in children and concluded that 58.8% of 4–6-year-olds, 84.7% of 7–9-year-olds, and 79.6% of 10–12-year-olds reported nocturnal fears. Mindell and Owens (2010) report in a more recent study that 64% of children ages 8–16 had reported nighttime fears. They describe a relationship between age and propensity to experience nighttime fears, in that 79% of children reported nocturnal fears versus 49% of adolescents. Less common are severe nighttime fears, reported in 20%–30% of children. For most children, nighttime fears can be conceptualized as a normal and benign aspect of childhood, stressful at times but with no appreciable long-term effects. However, if the child's experience of nighttime fears begins to interfere with his quantity and quality of sleep, or when found accompanying comorbid sleep or psychiatric disorders, even nighttime fears may have deleterious effects upon a child's physical and mental health, academic performance, impulse control and risk-taking behavior, and/or social functioning (Alfano & Gamble, 2009; Mindell & Owens, 2010; Kushnir & Sadeh, 2011). Children with nighttime fears also present with accompanying sleep disturbances, including difficulty falling asleep, frequent night wakings, and difficulty returning to sleep (Gordon, King, Gullone, Muris, & Ollendick, 2007a; Sadeh, 2005; Gordon, King, Gullone, Muris & Ollendick, 2007b; Blader, Koplewicz, Abikoff & Foley, 1997). Kushnir and Sadeh (2011) conducted an instrumental assessment of sleep using actigraphy and demonstrated that children with nighttime fears experience shorter periods of continuous sleep, more frequent night wakings, less true sleep time, and a decrease in sleep efficiency.

Nighttime fears are considered a normal part of development, typically surfacing around the ages of 3 to 6, as a child's cognitive development sets the stage for the realization of both real-world and imaginary harm (Stores, 2007). Younger children tend toward more imaginary fears such as monsters, whereas older children tend to fear burglars, robbers, or other potentially real home invaders or natural disasters like hurricanes or tornadoes. Children of all ages appear to be plagued by nocturnal fears of "the dark," daily stressors, and the welfare of loved ones. Typically, parental reassurance is enough to quell the fears and the child grows out of such nighttime fears by the end of grade school. However, as mentioned before, if severe and/or frequent enough, nighttime fears can affect a child's daytime functioning as well as that of family members (Keller, Buckhalt, & El-Sheikh, 2008).

Factors associated with pediatric nighttime fears in healthy children include trauma, stress, family conflict, and parental anxiety. Children with anxiety disorders (especially separation anxiety, generalized anxiety [previously *overanxious disorder of childhood*], and specific phobias) are much more likely to experience severe nighttime fears. Girls (73%) are also more likely to report nocturnal fears than their male (55%) peers (Mindell & Owens, 2010).

The presentation of nighttime fears varies across chronological and developmental age, as well as individual differences, but commonly includes bedtime resistance, prolonged sleep onset, night wakings, fearful behaviors, and frequent requests for items or actions from caregivers after bedtime. Extended bouts of crying and panic are commonplace. Graziano and Mooney (1980) describe bedtime as a "highly emotional and disruptive nightly event, with delays and battles often lasting well beyond midnight." These children may also manifest somatic complaints and/or diurnal fears. Often children's fears are alleviated by the presence of a parent or sibling; consequently the entire family system may well be affected by one child's nocturnal fears (Kushnir & Sadeh, 2011, 2012).

Nightmares

The experience of fear after the onset of sleep can be classified as nightmares or night terrors. Whereas nightmares are ubiquitous in the pediatric population with 75% of children reporting such an experience, night terrors are reported in only 1%–6% of children ages 4 to 12 (Mindell & Owens, 2010). Nightmares are considered scary dreams that awaken a child from REM sleep, whereas night terrors are described as "a sudden episode of terror (that) occurs during sleep, usually initiated by cry or loud scream that is accompanied by autonomic nervous system and behavioral manifestations of intense fear." Night terrors are also associated with at least one of the following: "1. Difficulty in arousing the person, 2. Mental confusion when awakened from the episode, 3. Amnesia (partial or complete) for the episode and/or Dangerous or potentially dangerous behaviors" (AASM, 2005).

Nightmares are quite common, with 87%–96% of 7–9–years-olds reported experiencing bad dreams sometimes or often (Muris, Merckelbach, & Gadet, & Moulaert, 2000). Many young children seek out their parents for support following a nightmare. Chronic nightmares are less frequent; with 24% of children aged 2–4 and 41% of children aged 6–10 experiencing nightmares for 3 months or more.

Parents of preschoolers indicate that only 1.9% to 3.9% of their children suffer from chronic nightmares. There is a decreasing prevalence with age, with 28% of 5–8-year-olds, 23% of 9–11-year-olds, and 10% of 12–14-year-olds reporting nightmares at least once every 6 months (Simonds, Parraga 1982). Prior to age 13, the prevalence rates of nightmares is roughly equal in boys and girls; however, after age 13 girls are much more likely to continue experiencing nightmares (Nielsen et al., 2000).

Like nocturnal fears, the content of a child's nightmare is dependent, in part, upon the child's neurocognitive development. Common childhood nightmares include being separated from one's parents, enduring physical harm from imaginary creatures like the boogeyman or "bad guys" from television, or stressful recent and/or impending events. Negative emotions such as fear, anxiety, sadness, anger, disgust, and embarrassment are associated with the experience of nightmares. Precipitating factors include prior nightmares, daytime stressors and anxiety, trauma, sleep deprivation, insomnia, and anxiety disorders. Certain medications like antidepressants, benzodiazepines, or psychostimulants effecting REM sleep may also increase the propensity for a child to suffer from nightmares (Stores, 2007).

When children experience nightmares they frequently seek out parental support, fear returning to sleep, and remember details from their frightening dreams. They are typically lucid enough to explain to their parent(s) portions of the dream and their accompanying emotions. Daytime features of children with chronic nightmares include bedtime resistance, nocturnal and/or diurnal fears, and other symptoms of anxiety such as excessive worrying, restlessness, and irritability (Stores, 2007; Mindell & Owens, 2010).

Nightmares of high frequency and/or intense severity may be classified as Nightmare Disorder (307.47) in the American Academy of Sleep Medicine's (AASM) *International Classification of Sleep Disorders: Diagnostic and Coding Manual*, 2nd edition (ICSD-2). A diagnosis of Nightmare Disorder must meet the following criteria:

A. Recurrent episodes of awakening from sleep with recall of intensely disturbing dream mentation, usually involving fear or anxiety, but also anger, sadness, disgust, and other dysphoric emotions.

B. Full alertness on awakening, with little confusion or disorientation; recall of sleep mentation is immediate and clear.

C. At least one of the following associated features is present:

1. Delayed return to sleep after the episodes
2. Occurrence of episodes in the latter half of the habitual sleep period. (AASM, 2005)

For the most part, parental reassurance, a nightlight, and/or security objects are all that is necessary to help a child who experiences nightmares. For preschool and school-age children, simple behavioral techniques can be used as well, such as retelling the dream with a humorous ending (cognitive restructuring) or providing "monster spray," "magic wands," dreamcatchers, or other protective items. Also, parents should utilize preventative measures such as limiting scary stimuli prior to bed (stories, movies, pictures, etc.), relaxation techniques and other stress-reducing activities, as well as ensuring that the child gets enough sleep every night. The deleterious effects of sleep deprivation on children include an increased propensity to experience these and other parasomnias (Kotagal, 2012). If such techniques do not alleviate the nightmares, referral to a mental health provider is warranted to rule out a psychiatric disorder, underlying stressors or trauma, as well as to obtain recommendations for more substantive behavioral strategies.

Nocturnal Fears and Nightmares in Preschool Children

As a child's imagination develops, so too does his or her arsenal of potential fears. Suddenly, being alone is stress-producing: "the dark" becomes a playground for the unseen and insidious. Nighttime fears are common among preschool children: 58.8% of 4_6-year-old children report nocturnal fears (Muris et al., 2001). These frequently interfere with going to sleep and staying asleep, and cause nocturnal awakenings. Persistent nocturnal anxiety has been associated with severe nighttime fears (Gordon et al., 2007a, 2007b; King et al., 1997; Muris et al., 2001; Sadeh, 2005). Although nighttime fears do not constitute a formal diagnostic entity, they can cause development of behavioral insomnia. Anything and everything can become scary: a well visit to the pediatrician can become the impetus for fears of blood, needles, strangers, and pain. A summer storm through the eyes of a four year-old may be akin to Armageddon, with thunder the death-knell warning of perilous winds and bolts of fire to come. As creative as their fears, so too are the preschoolers' manifestations of reassurance-seeking. Suddenly a child is thirsty, hungry, lonely, itchy, hot, cold, and, of course, has to go to the bathroom. Children are seeking the reassurance of their caregivers that they are safe and will continue to be safe once their eyes are closed and they drift off to sleep. Parental presence in the child's bedroom is a common strategy to deal with nighttime fears. Co-sleeping is another type of parental behavior aimed to reduce nocturnal anxiety and to provide reassurance. In some cases these strategies have been associated with positive outcomes (Johnson, 1991; Rath & Okum, 1995) and in some they have reinforced long-term co-sleeping (Medoff & Schaefer, 1993).

Most prevalence studies of nightmares concern children age 5 years or older. Studies of nightmares in preschoolers are based mainly on parental reports. Longitudinal studies of nightmares across different developmental stages are essentially absent. One small retrospective study indicated that 13.5% of preschool children have bad dreams at least once per week (Hawkins & Williams, 1992). Longitudinal logistic regression analysis models were used in a large study of bad dreams in preschool children to investigate prevalence, demographic characteristics, risk, and protective factors (Simard et al., 2008). The authors found lower than expected prevalence of mother-reported frequent bad dreams (1.3% to 3.9%). Early protective factors included parental practices favoring nurturance after nocturnal awakening. Risk factors included sleep-onset emotional nurturance, anxiousness, and difficult temperament (Simard et al., 2008).

Often children who experience recurrent bad dreams become afraid to go to sleep for fear of nightmares (Mindell & Owens, 2010), although the relationship between nightmares and insomnia has not been thoroughly studied in children.

Discussing the content of their nightmares can be beneficial if done during the day, as well as giving a child a sense of control over their fears. A preschooler can learn to laugh at the silly monster that once terrified her, or look forward to the next storm while he visualizes his kite flying through the tumultuous skies. Relaxation techniques, systematic desensitization, and cognitive behavioral modification can all be effectively used with preschoolers.

Nocturnal Fears and Nightmares in School-Age Children

As children develop, their awareness of the real world increases exponentially and with it, their realization of the numerous entities that can cause harm to them and their loved ones. A cross-sectional study of bad dreams showed a peak prevalence between 7 and 9 years with 87% to 95.7% of children reporting having bad dreams often or sometimes (Hawkins & Williams, 1992). Other studies estimated prevalence of bad dreams at 41% (Salzarulo & Chevalier, 1983) and 23% (Simonds & Parraga, 1982) among 6–10–year-olds and 9–11-year-olds, respectively.

Children at this age seem especially concerned about robbers, burglars, and other home invaders, as well as natural disasters including hurricanes and tornadoes (Mindell & Owens, 2010). They also succumb to fears about supernatural phenomena: witches, vampires, ghosts, and other beasties that may be lurking in the night. School-age children also begin to feel (and fear) social inequities, so performance anxiety related to academics, athletics, or social activities becomes relevant.

Nightmares reflect this variety of real-world fears as well as previous or upcoming stressors such as first sleepovers, impending exams, or being sent to the principal. Also, stories, movies, and books with frightening content are often played out in a child's dreams. Nocturnal fears manifest as bedtime resistance or refusal and reassurance-seeking in the form of repetitive requests for drinks, snacks, the addition or removal of blankets, special toys, nightlights, and so forth. In a recent study of school-age children with sleep problems and normal controls, bedtime resistance, sleep anxiety, night wakings and nighttime fears were significantly predictive of co-sleeping (Cortesi et al., 2008). Parental reassurance and reinforcement for appropriate coping strategies and limit setting are most beneficial for this age group.

Nocturnal Fears and Nightmares in Adolescents

Prevalence of nightmares and nocturnal fears decreases during adolescence, but it is important to consider the variability in reporting styles of adolescents (Simonds & Parraga, 1982; Nielsen et al., 2000). In a recent large survey conducted among 90,081 Japanese adolescents, the prevalence rate of nightmares was as high as 32.5% (Munezawa et al., 2011). Multiple logistic analyses revealed that female sex, use of alcohol, poor mental health, difficulty initiating sleep, low subjective sleep assessment, presence of excessive daytime sleepiness, and presence of sleep paralysis had higher odds ratios for nightmares.

Often teens will not report to their parents or health care providers anything they may consider to be a weakness or something they "should have" grown out of. Adolescents who report nocturnal fears and nightmares describe more future-oriented and abstract fears, such as college acceptance or "the unknown" (Mindell & Owens, 2010). Adolescents also remain concerned with academic, athletic, and social performance, which is reflected in the content of their nightmares. Adolescents often attempt to avoid sleeping by distracting themselves with television, computers, reading, and so forth. They may also use wake-promoting or sleep-inducing substances to avoid feeling sleepy and thus susceptible to their fears. Parental involvement should include a discussion of safety and the importance of sleep, limit setting, and reinforcement of appropriate coping strategies.

Anxiety Disorders and Sleep

Children with nighttime fears and/or nightmares often have comorbid sleep disruptions or disorders such as night terrors or behavioral insomnia, as well as psychiatric disorders such as anxiety, depression, and/or attention-deficit hyperactivity disorder (ADHD) (Alfano & Gamble, 2009). Many of these disorders share symptoms such as bedtime resistance. To treat a child effectively, diagnostic accuracy is paramount. Careful interviews with the child and parent(s), as well as the use of parental and self-reports, questionnaires, and sleep diaries, will help elucidate the diagnostic picture. If necessary, more objective measures such as polysomnography (PSG) or neuropsychological testing will help to delineate psychiatric and physiological symptoms (Sheldon, 2005). For instance, if a child is experiencing bedtime-related anxiety, it is important to ask specific questions regarding the nature of the anxiety: does it involve falling asleep or staying asleep? If so, it may be psychophysiologic insomnia (see Roane and Taylor, Chapter 22). Is the anxiety dream-related? If so, the child is more likely to be experiencing nightmares. Are the fears developmentally appropriate, short-lived, and benign? If so, it is likely nighttime fears. If the anxiety occurs during the day as well as night, then the child should be assessed for an anxiety disorder (Mindell & Owens, 2010; Alfano & Gamble, 2009).

Childhood psychiatric disorders are often found in children with sleep disorders and, similarly, children with sleep disturbances or disorders are often found to meet criteria for a psychiatric disorder as well. This bidirectional relationship between sleep and psychopathology is most commonly observed in childhood anxiety disorders: generalized anxiety disorder (GAD), previously known as *overanxious disorder of childhood*, separation anxiety, social anxiety, and post-traumatic stress disorder (PTSD) (Alfano & Gamble, 2009). In the last 10 years, research has shown that early childhood sleep disruptions maybe predictive of later emotional and behavioral symptoms and disorders, including anxiety and depression, inattention, and hyperactivity (Gregory et al., 2004; Gregory & O'Connor, 2002; Johnson et al., 2000).

Anxiety is the most common childhood psychiatric disorder, affecting up to 20% of children (Costello et al., 2005; Shaffer et al., 1996) and includes GAD, separation anxiety disorder, PTSD, panic disorder, social phobias (social anxiety disorder), agoraphobia, specific phobias, obsessive-compulsive disorder, acute stress disorder, and others. These disorders are concomitant with severe distress and morbidity and frequently are associated with significant disruptions in a child's home, school, and social lives. Children with anxiety disorders are more likely to suffer from mood and anxiety disorders later in life and are also at an increased risk for future suicide attempts and psychiatric hospitalizations (Pine et al., 1998). In children with sleep disorders, the most commonly associated comorbid anxiety disorders include GAD, separation anxiety disorder, and PTSD.

Alfano and colleagues (2007) found that 88% of children ages 6–17 with non-trauma-related anxiety disorders experience at least one sleep-related disturbance; however, the majority experienced three or more sleep problems (Alfano, Ginsgurg, & Kingery 2007). Insomnia, nightmares, and refusal/reluctance to sleep alone were the most frequently mentioned sleep disturbances in her study. She also found that 95% of parents whose children have been diagnosed with an anxiety disorder report comorbid sleep disturbances (Alfano et al., 2007).

Biological and environmental factors also influence the bidirectional relationship between sleep disorders and anxiety. It is well known that there is a genetic predisposition for psychiatric disorders in general to be passed from one generation to the next. In addition to a biological predisposition, childhood behaviors are also impacted by the environment in which the child is raised. For example, an anxious parent may be so overinvolved in their child's daily routines that the child may not learn independence. At bedtime this may result in the child never learning to self-soothe, manage developmentally appropriate fears and stressors, or even to develop the ability to identify when she becomes sleepy. When this child is confronted with a stressor she will not have developed an appropriate coping strategy and may likely react in an unhealthy and anxiety-producing manner. This child, physiologically predisposed to anxiety, now also has "learned" anxiety. There are also metabolic factors implicated in an anxious child's propensity to experience sleep disturbances. In Forbes' 2006 study, the dysregulation of the hypothalamic pituitary adrenal (HPA) loop was indicated in altering the timing and architecture of children's sleep, due to heightened cortisol levels just prior to sleep. Higher levels of cortisol were found in neither the depressed nor the control groups, indicating that the presence of extra cortisol may be a biological impetus for disorganized sleep in anxious children.

Generalized Anxiety Disorder/Overanxious Disorder of Childhood

The Forbes and colleagues' study (2008) describes the physiological changes that children with generalized anxiety disorder or overanxious disorder of childhood experience in sleep. These researchers followed children with anxiety disorders, depression, and a control group for 3 consecutive nights in a sleep lab and compared their polysomnography data. They found several differences between the groups. The children with anxiety had more nocturnal awakenings than the depressed children and less slow wave sleep than either the control group or the depressed children. Whereas the control group and the depressed children appeared to habituate to the sleep lab, the anxious children experienced greater sleep latency and took twice as long to fall asleep on the second night. They further found that sleep-related problems independently predict a child's functioning at home, after controlling for severity of anxiety (Alfano et al., 2007).

Separation Anxiety

It is normal for older infants to experience separation anxiety as their cognitive skills develop, often accompanied by increased bedtime resistance. It does not take long for the infant to realize, as object permanence crystallizes, that his parents still exist and will soon return. This realization often quells the fears of the older infant, and bedtime problems decrease again. However, if the child continues to experience separation anxiety his bedtime resistance will likely remain and evolve alongside his neurocognitive development (Mindell, Kuhn, Lewin, Meltzer, & Sadeh, 2006). Many children with separation anxiety experience sleep disturbances as well, including nightmares and nighttime fears. If a child's bedtime resistant behaviors are alleviated by the presence of the parent(s), then separation anxiety is most likely the cause of his resistance. Similarly, if the child engages in similar diurnal behaviors when he is isolated from his parent(s), the behavior is most likely caused by his separation anxiety. If the child's diurnal experience of anxiety does not directly involve the presence of his parent, than GAD is the most likely diagnosis.

Post-traumatic Stress Disorder (PTSD)

In both adults and children the experience of sleep disturbances following a traumatic event are common and include insomnia as well as parasomnias, such as nightmares, night terrors, sleep talking, and nocturnal enuresis. Sleep disturbances have been linked to numerous types of traumatic events in recent literature including war, sniper attacks, motor vehicle accidents, burn injuries, floods, and—the most common—childhood maltreatment and abuse (Charuvastra & Cloitre, 2009; Chimienti et al., 1989; Kravitz et al., 1993; Nader et al., 1990). Rimsza, Berg, and Locke (1988) found that childhood sexual abuse victims experienced sleep disturbances that correlated positively with both the duration of abuse as well as the age of abuse onset. Krakow et al. (2002) found in their longitudinal study that 10 years after the report of abuse, sleep disturbances correlated with depression and PTSD symptomology (see Spilsbury, Chapter 14). Interestingly, the abuse itself predicted the girls' sleep problems, even after controlling for symptoms of depression and PTSD. They purport it is the association between the environment in which most sexual abuse occurs and that in which sleep occurs (the bedroom, nighttime, sleep, the dark) that leads to sleep disturbances, because in order to achieve normal sleep one must feel an adequate sense of safety. Victims of sexual abuse are often deprived of this basic necessity, further sabotaging their sleep. Glod et al. (1997) found that childhood victims of trauma and/or abuse experience sleep disturbances whether they meet the criteria for PTSD or not.

Assessment of Nocturnal Fears and Anxiety in Children and Adolescents

Because inadequate sleep has been implicated in numerous psychiatric, medical, academic, and safety-related issues, it is imperative that clinicians learn to address sleep issues early and often throughout a child's development. Currently sleep disorders are frequently unrecognized and underreported (Ivanenko & Patwari, 2009), which underscores the need for primary care providers to obtain detailed and comprehensive sleep assessments. A full discussion of sleep assessment is beyond the scope of this chapter; however, a description of the various tools used in sleep diagnostics is discussed below. As mentioned previously, a thorough history and description of a child's sleep habits is imperative. Interviewing both the child and the parent(s) is necessary, as each reports their subjective experience of nighttime events. Parents tend to report problems that interrupt their own sleep, so they may be unaware of certain details regarding their child's sleep. Likewise, children often report experiences that their parents know nothing about. Parents of children with anxiety tend to report that their children experience more disruptive sleep than the children themselves report (Alfano, 2010; Forbes et al., 2008; Hudson et al., 2009). Parents and children may not view particular behaviors as problematic (i.e., snoring, inconsistent bedtimes, or limit setting). It is crucial to ask specific questions regarding sleep hygiene, bed and wake times, the time it takes a child to fall asleep (sleep latency), the difference between weekday and weekend sleep duration, night awakenings, time spent awake after sleep onset, and any other individualized information. Asking children and adolescents about their television viewing habits and the types of books they read and games they play can be a fruitful conversation when the child is experiencing nighttime fears or nightmares related to the content of such.

When assessing for sleep disorders, it is imperative to include neurodevelopmental, medical, and psychiatric data as well, as many conditions share symptoms with or exacerbate sleep disorders. Some medications like psychostimulants used to treat ADHD and selective serotonin reuptake inhibitors (SSRIs) used to treat anxiety and depression may disrupt sleep. A great accompaniment to a thorough history is a sleep diary. Have the child and/or parent (depending on age and developmental ability) complete a sleep diary for one to two weeks. Many of the aforementioned questions regarding timing of bed and sleep onset, wakings, and naps are answered in a graphical format to allow children and their parents to see the patterns of their sleep cycles.

Also of clinical utility is employing one of the many questionnaires available (see Spruyt, Chapter 18). These not only allow for comprehensive assessment across several fundamental domains in pediatric sleep, but also allow for longitudinal comparison over time in the same child. Judy Owens' *Children's Sleep Habits Questionnaire* (CHSQ; Owens et al., 2000a), the *Sleep Disturbance Scale for Children* (SDSC; Bruni et al., 1996), the *Pediatric Sleep Questionnaire* (PSQ; Chervin et al., 2000), and the *Sleep Disorder Inventory for Students* (SDIS; Lugienbuehl, 2004) are widely used measures for parental report. Owens' *Sleep Self Report* (SSR; Owens et al., 2000b) is a child report that corresponds with the CHSQ parental report. Other child-report sleep measures include the *School Sleep Habits Survey* (SSHS; Wolfson & Carskadon, 1998) and the *Pediatric Daytime Sleepiness Scale* (PDSS; Drake et al., 2003).

Sometimes the subjective ratings by the child and his parents are not enough to provide a comprehensive clinical picture of the child's sleep habits. If more objective data were required, for example in cases with a comorbid sleep-related breathing or movement disorder, actigraphy, polysomnography (PSG), or a multiple sleep latency test (MSLT) would provide such data. Actigraphy is a system for continuous monitoring of child movements used to estimate measures of sleep/wakefulness using a small device, typically worn on the wrist, for at least three consecutive 24-hour periods. Unlike actigraphy, PSG and MSLTs are typically performed in a sleep lab. PSG is a nocturnal sleep study which includes an electroencephalogram (EEG), electromyogram (EMG), and electro-oculogram (EOG), as well as measures of airflow, respiratory and abdominal efforts, oxygen saturation, end tidal CO^2 level, and limb muscle activity (Ivanenko & Massie, 2006). The MSLT is a diurnal test that assesses levels of daytime sleepiness by having a child take successive naps every two hours following their last morning awakening recorded on the PSG.

Treatment of Nocturnal Fears in Children and Adolescents

Like many other pediatric sleep disorders, nighttime fears and nightmares are treated nonpharmacologically. Cognitive and behavioral interventions include parental education regarding sleep hygiene, limit setting, and consistent bedtime routines, as well as specific approaches such as extinction and scheduled wakings. Therapy can help children acquire self-soothing and coping mechanisms that will prevent further distress and anxiety. Developmentally appropriate guidelines regarding sleep hygiene—bedtime, wake time, and nap times, usage of caffeine or other stimulants as well as evening use of television, video games, computers, and cell phones—should be reviewed with the child. The child should be an active participant in setting up a new bedtime routine. Graziano and Mooney's study on the reduction of nighttime fears in children ages 6–12 purports that parent-supervised self-control techniques, consisting of muscle relaxation, guided imagery, the recitation of "brave" self-statements and token reinforcement, significantly reduce children's experience of nighttime fears (Graziano & Mooney, 1980). McMenamy and Katz (1989) replicated the study with children aged 4–5 with similar results, indicating that training children in relaxation, self-guided coping skills, and guided imagery are effective treatments for those with severe nighttime fears. In their most recent study using both subjective and objective assessment of sleep with actigraphy, Kushnir and Sadeh (2012) demonstrated that simple doll interventions can reduce nocturnal fears and associated sleep disruptions. A full discussion of treatment is beyond the scope of this chapter; for further reading please see *Part 7: Prevention and Intervention* in this volume.

Parasomnias

There are currently two main classification systems of sleep disorders. In the psychiatric nosology, *DSM-IV*-TR defines parasomnias as "disorders characterized by abnormal behavioral or physiological events occurring in association with sleep, specific sleep stages, or sleep-wake transition," (DSM-IV–TR, 2000).

International Classification for Sleep Disorders, 2nd Edition (ICSD-2) defines parasomnias as "undesirable physical phenomena that occur predominantly during sleep" (AASM, 2005). According to ICSD-2, parasomnias are subdivided into four categories:

- Arousal disorders
- Sleep–wake transition disorders
- Parasomnias usually associated with REM sleep
- Other parasomnias

Most common parasomnias seen in children include the following sleep-related behaviors: sleepwalking, sleep talking, confusional arousals, night terrors, nightmares, bruxism, rhythmic movement disorder, and enuresis. The precise etiology of parasomnias remains unknown. However, genetic and developmental factors seem to play an important role in the pathophysiology of childhood parasomnias, along with strong environmental and psychological influences (Mahowald & Schenck, 1992).

Disorders of Arousal

Disorders of arousal usually occur from non-REM sleep and share some clinical characteristics. Impaired arousal from sleep has been proposed as a cause for these disorders. They are seen more frequently among young children and tend to resolve by adolescence, although some may persist into adulthood and throughout the life span (Klackenberg, 1987).

Sleepwalking

Sleepwalking is a common parasomnia, with reported episodes in approximately 15% of children and with 1% to 6% of children having frequent sleepwalking. Some children have nightly episodes of sleepwalking. The prevalence of sleepwalking peaks between ages 4 and 8 and gradually declines over the preadolescent and adolescent years of development (Anders & Eiben, 1997; Stores, 2009). Most studies have shown equal distribution of sleepwalking between sexes with one study indicating higher prevalence among boys (Petit et al., 2007).

Episodes of sleepwalking occur in NREM sleep, usually during slow wave sleep (SWS). Because most of the SWS is distributed during the first third of the night, sleepwalking tends to occur during the first 2 hours of sleep. Episodes may last up to 30 minutes. For younger children, the episodes may last only a few minutes. During the typical episode of sleepwalking the child gets out of bed and quietly walks around the bedroom or goes to the bathroom. Often sleepwalking is associated with urinating in unusual places like a bedroom closet or hallway. Older children may experience episodes of more complex behaviors with sleep eating, wandering around the house, or even getting out of the house. Sleepwalking can be accompanied by vocalization and children may even answer simple questions with no recollection of nocturnal events the next day.

Parents usually describe their children walking with eyes wide open but looking "confused." Children occasionally exhibit agitation or distress, especially if awakened from the sleepwalking episode. Sleepwalking can be potentially dangerous, as the child may fall down the stairs or even out of the window. It is also possible for an episode of somnambulism to become a confusional arousal, where the likelihood of accidental violence (to oneself or others) is much greater. There have been reports of accidental self-harm associated with sleepwalking, making safety precautions an important part of treatment intervention.

Sleep Terrors

Sleep terrors (*pavor nocturnus*) are somewhat less common than sleepwalking. Prevalence of sleep terrors has been difficult to study because parents often confuse them with nightmares. The prevalence of night terrors is estimated to be around 3% to 6% among pediatric patients, with a much lower prevalence rate in adolescents (Laberge & Tremblay et al., 2000). There are no consistent sex differences among children with night terrors.

Pathophysiology of night terrors is felt to represent an autonomic arousal with the admixture of neurophysiological features of wakefulness and NREM sleep, with behavioral agitation (Mahowald & Schenck, 2005). The child typically sits up in bed abruptly with glazed eyes and screams inconsolably. Tachycardia, flushing, rapid respiration, and diaphoresis may accompany this behavior. Attempts to comfort or awaken the child often only exacerbate agitation and trigger combative behaviors. Episodes of sleep terrors generally occur during SWS within the first third of the night. They are short in duration compared to confusional arousals and last between 30 seconds and 3 minutes.

Sleep terrors in susceptible children can be precipitated by anything that stimulates arousal from sleep, either intrinsically or environmentally. The examples of precipitating events include medical illness, psychological stress, noises, other sleep disorders like obstructive sleep apnea or certain medications. Sleep terrors can be very disruptive for family members who awaken to the child's screaming in the middle of the night. Children usually lie back down and fall asleep with little or no recollection of the episode upon waking in the morning.

Sleep terrors are brief in duration and rarely associated with self-harm, since children usually remain in bed. Attempts to awaken the child from a sleep terror may exacerbate agitation and precipitate combative behaviors while the child remains in a confused partially aroused state. Occasionally a sleep terror can progress into confusional arousal or sleepwalking with more potential for self-injury.

Confusional Arousals

Confusional arousals are frequently seen in children of young age and tend to be more prevalent in infants and toddlers. They are often misdiagnosed as nightmares or sleep terrors, as they have similar clinical presentations. However, there are some clinical characteristics that distinguish confusional arousals from other disorders of arousal. At the beginning of an episode, a child may moan or cry, then may start to thrash around and becomes increasingly agitated. Some children can get out of bed onto the floor, kicking and screaming during the episode. Episodes of confusional arousal resemble temper tantrums in younger children or can be perceived by parents as convulsive seizures. Parents are often alarmed by their child's apparent distress. The child is almost impossible to awaken and responds negatively, with more severe agitation or combativeness, to the parents' attempts to comfort him.

Confusional arousals, like other disorders of arousal, occur during the first third of the night during SWS and are associated with complete amnesia for the event on the next day. They last longer then sleep terrors, sometimes up to 45 minutes, causing significant distress for the family. The prevalence of confusional arousals was reported to be 17% in a group of children ages 3–13 years (Kotagal, 2009). The incidence of confusional arousals decreases with age, with fewer episodes reported during adolescence.

Sleep Inertia

Typically arising from deep SWS, incomplete awakenings have been also identified as sleep drunkenness or sleep inertia (Roth et al., 1972, Tassi & Muzet, 2000).

Sleep inertia refers to a period of impaired performance and reduced vigilance and represents a dissociative state following awakening from sleep (Roth et al., 1972; Dinges et al., 1989). Sleep inertia is a clinical phenomenon that may last from minutes to a few hours and is associated with impaired levels of alertness, confusion, and disorientation with elements of microsleep. It has been frequently observed among adolescents, especially in the context of sleep deprivation.

Sleep–Wake Transition Disorders

Sleep–wake transition disorders are defined as clinical conditions occurring on the transition from wakefulness to sleep, on transition from sleep to wakefulness, and on transition from one sleep stage to another sleep stage. There are four sleep disorders included in this category:

- Sleep talking
- Sleep starts
- Rhythmic movement disorder
- Nocturnal leg cramps

Sleep Talking

Sleep talking is extremely common among all ages, and often occurs during sleep–wake transitions. Sleep talking is defined as utterance of sounds during sleep without subjective awareness of the event. There are various degrees of severity in sleep talking, ranging from occasional vocalization like moaning in sleep to loud, frequent, nightly long speeches with elements of anger and hostility. The sleep-talking episode does not in itself involve physical movement, although sleep talking is often associated with sleepwalking or confusional arousal. It has been shown in a few studies that the prevalence of parent-reported sleep talking ranges from 55.5% among children ages 3–13 (Laberge et al., 2000) to 84% in preschoolers (Petit et al., 2007). While the incidence decreases as children age, it remains common in adulthood with 24% still reporting occasional episodes of sleep talking (Ohayon et al., 1997).

Polysomnographic studies demonstrated that sleep talking occurs in all sleep stages. A sleep study is not required to diagnose sleep talking, as this condition is observable and can be described by the parents. However, when it is associated with other sleep disorders, sleep talking my require polysomnographic monitoring in a sleep laboratory.

Sleep talking is more frequently seen among patients with psychopathology or under stress. Petit et al. (2007) demonstrated a connection between sleep talking and separation anxiety in children.

Rhythmic Movement Disorder

According to the ICSD-2 classification system, rhythmic movement disorder "comprises a group of stereotyped, repetitive movements involving large muscles, usually of the head and neck; the movements typically occur immediately prior to sleep onset and are sustained into light sleep" (AASM, 2005).

Rhythmic movements may occur during arousals from sleep and can be observed during stages of NREM sleep. The most common form of rhythmic movement disorder in children is head banging. The child may lie in a prone position, lifting the head and upper torso and forcibly banging the head into the pillow or mattress. Some children bang their heads against hard surfaces like a wall, floor, or bed rails, resulting in soft tissue damage.

Other forms of rhythmic movement disorder include head rolling with side-to-side head movements or body rolling that involves the full body rolling in bed. Body-rocking usually occurs in a sitting position or on hands and knees, rocking the entire body forward and backward. The frequency of movements usually ranges from 0.5 to 2 per second. Rhythmic vocalization like humming may sometimes accompany these movements. Some forms of rhythmic movements are seen in two-thirds of normal infants, with a gradual reduction in prevalence by age 4 years (Klackenburg, 1971). Environmental stress has been proposed as precipitating factor in susceptible individuals.

Traumatic injury is uncommon in rhythmic movement disorder; however, there have been cases of soft tissue injury reported. Violent movements can be very disturbing to other family members (Newell et al., 1999; Vetrugno & Montagna, 2011). Rhythmic movement disorder should be differentiated from other stereotypical movements in sleep like thumb sucking, tooth grinding, periodic limb movements in sleep, or epileptic seizures. Although not required, video recording and polysomnography can help with differential diagnosis of rhythmic movements disorder from other sleep-related disorders.

Parasomnias Usually Associated with REM sleep

Sleep related behaviors during REM sleep have been grouped together under this category and include the following clinical conditions that are seen in pediatric patients:

- Nightmares
- Sleep paralysis
- REM sleep–related behavior disorder

Nightmares and REM behavior disorder are discussed in this chapter due to their high prevalence among children and adolescents.

REM Behavior Disorder

Rapid eye movement behavior disorder (RBD) is a sleep-related phenomenon characterized by the intermittent loss of atonia (paralysis, which is a normal feature of REM sleep) accompanied by extreme motor activity and dream mentation. Patients with REM behavior disorder enact their dreams while remaining asleep. They may become very violent during the episode, kicking, punching, and throwing things around them, posing significant risk to themselves and others. RDB was originally described in adults with neurodegenerative disorders. However, there have been a number of cases indicating the presence of RDB in children and adolescents (Barros-Ferreira et al., 1975; Schenck et al., 1986; Herman et al., 1989; Turner & Allen, 1990).

RBD is a rare condition with the prevalence estimated to range from 0.38% to 0.50%. Prevalence of RDB is probably underreported because it can easily be misdiagnosed as a disorder of arousal like sleepwalking, confusional arousal, night terror or epilepsy due to the extreme and dramatic movements associated with it. The exact etiology of childhood RBD is not completely understood. Certain neurological conditions, medications, and alcohol use are thought to be predisposing factors (Schenck & Mahowald, 2002).

Diagnosis of RBD requires comprehensive clinical assessment and polysomnography. Patients frequently are able to recall dream content that corresponds to the types of behaviors observed during the RBD episode. Polysomnography usually reveals loss of atonia during REM sleep in patients with RDB.

RBD is also seen with other sleep disorders like narcolepsy, sleepwalking, sleep terrors, and periodic limb movements. Treatments for RBD should be diagnostically driven and frequently involve pharmacological interventions along with safety precautions and sleep hygiene training.

Other Parasomnias

This group of parasomnias includes clinical disorders that cannot be included into other categories of parasomnias and consist of the following conditions seen among children and adolescents:

- Sleep bruxism
- Sleep enuresis
- Sleep-related abnormal swallowing syndrome
- Nocturnal paroxysmal dystonia
- Primary snoring
- Infant sleep apnea
- Congenital central hypoventilation syndrome
- Sudden infant death syndrome
- Benign neonatal sleep myoclonus
- Other parasomnias not otherwise specified

Sleep enuresis and bruxism are the most prevalent disorders in children in this category of parasomnias. Sleep bruxism is tooth grinding and/or clenching that occurs in an episodic fashion throughout the night, usually during light stages of sleep. Sleep bruxism prevalence is reported to be as high as 20% among children who complain of headaches or pain in the face (Stores, 2007).

Sleep Enuresis

Enuresis is a parasomnia in which involuntary loss of urine occurs during sleep only (see Caldwell and Waters, Chapter 16). It is considered a normal behavior for children under age 5, due to normal maturational process of the central nervous system. According to the ICSD-2 (2005) diagnostic criteria, enuresis should be present at least twice per month in children between 3 and 6 years and at least once per month in older individuals to qualify as a disorder.

Children with primary enuresis have never been dry since birth; alternatively, if they have been dry for a period of at least 4 to 6 months and then begin to wet the bed, they are considered to have secondary enuresis. Occurrence of secondary enuresis is frequently associated with other medical, psychiatric, or sleep disorders (Mason & Pack 2007).

Prevalence of enuresis is estimated between 15% to 25% for children at age 5, with prevalence rate going down by approximately 15% for each year after 5 (Mason & Pack, 2007). Enuresis was found to be more common in boys than in girls (Petit et al., 2007). Enuresis can occur during stages 2 and 3 of NREM sleep, as well as REM sleep, with the majority of enuretic episodes occurring during the first half of the night. Although the exact causes of enuresis are unknown, several pathophysiological mechanisms of enuresis have been proposed including immature arousal system, insufficient release of antidiuretic hormone during sleep, and small functional bladder capacity.

Persistent enuresis may have a significant psychological impact on child's self-image and self-esteem and should be carefully evaluated and treated (Theunis et al., 2002).

Behavioral interventions have been shown to be most effective in the treatment of primary enuresis among pediatric patients. Enuretic alarm systems utilize behavioral conditioning as a therapeutic approach to achieve bladder control during sleep. For this system, an alarm signal goes off if any moisture is detected. This can help train the child to sense the need to urinate. Scheduled awakenings have been shown to decrease the incidence of enuresis. Parents are usually instructed to gently awaken their child and lead him to the bathroom in the middle of the night. Daytime bladder exercises, mental imagery, and hypnosis have also been helpful in reducing bedwetting episodes (Zaffanello, Giacomello, Brugnara, & Fanos, 2007). Pharmacological treatments have been used for those children who failed behavioral interventions and may include medications like desmopressin (DDAVP), imipramine, or oxybutynin. (Mathew, 2010).

Evaluation of Parasomnias

Evaluation of parasomnias should include a comprehensive medical, behavioral, developmental, and sleep history, and physical examination (Sheldon, 2005). Detailed and careful history of sleep-related behaviors should be obtained with the emphasis on usual time of occurrence, duration of the episode, description of movements and behaviors, presence of precipitating events, and amnesia of the event.

Patients should be assessed for daytime behavioral problems and developmental abnormalities; special emphasis should be placed on a sleep routine, sleep and wake schedule, sleeping arrangements, presence of daytime sleepiness, and sleep-related respiratory symptoms or movement abnormalities.

Polysomnography (PSG) is helpful in determining whether the disorder of arousal is secondary to another sleep disorder or is a physiological condition. For example, sleep apnea or periodic limb movements are frequently associated with disorders of arousal; epileptic seizures may also present with clinical features similar to parasomnias. Video or audio recording can be extremely helpful in documenting actual episodes (Stores, 2009). Video EEG or EEG telemetry can be used for differential diagnosis of epileptic seizures versus parasomnias.

Family history of parasomnias is an important part of the evaluation process, since parasomnias have family predisposition and tend to occur within several generations of the family (Lecendreux et al., 2003).

Association between Parasomnias and Psychiatric Disorders in Children and Adolescents

Children with psychiatric disorders are shown to have higher rates of parasomnias. Sleep terrors and sleepwalking were found more frequently among children with anxiety disorders, phobias, and suicidal ideation (Gau & Soong, 1999). Other studies have shown that sleepwalking and sleep terrors are correlated with separation anxiety, hyperactive-inattentive symptoms, as well as other disorders of arousal (Petit et al., 2007; Gau & Soong, 1999).

Prevalence of nocturnal enuresis is higher among children with psychiatric conditions. In a sample of 1155 children, Shreeram et al. (2009) found that those with enuresis had a 2.88 greater chance of having ADHD as compared to children without enuresis. Higher rates of enuresis have also been found in children with autism spectrum disorders (Miano et al., 2007).

Treatment of Parasomnias

Treatment for childhood arousal disorders includes both nonpharmacological and pharmacological interventions. Parents should be educated on the pathophysiology of parasomnias and reassured that nocturnal events that appear dramatic and frightening to them are benign in their course and will most likely resolve with age by later childhood or adolescence.

Parents should be instructed not to attempt to awaken or restrain their child in cases of confusional arousal or sleepwalking, and instead gently redirect the child back into bed.

It is critical to institute safety interventions to minimize the risk of injury that the episodes pose. These include sound alarms on the bed or door if the child gets up and begins to walk, locks on the windows and entry doors, gates in front of stairs, and so forth.

Implementing good sleep hygiene is crucial in treating parasomnias, with a consistent bedtime, elimination of caffeinated foods or drinks prior to bedtime, restricting access to television and other electronics at bedtime, and avoiding exercise late in the evening. It is very important to minimize risks of sleep deprivation in the managements of parasomnias. Behavioral intervention with scheduled awakenings has shown positive results for children who have regular episodes of parasomnia. Clinicians should instruct parents to awaken the child 15–30 minutes before the parasomnia typically occurs and then allow him to return to sleep. Scheduled awakenings should be repeated on a nightly basis for several weeks until parasomnias subside (Frank et al., 1997).

Since parasomnias frequently co-occur with other sleep disorders like restless legs syndrome, periodic limb movement disorder, and obstructive sleep apnea, the child should be evaluated and treated for comorbid primary sleep disorders.

When behavioral interventions along with the treatment for possible underlying medical or psychiatric conditions do not ameliorate disorders of arousal, medication can be considered. Benzodiazepines such as clonazepam have been shown to be effective when given approximately one hour before bedtime. Similarly, tricyclic antidepressants like imipramine can reduce the frequency of parasomnias (Mason & Pack, 2007).

Conclusion

Pediatric nighttime fears and nightmares are common from infancy through adolescence and are typically quite benign. In normally developing children they are relatively short-lived and remit with parental reassurance and simple behavioral strategies. When frequent or severe enough, nighttime fears and/or nightmares can interfere with a child's physical, social, and academic well-being, as well as create stress for his/her family members. Children with anxiety disorders, especially GAD, separation anxiety, and PTSD, have a higher rate of sleep disturbances and suffer the same deleterious results as those with severe and frequent nighttime fears and nightmares.

Parasomnias defined as dysfunctions associated with sleep, sleep states, and incomplete arousals from sleep manifest in different ways during childhood, with spontaneous remission frequently occurring by adolescence. There is a correlation between higher rates of parasomnias and psychopathology in children. Treatment for nighttime fears and parasomnias relies heavily upon cognitive and behavioral interventions such as extinction and scheduled awakenings. Children specifically suffering from severe nocturnal fears, persistent parasomnias, or anxiety may be treated pharmacologically as an adjunct to the cognitive-behavioral interventions.

Future Directions

Despite substantial progress in our current knowledge of the neurobiological mechanisms of sleep disorders, there is a significant gap in the understanding of sleep-related disorders in children and their impact on daytime functions and on overall psychological and physical development. These are several suggestions for future research directions in the area of parasomnias and nighttime fears:

– More epidemiological studies are needed to investigate the prevalence of nocturnal fears and parasomnias across different ages.

– Psychosocial and environmental factors, as well as developmental factors, should be further explored as part of the etiology of parasomnias and nocturnal fears.

– It is important to investigate the impact of parasomnias and nighttime fears on daytime neurobehavioral function of children and adolescents.

– Interface between parasomnias, nocturnal fears and psychopathology in pediatric patients should be studied across different stages of a child's development.

– Prospective, large-scale studies are needed to examine the impact of sleep-related behaviors on children's neuropsychological development.

– There should be studies investigating the effects of psychopharmacological agents used for the treatment of other psychiatric disorders on sleep-related behaviors.

– There is a clinical need to develop new, innovative, nonpharmacological treatment approaches to parasomnias and nocturnal fears with well-designed and controlled clinical trials to test the effectiveness of these interventions.

References

Alfano, C. A., Ginsgurg, G. S., & Kingery, J. N. (2007). Sleep-related problems among children and adolescents with anxiety disorders. *Journal of the American Academy of Child and Adolescent Psychiatry, 46*(2), 224–232.

Alfano, C. A., Gamble, A. L. (2009). The role of sleep in childhood psychiatric disorders. *Child Care Youth Forum, 38*, 327–340.

Alfano, C. A., Pina, A. A., Zerr, A. A., & Villalta, I. K. (2010). Pre-sleep arousal and sleep problems of anxiety-disordered youth. *Child Psychiatry and Human Development, 41*(2), 156–67.

American Academy of Sleep Medicine. (2005). *International Classification of Sleep Disorders: Diagnostic and Coding Manual* (2nd ed.). Westchester, IL: American Academy of Sleep Medicine.

American Psychiatric Association (2000). *Diagnostic and Statistical Manual of Mental Disorders, Fourth Edition Text Revision.* Washington, DC: American Psychiatric Association.

Anders, T., & Eiben, L. (1997). Pediatric sleep disorders: a review of the past 10 years. *Journal of the American Academy of Child and Adolescent Psychiatry, 36*(1), 9–20.

Barros-Ferreira, M., Chodkiewicz, J.-P., Lairy, G. C., Salzarulo, P. (1975). Disorganized relations of tonic and phasic events of REM sleep in a case of brain-stem tumour. *Electroencephography and Clinical Neurophysiology, 38*, 202–207.

Blader, J. C., Koplewicz, H. S., Abikoff, H., & Foley, C. (1997). Sleep problems of elementary school children: A community survey. *Archives of Pediatric and Adolescent Medicine, 151*, 473–480.

Bruni, O., Ottaviano, S., Guidetti, V., Romoli, M., Innocenzi, M., Cortesi, F., et al. (1996). The sleep disturbance scale for children (SDSC) construction and validation of an instrument to evaluate sleep disturbances in childhood and adolescence. *Journal of Sleep Research, 5*, 251–261.

Charuvastra, A., & Cloitre, M. (2009). Safe enough to sleep: Sleep disruptions associated with trauma, post-traumatic stress, and anxiety in children and adolescents. *Child and Adolescent Psychiatric Clinics of North America, 18*, 877–891.

Chervin, R. D. Hedger, K., Dillon, J. E., & Pituch, K.J. (2000). Pediatric Sleep Questionnaire (PSQ): Validity and reliability of scales for sleep-disordered breathing, snoring. Sleepiness, and behavioral problems. *Sleep Medicine, 1*, 21–32.

Chimienti, G., Nasr, J. A., Khalifeh, I. (1989). Children's reactions to war-related stress: Affective symptoms and behaviour problems. *Social Psychiatry and Psychiatric Epidemiology, 24*(6), 282–287.

Cortesi., F., Giannotti., F., Sebastiani., T., Vagnoni., C., Marioni., P. (2008). Cosleeping versus solitary sleeping in children with bedtime problems: Child emotional problems and parental distress. *Behavioral Sleep Medicine, 6*(2):89–105.

Costello, E. J., Egger, H., & Angold, A. (2005). 10-year research update review: The epidemiology of child and adolescent psychiatric disorders: I. Methods and public health burden. *Journal of the American Academy of Child and Adolescent Psychiatry, 44*, 972–986.

Dinges, D. F., Broughton, R. J. (1989). *Sleep and Alertness: Chronobiological, Behavioral and Medical Aspects of Napping* (p. 322). New York: Raven Press.

Drake, C., Nickel, C., Burduvali, E., Roth, T., Jefferson, C., & Pietro, B. (2003).The pediatric daytime sleepiness scale (PDSS): Sleep habits and school outcomes in middle-school children. *Sleep, 26*(4), 455–458.

Frank, N. C., Spirito, A., Stark, L., Owens-Stively, J. (1997). The use of scheduled awakenings to eliminate childhood sleepwalking. *Journal of Pediatric Psychology, 22,* 345–353.

Forbes, E. E., Bertocci, M. A., Gregory, A. M., Ryan, N. D., Axelson, D. A., Birmaher, B., et al. (2008). Objective sleep in pediatric anxiety disorders and major depressive disorder. *Journal of American Academy of Child and Adolescent Psychiatry, 47*(2), 148–155.

Gau, S., Soong, W. (1999). Psychiatric comorbidity of adolescents with sleep terrors or sleepwalking: a case-control. *Australian and New Zealand Journal of Psychiatry, 33,* 734–739.

Glod, C.A., Teicher, M. H., Hartman, C. R., & Harakal, B. S. (1997). Increased nocturnal activity and impaired sleep maintenance in abused children. *Journal of the American Academy of Child and Adolescent Psychiatry, 36,* 1236–1243.

Gordon, J., King, N. J., Gullone, E., Muris, P., & Ollendick, T. H. (2007a). Treatment of children's night-time fears: The need for a modern randomized controlled trial. *Clinical Psychology Review, 27,* 98–113.

Gordon, J., King, N. J., Gullone, E., Muris, P., & Ollendick, T. H. (2007b). Night-time fears of children and adolescents: Frequency, content, severity, harm, expectations, disclosure, and coping behaviours. *Behavioural Research and Therapy, 45,* 2464–2472.

Graziano, A. M., & Mooney, K .C. (1980). Family self-control instruction for children's nighttime fear reduction. *Journal of Consulting and Clinical Psychology, 48*(2), 206–213.

Gregory, A. M., Eley, T. C., O'Connor, T. G., & Plomin, R. (2004). Etiologies of associations between childhood sleep and behavioral problems in a large twin sample. *Journal of the American Academy of Child and Adolescent Psychiatry, 43,* 744–751.

Gregory, A. M., & O' Connor, T. G. (2002). Sleep problems in childhood: A longitudinal study of developmental change and association with behavioral problems. *Journal of the American Academy of Child and Adolescent Psychiatry, 41,* 964–971.

Hawkins, C., Williams, T. I. (1992). Nightmares, life events and behaviour problems in preschool children. *Child: Care, Health and Development,18,*117–128.

Herman, J. H., Blaw, M. E., & Steinberg, J. B. (1989). REM behavior disorder in a two year old male with evidence of brainstem pathology. *Sleep Research,18,* 242.

Hudson, J. L., Gradisar, M., Gamble, A., Schniering, C. A., & Rebelo, I. (2009). The sleep patterns and problems of clinically anxious children. *Behaviour Research and Therapy, 47,* 339–344.

Ivanenko, A., & Patwari, P. P. (2009). Recognition and management of pediatric sleep disorders. *Primary Psychiatry, 16*(2), 42–50.

Johnson, C. M. (1991). Infant and toddler sleep: A telephone survey of parents in one community. *Journal of Devopmental and Behavioral Pediatrics, 12,* 108–114.

Johnson, E. O., Chilcoat, H. D., & Breslau, N. (2000). Trouble sleeping and anxiety/depression in childhood. *Psychiatry Research, 94,* 93–102.

Keller, P. S., Buckhalt, J. A., & El-Sheikh, M. (2008). Links between family functioning and sleep. In A. Ivanenko (Ed.), *Sleep and Psychiatric Disorders in Children and Adolescents* (pp. 49–60). New York: Informa Healthcare.

King, N., Ollendick, T. H., & Tonge, B. J. (1997). Children's nighttime fears. *Clinical Psychology Reviews, 17,* 431–443.

Klackenburg, G. (1971). Rhythmic movements in infancy and early childhood. *Acta Pediatrica Scandinavia, 224* (suppl), 74.

Klackenberg, G. (1987). Incidence of parasomnias in children in a general population. In C. Guilleminault(Ed.), *Sleep and its Disorders in Children* (pp. 99–113). New York: Raven Press.

Kotagal, S. (2009). Parasomnias in childhood. *Sleep Medicine Reviews, 13*(2), 157–168.

Kotagal, S. (2012). Parasomnias, periodic limb movements and restless legs in children. In Barkoukis, Matheson, Ferber, & Doghramji (Eds.), *Therapy in Sleep Medicine*(pp. 475–484). Philadelphia: Elsevier.

Krakow, B., Schrader, R., Tandberg, D., Hollifield, M., Koss, M. P., Yau, C. L., & Cheng, D. T. (2002). Nightmare frequency in sexual assault survivors with PTSD. *Journal of Anxiety Disorders, 16*(2), 175–190.

Kravitz, M., McCoy, B. J., Tompkins, D. M., Daly, W., Mulligan, J., McCauley, R. L., et al. (1993). Sleep disorders in children after burn injury. *Journal of Burn Care Rehabilitation, 14*(1), 83–90.

Kushnir, J., & Sadeh, A. (2011). Sleep of preschool children with night-time fears. *Sleep Medicine, 12,* 870–874.

Kushnir, J., & Sadeh, A. (2012). Assessment of brief intervention for nighttime fears in preschool children. *European Journal of Pediatrics, 171,* 67–75.

Laberge, L., Tremblay, R. E., Vitaro, F., & Montplaisir, J. (2000). Development of parasomnias from childhood to early adolescence. *Pediatrics,106,* 67–74.

Lecendreux, M., Bassetti, C., Dauvilliers, Y., Mayer, G., Neidhart, E., & Tafti, M. (2003). HLA and genetic susceptibility to sleepwalking. *Molecular Psychiatry, 8,* 114–117.

Lugienbuehl, M. (2004). *Sleep Disorder Inventory for Students.* Clearwater, FL: Child Uplift, Inc.

Mahowald, M. W., & Schenck, C. H. (1992). Dissociated states of wakefulness and sleep. *Neurology, 42*(suppl 6), 44–51.

Mahowald, M. W., & Schenck C. H. (2005). Non-rapid eye movement sleep parasomnias. *Neurological Clinics, 23*(4), 1077–1106.

Mathew, J. L. (2010). Evidence-based management of nocturnal enuresis: An overview of systematic reviews. *Indian Pediatrics, 47*(9),777–780.

Mason, T. B. A., & Pack, A. I. (2007). Pediatric parasomnias. *Sleep 30*(2),141–151.

McMenamy, C., & Katz, R. C. (1989). Brief parent-assisted treatment for children's nighttime fears. *Developmental and Behavioral Pediatrics, 10,* 145–148.

Medoff, D., & Schaefer, C. E. (1993). Children sharing the parental bed: A review of the advantages and disadvantages of cosleeping. *Psychology: A Journal of Human Behavior, 30,* 1–9.

Miano, S., Bruni, O., Elia, M., Trovato, A., Smerieri, A., Verrillo, E., et al. (2007). Sleep in children with autistic spectrum disorder: A questionnaire and polysomnographic study. *Sleep Medicine, 9,* 64–70.

Mindell, J. A., Kuhn, B., Lewin, D. S., Meltzer, L. J., & Sadeh, A.; American Academy of Sleep Medicine. (2006). Behavioral treatment of bedtime problems and night wakings in infants and young children. *Sleep, 29*(10), 1263–1276.

Mindell, J. A., & Owens, J. A. (2010). *A Clinical Guide to Pediatric Sleep: Diagnosis and Management of Sleep Problems* (2nd ed). Philadelphia, PA: Wolters Kluwer/Lippincott, Williams, and Watkins.

Munezawa, T., Kaneita., Y., Osaki, Y., Kanda, H., Ohtsu. T., Suzuki. H., et al. (2011) Nightmare and sleep paralysis among Japanese adolescents: a nationwide representative survey. *Sleep Medicine, 12*(1), 56–64.

Muris, P., Merckelbach, H., Gadet, B., & Moulaert, V. (2000). Fears, worries, and scary dreams in 4- to 12-year-old children: their content, developmental pattern, and origins. *Journal of Child Psychology, 29*, 43–52.

Muris, P., Merckelbach, H., Ollendick, T.H., King, N.J., & Bogie, N. (2001). Children's night-time fears: Parent-child ratings of frequency, content, origins, coping behaviors and severity. *Behavioral Research and Therapy, 39*, 13–28.

Nader, K., Pynoos, R., Fairbanks, L., & Frederick C. (1990). Children's PTSD reactions one year after a sniper attack at their school. *American Journal of Psychiatry, 147*(11), 1526–1530.

Newell, K. M., Sprague, R. L., Pain, M. T., Deutsch, K. M., & Meinhold, P. (1999). Dynamics of self-injurious behaviors. *American Journal of Mental Retardation,104*,11–21.

Nielsen, T. A., Laberge, L., Tremblay, R., Vitaro, F., & Montplaisir, J.(2000). Development of disturbing dreams during adolescence and their relationship to anxiety symptoms. *Sleep, 23*,727–736.

Ohayon, M. M., Caulet, M., & Priest, R. G. (1997). Violent behavior during sleep. *Journal of Clinical Psychiatry,58*, 369–376.

Owens, J. A., Spirito, A., & McGuinn, M. (2000a). The children's sleep habits questionnaire (CSHQ): Psychometric properties of a survey instrument for school-aged children. *Sleep, 23*, 1–9.

Owens, J. A., Spirito, A., McGuinn, M., & Nobile, C. (2000b). Sleep habits and sleep disturbance in school-aged children. *Journal of Developmental and Behavioral Pediatrics, 21*, 27–36.

Petit, D., Touchette, E., Tremblay, R. E., Boivin, M., &Montplaisir, J. (2007). Dyssomnias and parasomnias in early childhood. *Pediatrics,119*(5), e1016–e1025.

Pine, D. S., Cohen, P., Gurley, D., Brook, J., & Ma, Y. (1998). The risk for early-adulthood anxiety and depressive disorders in adolescents with anxiety and depressive disorders. *Archives of General Psychiatry, 55*(1), 56–64.

Rath Jr., F. H., & Okum, M. E. (1995). Parents and children sleeping together: Cosleeping prevalence and concerns. *American Journal of Orthopsychiatry, 65*, 411–418.

Rimsza, M. E., Berg, R. A., & Locke, C. (1998). Sexual abuse: Somatic and emotional reactions. *Child Abuse and Neglect, 15*(3), 239–248.

Roth, B., Nevsimalova, S., & Rechtschaffen, A. (1972). Hypersomnia with sleep drunkenness. *Archives of General Psychiatry, 26*, 456–462.

Sadeh, A. (2005). Cognitive-behavioral treatment for childhood sleep disorders. *Clinical Psychology Review, 25*, 612–628.

Salzarulo, P., & Chevalier, A. (1983). Sleep problems in children and their relationship with early disturbances of the waking-sleeping rhythms. *Sleep, 6*, 47–51.

Schenck, C. H., Bundlie, S.,R, Smith, S. A., et al.(1986). REM behavior disorder in a 10 year old girl and aperiodic REM and NREM sleep movements in an 8 year old brother. *Sleep Research, 15*, 1986.

Schenck, C. H., & Mahowald, M. W. (2002). REM sleep behavior disorder: Clinical, developmental, and neuroscience perspectives 16 years after its formal identification in sleep. *Sleep, 25*(2), 120–138.

Shaffer, D., Fisher, P., Dulcan, M. K., & Davies, M. (1996). The NIMH diagnostic interview schedule for children version 2.3 (DISC-2.3). Description, acceptability, prevalence rates, and performance in the MECA study. Methods for the epidemiology of child and adolescent mental disorders study. *Journal of the American Academy of Child and Adolescent Psychiatry, 35*(86), 5–877.

Sheldon, S. (2005). The parasomnias. In S. H. Sheldon, R. Ferber, & M. H. Kryger (Eds.), *Principles and Practice of Pediatric Sleep Medicine* (pp. 305–316). Elsevier.

Shreeram, S., He, J., Kalaydjian, A., Brothers, S., & Merikangas, K. R. (2009). Prevalence of enuresis and its association with Attention-Deficit/Hyperactivity Disorder among U.S. children: Results from a nationally representative study. *Journal of the American Academy of Child and Adolescent Psychiatry, 48*(1), 35–41.

Simard, V., Nielsen, T. A., Tremblay, R. E., Boivin, M., & Montplaisir, J. Y.(2008) Longitudinal study of bad dreams in preschool-aged children: Prevalence, demographic correlates, risk and protective factors. *Sleep, 31*(1), 62–70.

Simonds, J. F., & Parraga, H. (1982). Prevalence of sleep disorders and sleep behaviors in children and adolescents. *Journal of the American Academy of Child and Adolescent Psychiatry, 21*, 383–388.

Stores, G. (2007). Parasomnias of childhood and adolescence. *Sleep Medicine Clinics, 2*, 405–417.

Stores, G. (2009). Aspects of parasomnias in childhood and adolescence. *Archives of Disease in Childhood, 94*,63–69.

Tassi, P., & Muzet, A. (2000) Sleep inertia. *Sleep Medicine Reviews*, 4341–4353.

Theunis, M., Van Hoecke, E., Paesbrugge, S., Hoebeke, P., & Van de Walle, J. (2002). Self-image and performance in children with nocturnal enuresis. *European Urology, 41*(6), 660–667.

Turner, R., & Allen, W. T. (1990). REM sleep behavior disorder associated with narcolepsy in an adolescent: A case report. *Sleep Research, 19*, 302.

Vetrugno, R., Montagna, P. (2011). Sleep-to-wake transition movement disorders. *Sleep Medicine, 12*(Suppl 2), S11-S16.

Wolfson, A. R., & Carskadon, M. A. (1998). Sleep schedules and daytime functioning in adolescents. *Child Development, 69*, 875–887.

Zaffanello, M., Giacomello, L., Brugnara, M., & Fanos, V. (2007). Therapeutic options in childhood nocturnal enuresis. *Minerva Urologica e Nefrologica, 59*(2), 199–205.

CHAPTER

25 Pediatric Sleep Apnea and Adherence to Positive Airway Pressure (PAP) Therapy

Kristen H. Archbold

Abstract

Obstructive sleep apnea (OSA) in children is a sleep disorder where the movement of air through the upper airway (nose, mouth, trachea) is decreased due to an obstruction that is most commonly caused by enlarged adenoids and tonsils. It results in disturbed and fragmented sleep and decreased levels of blood oxygenation. In turn, children with OSA can experience enuresis, growth retardation, and cognitive and behavioral difficulties. Treatment of pediatric OSA focuses on the removal of adenoid and tonsil tissues where applicable. Secondary treatment of OSA is continuous positive airway pressure (CPAP), which has a series of issues regarding adherence and use that could be addressed by cognitive-behavioral therapies or group therapy. Children with special medical conditions such as Trisomy 21, other genetic syndromes, and psychiatric illness are at increased risk for the development of OSA and should be closely monitored for the presence of the disease. Future directions include delving deeper into an understanding of how CPAP effectively treats OSA in children and strategies to improve adherence to CPAP therapy in the pediatric population.

Key Words: obstructive sleep apnea, sleep fragmentation, CPAP adherence, pediatrics

Introduction

Pathophysiology

The pathophysiology of obstructive sleep apnea is focused around anatomical and physiological issues that cause the diameter of the upper airway to be decreased. This decrease in diameter then results in a decreased ability to effectively move air in and out of the upper airway during sleep. Movement of air in and out of the upper airway can be impaired when the diameter of the airway is decreased and/or chest wall muscles cannot effectively support the increased work of breathing during sleep. Obstructive sleep apnea is associated with an inability to effectively move air in and out of the upper airway due to a decrease in airway diameter.

Pediatric obstructive sleep apnea (OSA) has been defined by the American Thoracic Society as a disorder of breathing during sleep where there are prolonged partial upper airway obstructions (hypopneas) and/or complete airway obstruction (obstructive apnea) events that disrupt sleep patterns and normal ventilation during sleep (Loughlin et al., 1996). Normal oxygen and carbon dioxide gas exchange becomes impaired, resulting in intermittent and repetitive decreased blood oxygenation levels (hypoxia) and frequent arousals from sleep caused by repeated disturbances throughout the sleep cycle.

The most common cause of OSA in children is enlarged adenoid and tonsillar tissues that block and subsequently decrease the diameter of the upper airway (Halbower & Marcus, 2003). Snoring, the most common symptom of OSA in children from infancy through adolescence, results from turbulence in airflow through a narrowed upper airway. Children who snore do not necessarily have OSA, but may have some degree of upper airway obstruction (primary snoring, upper airway resistance syndrome). However, snoring is not always present in obstructive sleep apnea and cannot be relied upon as a diagnostic hallmark in the absence of a polysomnographic (PSG) sleep study (Aurora et al., 2011).

Overweight and obesity are increasingly significant risk factors for OSA in children. The large increase in the proportion of obese children and adolescents is associated with increases in the incidence and prevalence of obstructive sleep apnea (Ross et al., 2009). This is a major public health concern, given the implications of both obesity and sleep apnea for metabolic and cardiovascular disorders (Kim et al., 2010; Silva et al., 2011).

This chapter will report and discuss the prevalence of OSA in the pediatric population, symptomatology, and also present a description of sleep staging and quantification. Discussion will then address current treatment strategies and the prevalence of OSA in special populations of children with different medical syndromes that can decrease airway diameter because of such issues as craniofacial malformations or enlarged tongue size.

Prevalence

Some reports suggest that between 1% and 3% of the pediatric population has obstructive sleep apnea, but investigators have found its symptoms in up to 16% of children (Archbold, Pituch, Panahi, & Chervin, 2002; Bixler et al., 2009). Whether this discrepancy is a result of underdiagnosis is not known. OSA affects boys and girls at the same rate throughout childhood, but it may be more prevalent in boys during the teenaged years as body mass index (BMI) and body composition change during puberty. African-American and socially disadvantaged children appear to be at a greater risk for developing OSA versus Hispanic or White children and also may be subject to underdiagnosis because of their African-American race or decreased access to health care (Boss, Smith, & Ishman, 2011; Mulvaney et al., 2006; Spilsbury et al., 2006).

Sleep Cycle Overview

At this point, a general description of sleep staging and scoring will be presented as evidence suggests that certain stages of sleep are associated with different patterns of symptoms in pediatric OSA.

Human sleep is commonly divided into 5 separate stages that progress from light (N1) to intermediate (N2) to very deep, sound sleep (N3). It is also grouped into classification of non-rapid eye movement (NREM sleep: N1, N2 & N3) and rapid eye movement (REM) sleep. Each stage of sleep is mainly quantified based on the frequency and rhythms of brain activity at any given point (Rechtschaffen & Kales, 1968).

During stage N1, the brain is resonating at a frequency of approximately 2–7 Hz, which is a relatively low-voltage and mixed-frequency electroencephalography (EEG) pattern. Stage N1 is relatively "light" sleep, whereby a person can be easily awoken. N1 sleep most often occurs in the transition from wake to stage N2 and usually accounts for 5% of total sleep time during a typical pediatric sleep cycle (Chokroverty, 1995; Mindell & Owens, 2003).

Stage N2 sleep is a bit deeper sleep and has hallmark EEG characteristics including sleep spindles and k-complexes (bursts of 12–14 Hz EEG activity). N2 sleep comprises the majority of usual pediatric sleep architecture, accounting for 45%–50% of the total sleep time throughout the sleep cycle (Chokroverty, 1995).

The deepest stage of human sleep is N3 sleep, where voltages are high-amplitude and slow-wave with EEG frequencies that range from 2–7 Hz. During N3 sleep, a child is not easily awoken and can be considered to be in "sound sleep." A child with average sleep patterns will experience approximately 25% of their total sleep time as N3 sleep (Mindell & Owens, 2003).

Rapid eye movement sleep, or REM sleep, is also known as "dreaming sleep" and is when most dreams that can be remembered upon awakening occur. EEG amplitude during REM sleep is low-voltage and mixed-frequency and usually comprises approximately 20% of the total sleep time during childhood (Mindell & Owens, 2003).

During a typical night of sleep, each one of the NREM and REM cycles occurs during a period of approximately 90–120 minutes. This is known as the sleep "cycle." During childhood, these sleep cycles occur approximately 4–6 times per night, depending on the total sleep time length (Mindell & Owens, 2003).

OSA is a sleep disorder that is associated with frequent arousals from sleep (i.e., shifting from a deeper to lighter stage of sleep), which result in fragmented sleep and prevent the child from experiencing a night of continuous sleep with normal smooth transitions from stage to stage. In addition to sleep fragmentation, OSA has a series of other characteristic symptoms that can be identified to document the presence of the disorder.

Symptoms of OSA

Primary nocturnal symptoms of OSA are the presence of snoring on most nights during the week, witnessed apneas (where a witness reports hearing or seeing a child stop breathing during his or her sleep), and needing to wake a child from sleep in order to get him or her to breathe again. Restless sleep has also been reported in children with OSA as a symptom of respiratory pauses. Observers report bedclothes twisted or disheveled in the morning, or the child preferring to sleep in awkward positions with the head back to facilitate patency of the upper airway (Brooks, 2005). To confirm a diagnosis of OSA, these subjective symptoms must be verified by polysomnography (PSG; full in-lab sleep study) in order to document the severity and frequency of the events.

As a result of decreased upper airway diameter, oxygen flow is also decreased in OSA. When oxygen flow is decreased, blood oxygen levels fall to greater than 70% of baseline in severe cases. This type of blood oxygen level decrease is known as *hypoxia*, a hallmark diagnostic symptom associated with OSA. During hypoxic events (apneas, hypopneas), levels of carbon dioxide build up in the bloodstream, which subsequently will cause an arousal from sleep in order to restore airflow within the upper airway (Katz & Marcus, 2005). In OSA, hypoxic events are repeated and intermittent and so are the subsequent arousals from sleep. Frequent arousals from sleep cause fragmentation of the sleep cycle so that a child with OSA is not getting a continuous pattern of sleep throughout the night. Frequent hypoxic events and arousals from sleep combine to purportedly produce the most commonly observed daytime behavior symptoms associated with OSA: inattention, impulsivity, and in some cases extreme daytime sleepiness.

In terms of behavioral symptoms of OSA, etiology seems to have a differential impact on daytime functioning in children. When overweight or obesity is the main cause of OSA, children are most likely to exhibit symptoms of excessive daytime sleepiness, failing or poor quality school work, behavioral problems, and falling asleep in class (Bourke et al., 2011; Gozal & Kheirandish-Gozal, 2009; Moore et al., 2009; Ross et al., 2009; Spruyt, Capdevila, Kheirandish-Gozal, & Gozal, 2009; Spruyt et al., 2006).

On the other hand, children with enlarged lymphoid tissues or other non–obesity-related OSA etiologies are more likely to display hyperactive and disruptive behaviors in school and at home than to appear excessively sleepy during the daytime (Dayyat, Kheirandish-Gozal, Sans Capdevila, Maarafeya, & Gozal, 2009). In fact, these symptoms may be severe enough as to mimic diagnostic criteria for a diagnosis of attention-deficit/hyperactivity disorder (ADHD; O'Brien et al., 2003).

Regardless of etiology, children with OSA can display patterns of inattention and disturbed social skills that may be similar to conduct disorder, oppositional defiant disorder, and other difficult behaviors (Blunden & Chervin; Chervin et al., 2002; Giordani et al., 2008; Kheirandish-Gozal, De Jong, Spruyt, Chamuleau, & Gozal; Montgomery-Downs, O'Brien, Holbrook, & Gozal, 2004). Snoring in the absence of full OSA is also associated with impaired scholastic and behavioral patterns (Chervin, Ruzicka, Archbold, & Dillon, 2005; Chervin et al., 2006; Melendres, Lutz, Rubin, & Marcus, 2004; Montgomery-Downs et al., 2004; O'Brien, Mervis, Holbrook, Bruner, Klaus, et al., 2004; also (see O'Brien, Chapter 29).

Other Symptoms Associated with OSA

Children with OSA may have enuresis due to the decreased amount of N3 sleep, the stage in which urine is concentrated due to the release of antidiuretic and growth hormones. Effective treatment of OSA often eliminates enuresis and may lead to growth spurts as a result of the increase amounts of N3 sleep and secretion of growth hormones (Chervin et al., 2006; Dillon et al., 2007; Caldwell and Waters, Chapter 26). When a child presents to a clinic with enuresis as a complaint, evaluation of OSA symptoms should be performed to determine if OSA could be present in the child.

OSA is also associated with inflammatory and altered metabolic processes in children (Gozal, Kheirandish-Gozal, Bhattacharjee, & Spruyt; Gozal, Kheirandish-Gozal, Serpero, Sans Capdevila, & Dayyat, 2007). Obese children with OSA have increased levels of systemic inflammation and increased platelet-leukocyte-endothelial processes that have both been associated with cardiovascular disease (Tauman, O'Brien, & Gozal, 2007). It is currently not known the extent to which OSA in childhood relates to the presence or potentiation of cardiovascular disease in adulthood. Future studies should attempt to address this issue.

Treatment of OSA

ADENOTONSILLECTOMY

Adenotonsillectomy is considered the first line of treatment for OSA and is considered curative in 60% of children ages 5–12. A landmark study (Gozal, 1998) found that scholastic performance (measured by year-end grades) improved by an entire grade level one year after adenotonsillectomy, compared with children with OSA who did not have adenotonsillectomy. Subsequent studies have consistently demonstrated the negative effects of persistent OSA in children. These include alteration of endothelial function and sleep architecture, decreased attention and mental flexibility, and impaired behavior patterns (Archbold, Giordani, Ruzicka, & Chervin, 2004; Bhattacharjee et al., 2010; Bourke et al., 2011; Chervin et al., 2003; Gozal et al.; O'Brien, Mervis, Holbrook, Bruner, Smith, et al., 2004).

Treatment of children who have OSA with adenotonsillectomy has led to decreases in serum c-reactive protein and other inflammatory biomarkers (Gozal & Kheirandish-Gozal, 2009). Recent data is emerging to show that following adenotonsillectomy, children improve in the areas of cognitive function and behavior (Dillon et al., 2007; Giordani et al., 2012) and sleep cycle continuity (Goodwin, Vasquez, Silva, & Quan, 2010).

OSA can persist in 21%–73% of children following surgery (Bhattacharjee et al., 2010; Chervin et al., 2006; Walker, Whitehead, & Gulliver, 2008; Wei et al., 2009) In particular, OSA most often persists in children older than 7 years of age, those who are obese, and those with chronic asthma (Bhattacharjee et al., 2010). These children are most likely to require use of continuous positive airway pressure (CPAP) to treat their OSA.

CONTINUOUS POSITIVE AIRWAY PRESSURE (CPAP)

Continuous positive airway pressure (CPAP) is a second-line treatment for OSA in children and effectively treats OSA when used for 6 hours at least 5 nights per week (Koontz, Slifer, Cataldo, & Marcus, 2003; Marcus et al., 1995). During CPAP use, positive pressure is generated by a small machine attached to a mask worn over the nose and/or mouth and blows air at a prescribed pressure that is required to maintain the patency of the upper airway. For obese and other children who are not candidates for adenotonsillar surgery, PAP therapy is the first line of treatment for OSA.

Remarkably little data are available to illustrate general CPAP treatment adherence patterns in children. Moreover, the use of PAP therapy in children less than 30 kilograms has yet to be approved by the United States Food and Drug Administration (FDA), making a prescription of PAP therapy off-label for treatment of OSA in smaller children. Furthermore, there are fewer than ten PAP masks that are specifically designed and FDA-approved for use in children and again, children who are less than 30 kilograms have few FDA-approved options at this point in time. Despite these therapeutic hurdles, PAP therapy is frequently prescribed to treat OSA in children of all ages.

Rates of adherence to PAP therapy in children have not been widely reported. Published studies available often include patients in their sample with developmental and/or genetic issues (i.e., Down syndrome, Chiari malformation, craniofacial malformation, etc.), which makes generalization of findings to normally developing populations difficult (Marcus et al., 2012; Marcus et al., 2006; O'Donnell, Bjornson, Bohn, & Kirk, 2006; Uong, Epperson, Bathon, & Jeffe, 2007).

Adherence to PAP therapy is generally measured and reported as the average numbers of hours per night of the week a PAP device is used. In a recent study (Marcus et al., 2012) an adherence rate of 201 ± 135 minutes of PAP use per night over a period of 24 ± 6 days per month was reported in a sample of 56 children. This translates to an average of about 3.5 hours per night of PAP use in children. Similar rates of adherence to PAP therapy have been reported by Marcus et. al., 2006, O'Donnell et al., 2006, and Uong et al, 2007.

One study has been published which recommends strategies for improvement of PAP adherence in children (Koontz et al., 2003). In the Koontz et al. (2003) study, children and their families were randomized into three groups: one received behavioral therapy that consisted of positive reinforcement, another received graduated exposure to PAP equipment, and a third received counterconditioning to use of PAP equipment with a distracting activity such as music. Children and caregivers that received an average of 6 behavioral therapy sessions had significantly increased times of PAP adherence versus those children who did not have behavioral therapy (Koontz et al., 2003).

Most of the other available data on strategies to investigate and improve PAP adherence have been researched and recommended for adults with OSA. Barriers to PAP adherence in adults include negative marital and employment status (Gagnadoux et al., 2011), low socioeconomic background (Billings et al., 2011; Tarasiuk, Reznor, Greenberg-Dotan, & Reuveni, 2012), Black race (Billings et al., 2011), practical problems with the equipment, and negative attitudes toward the treatment (Brostrom et al., 2010).

Barriers to PAP therapy in children may be similar to those reported in adults, including low socioeconomic background and Black race (Simon, Duncan, Janicke, & Wagner, 2012). Simon and colleagues (2012) have developed the *Adherence Barriers to CPAP Questionnaire* (ABCQ) that measures patient and caregiver perceived barriers to PAP use. Findings indicate that the most frequently endorsed barriers to PAP usage in children were: the child does not use the equipment when away from home; child does not use the equipment when not feeling well; child forgets to use the equipment; child does not feel like using PAP treatment; child just wants to forget about having OSA; and child is embarrassed about having to use PAP therapy (Simon et al., 2012). When children endorsed ABCQ items themselves, the most frequent issues were not wanting to use the machine when away from home and just wanting to forget about having OSA (Simon et al., 2012). Clearly, children have their own psychological profile of needs when it comes to usage of PAP therapy that clinicians should be aware of when attempting to support their patients' usage of PAP for OSA.

Cognitive-behavioral therapy may be effective to help with negative feelings relating to use of PAP therapy, and group settings could permit the sharing of experiences thereby reducing embarrassment or feelings of awkwardness where use of PAP therapy outside of the home is concerned (i.e., overnight sleepovers away from the family home). The use of the ABCQ as a screening device to assess areas of potential concern for adherence to PAP therapy may be of clinical utility when attempting to understand potential barriers to PAP usage in pediatric patients (Simon et al., 2012).

Children with developmental and genetic disabilities may be slower to adapt to PAP therapy than nondisabled children (O'Donnell et al., 2006). However, programs that focus on specialized desensitization processes prior to initiation of PAP therapy (i.e., sending the child home with PAP mask prior to initiation of therapy in order to wear the mask at home for increasing time intervals) have shown utility in populations of children with special cognitive needs (O'Donnell et al., 2006).

OTHER TREATMENTS FOR OSA IN CHILDREN

There is little evidence to support the use of dental appliances to treat OSA in children (Guilleminault, Quo, Huynh, & Li, 2008), but research is underway to assess the utility of upper palate distraction (use of dental bridgework to gradually expand the width of the upper palate) in children with OSA who have high-arched palates (Guilleminault et al., 2008). Maxillofacial surgery is used in some children to correct facial structures that contribute to a narrowed airway (i.e., micrognathia, retrognathia, genetic syndromes with facial morphologies), but other surgical procedures (i.e., uvulopalatalpharyngoplasty/UPPP) are not used in children who have normal craniofacial structure (Abad & Guilleminault, 2009). Though dental appliances may not be the ideal intervention in pediatric OSA, diet, exercise, and education regarding the effects of obesity on OSA and daily function are also important interventions (Fennig, 2006; Spruyt, Sans Capdevila, Serpero, Kheirandish-Gozal, & Gozal) and have additional health-related benefits.

Effecting weight loss in obese children has been shown to occur when interventions include high intensity exercise in conjunction with nutritional education (Doyle-Baker, Venner, Lyon, & Fung, 2011), when children can establish healthy relationships with an athletic trainer who focuses on improvements in physical ability rather than psychological improvements (Twiddy, Wilson, Bryant, & Rudolf, 2012) and when weight loss interventions are closely tailored to address alterations in family dynamics and characteristics (Frohlich, Pott, Albayrak, Hebebrand, & Pauli-Pott, 2011). While a complete review of strategies for promoting successful weight loss in obese children is beyond the scope of this chapter, certain components of behavioral interventions along these lines may succeed in promoting weight loss in obese children that, in turn, could help alleviate OSA symptomatology.

There is a great need for further study of all of the treatments for OSA, including weight loss in obese children and the ways in which treatment improves cognitive, physical, metabolic and cardiovascular health outcomes for children with OSA.

Special Pediatric Populations and OSA

Children with developmental disabilities and genetic syndromes (e.g., Trisomy 21, Prader-Willi Syndrome, craniofacial abnormalities) are generally at greater risk for OSA due to many factors, such as upper airway shape, alterations in airflow, and excessive weight gain that occurs with certain genetic profiles. Much has yet to be learned about the factors that place these children at increased risk for sleep disorders and the impact of sleep disorders on the developmental trajectory in these children. Nevertheless, it is important that health care providers pay special attention to the factors that may place these children at risk for OSA.

As many as 35% of children seen in pediatric psychiatric clinics have symptoms suggestive of OSA (Chervin & Archbold, 2001). Children with ADHD, oppositional defiant disorder (ODD), and conduct disorder (CD) are at increased risk for OSA (Dillon et al., 2007; Gaultney, Merchant, & Gingras, 2009). Although there is a need for extensive research on the best ways to address this problem, there is evidence that treatment of OSA with tonsillectomy eliminated problematic behaviors associated with ODD/CD diagnoses (Dillon et al., 2007). Although obstructive sleep apnea is not described on standard clinical algorithms used to identify and diagnose problems such as attention-deficit/hyperactivity disorder (Reynolds & Redline, 2010), the behavioral effects of OSA are often similar to those of ADHD. Children with ADHD and those with problematic daytime behavior patterns should always be screened for obstructive sleep apnea (Gaultney et al., 2009; Mehl et al., 2006; O'Brien & Gozal, 2004; O'Brien, Mervis, Holbrook, Bruner, Klaus, et al., 2004).

Conclusion

Obstructive sleep apnea (OSA) is a phenomenon that affects upwards of 3% of children worldwide. It is a disorder that results in fragmented sleep, reduced blood oxygen levels, and cognitive and behavioral difficulties. Treatment for OSA focuses on the removal of tonsil and adenoidal tissues where applicable. Subsequent use of continuous positive airway pressure (CPAP) therapy is indicated when surgery is not an option for treatment of the disorder. CPAP therapy has many hurdles to effective use in pediatric populations. Namely, children may not want to use the treatment when they are away from their homes overnight, nor do they want to admit to or think about having OSA. These issues can make adherence to CPAP therapy challenging. Other treatments for OSA in children may include weight reduction and maxillofacial distraction, but the effectiveness of these treatments remains unknown. Children with special medical conditions such as Trisomy 21 and other genetic disorders may be at increased risk for OSA and should be carefully screened for the disorder. Psychiatric populations of children may also have an increased frequency of diagnosis and should also be carefully assessed for the presence of OSA symptoms.

Future Directions

- Determining the effectiveness of PAP therapy in the treatment of pediatric OSA
- Development and assessment of interventions which promote adherence to PAP therapy in pediatric populations
- Exploring links between psychiatric illness and presence of OSA and how treatment for OSA may lead to improvement of behavior and mood in children with psychiatric illness

References

Abad, V. C., & Guilleminault, C. (2009). Treatment options for obstructive sleep apnea. *Current Treatment Options in Neurology, 11*(5), 358–367.

Archbold, K. H., Pituch, K. J., Panahi, P., & Chervin, R. D. (2002). Symptoms of sleep disturbances among children at two general pediatric clinics. *Journal of Pediatrics, 140*(1), 97–102.

Archbold, K. H., Giordani, B., Ruzicka, D. L., & Chervin, R. D. (2004). Cognitive executive dysfunction in children with mild sleep-disordered breathing. *Biological Research for Nursing, 5*(3), 168–176.

Aurora, R. N., Zak, R. S., Karippot, A., Lamm, C. I., Morgenthaler, T. I., Auerbach, S. H., et al.. (2011). Practice parameters for the respiratory indications for polysomnography in children. *Sleep, 34*(3), 379–388.

Bhattacharjee, R., Kheirandish-Gozal, L., Spruyt, K., Mitchell, R. B., Promchiarak, J., Simakajornboon, N., et al. (2010). Adenotonsillectomy outcomes in treatment of obstructive sleep apnea in children: A multicenter retrospective study. *American Journal of Respiratory and Critical Care Medicine, 182*(5), 676–683.

Billings, M. E., Auckley, D., Benca, R., Foldvary-Schaefer, N., Iber, C., Redline, S., et al. (2011). Race and residential socioeconomics as predictors of CPAP adherence. *Sleep, 34*(12), 1653–1658.

Bixler, E. O., Vgontzas, A. N., Lin, H. M., Liao, D., Calhoun, S., Vela-Bueno, A., et al. (2009). Sleep disordered breathing in children in a general population sample: Prevalence and risk factors. *Sleep, 32*(6), 731–736.

Blunden, S., & Chervin, R. D. (2010). Sleep, performance and behaviour in Australian indigenous and non-indigenous children: An exploratory comparison. *Journal of Paediatrics and Child Health, 46*(1–2), 10–16.

Boss, E. F., Smith, D. F., & Ishman, S. L. (2011). Racial/ethnic and socioeconomic disparities in the diagnosis and treatment of sleep-disordered breathing in children. *International Journal of Pediatric Otorhinolaryngology, 75*(3), 299–307.

Bourke, R., Anderson, V., Yang, J. S.; Jackman, A. R., Killedar, A., Nixon, G. M., et al. (2011). Cognitive and academic functions are impaired in children with all severities of sleep-disordered breathing. *Sleep Medicine, 12*(5), 489–496.

Brooks, L. J. (2005). *Obstructive Sleep Apnea Syndrome in Infants and Children: Clinical Features and Pathophysiology.* Philadelphia, PA: Elsevier Saunders.

Brostrom, A., Nilsen, P., Johansson, P., Ulander, M., Stromberg, A., Svanborg, E., & Fridlund, B. (2010). Putative facilitators and barriers for adherence to CPAP treatment in patients with obstructive sleep apnea syndrome: A qualitative content analysis. *Sleep Medicine, 11*(2), 126–130.

Chervin, R. D., & Archbold, K. H. (2001). Hyperactivity and polysomnographic findings in children evaluated for sleep-disordered breathing. *Sleep, 24*(3), 313–320.

Chervin, R. D., Archbold, K. H., Dillon, J. E., Panahi, P., Pituch, K. J., Dahl, R. E., & Guilleminault, C. (2002). Inattention, hyperactivity, and symptoms of sleep-disordered breathing. *Pediatrics, 109*(3), 449–456.

Chervin, R. D., Clarke, D. F., Huffman, J. L., Szymanski, E., Ruzicka, D. L., Miller, V., et al. (2003). School performance, race, and other correlates of sleep-disordered breathing in children. *Sleep Medicine, 4*(1), 21–27.

Chervin, R. D., Ruzicka, D. L., Archbold, K. H., & Dillon, J. E. (2005). Snoring predicts hyperactivity four years later. *Sleep, 28*(7), 885–890.

Chervin, R. D., Ruzicka, D. L., Giordani, B. J., Weatherly, R. A., Dillon, J. E., Hodges, E. K., et al. (2006). Sleep-disordered breathing, behavior, and cognition in children before and after adenotonsillectomy. *Pediatrics, 117*(4), e769–778.

Chokroverty, S. (1995). An overview of sleep. In S. Chokroverty (Ed.), *Sleep Disorders Medicine: Basic Science, Technical Considerations and Clinical Aspects* (pp. 7–16). Boston, MA: Butterworth-Heinemann.

Dayyat, E., Kheirandish-Gozal, L., Sans Capdevila, O., Maarafeya, M. M., & Gozal, D. (2009). Obstructive sleep apnea in children: Relative contributions of body mass index and adenotonsillar hypertrophy. *Chest, 136*(1), 137–144.

Dillon, J. E., Blunden, S., Ruzicka, D. L., Guire, K. E., Champine, D., Weatherly, R. A., et al. (2007). DSM-IV diagnoses and obstructive sleep apnea in children before and 1 year after adenotonsillectomy. *Journal of the American Academy of Child and Adolescent Psychiatry, 46*(11), 1425–1436.

Doyle-Baker, P. K., Venner, A. A., Lyon, M. E., & Fung, T. (2011). Impact of a combined diet and progressive exercise intervention for overweight and obese children: the B.E. H.I.P. study. *Applied Physiology, Nutrition, and Metabolism, 36*(4), 515–525.

Fennig, S. (2006). Can we treat morbid obese children in a behavioral inpatient program? *Pediatric Endocrinology Reviews, 3*(Suppl 4), 590–596.

Frohlich, G., Pott, W., Albayrak, O., Hebebrand, J., & Pauli-Pott, U. (2011). Conditions of long-term success in a lifestyle intervention for overweight and obese youths. *Pediatrics, 128*(4), e779–785.

Gagnadoux, F., Le Vaillant, M., Goupil, F., Pigeanne, T., Chollet, S., Masson, P., et al. (2011). Influence of marital status and employment status on long-term adherence with continuous positive airway pressure in sleep apnea patients. *PLoS One, 6*(8), e22503.

Gaultney, J. F., Merchant, K., & Gingras, J. L. (2009). Parents of children with periodic limb movement disorder versus sleep-disordered breathing report greater daytime mood and behavior difficulties in their child: The importance of using ICSD-2nd Edition criteria to define a PLMD study group. *Behavioral Sleep Medicine, 7*(3), 119–135.

Giordani, B., Hodges, E. K., Guire, K. E., Ruzicka, D. L., Dillon, J. E., Weatherly, R. A., et al. (2008). Neuropsychological and behavioral functioning in children with and without obstructive sleep apnea referred for tonsillectomy. *Journal of the International Neuropsychological Society, 14*(4), 571–581.

Giordani, B., Hodges, E. K., Guire, K. E., Ruzicka, D. L., Dillon, J. E., Weatherly, R. A., et al. (2012). Changes in neuropsychological and behavioral functioning in children with and without obstructive sleep apnea following tonsillectomy. *Journal of the International Neuropsychological Soceity, 18*(2), 212–222.

Goodwin, J. L., Vasquez, M. M., Silva, G. E., & Quan, S. F. (2010). Incidence and remission of sleep-disordered breathing and related symptoms in 6- to 17-year old children—the Tucson Children's Assessment of Sleep Apnea Study. *Journal of Pediatrics, 157*(1), 57–61.

Gozal, D. (1998). Sleep-disordered breathing and school performance in children. *Pediatrics, 102*(3 Pt 1), 616–620.

Gozal, D., Kheirandish-Gozal, L., Serpero, L. D., Sans Capdevila, O., & Dayyat, E. (2007). Obstructive sleep apnea and endothelial function in school-aged nonobese children: Effect of adenotonsillectomy. *Circulation, 116*(20), 2307–2314.

Gozal, D., & Kheirandish-Gozal, L. (2009). Obesity and excessive daytime sleepiness in prepubertal children with obstructive sleep apnea. *Pediatrics, 123*(1), 13–18.

Gozal, D., Kheirandish-Gozal, L., Bhattacharjee, R., & Spruyt, K. (2010). Neurocognitive and endothelial dysfunction in children with obstructive sleep apnea. *Pediatrics, 126*(5), e1161–1167.

Guilleminault, C., Quo, S., Huynh, N. T., & Li, K. (2008). Orthodontic expansion treatment and adenotonsillectomy in the treatment of obstructive sleep apnea in prepubertal children. *Sleep, 31*(7), 953–957.

Halbower, A. C., & Marcus, C. L. (2003). Sleep disorders in children. *Current Opinion in Pulmonary Medicine, 9*(6), 471–476.

Katz, E. S., & Marcus, C. L. (2005). *Diagnosis of Obstructive Sleep Apnea Syndrome in Infants and Children*. Philadelphia, PA: Elsevier Saunders.

Kheirandish-Gozal, L., De Jong, M. R., Spruyt, K., Chamuleau, S. A., & Gozal, D. (2010). Obstructive sleep apnoea is associated with impaired pictorial memory task acquisition and retention in children. *European Respiratory Journal, 36*(1), 164–169.

Kim, J., Bhattacharjee, R., Snow, A. B., Capdevila, O. S., Kheirandish-Gozal, L., & Gozal, D. (2010). Myeloid-related protein 8/14 levels in children with obstructive sleep apnoea. *European Respiratory Journal, 35*(4), 843–850.

Koontz, K. L., Slifer, K. J., Cataldo, M. D., & Marcus, C. L. (2003). Improving pediatric compliance with positive airway pressure therapy: The impact of behavioral intervention. *Sleep, 26*(8), 1010–1015.

Loughlin, G. M., Brouillette, R. T., Brooke, L. J., Carroll, J. L., Chipps, B. E., England, S. J., et al. (1996). Standards and indications for cardiopulmonary sleep studies in children (Vol. 153, p. 866, 1995). *American Journal of Respiratory and Critical Care Medicine, 153*(6), U54–U54.

Marcus, C. L., Ward, S. L., Mallory, G. B., Rosen, C. L., Beckerman, R. C., Weese-Mayer, D. E., et al. (1995). Use of nasal continuous positive airway pressure as treatment of childhood obstructive sleep apnea. *Journal of Pediatrics, 127*(1), 88–94.

Marcus, C. L., Rosen, G., Ward, S. L. D., Halbower, A. C., Sterni, L., Lutz, J., et al. (2006). Adherence to and effectiveness of positive airway pressure therapy in children with obstructive sleep apnea. *Pediatrics, 117*(3), E442–E451.

Marcus, C. L., Beck, S. E., Traylor, J., Cornaglia, M. A., Meltzer, L. J., DiFeo, N., et al. (2012). Randomized, double-blind clinical trial of two different modes of positive airway pressure therapy on adherence and efficacy in children. [Research Support, Non-U.S. Gov't]. *Journal of Clinical Sleep Medicine, 8*(1), 37–42.

Mehl, R. C., O'Brien, L. M., Jones, J. H., Dreisbach, J. K., Mervis, C. B., & Gozal, D. (2006). Correlates of sleep and pediatric bipolar disorder. *Sleep, 29*(2), 193–197.

Melendres, M. C., Lutz, J. M., Rubin, E. D., & Marcus, C. L. (2004). Daytime sleepiness and hyperactivity in children with suspected sleep-disordered breathing. *Pediatrics, 114*(3), 768–775.

Mindell, J. A., & Owens, J. A. (2003). *A Clinical Guide to Pediatric Sleep: Diagnosis and Management of Sleep Problems.* Philadelphia, PA: Lippincott Williams & Wilkins.

Montgomery-Downs, H. E., O'Brien, L. M., Holbrook, C. R., & Gozal, D. (2004). Snoring and sleep-disordered breathing in young children: Subjective and objective correlates. *Sleep, 27*(1), 87–94.

Moore, M., Kirchner, H. L., Drotar, D., Johnson, N., Rosen, C., Ancoli-Israel, S., & Redline, S. (2009). Relationships among sleepiness, sleep time, and psychological functioning in adolescents. *Journal of Pediatric Psychology, 34*(10), 1175–1183.

Mulvaney, S. A., Goodwin, J. L., Morgan, W. J., Rosen, G. R., Quan, S. F., & Kaemingk, K. L. (2006). Behavior problems associated with sleep disordered breathing in school-aged children—the Tucson Children's Assessment of Sleep Apnea study. *Journal of Pediatric Psychology, 31*(3), 322–330.

O'Brien, L. M., Holbrook, C. R., Mervis, C. B., Klaus, C. J., Bruner, J. L., Raffield, T. J., et al. (2003). Sleep and neurobehavioral characteristics of 5- to 7-year-old children with parentally reported symptoms of attention-deficit/hyperactivity disorder. *Pediatrics, 111*(3), 554–563.

O'Brien, L. M., & Gozal, D. (2004). Sleep in children with attention deficit/hyperactivity disorder. *Minerva Pediatrica, 56*(6), 585–601.

O'Brien, L. M., Mervis, C. B., Holbrook, C. R., Bruner, J. L., Klaus, C. J., Rutherford, J., et al. (2004). Neurobehavioral implications of habitual snoring in children. *Pediatrics, 114*(1), 44–49.

O'Brien, L. M., Mervis, C. B., Holbrook, C. R., Bruner, J. L., Smith, N. H., McNally, N., et al. (2004). Neurobehavioral correlates of sleep-disordered breathing in children. *Journal of Sleep Research, 13*(2), 165–172.

O'Donnell, A. R., Bjornson, C. L., Bohn, S. G., & Kirk, V. G. (2006). Compliance rates in children using noninvasive continuous positive airway pressure. *Sleep, 29*(5), 651–658.

Rechtschaffen, A., & Kales, A. (1968). *A Manual of Standardized Terminology, Techniques and Scoring System for Sleep Stages of Human Subjects.* Los Angeles: UCLA Brain Information Service/Brain Research Institute.

Reynolds, C. F., 3rd, & Redline, S. (2010). The DSM-v sleep-wake disorders nosology: An update and an invitation to the sleep community. *Journal of Clinical Sleep Medicine, 6*(1), 9–10.

Ross, K. R., Hart, M. A., Storfer-Isser, A., Kibler, A. M., Johnson, N. L., Rosen, C. L., et al. (2009). Obesity and obesity related co-morbidities in a referral population of children with asthma. *Pediatric Pulmonology, 44*(9), 877–884.

Silva, G. E., Goodwin, J. L., Parthasarathy, S., Sherrill, D. L., Vana, K. D., Drescher, A. A., & Quan, S. F. (2011). Longitudinal association between short sleep, body weight, and emotional and learning problems in Hispanic and Caucasian children. *Sleep, 34*(9), 1197–1205.

Simon, S. L., Duncan, C. L., Janicke, D. M., & Wagner, M. H. (2012). Barriers to treatment of paediatric obstructive sleep apnoea: Development of the adherence barriers to continuous positive airway pressure (CPAP) questionnaire. [Validation Studies]. *Sleep Medicine, 13*(2), 172–177.

Spilsbury, J. C., Storfer-Isser, A., Kirchner, H. L., Nelson, L., Rosen, C. L., Drotar, D., & Redline, S. (2006). Neighborhood disadvantage as a risk factor for pediatric obstructive sleep apnea. *Journal of Pediatrics, 149*(3), 342–347.

Spruyt, K., O'Brien, L. M., Macmillan Coxon, A. P., Cluydts, R., Verleye, G., & Ferri, R. (2006). Multidimensional scaling of pediatric sleep breathing problems and bio-behavioral correlates. *Sleep Medicine, 7*(3), 269–280.

Spruyt, K., Capdevila, O. S., Kheirandish-Gozal, L., & Gozal, D. (2009). Inefficient or insufficient encoding as potential primary deficit in neurodevelopmental performance among children with OSA. *Developmental Neuropsychology, 34*(5), 601–614.

Spruyt, K., Sans Capdevila, O., Serpero, L. D., Kheirandish-Gozal, L., & Gozal, D. (2010). Dietary and physical activity patterns in children with obstructive sleep apnea. *Journal of Pediatrics, 156*(5), 724–730, 730 e721–730 e723.

Tarasiuk, A., Reznor, G., Greenberg-Dotan, S., & Reuveni, H. (2012). Financial incentive increases CPAP acceptance in patients from low socioeconomic background. *PLoS One, 7*(3), e33178.

Tauman, R., O'Brien, L. M., & Gozal, D. (2007). Hypoxemia and obesity modulate plasma C-reactive protein and interleukin-6 levels in sleep-disordered breathing. *Sleep and Breathing, 11*(2), 77–84.

Twiddy, M., Wilson, I., Bryant, M., & Rudolf, M. (2012). Lessons learned from a family-focused weight management intervention for obese and overweight children. *Public Health Nutrition*, 1–8.

Uong, E. C., Epperson, M., Bathon, S. A., & Jeffe, D. B. (2007). Adherence to nasal positive airway pressure therapy among school-aged children and adolescents with obstructive sleep apnea syndrome. *Pediatrics, 120*(5), e1203–1211.

Walker, P., Whitehead, B., & Gulliver, T. (2008). Polysomnographic outcome of adenotonsillectomy for obstructive sleep apnea in children under 5 years old. *Otolaryngology – Head and Neck Surgery, 139*(1), 83–86.

Wei, J. L., Bond, J., Mayo, M. S., Smith, H. J., Reese, M., & Weatherly, R. A. (2009). Improved behavior and sleep after adenotonsillectomy in children with sleep-disordered breathing: Long-term follow-up. *Archives of Otolaryngology Head and Neck Surgery, 135*(7), 642–646.

CHAPTER

26 Nocturnal Enuresis

Patrina HY Caldwell *and* Karen Waters

Abstract

Nocturnal enuresis (bedwetting) is one of the most well-studied sleep disorders of childhood. This common condition occurs in up to 20% of school children. Although most children will outgrow their problem, nocturnal enuresis can persist into adulthood. Nocturnal enuresis is considered one of the parasomnias and is diagnosed when the night wetting persists beyond the age of 5 in a child who has attained daytime continence.

The etiology of nocturnal enuresis is multifactorial and occurs when the child is unable to arouse from sleep in response to a full bladder sensation, with excessive nocturnal urine production and/or reduced nocturnal bladder capacity commonly being a feature. An understanding of the physiology of sleep and the relationship between sleep arousal and nocturnal enuresis is a first step to understanding how treatments work. It will enable clinicians to identify the most appropriate treatment for each individual and appreciate why some children fail treatment.

Key Words: enuresis, nocturnal enuresis, bedwetting, children, incontinence, urinary incontinence, sleep

Introduction

Bedwetting (nocturnal enuresis) has long been recognized as a childhood disorder, with the earliest reference found in the Ebers papyrus of 1550 BC. Nocturnal enuresis was also mentioned in the first book of diseases of children in 1472 by Paulus Bagallardus of Padua (Salmon, 1975). This common condition not only affects the physical, psychological, and social well-being of the child, but also other members of the family.

Nocturnal enuresis is defined as persistent bedwetting occurring during sleep in a child age 5 or older. This chapter will examine factors that contribute to nocturnal enuresis and the relationship between nocturnal enuresis and sleep. It will also explore the impact of nocturnal enuresis on the child and family, and will discuss treatments used for managing this condition and analyze how they work.

Definitions

There are several terms used for bedwetting including *nocturnal enuresis* (the most commonly used term), *enuresis, sleep enuresis* and *intermittent nocturnal incontinence*. The American Psychiatric Association (APA) generally uses the term *enuresis*. The International Children's Continence Society (ICCS) recommends the use of standardized terminology; therefore, definitions in this chapter will conform to the standards recommended by the International Children's Continence Society and the term *nocturnal enuresis* or *enuresis* will be used.

Nocturnal enuresis is divided into primary and secondary enuresis, with children who have primary enuresis never having attained night dryness and secondary enuresis occurring after the child has attained night dryness for at least 6 months. The majority of enuretic children have primary nocturnal enuresis (Forsythe & Redmond, 1974). The distinction between primary and secondary nocturnal enuresis is important, since secondary nocturnal enuresis is more likely to be associated with a pathological etiology (Neveus et al., 2006).

Diagnostic Criteria

There are three commonly used diagnostic criteria for nocturnal enuresis: *The Diagnostic and Statistical Manual of Mental Disorders—IV-TR* (DSM-IV-TR), *The International Classification of Sleep Disorders, Revised* (ICSD), and the criteria developed by the International Children's Continence Society (ICCS). The different diagnostic criteria vary slightly, but common features for all are persistent wetting occurring during sleep in a child aged 5 years or older.

THE DIAGNOSTIC AND STATISTICAL MANUAL OF MENTAL DISORDERS

The DSM-IV-TR, published by the American Psychiatric Association, provides a classification for mental disorders. The DSM-IV-TR diagnostic criteria for enuresis are, "the repeated voiding of urine into the bed or clothes (whether involuntary or intentional)." The behavior needs to be clinically significant, with a wetting frequency of at least twice a week for at least 3 consecutive months or where it causes clinically significant distress or impairment in social, academic, or other functioning for the child who is developmentally 5 years of age or more. The behavior should not be due to the direct physiological effect of a substance (such as a diuretic) or a general medical condition (such as diabetes, spina bifida, or a seizure disorder).

THE INTERNATIONAL CLASSIFICATION OF SLEEP DISORDERS

The ICSD- Revised Diagnostic and Coding Manual, produced by the American Academy of Sleep Medicine, defines "sleep enuresis" as episodic involuntary voiding of urine during sleep at least twice per month in children aged 3–6 years and at least once per month in older individuals (American Sleep Disorders Association, 1997). The enuresis can be associated with medical or mental disorders such as diabetes, urinary tract infection, obstructive sleep apnea syndrome, epilepsy, or other disorders. A diagnostic polysomnography feature should include voiding during sleep in the absence of epileptic activity.

THE INTERNATIONAL CHILDREN'S CONTINENCE SOCIETY

The ICCS's *Standardization of Terminology Document* (Neveus et al., 2006), produced by the ICCS, a global multidisciplinary organization for professionals involved with lower urinary tract function and malfunction in children, define nocturnal enuresis as intermittent nocturnal incontinence in discrete episodes while asleep. It is both a symptom and a condition.

The ICCS also recommends that nocturnal enuresis be subgrouped into *monosymptomatic* or *non-monosymptomatic* nocturnal enuresis. Monosymptomatic nocturnal enuresis is not associated with any daytime urinary symptoms, and non-monosymptomatic nocturnal enuresis is associated with urgency, frequency, or daytime urinary incontinence. The distinction between monosymptomatic and non-monosymptomatic nocturnal enuresis is important for determining management. The most common form of nocturnal enuresis is primary monosymptomatic nocturnal enuresis (Forsythe & Redmond, 1974), although there is an argument that less than half the children with nocturnal enuresis are truly monosymptomatic (Neveus et al., 2010).

Factors that Contribute to Nocturnal Enuresis

Epidemiology

Nocturnal enuresis is common in childhood, with a prevalence rate of up to 20% for 5-year-olds, 7% for 7-year-olds, 5% for 10-year-olds, and 0.5–2% for adults (Bower, Moore, Shepherd, & Adams, 1996; Hirasing, van Leerdam, Bolk-Bennink, & Janknegt, 1997; Yeung et al., 2004). Most children outgrow their nocturnal enuresis, with an annual spontaneous remission rate of 14% until adulthood when the prevalence of nocturnal enuresis remains static (Yeung et al., 2004). Children with mild symptoms were more likely to outgrow their nocturnal enuresis, and adolescents and adults with nocturnal enuresis were more likely to have severe symptoms (Yeung, Sreedhar, Sihoe, Sit, & Lau, 2006). Nocturnal enuresis is also more common in boys, with a male to female ratio of 3:2 (Forsythe & Redmond, 1974).

Etiology

The etiology of nocturnal enuresis is multifactorial, with a complex interaction of genetic and environmental factors, although the exact mechanism of interaction is unknown. Proposed causes for nocturnal enuresis include delayed maturation of the micturition process, central nervous system immaturity and developmental delay (Järvelin, 1989), altered bladder physiology, psychiatric and behavioral disturbances, environmental factors, and genetic factors (Mikkelsen & Rapoport, 1980). The symptom of nocturnal enuresis is thought to be caused by interplay between the three major pathogenic mechanisms of defective sleep arousal, nocturnal bladder volume, and nocturnal urine production.

DEFECTIVE SLEEP AROUSAL

During sleep, an urge to void is experienced in non-enuretic children when the volume of urine produced reaches the bladder storage capacity, which results in the child waking to void (nocturia). This arousal response is defective in many enuretic children (Kawauchi et al., 1998; Wolfish, Pivik, & Busby, 1997), who show polysomnographic changes from deep sleep to light sleep during bladder contraction but without full awakening, resulting in wetting during sleep (Watanabe & Azuma, 1989). Children with severe nocturnal enuresis and bladder instability appear to have more frequent cortical arousals during bladder contractions but are unable to awaken completely (Yeung, Diao, & Sreedhar, 2008).

REDUCED NOCTURNAL BLADDER CAPACITY

Children with a defective arousal response who have a reduced nocturnal bladder capacity may develop enuresis when their overnight urine volume exceeds the bladder capacity. Usually these children will also exhibit daytime bladder symptoms (presenting as non-monosymptomatic nocturnal enuresis), but curiously some children have nocturnal detrusor overactivity despite normal daytime bladder function, resulting in urinary leakage only during sleep (Yeung et al., 2002).

NOCTURNAL POLYURIA

Nocturnal polyuria (high overnight urine production) can result in nocturnal enuresis in children with defective arousal when the volume of urine produced exceeds the bladder capacity (Norgaard, 1991). Nocturnal polyuria may be caused by excessive evening fluid intake. This commonly occurs in children who fluid-restrict for whatever reason during the day (including those who fluid-restrict because of concerns about daytime wetting) and then drink excessively in the evening because of thirst.

Nocturnal polyuria can also occur when there is an alteration in the daily circadian secretion of antidiuretic hormone (ADH, also known as arginine vasopressin) by the pituitary gland. In the non-enuretic child, ADH secretion is highest at night, causing the kidney to conserve water resulting in a reduction in overnight urine production, which explains why most people do not need to wake during the night to void. In about two-thirds of children with nocturnal enuresis there is a lower nocturnal level of ADH compared with non-enuretic children, resulting in the production of larger amounts of relatively dilute urine during sleep (Rittig, Knudsen, Norgaard, Pedersen, & Djurhuus, 1989), which increases the risk of nocturnal enuresis.

OTHER RISK FACTORS FOR NOCTURNAL ENURESIS

The risk of nocturnal enuresis is increased in children with sleep disordered breathing (discussed in detail later; Brooks & Topol, 2003), attention-deficit/hyperactivity disorder (Baeyens et al., 2005), and constipation (McGrath, Caldwell, & Jones, 2008; O'Regan, Yazbeck, Hamberger, & Schick, 1986). These cause nocturnal enuresis by their impact on arousal thresholds from sleep, bladder capacity, or overnight urine production (including through secretion of hormones relevant to urine production).

Nocturnal enuresis can also be an inherited disorder with a heterogeneous mode of inheritance, where several loci on different chromosomes have been identified to be associated with nocturnal enuresis. The odds for severe nocturnal enuresis are 3.63 times higher if the mother and 1.85 times higher if the father had a history of nocturnal enuresis (von Gontard, Heron, & Joinson, 2011).

The Relationship between Nocturnal Enuresis and Sleep

The two main relationships between nocturnal enuresis and sleep are the high arousal threshold noted in nocturnal enuresis and the link between nocturnal enuresis and sleep disordered breathing.

High Arousal Thresholds

Monosymptomatic nocturnal enuresis is considered a form of parasomnia because it meets the definition of disturbed behavior or experiences that occur exclusively or predominantly during sleep. However, children with enuresis do not have an increased incidence or association with other parasomnias such as sleepwalking or night terrors. The distribution of sleep architecture is also equivalent between children with nocturnal enuresis and controls. Thus, the major finding pertinent to sleep in children with nocturnal enuresis is that they have increased arousal thresholds.

Well-documented studies indicate that enuretic episodes occur in all sleep stages (Cohen-Zrubavel, Kushnir, Kushnir, & Sadeh, 2011). In this context, children with monosymptomatic nocturnal enuresis usually wet during the early phases of sleep. If episodes of enuresis occur early in the night they are more likely to occur during non-REM and slow wave sleep (SWS) than in REM sleep (although they are not directly linked to any specific sleep stage), since REM sleep tends to predominate in the early morning. The most likely explanation for why enuresis alarm therapy may precipitate sleepwalking or confusional arousal episodes is that confusional arousals with semi-purposeful behaviors arise out of slow wave sleep.

Normally, arousal and awakening from sleep occur prior to physiological phenomena such as cough, and pelvic visceral stimuli including colonic and bladder distension. By term, normally developing infants arouse before bladder emptying (Zotter, Sauseng, Kutschera, Mueller, & Kerbl, 2006). Bladder distension results in increased stimulation of the Barrington's nucleus (the Pontine micturition center) in the locus coeruleus, which is implicated in arousal (Rouzade-Dominguez, Curtis, & Valentino, 2001). Children with nocturnal enuresis are reported by parents to be difficult to arouse, and various methods have been used to demonstrate that the children have arousal deficits with additional evidence such as increased density of delta frequency in their sleep and electroencephalogram supporting a decreased arousability (Kaditis et al., 2011).

Yeung and others postulated that in a subgroup of enuretic patients the reduced arousability is due to an increased frequency of cortical stimulation from bladder instability that led to lightening of sleep and an increase in the proportion of light sleep, but not to full arousal (Yeung, Diao, & Sreedhar, 2008). Other studies including actigraphy, polysomnography, and self-reports from the children with nocturnal enuresis demonstrate more sleep disturbance in children with nocturnal enuresis, including: higher sleep latency and lower sleep efficiency (Ertan et al., 2009); increased sleep latency and increased frequency of actigraphic awakenings (Cohen-Zrubavel et al., 2011); or periodic limb movements (Dhondt et al., 2009). The postulated abnormality in these children is that frequent small sleep disturbances cause a reduction in deep sleep and/or sleep quality that reduces the child's capacity to fully awaken in response to a full bladder, resulting in enuresis. On actigraphy, the children have lower percentages of motionless sleep and shorter periods of continuous sleep, while questionnaire self-reports indicate poorer sleep quality and reduced sleep efficiency and a higher incidence of periodic limb movements leading to arousals, associated with increased cortical arousability. Together, these studies suggest that the increased arousal threshold is likely to be secondary to sleep deprivation (Cohen-Zrubavel et al., 2011). The increased arousal threshold in children with nocturnal enuresis may also reflect some delay in the maturation of brainstem arousal (Freitag, Röhling, Seifen, Pukrop, & von Gontard, 2006).

Sleep Disordered Breathing

Children with sleep disordered breathing, including habitual snoring reported on questionnaire and obstructive sleep apnea on polysomnography (Brooks & Topol, 2003), have a higher prevalence of nocturnal enuresis than controls who do not snore. In addition, children whose sleep disordered breathing is treated with adenotonsillectomy show improvement or resolution of their nocturnal enuresis, although those whose nocturnal enuresis improves are more likely to be non-monosymptomatic (Basha, Bialowas, Ende, & Szeremeta, 2005). The links between OSA and enuresis are not restricted to initiation or exacerbation of reduced arousability through sleep deprivation, but are also linked to increased urine output. The main hormones affected by OSA include natiuretic peptides (atrial natiuretic peptide, or ANP), aldosterone, and ADH. The large negative intrathoracic pressure swings that occur during OSA lead to increased venous return followed by acute right atrial distension. This causes increased ANP, a hormone that regulates blood volume and pressure, to be released from the wall of the right atrium. The ANP acts on the renal tubules to increase salt and water excretion. The hypoxia caused by the apneas also contributes to increased ANP secretion (Stone, Malone, Atwill, McGrigor, & Hill, 2008). There is a negative correlation between levels of ANP and ADH in patients with OSA (Ichioka et al., 1992) so that children with OSA have reduced levels of ADH correlated with higher urine volumes, both of which improve after successful adenotonsillectomy (Yue, Wang, Xu, Li, & Wang, 2009). Other sequelae of OSA that may result in increased urine production include hyperinsulinemia and type 2 diabetes.

Impact of Nocturnal Enuresis on the Child and Family

Despite its benign nature, nocturnal enuresis is a most frustrating and bothersome condition, which has significant impacts on the child and the child's family. Because of the stigmatizing nature of this condition, only one-third of families seek help to address the problem (Bower et al., 1996). Children are embarrassed and ashamed about their nocturnal enuresis and often decline sleepovers and overnight school excursions, fearing detection by their peers. At times, these children are subjected to bullying and ridicule. Nocturnal enuresis negatively affects children's self-esteem, interpersonal relationships, and quality of life (Warzak, 1993; Deshpande et al., 2011; Redsell & Collier, 2001; Morison, 1998). When nocturnal enuresis continues into adult life, the impact can be devastating (Stone, 1973).

Nocturnal enuresis can also affect other family members. There are increased costs and work associated with the purchase of continence products and with extra washing of bedclothes. Parents are often frustrated by the failure to attain night dryness and may feel guilty, anxious, and lose confidence in their parenting skills (Warzak, 1993). Some parents erroneously believe that the child intentionally wet the bed or is too lazy to go to the toilet at night, resulting in conflict with the child and a stressful home environment. Because bedwetting is outside of the child's conscious control, children can become frustrated by their lack of success despite trying and may appear defiant to attempts of treatment. Parents frustrated with the lack of success and apparent lack of effort by their child may respond by belittling the child or harsh punishment. There is a higher risk of emotional and physical abuse among enuretics (Schmitt, 1987; Warzak, 1993; Morison, 1998).

Management of Nocturnal Enuresis

ICCS recommends evaluation and treatment for children over 5 years of age with nocturnal enuresis (Neveus et al., 2010). Accurate assessment is essential, as it directs management.

Assessment

HISTORY TAKING

A thorough history is essential in the evaluation. It is important to identify the type of enuresis and also any risk factors which may contribute to the enuresis or treatment response.

As somatic and psychological comorbid conditions (such as urinary tract infections, diabetes mellitus and insipidus, stress, sexual abuse, and bladder dysfunction) are more common in secondary nocturnal enuresis (Neveus et al., 2010), these need to be sought in the history taking. It is also important to differentiate monosymptomatic and non-monosymptomatic nocturnal enuresis, as treatment for the daytime bladder symptoms should precede treatment for the nocturnal enuresis (Neveus et al., 2010).

PHYSICAL EXAMINATION

Physical examination in children with nocturnal enuresis is usually normal. Examination should include urinalysis (to identify urinary tract infection, kidney disease, and diabetes mellitus), examination of the spine (for neurological abnormalities such as spina bifida occulta), the abdomen (to assess for constipation), and the external genitalia (to assess for urogenital abnormalities). Rectal and genital examination is usually not necessary.

INVESTIGATION

A frequency volume chart (bladder diary) measuring the time and volume of all fluid intake and urine output in a 24-hour period is one of the most useful tools for assessing nocturnal enuresis. This is an assessment tool commonly used by continence clinicians, that can be used for any child who has been toilet trained. It provides objective, reliable data about the child's fluid intake, frequency of voiding during the day, bladder capacity (estimated from the volume of each void), and total overnight urine production. A urine culture to exclude a urinary tract infection is the only investigation indicated for nocturnal enuresis. An ultrasound of the child's kidneys and urinary tract is usually not warranted, unless there is a suggestion of underlying bladder dysfunction.

Treatment

Treatments for nocturnal enuresis target the three major pathogenic mechanisms—defective sleep arousal, nocturnal bladder volume, and nocturnal urine production. If a child and parents both desire the child to achieve nighttime continence, have a positive attitude to address the wetting problem, and are motivated to engage in treatment, they are much more likely to achieve success (Morison, 1998).

UROTHERAPY

Urotherapy is a term used to describe all forms of nonsurgical and nonpharmacological interventions used for treating micturition disorders (nocturnal enuresis and daytime urinary incontinence). This includes educating the child and family about the condition and the aim of treatment, as well as offering general advice about voiding (correct voiding

Table 26.1 History Taking (adapted with permission from Neveus et al., 2010).

Assess for type of enuresis: Primary or secondary? Monosymptomatic or non-monosymptomatic?	Look for causes of secondary nocturnal enuresis. Did occurrence of wetting coincide with any major event? Treat bladder symptoms first if non-monosymptomatic.
History of daytime voiding habits: Is there urgency, frequency, holding maneuvers? Is there an interrupted or weak urine stream, continuous urine leakage or the use of abdominal pressure to void?	Assess for bladder dysfunction which may need treatment or referral to a specialized center for further management .
History of nocturnal enuresis: How often does it occur? Does the child wake to void during the night?	Assess for severity of nocturnal enuresis and as a baseline to compare treatment response. Nocturia would indicate that the child is not extremely difficult to wake during the night.
History of fluid intake: Does the child drink adequate fluid? Does the child have a high evening fluid intake? Does the child drink too much caffeinated drinks?	Inadequate fluid intake can contribute to constipation. High evening fluid intake can cause nocturnal polyuria. Caffeine can cause bladder dysfunction in some children.
Assess for comorbid conditions: Does the child have constipation or fecal incontinence? Does the child have ADHD (attention-deficit/hyperactivity disorder)? Does the child have sleep disordered breathing?	Bladder and bowel function are closely interrelated. Treatment of bowel disorder is important for optimizing anti-enuretic therapy. Children with ADHD may need treatment for ADHD in parallel with anti-enuretic therapy. Relief of upper airway obstruction can improve nocturnal enuresis.
Assess for the general health of the child	Childhood illness including kidney disease and diabetes can affect bladder function and nocturnal enuresis.
What strategies have the family previously tried for their nocturnal enuresis?	If previous treatments have been tried, it is important to assess that they were used correctly.

postures and regular voiding [timed voiding], optimizing fluid intake [including ensuring adequate fluid intake during the day, minimizing night time fluid intake and minimizing caffeinated drinks such as cola and chocolate drinks], treating constipation, and ensuring adequate sleep (Neveus et al., 2006). Urotherapy aims to improve bladder function and compliance to treatment.

ALARM TRAINING

Enuresis alarm training is the most effective treatment for nocturnal enuresis and is the first-line treatment for it (Glazener, Evans, & Peto, 2005b). About two-thirds of children become dry with alarm training, and half sustain nighttime dryness after completion of alarm therapy (Glazener et al., 2005b). Enuresis alarms are used to train the child to withhold urination while asleep or to wake to void. They were used as early as 1938 by Mowrer (Mowrer & Mowrer, 1938). The earliest enuresis alarms were placed on the bed ("bell and pad alarms"), and rang in response to contact with urine. This underlying principle remains unchanged. The newer alarms are worn in the child's underpants ("body worn alarms"), and both types appear to be equally effective. Enuresis alarms address the poor arousal response in enuretics by conditioning the child to either wake to urinate when their bladder is full or withhold urination while they sleep. However, treatment failure commonly occurs when children fail to respond and awaken in response to the alarm stimuli. Alarms produce a gradual but more sustained improvement in bedwetting compared to other treatments (Glazener et al., 2005b). Overlearning (giving additional fluids at bedtime while continuing alarm training) can reinforce alarm training and further reduce relapse in a child who has initially responded to alarm therapy (Glazener et al., 2005b). Alarms are usually worn till the child achieves 14 consecutive dry nights.

DESMOPRESSIN

Desmopressin is second-line therapy for nocturnal enuresis. It is a synthetic analogue of antidiuretic hormone (arginine vasopressin, ADH) that is normally secreted by the pituitary gland during sleep. Desmopressin comes in a nasal spray, tablet, and lyophilisate (melt) formulation. It exerts an antidiuretic effect by increasing the water permeability of the collecting tubules in the kidney. A significant proportion of enuretics have inadequate ADH secretion and nocturnal polyuria, which can be treated with desmopressin (Rittig et al., 1989). Care needs to be observed when using desmopressin to ensure that fluid intake at night is not excessive, as this increases the risk of water intoxication. There is also some debate about whether desmopressin increases the arousability of children with nocturnal enuresis (Eggert, Fritz, Stecker, & Muller, 2004; Rahm, Schulz-Juergensen, & Eggert, 2010). When administered at bedtime, it rapidly helps to reduce the volume of urine produced overnight. On desmopressin, children have on average one fewer wet night per week, and 19% become dry on treatment. However, this response is not sustained on discontinuation of treatment (Glazener & Evans, 2002). Desmopressin is particularly useful when a rapid response is required (such as for overnight school excursions or sleepovers) and when alarm training is ineffective or difficult. It is also particularly useful when the total overnight urine volume produced is large. It is effective in children of all ages and is generally recommended for children aged 6 years and older. Desmopressin is sometimes used in conjunction with other therapies when there is treatment resistance. There is some suggestion that combination therapy using desmopressin and alarm training is more effective than alarm monotherapy (Glazener & Evans, 2002).

TRICYCLIC ANTIDEPRESSANTS

Tricyclic antidepressants (such as imipramine and amitriptyline) have been used to treat nocturnal enuresis since the 1970s. The mechanism of action is not known, although it is thought that the tricyclics may exert its anti-enuretic effect by an anticholinergic effect on the bladder and possibly also by its effect on the sleep center of the brain, improving arousability (Glazener, Evans, & Peto, 2003b). Children on tricyclics have on average one fewer wet night per week and about one-fifth become dry on treatment. However, like for desmopressin, the relapse rate on discontinuation of treatment is high (Glazener et al., 2003b). The major concern about using tricyclic antidepressants is the risk of significant adverse effects such as cardiotoxicity and hepatotoxicity in overdose. Given the availability of other, safer options, such as alarm training and desmopressin, tricyclics are now used as third-line therapy in nocturnal enuresis.

ANTICHOLINERGIC MEDICATIONS

In children with non-monosymptomatic nocturnal enuresis or nocturnal detrusor overactivity, anticholinergic medications can improve the bladder function by inhibiting bladder contractions and increasing bladder capacity. This is particularly helpful for enuretics with small bladder capacity who are resistant to therapy (Yeung et al., 2002). Anticholinergic medications commonly used for children include oxybutynin and tolterodine. Anticholinergics are also sometimes used in combination with alarm training or desmopressin for treating therapy-resistant nocturnal enuresis (Austin et al., 2008).

OTHER THERAPIES

Other therapies used for treating nocturnal enuresis include behavioral interventions such as lifting (parents taking the child to void during the night without waking them), waking (waking the child up to void during the night), rewards (rewarding the child for dry nights), bladder training (various daytime drinking and voiding programs aimed at increasing the bladder volume, including encouraging the child to drink and then to "hold on" and delay going to the toilet), dry bed training and full-spectrum home training (which involves the child getting up during the night to void and getting him or her to change their own bed after they have wet; Glazener & Evans, 2004a; Glazener, Evans, & Peto, 2004b), complementary and miscellaneous interventions such as hypnotherapy, acupuncture, and chiropractics (Glazener, Evans, & Cheuk, 2005a), and other medications (Glazener, Evans, & Peto, 2003a). There is currently insufficient evidence to demonstrate whether any of these treatments are effective.

Conclusion

Nocturnal enuresis is a common childhood sleep disorder that is largely a result of poor arousal to bladder contraction during sleep. As it is a benign condition that most children outgrow, it is reasonable to reassure parents of children aged 5 and below that no particular treatment is necessary. However, in older children and adolescents who are less likely to outgrow their condition, if the child is particularly distressed by the enuresis, or if it negatively affects the child's life (resulting in low self-esteem, bullying, and missed socializing opportunities such as sleepovers and school excursions), treatment is recommended. Treatments target the three major pathogenic mechanisms of poor arousal from sleep, nocturnal bladder volume, and nocturnal urine production. Behavioral therapy focusing on alarm training and urotherapy will improve treatment response. Although there are many available treatments, treatment failure is common. Many children find treatment overwhelming (particularly alarm training, which affects the sleep of the child and other family members), and support during treatment with strategies to improve compliance will help. A better understanding of what happens during sleep and why some children fail to wake when the bladder contracts will enable researchers and clinicians to improve current treatments for this devastating condition.

Future Directions

- Understanding why enuretic children have disordered arousal mechanisms during sleep
- Identifying what causes treatment failure for the various treatments used for nocturnal enuresis
- Understanding how enuresis alarms affect sleep stages and sleep quality
- Identifying therapies (including new medications and other behavioral approaches to improve sleep quality) which may improve arousal response and/or consolidate sleep.

References

American Sleep Disorders Association. (1997). *The International Classification of Sleep Disorders: Diagnostic and Coding Manual—Revised.* Rochester, MN: American Sleep Disorders Association.

Austin, P. F., Ferguson, G., Yan, Y., Campigotto, M. J., Royer, M. E., & Coplen, D. E. (2008). Combination therapy with desmopressin and an anticholinergic medication for nonresponders to desmopressin for monosymptomatic nocturnal enuresis: A randomized, double-blind, placebo-controlled trial. *Pediatrics, 122*(5), 1027.

Baeyens, D., Roeyers, H., Demeyere, I., Verte, S., Hoebeke, P., & Walle, J. V. (2005). Attention-deficit/hyperactivity disorder (ADHD) as a risk factor for persistent nocturnal enuresis in children: A two-year follow-up study. *Acta Paediatrica, 94*(11), 1619–1625.

Basha, S., Bialowas, C., Ende, K., & Szeremeta, W. (2005). Effectiveness of adenotonsillectomy in the resolution of nocturnal enuresis secondary to obstructive sleep apnea. *The Laryngoscope, 115*(6), 1101–1103.

Bower, W., Moore, K., Shepherd, R., & Adams, R. (1996). The epidemiology of childhood enuresis in Australia. *British Journal of Urology, 78*(4), 602–606.

Brooks, L. J., & Topol, H. I. (2003). Enuresis in children with sleep apnea. *Journal of Pediatrics, 142*(5), 515–518.

Cohen-Zrubavel, V., Kushnir, B., Kushnir, J., & Sadeh, A. (2011). Sleep and sleepiness in children with nocturnal enuresis. *Sleep, 34*(2), 191.

Deshpande, A. V., Craig, J. C., Smith, G. H. H., & Caldwell, P. H. Y. (2011). Factors influencing quality of life in children with urinary incontinence. *The Journal of Urology, 186* (3), 1048–1052.

Dhondt, K., Raes, A., Hoebeke, P., Van Laecke, E., Van Herzeele, C., & Vande Walle, J. (2009). Abnormal sleep architecture and refractory nocturnal enuresis. *The Journal of Urology, 182*(4), 1961–1966.

Eggert, P., Fritz, A., Stecker, B., & Muller, D. (2004). Desmopressin has an influence on the arousability of children with primary nocturnal enuresis. *The Journal of Urology, 171*(6), 2586–2588.

Ertan, P., Yilmaz, O., Caglayan, M., Sogut, A., Aslan, S., & Yuksel, H. (2009). Relationship of sleep quality and quality of life in children with monosymptomatic enuresis. *Child: Care, Health and Development, 35*(4), 469–474.

Forsythe, W., & Redmond, A. (1974). Enuresis and spontaneous cure rate. *Archives of Disease in Childhood, 49*(4), 259–263.

Freitag, C. M., Röhling, D., Seifen, S., Pukrop, R., & von Gontard, A. (2006). Neurophysiology of nocturnal enuresis: Evoked potentials and prepulse inhibition of the startle reflex. *Developmental Medicine & Child Neurology, 48*(04), 278–284.

Glazener, C. M., & Evans, J. H. (2002). Desmopressin for nocturnal enuresis in children. *Cochrane Database of Systematic Reviews*(3), CD002112.

Glazener, C. M. A., Evans, J. H. C., & Peto, R. E. (2003a). Drugs for nocturnal enuresis in children (other than desmopressin and tricyclics). *Cochrane Database of Systematic Reviews*(4), CD002238.

Glazener, C. M. A., Evans, J. H. C., & Peto, R. E. (2003b). Tricyclic and related drugs for nocturnal enuresis in children. *Cochrane Database of Systematic Reviews*(3), CD002117.

Glazener, C. M. A., & Evans, J. H. C. (2004a). Simple behavioural and physical interventions for nocturnal enuresis in children. *Cochrane Database of Systematic Reviews*(2), CD003637.

Glazener, C. M. A., Evans, J. H. C., & Peto, R. E. (2004b). Complex behavioural and educational interventions for nocturnal enuresis in children. *Cochrane Database of Systematic Reviews*(1), CD004668.

Glazener, C. M. A., Evans, J. H. C., & Cheuk, D. K. L. (2005a). Complementary and miscellaneous interventions for nocturnal enuresis in children. *Cochrane Database of Systematic Reviews*(2), CD005230.

Glazener, C. M. A., Evans, J. H. C., & Peto, R. E. (2005b). Alarm interventions for nocturnal enuresis in children. *Cochrane Database of Systematic Reviews*(2), CD002911.

Hirasing, R. A., van Leerdam, F. J. M., Bolk-Bennink, L., & Janknegt, R. A. (1997). Enuresis nocturna in adults. *Scandinavian Journal of Urology and Nephrology, 31*(6), 533–536.

Ichioka, M., Hirata, Y., Inase, N., Tojo, N., Yoshizawa, M., Chida, M., et al. (1992). Changes of circulating atrial natriuretic peptide and antidiuretic hormone in obstructive sleep apnea syndrome. *Respiration, 59*(3), 164–168.

Järvelin, M. R. (1989). Developmental history and neurological findings in enuretic children. *Developmental Medicine & Child Neurology, 31*(6), 728–736.

Kaditis, A. G., Chaidas, K., Alexopoulos, E. I., Varlami, V., Malakasioti, G., & Gourgoulianis, K. (2011). Effects of adenotonsillectomy on RR interval and brain natriuretic peptide levels in children with sleep apnea: A preliminary report. *Sleep Medicine 12*(7), 646–651..

Kawauchi, A., Imada, N., Tanaka, Y., Minami, M., Watanabe, H., & Shirakawa, S. (1998). Changes in the structure of sleep spindles and delta waves on electroencephalography in patients with nocturnal enuresis. *British Journal of Urology, 81*, 72–75.

McGrath, K. H., Caldwell, P. H. Y., & Jones, M. P. (2008). The frequency of constipation in children with nocturnal enuresis: A comparison with parental reporting. *Journal of Paediatrics and Child Health, 44*(1–2), 19–27.

Mikkelsen, E. J., & Rapoport, J. L. (1980). Enuresis: psychopathology, sleep stage, and drug response. *Urologic Clinics of North America, 7*(2), 361–377.

Morison, M. (1998). Parents' and young people's attitudes towards bedwetting and their influence on behaviour, including readiness to engage in and persist with treatment. *British Journal of Urology, 81*, 56–66.

Mowrer, O. H., & Mowrer, W. M. (1938). Enuresis: a method for its study and treatment. *American Journal of Orthopsychiatry, 8*, 436–459

Neveus, T., von Gontard, A., Hoebeke, P., Hjalmas, K., Bauer, S., Bower, W., et al. (2006). The standardization of terminology of lower urinary tract function in children and adolescents: report from the Standardisation Committee of the International Children's Continence Society. *Journal of Urology, 176*(1), 314–324.

Neveus, T., Eggert, P., Evans, J., Macedo, A., Rittig, S., Tekgül, S., et al. (2010). Evaluation of and treatment for monosymptomatic enuresis: a standardization document from the International Children's Continence Society. *The Journal of Urology, 183*(2), 441–447.

Norgaard, J. P. (1991). Pathophysiology of nocturnal enuresis. *Scandinavian Journal of Urology and Nephrology, 40*(Suppl 140), 1–35.

O'Regan, S., Yazbeck, S., Hamberger, B., & Schick, E. (1986). Constipation a commonly unrecognized cause of enuresis. *Archives of Pediatrics and Adolescent Medicine, 140*(3), 260.

Rahm, C., Schulz-Juergensen, S., & Eggert, P. (2010). Effects of desmopressin on the sleep of children suffering from enuresis. *Acta Paediatrica, 99*(7), 1037–1041.

Redsell, S., & Collier, J. (2001). Bedwetting, behaviour and self-esteem: A review of the literature. *Child: Care, Health And Development, 27*(2), 149–162.

Rittig, S., Knudsen, U., Norgaard, J., Pedersen, E. B., & Djurhuus, J. (1989). Abnormal diurnal rhythm of plasma vasopressin and urinary output in patients with enuresis. *American Journal of Physiology-Renal Physiology, 256*(4), F664–F671.

Rouzade-Dominguez, M. L., Curtis, A. L., & Valentino, R. J. (2001). Role of Barrington's nucleus in the activation of rat locus coeruleus neurons by colonic distension. *Brain Research, 917*(2), 206–218.

Salmon, M. A. (1975). An historical account of nocturnal enuresis and its treatment. *Proceedings of the Royal Society of Medicine, 68*(7), 443.

Schmitt, B. D. (1987). Seven deadly sins of childhood: Advising parents about difficult developmental phases. *Child Abuse & Neglect, 11*(3), 421–432.

Stone, H. (1973). Adult bedwetters and their problems: A road to homelessness. *The Cyrenians (Canterbury)*, 45–47.

Stone, J., Malone, P. S. J., Atwill, D., McGrigor, V., & Hill, C. M. (2008). Symptoms of sleep-disordered breathing in children with nocturnal enuresis. *Journal of Pediatric Urology, 4*(3), 197–202.

von Gontard, A., Heron, J., & Joinson, C. (2011). Family history of nocturnal enuresis and urinary incontinence: Results from a large epidemiological study. *The Journal of Urology. 185*(6), 2303–2306.

Warzak, W. J. (1993). Psychosocial implications of nocturnal enuresis. *Clinical Pediatrics, 32*(1 suppl), 38–40.

Watanabe, H., & Azuma, Y. (1989). A proposal for a classification system of enuresis based on overnight simultaneous monitoring of electroencephalography and cystometry. *Sleep, 12*(3), 257–264.

Wolfish, N. M., Pivik, R. T., & Busby, K. A. (1997). Elevated sleep arousal thresholds in enuretic boys: Clinical implications. *Acta Paediatrica, 86*(4), 381–384.

Yeung, C. K., Sit, F., To, L., Chiu, H., Sihoe, J., Lee, E., & Wong, C. (2002). Reduction in nocturnal functional bladder capacity is a common factor in the pathogenesis of refractory nocturnal enuresis. *BJU International, 90*(3), 302–307.

Yeung, C. K., Sihoe, J., Sit, F., Bower, W., Sreedhar, B., & Lau, J. (2004). Characteristics of primary nocturnal enuresis in adults: An epidemiological study. *BJU international, 93*(3), 341–345.

Yeung, C. K., Sreedhar, B., Sihoe, J. D. Y., Sit, F. K. Y., & Lau, J. (2006). Differences in characteristics of nocturnal enuresis between children and adolescents: A critical appraisal from a large epidemiological study. *BJU International, 97*(5), 1069–1073.

Yeung, C. K., Diao, M., & Sreedhar, B. (2008). Cortical arousal in children with severe enuresis. *New England Journal of Medicine, 358*(22), 2414–2415.

Yue, Z., Wang, M., Xu, W., Li, H., & Wang, H. (2009). Secretion of antidiuretic hormone in children with obstructive sleep apnea-hypopnea syndrome. *Acta Oto-laryngologica, 129*(8), 867–871.

Zotter, H., Sauseng, W., Kutschera, J., Mueller, W., & Kerbl, R. (2006). Bladder voiding in sleeping infants is consistently accompanied by a cortical arousal. *Journal of Sleep Research, 15*(1), 75–79.

PART 5

Consequences of Insufficient Sleep

CHAPTER

27 Children's Sleep and Internalizing and Externalizing Symptoms

Erika Bagley *and* Mona El-Sheikh

Abstract

This chapter reviews the growing literature on relations between sleep and externalizing and internalizing symptoms in school-age children. Included are studies that have examined a wide range of nonclinical sleep problems involving shorter duration, less optimal quality, and less consistent sleep schedules and their association with internalizing and externalizing symptoms, also within the nonclinical range. The primary goal of this chapter is to summarize and provide a synthesis of the extant literature that documents associations between sleep and adjustment. A secondary goal is to provide an overview of various conceptualizations and supportive research that may help explain the link or moderate associations between sleep and internalizing and externalizing symptoms. Most notably, the possible mediating role of emotion regulation is highlighted. Also considered are vulnerability and protective factors (e.g., individual differences) that can exacerbate or ameliorate adjustment problems in the context of poor sleep.

Key Words: sleep, adjustment, internalizing, externalizing, children

When a child acts out uncharacteristically, parents and strangers alike will wonder if that child needs sleep. The "cure-all" effects of sleep on children's problem behavior have been touted for generations; a straightforward association between sleep and adjustment seems intuitive. However, it has only been within the past decade that researchers have begun in earnest to measure, describe, and explain the link between sleep and adjustment in normally developing children. And, as is often the case, a critical examination of the association suggests that any simple, straightforward link is an illusion. Thoughtful research has revealed dynamic, bidirectional relationships between sleep and adjustment that are moderated by individual and contextual factors. The primary goal of this chapter is to summarize the current understanding of the associations between sleep and externalizing (e.g., aggression, conduct problems) and internalizing (e.g., depression, anxiety) symptoms in school-age children (5 to 11 years old). A secondary goal is to provide an overview of various conceptualizations and supportive research that may help explain the link between sleep and adjustment. Most notably, the possible mediating roles of emotion regulation and cognitive processes are highlighted; vulnerability and protective factors associated with sleep and adjustment are also discussed.

Sleep problems considered in this chapter are nonclinical, conceptualized along a continuum and indicated by shorter sleep duration, less optimal sleep quality, and less consistent schedules; we use the term *sleep duration* to refer to this construct in general and not as it pertains to its very specific meaning in actigraphy unless otherwise noted. We have included studies that used subjective (e.g., self or parent report) and/or objective (e.g., actigraphy) methods for estimating sleep, as each provides important information about different aspects of sleep and may be differentially related to adjustment in meaningful ways (Sadeh, 2011; Sadeh & Acebo, 2002). In addition, this chapter focuses on the relations between sleep and internalizing and externalizing symptoms in otherwise typically developing children. A more in-depth review of sleep in children with clinical diagnoses (e.g., depression or ADHD) is provided in separate chapters. (See Chapters 34 and 35)

Sleep and Adjustment: Documenting Associations

The greatest challenge to the study of relations between sleep and adjustment is the lack of complete understanding regarding the function of sleep and thus the mechanisms that may explain the link. As Sadeh noted in a 2007 review of the literature, research has been focused on demonstrating links between sleep and behavioral domains, and the majority of current research has continued in this vein. As a result, what we think we know about the role of sleep is mostly a result of observing the consequences of inadequate or problematic sleep. However, despite this limitation, documenting associations between sleep and adjustment across diverse samples and under a variety of conditions strengthens the assertion that sleep can contribute to internalizing and externalizing behavior problems.

How one chooses to measure a construct of interest is always a fundamental decision in social science research. However, when a construct can be assessed through multiple methods and includes various parameters, as is the case with sleep, the consideration of measurement becomes critical to interpretation. A wide range of sleep variables and different methodologies complicate the research related to the relation between sleep and adjustment and pose challenges to a straightforward synthesis of findings. Four sleep domains in nonclinical child sleep research are summarized in this chapter: sleep duration, sleep quality, variability of sleep schedules, and what we refer to as sleep difficulties (a diverse set of problems pertaining to falling asleep, staying asleep, and experiencing nightmares and parasomnias, which are typically reported by parents in the reviewed studies and may overlap with or result in shortened sleep or poor quality sleep). From the standpoint of research on relations between sleep and daytime adjustment, a more complete picture is revealed when multiple sleep parameters are assessed objectively and subjectively. Careful consideration of the similarities and differences across research utilizing different methodologies may allow for patterns to emerge and provide some insight into possible mechanisms for future research.

Sleep Duration

The amount of sleep a child attains on a nightly basis is probably the most salient aspect of sleep, and there exists a growing body of literature linking shorter sleep duration to adjustment problems using correlational and, to a lesser extent, experimental designs. Sleep duration has been assessed subjectively with single or a few questions that ask about the amount of sleep a child obtains on average and also has been calculated using parent or child report of bedtimes and wake times on a sleep diary kept for a week or longer. Further, this construct also has been assessed using objective means, often with actigraphy that measures movement during the night with a small wristwatch-like device and applies an algorithm to estimate sleep and waking. A nuance worth noting using actigraphy is that researchers are able to calculate both the sleep period (time elapsed between bedtime and waking) and total sleep minutes, which is the total minutes scored as sleep during the sleep period.

In correlational studies of sleep duration, the data collected on sleep are assumed to be a naturalistic sample of the amount of sleep a child typically receives and may relate to individual differences in sleep need, the ability to regulate sleep patterns, and external forces that shape the hours available for sleep. One of the earlier studies to examine links between children's sleep duration and adjustment employed actigraphy and gathered data on child behavior from both teachers and parents (Aronen, Paavonen, Fjallberg, Soininen, & Torronen, 2000). The sample included 49 primary school children ages 7 to 12 years and compared children with longer (mean of 9.6 hours), average (mean of 8.9 hours), and shorter (mean of 8 hours) total sleep minutes over the course of 3 nights. Significant group differences in the expected direction were found in mean levels of aggressive, delinquent, and inattentive behavior problems as reported by teachers; no significant associations were observed between sleep minutes and parent-reported behavior problems.

In a correlational study with similar aims, El-Sheikh and colleagues used actigraphy collected over the course of one week to examine links between fewer sleep minutes (defined as total number of minutes identified as sleep during the sleep period) and adjustment problems in school-age children (El-Sheikh, Erath, & Keller, 2007). With a sample of 167 children between the ages of

8 and 9, findings revealed that fewer sleep minutes were significantly associated with greater parent-reported externalizing problems and greater child-reported depressive symptoms while controlling for family socioeconomic status, gender, and ethnicity. Sample and methodological differences between studies likely underlie, at least in part, why sleep was related to parent-reported adjustment outcomes in this study but not in the aforementioned Aronen et al. (2000) study.

Using a single question, parent report of average sleep duration, Paavonen, Porkka-Heiskanen, and Lahikainen (2009) examined sleep as a correlate of behavioral problems reported by parents and teachers. In a sample of nearly 300 children 5 to 6 years old, the relations between sleep and behavior were stronger when using parent report of behavioral symptoms, showing that short sleep duration (5–9 hr) significantly increased the likelihood of inattention problems, internalizing behaviors, and total psychiatric symptoms on the Child Behavior Checklist (CBCL; Achenbach, 1991a). Using teacher report, only internalizing behaviors were related to sleep duration at a trend level. The lack of association for teacher report and significant findings for parent-reported behavior are in contrast to Aronen et al.'s (2000) findings in which significant associations between sleep duration and behavior problems were found based on teacher but not parent reports.

Avoiding some of the concerns related to reporter bias, in a separate study Paavonen and colleagues (2009) also examined the relations between sleep and inattentive and hyperactive symptoms in 7- to 8-year-old children using actigraphy. Children whose average sleep duration (i.e., time elapsed from sleep onset to waking) was below the 10th percentile (<7.7 hours) had significantly higher impulsivity scores and total attention-deficit/hyperactivity symptoms reported by parents. Further, controlling for demographic characteristics, child body mass, and other neurologic and somatic illnesses, short sleep duration predicted hyperactivity and impulsivity.

In a similar correlational study, Pesonen and colleagues (2010) considered the associations between actual sleep minutes, measured using actigraphy, and children's behavioral problems as rated by mothers and fathers using the CBCL. When considering sleep minutes on a continuum, no significant relations between sleep and behavior were found. However, when the authors looked at percentiles of sleep minutes significant associations were evident. Specifically, children who were in the 10th percentile for short sleep duration (less than 7.7 hours on average per night) were at higher risk for having maternal-reported behavioral problems, thought problems, and ADHD symptoms and paternal-reported rule breaking and externalizing symptoms.

Holley, Hill, and Stevenson (2011) considered the association between actigraphy-measured sleep variables and parent-reported behavior problems indexed via the Strengths and Difficulties Questionnaire in 6- to 11-year-old children (SDQ; Goodman, 1997). The SDQ was completed by parents and includes five subscales that assess emotional symptoms, conduct problems, hyperactivity, peer problems, and pro-social behavior. Variables were calculated for both the sleep period and sleep minutes (which excludes the time awake during the sleep period). The authors found significant relations only between conduct problems and sleep minutes, but not for sleep period or other adjustment variables. As these data were correlational, the direction of effects remains unclear but it is interesting to note that the researchers come to a similar conclusion as Sadeh, Gruber, and Raviv (2003) in their study of the impact of an experimental manipulation of sleep on neurobehavioral functioning that "just an hour" can make a significant difference in children's behavior. In addition, the fact that significant relations were observed only when considering sleep minutes suggests that research that relies solely on report of sleep onset and wake times or actigraphy to calculate total sleep period may fail to detect relations that might nevertheless exist.

Biggs, Lushington, van den Heuvel, Martin, and Kennedy (2011) examined associations between sleep duration and behavioral problems in a very large sample of over 1600 Australian children, ages 5 to 10. Using parent-reported sleep diaries, their results showed that while controlling for demographic characteristics, children who slept less than 10 hours per night (the sample's average duration) were at double the risk for scoring in the 95th percentile of the hyperactive subscale of the Strengths and Difficulties Questionnaire. These same children were not found to be at higher risk for internalizing symptoms, however.

In one of the few studies to consider longitudinal relations between objectively measured sleep and adjustment in childhood while controlling for autoregressive effects, El-Sheikh, Kelly, Buckhalt, and Hinnant (2010) reported that sleep period did not predict change in either internalizing or externalizing behavior problems over 2 years. Although findings revealed that longer sleep duration was negatively correlated with parent-reported internalizing symptoms, the cross-sectional association became nonsignificant after placing these variables within a larger model that included other sleep parameters, externalizing symptoms, and control variables of ethnicity and SES. Longitudinally, sleep duration at T1 (mean age 8.7 years) was not predictive of either internalizing or externalizing behavior problems at T2 (mean age 10.7 years), again as part of the larger model. Conversely, as will be discussed in the following sections, this study did find longitudinal relations for sleep predicting adjustment using other sleep parameters.

Sleep duration is arguably the most easily manipulated of the sleep parameters and, as a result, all of the studies in which sleep is experimentally manipulated (extended, restricted) assess effects of changes in sleep duration. As opposed to the research that has experimentally implemented total sleep deprivation in adults, the experimental protocols used with children are more modest and typically restrict sleep by an hour for a period of a week to a few weeks. Experimental studies eliminate concerns about the substantial number of confounding influences on sleep duration that also may be related to adjustment difficulties. However, as summarized by Beebe (2011) in his recent review of research on the effects of inadequate sleep on a broad range of outcomes for children and adolescents, very few experimental studies of sleep restriction in children exist and, unfortunately, even fewer have included behavioral measures that tap into effects of sleep on adjustment.

In the largest experimental study so far, Fallone, Acebo, Seifer, and Carskadon (2005) recruited 74 healthy children, ages 6 to 12, for participation in a 3-week home-based protocol that allowed for children to be assessed under baseline, restricted, or optimized sleep conditions (each for one week). Sleep restriction was age-based, such that time in bed was restricted to 8 hours for children in first and second grades and to 6.5 hours for children in third grade and above. Under the optimized sleep condition, all children were assigned to no fewer than 10 hours of time in bed per night. The experimental manipulation of sleep was validated by actigraphy and showed that relative to children's own baseline, the optimized sleep condition resulted in 39 minutes more sleep and the restricted sleep condition resulted in 139 minutes less sleep. Teachers rated children's behavior across these three conditions and findings showed that under restricted conditions, children displayed significantly more attention problems; however, children were not reported as more hyperactive or impulsive. On the contrary, children in the restricted sleep condition were more hypoactive in the classroom setting compared to their own baseline (possibly due to fatigue), and no significant differences were found between conditions on oppositional-aggressive behaviors.

Rather than restricting sleep, another approach to experimentally manipulating sleep duration is to enhance sleep in a group that has already demonstrated short sleep duration or other sleep problems. Melatonin, a naturally occurring hormone important for regulating the sleep–wake cycle, has been shown to be an effective treatment for symptoms of insomnia in children (Smits, Van Stel, Van Der Heijden, Meijer, Coenen, & Kerkhof, 2003) In the first study of its kind, van Maanen, Meijer, Smits, and Oort (2011) examined the effects of melatonin treatment on children's sleep duration and, in turn, on children's behavior. Their sample included children with an average age of 9 who were identified as having delayed dim-light melatonin onset, causing symptoms of sleep onset problems. These children were treated with melatonin following a standard protocol for 3 weeks, followed by a "half-dose week" and finally the "stop week"; behavioral measures were collected at the end of treatment and the final stop week. The results showed that melatonin treatment had significant effects on increasing sleep minutes measured with actigraphy, and those improvements in sleep duration were paralleled by improved behavior as reported by parents on the CBCL (total problem score). The effects of treatment were the strongest for the children with less severe problems with delayed melatonin onset at baseline. Although the subset of children with delayed dim-light melatonin onset may be unique in terms of the etiology of their sleep problems, this study represents an excellent example of the potential to examine the causal role of sleep on daytime behavior via experimental sleep enhancement.

Sleep Quality—Actigraphy-Based

Child sleep quality has been examined via objective and subjective measures. Because of the wide range of sleep quality parameters (e.g., lack of satisfaction, general disturbance, sleeps worse than other children) indexed by parent and child reports, we review the literature linking adjustment problems with questionnaire-based sleep quality variables later, under the heading of *Sleep Difficulties.*

In this section we review the small body of literature on associations between child adjustment and actigraphy-based sleep quality indices. Information regarding sleep quality obtained through actigraphy pertains to the frequency and duration of night wakening and activity levels during the sleep period and often includes sleep efficiency (% of motionless sleep); waking minutes after sleep onset, long wake episodes (usually > 5 min per episode); and the activity index (% of epochs with activity). Therefore, the variables typically associated with sleep quality reflect the extent to which a child maintains motionless sleep or quickly returns to sleep after a night waking. Of note is that some sleep variables such as latency may be classified in more than one category; in this chapter we review the literature pertaining to latency under the *Sleep Difficulties* heading.

Sadeh, Gruber, and Raviv (2002) examined the sleep of 135 children in 2nd, 4th, and 6th grades using actigraphy and considered associations between a variety of sleep parameters and parent report of child problem behaviors on the CBCL (Achenbach, 1991a). The authors calculated sleep percentage by dividing the number of minutes scored as sleep by the total number of minutes between sleep onset and waking. In this study, 25 of 135 children were considered poor sleepers based on low sleep percentage (90% or lower) and on average at least 3 awakenings per night that lasted at least 5 minutes each. "Poor sleepers" were rated by parents as significantly higher than "good sleepers" on delinquency and total problem behaviors. The findings were specific to externalizing behaviors, as no significant relations were found between sleep quality and internalizing problems, and specific to sleep quality as no relations were found between sleep duration and problem behaviors.

The work of El-Sheikh, Kelly, Buckhalt, and Hinnant (2010) provides a look at both correlational and longitudinal relations between sleep quality, as indexed by sleep efficiency, and adjustment. Participants were 176 children in 3rd grade at the first time point and in 5th grade at the follow-up. Children had their sleep assessed via actigraphy for a week at each time point, and parents reported on internalizing and externalizing symptoms using the Personality Inventory for Children (PIC; Lachar, 1982). Greater sleep efficiency in 3rd grade was correlated with both internalizing and externalizing behavior problems, and with only internalizing problems in 5th grade. However, when placed within a larger model that included all sleep parameters and control variables, there was no evidence that sleep efficiency predicted externalizing or internalizing behavior cross-sectionally. The authors did find evidence of an interaction between sleep efficiency and socioeconomic status (SES) cross-sectionally such that when sleep efficiency was low, children from low-SES backgrounds were especially at risk for higher externalizing symptoms.

El-Sheikh and colleagues (2010) also considered longitudinal relations between sleep efficiency and behavior problems. Surprisingly, the authors found that increases in sleep efficiency over 2 years predicted increases in externalizing problems from 3rd to 5th grade. Longitudinal relations between sleep quality and internalizing symptoms across time only existed for African-American children in the sample, such that increases in sleep efficiency were predictive of increases in internalizing problems. These findings were surprising in that high sleep efficiency is typically considered to reflect good biobehavioral regulation; however, it was found to predict increases in problem behaviors. A possible explanation for this finding may be that high sleep efficiency is a compensatory mechanism for insufficient sleep over time. This explanation is supported by the results of Sadeh, Gruber, and Raviv (2003), who found that children who had their sleep duration experimentally restricted actually experienced improvements in sleep efficiency and fewer night wakings. Therefore, high sleep efficiency in this observational study may reflect ongoing problems that children have had with attaining sufficient sleep and a corresponding high level of chronic partial sleep deprivation and sleep debt.

VARIABILITY IN SLEEP SCHEDULES

In addition to sleep duration and quality, the variability in sleep patterns is another sleep parameter that has shown significant associations with adjustment. Lower levels of variability in sleep schedules reflect higher stability and consistency in bedtime and wake time (or actual sleep onset and waking) on a night-to-night basis; variability in sleep schedules during week versus weekend nights has also been examined. Similar to sleep duration and quality, variability may reflect individual differences in biobehavioral regulation, but may also be strongly influenced by familial (e.g., routines, parental work schedules) and sociocultural factors (e.g., co-sleeping). In school-age children, in addition to variability over the week, variability between weekday and weekend sleep patterns may be meaningful in that it captures the differences in how a child sleeps under conditions that require a consistent wake time (e.g., school) and under less controlled conditions. It has been suggested that highly variable sleep patterns may have a stressing effect similar to jet lag, and variability might affect adjustment through detrimental effects on attention and neurohormonal stress response systems (Weissbluth, 1989). In addition to variability in sleep schedules, variability in sleep duration and other sleep parameters may influence children's functioning (Bates, Viken, Alexander, Beyers, & Stockton, 2002).

Testing this suggestion, Bates and colleagues (2002) considered the associations between sleep patterns (including variability in sleep duration and bedtimes) and school adjustments in 5-year-old children across 4 months. Mothers reported on child sleep using a daily diary method, and preschool teachers reported on children's positive and negative classroom behaviors. Bivariate correlations between sleep and adjustment revealed that both variability in sleep duration and bedtime over the course of 4 weeks were significantly positively associated with teacher report on the Problem Behavior Questionnaire (PBQ; Behar, 1977), which assesses school adjustment using items related to child compliance and externalizing behavior problems. Structural equation modeling suggested that family stress contributed to variability in children's sleep, which in turn significantly predicted school adjustment. Interestingly, variability in sleep onset and duration were more predictive of negative behaviors than total hours of sleep.

On the other hand, two studies discussed previously showing significant associations between sleep duration (defined as actual sleep time) and adjustment also found significant relations involving sleep variability. Specifically, Pesonen et al. (2010) considered variability in sleep duration between weekdays and weekends, as well as the variability in bedtime and waking time between weekdays and weekends. No significant associations were found between sleep variability and adjustment as reported by mothers on the CBCL; however, significant associations existed for father-reported adjustment. Results revealed that a 1.0 standard deviation increase in weekday-to-weekend irregularity in sleep duration was associated with a 0.2 standard deviation increase in internalizing and total problem scores, and the significance of these findings held even after controlling for actual bedtimes.

Biggs et al. (2011), also discussed earlier, found support for significant relations between inconsistent sleep schedules and behavioral difficulties on the Strengths and Difficulties Questionnaire (SDQ; Goodman, 1997). In their study, bedtime variability between weekdays and weekends was strongly associated with problem behaviors; children with a difference greater than 2 hours (more sleep on weekends) were at six times the likelihood of scoring in the 95th percentile on the hyperactivity subscale. Variability of bedtimes and wake times on school nights of at least 1 hour also increased the likelihood of scoring in the 95th percentile for hyperactivity and internalizing behaviors.

Sleep Difficulties

The largest body of literature in the area of children's sleep and adjustment pertains to sleep difficulties broadly construed. As a category, sleep difficulties as defined in this chapter are unique in that they refer to a diverse set of problems involving falling asleep, staying asleep, satisfaction with one's sleep, perceptions of sleeping worse than other children, and experiencing nightmares and parasomnias. In the pertinent literature, these are typically reported by parents and children and thus this section of the chapter relates, mostly yet not exclusively, to sleep problems based on such reports (the few studies on sleep latency obtained via actigraphy are reviewed in this section). Worth mentioning is that these problems may overlap with shorter sleep duration and poorer sleep quality.

The high proportion of studies that consider sleep difficulties broadly construed and adjustment is not surprising, because the CBCL and other adjustment measures that have been widely used to assess behavioral problems in normally developing children for decades also include items related to sleep. Researchers have created subscales from a variety of sleep items to examine relations between sleep problems and adjustment. Unfortunately, this research stands on somewhat tenuous ground because these "sleep problem subscales" were not intended or validated to be used in such a manner. In a recent 2011 publication, Gregory et al. addressed methodological concerns by comparing the pertinent CBCL items with well-validated methods, such as actigraphy and sleep diaries. The authors excluded two CBCL items related to parasomnias and specifically focused on four items in their analyses that may tap into sleep disturbance ("overtired," "sleeps less than most kids," "sleeps more than most kids," and "trouble sleeping"). The findings did not support clear coherence between these four CBCL items and other methodologies. For example, the "overtired" and "trouble sleeping" items were only weakly to moderately correlated with sleep latency measured using daily diary method or actigraphy. Overall, the authors concluded that the CBCL should not be the measure of choice, but may tap into some relevant aspects of sleep disturbance. Furthermore, it remains unclear how inclusion of the two items related to parasomnias ("nightmares" and "talks or walks in sleep") may further bias the results of studies that include all six CBCL items related to sleep. Given these caveats, it should be said that the use of CBCL sleep items has allowed for important questions to be addressed regarding sleep and adjustment in rich datasets (often longitudinal) that were not necessarily designed to examine sleep.

Gregory and O'Connor's (2002) study is an excellent example of an investigation that made use of the information available on sleep problems from all six items on the CBCL to investigate associations with behavioral problems. Using a prospective study of 490 children in adoptive and biological families, the authors examined longitudinal associations and developmental changes in associations from age 4 into mid-adolescence. First, authors did find evidence that sleep problems at age 4 predicted changes in depressive, anxious, aggressive, and attentional problems 11 years later. Testing the reciprocal effects, they did not find evidence that early behavioral problems predicted sleep problems in adolescence except in the case of attention problems. The authors also examined changes in the associations between sleep problems and behavior problems, finding that the relation between sleep and internalizing symptoms got stronger throughout childhood and into adolescence; no significant changes in associations existed for other types of behavioral problems.

In a very large sample of over 6000 children, Paavonen et al. (2002) examined the association between the severity of sleep problems and problem behaviors. They used an index of sleep problems, which comprised one item that is included on the child-report Children's Depression Inventory (CDI; Kovacs, 1985) and one item from the parent-report Rutter scale (Rutter, Tizard, & Whitmore, 1997) to create three groups representing children without sleep problems, with mild sleep problems, and with severe sleep problems. These items are limited in their scope and in a single question ask children about the extent to which they have "trouble" with sleep and parents about their child's "sleeping difficulty." Children with severe sleep problems, approximately 5% of the sample, were significantly more likely to display problematic internalizing, externalizing, and hyperactivity behaviors as rated by teachers, with odds ratios exceeding 2.0.

Given that parents are not always aware of problems that their children may have with sleep, children may be important sources of information about their own sleep difficulties. Using the 13-item Sleep Self-Report (SSR; Owens, Maxim, Nobile, McGuinn, & Msall, 2000), Gregory and Eley (2005) considered cross-sectional associations between sleep problems and child-reported anxiety symptoms assessed with the Screen for Child Anxiety-Related Emotional Disorders (SCARED; Birmaher et al.,1997). They found significant relations between specific sleep problems included on the SSR ("fight with parents about bedtime," "afraid to sleep alone," "afraid of dark," and "have nightmares") and the total anxiety score. Similarly, specific anxiety scales (somatic, separation anxiety, school phobia, and general anxiety) were significantly correlated with the total sleep problems score. Using linear regression and after controlling for other symptoms of anxiety, school phobias emerged as a significant statistical predictor of sleep problems. Although single-reporter bias may have influenced the results of this study, it also highlights the possibility that certain important factors in the association between sleep and adjustment may be best reported by the child.

Gregory, Rijsdjik, Dahl, McGuffin, and Eley (2006) used a twin study design to assess the contributions of genetic and environmental influences on the relation between sleep and internalizing problems in 8-year-old children. Questionnaires were used for self-report of anxiety and depressive symptoms and parent-report of children's sleep problems using the Child Sleep Habits Questionnaire (CSHQ; Owens, Spirito, McGuinn, & Nobile, 2000). The CSHQ incudes a wide range of sleep problems with subscales for bedtime resistance, sleep onset delay, sleep duration, sleep anxiety, night wakings, and parasomnias. Parent-reported sleep problems were associated with internalizing symptoms although, overall, stronger relations were observed between sleep problems and depression compared to anxiety symptoms. Further, by comparing the univariate and bivariate correlations across monozygotic and dizygotic twin pairs, the authors found evidence that the association between sleep problems and depression symptoms is heavily influenced by genetic factors, suggesting that there is some overlap between the genes that are important for depression and for sleep problems.

In another cross-sectional study, Coulombe, Reid, Boyle, and Racine (2010) examined associations between sleep and adjustment problems reported by both parents and teachers. This study is somewhat unique in that the authors also accounted for a number of shared risk factors, including gender, age, family income, maternal education, maternal negative affect, stressful life events, marital disharmony, and family functioning. Furthermore, they also controlled for comorbid symptoms to examine the unique associations between sleep and specific behavioral problems. Using subscales of both the parent-reported CBCL or the associated Teacher Report Form (TRF; Achenbach, 1991b), children's aggression, attention problems, and anxious/depressed mood were separately examined. To assess sleep problems the authors used five items from the parent-reported CBCL ("trouble sleeping," "sleeps less than other children," "nightmares," "talks or walks in sleep" and "sleeps more than other children"). In addition, one parent-reported item ("overtired") and two teacher-reported items ("overtired" and "sleeps in class") were used as indicators of inadequate sleep. Using hierarchical regression, the association between each parent-reported and teacher-reported behavioral problem and sleep problem were examined separately. Overall, the findings did show significant relations between some sleep variables and behavioral problems. Specifically, nightmares and trouble sleeping were related to parent, but not teacher, report of anxious/depressed mood. "Overtired" predicted all behavioral problems whether reported by parent or teacher. However, it should be noted that in this very conservative analytic strategy, which controlled for shared risk and co-occurring behavioral problems, the variance in behavior accounted for by sleep was quite small (up to 3%). By contrast, the shared risk and co-occurring symptoms accounted for 23%–53% of the variance in behavioral problems. Unfortunately, in this study the measurement of each sleep difficulty consisted of a single CBCL/TRF item, and the behavioral assessment came from the CBCL/TRF as well. It is not clear whether the measurement issues in this study had an impact on the results.

The work of Alfano and colleagues (2009) provides a more thorough assessment of relations between sleep problems and anxiety and depression symptoms. Specifically, they examined internalizing symptoms using the 47-item Revised Child Anxiety and Depression Scales (RCADS; Chorpita, Yim, Moffitt, Umemoto, & Francis, 2000), the 37-item Revised Children's Manifest Anxiety Scale (RCMAS; Reynolds & Richmond, 1978) and the Child Depression Inventory (CDI; Kovacs, 1985). A total sleep problem score was created by summing parent responses to four items from the CBCL ("overtired," "sleeps less than most children," "sleeps more than most children," and "trouble sleeping"), two from the RCADS ("trouble sleeping" and "tired a lot"), and one from the RCMAS ("worries when going to bed"). In a sample of 88 children ages 6 to 11, there was evidence that sleep disturbance is more closely associated with anxiety during childhood, whereas in adolescents ages 12–17 years the association was more evident for depression. The authors used hierarchical linear regression to show that during childhood, anxiety symptoms were associated with sleep problems while controlling for demographic characteristics and, importantly, depressive symptoms. Using a similar strategy, depressive symptoms were not associated with sleep problems while controlling for anxiety symptoms, suggesting some specificity to the relations between sleep and adjustment symptoms. In the case of this study, however, the use of the sum score for sleep problems precludes any conclusions about the unique contribution of different sleep difficulties to internalizing symptoms in childhood.

In a longitudinal study with over 500 children, Goodnight, Bates, Staples, Pettit, and Dodge (2007) used cross-domain latent growth curve modeling to test whether growth in sleep problems was related to growth in behavior problem trajectories in children from 5 to 9 years of age. This study is unique in that it is among the few that examined change in sleep problems as they relate to change in behavior problems. Parent report on the "overtired," "trouble sleeping," and "sleeps less than most children" items from the CBCL were used to assess sleep. Teachers reported on children's externalizing behavior problems. No main effects were found between sleep problems and behavior problems. Further, the authors also considered whether the relation between sleep problems and behavior was influenced by early resistance to control, and found that growth in sleep problems was positively associated with growth in externalizing behaviors only for children who were high on resistance to control. This finding highlights the importance of individual differences and moderator effects in the link between sleep and adjustment.

In addition to sleep duration and quality, El-Sheikh, Kelly, Buckhalt, and Hinnant (2010) also considered cross-sectional and longitudinal associations between adjustment and child-reported sleep problems (e.g., insufficient sleep as well as difficulty initiating and maintaining sleep) examined via the child report on the Sleep Habits Survey (SHS; Wolfson & Carskadon, 1998) and parent report using the Children's Sleep Habits Questionnaire (CHSQ). At both time points, when children were 8 and 10, bivariate correlations revealed that parent-reported and child-reported sleep/wake problems were associated with higher levels of parent- and child-related internalizing and externalizing symptoms. When placed in a larger model that included multiple sleep parameters and control variables, child-reported sleep/wake problems were positively associated with parent-reported internalizing symptoms—however, only for the children from lower SES backgrounds. When considering relations longitudinally, race/ethnicity was found to moderate the associations between sleep/wake problems and adjustment. Specifically, at higher levels of sleep problems, African-American children had higher predicted means for internalizing and externalizing behavior problems compared to European-American children; race/ethnic-related effects were not evident when sleep was more optimal. In addition to providing additional documentation of longitudinal associations between sleep and adjustment, the findings also raise interesting questions about biological, psychological, and/or contextual factors that may explain the vulnerability of children from poor or minority backgrounds to the effects of sleep on adjustment.

Finally, symptoms of sleep disordered breathing (e.g., snoring) have been shown to impact the sleep of children and be associated with externalizing behavior problems. A recent study by O'Brien et al. (2011) examined the cross-sectional associations between symptoms of sleep disordered breathing (in the nonclinical range) and bullying behavior in elementary school aged children. The authors found a significant positive relation between the child's score on the disordered breathing subscale and bullying behavior. Forty-two percent of children who were identified by the parent as participating in bullying behavior were at risk for sleep disordered breathing, while only 17.5% of nonbullying children had such risk. Although mono-reporter bias (most measures were parent-reported) and single time-point analyses are limitations of the study, this work broadens the scope of important outcomes to consider including peer relations and social adjustment.

Summary of Findings and Caveats

In consideration of the body of research that has documented associations within and across time between sleep and adjustment problems, a few conclusions can be drawn. First, there is substantial evidence to support the idea that sleep and adjustment are significantly associated during childhood in normally developing, nonclinical samples. This evidence comes from studies with community samples of children from many countries including United States, Finland, Australia, New Zealand, and Israel.

From longitudinal work, it appears that sleep is more likely to predict adjustment, rather than adjustment predicting sleep. Recent work by Kelly and El-Sheikh (2013), which utilized cross-lagged panel models to examine reciprocal relations between sleep and adjustment in 176 children from 8 to 13 years of age, came to a similar conclusion. In addition, findings from the study suggest that the influence of sleep on symptoms of depression and anxiety may be stronger during late childhood/early adolescence (ages 10–13) as opposed to middle childhood (ages 8–10). Future research of reciprocal relations between sleep and adjustment across developmental stages will be critical, as will examinations of these relations considered on a day-to-day basis to fully capture the transactional processes that may be at work. Further, the scarcity of longitudinal work leaves many questions unanswered about potential critical periods that may exist within childhood or how sleep and adjustment may interact differentially across various developmental periods. Looking forward, studies that include at least three waves of data would permit the examination of trajectories of growth and change in both sleep and adjustment and their association. So-called "change on change" analyses would be useful to describe the developmental course of the relation between sleep and adjustment and may also be used to understand individual differences in development. Similar research by Bub, Buckhalt, and El-Sheikh (2011) looking at relations between changes in sleep and changes in cognitive performance across 3 years has shown the importance of considering individual differences in the growth of sleep problems and promises to be an important next step in research with the increasing number of longitudinal studies in the field.

A critical review of the extant literature suggests that the associations between sleep and adjustment are rather nonspecific. Although not always the case, researchers have shown that the different parameters of sleep (i.e., duration, quality, variability, and difficulties broadly defined) collected using different methodologies are generally associated with both internalizing and externalizing symptoms. The lack of specificity may suggest that different parameters of sleep are associated even if they reflect different conceptual constructs (e.g., sleep duration measures are frequently correlated with quality measures). Nevertheless, relatively few studies have examined multiple sleep parameters as they relate to adjustment outcomes, and thus conclusions about such potentially differential associations are not tenable.

As other reviews have pointed out (Blunden, Hoban, & Chervin, 2006; Sadeh, 2007; Beebe, 2011), the overwhelming majority of studies linking sleep and adjustment are correlational. Experimental studies have the major advantage of reducing concerns over potential confounding variables, such as family stress, which may serve as third variables responsible for poor sleep and adjustment problems. Therefore, experimental studies are necessary to determine the causal role of sleep. Simultaneously, even experimental studies have limitations that make observational studies important as well. For example, the association between sleep and adjustment likely unfolds across time and may not be captured with the typical (and ethical) protocols for sleep restriction with children. Even when effects of experimental sleep restriction on daytime functioning are observed, the mechanisms that underlie the effects may not be the same as those that are the result of chronic sleep deprivation.

One major obstacle to experimental research is the ethical issues related to sleep restriction protocols in children. In response to the major concern regarding the possibility that sleep restriction could irreparably impact a child's development, sleep has only been modestly reduced for short periods. However, an alternative approach to dealing with these concerns would be to develop protocols that improve sleep and measure the benefits in experimental versus control groups. Given the large numbers of children who receive poor or inadequate sleep, it would not be difficult to recruit samples of children who would benefit from this type of intervention. Sadeh et al. (2003) showed that even modest extension of sleep could have significant effects on neurobehavioral functioning. Alternatively, research could capitalize on naturally occurring sleep deprivation. Finally, the wider use of longitudinal data will allow for statistical approaches, such as cross-lag analyses and growth curve modeling, which can better assess directionality of effects between sleep and adjustment while still using data from observational studies.

Across and within studies, sleep has been shown to be associated with internalizing, externalizing, and with both problem behaviors concurrently. Therefore, it is important for researchers in the field to address some of the same long-standing controversies regarding the conceptual and data analytic issues that exist for understanding adjustment in the context of comorbidity (Lilienfeld, 2003). Conceptually, the co-occurrence of internalizing and externalizing behavior problems in association with sleep could suggest several explanations. First, it is possible that different pathways underlie the associations for internalizing and externalizing symptoms; however, the research strategies used to date have not been capable of identifying unique processes. Conversely, internalizing and externalizing behavior problems may stem from deficits in a common ability, such as emotion regulation (Eisenberg et al., 2009), which could either be affected by or itself affect sleep (Dahl, 1996); the role of emotion regulation is discussed in more detail later in the chapter.

Apart from a few select studies (Gregory, Eley, O'Connor, & Plomin, 2004; Coulombe et al., 2010; El-Sheikh et al., 2010), the bulk of the literature on relations between sleep problems in typically developing children and their adjustment outcomes has not sought to examine the "pure" relations between sleep and individual dimensions of adjustment problems by controlling for externalizing behaviors when examining internalizing behaviors and vice versa. This approach is reasoned, because these behavior problems naturally co-occur and controlling would remove an important shared dimension of externalizing behaviors when examining internalizing symptoms and vice versa, thereby reducing the strength of associations. Nevertheless, in studies in which researchers are interested in identifying "pure" symptoms it may be useful to consider controlling for the co-occurrence of behavior problems to provide further clarity and explication of effects. Yet, the cost-benefit ratio of such controls and the particular research question under consideration ought to guide analyses.

Controlling for potential individual differences (age, gender, SES, body mass index, pubertal status, etc.) that may influence the relation between sleep and adjustment problems represents a more conservative approach to examining relations than studies that do not control for such potential confounds (Coulombe et al., 2010). Controls for possible influential variables across studies are very inconsistent, hindering comparisons across investigations. Improving the precision of analytic techniques and consistent application of controls across studies may serve the field by allowing for a greater synthesis of findings and deepening of understanding regarding relations between sleep and adjustment problems.

Pathways and Moderators of Effects in the Context of Sleep and Adjustment

Emotion Regulation

The very suggestion that sleep could play a causal role in the development of adjustment problems is exciting because it raises the possibility that improvements in sleep could lead to significant reductions in problem behavior. Indeed, limited longitudinal (Gregory & O'Connor, 2002; El-Sheikh et al., 2010) and experimental studies (Fallone et al., 2005; van Maanen et al., 2011) do support the suggestion that sleep predicts both internalizing and externalizing behavior problems. Dahl (1996; 1999; Dahl & Lewin, 2002) has written extensively on the close relationship between sleep and adjustment, suggesting that poor emotion regulation is a primary consequence of insufficient sleep. Emotion regulation, which involves both the evaluation of emotional cues and modulation of emotional and behavioral responses (Gross & Thompson, 2007), has been widely discussed as a risk factor for the development of internalizing and externalizing behavior (Cole & Deater-Deckard, 2009). Emotion regulation could provide a plausible explanation for how sleep could lead to internalizing and externalizing problems, as each has been suggested to result from poor effortful regulation of behavior and emotion (Eisenberg, et al., 2001).

Emotion regulation is thought to be largely dependent on processes of executive control, primarily located in the prefrontal cortex (PFC). Importantly, insufficient sleep has been shown to disrupt processes mediated in the PFC, including executive processes necessary for controlling emotion (Muzur, Pace-Schott, & Hobson, 2002). It is also thought that long-term sleep disruptions may have especially detrimental effects during childhood when the brain is undergoing rapid development. Jan and colleagues (2010) provide an excellent review of the research based on adult, child, and animal models showing how persistent sleep problems can cause permanent neuronal cellular stress and damage over time, which may result in long-term adverse socioemotional outcomes, especially when they occur during critical periods of brain development.

At the same time, initiating and maintaining sleep are important tasks for children that draw on emotional regulatory abilities and may stand in contrast to daytime challenges, which often involve a great deal of social engagement, interpretation of environmental cues, and the acquisition of new cognitive skills. In many societies, sleep regulation is a process that is highly scaffolded during infancy, but expectations for independent regulation of sleep increase rapidly during early childhood. Therefore, emotional regulation can also be seen as a predictor of sleep; however, research has yet to fully consider the complex reciprocal relations that likely exist.

Breakthroughs in understanding connections between sleep and emotion regulation may come from research that broadly considers interactions across cognitive, emotional, and physiological levels of functioning. For example, researchers in cognitive neuroscience have begun to describe the effects of sleep deprivation, particularly of REM sleep, on neurocognitive functioning (Walker & van der Helm, 2009). From this research it appears that sleep may play a vital role in the "way we process, consolidate, and buffer our daily [emotional] experiences" (Vandekerckhove & Cluydts, 2010). Specifically, studies using experimentally induced sleep deprivation in adults have shown that, as opposed to memories with neutral and positive affective content, negative memories were relatively resistant to the effects of sleep deprivation on retention (Phelps, 2004). Although this type of research certainly needs replication in children, one can start to make some hypotheses about how the tendency to forget positive information and remember negative information might play into the development of adjustment problems over time.

A promising area of research has sought to examine the effects of sleep on specific emotion regulatory processes. A recent study by Berger et al. (2011) shows the consequences of sleep restriction on the emotional experiences of toddlers. In an experimental design, normally developing 30–36-month-old children were assigned to napping and no nap conditions for an 11-day protocol. At the end of the protocol that resulted in sleep restriction for the toddlers in the no nap condition, researchers coded observations of facial responses to solvable and nonsolvable tasks to gauge emotionality. Children in the sleep restriction group showed more negativity to neutral and negative conditions, and less positivity to positive conditions, compared to children who were allowed time to nap daily. The authors concluded that as a result of sleep restriction, toddlers were neither able to take full advantage of positive experiences nor were they as adaptive in challenging contexts.

Not only may sleep influence the emotional experience of the child, but also may impact the ability of children to interpret the emotional experiences of those around them. In a sample of nearly 100 10-year-old children, Soffer-Dudek and colleagues (2011) considered the effect of sleep on the ability to process emotional information yearly for 3 years. On a cognitive neurobehavioral task, participants were tested on their ability to identify gender (neutral emotion) and emotion of presented faces. The authors found children with elevated night waking and decreasing sleep efficiency from 10–13 had poorer ability to accurately interpret emotional information, but poor sleep had no effect on the ability to process the neutral task. Taken together with the research from Berger et al. (2011), this work suggests that sufficient sleep is necessary for optimal social functioning, which in turn may be an important determinant of adjustment. A potentially fruitful avenue for research is explicating how the effects of insufficient sleep on daily interactions might play out to affect children's ability to manage emotional situations, and how less adaptive microtransactions on a day-to-day basis may place children at risk for long-term emotional and behavioral problems.

Consistent with the idea that poor regulation may underlie the association between sleep problems and adjustment, El-Sheikh and Buckhalt (2005) investigated the role of vagal regulation indexed by respiratory sinus arrhythmia, which is considered a measure of parasympathetic nervous system activity, and emotional intensity in predicting subjectively and objectively assessed sleep parameters in a small sample of 6- to 12-year-old children. Results showed that increased dispositional emotional intensity predicted fewer sleep minutes and increased night activity. Similarly, a lower level of vagal withdrawal, suggestive of less apt vagal regulation, was predictive of increased sleep problems as assessed through both subjective and actigraphy-based measures. The findings of this study suggest that children's emotionality and physiological regulation predict unique variance in the amount and quality of children's sleep. Given what is also known about the importance of these factors for overall adjustment (Thompson & Calkins, 1996), the findings may also shed light on how emotional and physiological dysregulation may mediate or moderate the association between sleep and adjustment.

The research considering relations between sleep and adjustment has almost solely focused on associations between poor sleep and poor adjustment to the exclusion of examining the effects of sleep on other, positive facets of socioemotional adjustment. This is unfortunate because, in the process, the field may be ignoring important protective mechanisms related to sleep. Instead of focusing on negative outcomes of insufficient sleep, Lemola et al. (2011) suggest another pathway for sleep to be related to children's adaptation by looking at the association between sleep and markers of positive adjustment (optimism and self-esteem) in 8- year-old children. While controlling for age, sex, body mass index, and parental education, they found a significant nonlinear relationship between sleep duration and optimism (inverse J-shaped curve). Although the cross-sectional nature of the study does not allow determination of direction of effects, it nonetheless supports the hypothesis that processes that occur during sleep may shape the lens through which daily interactions are interpreted.

Sleep as a Protective and Vulnerability Factor for Adjustment Problems

It is likely that the behavior of all children is not equally affected by sleep disturbance. However, few studies have examined interactions between sleep and other variables in the prediction of behavior problems (i.e., moderation effects). Consideration of variables that can enhance or ameliorate the risk for adjustment problems otherwise associated with sleep is imperative to clarify for whom and under which conditions sleep is likely to be associated with adjustment problems. Several studies investigated the role of sleep as a protective or vulnerability factor in the context of risk. Risk variables examined included individual differences (e.g., physiological regulation, gender) as well as familial (e.g., marital conflict) and socioeconomic factors (e.g., income, ethnicity, living environment). When examined in the context of risk variables (e.g., familial problems or economic disadvantage), such examinations are frequently based on the premise that aggregation of risk (e.g., sleep problems in conjunction with economic disadvantage) could exacerbate adjustment problems (Buckhalt, 2011; Marco & Wolfson, 2012).

Gender may be an important moderator of associations between sleep and adjustment. The previously mentioned Bub et al. (2011) study that considered change over time in sleep and cognitive performance demonstrated that across the three assessment points, girls were most sensitive to the negative effects of increases in sleepiness on verbal comprehension. El-Sheikh, Bub, Kelly, and Buckhalt (under review) has similarly examined the change over time in sleep and adjustment, again finding that gender moderated the association between sleep and adjustment, such that girls who had the greatest growth in sleepiness over the course of 3 years had the greatest increase in depressive symptoms over the same period of time. Going forward, considering gender and other important individual differences as moderators of the relations between sleep and adjustment will likely lead to a better understanding of who is at greatest risk.

Several studies have shown that better sleep can serve as a protective factor (or poor sleep can function as a vulnerability factor) in the context of risk. For example, in a longitudinal study of children at high genetic risk for depression, Silk et al. (2007) found that short sleep latency at the initial assessment (age 6–11), when none of the children were diagnosed with depression, predicted membership in the depression-resilient group in early adulthood (age 18–29). El-Sheikh, Hinnant, Kelly and Erath (2010) considered the moderating effect of sleep on the relation between maternal psychological control and children's depressive symptoms. The authors found that maternal psychological control was positively related to depressive symptoms, but only for children with poorer sleep. In the context of better sleep, children were protected against the negative effects of psychological control on their adjustment problems. Furthermore, as reviewed previously, SES and ethnicity interacted with sleep problems to predict adjustment problems and this association was more evident for either African Americans or children from lower SES backgrounds (El-Sheikh, Kelly et al., 2010). Furthermore, physiological regulation, indexed by respiratory sinus arrhythmia, has been shown to interact with sleep in the prediction of adjustment problems (El-Sheikh, Erath, & Keller, 2007) and poor sleep had its most pronounced links with adjustment problems for children with less optimal vagal regulation. However, this area of study is still very young and much more stands to be learned about moderation effects associated with individual differences and sleep as they relate to adjustment problems in children.

It is possible that common risk factors explain at least a portion of the association between sleep and adjustment. For example, a range of family-level factors with established links to children's adjustment have been shown to influence children's sleep. Using the NICHD Study of Early Childcare, Bell and Belsky (2008) examined a wide range of parent characteristics and their effect on the growth in sleep problems from age 8 to 11. Children who had an absent father or younger mother and experienced higher levels of maternal negativity, lower levels of maternal sensitivity, and less maternal–child closeness had greater growth in sleep problems over the course of the 3 years. Furthermore, other work has found that authoritative parenting (Johnson & McMahon, 2008) and attachment security (Keller & El-Sheikh, 2011) are both related to less problematic sleep in children. Finally, family conflict that is associated with worse developmental outcomes for children has also been shown in community samples to have detrimental effects on sleep (El-Sheikh, Buckhalt, Mize, & Acebo, 2006). Together, these studies suggest that the same family-level variables that have been shown to be potent predictors of adjustment in children also are significantly associated with sleep.

Future Directions

Research on links between children's sleep and adjustment is continuing to grow at a rapid pace, and one hopes that this will be accompanied by a thoughtful integration of findings. Gaining greater insight into the processes that occur during sleep will be critical to furthering the field and will allow the next generation of research to test hypotheses that result from this knowledge. The scarcity of longitudinal and experimental studies and the frequent use of non-nuanced measures to examine sleep problems in children are significant challenges to the field. However, the challenges imposed by understanding the complex relations between sleep and adjustment in children are offset by the potential rewards of this work. The following are recommendations for research that will help further understanding of the association between sleep and adjustment in children.

- Experimental studies that either restrict or enhance sleep are necessary to better assess the extent to which shorter-term sleep problems are *causally* linked to behavioral problems in children.
- Longitudinal studies are necessary to better understand the effects of chronic sleep problems, identify critical periods, and capture reciprocal relations between sleep and adjustment overtime. Such studies of sleep and adjustment should assess competence in other pertinent areas (e.g., social, academic) to capture possible cascading effects of sleep across multiple domains of functioning.
- A better understanding of risk factors for sleep problems in children could provide insights for intervention but also allow for improved methodology that would account for common

risk factors that contribute to both sleep and adjustment difficulties.

• Not all children are equally vulnerable to the negative effects of sleep on adjustment, nor are they equally likely to exhibit internalizing versus externalizing behavior problems; research should consider biological, psychological, and contextual factors that may moderate relations between sleep and adjustment.

• Researchers should consider utilizing existing theoretical models (e.g., emotion regulation, social information processing, etc.) that describe mechanisms and pathways leading to internalizing and/or externalizing behavior problems by exploring how, within those models, sleep may contribute to the development or maintenance of problem behaviors.

Acknowledgments

This work was supported in part by National Institutes of Health Grant R01-HL093246.

References

Achenbach, T. M. (1991a). *Manual for the Child Behavior Checklist/4–18 and 1991 Profile*. Burlington, VT: University of Vermont Department of Psychiatry.

Achenbach, T. M. (1991b). *Manual for the Teacher's Report Form and 1991 Profile*. Burlington, VT: University of Vermont Department of Psychiatry

Alfano, C. A., Zakem, A. H., Costa, N. M., Taylor, L. K. & Weems, C. F. (2009). Sleep problems and their relation to cognitive factors, anxiety, and depressive symptoms in children and adolescents. *Depression and Anxiety, 26*, 503–512.

Aronen, E. T., Paavonen, E. J., Fjallberg, M., Soininen, M., & Torronen, J. (2000). Sleep and psychiatric symptoms in school-age children. *Journal of the American Academy of Child & Adolescent Psychiatry, 39*, 502–508.

Bates, J. E., Viken, R. J., Alexander, D. B., Beyers, J., & Stockton, L. (2002). Sleep and adjustment in preschool children: Sleep diary reports by mothers related to behavior reports by teachers. *Child Development, 73*, 62–74.

Beebe, D. W. (2011). Cognitive, behavioral, and functional consequences of inadequate sleep in children and adolescents. *Pediatric Clinics of North America, 58*, 649–655.

Behar, L. B. (1977). The preschool behavior questionnaire. *Journal of Abnormal Child Psychology, 5*, 265–275.

Bell, B. G. & Belsky, J. (2008). Parents, parenting, and children's sleep problems: Exploring reciprocal effects. *British Journal of Developmental Psychology, 26*, 579–593.

Berger, R. H., Miller, A. L., Seifer, R., Cares, S. R., & LeBourgeois, M. K. (2011). Acute sleep restriction effects on emotion responses in 30- to 36-month-old children. *Journal of Sleep Research, 21*(3), 235–246.

Biggs, S. N., Lushington, K., van den Heuvel, C. J., Martin, A. J., & Kennedy, J. D. (2011). Inconsistent sleep schedules and daytime behavioral difficulties in school-age children. *Sleep Medicine, 12*, 780–786.

Birmaher, B., Kheterpal, S., Brent, D., Cully, M., Balash, L., Kaufman, J., et al. (1997). The screen for child anxiety related emotional disorders (SCARED): Scale construction and psychometric characteristics. *Journal of the American Academy of Child and Adolescent Psychiatry, 36*, 545–553.

Blunden, S., Hoban, T. F., & Chervin, R. D. (2006). Sleepiness in children. *Sleep Medicine Clinics, 1*, 105–118.

Bub, K. L., Buckhalt, J. A., & El-Sheikh, M. (2011). Children's sleep and cognitive performance: A cross-domain analysis of change over time. *Developmental Psychology, 47*(6), 1504–1514.

Buckhalt, J. (2011). Insufficient sleep and the socioeconomic status achievement gap. *Child Development Perspectives, 5*(1), 59–65.

Chorpita, B. F., Yim, L., Moffitt, C., Umemoto, L. A., & Francis, S. E. (2000). Assessment of symptoms of DSM-IV anxiety and depression in children: A revised child anxiety and depression scale. *Behavioral Research and Therapy, 38*, 835–855.

Cole, P. M. & Deater-Deckard, K. (2009). Emotion regulation, risk, and psychopathology. *The Journal of Child Psychology and Psychiatry, 50*, 1327–1330.

Coulombe, J. A., Reid, G. J., Boyle, M. H., & Racine, Y. (2010). Concurrent associations among sleep problems, indicators of inadequate sleep, psychopathology, and shared risk factors in a population-based sample of healthy Ontario children. *Journal of Pediatric Psychology, 35*, 790–799.

Dahl, R. E. (1996). The regulation of sleep and arousal: Development and psychopathology. *Development and Psychopathology, 8*, 3–27.

Dahl, R. E. (1999). The consequences of insufficient sleep for adolescents: Links between sleep and emotional regulation. *Phi Delta Kappan, 80*, 354–359.

Dahl, R. E. & Lewin, D. S. (2002). Pathways to adolescent health, sleep, regulation and behavior. *Journal of Adolescent Health, 31*, 175–184.

Eisenberg, N., Cumberland, A., Spinrad, T. L., Fabes, R. A., Shepard, S. A., Reiser, M., Murphey, B. C., et al. (2001). The relations of regulation and emotionality to children's externalizing and internalizing problem behavior. *Child Development, 72*, 1112–1134.

Eisenberg, N., Valiente, C., Spinrad, T., Cumberland, A., Liew, J., Zhou, Q., & Losoya, S. H. (2009). Longitudinal relations of children's effortful control, impulsivity, and negative emotionality to their externalizing, internalizing and co-occurring behavior problems. *Developmental Psychology, 45*, 988–1008.

El-Sheikh, M., & Buckhalt, J. (2005). Vagal regulation and emotional intensity predict children's sleep problems. *Developmental Psychobiology, 46*(4), 307–317.

El-Sheikh, M., Buckhalt, J., Mize, J., & Acebo, C. (2006). Marital conflict and disruption of children's sleep. *Child Development, 77*(1), 31–43.

El-Sheikh, M., Erath, S. A., & Keller, P. S. (2007). Children's sleep and adjustment: The moderating role of vagal regulation. *Journal of Sleep Research, 16*, 396–405.

El-Sheikh, M., Hinnant, J. B., Kelly, R. J., & Erath, S. (2010). Maternal psychological control and child internalizing symptoms: Vulnerability and protective factors across bioregulatory and ecological domains. *The Journal of Child Psychology and Psychiatry, 51*, 188–198.

El-Sheikh, M., Kelly, R. J., Buckhalt, J. A., & Hinnant, J. B. (2010). Children's sleep and adjustment over time: The role of socioeconomic context. *Child Development, 81*, 870–883.

Fallone, G., Acebo, C., Seifer, R., & Carskadon, M. A. (2005). Experimental restriction of sleep opportunity in children: Effects on teacher ratings. *Pediatrics, 28*, 1561–1567.
Goodman, R. (1997). The strengths and difficulties questionnaire: A research note. *Journal of Child Psychology and Psychiatry, 38*, 581–586.
Goodnight, J. A., Bates, J. E., Staples, A. D., Pettit, G. S., & Dodge, K. A. (2007). Temperamental resistance to control increases the association between sleep problems and externalizing behavior development. *Journal of Family Psychology, 21*, 39–48.
Gregory, A. M. & O'Connor, T. G. (2002). Sleep problems in childhood: A longitudinal study of developmental change and association with behavioral problems. *Journal of the American Academy of Child and Adolescent Psychiatry, 41*, 964–971.
Gregory, A. M., Eley, T. C., O'Connor, T., & Plomin, R. (2004). Etiologies of associations between childhood sleep and behavioral problems in a large twin sample. *Journal of the American Academy of Child and Adolescent Psychiatry, 43*, 744–751.
Gregory, A. M., & Eley, T. C. (2005). Sleep problems, anxiety and cognitive style in school-aged children. *Infant and Child Development, 14*, 435–444.
Gregory, A. M., Rijsdjik, F. V., Dahl, R. E., McGuffin, P., & Eley, T. C. (2006). Associations between sleep problems, anxiety and depression in twins at 8 years of age. *Pediatrics, 118*, 1124–1132.
Gregory, A. M., Cousings, J. C., Forbes, E. E., Trubnik, L., Ryan, N. D., Axelson, D. A., Birmaher, B., et al. (2011). Sleep items in the child behavior checklist: A comparison with sleep diaries, actigraphy, and polysomnography. *Journal of the American Academy of Child & Adolescent Psychiatry, 50*, 499–507.
Gross, J. J., & Thompson, R. A. (2007). Emotion regulation conceptual foundations. In J. J. Gross (Ed.), *Handbook of Emotion Regulation* (pp. 2–24). New York: Guilford.
Holley, S., Hill, C. M., & Stevenson, J. (2011). An hour less sleep is a risk factor for childhood conduct problems. *Child: Care, Health and Development, 37*, 563–570.
Jan, J. E., Reiter, R. J., Bax, M., Ribrary, U., Freeman, R. D., & Wasdell, M. B. (2010). Long-term sleep disturbances in children: A cause of neuronal loss. *European Journal of Pediatric Neurology, 14*, 380–390.
Johnson, N., & McMahon, C. (2008). Preschoolers' sleep behavior: Associations with parental hardiness, sleep related cognitions and bedtime interactions. *The Journal of Child Psychology and Psychiatry,49*, 765–773.
Keller, P., & El-Sheikh, M. (2011). Children's emotional security and sleep: Longitudinal relations and directions of effects. *The Journal of Child Psychology and Psychiatry, 52*, 64–71.
Kelly, R. J., & El-Sheikh, M. (2013, April). Reciprocal relations between sleep and adjustment among youth over time. In A. Fuligni (Chair), *New insights into teen sleep*. Symposium presented at the biennial meeting of the Society for Research in Child Development, Seattle, WA.
Kovacs, M. (1985). The Children's Depression Inventory. *Psychopharmacology Bulletin, 21*, 995–998.
Lachar, D. (1982). *The Personality Inventory for Children*. Los Angeles: Western Psychological Services.
Lemola, S., Raikkonen, K., Scheier, M. F., Matthews, K. A., Pesonen, A., Heinonen, K., et al. (2011). Sleep quantity, quality and optimism in children. *Journal of Sleep Research, 20*, 12–20.
Lilienfeld, S. O. (2003). Comorbidity between and within childhood externalizing and internalizing disorders: Reflections and directions. *Journal of Abnormal Child Psychology, 31*, 285–291.
Muzur, A., Pace-Schott, E. F., & Hobson, J. A. (2002). The prefrontal cortex in sleep. *Trends in Cognitive Sciences, 6*, 475–481.
O'Brien, Lucas, N. H., Felt, B. T., Hoban, T. F., Rudzicka, D. L., Jordan, R., et al. (2011). Aggressive behavior, bullying, snoring, and sleepiness in schoolchildren. *Sleep Medicine, 12*(7), 652–658.
Owens, J. A., Maxim, R., Nobile, C., McGuinn, M., & Msall, M. (2000). Parental and self-report of sleep in children with attention-deficit/hyperactivity disorder. *Archives of Pediatrics and Adolescent Medicine, 154*, 549–555.
Owens, J. A., Spirito, A., McGuinn, M., & Nobile, C. (2000). The children's sleep hábits questionnaire (CSHQ): Psychometric properties of a survey instrument for school-aged children. *Sleep, 23*, 1043
Paavonen, E. J., Almquist, F., Tamminen, T., Moilanen, I., Piha, J., Rasanen, E., & Aronen, E.T. (2002). Poor sleep and psychiatric symptoms at school: An epidemiological study. *European Child & Adolescent Psychiatry, 11*, 10–17.
Paavonen, E. J., Raikkonen, K., Lahti, J., Konsi, N., Heinonen, K., Pesonen, A., et al. (2009). Short sleep duration and behavioral symptoms of attention-deficit/hyperactivity disorder in healthy 7- to 8- year-old children. *Pediatrics, 123*, e857–e864.
Paavonen, E. J., Porkka-Heiskanen, T., & Lahikainen, A. R. (2009). Sleep quality, duration and behavioral symptoms among 5–6 year old children. *European Child and Adolescent Psychiatry, 18*, 747–754.
Pesonen, A., Raikkonen, K., Paavonen, E. J., Heinonen, K., Komsi, N., Lahti, J., et al. (2010). Sleep duration and regularity are associated with behavioral problems in 8-year-old children. *International Journal of Behavioral Medicine, 17*, 298–305.
Phelps, E. A. (2004). Human emotion and memory: Interactions of the amygdale and hippocampal complex. *Current Opinions in Neurobiology, 14*, 198–202.
Reynolds, C. R., & Richmond, B. O. (1978). What I think and feel: A revised measure of children's manifest anxiety. *Journal of Abnormal Child Psychology, 6*, 271–280.
Rutter, M., Tizard, J. R., & Whitmore, K. (Eds). (1997). *Education, Health and Behavior*. London: Longman.
Sadeh, A., & Acebo, C. (2002). The role of actigraphy in sleep medicine. *Sleep Medicine Reviews, 6*, 113–124.
Sadeh, A., Gruber, R., & Raviv, A. (2002). Sleep, neurobehavioral functioning, and behavior problems in school-age children. *Child Development, 73*, 405–417.
Sadeh, A., Gruber, R., & Raviv, A. (2003). The effects of sleep restriction and extension in school-age children: What a difference a hour makes. *Child Development, 74*, 444–455.
Sadeh, A. (2007). Consequences of sleep loss or sleep disruption in children. *Sleep Medicine Clinics, 2*, 513–520.
Sadeh, A. (2011). The role and validity of actigraphy in sleep medicine: An update. *Sleep Medicine Reviews, 15*, 259–267.
Silk, J. S., Vanderbilt-Adriance, E., Shaw, D. S., Forbes, E. E., Whalen, D. J., Ryan, N. D., & Dahl, R. E. (2007). Resilience among children and adolescents at risk for depression: Mediation and moderation across social and neurobiological contexts. *Development and Psychopathology, 19*, 841–865.
Smits, M. G., Van Stel, H. F., Van Der Heijden, K. B., Meijer, A. M., Coenen, A. M., & Kerkhof, G. A. (2003). Melatonin improves health status and sleep in children with idiopathic

chronic sleep-onset insomnia: A randomized placebo-controlled trial. *Journal of the American Academy of Child and Adolescent Psychiatry, 42,* 1286–1293.

Soffer-Dudek, N., Sadeh, A., Dahl, R. E., & Rosenblat-Stein, S. (2011). Poor sleep quality predicts deficient emotion information processing over time in early adolescence. *Sleep, 34,* 1499–1508.

Vandekerckhove, M., & Cluydts, R. (2010). The emotional brain and sleep: An intimate relationship. *Sleep Medicine Reviews, 14,* 219–226.

van Maanen, A., Meijer, A. M., Smits, M. G., & Oort, F. J. (2011). Termination of short term melatonin treatment in children with delayed Dim Light Melatonin Onset: Effects on sleep, health, behavior problems, and parenting stress. *Sleep Medicine, 12,* 875–879.

Walker, M. P., & van der Helm, E. (2009). Overnight therapy? The role of sleep in emotional brain processing. *Psychological Bulletin, 135,* 731–748.

Weissbluth, M. (1989). Sleep-loss stress and temperamental difficultness: Psychological processes and practical considerations. In G. A. Kohnstamm, J. E. Bates, & M. K. Rothbart (Eds.), *Temperament in Childhood* (pp. 357–375). Chichester, UK: Wiley.

Wolfson, A. R., & Carskadon, M. A. (1998). Sleep schedules and daytime functioning in adolescents. *Child Development, 69,* 875–887.

CHAPTER

28 Sleep in Preschoolers: School Readiness, Academics, Temperament, and Behavior

Victoria J. Molfese, Kathleen Moritz Rudasill, *and* Dennis L. Molfese

Abstract

Kindergarten readiness is characterized by important achievements in the acquisition of content knowledge and development of self-regulation skills—effortful control and executive function—needed for controlled and focused behaviors. Development of these readiness skills begins in the preschool period, and there is now strong evidence that these preschool skills are critically important for children's academic performance in kindergarten and through elementary grades. Therefore, the focus of this chapter is on the preschool and early elementary periods (kindergarten through third grade) and the roles that sleep habits and sleep problems play in the development of cognitive skills, temperament, and executive functions. Research models, methods, measures and findings reported in published literature involving young children are reviewed and integrated into a framework identifying the influence of sleep on children's skills and behaviors and suggesting that, at least for temperament, child characteristics may influence sleep.

Key Words: self-regulation, effortful control, executive function, cognitive skills, school readiness, sleep habits, sleep disordered breathing, actigraphy, sleep questionnaire, sleep log

Introduction

Kindergarten is an important developmental transition for children, as it represents the first year of formal education and the point at which most children are first evaluated for school readiness. School readiness has many different definitions, but often this term refers to the social-emotional, physical, behavioral, and cognitive skills children need to learn and function successfully in school. Children's school readiness is also related to the mechanisms and readiness of their families, communities, and schools to support and prepare young children to learn in school (Getting Ready, 2005). Thus, the skills and support mechanisms that children bring with them to kindergarten are critical to academic success. This reality has motivated intense interest in the preschool period as researchers, parents, educators, and policy makers seek to better understand how to enable children to succeed in school.

The importance of kindergarten readiness skills is highlighted by clear evidence that the cognitive skills children develop through participation in high quality preschool education programs influence their academic proficiencies when measured at kindergarten entry and in later grades (Denton & West, 2002; National Association of the Education of Young Children and National Council of Teachers of Mathematics, 2002). Indeed, there is growing evidence that the development of conventional reading and mathematics skills are linked with specific emergent or precursor cognitive skills developed in the preschool period. For reading, the important cognitive skills include alphabetic knowledge, phonological awareness and short-term memory, rapid automatized naming, and writing (National Early Literacy Panel, 2008). For mathematics, the important cognitive skills for young children include understanding the concepts and processes involving number, relations, and operations (National Research Council, 2009). Yet, there is a growing awareness that school readiness requires more than emergent content knowledge. Children need to begin to develop the self-regulation skills that will enable them to successfully transition from prekindergarten to kindergarten and elementary classrooms. Boyd and colleagues describe these self-regulation skills as the ability to "pay attention, remember information on purpose (and) function socially by getting along with others, and delaying gratification" (p. 2, Boyd, Barnett, Bodrova, Leong, & Gomby, 2005). Self-regulation has been conceptualized as both temperamentally and cognitively based; however, they are not interchangeable constructs. In a recent article, Liew (2011) conceptualized effortful control and executive functions as distinct constructs that are also overlapping and complementary. Temperamental self-regulation, or effortful control, is biologically based yet evolves through interaction with environmental forces. Cognitive self-regulation, or executive function, encompasses higher-order skills that are neurologically based, begin to develop in early childhood, and are malleable via training or intervention (Liew, 2011). School readiness, then, is a combination of the development of cognitive skills as well as the development of self-regulation skills needed for the controlled and focused behaviors that contribute to early academic performance.

Sleep in Early Childhood

The focus on this chapter is on sleep in preschool children and how this relates to their school readiness, academics, temperament, and daytime. There is a growing body of research on the characteristics of sleep in this age group. It is estimated that the average 3- to 6-year-old child requires 10 to 12 hours of nighttime sleep (Bates, Viken, Alexander, Beyers, & Stockton, 2002; National Sleep Foundation, 2004; Thiedke, 2001). However, there is some uncertainty regarding how much sleep young children are actually getting at night. Sleep duration is often measured in two ways. One way involves the use of parent logs to record day-by-day information across a specific period of time, such as a week. Typical information includes daily bedtime and rise time, but sleep logs can also contain information on hourly periods across nighttime, such as between 6 pm and 6 am, in which the parent may be asked to report on whether the child is "out of bed," "in bed," and "asleep." Actigraphs also are used to measure sleep duration (see Horne and Biggs, Chapter 16). Actigraphs are small, portable devices that sense physical motion and record information useful for determining sleep onset time, sleep offset time, sleep duration, true sleep time (sleep duration with night wakefulness subtracted), sleep efficiency (ratio between true sleep time and sleep duration), longest sleep interval (longest continuous period scored as true sleep without identified wakening), activity level (level of activity during true sleep), and number of arousals during the night. These two sources of information on children's sleep can be compared.

In our research (Dayyat, Spruyt, Molfese, & Gozal, 2011) with 110 typically developing children aged 3 to 9.5 years old (M = 6.6 years), sleep duration data were obtained using parent sleep logs and actigraphs. Sleep duration across a 1-week period averaged 8.17 hours based on actigraph data and 10.10 hours when sleep log data were used. On average, parent sleep logs overestimated sleep duration by 111 minutes when compared to actigraph data. It appears that actigraphy might provide more accurate measures of sleep duration, but the use of daily sleep logs and sleep questionnaires provide additional information from parents about a variety of dimensions of young children's sleep (e.g., sleep disruptions related to illness or specific sleep habits related to sleeping arrangements) that are needed to obtain a fuller understanding of sleep and sleep impacts on behavior.

There is evidence in a growing number of studies that many young children experience sleep problems such as snoring or difficulty breathing, difficulty getting to sleep at night, night awakenings, and daytime sleepiness. This is concerning because children with sleep problems are characterized by more health and behavior problems and with higher rates of attention-deficit/hyperactivity disorder (Hiscock, Canterford, Ukoumunne, & Wake, 2007; V. Molfese, 2008). Hiscock et al. (2007) used parental reports to document sleep behaviors and behavioral sequelae in a nationally representative sample of Australian preschool children (4 to 5 years of age). They report that nearly 20% of children had mild and 14% had moderate to severe sleep problems. Compared to children without sleep problems, those with sleep problems were more likely to have physical and psychosocial problems and to have problems related to conduct, peer relations, emotions, hyperactivity/inattention, and prosocial behaviors. Sleep problems also are negatively associated with children's learning and behavior (Archbold, Giordani, Ruzicka, & Chervin, 2004;

Blunden, Lushington, & Kennedy, 2001; O'Brien & Gozal, 2004; Sadeh, Gruber, & Raviv, 2003). Understanding how this essential, biologically based behavior of sleep influences young children's cognitive skills and self-regulatory behaviors enables a broader conceptualization of the critical elements that influence education in early childhood.

Sleep Insufficiency

Sleep insufficiency, or not sleeping enough to be fully alert the next day, in childhood has been ascribed to a variety of conditions, including sleep disordered breathing (SDB) and poor sleep habits (SH). SDB is a condition marked by periodic apnea and intermittent hypoxia that is a relatively common occurrence in children who are otherwise healthy. The symptoms of SDB include nighttime restlessness, daytime sleepiness and, most often, habitual snoring. While reports of snoring history are not sufficient for a diagnosis of SDB, snoring is reliably present in sleep study–based diagnoses of obstructive sleep apnea (OSA); indeed, snoring indicates the presence of increased upper airway resistance, a distinctive symptom of SDB (Kuehni, Strippoli, Chauliac & Silverman, 2008; Carroll, McColley, Marcus & Loughlin, 1995). In population-based studies, parents report symptoms of SDB in 9% to 25% of preschool children (Ali, Pitson & Strandling, 1993, 1994; Castronovo, Zucconi, Nosetti, Marazzini, Hensley, Vegia, et al., 2003; Gottlieb Vezina, Chase, Lesko, Heeren, Wesse-Mayer, et al., 2003; Hiscock et al., 2007; Montgomery-Downs, Jones, Molfese, & Gozal, 2003).

Sleep Insufficiency and Sleep Habits

Sleep insufficiency may also arise due to problems related to the child's resistance to going to bed/sleep, multiple nighttime awakenings that require parental interactions, difficulty initiating or maintaining sleep, fears associated with sleeping, and a child's poor sleep schedule. The most common sleep problems of young children are frequent nighttime awakenings and difficulty initiating sleep (Sadeh, Mindell, Luedtke & Wiegand, 2009). Sleep problems such as these are described as poor sleep habits (SH). Poor SH are associated with "daily living activities that are inconsistent with the maintenance of good quality sleep and full daytime alertness," according to the *International Classification of Sleep Disorders, Revised* (ICSD, 2005, p. 18). SH is used here to refer to poor sleep habits that lead to insufficient nighttime sleep due to a variety of reasons that may contribute to non-optimal daytime performance. An estimated 10% to 66% of 4- to 5-year-old children experience one or more SH problems (Hiscock et al., 2007; Johnson & McMahon, 2008; Ottaviano, Giannotti, Cortesi, Bruni, & Ottaviano, 1996; Goodlin-Jones, Tang, Liu, & Anders, 2009; Pollock, 1994; Tikotzky & Sadeh, 2001). Children characterized by SH problems in the infancy/toddler period are likely to have SH problems later in the preschool period (Lam, Hiscock, & Wake, 2003; Kataria, Swanson & Trevathan, 1987; Zuckerman, Stevenson, & Bailey, 1987).

Sleep and Cognitive Skills

Studies of sleep behaviors in young children have shown the effects of sleep on cognitive skills (see Blunden et al., 2001 for a review, and O'Brien, Chapter 29). For example, Jones (2006) studied 448 preschool and school-age children (ages 3 to 8 years) in an investigation of the relation between SH, literacy activities in the home, and children's verbal, nonverbal, language, and visual-spatial skills. Parents completed a sleep questionnaire (Gozal, 1998; Montgomery-Downs, O'Brien, Holbrook, & Gozal, 2004) and a home literacy environment questionnaire (the STIM Q: Dreyer, Mendelsohn, & Tamis-LeMonda, 1996) that asked about literacy materials in the home, parent–child reading activities, availability of language-related toys and materials, and reading-related activities. SH was measured using items from the sleep questionnaire reflecting sleeping arrangements (sleep alone, sleep with one to more than three others), sleep duration (4–5, 6–7, 8–9, 10–11, more than 11 hours, bedtime/wake times), and sleep behaviors and symptoms of sleep disorders. The verbal and nonverbal cognitive skills outcome measures were assessed using Differential Abilities Scale scores (DAS: Elliott, 1990), and the language and visual-spatial skills were assessed using the Developmental Neuropsychological Assessment (NEPSY: Korkman, Kirk, & Kemp, 1998). The children's cognitive skills were related to the quality of home literacy environment, but the effects of the home literacy environment were mediated by SH. A strong correlation ($r = .78$) was found between SH and the home literacy environment in contrast to the weaker relation between SH and cognitive skills ($r = .22$). These findings were interpreted as showing that home literacy environment and SH together play important roles in the development of cognitive skills of young children. In a follow-up to this study, Dayyat and colleagues reported on race differences in the measures (Dayyat, Newland,

Bennett, Gozal, Spruyt, Molfese, & Jones, 2010). When compared to White parents, parents of African-American children reported lower scores on all the measures of the home literacy activities except the reading subscale and on the SH measures, and these scores were related to the children's performance on the cognitive assessments. A structural equation model revealed that SH and the home literacy environment mediated the relation between race and cognitive scores.

V. Molfese and colleagues investigated the relation between SH (sleep duration, bedtime and rise time), children's problem behaviors using items from the Child Behavior Checklist (CBCL: Achenbach & Rescorla, 2000), and children's learning of letter names in preschool, an important emergent cognitive skill known to predict conventional reading at school age (Molfese, Beswick, Molnar, Jacobi-Vessels, & Gozal, 2007). The children in the study were 4 year olds from high-poverty families who were enrolled in Head Start or public prekindergarten programs. Parents completed a sleep questionnaire (Gozal, 1998; Montgomery-Downs et al, 2004), as well as eight questions from the CBCL to obtain information about concentration, hyperactivity, confused behavior, involvement with others, predictable behavior, frustration tolerance, cooperation, and energy level of the child. The study investigated whether the gains children made across the school year in learning letter names were related to their sleep habits and the presence of behaviors that might interfere with classroom learning. The results showed that children making small gains in letter identification across the school year (fall to spring gains of 0–3 letters out of a total of 15 letters) were characterized by shorter sleep durations (less than 10 hours) and more problem behaviors (scores of "very true" on two or more of eight behaviors) compared to children making big gains (fall to spring gains of 4 or more letters). In this study, the association of risk conditions related to sleep duration and evaluations of problem behaviors show combined relations to children's alphabet learning.

In some studies, direct links between sleep behaviors and measures of cognitive skills have not been found. In one of our studies (Montgomery-Downs et al., 2004), we investigated the relation between sleep behaviors and general cognitive skills in a group of 67 children (28 males, 39 females) aged 42 to 59 months (M = 50.52 months) who were at academic risk due to family poverty. The children were enrolled in Head Start and public prekindergarten programs and were assessed on verbal, nonverbal, and overall cognitive skills using the DAS. The children's parents completed a sleep questionnaire (Gozal, 1998; Montgomery-Downs et al., 2004) that requested information about the child's typical bedtime and rise times, duration of sleep, and sleep behaviors and questions related to SDB, such as snoring frequency and loudness. The sleep questionnaire also included questions about the child's health history (the presence of allergies, asthma, poor appetite, ear infections, frequent colds/flu, constant runny nose, vision and hearing problems) and eight questions from the CBCL (Achenbach & Rescorla, 2000) that asked parents to report on their child's characteristic levels of activity. We expected to find that children grouped (high, low) based on sleep behavior scores reflecting SH (e.g., less than 10 hours of night time sleep, bedtime after 9 pm, and rise time before 7 am) and SDB (snoring frequency and loudness) would evidence differences in their cognitive performance. This expectation was supported for the children with high SDB scores, who had significantly lower DAS verbal, nonverbal, and overall cognitive scores compared to children with low SDB scores. However, group differences were not found when children were grouped based on SH scores. While the lack of relation between SH and cognitive scores might be due to the relatively few SH items on the questionnaire (7 items compared to 17 items for SDB), it is clear that sleep problems reflecting SDB were related to the measures of cognitive skills.

Results from a larger longitudinal study of Australian children reported by Hiscock et al. (2007) showed that a parental report of SH was not related to children's cognitive skills. In that study, parents evaluated their 4- to 5-year-old children's sleep according to whether they considered their children to have a sleep problem. Parents provided holistic ratings of their children's sleep as reflecting "no, mild, moderate, or severe" problems. Children were assessed on receptive vocabulary (Peabody Picture Vocabulary Test III, Dunn and Dunn, 1997) and performance on a cognitive assessment (*Who am I*; de Lemnos & Doig, 1999) that included items related to literacy and numeracy skills. No association was found between the parent ratings of sleep problems and cognitive performance. However, these findings might well be due to using the holistic evaluations of sleep rather than using a questionnaire containing a series of questions about different types of sleep behaviors and a range for evaluating the magnitudes of those behaviors.

Other researchers studying older children (9 to 14 years of age) have reported somewhat mixed results in relating sleep measures to different measures of cognitive skills. In the study by Meijer, Habekothe, and van den Wittenboer (2000), 449 children completed questionnaires related to time in bed and sleep quality. The children also participated in an attention task and answered a questionnaire about school functioning. The researchers reported that the sleep questionnaire responses were not related to performance on the visual attention task but were associated with general school functioning, and suggested that the lack of relation between sleep and the attention task might have been due to the nature of the task, which was short and relatively simple.

Indicators of Sleep Disordered Breathing and Behavior Problems

There is strong evidence linking symptoms of SDB and SH with problem behaviors of young children that are likely to influence learning in the classroom, particularly hyperactivity and inattention. In a study of a general pediatric population involving 866 children, Chervin, Hedger Archbold, et al. (2002) reported that 2- to 13.9-year-old children characterized by habitual snoring, daytime sleepiness, and overall SDB traits were more likely to be rated by their parents as inattentive and hyperactive on two scales, one derived from the *Diagnostic and Statistical Manual of Mental Disorders IV* (American Psychiatric Association, 2000) and the other from the Conners Parent Rating Scale (Conners & Barkley, 1985). The predicted association between snoring and hyperactivity was particularly strong among boys who were younger than 8 years old. Similarly, Ali and colleagues (1994) studied a longitudinal sample of children across two time points—Time 1 when they were 4 to 5 years of age (N = 782) and Time 2 when they were 6.5 to 7.5 years old (N = 507). These researchers reported that prevalence of habitual snoring remained the same (roughly 12%) across the time span, as did the prevalence of ratings of children as hyperactive (20% to 24%). Interestingly, the researchers reported on cases of children who were habitual snorers at Time 1 but were no longer snoring at Time 2 (around 50% of the cases resolved) and children who were not reported as habitual snorers at Time 1 but who were reported as snoring at Time 2 (around 6% of the children). At both time points, children rated as habitual snorers also received high ratings on hyperactivity.

Gottlieb and colleagues (2003) report similar links between parents' ratings of child SBD behaviors and behaviors in 5-year-olds in a population-based sample of 205 children (Gottlieb et al., 2003). Parents completed the Conners Parent Rating Scale (1997) to evaluate attention deficit/hyperactivity and other problem behaviors. Children with SDB symptoms were significantly different from children without SBD symptoms on the ADHD Index and cognitive/inattention scales, but not on the hyperactivity scale. Montgomery-Downs et al. (2003) studied a community sample of 101 children ranging in age from 3 to 5 years (M = 4.2 years) from low-income families. Children were evaluated for risk for SDB based on parental reports from a sleep questionnaire using two indicators: the presence of habitual snoring (3 or more days per week), and snoring loudness (ranging from medium to extremely loud). Children at risk for SDB were more likely to be evaluated by their parents as evidencing symptoms of ADHD or hyperactivity.

Barnes, Huss, Garrod, et al. (2009) have also examined sleep quality and behaviors in 44 children aged 4 to 8 years (M = 6.92). Based on the results of parental reports from a sleep questionnaire and follow-up polysomnography, the children were identified as either "rarely" or "occasionally" snoring or as never snoring (the control group). While the snoring children did not meet diagnostic criteria for SDB, parents rated these children as having more behavioral problems than control children. The snoring children scored higher on Conners Parent Rating Scales-Revised: Long (Conners, 2000) subscales for restlessness, cognitive problems/inattention, ADHD inattentive subtype, and ADHD combined subtype. Half of the snoring children scored one standard deviation or more above average on one or more subscales. The participants also took part in an "oddball" attention task that included the recording of event-related potentials (ERPs). Children exhibiting snoring showed evidence of altered brain processing beginning very early in the brain response. The oddball task was more cognitively demanding for the snoring children, whose brain responses reflected more delayed and effortful processing. In contrast, control children who were reported to never snore processed the tones more quickly, engaging higher brain regions at an earlier latency than snorers. Interestingly, there were no significant differences between snoring and control children in the number of correct responses or the average reaction time for correct responses during the oddball task. The attention resources of the snoring children that were allocated to the processing of novel stimuli appear to be sufficient for behavioral responding, but required more effortful brain processing compared to control children.

Sleep Habits and Behavior Problems

SH problems also are associated with daytime sleepiness and problem behaviors. Goodlin-Jones et al. (2009) studied a sample of 3- to 4-year-old typically developing children (N = 69) as well as children with autism (N = 68) and children with developmental delays (N = 57). Actigraphs were used to measure sleep patterns, and parental questionnaire responses (Children's Sleep Habits Questionnaire: Owens, Spirito, & McGuinn, 2000) were used to measure sleep problems such as parasomnias (sleepwalking/talking, night terrors, bedwetting, restless legs) and SDB. Daytime sleepiness was measured using parental responses to questions about their child falling asleep in everyday situations, and behavior problems were measured using the CBCL (Achenbach & Rescorla, 2000). After controlling for diagnostic group and developmental age, significant associations were found between SH, CBCL behavior problem scores, and daytime sleepiness. Interestingly, children whose parents reported that they currently had a sleep problem were more likely to fall asleep during their laboratory visit when given an opportunity to rest.

Witcher, Gozal, Molfese, and Crabtree (2007) investigated the relationship between SH, SDB, and problem behaviors in a sample of 100 children aged 5 to 8 years (M = 6.87 years). Parents of the children completed the Children's Sleep Hygiene Scale (CSHS; Harsh, Easley & LeBourgeois, 2002) that included questions on sleep behaviors rated on a six-point scale and the Conners Parent Rating Scales-Revised (CPRS-R: Conners & Barkley, 1985), which uses a seven-point scale for ratings of physiological, cognitive, emotional, and bedtime routines. SDB status of the children was determined based on parental reports that the children "frequently" to "almost always" snored at night. A comparison group of 30 children (M = 7.44 years) whose parents reported that they "never" snored at night was also studied. In the SDB group, the overall SH score was strongly and negatively correlated with many of the CPRS-R subscales, including the ADHD Index. No such relations were found between the SH and the CPRS-R scores in the control group. The children with SDB had poorer SH, which also was related to high ratings on daytime behavior problems. The findings were interpreted as showing that children at risk for SDB may be more likely to develop daytime behavior problems related to poor SH.

Bates and colleagues (2002) studied a community sample of 202 4- to 5-year-old children. Parents completed sleep logs recording daily sleep and rise times, and sleep disruptions characterized by measures related to SH, such as total sleep, amount and variability in nighttime sleep, bedtime variability and late bedtimes. Teachers evaluated school adjustment using the Preschool Adjustment Questionnaire (Jewsuwan, Luster & Kostelnik, 1993) and the Preschool Behavior Questionnaire (Behar, 1977). Children who were reported by their teachers as having more behavioral and adjustment problems in preschool also had more sleep disruptions. This relation was seen even when characteristics that might influence children's sleep problems, such family stress and family management practices, were factored out. Touchette and colleagues conducted a large longitudinal study involving over 2000 families and used parental reports to obtain yearly measures of nighttime sleep duration on children between 2.5 and 5 years of age and quarterly reports on children's hyperactive behaviors between 1.5 and 5 years of age (Touchette, Cote, Petit, Liu, Boivin, Falissard, et al., 2009). Significant associations were reported between persistent short nighttime sleep durations and high incidence of hyperactive behaviors. Although the study is correlational, the authors suggest that it is hyperactivity that interferes with nighttime sleep duration rather than sleep problems leading to hyperactivity.

The Touchette et al. interpretation is interesting because other researchers studying children with SBD report that treatment involving adenotonsillectomy (removal of adenoids and tonsils) resulted in significant improvements in children's behaviors, including reduction in reported hyperactivity and other externalizing behaviors and/or internalizing behaviors (Ali, Pitson, Stradling, 1996; Friedman, Hendeles-Amitai, Kozminsky, Leiberman, Friger, Tarasiuk & Tal, 2003; Mitchell & Kelly, 2005, 2007; Wei, Bond, Mayo, Smith, Reese, & Weatherly, 2009) as well as significant improvements in school performance measured by grades (Gozal, 1998; O'Brien & Gozal, 2002). While dramatic improvements are reported for children with SDB following adenotonsillectomy, not all children show improvements (Mitchell, 2007), which might be due to the presence of AHDH as suggested by Touchette et al. (2009) and Hiscock et al. (2007). However, compelling evidence reported by Hiscock et al. (2007) on the changing relations between symptoms of SBD and the resolution of these symptoms, and the presence or absence of hyperactive behaviors, reflects the interdependence of these two variables.

Temperament

Temperament is an individual's general style of responding to stimuli in the environment and refers to constitutionally based individual differences in *reactivity* and *regulation* (Rothbart, Derryberry, & Hershey, 2000). According to Rothbart and Derryberry (1981), temperament is *constitutional* because it is, "the relatively enduring biological makeup of the [individual], influenced over time by heredity, maturation, and experience" (p. 40). There is ample support for the stability of temperament through early elementary school and beyond (Caspi & Silva, 1995; Kagan, Resnick, Snidman, Gibbons, & Johnson, 1988; Resnick, Kagan, Snidman, Gersten, Baak, & Rosenberg, 1986; Rimm-Kaufman & Kagan, 2005; Rothbart & Posner, 2005), and its evolution from environmental influences.

Temperament is often conceptualized as a two-system construct: one system is a reaction to stimuli in the environment (reactivity), and the other system is the regulatory function that operates on reactivity (regulation) (Rothbart & Posner, 2005). A child's ability to regulate may be most critical for success in school and, therefore, relevant when considering the influence of sleep and early academic performance. Temperamental regulation comprises the ability to both *focus* and *shift* attention, and to inhibit reactions that are not appropriate. Together, these skills are often termed *effortful control*, "the ability to inhibit a dominant response to perform a subdominant response" (p. 137, Rothbart & Bates, 1998) and are considered to be indicators of school readiness skills, such as attention, task persistence, and constraint. To illustrate, a child who displays high effortful control in the classroom will be focused on the teacher during classroom instruction and on task during class activities. Children experience rapid growth in regulation from age 4 to 7 years, concurrent with their transition to formal school (Rothbart & Bates, 2006).

Temperament, Academic Achievement, and Sleep

There is a long history of researchers investigating relations between temperament and school performance, and a growing literature that relates temperament and sleep habits. For example, research relating temperament and school performance shows that children's effortful control has implications in the classroom, as it is associated with the ability to persist on difficult tasks, work in the face of distractions, follow classroom rules, inhibit inappropriate behaviors, and attend to classroom activities (Alexander, Entwisle, & Dauber, 1993; Kendall, 1993; Veldman &Worsham, 1983). Recent research by Rudasill, Gallagher, and White (2010) shows that children rated by mothers as having higher levels of attentional focusing on the Children's Behavior Questionnaire (CBQ: Rothbart, Ahadi, Hershey, & Fisher, 2001) at age 4.5 years performed better on standardized reading and mathematics tests in 3rd grade than their peers with lower attention ratings. Findings also indicated that attentional focusing buffered children from the negative effects of classrooms with low levels of emotional support. Martin and Holbrook (1985) examined the relationship between teacher ratings of 1st-grade children's temperament using the Temperament Assessment Battery (Martin, 1984) and their academic achievement (using grades and standardized test scores on the American School Achievement Test). They found more persistence and less distractibility were significantly and positively related to grades and standardized achievement scores. Nelson, Martin, Hodge, Havill, and Kamphaus (1999) examined associations between children's parent-rated temperament using the Temperament Assessment Battery for Children (Martin, 1988) at age 5 and their teacher-rated school performance using the Behavior Assessment System for Children (Reynolds & Kamphaus, 1992) in 3rd grade. Children's poor self-regulation was positively linked to school performance problems (e.g., failure to complete assignments, difficulty following directions). Taken together, existing research shows clear links between children's temperamental regulation and academic achievement in early elementary school.

Temperament and Sleep

Links between temperament and sleep have been identified in the literature (Ednick, Cohen, McPhail, Beebe, Simakajornboon, & Amin, 2009; Goodnight, Bates, Staples, Pettit, & Dodge, 2007; Hall, Zubrick, Silburn, Parsons, & Kurinczuk, 2007; Sakimura, Dang, Ballard, & Hansen, 2008; Simard, Nielsen, Tremblay, Boivin, & Montplaisir, 2008). Yet it remains unclear whether temperament influences sleep, sleep influences temperament, or there is a bidirectional relationship between the two. Given the conceptualization of temperament as biologically based individual differences in reactivity and regulation (Rothbart & Bates, 2006) that inform affect, attention, and behavior (Rothbart, Ahadi, & Evans, 2000), it seems natural to expect temperament to influence sleep. Indeed, Scher, Hall, Zaidman-Zait, and Weinberg (2010) and Sadeh, Lavie, and Scher (1994) have found support for this relationship. For example, a child who is highly sensitive may be more likely to experience sleep disruptions from fears or environmental noises (Carey, 2005). On the other hand, the regulatory component of temperament develops across time, particularly during early childhood, in part as a result of children's experiences (Rothbart & Bates, 2006). In this way, sleep may be conceptualized as contributing to downstream regulatory development. For instance, a tired child is more likely to display inappropriate classroom behavior than a child who is properly rested (Lavigne, Arend, Rosenbaum, & Smith, 1999; Owens-Stively et al., 1997). Indeed, temperament is dynamic and temperamental predispositions are not blueprints for outcomes, but rather risk or protective factors that interact with other environmental features leading to outcomes. Therefore, it is critical to consider temperament when seeking to understand associations between sleep and self-regulation, as literature supports temperament as a predictor (e.g., Novosad, Freudigman, & Thoman, 1999), an outcome (Ednick et al., 2009), and a moderator (Goodnight et al., 2007) of sleep in childhood.

Concurrent Associations between Sleep and Temperamental Self-Regulation

Several studies have shown connections between mother reports of temperament (particularly negative emotionality) and mother reports of sleep problems in children from preschool to 8 years (Carey, 1974; Owens-Stively et al., 1997; Sadeh et al., 1994; Schaefer, 1990; Van Tassel, 1985; Weissbluth, Davis, & Poncher, 1984; Weissbluth & Liu, 1983; Zuckerman et al., 1987). For example, a recent study with 27 healthy toddlers aged 12–36 months was reported by Scher and colleagues (2010) to show clear associations between sleep quality measured with actigraphy over 3 nights and self-regulatory behavior in daycare based on two measures: parent reports on the Toddlers' Behavior Assessment Questionnaire (Goldsmith, 1996) and teacher reports on the Teacher Daily Report (Bates et al., 2002). Children with more efficient sleep (i.e., less fragmented) had less anger and more inhibitory control, based on parent report.

Ward, Gay, Alkon, Anders, and Lee (2008) studied 54 children ages 3 to 5 years in full-time daycare. Researchers examined cortisol levels as correlates of problematic napping. Actigraph information was collected on children for 3 consecutive nights. In addition, parents completed a sleep diary and the Children's Sleep Habits Questionnaire (Bloom, Owens, McGuinn, Nobile, Schaeffer, & Alario, 2002). Observers measured naptime sleep behaviors at daycare during 15-minute intervals across a 2.5-hour period. Children were coded during this period as sleeping, lying still, restless, or receiving teacher attention. Salivary cortisol was collected in the morning and after naptime on two consecutive days. Parents completed a short-form of the CBQ (Rothbart et al., 2001) to assess children's temperament. Parents rated problem nappers as higher in negative affect and lower in effortful control than nonproblem nappers.

Bruni, Ferini-Strambi, Russo, et al. (2006) examined connections between sleep quality and children's academic skills and temperament with a sample of 264 older children, ages 8 to 11 years. Sleep quality was assessed through parent report on the Sleep Disturbance Scale for Children, a 26-item scale querying parents on children's sleep behavior and problems over the past 6 months. Academic skills were assessed with teacher report on four items measuring reading ability, reading comprehension, mathematics, and executive ability. Academic behavior was measured via teacher report on the Teacher Temperament Questionnaire (Thomas & Chess, 1977). Results indicated that sleep quality was negatively related to task orientation, a temperament dimension where a higher score suggests a child has better skills at paying attention and staying on task. In addition, poorer sleep was a negative predictor of academic skills. Together, these studies provide support for *concurrent* associations between sleep and children's self-regulation. However, the correlational nature of these studies leaves the direction of this relationship unclear.

Longitudinal Studies of Sleep and Temperamental Self-Regulation

Mounting evidence points to the likelihood that indicators of sleep problems measured early in life are related to temperamental regulation measured in later childhood or adolescence. For example, a recent longitudinal study of 25 mothers and their children by Van den Bergh and Mulder (2012) examined fetal transitions from quiet to active sleep as measured by 2-hour monitoring of fetal activity when mothers were near the end of gestation. When the children were 8 to 9 years old, and again when they were 12 to 14 years old, mother reports of their children's effortful control were obtained using the CBQ (Rothbart et al., 2001) and the Early Adolescence Temperament Questionnaire (Capaldi & Rothbart, 1992). Faster fetal transitions (i.e., greater sleep maturity) from quiet to active sleep predicted better effortful control, above and beyond the effects of other correlates of self-regulation such as maternal education, as well as the effects of maternal age, use of alcohol or tobacco during pregnancy, neonatal birth weight, and 5-minute Apgar scores. This evidence suggests that effortful control and sleep maturity may stem from the same mechanism. Rather than one influencing the other, it is possible that they amplify each other.

Zuckerman et al. (1987) studied 308 mothers and their children from age 8 months to 3 years. Sleep difficulties at 8 months were assessed with a semistructured interview with mothers querying infant sleep behavior over the previous 7 days and at age 3 years, behavioral outcomes were assessed with mother reports on the Behavioral Screening Questionnaire (BSQ: Richman & Graham, 1971), without the sleep items. The BSQ items measured behaviors such as peer and sibling relationships, attention span, activity level, difficulty in management, temper tantrums, and fears. Children with persistent sleep problems (i.e., problems at both 8 months and 3 years) were more likely to have self-regulation problems at 3 years; specifically, these children were more likely to be rated as difficult to manage and to have more temper tantrums than children with sleep problems at 8 months only.

Gregory and O'Connor (2002) provide evidence of sleep problems as influencing later issues with self-regulation, as measured with the CBCL with a sample of 490 children and their parents. Sleep problems at 4 years of age measured with parent report on the sleep problems scale of the CBCL were positively related to attention and aggression problems in mid-adolescence (using attention and aggression scale items of the CBCL) after controlling for sex, measures of attention or aggression at 4 years of age, and adoptive status. Although these studies cannot definitively point to sleep problems as causing self-regulatory difficulties, their longitudinal nature provides temporal evidence to support this direction of effects.

TEMPERAMENT AS A MODERATOR OR MEDIATOR OF SLEEP AND SELF-REGULATION

It has been proposed that sleep problems amplify traits that are indicative of more difficult temperament (Novosad et al., 1999). Goodnight et al. (2007) examined resistance to control, a temperament construct conceptualized as encompassing both reactivity and regulation, as a moderator of the association between sleep difficulties and downstream externalizing behaviors. With a longitudinal sample of 556 children followed from 5 to 9 years of age, Goodnight et al. (2007) found childhood resistance to control, rated by mothers when children were approximately 5 years old using the Retrospective Infant Characteristics Questionnaire (Bates, Pettit, Dodge, & Ridge, 1998), was positively related to parent-reported sleep problems using three items from the CBCL at 5, 6, and 8 years of age. Sleep problems were also positively related to externalizing behaviors, as reported by teachers using the CBCL, at ages 5 to 9 years. For children with higher levels of resistance to control at age 5, the link between growth in sleep problems and externalizing behavior was stronger than for children with lower levels of resistance to control at age 5.

Indicative of the uncertainty in the field as to whether temperament is a predictor or result of sleep problems, Reid, Hong, and Wade (2009) investigated temperamental difficulty as a predictor of sleep problems and emotional/behavioral problems. Thus, Reid et al. (2009) conceptualized temperament as a predictor of sleep problems, sleep problems as predictors of self-regulation, and difficult temperament as a predictor of behavior problems including those characteristics of self-regulatory challenges such as impulsivity and inattention. With a large sample of 3050 children ages 2 and 3 years, Reid et al. (2009) used parent report on CBCL to assess emotional and behavioral problems of children, such as clinginess, sadness, impulsivity, and inattention. Parents rated children's problems in getting to sleep and staying asleep with four items measuring trouble falling and staying asleep. Difficult temperament was assessed based on parent report on 10 items from the Infant Characteristics Questionnaire (Bates, Freeland, & Lounsbury, 1979). Difficult temperament was found to be a predictor of both sleep problems and emotional/behavioral problems. Difficult temperament also was significantly associated with both emotional and behavioral problems, and sleep problems were significantly associated with both emotional and behavioral problems. In addition, difficult temperament was a positive predictor of behavior problems.

Together, these studies highlight the complexity of children's sleep and temperamental regulation, suggesting that they bidirectionally influence each other while simultaneously setting the stage for amplified effects in conditions where sleep or temperamental regulation is less than optimal.

Sleep and Preschool Executive Function Skills

There is a large body of research investigating the role that executive function (EF) skills play in problem solving and task performance (see O'Brien, Chapter 29). Executive function skills include the ability to initiate, shift, inhibit, and sustain attention, as well as to plan, organize, and develop strategies or rules. An extensive research literature links EF skills and neuropsychological (brain region) functioning and identifies developmental changes in EF skills with notable changes occurring between 2 and 5 years (e.g., Baddeley, 1998; Zelazo & Muller, 2002). Indeed, it is now evident that EF skills in the preschool years resemble those of older children and that EF skills are directly linked to academic performance (e.g., Espy, McDiarmid, Cwik, Senn, Hamby, & Stalets, 2004; Klein & Bisanz, 2000). The early childhood years appear to constitute a unique period of development in which sleep adequacy may be particularly important to brain functioning, especially in the prefrontal cortex (Gozal, Row, Schurr, & Gozal 2001). A theoretical framework has linked the effects of sleep to prefrontal cortex function, a particularly important brain region due to its involvement in executive function and other complex cognitive skills (Horne, 1988; Harrison & Horne, 1997; Sadeh, Gruber, & Raviv, 2002). Indeed, since the prefrontal cortex matures later than other cortical regions, it is possible that differences in the rates of maturation of different brain regions enhance the vulnerability of the prefrontal cortex to the effects of sleep deprivation (Fuster, 1997).

Molfese, Gozal, and Molfese (2004) have engaged in several investigations of the impact of sleep on brain processes and behaviors in community samples of typically developing young children (6 to 9 years of age). The purpose of these studies was to gain information from manipulating sleep adequacy through "mild sleep loss"—defined in these studies is a 1-hour reduction in sleep time per night for one week. Children frequently face mild sleep restrictions due to a host of pressures, such as demands of homework, school activities, peer interactions, and family activities. These events work to reduce the number of hours of nighttime sleep that children experience from day to day or week to week, as well as children's sleep schedules. In such cases, sleep restriction usually arises from late bedtimes rather than from early rise times. Sleep restriction is hypothesized to result in sleep insufficiencies that impact the child's ability to attend to classroom studies or other activities that place heavy processing demands on the child's cognitive abilities and increase incidence of poor task performance, acting out, and restless behaviors. Increases in processing demands related to sleep restriction were studied by examining children's performance during two study phases. Phase one was a 1-week baseline period in which children followed their typical sleep routines. This baseline phase was followed by the second phase during the following week in which the children's sleep routine was restricted by 1 hour per night for 1 week. During this phase children went to bed 1 hour later than they did when they followed their usual sleep routine but the children got up at the same time, effectively reducing their sleep duration. This sleep-time, rise-time routine is "family friendly," because by utilizing the children's usual rise time family routines can be maintained in the mornings when children must depart for school/daycare and parent(s) must depart for work. Children's compliance with the study phases were verified in this research using sleep logs kept by parents and actigraphs worn by children that record a variety of sleep and activity measures.

Molfese, Ivanenko, Fonaryova Key, et al. (2012) used this methodology to study six children ranging in age from 6.6 to 8.3 years. The children underwent polysomnographic screening to establish that their sleep patterns were normal and then participated in the two phases of the study. The impact of typical sleep compared to restricted sleep on brain processing was investigated using event-related potentials (ERPs). These ERPs were recorded using a geodesic 128 high-density array electrode net that measured brain responses evoked during the children's performance on three tasks that varied in processing demands. Task 1 utilized the standard oddball paradigm (Sangal & Sangal, 1997) known to measure attention-related neurocognitive components. The oddball paradigm is based on the detection of infrequent tones (1000 Hz tones presented on 30% of trials) that appear among a series of frequent tones (1500 Hz tones presented on 70% of trials). Task 2 involved a simple speech perception task in which six consonant-vowel (CV) syllables (ba, da, ga, bu, du, gu) were used to measure auditory discrimination (D. Molfese, 1978). Task 3 used a Directional Stroop paradigm to measure two executive function skills—working memory and inhibitory control

(Davidson, Cruess, Diamond, O'Craven, & Savoy, 1999). The Directional Stroop paradigm is specifically designed for young children who cannot read and is a nonreading form of the classic Stroop task (Stroop, 1935) that involves reading color words correctly regardless of the color of the printed word. The Directional Stroop task has three conditions: in the congruent condition, the child presses a button on the same side of the display that a stimulus appears (e.g., a gray circle presented on the right side of the screen requires pressing the right button); in the incongruent condition, the child presses a button on the opposite side of the display when a different stimulus is presented (e.g., a striped circle on the right side of the screen requires pressing a button on the left); and in the mixed condition there are randomly ordered presentations of congruent and incongruent trials. Changes in ERP brain responses following the 1-week baseline condition were compared to ERP responses following the 1-week restricted sleep condition. Overall, the pattern of ERP activation showed reductions in ERP amplitudes across brain regions for all tasks following the week of restricted sleep. The most marked changes were noted for the Directional Stroop task on the mixed condition, which has the most processing demands. Marked decreases in ERP activation were particularly identifiable, and were interpreted as reflecting impairments in the children's abilities to respond to heavy demands on memory, attention, and inhibitory skills following sleep restriction.

A second study (Osborne, Romas, Gozal, Molfese, & Molfese, 2008) examined the effects of sleep restriction on the performance of 25 children between 5 and 8 years old (M = 6.69 years) on a visual attention task. The NEPSY (Korkman et al., 1998) visual attention task is appropriate for children aged 5 to 12 years and is designed to measure the speed and accuracy with which a child can scan an array and locate a target. Children also participated in the Directional Stroop (described above), in which 128 high-density array electrode nets were used to record brain processing during the task. Results showed no differences due to sleep restriction on the visual attention tasks, possibly because the task demands were not sufficiently complex, but there were differences in the expected direction in brain responses during the Directional Stroop task. Specifically, children generated larger positive amplitude peaks during the mixed condition over the frontal and central brain regions, while generating larger negative peaks over parietal and occipital brain regions. The increases in the amplitudes of the peak brain waves reflect increases in brain activation due to the task condition. These findings confirmed the earlier findings that sleep loss negatively impacts the cognitive functioning of children engaged in tasks with high demands on working memory and inhibition.

Barnes, Gozal, and Molfese (2012) studied 14 children (9 females) aged 4 to 8 years (M = 6.2 years) with suspected obstructive sleep apnea (OSA) and 14 matched controls. All children underwent several assessments, including overnight polysomnography to verify sleep classification as OSA or control, neurocognitive testing on the scales within the NEPSY domains of attention/executive function and memory and learning, as well as participation in the Directional Stroop test while ERPs were recorded. Children with OSA were found to score significantly lower on NEPSY subtests. The ERP responses during the Directional Stroop task were found to reflect increased activation across more brain areas, possibly reflecting more effortful processing relative to the controls. Further, the ERP variables were found to be related to group differences (OSA versus controls) in scores on NEPSY.

Gottlieb and colleagues (2003) also investigated the relation between SBD and young children's performance on executive function tasks. They studied 5-year-old children with and without parental reports of SBD (habitual snoring, loud or noisy breathing, and witnessed apneas). The NEPSY assessments in the attention and executive core domain (tower, auditory attention, visual attention) and the memory core domain (memory for faces, memory for names, and narrative memory) were used along with a continuous performance test (Catch the Cat) as a measure of sustained attention. The children also completed the Wechsler Preschool and Primary Scale of Intelligence, Revised (WPPSI-R: Wechsler, 1989). The children with SBD had significantly poorer scores on all of the NEPSY measures, as well as lower scores on the WPPSI, but not on the continuous performance test. These findings reinforce the important connections between SBD and performance on assessments of executive function as well as on assessments of the general cognitive skills reflected in tests of intelligence.

Other researchers have investigated the relations between quality and quantity of sleep and performance on working memory tests. Working memory refers to the ability to hold information in mind and work with it to relate one idea to another, doing mental problem solving, or holding a string of facts in memory. Steenari, Vuontela, Paavonen, Carlson,

Fjällberg, and Arone (2003) studied a nonclinical sample of 60 children ranging in age from 6 to 13 years (M = 9.9 years). Measures of sleep quality and quantity were determined from actigraphy and parents kept logs of sleep and wake times. Children wore the actigraph for a 3-day period beginning one day before participation in the working memory tasks, and continuously until the task participation was completed. The working memory tasks were visual and auditory versions of the n-back task with three different memory load levels. In n-back tasks, children hear a list (e.g., a string of letters or numbers) and must repeat the item corresponding to "n" steps earlier in the list. Both low sleep efficiency and long sleep latency were associated with poorer performance on the working memory tasks. Shorter sleep time was related to poorer performance on the memory tasks but only at the most difficult level.

The findings from both studies show that brain processing is less than optimal during periods of even minor sleep reduction or shorter sleep time. Mild sleep restriction procedures may mimic conditions occurring in children's real lives and appear to impose substantial alterations in brain responses on cognitive tasks with increasing processing demands. The long-term implications of sleep restrictions or short sleep time on synaptic organization and function during critical periods of brain development are currently unknown. However, the findings described here provide initial insights and a major impetus to investigate this important topic further.

Conclusions

The studies reviewed in this chapter were selected to highlight our understanding of how sleep habits and sleep problems are related to the cognitive skills and the controlled and focused behaviors that are important for young children's success in school. The articles reviewed have included young children, roughly 3- to 8-year-olds, and their families in their studies of sleep problems, including snoring and sleep disordered breathing (SDB), and sleep habits that result in sleep insufficiency. From these studies there is a preponderance of evidence that sleep problems and sleep habits are associated with health and behavior problems such as hyperactivity, inattention, and school adjustment, and with poorer cognitive skills. However, there also is evidence across studies that the associations are not always straightforward. For example, not all of the studies reviewed show the expected relations between poor sleep habits and poor cognitive performance, although the link between SDB and poor cognitive performance is more consistent. Several studies report that sleep habits in combination with other variables (such as activities in the home environment) influence children's performance on the cognitive measures. Investigations of the relations between temperamental self-regulation and sleep provide evidence of concurrent and predictive associations, as well as evidence of bidirectional effects on measures of children's behavior problems. Studies indicate that the specific measures used to document sleep habits and SDB influence findings such that the use of more detailed questionnaires and combinations of measures of sleep (e.g., questionnaires, sleep diaries or logs, actigraphs, and polysomnography) are more consistently related to the children's task performance than those employing holistic evaluations or questionnaires with few items. Results from some studies showed that the effects of mild sleep restriction are detectable in measures of brain processing reflecting increased processing effort and poorer performance on executive function tasks involving working memory, inhibitory control, and attention. While the work reviewed here strongly suggests that young children's sleep influences their cognitive skills and behaviors, there is still much to be learned in order for a coherent picture to emerge.

Future Directions

There is a growing interest in and understanding of the preschool period as a critical developmental period with implications for academic performance in kindergarten and the early elementary grades. Yet, just as development in the preschool period is related to and often predictive of development in subsequent periods, so too is the development in infancy and toddlerhood (or roughly from the age at which motor skills develop that enable the child to have more independent explorations), which are critical parts of the developmental progression. There is still relatively little published sleep research on infants and toddlers. The critical importance of this developmental period is related to the rapid growth of cognitive and motor skills as well as changes in self-regulation behaviors and sleep habits. However, few studies have been published that explore longitudinal and predictive relations between early sleep habits and temperamental and cognitive self-regulation.

A study by Bernier, Carlson, Bordeleau and Carrier (2010) demonstrates the importance of the infancy and toddlerhood period in understanding how sleep influences cognitive skills and self-regulatory behaviors. In this study, 60 typically developing infants were studied across three time points: 12 to 13 months, 18 months, and 26 months of age. Parent sleep diaries provided information on sleep habits (total sleep duration, percentage of total sleep occurring at nighttime [between 7 pm and 7 am], and nighttime awakenings). Infants participated in age-appropriate executive function tasks designed to tap working memory at 18 months of age, working memory, inhibitory control, and set-shifting at 26 months of age; general cognitive functioning Bayley Scales of Infant Development (Bayley, 1993) at 12 months of age; and expressive language skills (MacArthur Communicative Development Inventory; Fenson, Dale, Reznick, Bates, Thal, & Pethick, 1994) at 18 and 26 months. The authors report that children with more nighttime sleep duration and fewer night awakenings performed better on the EF tasks but not the general cognitive and language skills assessments. Thus, in this study sleep was associated with the specialized cognitive skills that are known to involve frontal and prefrontal brain areas. Sleep appears to affect the development of brain structures in these critical brain regions, with detectable effects beginning in the first two years of life. As Bernier et al. (2010) note, these early impacts of sleep on executive functions "(set) in motion a cascade of neural effects that may carry substantial implications for later executive functioning" and, we would argue, further implications for subsequent cognitive development and school achievement. Research involving infants and toddlers is needed to gain a more complete understanding of the relations between sleep, self-regulation, cognitive skills, and subsequent academic achievement. Such research might address questions such as:

- Are the measures of sleep habits and sleep problems that have been used in studies of older children and adults valid measures in infancy and toddlerhood?
- Do infant and toddler sleep measures reflect concurrent and predictive associations with specific cognitive skills or specific components of self-regulation?
- Can sleep measures be used to investigate the neural mechanisms by which sleep influences early cognitive and self-regulation skills?

These and other important research questions are opportunities for future research.

References

Achenbach, T. M., & Rescorla, L. A. (2000). *Manual for ASEBA Preschool Forms & Profiles.* Burlington, VT: University of Vermont, Research Center for Children, Youth, & Families.

Alexander, K. L., Entwisle, D. R., & Dauber, S. L. (1993). First-grade classroom behavior: Its short- and long-term consequences for school performance. *Child Development, 64,* 801–814.

Ali, N., Pitson, D., & Stradling, J. (1993). Snoring, sleep disturbance and behavior in 4–5 year olds. *Archives of Disease in Childhood, 68,* 360–366.

Ali, N., Pitson, D., & Stradling, J. (1994). Natural history of snoring and related behavior problems between the ages of 4 and 7 years. *Archives of Disease in Childhood, 71,* 74–76.

Ali N., Pitson D., & Stradling, J. (1996). Sleep disordered breathing: Effects of adenotonsillectomy on behavior and psychological functioning. *European Journal of Pediatrics 155,* 56–62.

American Psychiatric Association. (2000). *Diagnostic and Statistical Manual of Mental Disorders* (4th ed.). Washington, DC: American Psychiatric Association.

Archbold K. H., Giordani B., Ruzicka, D. L., & Chervin, R. D. (2004). Cognitive executive dysfunction in children with mild sleep-disordered breathing. *Biological Research for Nursing. 5,* 168–176.

Baddeley, A., (1998). The central executive: A concept and some misconceptions. *Journal of the International Neuropsychological Society, 4,* 523–526.

Barnes, M. E., Huss, E. A., Garrod, K. N., Van Raay, E., Dayyat, E., Gozal, D., & Molfese, D. L. (2009). Impairments in attention in occasionally snoring children: An event-related potential study. *Developmental Neuropsychology, 34*(5), 629–649.

Barnes, M. E., Gozal, D., & Molfese, D. L. (2012). Attention in children with obstructive sleep apnea: An event-related potentials study. *Sleep Medicine, 13*(4), 368–377.

Bates, J., Viken, R., Alexander, D., Beyers, J., & Stockton, L. (2002). Sleep and adjustment in preschool children: Sleep diary reports by mothers relate to behavior reports by teachers. *Child Development, 73,* 62–74.

Bates, J. E., Freeland, C. A., & Lounsbury, M. L. (1979). Measurement of infant difficultness. *Child Development, 50,* 797–803.

Bates, J. E., Pettit, G. S., Dodge, K. A., & Ridge, B. (1998). Interaction of temperamental resistance to control and restrictive parenting in the development of externalizing behavior. *Developmental Psychology, 34,* 982–995.

Bayley, N. (1993). *Bayley Scales of Infant Development* (2nd Ed.) New York: Psych Corp.

Behar, L. (1977). The Preschool Behavior Questionnaire. *Journal of Abnormal Child Psychology, 5*(3), 265–275.

Bernier, A., Carlson, S. M., Bordeleau, S., & Carrier, J. (2010). Relations between physiological and cognitive regulatory systems: Infant sleep regulation and subsequent executive functioning. *Child Development, 81,* 1739–1752.

Bloom, B. J., Owens, J. A., McGuinn, M., Nobile, C., Schaeffer, L., & Alario, A. J. (2002). Sleep and its relationship to pain, dysfunction, and disease activity in juvenile rheumatoid arthritis. *Journal of Rheumatology, 29,* 169–173.

Blunden, S., Lushington, K., & Kennedy, D. (2001). Cognitive and behavioral performance in children with sleep-related obstructive breathing disorders. *Sleep Medicine, 5,* 447–461.

Boyd, J., Barnett, W. S., Bodrova, E., Leong, D. J., & Gomby, D. (2005). Promoting children's social and emotional development through preschool. New Brunswick, NJ: NIERR. Retrieved September 19, 2010 from http://nieer.org/resources/policyreports/report7.pdf.

Bruni, O., Ferini-Strambi, L., Russo, P. M., Antignani, M., Innocenzi, M., Ottaviano, P., et al. (2006). Sleep disturbances and teacher ratings of school achievement and temperament in children. *Sleep Medicine, 7*, 43–48.

Capaldi, D. M., & Rothbart, M. K. (1992). Development and validation of an early adolescent temperament measure. *Journal of Early Adolescence, 12*, 153–173.

Carey, W. B. (1974). Night waking and temperament in infancy. *Journal of Pediatrics, 84*, 756–758.

Carey, W. B. (2005). *Understanding Your Child's Temperament.* New York: MacMillan.

Carroll J., McColley S., Marcus C., & Loughlin, G. (1995). Inability of clinical history to distinguish primary snoring from obstructive sleep apnea syndrome in children. *Chest, 108*, 610–618

Caspi, A., & Silva, P. A. (1995). Temperament qualities at age three predict personality traits in young adulthood: Longitudinal evidence from a birth cohort. *Child Development, 66*, 486–498.

Castronovo, V., Zucconi, M., Nosetti, L., Marazzini, C., Hensley, M., Vegia, F., et al. (2003). Prevalence of habitual snoring and sleep-disordered breathing in preschool-aged children in an Italian community. *Journal of Pediatrics, 142*, 364–365.

Chervin, R., Hedger Archbold, K., Dillon, J., Panahi, P., Pituch, K., Dahl, R., & Guilleminault, C. (2002). Inattention, hyperactivity, and symptoms of sleep-disordered breathing. *Pediatrics, 109*, 449–456.

Conners, C. K. (1997). *Conners Rating Scales–Revised.* North Tonawanda, NY: Multi-Health Systems Publishing.

Conners, C. K. (2000). *Conners Rating Scales–Revised Technical Manual.* North Tonawanda, NY: Multi-Health Systems, Inc.

Conners, C. K., & Barkley, R. A. (1985). Rating scales and checklists for child psychopharmacology. *Psychopharmacology Bulletin, 21*, 809–868.

Dayyat, E., Newland, J., Bennett, J., Gozal, D., Spruyt, K., Molfese, V., & Jones, V. F. (2010). *Child Development: Forty winks and a fairy tale!* Paper presented at the Black Family in America Conference, Louisville, KY.

Dayyat, E., Spruyt, K., Molfese, D., & Gozal, D. (2011). Sleep estimates in children: Parental versus actigraphic assessment. *Nature and Science of Sleep, 3*, 1–9.

Davidson, M., Cruess, L., Diamond, A., O'Craven, K. M., & Savoy, R. L. (1999). *Comparison of executive functions in children and adults using directional Stroop tasks.* Presented at Biennial Meeting of the Society for Research in Child Development, April, Albuquerque, NM, April 1999.

de Lemnos, M., & Doig, B. (1999) Who Am I: Developmental Assessment Manual. Melbourne, Australia: Australian Council for Education Research. *Archives Of Otolaryngology—Head & Neck Surgery, 128*, 489–496.

Denton, K., & West, J. (2002). Children's reading and mathematics achievement in kindergarten and first grade. Washington, DC: U.S Department of Education, National Center for Education Statistics.

Dreyer, B. P., Mendelsohn, A. L., & Tamis-LeMonda, C. S. (1996). Assessing the child's cognitive home environment through parental report: Reliability and validity. *Early Development and Parenting, 5*, 271–287.

Dunn, L. & Dunn, L. (1997). *Peabody Picture Vocabulary Test* (3rd ed). Circle Pines, MN: American Guidance Service.

Ednick, M., Cohen, A., McPhail, G. L., Beebe, D., Simakajornboon, N., & Amin, R. S. (2009). A review of the effects of sleep during the first year of life on cognitive, psychomotor, and temperament development. *Sleep, 32*, 1449–1458.

Elliott, C. (1990). *Differential Ability Scales: Introductory and Technical Handbook.* New York: Psychological Corporation; Harcourt Brace Jovanovich, Inc.

Espy, K. A., McDiarmid, M. D., Cwik, M. F., Senn, T. E., Hamby, A., & Stalets, M. M. (2004). The contributions of executive functions to emergent mathematic skills in preschool children. *Developmental Neuropsychology, 26*(1), 465–486.

Fenson, L., Dale, P. S., Reznick, J. S., Bates, E., Thal, D. J., & Pethick, S. J. (1994). Variability in early communicative development. *Monographs of the Society for Research in Child Development, 59*, 242.

Friedman, B., Hendeles-Amitai, A., Kozminsky, E., Leiberman, A., Friger, M., Tarsiuk, A., & Tal, A. (2003). Adenotonsillectomy improves neurocognitive function in children with obstructive sleep apnea syndrome. *Sleep, 26*, 999–1005.

Fuster, J. (1997). *The Prefrontal Cortex: Anatomy, physiology, and neuropsychology of the frontal lobes* (3rd Ed.). Philadelphia: Lippencott-Raven.

Getting Ready: Findings from the National School Readiness Indicators Initiative (2005). Retrieved April 15, 2013 from www.gettingready.org/matriarch/MultiPiecePage.asp_Q_PageID_E_318_A_PageName_E_NationalSchoolReadinessIndicators

Goldsmith, H. H. (1996). Studying temperament via construction of the Toddlers' Behavior Assessment Questionnaire. *Child Development, 67*, 218–325.

Goodlin-Jones, B., Tang, K., Liu, J., & Anders, J. F., (2009). Sleep problems, sleepiness and daytime behavior in preschool-age children. *Journal of Child Psychology and Psychiatry, 50*, 1532–1540.

Goodnight, J. A., Bates, J. E., Staples, A. D., Pettit, G. S., & Dodge, K. A. (2007). Temperamental resistance to control increases association between sleep problems and externalizing behavior development. *Journal of Family Psychology, 21*, 39–48.

Gottlieb, D., Vezina, R., Chase, C., Lesko, S., Heeren, T., Wesse-Mayer, D., et al. (2003). Symptoms of sleep-disordered breathing in 5-year-old children are associated with sleepiness and problem behaviors. *Pediatrics, 112*, 870–877.

Gozal, D. (1998). Sleep disordered breathing and school performance in children. *Pediatrics, 192*, 616–620.

Gozal E., Row, B., Schurr A., & Gozal D. (2001). Developmental differences in cortical and hippocampal vulnerability to intermittent hypoxia in the rat. *Neuroscience Letters, 305*, 197–201.

Gregory, A. M., & O'Connor, T. G. (2002). Sleep problems in childhood: A longitudinal study of developmental change and association with behavioral problems. *Journal of the American Academy of Child and Adolescent Psychiatry, 41*, 964–971.

Hall, W. A., Zubrick, S. R., Silburn, S. R., Parsons, D. E., & Kurinczuk, J. J. (2007). A model for predicting behavioral sleep problems in a random sample of Australian preschoolers. *Infant and Child Development, 16*, 509–523.

Harrison, Y., & Horne, J. (1997). Sleep deprivation affects speech. *Sleep, 10*, 871–877.

Harsh, J. R., Easley, A., & LeBourgeois, M. K. (2002). A measure of sleep hygiene. *Sleep, 25,* A316.

Hiscock, H., Canterford, L., Ukoumunne, O. C, & Wake, M. (2007). Adverse associations of sleep problems in Australian preschoolers: national population study. *Pediatrics, 119,* 86–93.

Horne, J. (1988). Sleep loss and "divergent" thinking ability. *Sleep, 11,* 528–536.

Jewsuwan, R., Luster, T., & Kostelnik, M. (1993). The relation between parents' perceptions of temperament and children's adjustment to preschool. *Early Childhood Research Quarterly, 8,* 33–51.

Johnson, N., & McMahon, C. (2008). Preschoolers' sleep behavior: Associations with parental hardiness, sleep-related cognitions and bedtime interactions *Journal of Child Psychology and Psychiatry, 49*(7), 765–773.

Jones, V. F. (2006) *Sleep hygiene as a mediator of the home literacy environment to affect children's neurocognitive function.* Unpublished doctoral dissertation. Louisville, KY: University of Louisville.

Kagan, J., Resnick, J. S., Snidman, N., Gibbons, J., & Johnson, M. O. (1988). Childhood derivatives of inhibition and lack of inhibition to the unfamiliar. *Child Development, 59,* 1580–1589.

Kataria, S., Swanson, M., & Trevathan, G. (1987). Persistence of sleep disturbances in preschool children. *Journal of Pediatrics, 110,* 642–646.

Kendall, P. C. (1993). Cognitive-behavioral therapies with youth: Guiding theory, current status, and emerging developments. *Journal of Consulting and Clinical Psychology, 61,* 235–247.

Klein, J. S., & Bisanz, J. (2000). Preschoolers doing arithmetic: The concepts are willing but the working memory is weak. *Canadian Journal of Educational Psychology, 54,* 105–116.

Korkman, M., Kirk, U., & Kemp, S. (1998). *NEPSY: A Developmental Neuropsychological Assessment.* San Antonio, TX: Psychological Corporation.

Kuehni, C. E., Strippoli, M-P. F., Chauliac, E. S. & Silverman, M. (2008). Snoring in preschool children: Prevalence, severity and risk factors. *European Respiration Journal, 31,* 326–333.

Lam, P., Hiscock, H., & Wake, M. (2003). Outcomes of infant sleep problems: A longitudinal study of sleep, behavior, and maternal well-being. *Pediatrics, 111,* 203–207.

Lavigne, J., Arend, R., Rosenbaum, D., Smith, A., Weissbluth, M., Binns, H. J., & Christoffel, K. (1999). Sleep and behavior problems among preschoolers. *Journal of Developmental and Behavioral Pediatrics, 20,* 164–169.

Liew, J. (2011). Effortful control, executive functions, and education: Bringing self-regulatory and social-emotional competencies to the table, *Child Development Perspectives,* DOI: 10.1111/j.1750-8606.2011.00196.x.

Martin, R. P. (1984). *The Temperament Assessment Battery: Interim manual.* Athens, GA: Developmental Metrics.

Martin, R. P., & Holbrook, J. (1985). Relationship of temperament characteristics to the academic achievement of first-grade children. *Journal of Psychoeducational Assessment, 3,* 131–140.

Martin, R. P. (1988). *The Temperament Assessment Battery for Children.* Brandon, VT: Clinical Psychology Publishing Co.

Meijer, A., Habekothe, H., & Van Den Wittenboer, G. (2000). Time in bed, quality of sleep and school functioning of children. *Journal of Sleep Research, 9,* 145–153

Mitchell, R. B. (2007). Adenotonsillectomy for obstructive sleep apnea in children: Outcome evaluated by pre- and postoperative polysomnography. *Laryngoscope, 117*(10), 1844–1854.

Mitchell, R.B., & Kelly, J. (2005). Outcome of adenotonsillectomy for obstructive sleep apnea in children under 3. *Journal of Otorhinolaryngology Head and Neck, 137*(1), 681–684.

Mitchell, R. B., & Kelly, J. (2007). Outcomes and quality of life following adenotonsillectomy for sleep-disordered breathing in children. *Journal of Otorhinolaryngology and its Related Specialties, 69*(6), 345–348.

Molfese, D. (1978). Neuroelectrical correlates of categorical speech perception in adults. *Brain and Language, 5,* 25–35.

Molfese, D. L., Gozal, D., & Molfese, V., (2004) *Sleep and Psychophysiological Function in Children.* NIH: National Heart, Lung, and Blood Institute

Molfese, D. L., Ivanenko, A., Fonaryova Key, A., Roman, A., Molfese, V.J., O'Brien, L., et al. (2012). A one-hour sleep restriction affects brain processing in young children across tasks: Evidence from brain recordings.

Molfese, V., Beswick, J., Molnar, A., Jacobi-Vessels, J., & Gozal, D. (2007). The impacts of sleep duration, problem behaviors and health status on letter knowledge in pre-kindergarten children. *Child Health and Education: An Interdisciplinary Journal, 1,* 41–53.

Molfese, V. (2008). *Health, Behavior and Sleep Habits & Learning Disabilities.* Presentation at the School of Public Health Roundtable. University of Louisville, Louisville, KY.

Montgomery-Downs, H., Jones, V. F., Molfese, V., & Gozal, D. (2003). Snoring in preschoolers: Associations with sleepiness, ethnicity and learning. *Clinical Pediatrics, 42,* 719–726.

Montgomery-Downs H, Molfese V, Bonebright, T, Modglin A, Walker J, Neamon J, & Gozal D (June, 2004). Contributions of child sleep characteristics, biomedical risks, activities in the home, and maternal learning history to the development of phonological sensitivity and lexical retrieval in preschool children. Poster Presented at the 18th Annual Meeting of the Associated Professional Sleep Societies, Philadelphia, Pennsylvania.

Montgomery-Downs, H., O'Brien, L., Holbrook, C., & Gozal, D. (2004). Snoring and sleep-disordered breathing in young children: Subjective and objective correlates. *Sleep, 27,* 87–94.

National Association for the Education of Young Children & National Council of Teachers of Mathematics. (2002). *Early childhood mathematics: Promoting good beginnings.* Retrieved April 15, 2013 from http://oldweb.naeyc.org/about/positions/psmath.asp

National Early Literacy Panel (2008) (Eds.). *Developing early literacy: Report of the National Early Literacy Panel.* Washington, DC: National Institute for Literacy.

National Research Council. (2009). *Mathematics Learning in Early Childhood: Paths Toward Excellence and Equity.* Washington, DC: The National Academies Press.

National Sleep Foundation. (2004). Sleep in America poll. Retrieved 6/01-04 from: www.sleepfoundation.org.

Nelson, B., Martin, R. P., Hodge, S., Havill, V., & Kamphaus, R. (1999). Modeling the prediction of elementary school adjustment from preschool temperament. *Personality and Individual Differences, 26,* 687–700.

Novosad, C., Freudigman, K., & Thoman, E. B. (1999). Sleep patterns in newborns and temperament at 8 months: A preliminary study. *Journal of Developmental and Behavioral Pediatrics, 20,* 99–105.

O'Brien, L., & Gozal, D. (2004). Neurocognitive dysfunction and sleep in children: From human to rodent. *Pediatric Clinics of North America, 51*, 187–202.

Osborne, C., Romas, R., Gozal, D., Molfese, V., & Molfese, D. L. (April, 2008). *Sleep Restriction Affects Children's Performance on Visual Attention Task.* Conference on Human Development, Indianapolis, IN.

Ottaviano, S., Giannotti, F., Cortesi, F., Bruni, O., & Ottaviano, C. (1996). Sleep characteristics in healthy children from birth to 6 years of age in the urban area of Rome. *Sleep, 19*, 1–3.

Owens, J. A., Spirito, A., & McGuinn, M. (2000). The Children's Sleep Habits Questionnaire (CSHQ): Psychometric properties of a survey instrument for school-aged children. *Sleep, 23*, 1043–1051.

Owens-Stively, J., Frank, N., Smith, A., Hagino, O., Spirito, A., Arrigan, M., & Alario, A. J. (1997). Child temperament, parenting discipline style, and daytime behavior in childhood sleep disorders. *Journal of Developmental and Behavioral Pediatrics, 18*, 314–321.

Pollock, J. (1994). Night-waking at five years of age: Predictors and prognosis. *Journal of Child Psychology and Psychiatry, 35*, 699–708.

Reid, G. J., Hong, R. Y., & Wade, T. J. (2009). The relation between common sleep problems and emotional and behavioral problems among 2- and 3-year-olds in the context of known risk factors for psychopathology. *Journal of Sleep Research, 18*, 49–59.

Resnick, J. S., Kagan, J. J., Snidman, N., Gersten, M., Baak, K., & Rosenberg, A. (1986). Inhibited and uninhibited children: A follow-up study. *Child Development, 57*(3), 660–680.

Reynolds, C. R., & Kamphaus, R. W. (1992). The Behavior Assessment System for Children. Circle Pines, MN: American Guidance Services.

Richman, N., & Graham, P. (1971). A behavioral screening questionnaire for use with 3-year-old children. *Journal of Child Psychology and Psychiatry, 12*, 5–33.

Rimm-Kaufman, S. E., & Kagan, J. (2005). Infant predictors of kindergarten behavior: The contribution of inhibited and uninhibited temperament types. *Behavioral Disorders, 30*, 329–345.

Rothbart, M. K., & Derryberry, D. (1981). Development of individual differences in temperament. In M. E. Lamb & A. L. Brown (Eds.), *Advances in Developmental Psychology, Vol. 1* (pp. 37–86). Hillsdale, NJ: Erlbaum.

Rothbart, M. K., & Bates, J. E. (1998). Temperament. In W. Damon & N. Eisenberg (Eds.), *Handbook of Child Psychology: Social, emotional, and personality development* (5th ed., Vol. 3, pp. 105–176). New York: John Wiley & Sons, Inc.

Rothbart, M. K., Ahadi, S. A., & Evans, D. E. (2000). Temperament and personality: Origins and outcomes. *Journal of Personality and Social Psychology, 78*, 122–135.

Rothbart, M. K., Derryberry, D., & Hershey, K. L. (2000). Stability of temperament in childhood: Laboratory infant assessment to parent report at seven years. In V. J. Molfese & D. L. Molfese (Eds.), *Temperament and Personality Development Across the Life Span* (pp. 85–119). Hillsdale, NJ: Erlbaum.

Rothbart, M. K., Ahadi, S. A., Hershey, K. L., & Fisher, P. (2001). Investigations of temperament from three to seven years: The Children's Behavior Questionnaire. *Child Development, 72*, 1392–1408.

Rothbart, M. K., & Posner, M. I. (2005). Genes and experience in the development of executive attention and effortful control. *New Directions for Child and Adolescent Development, 109*, 101–108.

Rothbart, M. K., & Bates, J. E. (2006). Temperament. In W. Damon & N. Eisenberg (Eds.), *Handbook of Child Psychology: Social, Emotional, and Personality Development* (6th ed., Vol. 3, pp. 99–166). New York: John Wiley & Sons, Inc.

Rudasill, K. M., Gallagher, K., & White, J. M. (2010). Contributions of children's temperament and classroom emotional support to academic outcomes in elementary school. *Journal of School Psychology, 48*, 113–134.

Sadeh, A., Lavie, P., & Scher, A. (1994). Sleep and temperament: Maternal perceptions of temperament in sleep-disturbed toddlers. *Early Education and Development, 5*, 311–322.

Sadeh, A., Gruber, R., & Raviv, A., (2002). Sleep, neurobehavioral functioning, and behavior problems in school-aged children. *Child Development, 73*, 405–417.

Sadeh, A., Gruber, R., & Raviv, A. (2003). The effects of sleep restriction and extension on school-age children: What a difference an hour makes. *Child Development, 74*, 444–455.

Sadeh, A., Mindell, J. A., Luedtke, K. & Wiegand, B. (2009). Sleep and sleep ecology in the first 3 years: A web-based study. *Journal of Sleep Research, 18*, 60–73.

Sakimura, J. N., Dang, M. T., Ballard, K. B., & Hansen, R. L. (2008). Cognitive and temperament clusters in 3-to 5-year-old children with aggressive behavior. *Journal of School Health, 78*, 38–45.

Sangal, R., & Sangal, J. (1997). Abnormal visual P300 latency in obstructive sleep apnea does not change acutely upon treatment with CPAP. *Sleep, 20*, 702–704.

Schaefer, C. E. (1990). Night waking and temperament in early childhood. *Psychological Reports, 67*, 192–194.

Scher, A., Hall, W. A., Zaidman-Zait, A., & Weinberg, J. (2010). Sleep quality, cortisol levels, and behavioral regulation in toddlers. *Developmental Psychobiology, 52*, 44–53.

Simard, V., Nielsen, T. A., Tremblay, R. E., Boivin, M., & Montplaisir, J. Y. (2008). Longitudinal study of bad dreams in preschool-aged children: Prevalence, demographic correlates, risk and protective factors. *Sleep, 31*, 62–70.

Steenari, M.-J., Vuontela, V., Paavonen, E. J., Carlson, S., Fjällberg, M., & Arone, E. T. (2003). Working memory and sleep in 6- to 13-year-old school children. *Journal of the American Academy of Child and Adolescent Psychiatry, 42*, 85–92.

Stroop, J. R. (1935) Studies of interference in serial verbal reactions. *Journal of Experimental Psychology, 18*, 643–662.

The International Classification of Sleep Disorders—Revised (2005). Rochester, MN: American Academy of Sleep Medicine.

Thiedke, C. (2001). Sleep disorders and sleep problems in children. *American Family Physician, 63*, 277–284.

Thomas, A., & Chess, S. (1977). *Temperament and Development.* Oxford, England: Brunner/Mazel.

Tikotzky, L., & Sadeh, A. (2001). Sleep patterns and sleep disruptions in kindergarten children. *Journal of Clinical Child Psychology, 30*, 581–591.

Touchette, E., Cote, S. M., Petit, D., Liu, X., Boivin, M., Falissard, B., et al. (2009) Short nighttime sleep-duration and hyperactivity trajectories in early childhood. *Pediatrics, 124*, e985–e993.

Van den Bergh, B. R. H., & Mulder, E. J. H. (2012). Fetal sleep organization: A biological precursor of self-regulation in childhood and adolescence? *Biological Psychology, 89,* 584–590.

Van Tassel, E. B. (1985). The relative influence of child and environmental characteristics on sleep disturbances in the first and second years of life. *Developmental and Behavioral Pediatrics, 6,* 81–86.

Veldman, D. J., & Worsham, M. (1983). Types of student classroom behavior. *Journal of Educational Research, 76,* 204–209.

Ward, T. M., Gay, C., Alkon, A., Anders, T.F. & Lee, K.A. (2008). Nocturnal sleep and daytime nap behaviors in relation to salivary cortisol levels and temperament in preschool-age children attending child care. *Biological Research for Nursing, 9,* 244–253.

Wechsler, D. (1989). *Wechsler Preschool and Primary Scale of Intelligence—Revised.* San Antonio, TX: The Psychological Corporation.

Wei, J. L., Bond, J., Mayo, M. S., Smith, H. J., Reese, M., & Weatherly, R. A. (2009). Improved behavior and sleep after adenotonsillectomy in children with sleep-disordered breathing. *Archives of Otolaryngology Head and Neck Surgery, 135*(7), 642–646.

Weissbluth, M. & Liu, K. (1983)Sleep patterns, attention span, and infant temperament. *Journal of Developmental Behavioral Pediatrics, 4*(1), 34–36.

Weissbluth, M., Davis, A. T., & Poncher, J. (1984). Night waking in 4- to 8-month-old infants. *The Journal of Pediatrics, 104,* 477–480.

Witcher, L., Gozal, D., Molfese, D. L., & Crabtree, V. (2007). *Sleep Hygiene and Problem Behaviors in Children.* Poster presented at the Annual meeting of Associated Professional Sleep Societies, Minneapolis, MN.

Zelazo, P., & Muller, U. (2002). Executive function in typical and atypical development. In U. Goswami (Ed.), *Handbook of Childhood Cognitive Development* (pp. 445–460). Oxford: Blackwell.

Zuckerman, B., Stevenson, J., & Bailey, V. (1987). Sleep problems in early childhood: Continuities, predictive factors and behavioral correlates. *Pediatrics, 80,* 664–671.

CHAPTER

29 Neurocognitive Implications

Louise M. O'Brien

Abstract

Childhood sleep disruption is highly prevalent in today's society due to multiple school and personal demands, clinical sleep disorders, and family schedules. Accumulating literature suggests that sleep disruption is associated with multiple behavioral, emotional, and cognitive deficits. Clearly, insults during childhood that affect learning and academic performance have great potential to impact educational achievement and subsequent career direction later in life. Although longitudinal studies are lacking and it is currently unclear whether sleep disruption truly causes cognitive deficits, small studies suggest that treating the underlying sleep disorder may improve cognitive ability. If so, poor sleep during the childhood years could have a major impact on public health. This chapter will review current literature that has investigated the associations between sleep disruption and cognition in children.

Key Words: intelligence, memory, executive function, sleep disruption, sleep disordered breathing

Introduction

In recent years there has been a focus on the consequences of poor sleep in children. Sleep disruption, whether attributable to a clinical sleep disorder, a medical disorder, or to poor sleep hygiene, is associated with a wide range of behavioral, cognitive, emotional, and cardiovascular outcomes (Bhattacharjee, Kim, Kheirandish-Gozal, & Gozal, 2011; O'Brien, 2009). Academic achievement may also be affected, which has a potentially long-term impact on future success (Beebe, 2011). Over the past several decades the amount of time that children devote to sleeping has declined, likely related to demanding school schedules, after-school activities, and significant use of technology in the bedroom. Moreover, in parallel with the reduction in sleep duration, the prevalence of obesity has risen across age groups (Van Cauter & Knutson, 2008). Obesity has been postulated to be a direct consequence of sleep restriction (Knutson, Spiegel, Penev, & Van Cauter, 2007; Landhuis, Poulton, Welch, & Hancox, 2008) and it is also a significant risk factor for obstructive sleep apnea. Unsurprisingly, poor sleep in childhood has a significant impact on parental sleep and thus subsequent family functioning. Pediatric sleep disturbances affect a large proportion of families (Owens, 2008) yet few health care providers are equipped with the knowledge or training to screen, identify, and treat such problems. Adequate sleep is considered essential for development and while multiple studies have shown associations with poor school performance and neurocognitive assessments—see Beebe, 2011, for a comprehensive review—the particular cognitive domains affected by poor sleep are not well characterized in children. This chapter will focus on neurocognitive consequences of sleep disruption in children.

Prevalence of Sleep Disruption

As reviewed in earlier chapters, sleep problems are common in children. Although highly prevalent—with estimates suggesting around 25%

of all children (Blunden et al., 2004; Owens, 2008)—such difficulties are rarely queried at pediatric visits nor brought up by the parents (Blunden et al., 2004). Data from the National Sleep Foundation's Sleep In America Poll 2004 (www.sleepfoundation.org), a telephone survey of a representative sample of the United States, found that 70% of parents reported sleep difficulties in their child at least a few nights per week but <15% were asked about a sleep problem by their pediatrician. In addition, approximately one-third of parents reported that their child sleeps less than the parent believes they should. Lack of awareness of appropriate sleep durations and difficulty in recognition of clinical sleep disorders such as obstructive sleep apnea, restless leg syndrome, insomnia, circadian rhythm disorder, or even narcolepsy, suggests that a large proportion of children have unrecognized sleep deprivation or disruption. Such disruption has been shown to be associated with many morbidities including cognitive dysfunction.

Cognition

There are many definitions of cognition. For the purposes of this chapter, cognition is defined as a mental process by which knowledge and comprehension are acquired. This includes awareness, perception, intuition, thinking, remembering, reasoning, and problem solving. These are higher-level functions of the brain and encompass language, imagination, perception and planning. One of the fundamental roles of sleep is believed to be in learning, memory consolidation, and brain plasticity (Walker, 2009), and thus sleep disruption has the potential to impair cognition during wake.

Memory

There are now a wealth of data on the associations between sleep and memory, mostly from adult subjects. Evidence is strongly supportive of a role for sleep in memory and in the underlying neural plasticity of animals and humans (Stickgold & Walker, 2005a, 2005b; Walker & Stickgold, 2006). Few studies exist in children and most of these focus on memory impairment as a consequence of sleep disordered breathing (see later in this chapter for a full discussion). The term "memory" is rather broad since it includes several distinct abilities that can be tested individually and can be selectively impaired. Memory is typically classified as a distinction between declarative and nondeclarative memory (Squire & Zola, 1996). Declarative memory—fact-based memory—can be subcategorized as episodic memory (memory for past events) and semantic memory (memory for general knowledge) (Tulving, 1985). In contrast, nondeclarative memory may be considered nonconscious and includes procedural memory, the learning of habits and skills, as well as priming, or perceptual memory. In addition, there is also working memory, a form of short-term memory for manipulation of information in order to perform tasks such as reasoning and comprehension (Becker & Morris, 1999). The cognitive processes involved include the executive and attention control of short-term memory, which provides for the integration, processing, and retrieval of information.

Executive Function

Executive function is essentially a cognitive system that controls and manages other cognitive processes, such as planning, working memory, attention, problem solving, verbal reasoning, inhibition, mental flexibility, and multitasking (Lezak, 1995). The term *executive function* is used to describe the ability to develop and sustain an organized and flexible approach to problem solving (Goldberg, 2001; Lezak, 1995). Executive functions are located primarily in the prefrontal areas of the frontal lobe, particularly the prefrontal cortex. Such areas have many connections with other areas of the brain.

Intelligence

The term *cognition* is often used interchangeably with *intelligence* although they are not the same. Cognitive processes typically show an age-dependent performance increase, whereas intelligence typically refers to developmental differences between individuals (Anderson, 2005). Furthermore, cognitive processes can be influenced by intelligence. While lower-order cognitive processes, which include perceptual motor learning, visual short-term memory, and selective attention, can be measured by tasks such as reaction times or problem solving, intelligence, on the other hand, is indirectly inferred via psychometric testing. A detailed discussion of the associations between sleep, cognition, and intelligence is beyond the scope of this chapter but can be found in a recent article (Geiger, Achermann, & Jenni, 2010).

Neurocognitive Assessment

Most forms of cognition involve multiple cognitive functions working together. Nonetheless, tests can be organized into broad categories based on the particular cognitive function that they assess.

Of note, different aspects or different versions of the same test may be used to assess different cognitive functions. The main cognitive domains include intelligence, memory, language, visuospatial, attention, and executive functions. Each one of these domains has been shown to be impacted by sleep disruption and will be summarized below. Commonly used neurocognitive tests are shown in Table 29.1.

Sleep Deprivation and Restriction

The vast majority of literature regarding sleep deprivation and restriction has come from studies of adults (Pilcher & Huffcutt, 1996; Reynolds & Banks, 2010). Of note, sleep fragmentation is now believed to exert a similar effect on daytime function as does sleep deprivation (Bonnet & Arand, 2003). With today's 24-hour lifestyle and social media use even in young children, there is likely to be a huge

Table 29.1 Summary of Frequently Used Neurocognitive Tests

Test	Description
Children's Memory Scale (CMS)	Validated measure of general, verbal, and visual memory.
Continuous Performance Test (CPT)	Can be visual and/or auditory. Validated computer test to assess attention, impulsivity, vigilance, and executive functions. Common CPTs include the Conners CPT, the Integrated Visual and Auditory CPT (IVA), and the Test of Variables of Attention (TOVA). The TOVA is often used in the diagnosis of attention-deficit/hyperactivity disorder.
Developmental Neuropsychological Assessment (NEPSY)	Validated series of neuropsychological tests across several domains, designed to test cognitive functions not typically covered by general ability or achievement batteries. Domains include attention/executive function, language, sensorimotor, visuospatial, learning, and memory.
Differential Ability Scales (DAS)	Validated scale which measures a variety of cognitive abilities including verbal and visual working memory, immediate and delayed recall, visual recognition and matching, processing and naming speed, phonological processing, and understanding of basic number concepts.
Kaufmann Assessment Battery for Children (K-ABC)	Validated tool for assessing cognitive ability and mental processing, with minimal language requirements.
Peabody Picture Vocabulary Test (PPVT)	Validated tool for assessing verbal intelligence
Stanford-Binet Intelligence Scale	Validated intelligence/IQ test designed to test intelligence in four areas including verbal reasoning, quantitative reasoning, abstract and visual reasoning, and short-term memory skills.
Test of Everyday Attention for Children, The (TEA–Ch)	Measure to assess the ability of children to selectively attend, sustain, divide, and switch attention.
Wechsler Individualized Achievement Test (WIAT)	Tool to assess the academic achievement of children, adolescents, college students, and adults.
Wechsler Intelligence Scale for Children 3rd edition (WISC-III)	Validated intelligence/IQ test that does not require reading or writing. Includes full scale IQ as well as verbal and performance IQ.
Wechsler Preschool and Primary Scale of Intelligence 3rd edition (WPPSI-III)	Validated intelligence/IQ test for young children. Includes full scale IQ as well as verbal and performance IQ.
Wide Range Assessment of Memory and Learning (WRAML-2)	Tool to assess memory function in children, adolescents, and adults. Includes a general memory index as well as a verbal and visual memory, and an attention/concentration index.

personal, societal, and economic impact of insufficient sleep on behavior, emotional regulation, and cognition at critical developmental periods. Insufficient sleep can result from socially induced reduction of sleep time that occurs in many children related to homework requirements, after-school activities, increased television, cellphone, and social media usage (see Gradisar and Short, Chapter 11). Insufficient sleep in children has been shown to compromise school performance with poorer learning, memory, and attention, and unfortunately occurs at a time when successful academic performance is essential; for review see Beebe, 2011. Furthermore, there are many homes where both parents need to work, and good childhood sleep hygiene practices are often overlooked while juggling work, shifts, and raising a family.

Most work on pediatric sleep deprivation, restriction, and fragmentation has been conducted on older children and adolescents; however, there are several reports that suggest sleep in both preterm and term newborns is correlated with mental development later in infancy (Beckwith & Parmelee, 1986; Borghese, Minard, & Thoman, 1995; Freudigman & Thoman, 1993; Piteo, Kennedy, et al., 2011; Piteo, Lushington et al., 2011; Scher, Steppe, & Banks, 1996). Although a recent study did not find a relationship between infant sleep and cognitive development at 12 months, it did find a relationship with emotional regulation (Spruyt et al., 2008). Infant sleep regulation using parent sleep diary at 12 and 18 months old and subsequent executive functions at 18–26 months old found that higher proportions of total sleep occurring at night at both 12 and 18 months of age were related to better performance on executive tasks, especially those involving a strong impulse control component (Bernier, Carlson, Bordeleau, & Carrier, 2010). Most associations were independent of family socioeconomic status, prior mental development, and concurrent verbal ability. These findings add to previous results with school-age children in suggesting that sleep favors the development of higher-order cognitive functions requiring prefrontal cortex involvement, with the possibility that sleep–wake may be independently related to later neurocognitive development. However, there is currently insufficient data to conclude that a causal relationship exists. For a review on this topic the reader is referred to Ednick et al., 2009.

Few studies have investigated the relationships between sleep and cognition in young preschool children. In one study of almost 1500 young children between the ages of 2–6 years, short sleep duration, especially before the age of 41 months, was associated with externalizing problems and lower cognitive performance on neurodevelopmental tests at school entry (Touchette et al., 2007). Specifically, after adjustment for covariates, short sleep duration in early childhood tripled the risk for low performance on the Peabody Picture Vocabulary Test, a test of receptive vocabulary, and more than doubled the risk for scoring low on a block design test to evaluate nonverbal intellectual skills. The authors postulated that language acquisition and consolidation of new words into memory may be significantly impaired by chronic short sleep duration throughout childhood and further suggested that there may be a critical window for cognitive development that may be jeopardized by short sleep duration.

Subsequent work has shown that there are strong associations between sleep disturbances in kindergarten and failure to qualify for first grade (Ravid, Afek, Suraiya, Shahar, & Pillar, 2009a). In addition, children who failed 1st-grade achievement tests were more likely to have sleep disturbance such as increased sleep latency, increased arousals, and lower sleep efficiency compared to other children (Ravid, Afek, Suraiya, Shahar, & Pillar, 2009b). In the latter study, significant positive correlations were found between sleep quality and quantity with continuous performance tests of attention and IQ, and significant negative correlations were found with nocturnal awakenings and sleep latency. Notably, children with sleep disturbances suggestive of insomnia or parasomnias had significantly lower performance IQ, verbal IQ, and global IQ, and shorter attention span. Excessive daytime sleepiness was also associated with lower intelligence test scores. Perhaps somewhat counterintuitive is the finding that greater daytime napping in young children is associated with worse cognitive performance (Lam, Mahone, Mason, & Scharf, 2011). However, this study also found that daytime napping was negatively associated with nighttime sleep, suggesting that perhaps greater nighttime sleep facilitates cognitive performance and reduces the need for daytime napping, after accounting for developmental stage.

The majority of work on reduced sleep time and associated daytime sleepiness and cognitive dysfunction has been conducted in school-age children and adolescents. In a large community study of 1000 elementary school children, designed to investigate sleep quality and quantity, Kahn et al. (1989) found that those with parentally reported poor sleep had worse academic performance and 21%

had failed one or more years at school compared to those without reported sleep difficulties. These findings have been supported in subsequent work where later bedtimes and shorter sleep duration were associated with lower academic achievement in high school students (Wolfson & Carskadon, 1998). Even among students without a history of academic difficulty, reduction of sleep opportunity has a direct effect on teacher-rated academic performance (Fallone, Acebo, Seifer, & Carskadon, 2005; see Buckhalt, Chapter 21; Molfese, Rudasill and Molfese, Chapter 28; and Au, Appleman, and Stavitsky, Chapter 38).

Objective measures of sleep using actigraphy confirm a high prevalence of fragmented sleep in 2nd–6th-grade students, with almost one-fifth of children found to have sleep fragmentation (Sadeh, Raviv, & Gruber, 2000). Children with fragmented sleep demonstrate lower performance on neurobehavioral measures, particularly those associated with more complex tasks such as a continuous performance test and a symbol-digit substitution test, a test of declarative memory (Sadeh, Gruber, & Raviv, 2002). Longer sleep latency and poor sleep efficiency have been associated with worse auditory and visual working memory at all memory loads in children between 6–13 years (Steenari et al., 2003). However, shorter sleep duration was associated with lower working memory only at the highest load, suggesting that sleep quality rather than duration is related to working memory. Even a single night of sleep restriction (5 hours in bed compared to 11 hours in bed) has shown deficits on measures of verbal creativity and the Wisconsin Card Sorting Test, a measure of executive function (Randazzo, Muehlbach, Schweitzer, & Walsh, 1998). No deficits were found on less complex memory tasks, implying that higher cognitive functions may be more sensitive to sleep disruption. A study of a 4-hour sleep restriction in 8–15-year-olds did not find any impact on sustained attention, although children were more sleepy and had increased behavioral inattention (Fallone, Acebo, Arnedt, Seifer, & Carskadon, 2001). Notably, one extra hour of sleep extension has been shown to improve reaction time as well as well as a digit forward memory test (Sadeh, Gruber, & Raviv, 2003).

Several studies have assessed the effects of sleep restriction on memory. In children aged 11–13 years, the impact of a single night of restricted sleep (4 hours) was investigated (Carskadon, Harvey, & Dement, 1981a). This study found no significant effects on declarative memory (short-term recall of words) and other tasks of cognition and attention, but another study from the same authors (Carskadon, Harvey, & Dement, 1981b) found a significant reduction in working memory following total sleep deprivation. The authors concluded from this that children appear to tolerate a single night of sleep restriction relatively well, and that relevant differences might only emerge after prolonged periods of restricted sleep or total sleep deprivation. To date, most studies support the hypothesis that sleep facilitates both working memory and memory consolidation in children and adolescents, with complex tasks involving higher cognitive functions showing a stronger decline than simple tasks following sleep restriction and deprivation (Kopasz et al., 2010).

Of particular concern in today's 24–7 environment, electronic media use has become highly prevalent even in very young children. Data from the National Sleep Foundation's 2006 Sleep In America Poll (www.sleepfoundation.org) showed that almost all adolescents (97%) have at least one source of electronic media in their bedroom (see Gradisar and Short, Chapter 11). Even a significant proportion of primary school children are reported to have televisions or computers in their bedrooms (S. Li et al., 2007; Oka et al., 2008). In a study of 5–6-year-olds, even the number of hours that the television was switched on during a child's waking hours when the child was not actively viewing was inversely correlated with sleep duration (Paavonen, Pennonen, Roine, Valkonen, & Lahikainen, 2006). In addition, such passive exposure was associated with disorders of initiating and maintaining sleep, as well as overall sleep difficulty. Computer game playing has been associated with sleep difficulties such as increased sleep onset latency and less slow wave sleep with subsequent deficits in verbal memory performance (Dworak, Schierl, Bruns, & Struder, 2007). Strong emotional responses during computer or video game playing could influence memory consolidations, since recently acquired knowledge is sensitive during the subsequent consolidation period (Maquet, 2001). However, the content of the media may be more influential than the media itself, as negative associations between total electronic media use and academic achievement are abolished when other factors such as socioeconomic status and media content are taken into account (Schmidt & Vandewater, 2008). Nonetheless, data generally support a negative effect of media use on childhood sleep (Cain & Gradisar, 2010) with associated worsened cognitive performance (Dworak et al., 2007; see Gradisar and Short, Chapter 11).

Delayed Sleep Phase

Optimal sleep occurs when the internal circadian cycle is aligned with the external sleep–wake schedule and when this alignment becomes destabilized, circadian rhythm sleep disorders can occur. Delayed sleep phase disorder is a common circadian disorder, particularly in adolescent children, where the sleep period is delayed in relation to the required or desired sleep–wake times. Biologically, during development as children reach puberty there is a natural tendency to fall asleep at later times with the subsequent increased difficulty in waking early. Puberty is associated with a phase preference for eveningness (owl), as opposed to morningness (lark) (Carskadon, Vieira, & Acebo, 1993) and delayed sleep phase syndrome may be an extreme variant of these developmental shifts (see Carskadon and Tarokh, Chapter 8). Indeed, anecdotally, the vast majority of adolescents have great difficulty waking for school and many are unable to wake without the help of a parent.

Adolescents, including children with delayed sleep phase syndrome, often have difficulty with daytime sleepiness, behavior, and emotional regulation, and several studies show that this is extended to poor school achievement, attention deficit, and conduct disorder, as well as adolescent risk-taking behaviors (Cardinali, 2000; Giannotti, Cortesi, Sebastiani, & Ottaviano, 2002; Holm et al., 2009; Ming et al., 2011; O'Brien & Mindell, 2005). Many adolescents with delayed sleep phase are labeled as having behavioral problems, but if they are allowed to sleep until later in the morning their symptoms abate (Millman, 2005).

Since the biological delay in the circadian system of adolescents coupled with early school start times has been associated with impaired school performance, school start times have come under scrutiny. There is a growing literature regarding the timing of the school day in middle school and high school students, and several studies suggest that more time in bed is related to better school grades (Wolfson & Carskadon, 2003). In a group of 800 preadolescents, children who started school before 7:15 am were compared to those who started at 8:00 am. Daytime sleepiness, dozing off in class, and attention and concentration problems were more frequent in children who started class earlier (Epstein, Chillag, & Lavie, 1998). Similarly, in a study of over 3000 students, those reporting B grades or better were more likely to go to bed between 10–50 minutes earlier and obtain 17–33 minutes more sleep than their peers who obtained C grades or below (Wolfson & Carskadon, 1998). In a groundbreaking study of 18,000 children conducted over 5 years and designed to investigate the impact of delayed school start times, children were followed from 2 years before until 3 years after schools delayed start times from 7:15am to 8:40am (Wahlstrom, 2002). Multiple improvements were observed, from decreases in tardiness to increases in graduation rates, improved academic performance, and higher morale. These findings underscore the serious impact of early school start times on children's and adolescent's school performance, yet the majority of schools still have start times that are not conducive to good performance. For reviews see O'Malley & O'Malley, 2008, and Wolfson & Carskadon, 2003.

Sleep Disordered Breathing

While experimental studies of sleep deprivation have provided important data, the vast majority of information regarding the effects of sleep disturbance on cognition in children is from studies of sleep disordered breathing (SDB). Studies of the associations between SDB and behavioral difficulties are vast and demonstrate robust associations (Beebe, 2006; O'Brien, 2008) but the cognitive impact of SDB is less well understood.

Intelligence

Although many studies have investigated the intelligence quotient (IQ) in children with SDB, the findings are inconsistent. Multiple studies report lower IQ scores in children with SDB compared to controls, although these scores are typically still within the normal range (Beebe et al., 2004; Blunden, Lushington, Kennedy, Martin, & Dawson, 2000; Bourke et al., 2011; Emancipator et al., 2006; Ezzat, Fawaz, & Abdelrazek, 2010; Friedman et al., 2003; Gottlieb et al., 2004; Halbower et al., 2006; Kaemingk et al., 2003; Kennedy et al., 2004; Kohler et al., 2009; Miano et al., 2011; Montgomery-Downs, Crabtree, & Gozal, 2005; O'Brien et al., 2004a, 2004b; Suratt et al., 2006). A recent study of snoring children awaiting adenotonsillectomy found that, compared to healthy controls, snorers had a 10-point reduction in IQ (Kohler et al., 2009). While this may not be clinically relevant in a child with a high IQ, the implications are obvious in a child functioning at a lower level. Nonetheless, although several studies have failed to find overall differences in full-scale IQ (Aronen et al., 2009; Calhoun et al., 2009; Hill et al., 2006; Lewin, Rosen, England, &

Dahl, 2002) some find lower scores for verbal IQ (language skills) in children with SDB (Aronen et al., 2009; Lewin et al., 2002). Notably, one study (Emancipator et al., 2006) found an attenuation of effects between SDB and cognition once socioeconomic status was accounted for, which supports earlier work demonstrating that socioeconomic status is a consistent and independent predictor of performance (Chervin et al., 2003). Furthermore, stronger associations in preterm children suggest that birth outcomes may also play an important role in these relationships (Emancipator et al., 2006).

Nonetheless, a fundamental problem with the use of composite IQ tests is that they measure a child's combined performance across a variety of tasks and fail to address critical domains of cognition (Lezak, Howieson, & Loring, 2004).

Of particular interest, one group of investigators argued that score differences from standardized vocabulary tests—a measure of IQ—in children with and without SDB are equivalent to the impact of lead exposure (Suratt et al., 2007). These authors noted that vocabulary tests are the single best predictor of general cognitive functioning and are a strong predictor of academic success. The implications are potentially of great significance for future career achievements. Although ability to stay on task and pay attention in class may underlie learning ability, biological contributors including socioeconomic status, genetics, and obesity also play a role in cognitive outcomes (Beebe, Ris, Kramer, Long, & Amin, 2010; Montgomery-Downs, Jones, Molfese, & Gozal, 2003; Spruyt & Gozal, 2011).

Memory

Differences in memory have been found in children with SDB, although results are inconsistent with several studies failing to find evidence for memory impairment (Blunden, Lushington, Lorenzen, Martin, & Kennedy, 2005; O'Brien et al., 2004a, 2004b;). In one study, memory was found to be impaired in children with SDB with a dose-response effect (Rhodes et al., 1995) although, in general, most studies that find differences in memory do not find a dose-response (Kaemingk et al., 2003; Kennedy et al., 2004; Kheirandish-Gozal, De Jong, Spruyt, Chamuleau, & Gozal, 2010). Inconsistencies in memory findings are likely related to the type of memory measured (such as verbal memory or working memory). Interestingly, recent data in children with varying degrees of SDB severity found that working memory was impaired compared to controls by parental report, but not when an objective measure of working memory was utilized (Biggs et al., 2011). The authors found that parents of children with less severe SDB appeared to have a tendency to overestimate the level of working memory deficit, and postulated that this may be a reflection of behavior. They suggested that this raises the possibility that observation of working memory deficits may be somewhat dependent on the assessment method, and children with SDB may not be as impaired as previously thought. Further limitations to memory assessments are that many reports provide only a cumulative memory score rather than addressing specific processes involved in memory acquisition.

In a recent study (Kheirandish-Gozal et al., 2010) 54 children with varying degrees of SDB and 17 controls completed a pictorial memory task and had their recall assessed both immediately and the following day. Memory recall on both occasions was impaired in children with SDB and the latter children also exhibited declines in recall performance that were absent in controls, suggesting that those with SDB require more time and additional learning opportunities to reach immediate and longer-term recall performance. Furthermore, it has been suggested that children with SDB may have slower information processing and/or secondary memory problems and that inefficient encoding may account for the primary deficit (Spruyt, Capdevila, Kheirandish-Gozal, & Gozal, 2009). This is supportive of data from an investigation of event-related potentials, which found no performance deficits on standard measures of attention and memory but did find changes in basic perceptual processes that provide a foundation for the development of higher-order functions (Key, Molfese, O'Brien, & Gozal, 2009). Additional research is clearly required in order to understand the SDB-related impact on memory processes in children.

Academic Performance

Academic performance can be assessed by various means including mathematical abilities, spelling, reading, writing, and overall school grade. Studies have shown that symptoms of SDB in young children are associated with lower grades in mathematics, spelling, reading, and science (Kim, Lee, Lee, Hong, & Cho, 2011; Ravid et al., 2009b; Urschitz et al., 2005) even when intermittent hypoxemia is absent (Urschitz et al., 2003). In 1st-grade children, a 6–9-fold increase in gas-exchange abnormalities was found in those with poor school performance (Gozal, 1998). The presence of hypoxemia may affect the threshold of respiratory events associated with performance deficits, as the threshold for respiratory disturbances associated with learning problems may be lower in the presence of hypoxemia (Goodwin et al., 2003). Children with SDB have been found to perform lower than controls on a phonological processing test (Lundeborg, McAllister, Samuelsson, Ericsson, & Hultcrantz, 2009; O'Brien, 2004a,b) which measures phonological awareness, a skill that is critical for learning to read. However, not all studies find an association with SDB and academic achievement, particularly when other confounders such as socioeconomic status and preterm birth are accounted for (Chervin et al., 2003; Emancipator et al., 2006; Kaemingk et al., 2003; Mayes, Calhoun, Bixler, & Vgontzas, 2008).

Interestingly, symptoms of SDB in early childhood have been associated with future risk for poor performance in middle school (Gozal & Pope, 2001), again suggesting that there may be a window of vulnerability whereby an insult at a key developmental time period may manifest phenotypically later on. A recent carefully matched study found a complex verbal skill profile in children with SDB (Honaker, Gozal, Bennett, Capdevila, & Spruyt, 2009). Preschool children with SDB had difficulties in processing information with increasing linguistic complexity, whereas the school-age children had reduced vocabulary ability/knowledge. The authors postulated that their findings may support a longitudinal adverse effect of SDB. Notably, the vast majority of current literature does not include adolescents, a developmental stage where challenges differ considerably from those of young children and where SDB-associated behavioral difficulties may result in significant impairment in school performance at a critical time for future success (Beebe et al., 2010). In addition to verbal problems, poor academic achievement may also be affected by inattention difficulties due to the complex brain associations involved. Measurement of school performance is inherently difficult, and the role of SDB difficult to tease out, as it really represents a number of factors that include age, SES, home environment, genetics, behavior, and cognition (Beebe et al., 2010).

Executive Functions and Higher Cognitive Reasoning

As mentioned earlier, executive function encompasses cognitive processes that are crucial for normal psychological and social development (Lezak, 1995). Executive function is complex and it is difficult to isolate certain executive functions from other cognitive abilities; nonetheless, executive dysfunction is found in many studies of pediatric SDB, particularly in school-age children with SDB compared to controls (Archbold, Giordani, Ruzicka, & Chervin, 2004; Beebe et al., 2004; Halbower et al., 2006; Lewin et al., 2002). Even snoring preschool children have substantially lower performance on executive function dimensions such as inhibition, working memory, and planning (Karpinski, Scullin, & Montgomery-Downs, 2008). The latter study was the first to include a multidimensional conceptualization (e.g., planning, inhibition, working memory) and work relating executive function to SDB in preschool populations. As expected, performance on the planning, inhibition, and working memory dimensions of executive functions all showed marked improvements between the ages of 3 and 5 years. Notably, children with parent-reported risk for SDB performed significantly lower on each executive function dimension. These findings underscore the need to identify SDB risk in young children. The importance of executive dysfunction and the involvement of the prefrontal cortex in SDB was recently reviewed (Beebe & Gozal, 2002) and a model linking sleep disruption, hypoxemia, and disruption of the prefrontal cortex has been proposed.

Does SDB Cause Cognitive Deficits in Children?

Most studies in the literature provide cross-sectional data on associations between SDB and cognition. While the growing number of such studies appears to support a relationship between SDB and cognitive dysfunction, cross-sectional data cannot in itself prove that a causal relationship exists. This question can only be addressed by data from randomized controlled intervention trials. To date, no such studies have been published although a multicenter randomized controlled trial to address these issues is currently underway (Redline et al., 2011).

Current data in support of a causal relationship come from both longitudinal and interventional studies. In 2001 Gozal and Pope (Gozal & Pope, 2001) showed that middle school children with academic performance in the lowest 25% of their class were more likely to have snored during their preschool years and to have required adenotonsillectomy for snoring compared with schoolmates in the top 25% of class. These findings support the hypothesis that SDB-associated cognitive morbidity may be only partially reversible or that a "learning debt" may develop with SDB during early childhood and impair subsequent school performance.

The same group (Gozal, 1998) also conducted one of the first studies to assess the impact of sleep-associated gas exchange abnormalities on school academic performance in 1st-grade children. Two hundred ninety-seven 1st-grade children whose school performance was in the lowest 10th percentile of their class ranking were screened for SDB using a parental questionnaire and a single night recording of pulse oximetry and transcutaneous partial pressure of carbon dioxide. Parents of children with sleep-associated gas exchange abnormalities were encouraged to seek medical intervention. School grades of all children for the school year preceding and after the overnight study were obtained. Gas exchange abnormalities were found in 18% of children, approximately half of whom underwent adenotonsillectomy, and the others declined intervention. At follow-up in second grade, overall mean grades increased from 2.4 to 2.9 in those who underwent treatment, but no significant changes occurred in those who did not seek treatment (mean grades in 1st and 2nd grade were 2.4 and 2.5, respectively). These data were the first to suggest that a subset of children with poor academic performance could have SDB and may benefit from prospective medical evaluation and treatment.

Subsequently, there have been a number of small treatment intervention studies showing that cognitive function in preschool and school-age children with SDB appears to improve to control levels 6–12 months following adenotonsillectomy on multiple subtests including general conceptual ability, verbal and nonverbal ability, phonological processing and naming (Montgomery-Downs et al., 2005), IQ (Ezzat et al., 2010), cognitive attention index as measured by continuous performance assessment (Chervin et al., 2006), visual attention and processing speed (Hogan, Hill, Harrison, & Kirkham, 2008), matrix analogies, sequential and simultaneous processing scales, and mental processing scales, with medium to large effect sizes (Friedman et al., 2003).

However, not all studies report significant improvement in cognitive measures, including cognitive attention (Galland, Dawes, Tripp, & Taylor, 2006; Li, Huang, Chen, Fang, & Lee, 2006). A recent study from Australia of 44 snoring children aged 3–12 years compared to 48 controls showed a wide range of cognitive deficits at baseline, including IQ, language, and executive function, which did not improve to control levels following adenotonsillectomy (Kohler et al., 2009). The magnitude of the deficits persisted at the 6-month follow-up with a mean full scale IQ difference of 10 points between children with SDB and controls. Furthermore, the fluid reasoning, knowledge, quantitative reasoning, visuospatial, and working memory composite scores, as well as corresponding verbal and nonverbal subtest scores, were all significantly reduced in children with SDB compared to controls at both baseline and follow-up. In general, effects were greatest for the verbal component of tests, and specifically for measures of knowledge and working memory. Moreover, composite scores for attention/executive function (specifically planning, inhibition, auditory and visual attention), language (phonological processing), sensorimotor function, and memory (especially narrative memory) were significantly reduced in children with SDB at both baseline and follow-up. The finding that measures of executive function remain significantly lower in children with SDB following adenotonsillectomy compared to controls is supported by another study (Hogan et al., 2008). Figure 29.1 summarizes the effect sizes across several studies for changes in cognitive measures after surgical intervention for SDB.

These findings may be somewhat unexpected given the increasing number of studies showing improvement to control levels as described above. Nonetheless, it has been shown that children undergoing adenotonsillectomy for non-SDB reasons as well as SDB perform worse on specific cognitive measures such as short-term attention, visuospatial ability, memory, and arithmetic academic achievement compared to controls (Giordani et al., 2008). Of note, comparisons between the two surgical groups and controls revealed that those undergoing intervention for non-SDB reasons had larger and more consistent deficits across tests than did those who had adenotonsillectomy for SDB. Interestingly, children who were undergoing surgery for non-SDB reasons showed significantly lower ability in the matrices subtest than did children undergoing surgery for SDB. The authors postulated that this finding may reflect a combination of factors including age, daytime sleepiness, and measures of SDB that are not apparent on polysomnography and that require more sensitive methodologies.

The same authors (Giordani et al., 2012) recently provided data on a comprehensive 1-year follow up of neuropsychological outcomes in children who underwent adenotonsillectomy for both SDB and non-SDB reasons. These data extend the findings of the original cohort previously discussed

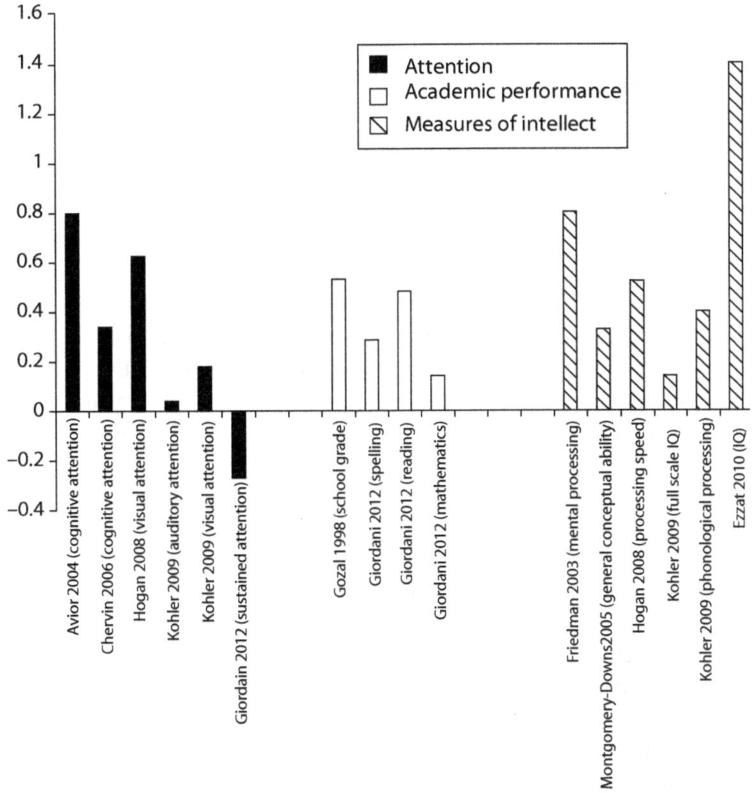

Figure 29.1 Summary of Effect Sizes for Changes in Several Key Cognitive Abilities following Adenotonsillectomy.

(Giordani et al., 2008). Results of the 1-year follow up were mixed in regards to academic and cognitive achievement between both groups undergoing adenotonsillectomy after controlling for developmental and retest issues (Giordani et al., 2012). For verbal ability there was a decline rather than an increase in children's performance, with small to moderate effect size; visuospatial ability showed no increase post-intervention; matrices showed an improvement for the non-SDB group but not for the SDB group post-treatment. Regarding executive function, although lower mean scores in both adenotonsillectomy groups were not significantly different from controls at baseline, both groups significantly increased their ability at 1 year, with moderate effect size. Similarly, academic achievement, spelling, reading, reading comprehension, and mathematics demonstrated significant improvements after intervention for both adenotonsillectomy groups, with small to large effect sizes. Overall, although cognitive abilities in general improved across both groups of children who underwent adenotonsillectomy (despite some declines), the initial hypothesis that improvements would be most evident in children with objective evidence of SDB was not consistently confirmed. Given these findings, the authors suggested that concern about the public health burden of childhood SDB, or adenotonsillar hypertrophy more generally, may be much larger than may have been expected based on previous literature that focuses only on children with clearly abnormal baseline measures of cognition. Furthermore, they advocate that effective treatment of SDB could conceivably mean the difference between average and excellent school performance for one child, or between excellent and exceptional performance for another. Clearly such differences in childhood have the potential to translate into significant lifetime impact for adults.

Potential Mechanisms

The majority of work regarding mechanisms of cognitive morbidity in pediatric sleep disruption has focused on SDB and its main components of sleep fragmentation and hypoxemia. The latter likely impact the prefrontal cortex, an area of the brain implicated in planning complex cognitive behavior and executive functions, of which a recent model has been proposed (Beebe & Gozal, 2002). This model suggests that hypoxemia and sleep fragmentation may alter the neurochemical substrate of the prefrontal cortex, which then manifests as executive dysfunction. Hypoxemia is known to impair cognition regardless of the presence of SDB (Bass et al., 2004). Animal models demonstrate that intermittent hypoxia during sleep induce neuronal cell loss and impair spatial memory (Gozal, Daniel, & Dohanich, 2001; Nair, Dayyat, Zhang, Wang, & Gozal, 2011; Row, 2007) and that early development may be a particularly vulnerable time (Row, Kheirandish, Neville, & Gozal, 2002). Interestingly, data from a brain imaging study have shown that neuronal metabolites are altered in children with SDB in the hippocampal and right frontal cortical regions (Halbower et al., 2006), the very areas that are implicated in executive function and cognition.

Sleep fragmentation or deprivation, however, do not exclusively affect those with SDB; indeed, non-SDB related sleep disruption has been shown to impact cognition in several studies (Randazzo et al., 1998; Sadeh et al., 2002, 2003; Steenari et al., 2003). Sleep disruption is associated with inflammatory markers (Clinton, Davis, Zielinski, Jewett, & Krueger, 2011; Meier-Ewert et al., 2004; Vgontzas et al., 2004) and rodent models show associations with sleep deprivation and oxidative stress (Silva et al., 2004), hippocampal-dependent learning (Hairston et al., 2005; Nair, Zhang, et al., 2011), and dysfunction of systems that are involved in learning, goal direction, and attention (Hanlon, Andrzejewski, Harder, Kelley, & Benca, 2005).

Conclusion

There is a growing literature suggesting that sleep disruption, whether due to sleep deprivation/restriction or SDB, is associated with cognitive deficits in children across the age spectrum. Current data are mixed with regards to the reversibility of such dysfunction, perhaps due to brain plasticity or genetic/environmental interactions. Despite the current lack of definitive data in the form of randomized controlled trials, in light of increasing cross-sectional and treatment studies it would seem pertinent to ensure that education and awareness regarding good sleep practices reaches health care providers, parents, and children themselves.

Future Directions

- Does sleep disruption cause cognitive deficits? While there are growing clinical data suggesting that this may be the case in some cognitive functions, findings are relatively inconclusive. For nonrespiratory sleep disruption the data are currently inadequate to make firm conclusions. Similarly, although there are significantly more data on the relationship between SDB and cognitive outcome, existing findings are not clear enough to confirm a causal relationship. There is an urgent need to perform randomized controlled trials, one of which is currently underway (Redline et al., 2011). The results of this trial will be a significant step forward for the field.
- A further limitation to current knowledge is the lack of longitudinal studies that assess children across development. This is important, since there are a number of animal and human studies that suggest a developmental window of vulnerability where an early insult may not manifest until a later age. The currently available cross-sectional data would miss these potential associations.
- More translational studies are clearly warranted, and should be a research priority, in order to understand the biological mechanisms and neural substrates that explain how sleep disruption may cause cognitive dysfunction. Results from translational studies would play a major role in the development of appropriate interventions, which could have substantial public health impact.

References

Anderson, M. (2005). *Marrying Intelligence and Cognition—a Developmental View.* New York: Cambridge University Press.

Archbold, K. H., Giordani, B., Ruzicka, D. L., & Chervin, R. D. (2004). Cognitive executive dysfunction in children with mild sleep-disordered breathing. *Biological Research for Nursing, 5*(3), 168–176.

Aronen, E. T., Liukkonen, K., Simola, P., Virkkula, P., Uschakoff, A., Korkman, M., et al. (2009). Mood is associated with snoring in preschool-aged children. *Journal of Developmental and Behavioral Pediatrics, 30*(2), 107–114.

Bass, J. L., Corwin, M., Gozal, D., Moore, C., Nishida, H., Parker, S., et al. (2004). The effect of chronic or intermittent hypoxia on cognition in childhood: A review of the evidence. *Pediatrics, 114*(3), 805–816.

Becker, J. T., & Morris, R. G. (1999). Working memory(s). *Brain and Cognition, 41*(1), 1–8.

Beckwith, L., & Parmelee, A. H., Jr. (1986). EEG patterns of preterm infants, home environment, and later IQ. *Child Development, 57*(3), 777–789.

Beebe, D. W., & Gozal, D. (2002). Obstructive sleep apnea and the prefrontal cortex: Towards a comprehensive model linking nocturnal upper airway obstruction to daytime cognitive and behavioral deficits. *Journal of Sleep Research, 11*(1), 1–16.

Beebe, D. W., Wells, C. T., Jeffries, J., Chini, B., Kalra, M., & Amin, R. (2004). Neuropsychological effects of pediatric obstructive sleep apnea. *Journal of the International Neuropsychological Society, 10*(7), 962–975.

Beebe, D. W. (2006). Neurobehavioral morbidity associated with disordered breathing during sleep in children: A comprehensive review. *Sleep, 29*(9), 1115–1134.

Beebe, D. W., Ris, M. D., Kramer, M. E., Long, E., & Amin, R. (2010). The association between sleep disordered breathing, academic grades, and cognitive and behavioral functioning among overweight subjects during middle to late childhood. *Sleep, 33*(11), 1447–1456.

Beebe, D. W. (2011). Cognitive, behavioral, and functional consequences of inadequate sleep in children and adolescents. *Pediatric Clinics of North America, 58*(3), 649–665.

Bernier, A., Carlson, S. M., Bordeleau, S., & Carrier, J. (2010). Relations between physiological and cognitive regulatory systems: Infant sleep regulation and subsequent executive functioning. *Child Development, 81*(6), 1739–1752.

Bhattacharjee, R., Kim, J., Kheirandish-Gozal, L., & Gozal, D. (2011). Obesity and obstructive sleep apnea syndrome in children: A tale of inflammatory cascades. *Pediatric Pulmonology, 46*(4), 313–323.

Biggs, S. N., Bourke, R., Anderson, V., Jackman, A. R., Killedar, A., Nixon, G. M., et al. (2011). Working memory in children with sleep-disordered breathing: Objective versus subjective measures. *Sleep Medicine, 12*(9), 887–891.

Blunden, S., Lushington, K., Kennedy, D., Martin, J., & Dawson, D. (2000). Behavior and neurocognitive performance in children aged 5–10 years who snore compared to controls. *Journal of Clinical and Experimental Neuropsychology, 22*(5), 554–568.

Blunden, S., Lushington, K., Lorenzen, B., Ooi, T., Fung, F., & Kennedy, D. (2004). Are sleep problems under-recognised in general practice? *Archives of Disease in Childhood, 89*(8), 708–712.

Blunden, S., Lushington, K., Lorenzen, B., Martin, J., & Kennedy, D. (2005). Neuropsychological and psychosocial function in children with a history of snoring or behavioral sleep problems. *The Journal of Pediatrics, 146*(6), 780–786.

Bonnet, M. H., & Arand, D. L. (2003). Clinical effects of sleep fragmentation versus sleep deprivation. *Sleep Medicine Reviews, 7*(4), 297–310.

Borghese, I. F., Minard, K. L., & Thoman, E. B. (1995). Sleep rhythmicity in premature infants: Implications for development status. *Sleep, 18*(7), 523–530.

Bourke, R., Anderson, V., Yang, J. S., Jackman, A. R., Killedar, A., Nixon, G. M., et al. (2011). Cognitive and academic functions are impaired in children with all severities of sleep-disordered breathing. *Sleep Medicine, 12*(5), 489–496.

Cain, N., & Gradisar, M. (2010). Electronic media use and sleep in school-aged children and adolescents: A review. *Sleep Medicine, 11*(8), 735–742.

Calhoun, S. L., Mayes, S. D., Vgontzas, A. N., Tsaoussoglou, M., Shifflett, L. J., & Bixler, E. O. (2009). No relationship between neurocognitive functioning and mild sleep disordered breathing in a community sample of children. *Journal of Clinical Sleep Medicine, 5*(3), 228–234.

Cardinali, D. (2000). The human body circadian: How the biological clock influences sleep and emotion. *Neuroendocrinolical Letters, 21*, 9–15.

Carskadon, M. A., Harvey, K., & Dement, W.C. (1981a). Acute restriction of nocturnal sleep in children. *Perceptual and Motor Skills, 53*, 103–114.

Carskadon, M. A., Harvey, K., & Dement, W. C. (1981b). Sleep loss in young adolescents. *Sleep, 4*(3), 299–312.

Carskadon, M. A., Vieira, C., & Acebo, C. (1993). Association between puberty and delayed phase preference. *Sleep, 16*(3), 258–262.

Chervin, R. D., Clarke, D. F., Huffman, J. L., Szymanski, E., Ruzicka, D. L., Miller, V., et al. (2003). School performance, race, and other correlates of sleep-disordered breathing in children. *Sleep Medicine, 4*(1), 21–27.

Chervin, R. D., Ruzicka, D. L., Giordani, B. J., Weatherly, R. A., Dillon, J. E., Hodges, E. K., et al. (2006). Sleep-disordered breathing, behavior, and cognition in children before and after adenotonsillectomy. *Pediatrics, 117*(4), e769–778.

Clinton, J. M., Davis, C. J., Zielinski, M. R., Jewett, K. A., & Krueger, J. M. (2011). Biochemical regulation of sleep and sleep biomarkers. *Journal of Clinical Sleep Medicine, 7*(5 Suppl), S38–42.

Dworak, M., Schierl, T., Bruns, T., & Struder, H. K. (2007). Impact of singular excessive computer game and television exposure on sleep patterns and memory performance of school-aged children. *Pediatrics, 120*(5), 978–985.

Ednick, M., Cohen, A. P., McPhail, G. L., Beebe, D., Simakajornboon, N., & Amin, R. S. (2009). A review of the effects of sleep during the first year of life on cognitive, psychomotor, and temperament development. *Sleep, 32*(11), 1449–1458.

Emancipator, J. L., Storfer-Isser, A., Taylor, H. G., Rosen, C. L., Kirchner, H. L., Johnson, N. L., et al. (2006). Variation of cognition and achievement with sleep-disordered breathing in full-term and preterm children. *Archives of Pediatrics & Adolescent Medicine, 160*(2), 203–210.

Epstein, R., Chillag, N., & Lavie, P. (1998). Starting times of school: Effects on daytime functioning of fifth-grade children in Israel. *Sleep, 21*(3), 250–256.

Ezzat, W. F., Fawaz, S., & Abdelrazek, Y. (2010). To what degree does adenotonsillectomy affect neurocognitive performance in children with obstructive sleep apnea hypopnea syndrome due to adenotonsillar enlargement? *ORL: Journal for Oto-Rhino-Laryngology and its Related Specialties, 72*(4), 215–219.

Fallone, G., Acebo, C., Arnedt, J. T., Seifer, R., & Carskadon, M. A. (2001). Effects of acute sleep restriction on behavior, sustained attention, and response inhibition in children. *Perceptual and Motor Skills, 93*(1), 213–229.

Fallone, G., Acebo, C., Seifer, R., & Carskadon, M. A. (2005). Experimental restriction of sleep opportunity in children: Effects on teacher ratings. *Sleep, 28*(12), 1561–1567.

Freudigman, K. A., & Thoman, E. B. (1993). Infant sleep during the first postnatal day: An opportunity for assessment of vulnerability. *Pediatrics, 92*(3), 373–379.

Friedman, B. C., Hendeles-Amitai, A., Kozminsky, E., Leiberman, A., Friger, M., Tarasiuk, A., & Tal, A. (2003). Adenotonsillectomy improves neurocognitive function in children with obstructive sleep apnea syndrome. *Sleep, 26*(8), 999–1005.

Galland, B. C., Dawes, P. J., Tripp, E. G., & Taylor, B. J. (2006). Changes in behavior and attentional capacity after adenotonsillectomy. *Pediatric Research, 59*(5), 711–716.

Geiger, A., Achermann, P., & Jenni, O. G. (2010). Sleep, intelligence and cognition in a developmental context: differentiation between traits and state-dependent aspects. *Progress in Brain Research, 185*, 167–179.

Giannotti, F., Cortesi, F., Sebastiani, T., & Ottaviano, S. (2002). Circadian preference, sleep and daytime behaviour in adolescence. *Journal of Sleep Research, 11*(3), 191–199.

Giordani, B., Hodges, E. K., Guire, K. E., Ruzicka, D. L., Dillon, J. E., Weatherly, R. A., et al. (2008). Neuropsychological and behavioral functioning in children with and without obstructive sleep apnea referred for tonsillectomy. *Journal of the International Neuropsychological Society, 14*(4), 571–581.

Giordani, B., Hodges, E. K., Guire, K. E., Ruzicka, D. L., Dillon, J. E., Weatherly, R. A., et al. (2012). Changes in neuropsychological and behavioral functioning in children with and without obstructive sleep apnea following tonsillectomy. *Journal of the International Neuropsychological Society 18*(2), 212–222.

Goldberg, E. (2001). *The Executive Brain: Frontal Lobes and the Civilized Mind.* Oxford: Oxford University Press.

Goodwin, J. L., Kaemingk, K. L., Fregosi, R. F., Rosen, G. M., Morgan, W. J., Sherrill, D. L., & Quan, S. F. (2003). Clinical outcomes associated with sleep-disordered breathing in Caucasian and Hispanic children—the Tucson Children's Assessment of Sleep Apnea study (TuCASA). *Sleep, 26*(5), 587–591.

Gottlieb, D. J., Chase, C., Vezina, R. M., Heeren, T. C., Corwin, M. J., Auerbach, S. H., et al. (2004). Sleep-disordered breathing symptoms are associated with poorer cognitive function in 5-year-old children. *The Journal of Pediatrics, 145*(4), 458–464.

Gozal, D. (1998). Sleep-disordered breathing and school performance in children. *Pediatrics, 102*(3 Pt 1), 616–620.

Gozal, D., Daniel, J. M., & Dohanich, G. P. (2001). Behavioral and anatomical correlates of chronic episodic hypoxia during sleep in the rat. *The Journal of Neuroscience, 21*(7), 2442–2450.

Gozal, D., & Pope, D. W., Jr. (2001). Snoring during early childhood and academic performance at ages thirteen to fourteen years. *Pediatrics, 107*(6), 1394–1399.

Hairston, I. S., Little, M. T., Scanlon, M. D., Barakat, M. T., Palmer, T. D., Sapolsky, R. M., & Heller, H. C. (2005). Sleep restriction suppresses neurogenesis induced by hippocampus-dependent learning. *Journal of Neurophysiology, 94*(6), 4224–4233.

Halbower, A. C., Degaonkar, M., Barker, P. B., Earley, C. J., Marcus, C. L., Smith, P. L., et al. (2006). Childhood obstructive sleep apnea associates with neuropsychological deficits and neuronal brain injury. *PLoS Medicine, 3*(8), e301.

Hanlon, E. C., Andrzejewski, M. E., Harder, B. K., Kelley, A. E., & Benca, R. M. (2005). The effect of REM sleep deprivation on motivation for food reward. *Behavioural Brain Research, 163*(1), 58–69.

Hill, C. M., Hogan, A. M., Onugha, N., Harrison, D., Cooper, S., McGrigor, V. J., et al. (2006). Increased cerebral blood flow velocity in children with mild sleep-disordered breathing: A possible association with abnormal neuropsychological function. *Pediatrics, 118*(4), e1100–1108.

Hogan, A. M., Hill, C. M., Harrison, D., & Kirkham, F. J. (2008). Cerebral blood flow velocity and cognition in children before and after adenotonsillectomy. *Pediatrics, 122*(1), 75–82.

Holm, S. M., Forbes, E. E., Ryan, N. D., Phillips, M. L., Tarr, J. A., & Dahl, R. E. (2009). Reward-related brain function and sleep in pre/early pubertal and mid/late pubertal adolescents. *The Journal of Adolescent Health, 45*(4), 326–334.

Honaker, S. M., Gozal, D., Bennett, J., Capdevila, O. S., & Spruyt, K. (2009). Sleep-disordered breathing and verbal skills in school-aged community children. *Developmental Neuropsychology, 34*(5), 588–600.

Kaemingk, K. L., Pasvogel, A. E., Goodwin, J. L., Mulvaney, S. A., Martinez, F., Enright, P. L., et al. (2003). Learning in children and sleep disordered breathing: findings of the Tucson Children's Assessment of Sleep Apnea (tuCASA) prospective cohort study. *Journal of the International Neuropsychological Society, 9*(7), 1016–1026.

Kahn, A., Van de Merckt, C., Rebuffat, E., Mozin, M. J., Sottiaux, M., Blum, D., & Hennart, P. (1989). Sleep problems in healthy preadolescents. *Pediatrics, 84*(3), 542–546.

Karpinski, A. C., Scullin, M. H., & Montgomery-Downs, H. E. (2008). Risk for sleep-disordered breathing and executive function in preschoolers. *Sleep Medicine, 9*(4), 418–424.

Kennedy, J. D., Blunden, S., Hirte, C., Parsons, D. W., Martin, A. J., Crowe, E., et al. (2004). Reduced neurocognition in children who snore. *Pediatric Pulmonology, 37*(4), 330–337.

Key, A. P., Molfese, D. L., O'Brien, L., & Gozal, D. (2009). Sleep-disordered breathing affects auditory processing in 5–7-year-old children: Evidence from brain recordings. *Developmental Neuropsychology, 34*(5), 615–628.

Kheirandish-Gozal, L., De Jong, M. R., Spruyt, K., Chamuleau, S. A., & Gozal, D. (2010). Obstructive sleep apnoea is associated with impaired pictorial memory task acquisition and retention in children. *The European Respiratory Journal, 36*(1), 164–169.

Kim, J. K., Lee, J. H., Lee, S. H., Hong, S. C., & Cho, J. H. (2011). School performance and behavior of Korean elementary school students with sleep-disordered breathing. *The Annals of Otology, Rhinology, And Laryngology, 120*(4), 268–272.

Knutson, K. L., Spiegel, K., Penev, P., & Van Cauter, E. (2007). The metabolic consequences of sleep deprivation. *Sleep Medicine Reviews, 11*(3), 163–178.

Kohler, M. J., Lushington, K., van den Heuvel, C. J., Martin, J., Pamula, Y., & Kennedy, D. (2009). Adenotonsillectomy and neurocognitive deficits in children with sleep disordered breathing. *PloS One, 4*(10), e7343.

Kopasz, M., Loessl, B., Hornyak, M., Riemann, D., Nissen, C., Piosczyk, H., & Voderholzer, U. (2010). Sleep and memory in healthy children and adolescents—a critical review. *Sleep Medicine Reviews, 14*(3), 167–177.

Lam, J. C., Mahone, E. M., Mason, T., & Scharf, S. M. (2011). The effects of napping on cognitive function in preschoolers. *Journal of developmental and behavioral Pediatrics, 32*(2), 90–97.

Landhuis, C. E., Poulton, R., Welch, D., & Hancox, R. J. (2008). Childhood sleep time and long-term risk for obesity: A 32-year prospective birth cohort study. *Pediatrics, 122*(5), 955–960.

Lewin, D. S., Rosen, R. C., England, S. J., & Dahl, R. E. (2002). Preliminary evidence of behavioral and cognitive sequelae of obstructive sleep apnea in children. *Sleep Medicine, 3*(1), 5–13.

Lezak, M. (1995). *Neuropsychological Assessment.* New York: Oxford University Press.

Lezak, M. D., Howieson, D.B., Loring D.W. (2004). *Neuropsychological Assessment* (4th ed.). New York: Oxford University Press.

Li, H. Y., Huang, Y. S., Chen, N. H., Fang, T. J., & Lee, L. A. (2006). Impact of adenotonsillectomy on behavior in children with sleep-disordered breathing. *The Laryngoscope, 116*(7), 1142–1147.

Li, S., Jin, X., Wu, S., Jiang, F., Yan, C., & Shen, X. (2007). The impact of media use on sleep patterns and sleep disorders among school-aged children in China. *Sleep, 30*(3), 361–367.

Lundeborg, I., McAllister, A., Samuelsson, C., Ericsson, E., & Hultcrantz, E. (2009). Phonological development in children with obstructive sleep-disordered breathing. *Clinical Linguistics & Phonetics, 23*(10), 751–761.

Maquet, P. (2001). The role of sleep in learning and memory. *Science, 294*(5544), 1048–1052.

Mayes, S. D., Calhoun, S. L., Bixler, E. O., & Vgontzas, A. N. (2008). Nonsignificance of sleep relative to IQ and neuropsychological scores in predicting academic achievement. *Journal of Developmental and Behavioral Pediatrics, 29*(3), 206–212.

Meier-Ewert, H. K., Ridker, P. M., Rifai, N., Regan, M. M., Price, N. J., Dinges, D. F., & Mullington, J. M. (2004). Effect of sleep loss on C-reactive protein, an inflammatory marker of cardiovascular risk. *Journal of the American College of Cardiology, 43*(4), 678–683.

Miano, S., Paolino, M. C., Urbano, A., Parisi, P., Massolo, A. C., Castaldo, R., & Villa, M. P. (2011). Neurocognitive assessment and sleep analysis in children with sleep-disordered breathing. *Clinical Neurophysiology, 122*(2), 311–319.

Millman, R. P. (2005). Excessive sleepiness in adolescents and young adults: Causes, consequences, and treatment strategies. *Pediatrics, 115*(6), 1774–1786.

Ming, X., Koransky, R., Kang, V., Buchman, S., Sarris, C. E., & Wagner, G. C. (2011). Sleep insufficiency, sleep health problems and performance in high school students. *Clinical Medicine Insights. Circulatory, Respiratory and Pulmonary Medicine, 5*, 71–79.

Montgomery-Downs, H. E., Jones, V. F., Molfese, V. J., & Gozal, D. (2003). Snoring in preschoolers: Associations with sleepiness, ethnicity, and learning. *Clinical Pediatrics, 42*(8), 719–726.

Montgomery-Downs, H. E., Crabtree, V. M., & Gozal, D. (2005). Cognition, sleep and respiration in at-risk children treated for obstructive sleep apnoea. *The European Respiratory Journal, 25*(2), 336–342.

Nair, D., Dayyat, E. A., Zhang, S. X., Wang, Y., & Gozal, D. (2011). Intermittent hypoxia-induced cognitive deficits are mediated by NADPH oxidase activity in a murine model of sleep apnea. *PloS One, 6*(5), e19847.

Nair, D., Zhang, S. X., Ramesh, V., Hakim, F., Kaushal, N., Wang, Y., & Gozal, D. (2011). Sleep fragmentation induces cognitive deficits via nicotinamide adenine dinucleotide phosphate oxidase-dependent pathways in mouse. *American Journal of Respiratory and Critical Care Medicine, 184*(11), 1305–1312.

O'Brien, L. M., Mervis, C. B., Holbrook, C. R., Bruner, J. L., Klaus, C. J., Rutherford, J., et al. (2004a). Neurobehavioral implications of habitual snoring in children. *Pediatrics, 114*(1), 44–49.

O'Brien, L. M., Mervis, C. B., Holbrook, C. R., Bruner, J. L., Smith, N. H., McNally, N., et al. (2004b). Neurobehavioral correlates of sleep-disordered breathing in children. *Journal of Sleep Research, 13*(2), 165–172.

O'Brien, E. M., & Mindell, J. A. (2005). Sleep and risk-taking behavior in adolescents. *Behavioral Sleep Medicine, 3*(3), 113–133.

O'Brien, L. M. (2008). Neurocognitive and Behavioral Consequences of Sleep Disordered Breathing in Children. In A. Ivanenko (Ed.), *Sleep and Psychiatric Disorders in Children and Adolescents*. (pp. 149–161). New York: Informa Healthcare USA, Inc.

O'Brien, L. M. (2009). The neurocognitive effects of sleep disruption in children and adolescents. *Child and Adolescent Psychiatric Clinics of North America, 18*(4), 813–823.

Oka, Y., Suzuki S., Inoue, Y. (2008). Bedtime activities, sleep environment, and sleep/wake patterns of Japanese elementary school children. *Behavioral Sleep Medicine, 6*(4), 220–233.

O'Malley, E. B., O'Malley, M. B. (2008). School start time and its impact on learning and behavior. In A. Ivanenko (Ed.), *Sleep and Psychiatric Disorders in Children and Adolescents* (pp. 79–94). New York: Informa Healthcare.

Owens, J. (2008). Classification and epidemiology of childhood sleep disorders. *Primary Care, 35*(3), 533–546, vii.

Paavonen, E. J., Pennonen, M., Roine, M., Valkonen, S., & Lahikainen, A. R. (2006). TV exposure associated with sleep disturbances in 5- to 6-year-old children. *Journal of Sleep Research, 15*(2), 154–161.

Pilcher, J. J., & Huffcutt, A. I. (1996). Effects of sleep deprivation on performance: A meta-analysis. *Sleep, 19*(4), 318–326.

Piteo, A. M., Kennedy, J. D., Roberts, R. M., Martin, A. J., Nettelbeck, T., Kohler, M. J., & Lushington, K. (2011). Snoring and cognitive development in infancy. *Sleep Medicine, 12*(10), 981–987.

Piteo, A. M., Lushington, K., Roberts, R. M., Martin, A. J., Nettelbeck, T., Kohler, M. J., & Kennedy, J. D. (2011). Parental-reported snoring from the first month of life and cognitive development at 12 months of age. *Sleep Medicine, 12*(10), 975–980.

Randazzo, A. C., Muehlbach, M. J., Schweitzer, P. K., & Walsh, J. K. (1998). Cognitive function following acute sleep restriction in children ages 10–14. *Sleep, 21*(8), 861–868.

Ravid, S., Afek, I., Suraiya, S., Shahar, E., & Pillar, G. (2009a). Kindergarten children's failure to qualify for first grade could result from sleep disturbances. *Journal of Child Neurology, 24*(7), 816–822.

Ravid, S., Afek, I., Suraiya, S., Shahar, E., & Pillar, G. (2009b). Sleep disturbances are associated with reduced school achievements in first-grade pupils. *Developmental Neuropsychology, 34*(5), 574–587.

Redline, S., Amin, R., Beebe, D., Chervin, R. D., Garetz, S. L., Giordani, B., et al. (2011). The Childhood Adenotonsillectomy Trial (CHAT): Rationale, design, and challenges of a randomized controlled trial evaluating a standard surgical procedure in a pediatric population. *Sleep, 34*(11), 1509–1517.

Reynolds, A. C., & Banks, S. (2010). Total sleep deprivation, chronic sleep restriction and sleep disruption. *Progress in Brain Research, 185*, 91–103.

Rhodes, S. K., Shimoda, K. C., Waid, L. R., O'Neil, P. M., Oexmann, M. J., Collop, N. A., & Willi, S. M. (1995). Neurocognitive deficits in morbidly obese children with obstructive sleep apnea. *The Journal of Pediatrics, 127*(5), 741–744.

Row, B. W., Kheirandish, L., Neville, J. J., & Gozal, D. (2002). Impaired spatial learning and hyperactivity in developing rats exposed to intermittent hypoxia. *Pediatric Research, 52*(3), 449–453.

Row, B. W. (2007). Intermittent hypoxia and cognitive function: implications from chronic animal models. *Advances in Experimental Medicine and Biology, 618*, 51–67.

Sadeh, A., Raviv, A., & Gruber, R. (2000). Sleep patterns and sleep disruptions in school-age children. *Developmental Psychology, 36*(3), 291–301.

Sadeh, A., Gruber, R., & Raviv, A. (2002). Sleep, neurobehavioral functioning, and behavior problems in school-age children. *Child Development, 73*(2), 405–417.

Sadeh, A., Gruber, R., & Raviv, A. (2003). The effects of sleep restriction and extension on school-age children: What a difference an hour makes. *Child Development, 74*(2), 444–455.

Scher, M. S., Steppe, D. A., & Banks, D. L. (1996). Prediction of lower developmental performances of healthy neonates by neonatal EEG-sleep measures. *Pediatric Neurology, 14*(2), 137–144.

Schmidt, M., & Vandewater, E. A. (2008). Media and attention, cognition, and school achievement. *The Future of Children, 18*(1), 63–85.

Silva, R. H., Abilio, V. C., Takatsu, A. L., Kameda, S. R., Grassl, C., Chehin, A. B., et al. (2004). Role of hippocampal oxidative stress in memory deficits induced by sleep deprivation in mice. *Neuropharmacology, 46*(6), 895–903.

Spruyt, K., Aitken, R. J., So, K., Charlton, M., Adamson, T. M., & Horne, R. S. (2008). Relationship between sleep/wake patterns, temperament and overall development in term infants over the first year of life. *Early Human Development, 84*(5), 289–296.

Spruyt, K., Capdevila, O. S., Kheirandish-Gozal, L., & Gozal, D. (2009). Inefficient or insufficient encoding as potential primary deficit in neurodevelopmental performance among children with OSA. *Developmental Neuropsychology, 34*(5), 601–614.

Spruyt, K., & Gozal, D. (2011). A mediation model linking body weight, cognition, and sleep disordered breathing. *American Journal of Respiratory and Critical Care Medicine, 185*(2), 199–205.

Squire, L. R., & Zola, S. M. (1996). Structure and function of declarative and nondeclarative memory systems. *Proceedings of the National Academy of Sciences of the United States of America, 93*(24), 13515–13522.

Steenari, M. R., Vuontela, V., Paavonen, E. J., Carlson, S., Fjallberg, M., & Aronen, E. (2003). Working memory and sleep in 6- to 13-year-old schoolchildren. *Journal of the American Academy of Child and Adolescent Psychiatry, 42*(1), 85–92.

Stickgold, R., & Walker, M. P. (2005a). Memory consolidation and reconsolidation: What is the role of sleep? *Trends in Neurosciences, 28*(8), 408–415.

Stickgold, R., & Walker, M. P. (2005b). Sleep and memory: The ongoing debate. *Sleep, 28*(10), 1225–1227.

Suratt, P. M., Peruggia, M., D'Andrea, L., Diamond, R., Barth, J. T., Nikova, M., et al. (2006). Cognitive function and behavior of children with adenotonsillar hypertrophy suspected of having obstructive sleep-disordered breathing. *Pediatrics, 118*(3), e771–781.

Suratt, P. M., Barth, J. T., Diamond, R., D'Andrea, L., Nikova, M., Perriello, V. A., Jr., et al. (2007). Reduced time in bed and obstructive sleep-disordered breathing in children are associated with cognitive impairment. *Pediatrics, 119*(2), 320–329.

Touchette, E., Petit, D., Seguin, J. R., Boivin, M., Tremblay, R. E., & Montplaisir, J. Y. (2007). Associations between sleep duration patterns and behavioral/cognitive functioning at school entry. *Sleep, 30*(9), 1213–1219.

Tulving, E. (1985). How many memory systems are there? *American Psychology, 40*, 385–389.

Urschitz, M. S., Guenther, A., Eggebrecht, E., Wolff, J., Urschitz-Duprat, P. M., Schlaud, M., & Poets, C. F. (2003). Snoring, intermittent hypoxia and academic performance in primary school children. *American Journal of Respiratory and Critical Care Medicine, 168*(4), 464–468.

Urschitz, M. S., Wolff, J., Sokollik, C., Eggebrecht, E., Urschitz-Duprat, P. M., Schlaud, M., & Poets, C. F. (2005). Nocturnal arterial oxygen saturation and academic performance in a community sample of children. *Pediatrics, 115*(2), e204–209.

Van Cauter, E., & Knutson, K. L. (2008). Sleep and the epidemic of obesity in children and adults. *European Journal of Endocrinology/European Federation of Endocrine Societies, 159*(Suppl 1), S59–66.

Vgontzas, A. N., Zoumakis, E., Bixler, E. O., Lin, H. M., Follett, H., Kales, A., & Chrousos, G. P. (2004). Adverse effects of modest sleep restriction on sleepiness, performance, and inflammatory cytokines. *The Journal of Clinical Endocrinology and Metabolism, 89*(5), 2119–2126.

Wahlstrom, K. (2002). Changing times: Findings from the first longitudinal study of later high school start times. *NASSP Bulletin, 86*, 633.

Walker, M. P., & Stickgold, R. (2006). Sleep, memory, and plasticity. *Annual review of psychology, 57*, 139–166.

Walker, M. P. (2009). The role of sleep in cognition and emotion. *Annals of the New York Academy of Sciences, 1156*, 168–197.

Wolfson, A. R., & Carskadon, M. A. (1998). Sleep schedules and daytime functioning in adolescents. *Child Development, 69*(4), 875–887.

Wolfson, A. R., & Carskadon, M. A. (2003). Understanding adolescents' sleep patterns and school performance: A critical appraisal. *Sleep Medicine Reviews, 7*(6), 491–506.

CHAPTER

30

Weight Control and Obesity

Chantelle N. Hart, Nicola Hawley, Elizabeth Kuhl, *and* Elissa Jelalian

Abstract

Over the past several years, there has been considerable interest in the association between children's sleep duration and obesity risk. Mounting epidemiological evidence suggests that short sleep is associated with concurrent and prospective risk of obesity during childhood. Studies have further suggested plausible mediators for the sleep–weight association, including hormones and eating and activity behaviors. Despite the convincing data, no pediatric experimental or treatment studies targeted at changing sleep length have been published. Thus, whether short sleep causes weight gain or changes in children's weight status remains unknown. Beyond sleep duration, there is also evidence for an association between obesity and sleep disordered breathing (SDB) in children with some evidence that weight loss may improve SDB symptoms. The present chapter reviews the extant literature on the association between pediatric sleep duration and obesity risk, the association between pediatric obesity and SDB, and concludes with suggestions for future research.

Key Words: sleep duration, insufficient sleep, sleep disordered breathing, obesity, dietary intake, sedentary activity, physical activity

Introduction

Insufficient sleep, which can be due to short sleep duration and/or poor quality of sleep (Knutson, 2012), has been associated with a number of deleterious effects in children and adolescents, including cognitive and behavioral impairments (Beebe, 2011) and increased risk-taking behaviors (see Hershner, Chapter 31). Although these consequences of insufficient sleep have been well documented, less is known regarding how sleep may impact health. Of particular interest over the past several years is the role that insufficient sleep may play in the current obesity epidemic. This interest has been spurred by epidemiological studies with children and adolescents, as well as experimental investigations with adults, which suggest not only an association between short sleep and increased obesity risk, but also point to possible mechanisms through which sleep duration may impact obesity status. In addition, mounting evidence demonstrates an association between pediatric obesity and sleep disordered breathing (SDB). The present chapter will review the extant literature on the association between insufficient sleep and weight status in children and adolescents and discuss possible implications for treatment of SDB. Limitations of studies conducted thus far and areas in need of future research will also be reviewed.

Pediatric Obesity: Definition and Significance

Pediatric obesity has risen dramatically in recent decades to become a worldwide epidemic. The most current prevalence reported in the United States, in 2009–2010, indicates that 31.8% (95% Confidence Interval, [CI]: 29.8–33.7) of children aged 2–19 years were overweight or obese (body mass index [BMI] ≥ 85th percentile) based on sex-specific Centers for Disease Control and Prevention (CDC) 2000 BMI-for-age references (Ogden, Carroll, Kit, & Flegal, 2012). Obesity (BMI ≥ 95th percentile) was present in 16.9% (95% CI: 15.4–18.4) of this age group, with males and children from ethnic minority backgrounds at slightly elevated risk (Ogden et al., 2012). The most current estimates for the global prevalence of childhood overweight and obesity were made in 2004 when it was estimated that 150–160 million school-age children (5–17 years) were overweight (85th ≤ BMI < 95th percentile for age and sex), with 35–40 million of these children classified as obese using the established International Obesity Task Force cut-offs (Cole, Bellizzi, Flegal, & Dietz, 2000; Wang & Lobstein, 2006). Despite recent suggestions for a plateau in the US obesity rate, revising these global estimates today would likely show an even greater proportion of children to be overweight or obese based on trends reported in both developed (Ogden et al., 2012; Stamatakis, Zaninotto, Falaschetti, Mindell, & Head, 2010) and developing nations (Gupta, Goel, Shah, & Misra, 2012).

Obesity in childhood carries a number of health risks both immediate and long term. Immediate risks include high blood pressure (Daniels, 2006; Freedman, Dietz, Srinivasan, & Berenson, 1999), high cholesterol and dyslipidemia (Freedman et al., 1999; McMurray, Harrell, Levine, & Gansky, 1995), as well as impaired glucose tolerance, insulin resistance, and type II diabetes (Cruz et al., 2005; Daniels, 2006; Hannon, Rao, & Arslanian, 2005; Sinha et al., 2002; Valente, Strong, & Sinaiko, 2001) or clustering of multiple risk factors (Nathan & Moran, 2008). Musculoskeletal problems (Wearing, Hennig, Byrne, Steele, & Hills, 2006), gallstones (Cuevas, Miquel, Reyes, Zanlungo, & Nervi, 2004; Lugo-Vicente, 1997) and nonalcoholic fatty liver disease (Fishbein, Miner, Mogren, & Chalekson, 2003; Roberts, 2005) are other potential health risks. Longitudinal studies have shown that overweight and obese children are more likely to become obese adults than their normal weight peers. Approximately one-third of children who are overweight and approximately half of adolescents who are overweight become obese adults (Power, Lake, & Cole, 1997; Serdula et al., 1993).

Of particular relevance to the focus of this chapter is that the increasing prevalence in pediatric obesity over the past 20–30 years has been associated with an increased prevalence in SDB and obstructive sleep apnea (OSA). More specifically, while the prevalence of OSA in the general pediatric population is estimated at 2% to 6% (Daftary & Kotagal, 2010; Guilleminault, Lee, & Chan, 2005), one study found the prevalence of OSA in children who are overweight or obese to range from 19%–41% (Verhulst et al., 2007). An additional study found that after controlling for family history of SDB, those children with a BMI > 28 kg/m^2 were at almost a five-fold increased risk for SDB compared to children with BMIs ≤ 28 kg/m^2 (Redline et al., 1999). The association between obesity and SDB is compounded by the decreased success of adenotonsillectomy (T&A) among children who are obese (Costa & Mitchell, 2009) and, in turn, the increased risk of weight gain following the procedure (Jeyakumar, Fettman, Armbrecht, & Mitchell, 2011; Roemmich et al., 2006; Soultan, Wadowski, Rao, & Kravath, 1999). Taken together with the fact that SDB is associated with possible metabolic dysfunction as well as cardiovascular disease risk factors (Witmans & Young, 2011), along with the documented medical risks of obesity noted above, the need to enhance current treatment approaches for obesity is clear.

Beyond medical risks, the detriment of obesity on psychosocial functioning is evident as well. Numerous studies have documented significantly lower health-related quality of life for obese youth compared to their healthy weight peers by both child self-report and parent proxy report (Tsiros et al., 2009). Social functioning appears to be particularly impaired, with as many as 30%–90% of obese youth reportedly experiencing weight-based teasing from peers (Griffiths, Wolke, Page, & Horwood, 2006; Neumark-Sztainer et al., 2002; Neumark-Sztainer, Story, & Faibisch, 1998). Findings that peer victimization may begin as early as age 3 (Holub, 2008; Margulies, Floyd, & Hojnoski, 2008) are particularly concerning, given the potential negative impact on social and emotional development. Even more surprising is that 34%–47% of obese youth may also be recipients of weight-based teasing by family members (Neumark-Sztainer et al., 2002). Behavioral problems, depression, anxiety, higher body dissatisfaction, and lower self-worth have also been noted in treatment-seeking obese children and adolescents compared to non–treatment-seeking obese and healthy weight youth (Wardle & Cooke, 2005). Collectively this evidence highlights the urgency of developing effective obesity prevention and intervention programs for children and adolescents.

It is believed that obesity results from an energy imbalance (i.e., greater energy intake than what is expended). Thus effective pediatric obesity prevention and treatment approaches have typically targeted both sides of this equation: eating and activity behaviors. Although evidence to date suggests that prevention approaches, particularly ones that target both eating and activity behaviors, are promising (Brown & Summerbell, 2009) and behavioral interventions for treatment of obesity are effective (Oude Luttikhuis et al., 2009; Epstein, Valoski, Wing, & McCurley, 1994), these efforts do not typically yield large enough weight losses to help most children achieve healthy weight status. The identification of novel, modifiable behaviors that can impact weight status is thus of high interest, as they may enhance efforts to achieve this goal (Keith et al., 2006).

Children's nocturnal sleep length has been identified as one such novel target (Keith et al., 2006) for several reasons. Paralleling increasing rates of obesity in recent years are decreases in children's reported sleep duration (Dollman, Ridley, Olds, & Lowe, 2007; Iglowstein, Jenni, Molinari, & Largo, 2003; Matricciani, Olds, & Petkov, 2011). In addition, mounting epidemiological evidence supports an association between insufficient sleep and obesity risk in children and adolescents (Cappuccio et al., 2008; Chen, Beydoun, & Wang, 2008). These findings taken together with experimental studies with adults, which document potential changes in appetite-regulating hormones that would favor increased food intake upon insufficient sleep (Brondel, Romer, Nougues, Touyarou, & Davenne, 2010; St-Onge et al., 2011), make a compelling argument for the role that insufficient sleep may play in the current pediatric obesity epidemic. Epidemiological evidence for the association between sleep and weight status will be reviewed below.

Pediatric Epidemiological Studies Assessing Short Sleep and Weight Status

A number of epidemiological studies have now considered the association between children's sleep length and obesity risk, both concurrently and prospectively. Meta-analyses of these studies demonstrate that shorter sleep duration in childhood is associated with a 58%–89% increased risk of obesity (Cappuccio et al., 2008; Chen et al., 2008). Although these studies are not without limitations, the consistency in findings across racial and ethnic groups and children of all ages is striking (Hart, Cairns, & Jelalian, 2011). It is particularly compelling given that findings typically persist after statistical control for relevant confounding factors (Hart et al., 2011). Highlights of study findings to date are provided below. In addition, the reader is referred to a number of recent reviews and meta-analyses for additional details on studies to date (Cappuccio et al., 2008; Chen et al., 2008; Hart et al., 2011; Patel & Hu, 2008).

Cross-Sectional Studies

With few exceptions, cross-sectional studies conducted worldwide have reported negative associations between sleep duration and obesity in children. Our own review of the pediatric literature (Hart et al., 2011) identified 24 original empirical studies of sleep and weight status in children from birth to 18 years. While the methodology employed to measure sleep duration, the referent values for short sleep, the obesity classification used, and the confounders controlled for varied between studies, the vast majority reported significant negative associations between sleep duration and obesity risk.

After controlling for several potential confounders Sekine et al. (2002) reported that obesity risk in 6–7-year-olds sleeping less than 8 hours/night was nearly triple that of those sleeping 10 hours or more/night (OR: 2.87 [1.61–5.05]). Eisenmann et al. (2006) found consistent results for children 7–15 years old (OR: 3.06 [2.11–4.46]) using the same referent values. Wing et al. (2009) showed that 5–15-year-olds sleeping less than 8 hours/night were at greater risk for overweight or obesity than their peers who slept for 10 or more hours/night during the week (OR: 1.74 [1.23–2.45]), while Ozturk et al. (2009) replicated these findings in boys only (OR: 2.06 [1.31–2.72]).

While the majority of cross-sectional studies rely on parent report for sleep duration (or self-reported sleep duration in older children), actigraphy has been used to assess sleep duration in two studies. Although they used only a single night of actigraphy recording, Nixon and colleagues (2008) reported a three-fold increase in obesity risk in 7-year-olds sleeping less than 9 hours/night compared to those sleeping longer. Also using only a single recording night with actigraphy, Gupta, Mueller, Chan, and Meininger (2002) reported that obese adolescents slept less than their non-obese peers, and that for each additional hour of sleep obesity risk was reduced by 80% after controlling for behavioral and demographic variation.

Several recent studies have also considered the relationship between sleep and other measures of body composition. Having a shorter sleep duration is associated in several pediatric studies with greater waist circumference (Chaput & Tremblay, 2007;

Eisenmann, Ekkekakis, & Holmes, 2006; Hitze et al., 2009; Ozturk et al., 2009; Yu et al., 2007). Shorter-sleeping 5–7-year-old children have been shown in two studies to have higher percentages of body fat as assessed using bioelectrical impedance analysis (Nixon et al., 2008; von Kries, Toschke, Wurmser, Sauerwald, & Koletzko, 2002), while shorter-sleeping 7–9–year-olds, whose percentage body fat was estimated with skinfolds, were also at greater risk (Padez et al., 2009). Adolescent girls sleeping less have also been shown to have greater total and truncal body fat and less lean mass when body composition was assessed using dual-energy x-ray absorptiometry (Yu et al., 2007).

Prospective Studies

Prospective studies have demonstrated temporal associations between sleep duration and obesity risk. One study found that for children 0–4 years (but not 5–13 years), sleeping less at night was associated with increased risk of overweight and obesity 5 years later (Bell & Zimmerman, 2010). Additional prospective studies with older children have found significant associations between sleep duration during middle childhood and obesity risk in adolescence (Seegers et al., 2011) and adulthood (Landhuis, Poulton, Welch, & Hancox, 2008). Furthermore, Snell and colleagues (2007) found that irrespective of age at baseline (3–12 years), there was a 0.75 kg/m^2 decrease in BMI at 5-year follow-up for each additional hour slept at baseline (Snell, Adam, & Duncan, 2007).

Additional studies assessed the influence of consistent short sleep on future obesity risk. The first found that children who were consistently short sleepers from 2.5 to 6 years of age had almost a three-fold increased risk of obesity when they were 6 years old (Touchette et al., 2008). A more recent study found similar results. Consistent short sleep duration between 1.5 and 2 years was associated with development of a greater amount of fat mass (FM) during childhood independent of early life factors (gestational age, weight status in infancy, feeding) and socioeconomic factors (FM measured at 7 years; Diethelm, Bolzenius, Cheng, Remer, & Buyken, 2011). There was no effect for either BMI or fat-free mass in this study.

Potential Mechanisms Linking Short Sleep Duration and Obesity Risk

Several reviews have outlined the potential pathways linking short sleep with obesity risk (Hart et al., 2011; Knutson & Van Cauter, 2008; Patel & Hu, 2008). These include changes that may occur within the neuroendocrine system, potential changes in food intake and energy expenditure (via changes in both physical activity and sedentary behaviors), and additional underlying factors that may simultaneously affect change in both sleep duration and weight status. Each of these areas will be reviewed below.

Neuroendocrine Changes

Perhaps the best-supported pathway between sleep duration and weight status is a neuroendocrine pathway in which changes in sleep duration are associated with changes in the secretion of hormones associated with eating behaviors and obesity risk. Several experimental studies have assessed this pathway by comparing partial sleep restriction with rested conditions (Knutson, Spiegel, Penev, & Van Cauter, 2007; Schmid, Hallschmid, Jauch-Chara, Born, & Schultes, 2008; Spiegel, Leproult et al., 2004; Spiegel, Tasali, Penev, & Van Cauter, 2004). To date, these studies have typically been conducted with healthy young adults, with no published experimental studies, to our knowledge, being done with children. Although these findings are from experimental studies with adult samples, it is important to highlight main findings in an effort to identify mechanisms that could translate to pediatric populations.

Compared to rested conditions, partial sleep restriction (e.g., 4–5 hours/night) in adults is associated with a number of neuroendocrine changes including decreased glucose tolerance and thyrotropin concentrations, elevations in evening cortisol concentrations, and increased activity of the sympathetic nervous system (Spiegel, Leproult, & Van Cauter, 1999). The hormones leptin and ghrelin, which are associated with the regulation of hunger and appetite (Cummings, 2006; Levin et al., 2006), are also influenced by sleep duration (Mullington et al., 2003; Shea, Hilton, Orlova, Ayers, & Mantzoros, 2005; Spiegel, Leproult et al., 2004; Spiegel, Tasali et al., 2004; Taheri, Lin, Austin, Young, & Mignot, 2004).

Extant epidemiological studies with children suggest that short sleep may be associated with similar hormonal profiles as found in adults (Flint et al., 2007; Tian et al., 2010; Verhulst et al., 2008). For example, children who were reported to be shorter sleepers evidenced higher fasting C-peptide (Verhulst et al., 2008) and increased risk for hyperglycemia (Tian et al., 2010), and insulin resistance (Flint et al., 2007) than their more rested counterparts.

Furthermore, Bornhorst and colleagues (2012) found that when a negative association between sleep duration and BMI status was identified in children, insulin levels attenuated this significant association—particularly for children with higher weight status. This suggests that insulin may, in part, mediate the association between sleep duration and BMI status. Finally, an additional study found that children with shorter and more variable sleep had higher C-reactive protein levels, and altered insulin and low density lipoprotein (Spruyt, Molfese, & Gozal, 2011). In sum, although these correlational studies parallel findings from experimental studies with adults they are limited because of their cross-sectional designs, which cannot demonstrate actual changes in hormones due to changes in sleep.

Both Sides of the Energy Balance Equation: Eating and Activity Behaviors

Given strong evidence from these experimental studies that partial sleep restriction may promote increased food intake, recent studies have begun to explore eating behaviors. Similar to our understanding of the neuroendocrine changes associated with sleep duration, experimental research regarding eating behaviors has focused on adults. In short, these findings have been mixed with two experimental studies finding no effect of sleep duration on food intake (Benedict et al., 2011; Schmid et al., 2009), and three other studies finding that partial sleep deprivation was associated with increased ad libitum food intake when compared with a rested condition (Brondel et al., 2010; Markwald et al., 2013; St-Onge et al., 2011); there was an associated increase in weight during the sleep restriction condition in one of these studies (Markwald et al., 2013). An additional laboratory-based study found mixed results for partial sleep restriction on food intake. Although there were no changes in overall energy intake from meals between the partial restriction and rested conditions, there was a greater intake of calories from snacks upon partial sleep deprivation (Nedeltcheva et al., 2009).

Two experimental studies have been conducted with adolescents. Similar to studies with adults, findings have been mixed. In one study, compared to a rested condition, sleep restriction was associated with decreased caloric intake at an ad libitum meal in adolescent males (Klingenberg et al., 2012). The second study, which was conducted with adolescent males and females found that, compared to a rested condition, sleep restriction was associated with a reported increased intake in foods high in glycemic index and load, but no overall differences in reported caloric intake (Beebe et al., in press). Despite these studies with adolescents and adults, to our knowledge no published experimental studies have been conducted with school-age children or younger. Recent correlational work suggests that short sleep duration may be associated with less healthy eating behaviors, and certain eating behaviors may mediate the association between sleep and weight status. One study that measured sleep with actigraphy found that adolescents with shorter weekday sleep reported consuming a higher percentage of calories from fat and lower percentage from carbohydrates (Weiss et al., 2010). Shorter reported sleep has also been associated with greater food cravings (Landis, Parker, & Dunbar, 2009), greater consumption of energy-dense foods (particularly on weekends, and for males; Westerlund, Ray, & Roos, 2009), inadequate consumption of fruits, vegetables, and fish (Garaulet et al., 2011; Tatone-Tokuda et al., 2011), and greater intake of sugar-sweetened drinks/less intake of milk products (Tatone-Tokuda et al., 2011).

Less attention has been paid to the other side of the energy balance equation: energy expenditure, yet it has been hypothesized that individuals who are chronically partially sleep-deprived may hold less of a propensity to be active (Reilly & Edwards, 2007). It also makes intuitive sense that insufficient nocturnal sleep could result in greater daytime sleepiness, which could lead to increased time spent in sedentary activities such as watching television. Two experimental studies with adults demonstrated that partial sleep restriction, compared to a rested condition, was associated with decreased physical activity/energy expenditure (Benedict et al., 2011; Schmid et al., 2009). Similar to eating behaviors, others have not found an association between partial sleep restriction and energy expenditure (St-Onge et al., 2011).

Beyond these experimental findings with adults, there is considerable evidence from pediatric studies that greater television viewing and having a television in the bedroom is associated with less sleep and with greater difficulties with sleep both concurrently and prospectively (Owens et al., 1999; Thompson & Christakis, 2005; Van den Bulck, 2004; Johnson, Cohen, Kasen, First, & Brook, 2004; see Gradisar and Short, Chapter 11). Less is known regarding the association between sleep duration and children's engagement in subsequent physical activity. One study with adolescents found that those who reported sleeping more also reported exercising more regularly (Chen, Wang, & Jeng, 2006), while a second study found no effect for measured sleep length on activity level (Gupta et al., 2002). Thus, although there is some signal for an association between children's sleep duration and engagement in sedentary and physical activity, the strength of this signal is unclear. Furthermore, it is possible that activity level underlies difficulties with both sleep and weight rather than mediating this association (e.g., watching more television leads to increased sleep disturbance and increased weight difficulties). However, more work is needed to delineate the true role of activity in the sleep-weight relationship.

Review of Study Limitations and Areas for Future Research

With few notable exceptions studies have consistently found that insufficient or short sleep duration is associated with an increased risk for obesity. Consistency in study findings across heterogeneous groups varying in age, sex, race, ethnicity, and nationality is striking. Furthermore, the persistence of a significant finding despite statistical control for a number of potential confounding factors suggests that there is a strong signal between children's sleep length and risk for being overweight or obese. Despite this impressive consistency, a number of study limitations are important to note.

First, from a methodological perspective, previous pediatric studies have relied heavily upon observational studies (Cappuccio et al., 2008. Hart et al., 2011; Hart, Kuhl, & Jelalian, 2012; Nielsen, Danielsen, & Sorensen, 2010). Although prospective studies can help to establish associations between short sleep and higher weight status, they cannot demonstrate that if a child were to sleep more he/she would either lose weight or maintain his/her current weight status. Self-report has also been the primary mode of collecting data regarding children's sleep duration, which is only moderately associated with objective assessments of sleep (Lockley, Skene, & Arendt, 1999). Additionally, it is important to note that some studies have not found an association between sleep duration and obesity status (Hiscock, Scalzo, Canterford, & Wake, 2011) or have found that the significance of findings either remitted once confounding factors were accounted for (Hassan, Davis & Chervin, 2011) or varied based on how sleep was measured (Knutson & Lauderdale, 2007). It has also been noted that sleep needs may vary from one individual to the next (Gozal & Kheirandish-Gozal, 2012), which may have important implications for interpretation of study findings to date. Finally, the pathways of the sleep–obesity relationship remain largely unclear, especially within pediatric samples.

A favored interpretation of observational findings is that we should begin to enhance sleep duration to help combat the obesity epidemic (Ayas, 2010; Sivak, 2006). Unfortunately, due to limitations noted above, epidemiological findings cannot effectively argue for a sleep intervention to help with weight control. Findings do provide sufficient evidence to suggest that this line of research is important to pursue and presents a unique opportunity for building the necessary research foundation for an innovative approach to weight control. Key questions that could help shape intervention development are outlined below.

What Sleep Variables Should We Target in Interventions Aimed at Decreasing Obesity Risk?

Although extant pediatric studies only support associations (rather than a causal relationship) between sleep and weight, when considered in light of experimental studies with adults the argument that enhancing sleep could help with weight control is more compelling. The vast majority of studies conducted to date have focused on sleep duration. Thus, investigating the role of duration of sleep—particularly through experimental manipulation and/or intervention—on weight and weight-related behaviors is important. Beyond sleep duration, recent studies have begun to explore the potential effect of additional sleep variables, including sleep timing and variability, on weight status (Maddah, Rashidi, Mohammadpour, Vafa, & Karandish, 2009; Olds, Blunden, Dollman, & Maher, 2010; Sekine, Yamagami, Hamanishi, et al., 2002; Sekine, Yamagami, Handa et al., 2002). Exploration of the potential influence of these variables is supported by findings from animal models suggesting that circadian clocks play an important role in metabolism and obesity (Bray & Young, 2007), and from emerging data from adult experimental studies, which suggest circadian influences on hunger and appetite (Scheer, Morris, & Shea, 2013) and increased food intake (Markwald et al., 2013). It has also been suggested that changes in sleep duration, which are often accounted for by earlier bedtimes, may also reflect a better alignment with endogenous circadian rhythms. Findings from pediatric studies suggest that later bedtimes (as opposed to rise times) are associated with increased obesity risk (Maddah et al., 2009; Olds et al., 2010; Sekine, Yamagami,

Handa, et al., 2002; Snell et al., 2007). They have also found that irregular sleep habits are associated with obesity risk, be it weekday/weekend sleep variability being associated with concurrent obesity risk (Spruyt et al., 2011) or parent report of irregular sleeping habits predicting their child's obesity risk in young adulthood (Al Mamun et al., 2007). Finally, there is evidence suggesting that "catching up" on sleep on weekends and/or holidays may be protective against a higher weight status (Lytle, Pasch, & Farbakhsh, 2011; Wing, Li, Li, Zhang, & Kong, 2009).

Accumulating evidence suggests that duration of sleep may not be the only sleep factor associated with pediatric obesity risk. Rather, it may be important to assess how changing a number of sleep-related factors affects children's weight status. In particular, it will be interesting to try and reconcile the potential benefit of "catching up" on sleep on weekends/holidays with the benefit of regularity of sleep, given that each may be associated with particular benefits for weight status (Hart et al., 2011; Hart et al., 2012). It may be that a balance is needed between maintaining some consistency in an effort to promote good sleep hygiene practices while also allowing for limited sleep extension when children's schedules allow (such as on weekends and holidays).

Should We Consider Targeting Possible Factors that May Underlie Problems with Sleep and Obesity?

Several pathways linking short sleep with obesity status have been hypothesized, including the possibility that a shared underlying factor exerts simultaneous influence on both sleep duration and weight. Thus, it is possible that we should intervene on some third factor that could affect change in both sleep and weight simultaneously. In this way, short sleep and obesity should be considered comorbid conditions that could benefit from a common intervention (Hart et al., 2011; Hart & Jelalian, 2008).

Parenting styles have been associated with both sleep and weight status (Adam et al., 2007; Arredondo et al., 2006; Meltzer & Montgomery-Downs, 2011; Sleddens et al., 2011). Furthermore, empirically supported treatment approaches for both sleep difficulties and behavioral weight loss intervene upon common parenting variables, including positive reinforcement, effective limit setting, and self-monitoring (Hart et al., 2011; Hart & Jelalian, 2008). In addition, there is evidence from a recent intervention designed to decrease obesity risk in infants that targeting parenting practices could be effective for promoting healthy weight status (Paul et al., 2011). Although part of a multicomponent intervention, one core intervention component in this study included the provision of skills to help parents soothe their child in an effort to minimize non–hunger-related feeding and maximize sleep. When incorporated with other parenting skills aimed at appropriate feeding behaviors, the combined intervention showed promise at effectively lowering weight status at 1 year (Paul et al., 2011).

Who Should Be Targeted in Sleep Interventions?

A number of studies to date have not only suggested that different sleep variables may be important to target in future investigations, but also that certain groups of individuals may particularly benefit from sleep interventions. Two groups seem to stand out the most: younger children and males. Reviews and meta-analyses demonstrate that the association between sleep duration and obesity risk is stronger and more consistent in younger age groups (Cappuccio et al., 2008; Patel & Hu, 2008). Thus, interventions targeted at younger children may reap greater benefits than those targeting older children and adolescents.

Similarly, a meta-analysis found a stronger association between sleep duration and obesity in boys than in girls (Chen et al., 2008). However, subsequent studies have been mixed (Ozturk et al., 2009; Tatone-Tokuda et al., 2011; Hitze et al., 2009; Sun, Sekine, & Kagamimori, 2009). It is possible that the noted effects for younger age and male gender may reflect an underlying influence of pubertal status on the sleep–weight association (Hart et al., 2012). However, this remains unknown at this time.

What is the Impact of Weight Loss on Improving Treatment and Overall Health Outcomes for Children with Comorbid Obesity and SDB?

Given the association between obesity and SDB, including the risk of weight gain following adenotonsillectomy, it is important to consider whether weight loss treatment could be an effective treatment option for children with comorbid obesity and SDB. Although evidence is sparse, there is some data suggesting that weight loss treatment may be effective at decreasing SDB symptoms in obese children (Van Hoorenbeeck et al., 2012; Verhulst, Franckx, Van Gaal, De Backer, & Desager, 2009).

Specifically, in children 10–18 years old, one study found a 71% remission rate in SDB following a residential weight loss program (Van Hoorenbeeck et al., 2012). A second study conducted by the same group found that a residential weight loss program was also effective at reducing SDB symptoms in adolescents. In that study, 62% of adolescents who had SDB prior to treatment no longer had SDB following residential weight loss treatment (Verhulst et al., 2009). It is important to note that both studies were conducted in residential settings where weight losses are much higher than what is seen in standard behavioral treatment (SBT) for weight loss. Thus, it is likely that SBT for weight loss will not have as large an impact on SDB symptoms. Nevertheless, the promise of weight loss in treatment of SDB deserves further study.

Conclusions

Epidemiological studies demonstrate that inadequate sleep is associated with increased risk of obesity in children. Additional work suggests that short sleep is associated with neuroendocrine profiles concomitant with increased weight status, as well as eating and activity behaviors that favor increases in adiposity. Despite the consistency in findings, it is still unclear whether enhancing children's sleep could have a significant impact on our current obesity epidemic and consequent potential increase in pediatric SDB. However, a number of avenues appear worthy of future exploration, including the potential role of parenting behaviors in promoting both longer sleep and decreased obesity risk, the utility of not only enhancing sleep duration, but also minimizing variability (while maximizing the ability to "catch up" on sleep when needed), and consideration of targeted sleep intervention approaches (i.e., directed at younger children and males) to decrease obesity risk. It is clear that the field is at a point where we need to move beyond correlations. What remains unknown is how significant an impact enhancing sleep will have on effecting changes in children's weight.

Future Directions

- What effect will enhancing sleep duration have on changes in children's weight and/or obesity status?
- What additional underlying factors might account for the association evidenced between sleep duration and obesity risk?
- Other than sleep duration, are there additional sleep parameters that might influence obesity risk?
- Who will benefit the most from interventions to enhance sleep duration?

References

Adam, E. K., Snell, E. K., & Pendry, P. (2007). Sleep timing and quantity in ecological and family context: a nationally representative time-diary study. *Journal of Family Psychology, 21*(1), 4–19.

Al Mamun, A., Lawlor, D. A., Cramb, S., O'Callaghan, M., Williams, G., & Najman, J. (2007). Do childhood sleeping problems predict obesity in young adulthood? Evidence from a prospective birth cohort study. *American Journal of Epidemiology, 166*(12), 1368–1373.

Arredondo, E. M., Elder, J. P., Ayala, G. X., Campbell, N., Baquero, B., & Duerksen, S. (2006). Is parenting style related to children's healthy eating and physical activity in Latino families? *Health Education Research, 21*(6), 862–871.

Ayas, N. T. (2010). If you weigh too much, maybe you should try sleeping more. *Sleep, 33*, 143–144.

Beebe, D. W. (2011). Cognitive, behavioral, and functional consequences of inadequate sleep in children and adolescents. *Pediatric Clinics of North America, 58*(3), 649–665.

Beebe D. W., Simon S, Summer S, Hemmer S, Strotman D, Dolan LM. (2013). Dietary intake following experimentally restricted sleep in adolescents. *Sleep, 36,* 827–834.

Bell, J. F., & Zimmerman, F. J. (2010). Shortened nighttime sleep duration in early life and subsequent childhood obesity. *Archives of Pediatrics and Adolescent Medicine, 164*(9), 840–845.

Benedict, C., Hallschmid, M., Lassen, A., Mahnke, C., Schultes, B., Schioth, H. B., et al. (2011). Acute sleep deprivation reduces energy expenditure in healthy men. *American Journal of Clinical Nutrition, 93*(6), 1229–1236.

Bornhorst, C., Hense, S., Ahrens, W., Hebestreit, A., Reisch, L., Barba, G., von Kries, R., & Bayer, O., on behalf of the IDEFICS Consortium (2012). From sleep duration to childhood obesity-what are the pathways? *European Journal of Pediatrics, 171*, 1029–1038.

Bray, M. S., & Young, M. E. (2007). Circadian rhythms in the development of obesity: potential role for the circadian clock within the adipocyte. *Obesity Reviews, 8*(2), 169–181.

Brondel, L., Romer, M. A., Nougues, P. M., Touyarou, P., & Davenne, D. (2010). Acute partial sleep deprivation increases food intake in healthy men. *American Journal of Clinical Nutrition, 91*(6), 1550–1559.

Brown, T., & Summerbell, C. (2009). Systematic review of school-based interventions that focus on changing dietary intake and physical activity levels to prevent childhood obesity: an update to the obesity guidance produced by the National Institute for Health and Clinical Excellence. *Obesity Reviews, 10*(1), 110–141.

Cappuccio, F. P., Taggart, F. M., Kandala, N. B., Currie, A., Peile, E., Stranges, S., et al. (2008). Meta-analysis of short sleep duration and obesity in children and adults. *Sleep, 31*(5), 619–626.

Chaput, J. P., & Tremblay, A. (2007). Does short sleep duration favor abdominal adiposity in children? *International Journal of Pediatric Obesity, 2*(3), 188–191.

Chen, M. Y., Wang, E. K., & Jeng, Y. J. (2006). Adequate sleep among adolescents is positively associated with health status and health-related behaviors. *BMC Public Health, 6*, 59.

Chen, X., Beydoun, M. A., & Wang, Y. (2008). Is sleep duration associated with childhood obesity? A systematic review and meta-analysis. *Obesity (Silver Spring), 16*(2), 265–274.

Cole, T. J., Bellizzi, M. C., Flegal, K. M., & Dietz, W. H. (2000). Establishing a standard definition for child overweight and obesity worldwide: international survey. *British Medical Journal, 320*(7244), 1240–1243.

Costa, D. J., & Mitchell, R. (2009). Adenotonsillectomy for obstructive sleep apnea in obese children: a meta-analysis. *Otolaryngology – Head and Neck Surgery, 140*(4), 455–460.

Cruz, M. L., Shaibi, G. Q., Weigensberg, M. J., Spruijt-Metz, D., Ball, G. D., & Goran, M. I. (2005). Pediatric obesity and insulin resistance: chronic disease risk and implications for treatment and prevention beyond body weight modification. *Annual Review of Nutrition, 25*, 435–468.

Cuevas, A., Miquel, J. F., Reyes, M. S., Zanlungo, S., & Nervi, F. (2004). Diet as a risk factor for cholesterol gallstone disease. *Journal of the American College of Nutrition, 23*(3), 187–196.

Cummings, D. E. (2006). Ghrelin and the short- and long-term regulation of appetite and body weight. *Physiology & Behavior, 89*(1), 71–84.

Daftary, A. S., & Kotagal, S. (2010). Treatment of childhood obstructive sleep apnea. *Current Treatment Options in Neurology, 12*(5), 369–378.

Daniels, S. R. (2006). The consequences of childhood overweight and obesity. *Future Child, 16*(1), 47–67.

Diethelm, K., Bolzenius, K., Cheng, G., Remer, T., & Buyken, A. E. (2011). Longitudinal associations between reported sleep duration in early childhood and the development of body mass index, fat mass index and fat free mass index until age 7. *International Journal of Pediatric Obesity, 6*(2–2), e114–123.

Dollman, J., Ridley, K., Olds, T., & Lowe, E. (2007). Trends in the duration of school-day sleep among 10- to 15-year-old South Australians between 1985 and 2004. *Acta Paediatrica, 96*(7), 1011–1014.

Eisenmann, J. C., Ekkekakis, P., & Holmes, M. (2006). Sleep duration and overweight among Australian children and adolescents. *Acta Paediatrica, 95*(8), 956–963.

Epstein, L. H., Valoski, A., Wing, R. R., & McCurley, J. (1994). Ten-year outcomes of behavioral family-based treatment for childhood obesity. *Health Psychology, 13*(5), 373–383.

Fishbein, M. H., Miner, M., Mogren, C., & Chalekson, J. (2003). The spectrum of fatty liver in obese children and the relationship of serum aminotransferases to severity of steatosis. *Journal of Pediatric Gastroenterology and Nutrition, 36*(1), 54–61.

Flint, J., Kothare, S. V., Zihlif, M., Suarez, E., Adams, R., Legido, A., et al. (2007). Association between inadequate sleep and insulin resistance in obese children. *Journal of Pediatrics, 150*(4), 364–369.

Freedman, D. S., Dietz, W. H., Srinivasan, S. R., & Berenson, G. S. (1999). The relation of overweight to cardiovascular risk factors among children and adolescents: the Bogalusa Heart Study. *Pediatrics, 103*(6 Pt 1), 1175–1182.

Garaulet, M., Ortega, F. B., Ruiz, J. R., Rey-Lopez, J. P., Beghin, L., Manios, Y., et al. (2011). Short sleep duration is associated with increased obesity markers in European adolescents: effect of physical activity and dietary habits. The HELENA study. *International Journal of Obesity (London), 35*(10), 1308–1317.

Gozal, D., & Kheirandish-Gozal, L. (2012). Childhood obesity and sleep: Relatives, partners or both?—A critical perspective on the evidence. *Annals of the New York Academy of Sciences, 1264*, 135–141.

Griffiths, L. J., Wolke, D., Page, A. S., & Horwood, J. P. (2006). Obesity and bullying: different effects for boys and girls. *Archives of Disease in Childhood, 91*(2), 121–125.

Grow, H. M., Cook, A. J., Arterburn, D. E., Saelens, B. E., Drewnowski, A., & Lozano, P. (2010). Child obesity associated with social disadvantage of children's neighborhoods. *Social Science & Medicine, 71*(3), 584–591.

Guilleminault, C., Lee, J. H., & Chan, A. (2005). Pediatric obstructive sleep apnea syndrome. *Archives of Pediatrics and Adolescent Medicine, 159*(8), 775–785.

Gupta, N., Goel, K., Shah, P., & Misra, A. (2012). Childhood obesity in developing countries: Epidemiology, determinants, and prevention. *Endocrinology Reviews, 33*(1), 48–70.

Gupta, N. K., Mueller, W. H., Chan, W., & Meininger, J. C. (2002). Is obesity associated with poor sleep quality in adolescents? *American Journal of Human Biology, 14*(6), 762–768.

Hannon, T. S., Rao, G., & Arslanian, S. A. (2005). Childhood obesity and type 2 diabetes mellitus. *Pediatrics, 116*(2), 473–480.

Hart, C. N., & Jelalian, E. (2008). Shortened sleep duration is associated with pediatric overweight. *Behavioral Sleep Medicine, 6*(4), 251–267.

Hart, C. N., Cairns, A., & Jelalian, E. (2011). Sleep and obesity in children and adolescents. *Pediatric Clinics of North America, 58*(3), 715–733.

Hart, C.N., Kuhl, E., & Jelalian, E. (in press). Short sleep and obesity risk in children. In: P. Shiromani, T. Horvath, S. Redline, and E. van Cauter (Eds.) *Sleep Loss and Obesity: Intersecting Epidemics,* New York: Springer.

Hassan, F., Davis, M. M., & Chervin, R. D. (2011). No independent association between insufficient sleep and childhood obesity in the National Survey of Children's Health. *Journal of Clinical Sleep Medicine, 7*(2), 153–157.

Hiscock, H., Scalzo, K., Canterford, L., & Wake, M. (2011). Sleep duration and body mass index in 0–7-year olds. *Archives of Disease in Childhood, 96*(8), 735–739.

Hitze, B., Bosy-Westphal, A., Bielfeldt, F., Settler, U., Plachta-Danielzik, S., Pfeuffer, M., et al. (2009). Determinants and impact of sleep duration in children and adolescents: Data of the Kiel Obesity Prevention Study. *European Journal of Clinical Nutrition, 63*(6), 739–746.

Holub, S. C. (2008). Individual differences in the anti-fat attitudes of preschool-children: The importance of perceived body size. *Body Image, 5*(3), 317–321.

Iglowstein, I., Jenni, O. G., Molinari, L., & Largo, R. H. (2003). Sleep duration from infancy to adolescence: Reference values and generational trends. *Pediatrics, 111*(2), 302–307.

Jeyakumar, A., Fettman, N., Armbrecht, E. S., & Mitchell, R. (2011). A systematic review of adenotonsillectomy as a risk factor for childhood obesity. *Otolaryngology – Head and Neck Surgery, 144*(2), 154–158.

Johnson, J. G., Cohen, P., Kasen, S., First, M. B., & Brook, J. S. (2004). Association between television viewing and sleep problems during adolescence and early adulthood. *Archives of Pediatrics and Adolescent Medicine, 158*(6), 562–568.

Keith, S. W., Redden, D. T., Katzmarzyk, P. T., Boggiano, M. M., Hanlon, E. C., Benca, R. M., et al. (2006). Putative contributors to the secular increase in obesity: Exploring the roads less traveled. *International Journal of Obeseity (London), 30*(11), 1585–1594.

Klingenberg L, Chaput JP, Holmback U, Jennum P, Astrup A, & Sjodin A. (2012). Sleep restriction is not associated with a positive energy balance in adolescent boys. *The American Journal of Clinical Nutrition, 96*, 240–248.

Knutson, K. L., & Lauderdale, D. S. (2007). Sleep duration and overweight in adolescents: Self-reported sleep hours versus time diaries. *Pediatrics, 119*(5), e1056–1062.

Knutson, K. L., Spiegel, K., Penev, P., & Van Cauter, E. (2007). The metabolic consequences of sleep deprivation. *Sleep Medicine Reviews, 11*(3), 163–178.

Knutson, K. L., & Van Cauter, E. (2008). Associations between sleep loss and increased risk of obesity and diabetes. *Annals of the New York Academy of Sciences,* 1129, 287–304.

Knutson, K. L. (2012). Does inadequate sleep play a role in vulnerability to obesity? *American Journal of Human Biology, 24*(3), 361–371.

Landhuis, C. E., Poulton, R., Welch, D., & Hancox, R. J. (2008). Childhood Sleep Time and Long-term risk for obesity: A 32-year prospective birth cohort study. *Pediatrics, 122*(5), 955–960.

Landis, A. M., Parker, K. P., & Dunbar, S. B. (2009). Sleep, hunger, satiety, food cravings, and caloric intake in adolescents. *Journal of Nursing Scholarship, 41*(2), 115–123.

Levin, F., Edholm, T., Schmidt, P. T., Gryback, P., Jacobsson, H., Degerblad, M., et al. (2006). Ghrelin stimulates gastric emptying and hunger in normal-weight humans. *Journal of Clinical Endocrinology & Metabolism, 91*(9), 3296–3302.

Lockley, S. W., Skene, D. J., & Arendt, J. (1999). Comparison between subjective and actigraphic measurement of sleep and sleep rhythms. *Journal of Sleep Research, 8*(3), 175–183.

Lugo-Vicente, H. L. (1997). Trends in management of gallbladder disorders in children. *Pediatric Surgery International, 12*(5–6), 348–352.

Lytle, L. A., Pasch, K. E., & Farbakhsh, K. (2011). The relationship between sleep and weight in a sample of adolescents. *Obesity (Silver Spring), 19*(2), 324–331.

Maddah, M., Rashidi, A., Mohammadpour, B., Vafa, R., & Karandish, M. (2009). In-school snacking, breakfast consumption, and sleeping patterns of normal and overweight Iranian high school girls: a study in urban and rural areas in Guilan, Iran. *Journal of Nutrion Education and Behavior, 41*(1), 27–31.

Margulies, A. S., Floyd, R. G., & Hojnoski, R. L. (2008). Body size stigmatization: an examination of attitudes of African American preschool-age children attending Head Start. *Journal of Pediatric Psychology, 33*(5), 487–496.

Markwald, R. R., Melanson, E. L., Smith, M. R., Higgins, J., Perreault, L., Eckel, R. H., & Wright, Jr., K. P. (2013). Impact of insufficient sleep on total daily energy expenditure, food intake, and weight gain. *Proceedings of the National Academy of Sciences, 110,* www.pnas.org/cgi/doi/10.1073/pnas.1216951110.

Matricciani, L., Olds, T., & Petkov, J. (2011). In search of lost sleep: Secular trends in the sleep time of school-aged children and adolescents. *Sleep Medicine Reviews, 16*(3), 203–211.

McMurray, R. G., Harrell, J. S., Levine, A. A., & Gansky, S. A. (1995). Childhood obesity elevates blood pressure and total cholesterol independent of physical activity. *International Journal of Obesity and Related Metabolic Disorders, 19*(12), 881–886.

Meltzer, L. J., & Montgomery-Downs, H. E. (2011). Sleep in the family. *Pediatric Clinics of North America, 58*(3), 765–774.

Mullington, J. M., Chan, J. L., Van Dongen, H. P., Szuba, M. P., Samaras, J., Price, N. J., et al. (2003). Sleep loss reduces diurnal rhythm amplitude of leptin in healthy men. *Journal of Neuroendocrinology, 15*(9), 851–854.

Nathan, B. M., & Moran, A. (2008). Metabolic complications of obesity in childhood and adolescence: More than just diabetes. *Current Opinion in Endocrinology, Diabetes and Obesity, 15*(1), 21–29.

Nedeltcheva, A. V., Kilkus, J. M., Imperial, J., Kasza, K., Schoeller, D. A., & Penev, P. D. (2009). Sleep curtailment is accompanied by increased intake of calories from snacks, *American Journal of Clinical Nutrition, 89*, 126–133.

Neumark-Sztainer, D., Story, M., & Faibisch, L. (1998). Perceived stigmatization among overweight African-American and Caucasian adolescent girls. *Journal of Adolescent Health, 23*(5), 264–270.

Neumark-Sztainer, D., Falkner, N., Story, M., Perry, C., Hannan, P. J., & Mulert, S. (2002). Weight-teasing among adolescents: Correlations with weight status and disordered eating behaviors. *International Journal of Obesity and Related Metabolic Disorders, 26*(1), 123–131.

Nielsen, L. S., Danielsen, K. V., & Sorensen, T. I. (2010). Short sleep duration as a possible cause of obesity: Critical analysis of the epidemiological evidence. *Obesity Reviews, 12*(2), 78–92.

Nixon, G. M., Thompson, J. M., Han, D. Y., Becroft, D. M., Clark, P. M., Robinson, E., et al. (2008). Short sleep duration in middle childhood: Risk factors and consequences. *Sleep, 31*(1), 71–78.

Ogden, C. L., Carroll, M. D., Kit, B. K., & Flegal, K. M. (2012). Prevalence of obesity and trends in body mass index among US children and adolescents, 1999–2010. *Journal of the American Medical Association, 307*(5), 483–490.

Olds, T., Blunden, S., Dollman, J., & Maher, C. A. (2010). Day type and the relationship between weight status and sleep duration in children and adolescents. *Australian and New Zealand Journal of Public Health, 34*(2), 165–171.

Oude Luttikhuis, H., Baur, L., Jansen, H., Shrewsbury, V. A., O'Malley, C., Stolk, R. P., et al. (2009). Interventions for treating obesity in children. *Cochrane Database System Reviews*(1), CD001872.

Owens, J., Maxim, R., McGuinn, M., Nobile, C., Msall, M., & Alario, A. (1999). Television-viewing habits and sleep disturbance in school children. *Pediatrics, 104*(3), e27.

Ozturk, A., Mazicioglu, M., Poyrazoglu, S., Cicek, B., Gunay, O., & Kurtoglu, S. (2009). The relationship between sleep duration and obesity in Turkish children and adolescents. *Acta Paediatrica, 98*(4), 699–702.

Padez, C., Mourao, I., Moreira, P., & Rosado, V. (2009). Long sleep duration and childhood overweight/obesity and body fat. *American Journal of Human Biology, 21*, 371–376.

Patel, S. R., & Hu, F. B. (2008). Short sleep duration and weight gain: A systematic review. *Obesity (Silver Spring), 16*(3), 643–653.

Paul, I. M., Savage, J. S., Anzman, S. L., Beiler, J. S., Marini, M. E., Stokes, J. L., et al. (2011). Preventing obesity during infancy: A pilot study. *Obesity (Silver Spring), 19*(2), 353–361.

Power, C., Lake, J. K., & Cole, T. J. (1997). Measurement and long-term health risks of child and adolescent fatness. *International Journal of Obesity and Related Metabolic Disorders, 21*(7), 507–526.

Redline, S., Tishler, P. V., Schluchter, M., Aylor, J., Clark, K., & Graham, G. (1999). Risk factors for sleep-disordered breathing in children. Associations with obesity, race, and respiratory problems. *American Journal of Respiratory and Critical Care Medicine, 159*(5 Pt 1), 1527–1532.

Reilly, T., & Edwards, B. (2007). Altered sleep-wake cycles and physical performance in athletes. *Physiology & Behavior, 90*(2–3), 274–284.

Roberts, E. A. (2005). Non-alcoholic fatty liver disease (NAFLD) in children. *Frontiers in Bioscience, 10*, 2306–2318.

Roemmich, J. N., Barkley, J. E., D'Andrea, L., Nikova, M., Rogol, A. D., Carskadon, M. A., et al. (2006). Increases in overweight after adenotonsillectomy in overweight children with obstructive sleep-disordered breathing are associated with decreases in motor activity and hyperactivity. *Pediatrics, 117*(2), e200–208.

Scheer, F. A. J. L., Morris, C. J., & Shea, S. A. (2013). The internal circadian clock increases hunger and appetite in the evening independent of food intake and other behaviors. *Obesity, 21*, 421–423.

Schmid, S. M., Hallschmid, M., Jauch-Chara, K., Born, J., & Schultes, B. (2008). A single night of sleep deprivation increases ghrelin levels and feelings of hunger in normal-weight healthy men. *Journal of Sleep Research, 17*(3), 331–334.

Schmid, S. M., Hallschmid, M., Jauch-Chara, K., Wilms, B., Benedict, C., Lehnert, H., et al. (2009). Short-term sleep loss decreases physical activity under free-living conditions but does not increase food intake under time-deprived laboratory conditions in healthy men. *American Journal of Clinical Nutrition, 90*(6), 1476–1482.

Seegers, V., Petit, D., Falissard, B., Vitaro, F., Tremblay, R. E., Montplaisir, J., et al. (2011). Short sleep duration and body mass index: A prospective longitudinal study in preadolescence. *American Journal of Epidemiology, 173*(6), 621–629.

Sekine, M., Yamagami, T., Hamanishi, S., Handa, K., Saito, T., Nanri, S., et al. (2002). Parental obesity, lifestyle factors and obesity in preschool children: Results of the Toyama Birth Cohort study. *Journal of Epidemiology/Japan Epidemiological Society, 12*(1), 33–39.

Sekine, M., Yamagami, T., Handa, K., Saito, T., Nanri, S., Kawaminami, K., et al. (2002). A dose-response relationship between short sleeping hours and childhood obesity: Results of the Toyama Birth Cohort Study. *Child: Care, Health and Development, 28*(2), 163–170.

Serdula, M. K., Ivery, D., Coates, R. J., Freedman, D. S., Williamson, D. F., & Byers, T. (1993). Do obese children become obese adults? A review of the literature. *Prevention Medicine, 22*(2), 167–177.

Shea, S. A., Hilton, M. F., Orlova, C., Ayers, R. T., & Mantzoros, C. S. (2005). Independent circadian and sleep/wake regulation of adipokines and glucose in humans. *Journal of Clinical Endocrinology & Metabolism, 90*(5), 2537–2544.

Shi, Z., Taylor, A. W., Gill, T. K., Tuckerman, J., Adams, R., & Martin, J. (2010). Short sleep duration and obesity among Australian children. *BMC Public Health, 10*, 609.

Shrewsbury, V., & Wardle, J. (2008). Socioeconomic status and adiposity in childhood: A systematic review of cross-sectional studies 1990–2005. *Obesity (Silver Spring), 16*(2), 275–284.

Sinha, R., Fisch, G., Teague, B., Tamborlane, W. V., Banyas, B., Allen, K., et al. (2002). Prevalence of impaired glucose tolerance among children and adolescents with marked obesity. *New England Journal of Medicine, 346*(11), 802–810.

Sivak M. (2006). Sleeping more as a way to lose weight. *Obesity Reviews, 7*, 295–296.

Sleddens, E. F., Gerards, S. M., Thijs, C., de Vries, N. K., & Kremers, S. P. (2011). General parenting, childhood overweight and obesity-inducing behaviors: a review. *International Journal of Pediatric Obesity, 6*(2–2), e12–27.

Snell, E. K., Adam, E. K., & Duncan, G. J. (2007). Sleep and the body mass index and overweight status of children and adolescents. *Child Development, 78*(1), 309–323.

Soultan, Z., Wadowski, S., Rao, M., & Kravath, R. E. (1999). Effect of treating obstructive sleep apnea by tonsillectomy and/or adenoidectomy on obesity in children. *Archives of Pediatrics and Adolescent Medicine, 153*(1), 33–37.

Spiegel, K., Leproult, R., & Van Cauter, E. (1999). Impact of sleep debt on metabolic and endocrine function. *Lancet, 354*(9188), 1435–1439.

Spiegel, K., Leproult, R., L'Hermite-Baleriaux, M., Copinschi, G., Penev, P. D., & Van Cauter, E. (2004). Leptin levels are dependent on sleep duration: Relationships with sympathovagal balance, carbohydrate regulation, cortisol, and thyrotropin. *Journal of Clinical Endocrinology & Metabolism, 89*(11), 5762–5771.

Spiegel, K., Tasali, E., Penev, P., & Van Cauter, E. (2004). Brief communication: Sleep curtailment in healthy young men is associated with decreased leptin levels, elevated ghrelin levels, and increased hunger and appetite. *Annals of Internal Medicine, 141*(11), 846–850.

Spruyt, K., Molfese, D. L., & Gozal, D. (2011). Sleep duration, sleep regularity, body weight, and metabolic homeostasis in school-aged children. *Pediatrics, 127*(2), e345–352.

St-Onge, M. P., Roberts, A. L., Chen, J., Kelleman, M., O'Keeffe, M., RoyChoudhury, A., et al. (2011). Short sleep duration increases energy intakes but does not change energy expenditure in normal-weight individuals. *American Journal of Clinical Nutrition, 94*(2), 410–416.

Stamatakis, E., Zaninotto, P., Falaschetti, E., Mindell, J., & Head, J. (2010). Time trends in childhood and adolescent obesity in England from 1995 to 2007 and projections of prevalence to 2015. *Journal of Epidemiology & Community Health, 64*(2), 167–174.

Sun, Y., Sekine, M., & Kagamimori, S. (2009). Lifestyle and overweight among Japanese adolescents: the Toyama Birth Cohort Study. *Journal of Epidemiology/Japan Epidemiological Society, 19*(6), 303–310.

Taheri, S., Lin, L., Austin, D., Young, T., & Mignot, E. (2004). Short sleep duration is associated with reduced leptin, elevated ghrelin, and increased body mass index. *PLoS Med, 1*(3), e62.

Tatone-Tokuda, F., Dubois, L., Ramsay, T., Girard, M., Touchette, E., Petit, D., et al. (2011). Sex differences in the association between sleep duration, diet and body mass index: a birth cohort study. *Journal of Sleep Research, 21*(4), 448–460.

Thompson, D. A., & Christakis, D. A. (2005). The association between television viewing and irregular sleep schedules among children less than 3 years of age. *Pediatrics, 116*(4), 851–856.

Tian, Z., Ye, T., Zhang, X., Liu, E., Wang, W., Wang, P., et al. (2010). Sleep duration and hyperglycemia among obese and nonobese children aged 3 to 6 years. *Archives of Pediatrics and Adolescent Medicine, 164*(1), 46–52.

Touchette, E., Petit, D., Tremblay, R. E., Boivin, M., Falissard, B., Genolini, C., et al. (2008). Associations between sleep duration patterns and overweight/obesity at age 6. *Sleep, 31*(11), 1507–1514.

Tsiros, M. D., Olds, T., Buckley, J. D., Grimshaw, P., Brennan, L., Walkley, J., et al. (2009). Health-related quality of life

in obese children and adolescents. *International Journal of Obesity (London), 33*(4), 387–400.
Valente, A. M., Strong, W., & Sinaiko, A. R. (2001). Obesity and insulin resistance in young people. *American Heart Journal, 142*(3), 440–444.
Van Cauter, E., & Spiegel, K. (1999). Sleep as a mediator of the relationship between socioeconomic status and health: a hypothesis. *Annals of the New York Academy of Sciences, 896*, 254–261.
Van den Bulck, J. (2004). Television viewing, computer game playing, and Internet use and self-reported time to bed and time out of bed in secondary-school children. *Sleep, 27*(1), 101–104.
Van Hoorenbeeck, K., Franckx, H., Debode, P., Aerts, P., Wouters, K., Ramet, J., et al. (2012). Weight loss and sleep-disordered breathing in childhood obesity: Effects on inflammation and uric acid. *Obesity (Silver Spring), 20*(1), 172–177.
Verhulst, S. L., Schrauwen, N., Haentjens, D., Suys, B., Rooman, R. P., Van Gaal, L., et al. (2007). Sleep-disordered breathing in overweight and obese children and adolescents: Prevalence, characteristics and the role of fat distribution. *Archives of Disease in Childhood, 92*(3), 205–208.
Verhulst, S. L., Schrauwen, N., Haentjens, D., Rooman, R. P., Van Gaal, L., De Backer, W. A., et al. (2008). Sleep duration and metabolic dysregulation in overweight children and adolescents. *Archives of Disease in Childhood, 93*(1), 89–90.
Verhulst, S. L., Franckx, H., Van Gaal, L., De Backer, W., & Desager, K. (2009). The effect of weight loss on sleep-disordered breathing in obese teenagers. *Obesity (Silver Spring), 17*(6), 1178–1183.
von Kries, R., Toschke, A. M., Wurmser, H., Sauerwald, T., & Koletzko, B. (2002). Reduced risk for overweight and obesity in 5- and 6-y-old children by duration of sleep—a cross-sectional study. *International Journal of Obesity, 26*(5), 710–716.
Wang, Y., & Lobstein, T. (2006). Worldwide trends in childhood overweight and obesity. *International Journal of Pediatric Obesity, 1*(1), 11–25.
Wardle, J., & Cooke, L. (2005). The impact of obesity on psychological well-being. *Best Practice & Research: Clinical Endocrinology & Metabolism, 19*(3), 421–440.
Wearing, S. C., Hennig, E. M., Byrne, N. M., Steele, J. R., & Hills, A. P. (2006). The impact of childhood obesity on musculoskeletal form. *Obesity Reviews, 7*(2), 209–218.
Weiss, A., Xu, F., Storfer-Isser, A., Thomas, A., Ievers-Landis, C. E., & Redline, S. (2010). The association of sleep duration with adolescents' fat and carbohydrate consumption. *Sleep, 33*(9), 1201–1209.
Westerlund, L., Ray, C., & Roos, E. (2009). Associations between sleeping habits and food consumption patterns among 10–11-year-old children in Finland. *British Journal of Nutrition, 102*(10), 1531–1537.
Wing, Y. K., Li, S. X., Li, A. M., Zhang, J., & Kong, A. P. (2009). The effect of weekend and holiday sleep compensation on childhood overweight and obesity. *Pediatrics, 124*(5), e994-e1000.
Witmans, M., & Young, R. (2011). Update on pediatric sleep-disordered breathing. *Pediatric Clinics of North America, 58*(3), 571–589.
Yu, Y., Lu, B. S., Wang, B., Wang, H., Yang, J., Li, Z., et al. (2007). Short sleep duration and adiposity in Chinese adolescents. *Sleep, 30*(12), 1688–1697.

CHAPTER

31 Impact of Sleep on the Challenges of Safe Driving in Young Adults

Shelley Hershner

Abstract

Driving may well be the most dangerous activity for young adults. In 2007, motor vehicle crashes were the leading cause of death among 13–19-year-olds in the United States (Insurance Institute for Highway Safety, 2009). Contributing factors for this high rate of accidents include: driving inexperience, age of licensing, high risk driving situations, presence of passengers, substance use, drowsy driving, and risk-taking behaviors. This chapter will review the literature on certain key aspects of driving performance with an emphasis on how sleep deprivation, drowsy driving, and sleep may impact driving performance.

Key Words: adolescents, teenagers, drowsy driving, motor vehicle accidents (mvas), risk-taking behaviors, sleep deprivation, circadian rhythms, alcohol, driving

Introduction

Driving is an inherently dangerous activity for everyone but is especially perilous to teenagers; during 2009, 3466 teenagers (ages 13–19) died in the United States from motor vehicle accidents (MVAs; Insurance Institute for Highway Safety, 2009). In 2006, car accidents resulted in the death of a teenager every hour during the weekend days and every two hours during weekdays. (National Highway Traffic Safety Administration). There are many reasons for the increased risk of motor vehicle accidents and deaths in this population. Teenage drivers are inexperienced and may drive in high-risk situations including driving at night and with distractions both in the form of passengers and technology, including the use of cell phones, texting, and global positioning devices. Sleep is a risk factor that is not often considered in the risk analysis of teenage driving. Sleep deprivation and drowsy driving increase the risk of motor vehicle accidents. Certain times of the day and night, which may relate to circadian system, may also increase the risk of accidents. Additionally, sleep deprivation may change risk-taking behaviors and contribute to the use of substances such as alcohol that worsen driving performance. This chapter will review some of the non-sleep-related risk factors for motor vehicle accidents, explore in greater depth the causes of sleep deprivation and how it impacts driving safety, and look at the legal implications of drowsy driving. Potential interventions including driver education and prolonged driving training, as well as unexpected interventions such as changing school start times, will also be reviewed.

Teenager drivers are hazardous both to themselves and to other drivers, as approximately 20% of all passenger fatalities involve a teenage driver (Insurance Instiitute for Highway Safety, 2005). Teenagers have a disproportionately high percentage of motor vehicle accidents, as young adults aged 15–20 years-old account for 8.4% of the population but 11.6% of MVAs. Although the frequency of motor vehicle–related fatalities and accidents are concerning, overall fatalities in young adults have decreased by 15% from 2008 and by 60% from the 1960s.

Factors that Increase the Risk of an Accident

Psychosocial Issues

Several defining features of MVAs relate to the psychosocial circumstances of adolescents (Shope, 2006). Weekends are the riskiest days, as 54% of MVAs occurred on Friday, Saturday, or Sunday (Insurance Institute for Highway Safety, 2006a). Half of accidents occur between the hours of 6:00 pm and 3:00 am. Many accidents are in context of socializing; 62% of teenage passenger deaths occurred in vehicles driven by another teenager, most within 5 miles (66%) of home with the purpose of the trip for socializing with friends or family (Braitman, Kirley, McCartt, & Chaudhary, 2008). Passengers increase the risk of a crash, although this is not a consistent finding in the literature (Hutchens, Senserrick, Jamieson, Romer, & Winston, 2008; Preusser, Ferguson, & Williams, 1998; Williams, 2003). Half of all MVA deaths of 16–17-year-olds occurred when passengers under 20 years of age were present without an adult (Williams & Ferguson, 2002). Males were 27% more likely to have an accident if three or more passengers were present in the vehicle. In this study, passengers in the car did not increase the risk for women (Rice, Peek-Asa, & Kraus, 2003). The presence of females as passengers may decrease the risk of MVAs (Simons-Morton et al., 2011).

High-Risk Driving Situations

Driver distractions from using cell phones and texting escalate the risk of crashes (Beede & Kass, 2006; Kass, Cole, & Stanny, 2007). Eighteen percent of teen accidents are thought to be due to driver distraction (National Highway Traffic Safety Administration, 2011). Alcohol, not surprisingly, augments the risk of an MVA significantly, as does driving in wet conditions and at higher speeds (Preusser et al., 1998; Rice et al., 2003). Age and inexperience are also factors. Teenagers are most likely to be involved in a motor vehicle accident immediately after licensure, which is typically between the ages of 16–18 years of age in the United States and at 18 years of age in other countries. The highest risk of accidents is at age 16 (Williams, 2003). In fact, the crash rate per mile driven is twice as high for 16-year-olds as it is for 18–19-year-olds (Insurance Institute for Highway Safety, 2009). The first month of driving may be the riskiest period, with self-reported accidents of 2.3 per 10,000 miles traveled; this declined to 0.5 crashes per 10,000 miles 11 months after licensure (McCartt, Shabanova, & Leaf, 2003). Males have more overall accidents than females, with an odds ratio of 3.3 (CI = 1.8–6.1 $p<.0001$), and males account for two out of every three teenagers killed (Insurance Institute for Highway Safety, 2006 (Insurance Institute for Highway Safety, 2009; Pizza et al., 2010). When accident rates are calculated by person miles driven (PMD), women may have more accidents compared to males (Rice et al., 2003). In Michigan, teenage males have 14.9 accidents per 100,000 PMD compared to 22.5 for female teenage drivers (Shope & Bingham, 2008). To contrast, in adult drivers (aged 45–65) men averaged 6.2 per 100,000 PMD versus women's 12.8.

Smoking

Smoking increases the risk of MVAs. In a telephone survey of drivers aged 14–22 years, smokers had a 54% greater odds of involvement in a car accident than nonsmokers (Hutchens et al., 2008). After controlling for gender, race, ethnicity, income, length of licensure, and geography, current cigarette smokers (smoked cigarettes in the last 30 days) were twice as likely to be involved in a crash. Smoking marijuana was also associated with a higher risk (36%) of crashes. Even after taking into account other general health-risk behaviors, (drinking alcohol and nonuse of seat belts) current smoking (both cigarettes and marijuana) had a strong association with crash risk. Why smoking impacts driving performance is not known, but may correlate to distractibility, one-handed steering (in order to hold the cigarette), an effect of nicotine (direct toxicity), increased propensity for risk-taking, or other unknown confounders. As smoking cigarettes and marijuana are both modifiable risk factors, further research is needed to better understand the relationship with smoking and crash risk.

Alcohol

All states and the District of Columbia have 21-year-old minimum drinking-age laws, with "alcohol-impaired" defined as a blood alcohol concentration (BAC) of 0.08 grams per deciliter (g/dL). In 2009, 28% of the young drivers (15 to 20 years old) killed in crashes had a BAC of .08 g/dL or higher (National Highway Traffic Safety Administration, 2009). Teenagers drink and drive less often than adults, but their risk of a related MVA is higher for all blood alcohol levels (Williams, 2003; Zador, Krawchuk, & Voas, 2000). Students in grades 9–12 admit to a lifetime alcohol use of 47.9% and current use of 30.4%. Alcohol-impaired driving was reported by 13.9%. Thirty-four percent of teenagers were a passenger with a driver that had consumed alcohol (Nelson, Naimi, Brewer, & Nelson, 2009). In a study of Italian teenagers, 14% of teenagers involved in a crash believed that alcohol was causative (Pizza et al., 2010).

Drowsy Driving:

Sleep, sleep deprivation, and daytime sleepiness are not often considered among the typical adolescent risk factors for motor vehicle accidents. But these underappreciated risk factors are significant and can have considerable impact on daytime sleepiness and driving performance. Most importantly, these sleep factors may be modifiable; reducing sleep deprivation and improving daytime alertness may decrease accidents.

Drowsy driving is prevalent among adolescents and young adults and is associated with increased fatal and nonfatal accidents. In the 2011 *Sleep in America Poll*, 30% of 13–18-year-olds and 66% of adults aged 19–29 admitted drowsy driving within the last month (National Sleep Foundation, 2011). By the 12th grade, 62% of students are driving daily, with 9% having fallen asleep at the wheel (National Sleep Foundation, 2006). Sleepiness while driving increases the risk of an accident two-fold (Pizza et al., 2010).

Etiology of Sleep Deprivation

To better understand drowsy driving, it is important to understand the etiology of drowsiness in this demographic. Drowsiness can occur for multiple reasons, including sleep deprivation, sleep disorders, and normal circadian rhythms. As discussed in detail in Chapters 8, 17, and 23, daytime sleepiness and inadequate sleep are common among teenagers. Most (61%) get less than 8 hours of sleep, while 59% wake non-refreshed in the morning (National Sleep Foundation, 2011). Concurrently, as young adults curtail their sleep they have an actual increase in sleep requirement (Carskadon, 1990). In a study by Oginska and Pokorski (2006), 36% of adolescents and 50% of college students admit having daytime sleepiness compared 36% of adults. Sleep deprivation is not the only cause of daytime sleepiness; sleep disorders and circadian rhythms may also contribute.

Circadian and Homeostatic Factors

Several factors work synergistically to place adolescents at risk for sleep deprivation and daytime sleepiness (see Carskadon, Chapter 8). Adolescents have a delayed circadian preference. The nocturnal preference, or shift of the circadian system to a later time, has been associated with puberty. The circadian system is an endogenous oscillating rhythm that helps to regulate sleep/wake cycles, feeding, and hormonal secretions. Melatonin, secreted by the pineal gland, helps regulate and entrain the circadian rhythm to the environment. Light, even as low 200–300 lux (room lights) can suppress endogenous melatonin (Zeitzer, Dijk, Kronauer, Brown, & Czeisler, 2000). This is important, as young adults often use technology prior to sleep. The other major component of the sleep/wake cycle is the homeostatic sleep drive. This process is conceptualized as a sleep drive, meaning the longer the period of wakefulness the stronger the drive to sleep. The interaction of these two systems is termed the *Two-Process Model* of sleep regulation (Borbely, 1982). Adolescents' nocturnal preference correlates with physical development as ascertained by their Tanner stage (Trockel, & Taylor, 2009; Carskadon, Vieira, & Acebo, 1993). In other words, physically more mature adolescents have a preference for later activities and bedtimes. The typical adult circadian period is 24.1 hours, compared to an adolescent's circadian period of 24.27 hours (Crowley, Acebo, & Carskadon, 2007; O'Brien & Mindell, 2005). This longer circadian period, or intrinsic day, allows the circadian system to more easily shift to later times. Sleep latency, which is a measure of sleep pressure or the homeostatic sleep drive, is also dependent upon physical maturity: subjects with a Tanner stage of 1 fall asleep faster than subjects with a Tanner stage 5 (Taylor, Jenni, Acebo, & Carskadon, 2005). The net effect of these physiologic changes appears to contribute to the nocturnal preference that develops during adolescence.

Sleep patterns from adolescence to adulthood

Exactly when this nocturnal preference or "night owl" tendency diminishes remains unclear (see Thacher, Chapter 40). When sleep patterns were evaluated longitudinally for 10 years, weekday bedtimes delayed until around 19 years of age (Thorleifsdottir, Bjornsson, Benediktsdottir, Gislason, & Kristbjarnarson, 2002). Weekend bedtimes remained late until the early 20s when it started to shift to earlier bedtimes. Across the transition from high school to college, a significant delay in bedtime was reported with college students going to bed 75 minutes later than high school students (Lund, Reider, Whiting, & Prichard, 2010). This delayed school-night bedtime continued until the junior and senior years of college.

Oversleeping or catch-up sleep on the weekend is a hallmark of a delayed circadian sleep phase. Sleep duration is normal when a person is on his or her preferred sleep schedule without external obligations such as morning employment or classes. Individuals with a delayed sleep phase often have inadequate sleep during the week and sleep later on the weekend to catch up on missed sleep. This delayed circadian rhythm and early-morning school start time can cause insufficient sleep leading to drowsy driving.

Drowsy Driving

Insufficient Sleep

Adolescents 14–22 years of age who sleep less than 8 hours per night have a 28% increased risk of an MVA (Hutchens et al., 2008). Nighttime driving is risky for all drivers, but the risk is much more pronounced in drivers under 25 years of age, with increased risk during later hours (Williams, 2003). Among 16–17-year-olds in California, an 86% increased risk of accidents occurred between the hours of 12:00–2:00 am compared to 8:00–10:00 pm (Rice et al., 2003). Early morning hours of 4:00–6:00 am have an astounding 929% increased risk (OR 9.29). This high risk in the early morning hours may signify both circadian factors and acute sleep deprivation. Details of individual accidents were not provided, but very early mornings may reflect near 24 hours of sleep deprivation as young adults with "all-nighters" are returning to home, work, or school. Vigilance decreases in the early morning hours and this effect can be augmented by alcohol (Lucidi, Devoto, Bertini, Braibanti, & Violani, 2002). The higher frequency of accidents during typical school commute times may relate to the higher number of students driving from school to work or extracurricular activities (Hellinga, McCartt, & Mandavilli, 2007). The overall trend for increased accidents with later hours may be the result of several different factors including drowsiness, sustained wakefulness, and circadian patterns.

School Start Time

Further elucidating the association between high school start time and MVAs (see Au, Appleman, and Stavitsky, Chapter 38), a school with an earlier start time had a higher community accident rate among 16–18-year-olds when compared to a school with a later start time (Vorona et al., 2011). Accidents were most common between 7:00–8:00 am and 2:00–5:00 pm coinciding with the commutes to school and to after-school activities. The increased rate of accidents in the morning might also be a manifestation of sleep inertia, while the afternoon rise might be indicative of increased sleepiness due to circadian rhythms. A change as small as 30 minutes later in school start times decreased teenage crash rates (Danner & Phillips, 2008). Other studies have shown this small change can decrease daytime sleepiness and increase sleep duration (Owens, 2010). These studies denote a relationship between MVAs and school start time but do not provide a causal relationship.

Emerging adults are also at risk for drowsy driving. Among 1039 undergraduate students in one survey, 16% reported falling asleep while driving and 2% had had a motor vehicle accident due to sleepiness. Men were more likely to fall asleep than women (16% vs. 14%) (Taylor & Bramoweth, 2010). A school in Utah had 86 student deaths due to motor vehicle accidents in a 15-year period; dozing/sleepiness was thought to be causative in 44%–72% of the cases. When asked about their "closest call" for a motor vehicle accident due to sleepiness, freshman and sophomore college students were at greatest risk. Peak hours were between 11:00 pm and 1:00 am; 40% of the events occurred within the first hour of driving. Nearly half (48%) of students had a less intense dozing episode during the same drive, while 68% of students continued their drive (Lindsay, Hanks, Hurley, & Dane, 1999). Teenagers also minimize or ignore drowsiness while driving, as 81% kept driving despite feeling sleepy (Pizza et al., 2010). It may be that young adults minimize the warning signs of drowsiness.

Sleep Deprivation and Alcohol

Sustained wakefulness can impair driving performance to an extent similar to that produced by blood alcohol levels. Sustained wakefulness of 17 hours was equivalent to a blood alcohol level of 0.05%, and 24 hours was equivalent to 0.1% (Dawson & Reid, 1997). The legal level for intoxication is 0.08% in most of the United States, while other countries are quite variable, ranging from 0.0 (below detection) up to to 0.8% (International Center For Alcohol Policies, 2013). Similar finding were reported in males ages 19–35 years where 18.5 and 21 hours of wakefulness produced changes in driving performance similar to 0.05% and 0.08% blood alcohol concentration. Alcohol, when compared to prolonged wakefulness, produced greater changes in speed deviation and off-road occurrences. Prolonging wakefulness even as little as 3 hours (equivalent to 18.5 hours of wakefulness) can impair driving to a similar extent as alcohol (Arnedt, Wilde, Munt, & MacLean, 2001). Sleep restriction in combination with alcohol has a synergistic effect on driving performance. To evaluate these effects, young male college students were sleep-restricted to 4 hours in bed; they then consumed alcohol until they attained blood BACs of 0.025 g/dL or 0.035 g/dL (Vakulin et al., 2007). These blood alcohol levels can be achieved with about one drink in most individuals and are below the legal limit of 0.08%. A simulated driving task at 2:00 pm monitored crashes, speed variability, and deviations. Crashes occurred in 23% and 33% of the subjects (BAC = 0.025g/dL and 0.035 g/dL respectively).

Alcohol consumption in young adults is common. Surveys have reported that 46% of teenagers have consumed alcohol (McKnight-Eily et al., 2011). Emerging adults often drink alcohol, and driving after drinking is commonplace; up to 34% of students reported driving after drinking within the past 30 days (American College Health Association, 2007). The combination of sleep deprivation and drinking may be especially common in college students, as they may be sleep-deprived after studying for exams and are more likely to drink alcohol. The dangerous combination of sleep deprivation with alcohol could compromise driving performance even in young adults who are not legally intoxicated. Alcohol may also impair the ability to predict crash risk. University students from Australia were sleep-restricted to 5 hours time in bed and provided alcohol to a mean alcohol concentration of 0.35 ± 0.015g/dl. When compared to sleep deprivation alone, low-dose alcohol decreased female participants' ability to predict crashes from 85% to 38%. Sleep-deprived men's ability to predict crash risk was substantially less than sleep-deprived women's (37% compared to 85%) and the addition of alcohol to sleep deprivation produced essentially no change in men's performance (33%; Banks, Catcheside, Lack, Grunstein, & McEvoy, 2004).

Changes in Driving Performance with Sleep Deprivation

Simulated Driving

Driving while sleepy causes several changes in driving performance. During driving simulation, prolonged wakefulness increases speed variability, tracking variability, and off-road events, although to a lesser extent than alcohol. Sleepy drivers showed worse vehicle control the longer they drove (Paul, 2005). Sleepiness causes a decrease in awareness of the environment and a slower reaction time; an average reaction time during alertness is 100–400 milliseconds, which decreased during sleepiness to 800–1200 milliseconds or longer (Culp, Gindy, & Haque, 2008). The addition of alcohol to sleep deprivation can increase lane variability and the presence of theta waves in the EEG (Horne, Reyner, & Barrett, 2003).

Microsleep Episodes

Microsleep episodes are changes in the electroencephalogram (EEG) frequency from the alpha rhythm (8–13 Hz) to the theta rhythm (4–7 Hz) lasting 3–14 seconds. It indicates a brief sleep onset and is characterized clinically by loss of attention and blank stares (Boyle, Tippin, Paul, & Rizzo, 2008). Microsleep episodes are associated with impaired ability to respond appropriately to the driving situation and increased lane and speed variability (Paul 2005). They have been associated with poor simulated driving performance (Risser, Ware, & Freeman, 2000). During driving simulation, microsleep episodes accompany a concurrent decrease in speed as subjects fail to maintain control over the accelerator pedal. Although not meeting the strict criteria for a microsleep episode, brief 3- second or longer changes in the EEG to a mix of increased alpha and theta can be associated with attention lapses (Risser et al., 2000).

Determining Sleep Onset

Understanding the onset of sleep is important when reviewing the risks of drowsy driving and potential interventions. During a polysomnogram, sleep onset is defined as the start of the first epoch scored as any stage other than wakefulness; normally this is stage 1 (N1) sleep (Iber, Ancoli-Israel, Chesson, & Quan, 2007). The EEG consists of low-amplitude theta activity (4–7 Hz) with slow eye movements and possibly the presence of vertex waves. Slow eye movements are conjugate, regular sinusoidal eye movements. However, this definition of sleep onset depends on the presence of an EEG and is rarely practical in real world driving circumstances. Other markers of sleep onset are of interest for both research and as possible interventions. One such marker of sleep onset is the decrease in eyelid movements and the emergence of slow rolling eye movements (SEM) during the transition from wakefulness to sleep (Atienza, Cantero, Stickgold, & Hobson, 2004). The presence of SEM correlates with

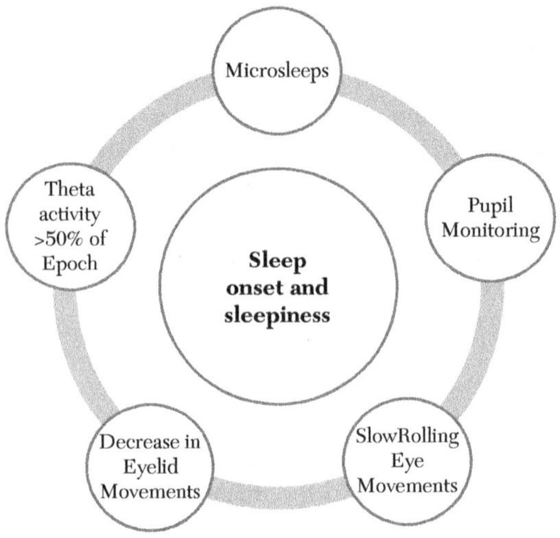

Figure 31.1 Sleep Onset and Sleepiness: Potential Options to Determine Sleep Onset and Decreased Alertness in Drivers

(Akerstedt & Gillberg, 1990; Atienza, Cantero, Stickgold, & Hobson, 2004; Iber, Ancoli-Israel, Chesson, & Quan, 2007), 2007; Kryger MH., 2011; Mitler & Miller, 1996).

decreased alertness (Akerstedt & Gillberg, 1990). Microsleep episodes can indicate sleep onset, but detecting them also requires the presence of an EEG. Pupillography may be an option to evaluate sleep onset in drivers (Kryger & Dement, 2011; Mitler & Miller, 1996). At the transition to sleep, parasympathetic activation constricts the pupil. Sleepiness is also associated with pupil size instability and speed of constriction. How pupillography could translate into monitoring drivers while driving is not clearly known, but monitoring pupil size could help alert drivers of potential drowsiness (see figure 31.1).

Risk-Taking Behaviors and Sleep Deprivation

Risk taking and sensation seeking behaviors increase MVAs in adolescence (Shope & Bingham, 2008; Shope, Raghunathan, & Patil, 2003). As a delay in the circadian system is linked to puberty, so are risk-taking behaviors, sensation seeking, and novelty seeking (Dahl, 2008). Physiologic changes interact with psychological and social factors, increasing risk-taking behaviors. Adolescents may not become immune to fear, but instead be more motivated to act boldly to enhance their social context. Developmentally, there also may be enhanced reward processing in the adolescent's brain when compared to the brain of an adult. Less activation is noted in the frontal cortex, an area responsible for executive function and self-control (Shope, 2006). Executive function is the ability to recognize future consequences resulting from current actions and to choose actions and modulate social responses (Pharo, Sim, Graham, Gross, & Hayne, 2011). The net sum of these factors is that adolescents may not be more risk prone, but rather more vulnerable to emotional influences affecting their risk while making decisions (Steinberg, 2004).

Sleep may also impact risk-taking behaviors. Some aspects of risk-taking behaviors may also be about sensation seeking and loss of self-regulation (Steinberg, 2004). Sleep deprivation may have an effect on the prefrontal cortex impairing executive function and resultant decision making and self-control (Catrett & Gaultney, 2009; Horne, 1993). Sleep deprivation and poor sleep quality can increase irritability, aggression, and impulsivity. In a survey of incarcerated juvenile and young adult males offenders, less total sleep was associated with increased aggression and impulsivity (Ireland & Culpin, 2006). Poor sleep quality predicted hostility. It is not implausible that increased aggression and hostility may exacerbate risky driving behaviors of speeding, lane changing, and failing to maintain distance between vehicles.

Risk-taking Behaviors, Substance Use, and Sleep

Risk-taking behaviors are prevalent in young adults with reported use of alcohol (46%–81%), marijuana (20%–47%), cigarette (21%–70%), and sexual behaviors (35%–49%; Kann et al., 2000; McKnight-Eily et al., 2011; O'Brien & Mindell, 2005). As students progress through high school, less sleep is obtained on school nights; in other words, 12th-graders get less sleep than 9th-graders 6.58 versus 7.44 hours; O'Brien & Mindell, 2005). Risk-taking behaviors also mirror these results, with increased risky behaviors of tobacco, alcohol, and marijuana use, and sexual behaviors in higher grades. Correlating total sleep time and risk-taking behaviors showed only a limited relationship with alcohol use and sexual behaviors. Students who slept less than 6 hours and 45 minutes on school nights were more likely to use alcohol than students who slept at least 8 hours and 25 minutes. Weekend delay is the difference between self-reported weekend bedtime and school bedtime defined as: low $\leq$ 1 hour, moderate 1–2 hours, and high$\geq$2 hours. A larger weekend delay correlated with risk-taking behaviors of substance use (alcohol, marijuana, tobacco, drugs) and safety and sexual behaviors. Catch-up sleep on the weekends was not connected with increased risk-taking behaviors.

This relationship between sleep and risk-taking behaviors is supported by other studies. In a survey of 12,154 students, many engaged in risky behaviors with 46% reporting alcohol, 20.9% marijuana, and 21.2% cigarette use (McKnight-Eily et al., 2011). Insufficient sleep on school nights (<8 hours) correlated to a 64% increased risk of alcohol, 52% marijuana, and 67% cigarette use. In a large population survey, the presence of possible insomnia correlated with increased risk of cigarette use, drinking and driving, and delinquency (Catrett & Gaultney, 2009) (see Table 31.1 and Figure 31.2).

Sleep Deprivation and Impulsivity

Not all studies support increased risk-taking in association with sleep deprivation. The Balloon Analogue Risk Task (BART) is designed to evaluate risk-taking and impulsive behaviors. Participants "pump-up a series of balloons" on a computer, with each pump being worth a specific amount of money. As the balloon expands more money is accumulated, but at the risk that the balloon would occasionally explode with a resultant loss of the accumulated money; therefore, more pumps are an indicator of greater risk-taking behaviors (Acheson, Richards, & de Wit, 2007). The majority of participants in this study were college students in their early 20s. Participants were sleep deprived for 24–36 hours. Significant gender differences were found: sleep deprivation decreased risk taking in women, but not men. Sleep deprivation has been shown to increase impulsivity to negative stimuli such that there was failure to inhibit a response. In the Go/No Go task, participants were presented words that were neutral or emotional in content: emotional words were positive (smile) or negative (frown). Sleep-deprived participants failed to inhibit a response to negative word stimuli. A possible physiologic explanation for the failure of inhibiting a response is that the prefrontal cortex, responsible for executive function, is diminished by sleep deprivation (Thomas et al., 2000; Yoo, Gujar, Hu, Jolesz, & Walker, 2007).

Care is needed interpreting these results, as these studies are not on adolescents but primarily young adults, and it is possible that adolescents may have a different impulsive response to sleep deprivation. These results do not prove a causal relationship between risk-taking behaviors, sleep, and sleep behaviors. It could be that young adults with a more erratic sleep schedule are more susceptible to risky behaviors, have less parental involvement, or there are unmeasured, unknown confounding variables.

Obstructive Sleep Apnea and Driving Risk

Obstructive sleep apnea can compromise driving performance, with an increase in accidents. In adults, obstructive sleep apnea with an apnea-hypopnea (AHI) of 10 or higher had an odds ratio of 6.3 for an accident compared to subjects without obstructive sleep apnea (Tiran-Santos, Jimenez-Gomez, et al. 1999). Severe obstructive sleep apnea (AHI > 30) is associated with a 2-fold increase in MVAs (Aldrich, 1989). These findings are supported by a large meta-analysis which also indicated a 2–3-fold increase in accidents (Ellen et al., 2006). These studies need to be interpreted with restraint as they are on adults, some of whom report being professional drivers; therefore, the results may not

Table 31.1 Prevalence and likelihood of health risk behaviors for students with <8 hours of school night sleep (McKnight-Eily et al., 2011). Adjusted for sex, age, and race/ethnicity.

	Percent of students	Adjusted Odds Ratio	Confidence Interval and p value
Alcohol use	50.3	1.64	(1.46–1.84) p = 0.00
Cigarette use	24.0	1.67	(1.45–1.93) p = 0.00
Marijuana use	23.3	1.52	(1.31–1.76) p = 0.00
Currently sexually active	39.1	1.41	(1.25–1.59) p = 0.00
Drank soda> 1 day	35.7	1.14	(1.03–1.28) p = 0.02
Physical fight in the last year	36.9	1.40	(1.24–1.60) p = 0.00
Felt sad or hopeless	31.1	1.62	(1.43–1.84) p = 0.00
Considered or attempted suicide	16.8	1.86	(1.60–2.16) p = 0.00

McKnight-Eily et al. (2011).

be directly applicable to young adults for several reasons: *(1)* the accident risk is higher in younger subjects, regardless of the presence of a sleep disorder; *(2)* professional drivers have more driving training than young adults; *(3)* adults and professional drivers commute more miles than young adults; *(4)* obstructive sleep apnea in teenagers can be defined by different criteria, either as an adult or as a child (Iber, Ancoli-Israel, Chesson, & Quan, 2007). Therefore, the best interpretation may be that the presence of obstructive sleep apnea in young adults will increase the risk of MVAs but to what degree is difficult to quantify.

In a study comparing untreated obstructive sleep apnea, 24 hours of sleep deprivation, and alcohol consumption, obstructive sleep apnea participants when treated had improvements in steering error, mean reaction time, and off-road events (Hack, Choi, Vijayapalan, Davies, & Stradling, 2001). As a comparison, untreated obstructive sleep apnea participants had steering performance that ranged between that of normal subjects consuming alcohol and sleep deprived participants.

Legal Implications of Drowsy Driving

Drowsy driving is a considerable public health issue with mounting attention in the media and the medical literature. The legal ramifications of drowsy driving have changed in recent years; within the United States, many states have developed legislation to combat this growing problem with increasingly strict consequences for drowsy driving. Below are some examples of current legislation in the United States, some enacted and others under consideration.

The Junior Operators' Bill from Massachusetts is a version of graduated driving licensure that was developed after the Drowsy Driving Law of 2005 failed to be passed; it went into effect January 2007. Graduated driving licensure is a program where independent driving occurs in stages; for example, teenagers may be able to drive only during certain hours and without passengers. After a certain time, these restrictions are lifted and the driver has unrestricted driving privileges. The Junior Operator's Bill limits some higher-risk driving situations. No driving is allowed from 12:30 to 5:30 am and it prohibits the use of mobile electronic devices (i.e., cell phones) for operators under the age of 18 while driving. Steep penalties, including a suspended license and fees, may occur if a junior operator is found talking on a cell phone or writing, sending, or reading text messages while operating a motor vehicle. Additionally, the law mandates that drivers' education courses will include the effects of sleep deprivation on driving performance (Transportation, 2012; Massachusetts Department of Transportation, 2012) (see table 31.2).

The Drowsy Driving Act of 2011, submitted from Massachusetts, is not yet in effect. It is also referred to as "Rob's Law," in memory of Major Robert Raneri, a US Army Reserve officer who was killed on June 26, 2002, by an admitted drowsy driver. The 19-year-old driver admitted that he had stayed up all night playing video games. Despite the accident resulting in a death, the driver was sentenced only to a misdemeanor since drugs and alcohol were not involved in the accident. In part, the provisional law states (The Commonwealth of Massachusetts, 2011; Sleep Research Society):

> [A driver] who has fallen asleep while operating a motor vehicle, or who was impaired by drowsiness of which the person was aware or could reasonably be expected to be aware shall be punished by a fine of not less than $500 nor more than $5,000 or by imprisonment for not more than 2 1/2 years, or both such fine and imprisonment. Evidence that the operator of a motor vehicle was awake for at least 22 of the 24 hours prior to said operation of a motor vehicle or at least 140 hours of the 168 hours prior to said operation of a motor vehicle that is involved in a crash that results in death, debilitating injury, or property damage in excess of $50,000, shall constitute sufficient evidence to conclude that said motor vehicle operator was impaired by drowsiness.

Maggie's Law, from the state of New Jersey, was passed after the death of 20-year old college student Maggie McDonnell, who was killed when a driver crossed three lanes of highway traffic and hit her car head-on (Grunstein & Rogers, 2005). The male driver admitted he had been awake for 30 hours, but lack of sleep was not considered a "crime" at that time; therefore, he received only a suspended jail sentence and $200 fine. "Maggie's Law "establishes driving while fatigued as recklessness under vehicular homicide statute (State of New Jersey 210th Legislature, 2002). For this state law, driving while fatigued is defined as "being without sleep for 24 continous hours" and can result in up to 10 years in jail and up to $100,000 in fines.

Since May 1, 2010, New Jersey has required all drivers younger than 21 with learner's permits or probationary licenses to display red reflective decals on their license plates when they drive (Lockwood,

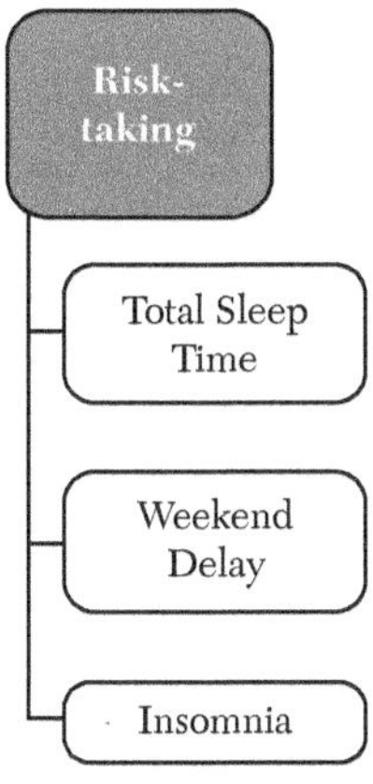

Figure 31.2 Sleep Variables Related to Increased Risk-Taking Behaviors: Increased risk-taking behaviors were seen for decreased total sleep time, depending on the study less than 6.45–8 hours. Weekend delay is the difference between weekend bedtime and school bedtime. Increased weekend delay of ≥2 hours was associated with more risk-taking behaviors when compared to subjects with a weekend delay of < 1 hour (Catrett & Gaultney, 2009; McKnight-Eily et al., 2011; O'Brien & Mindell, 2005).

2010; Insurance Institute for Highway Safety, December 15, 2011). It is a part of "Kyleigh's Law," named after a teenager who was killed while riding as a passenger. It appears that the decals are frequently not used, nor is the law enforced, as surveys of high school students showed that only 25%–64% of high school students displayed the red decal (see figure 31.3).

Potential Interventions to Reduce Motor Vehicle Accidents

Driving is a complex activity and mastery takes time, maturity, physical, social, and psychological skills. Reducing the rate of teen accidents is hampered by a lack of data on effective interventions. This section will focus on interventions that may decrease drowsiness while driving and will discuss a few brief non-sleep based interventions (Graham & Gootman, 2008). Inadequate sleep is common among young adults and is known to worsen driving performance; therefore, one possible intervention to reduce accidents is to decrease young adults' sleep deprivation. There are some intriguing trends in the literature that suggest modifying school start time may be an effective intervention. A change in one particular high school's start time from 7:30 am to 8:30 am increased sleep duration and decreased teenage average crash rates by 16.5% in the 2 years following the time change. In comparison, the teen crash rate increased by 7.8% in the concurrent time period for the rest of the state (Danner & Phillips, 2008). Two communities in Virginia with significantly different high school start times had different rates of MVAs. The community with a 75–80-minute earlier start time had 4.5 times more crashes among 16–18-year-olds in the community compared to the school with a later start time (Vorona et al., 2011). More definitive research is needed to determine if a later high school start time would decrease accident rates. Knowledge of the effects

Table 31.2 Penalties for violations of Junior Operators' Bill (Massachusetts Registry of Motor Vehicles, 2012)

Violation	1st offense	2nd offense	3rd offense
Passenger Restriction	60 day suspension $100 reinstatement fee	180 day suspension Driver Attitudinal Retraining Course $100 fee	1 year suspension Driver Attitudinal Retraining Course Full Exam $100 fee
Time Restriction Violation 12:30 am-5am	60 day suspension $100 fee	180 day suspension Driver Attitudinal Retraining Course $100 fee	1 year suspension Driver Attitudinal Retraining Course Full Exam $100 fee
Operating to Endanger/ Recklessly or Negligent	180 day suspension $500 fee	1 year suspension $500 fee	1 year suspension $500 fee
Drag-Racing	1 year suspension Driver Attitudinal Retraining Course $500 fee	3 year suspension Driver Attitudinal Retraining Course $1000 fee	3 year suspension Driver Attitudinal Retraining Course $1000 fee
Speeding	90 day suspension Driver Attitudinal Retraining Course $500 fee	1 year suspension Driver Attitudinal Retraining Course $500 fee	1 year suspension Driver Attitudinal Retraining Course $500 fee

Massachusetts Registry of Motor Vehicles. (2012). *JOL License and Permit Violations and Penalties*. Commonwealth of Massachusetts Retrieved from on 4/15/2013 http://www.massrmv.com/rmv/jol/jol_penalties_chart.htm and http://www.massrmv.com/rmv/jol/index.htm.

of drowsy driving may decrease the incidence of drowsy driving. Driving training courses educate most (69%) adolescents to the consequences of drowsy driving (National Sleep Foundation, 2006). However knowledge of the risks of drowsy driving may not be adequate to change behavior. A study of college students found that 68% of young adults continued to drive despite having a near-accident on that same drive (Lindsay et al., 1999). Since obstructive sleep apnea can worsen driving safety, it can be presumed that treatment of obstructive sleep apnea would improve driving. There are no studies on young adults to conform this, but treatment of obstructive sleep apnea improves driving performance in adults to some degree, although abnormalities may still be present with driving simulation (George, 2001; Hack et al., 2001; Sassani et al., 2004; Vakulin et al., 2011). Caution is needed in interpreting these results as they again pertain to adult subjects.

Graduated Driving Licensing

Graduated Driving Licensing (GDL) allows driving independence to occur in stages before a full unrestricted license is obtained. In practice, novice drivers progress from less risky to more risky driving situations (Foss, R. & Evenson, 1999). The general framework is supervised driving for a period of time, progression to unsupervised driving with specific limitations (i.e., no passengers, no nighttime driving) and the final stage of unrestricted licensure. These programs address some specific situations that increase the risk of MVAs such as limiting the presence of passengers and prohibiting nighttime driving. It may also address behavioral and development aspects with a graduated and conceivably longer time frame before an unrestricted license. In other words, more time may lead to more maturity and better decision-making ability. There is considerable variability among different graduated driving license programs among different states in the United States and other countries. This variability makes analysis of effectiveness problematic, but results are promising with an 8% reduction in crashes in New Zealand and a 5% reduction in Maryland after enactment. In North Carolina, the GDL reduced fatal crashes by 57%, nighttime crashes by 43%, and daytime crashes by 20% (Foss, Feaganes, & Rodgman, 2001).

Technology to Monitor Driving Performance

Technological advancements are being designed that may allow both monitoring for poor driving performance and potential interventions to avoid an accident. In general, these are research based and may not be commercially available. A lane departure warning system monitors the position of the vehicle within the lane; a warning is given if the vehicle appears to be leaving the lane or roadway. SafeTRAC is an example of this technology (Federal Motor Carrier Safety Administration, 2013; Shropshire, 2006). Slow eye movements and eye blinking can herald the onset of sleep. PERCLOSE monitors the proportion of time in a minute that the eyes are 80% closed. Studies have used this in association with various software systems to try to design an effective warning system. Other devices have evaluated the driver's steering angle; when drowsiness occurs the algorithm can detect the presence of prolonged pause before a correction in the driver's steering. AWAKE (the effective Assessment of driver vigilance and Warning According to traffic risK Estimation) is a multisensor approach evaluating both traffic and the driver's performance (Wang, Q. 2006). It monitors, in part, speed, eyelid movement, lane tracking, changes in steering grip and vehicle position, while also monitoring the current traffic risk from maps, anti-collision devices, driver gaze sensors, and odomotor readings. Monitoring both car and driver components are utilized to create the warning system. Artificial Neural Networks (ANN) is a complex of interconnected processing elements that are meant to function like a neuron, hence the "neural" name. Driver drowsiness detection occurs in a complex network that in part analyzes steering angle. On a simulated driving course, the AWAKE network was able to classify driving performance into drowsy and nondrowsy with 89.9% accuracy. It detected drowsy driving 3.5 minutes before a crash occurred on the simulated course (Sayed & Eskandarian, 2001).

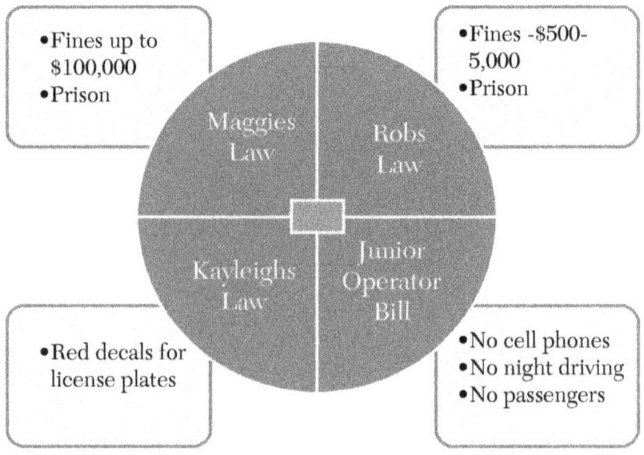

Figure 31.3 Legal Implications for Drowsy Driving (Grunstein & Rogers, 2005; Lockwood, 2010)

Table 31.3 Potential interventions for drowsy driving (Foss and Evenson 1999; Culp, El Gindy et al. 2008; Danner & Phillips, 2008)

Intervention for drowsy driving
Graduated driving licensure
Drivers education on affects of drowsy driving
Later school start times
Technology to monitor drowsy driving
Enhanced safety features of vehicles

Culp, Gindy, & Haque (2008).
Danner, F. & Phillips, B. (2008). Adolescent sleep, school start times, and teen motor vehicle crashes." *Journal of clinical sleep medicine: JCSM: official publication of the American Academy of Sleep Medicine, 4*(6), 533–535.
Foss, R., & Evenson, K. (1999). Effectiveness of graduated driver licensing in reducing motor vehicle crashes. *American Journal of Preventive Medicine, 16*(1, Supplement 1), 47–56.

Automotive manufacturers have developed collision-avoidance technology, also termed *forward collision warning systems*, which are available in some models. Each company's system has different features, but some can signal if the driver is following another car too closely or if a lane change occurs without proper preceding signals. The system can be primed in high-risk driving situations so that seat belts and the braking system are more effective (Bosch, 2010; Danielson, 2008; Ford Media.com, 2009). Further research is essential to evaluate the effectiveness of these technologies (see Table 31.1).

Conclusion

Driving in young adults has an unacceptably high rate of motor vehicle accidents and deaths. Driving is a complex task with many variables contributing to the risk of accidents, including physiological, neurocognitive, and psychosocial factors. Improving sleep is not often considered as an area for potential interventions because sleep deprivation and sleep disorders may not be considered as risk factors for accidents. Key sleep-related factors for increased risk of accidents are young adults' sleep duration, the detrimental effect of prolonged wakefulness on driving performance, and the circadian influences change on to of heightened risk of accidents during the early morning hours. Sleep may also influence less tangible risk factors such as risk-taking behaviors and substance use.

Effective interventions to reduce accident risk need to be developed and instituted. The timing of school classes can influence the amount of sleep teenagers obtain, and delaying the start of high school may decrease the community rate of accidents among teenagers. More states and countries need to develop graduated licensure programs, as these have been shown to decrease accidents. Since graduated licensure programs are so variable, research is needed to determine which key features (limiting passengers, night driving, and age of licensure) are most effective. Alerting drivers to the effects of drowsiness is vital, as it appears many young adults continue to drive despite feeling drowsy. Advances in technology may become an asset, as cars of the future are able to analyze and intervene when dangerous driving patterns are present. Future research is vital to better understand modifiable risk factors as they pertain to sleep and sleep disorders and to develop effective interventions for the serious public health issue of drowsy driving and accidents in young adults.

Future Directions

- Further research is needed to determine if a later school start would decrease motor vehicle accidents in young adults.
- Investigation into the increased rate of motor vehicle accidents around the start and end of school is crucial, as there may be certain transportation modalities, such as busing, that are optimal for safety of students.
- The development of cost-effective technology that can analyze driving patterns and behaviors and potentially intervene during the presence of concerning or hazardous driving behaviors (increased lane variability, speed, and tracking) is needed.
- The presence of gender differences with risk-taking behaviors and individuals ability for risk self-warrants further research.

References

Acheson, A., Richards, J. B., & de Wit, H. (2007). Effects of sleep deprivation on impulsive behaviors in men and women. *Physiology & Behavior, 91*(5), 579–587.
Akerstedt, T., & Gillberg, M. (1990). Subjective and objective sleepiness in the active individual. [Research Support, Non-U.S. Gov't]. *The International Journal of Neuroscience, 52*(1–2), 29–37.
Aldrich, M. S. (1989). Automobile accidents in patients with sleep disorders. *Sleep, 12*(6), 487–494.
Arnedt, J. T., Wilde, G. J. S., Munt, P. W., & MacLean, A. W. (2001). How do prolonged wakefulness and alcohol compare in the decrements they produce on a simulated driving task? *Accident Analysis & Prevention, 33*(3), 337–344.
American College Health Association. (2007). National college health assessment Spring 2006 Reference Group data report. *Journal of American College Health, 55*(4), 195–206.

Atienza, M., Cantero, J. L., Stickgold, R., & Hobson, J. A. (2004). Eyelid movements measured by Nightcap predict slow eye movements during quiet wakefulness in humans. *Journal of Sleep Research, 13*(1), 25–29.

Banks, S., Catcheside, P., Lack, L., Grunstein, R. R., & McEvoy, R. D. (2004). Low levels of alcohol impair driving simulator performance and reduce perception of crash risk in partially sleep deprived subjects. *Sleep, 27*(6), 1063–1067.

Beede, K. E., & Kass, S. J. (2006). Engrossed in conversation: The impact of cell phones on simulated driving performance. *Accident Analysis and Prevention, 38*(2), 415–421.

Borbely, A. (1982). A two process model of sleep regulation. *Human Neurobiology, 3*, 195–204.

Bosch. (2010). Bosch predictive emergency braking system goes into series production from Retrieved March 30, 2012, from http://www.bosch-presse.de/presseforum/details.htm?txtID=4570&locale=en.

Boyle, L. N., Tippin, J., Paul, A., & Rizzo, M. (2008). Driver performance in the moments surrounding a microsleep. *Transportation Research Part F: Traffic Psychology and Behaviour, 11*(2), 126–136.

Braitman, K. A., Kirley, B. B., McCartt, A. T., & Chaudhary, N. K. (2008). Crashes of novice teenage drivers: Characteristics and contributing factors. *Journal of Safety Research, 39*(1), 47–54.

Carskadon M. A. (1990). Patterns of sleep and sleepiness in adolescents. *Pediatrician, 17*(1), 5–12.

Carskadon, M. A., Vieira, C., & Acebo, C. (1993). Association between puberty and delayed phase preference. *Sleep, 16*(3), 258–262.

Catrett, C. D., & Gaultney, J. F. (2009). Possible insomnia predicts some risky behaviors among adolescents when controlling for depressive symptoms. *The Journal of Genetic Psychology, 170*(4), 287–309.

The Commonwealth of Massachusetts. (2011). *Bill S.1773: An Act relative to drowsy driving*. Retrieved on 2/13/2012 from http://www.malegislature.gov/Bills/187/Senate/S01773

Crowley, S. J., Acebo, C., & Carskadon, M. A. (2007). Sleep, circadian rhythms, and delayed phase in adolescence. *Sleep Medicine, 8*(6), 602–612.

Culp, J., Gindy, E., & Haque, A. (2008). Driver alertness monitoring techniques: a literature review. *International Journal of Heavy Vehicle Systems, 15*(2/3/4), 255–271.

Dahl, R. (2008). Biological, developmental and neurobiological factors relevant to adolescent driving risks. *American Journal of Preventive Medicine 35*, s278–S284.

Danner, F., & Phillips, B. (2008). Adolescent sleep, school start times, and teen motor vehicle crashes. *Journal of Clinical Sleep Medicine, 4*(6), 533–535.

Dawson, D., & Reid, K. (1997). Fatigue, alcohol and performance impairment. *Nature, 388*(6639), 235–235.

Ellen, R. L., Marshall, S. C., Palayew, M., Molnar, F. J., Wilson, K. G., & Man-Son-Hing, M. (2006). Systematic review of motor vehicle crash risk in persons with sleep apnea. [Review]. *Journal of Clinical Sleep Medicine, 2*(2), 193–200.

Federal Motor Carrier Safety Administration. (2013). Pilot Test of Fatigue Management Technologies-Final Report. Retrieved on 4/30/2013 from https://www.fmcsa.dot.gov/facts-research/research-technology/publications/pilot-test/fmt-selected-for-study.htm

Ford Media.com. (2009). Ford's Latest Safety Brakethrough—Collision Warning with Brake Support—Coming in 2009. Retrieved March 30, 2012, from http://media.ford.com/article_display.cfm?article_id=29188.

Foss, R., & Evenson, K. (1999). Effectiveness of graduated driver licensing in reducing motor vehicle crashes. *American Journal of Preventive Medicine, 16*(1, Supplement 1), 47–56. 3

Foss, R. D., Feaganes, J. R., & Rodgman, E. A. (2001). Initial effects of graduated driver licensing on 16-year-old driver crashes in North Carolina. *Journal of the American Medical Association, 286*(13), 1588–1592.

George, C. F. (2001). Reduction in motor vehicle collisions following treatment of sleep apnoea with nasal CPAP. *Thorax, 56*(7), 508–512.

Graham, R., & Gootman, J. A. (2008). Preventing teen motor crashes: Contributions from the behavioral and social sciences and summary of the report of the national research council and institute of medicine. *American Journal of Preventive Medicine, 35*(3, Supplement), S253–S257.

Grunstein, R. R., & Rogers, N. L. (2005). Medical work hours: Time for a Maggie's Law for doctoring? [Editorial]. *Internal Medicine Journal, 35*(5), 269–271.

Hack, M. A., Choi, S. J., Vijayapalan, P., Davies, R. J., & Stradling, J. R. (2001). Comparison of the effects of sleep deprivation, alcohol and obstructive sleep apnoea (OSA) on simulated steering performance. *Respiratory Medicine, 95*(7), 594–601.

Hellinga, L. A., McCartt, A. T., & Mandavilli, S. (2007). Temporal patterns of crashes of 16-to 17-year-old drivers in Fairfax County, Virginia. [Research Support, Non-U.S. Gov't]. *Traffic Injury Prevention, 8*(4), 377–381.

Horne, J. A. (1993). Human sleep, sleep loss and behavior—Implications for the prefrontal cortex and psychiatric-disorder. *British Journal of Psychiatry, 162*, 413–419.

Horne, J. A., Reyner, L. A., & Barrett, P. R. (2003). Driving impairment due to sleepiness is exacerbated by low alcohol intake. *Occupational and Environmental Medicine, 60*(9), 689–692.

Hutchens, L., Senserrick, T. M., Jamieson, P. E., Romer, D., & Winston, F. K. (2008). Teen driver crash risk and associations with smoking and drowsy driving. *Accident Analysis & Prevention, 40*(3), 869–876.

Iber, C., Ancoli-Israel, S., Chesson, A., & Quan, S. F. (Eds.). (2007). *The AASM Manual for the Scoring of Sleep and Associated Events: Rules, Terminology and Technical Specifications* (1st ed.). Westchester, Illinois.: American Academcy of Sleep Medicine.

Insurance Instituite for Highway Safety. (2005). Fatality Facts: Teenagers. Retrieved on 2/21/2012 from http://www.iihs.org/research/fatality.aspx?topicName=Teenagers&year=2005

Insurance Institute for Highway Safety. (2006). Fatality Facts 2006:Teenagers. Retrieved on 2/13/2012 from http://www.iihs.org/research/fatality.aspx?topicName=teenagers&year=2006

Insurance Institute for Highway Safety. (2009). Fatality Facts 2009: Teenagers. Retrieved on 1/18/2012 from http://www.iihs.org/research/fatality.aspx?topicName=Teenagers&year=2009

Insurance Institute for Highway Safety. (Dec. 15, 2011). Teen Drivers: New Jersey decal laws aids enforcement but not compliance with GDL laws. *Vol. 46, No. 11*, 1–8. Retrieved on 2/13/2012 from http://www.iihs.org/externaldata/srdata/docs/sr4611.pdf

International Center For Alcohol Policies. (2013). Blood Alcohol Concentration (BAC) Limits Worldwide. Retrieved on 4/15/2013 from http://www.icap.org/PolicyIssues/DrinkingandDriving/BACTable/tabid/199/Default.aspx

Ireland, J. L., & Culpin, V. (2006). The relationship between sleeping problems and aggression, anger, and impulsivity in a population of juvenile and young offenders. *Journal of Adolescent Health, 38*(6), 649–655.

Kann, L., Kinchen, S. A., Williams, B. I., Ross, J. G., Lowry, R., Grunbaum, J. A., & Kolbe, L. J. (2000). Youth Risk Behavior Surveillance—United States, 1999. State and local YRBSS Coordinators. *The Journal of School Health, 70*(7), 271–285.

Kass, S. J., Cole, K. S., & Stanny, C. J. (2007). Effects of distraction and experience on situation awareness and simulated driving. *Transportation Research Part F-Traffic Psychology and Behaviour, 10*(4), 321–329.

Kryger, M. H., Roth, T., & Dement, W. C. (Eds.). (2011). *Principles and Practice of Sleep Medicine*. St. Louis: Elsevier.

Lindsay, G. A., Hanks, W. A., Hurley, R. D., & Dane, S. (1999). Descriptive epidemiology of dozing and driving in a college student population. *Journal of American College Health, 47*(4), 157–162.

Lockwood, J. (2010). Kyleigh's Law requires license decals for young N.J. drivers. Retrieved on 3/1/2012 from http://www.nj.com/news/index.ssf/2010/04/kyleighs_law_requiring_license.html

Lucidi, F., Devoto, A., Bertini, M., Braibanti, P., & Violani, C. (2002). The effects of sleep debt on vigilance in young drivers: An education/research project in high schools. *Journal of Adolescence, 25*(4), 405–414.

Lund, H. G., Reider, B. D., Whiting, A. B., & Prichard, J. R. (2010). Sleep patterns and predictors of disturbed sleep in a large population of college students. *Journal of Adolescent Health, 46*(2), 124–132.

Massachusetts Department of Transportation. (2012). Registry of Motor Vehicles, Junior Operator License Retrieved April 2, 2012, from http://www.mass.gov/rmv/jol/index.htm

McCartt, A. T., Shabanova, V. I., & Leaf, W. A. (2003). Driving experience, crashes and traffic citations of teenage beginning drivers. *Accident Analysis and Prevention, 35*(3), 311–320.

McKnight-Eily, L. R., Eaton, D. K., Lowry, R., Croft, J. B., Presley-Cantrell, L., & Perry, G. S. (2011). Relationships between hours of sleep and health-risk behaviors in US adolescent students. *Preventive Medicine, 53*(4–5), 271–273.

Mitler, M. M., & Miller, J. C. (1996). Methods of testing for sleepiness [corrected]. [Review]. *Behavioral Medicine, 21*(4), 171–183.

National Highway Traffic Safety Administration. (2009). Traffic Safety Facts 2009: Young Drivers. Retrieved April 1, 2012 from http://www-nrd.nhtsa.dot.gov/Pubs/811400.pdf doi:DOT HS 811 400.

National Highway Traffic Safety Administration. (2011). *Teen Distracted Driver* Data. Retrieved April 25, 2012, from http://www-nrd.nhtsa.dot.gov/Pubs/811462.pdf.

National Highway Traffic Safety Administration. *Teen Drivers—Additional Resources*. Retrieved April 25, 2012, from http://www.nhtsa.gov/Driving+Safety/Teen+Drivers/Teen+Drivers+-+Additional+Resources.

National Sleep Foundation. (2006). *Teens and Sleep*. Arlington, VA National Sleep Foundation. Retrieved on 3/1/2012 from http://www.sleepfoundation.org/article/sleep-america-polls/2006-teens-and-sleep..

National Sleep Foundation. (2011). *Sleep in America: Technology Use and Sleep*. Arlington VA.: Retrieved on 2/13/2012 from http://www.sleepfoundation.org/article/sleep-america-polls/2011-communications-technology-use-and-sleep.

Nelson, D. E., Naimi, T. S., Brewer, R. D., & Nelson, H. A. (2009). State alcohol-use estimates among youth and adults, 1993–2005. *American Journal of Preventive Medicine, 36*(3), 218–224.

O'Brien, E. M., & Mindell, J. A. (2005). Sleep and risk-taking behavior in adolescents. *Behavioral Sleep Medicine, 3*(3), 113–133.

Oginska, H., & Pokorski, J. (2006). Fatigue and mood correlates of sleep length in three age-social groups: School children, students, and employees. *Chronobioogyl International, 23*(6), 1317–1328.

Owens, J. A. (2010). Impact of delaying school start time on adolescent sleep, mood, and behavior. *Archives of Pediatrics & Adolescent Medicine, 164*(7), 608–614.

Paul, A., Boyle, L., Boer, E., Tippin, J., & Rizzo, M. (2005). Variablity of driving perfromance during microsleeps. Retrieved on 3/1/2012 from http://drivingassessment.uiowa.edu/DA2005/PDF/04_AmitPaul_LBoyleformat.pdf

Pharo, H., Sim, C., Graham, M., Gross, J., & Hayne, H. (2011). Risky business: Executive function, personality, and reckless behavior during adolescence and emerging adulthood. [Research Support, Non-U.S. Gov't]. *Behavioral Neuroscience, 125*(6), 970–978.

Pizza, F., Contardi, S., Antognini, A. B., Zagoraiou, M., Borrotti, M., Mostacci, B., et al. (2010). Sleep quality and motor vehicle crashes in adolescents. *Journal of Clinical Sleep Medicine, 6*(1), 41–45.

Preusser, D. F., Ferguson, S. A., & Williams, A. F. (1998). The effect of teenage passengers on the fatal crash risk of teenage drivers. *Accident Analysis & Prevention, 30*(2), 217–222.

Rice, T. M., Peek-Asa, C., & Kraus, J. F. (2003). Nighttime driving, passenger transport, and injury crash rates of young drivers. *Injury Prevention, 9*(3), 245–250.

Risser, M. R., Ware, J. C., & Freeman, F. G. (2000). Driving simulation with EEG monitoring in normal and obstructive sleep apnea patients. *Sleep, 23*(3), 393–398.

Sassani, A., Findley, L. J., Kryger, M., Goldlust, E., George, C., & Davidson, T. M. (2004). Reducing motor-vehicle collisions, costs, and fatalities by treating obstructive sleep apnea syndrome. *Sleep, 27*(3), 453–458.

Sayed, R., & Eskandarian, A. (2001). Unobtrusive drowsiness detection by neural network learning of driver steering. *Proceedings of the Institution of Mechanical Engineers Part D-Journal of Automobile Engineering, 215*(D9), 969–975.

Shope, J. T., Raghunathan, T. E., & Patil, S. M. (2003). Examining trajectories of adolescent risk factors as predictors of subsequent high-risk driving behavior. *Journal of Adolescent Health, 32*(3), 214–224.

Shope, J. T. (2006). Influences on youthful driving behavior and their potential for guiding interventions to reduce crashes. *Injury Prevention, 12*, 9–14.

Shope, J. T., & Bingham, C. R. (2008). Teen driving—Motor-vehicle crashes and factors that contribute. *American Journal of Preventive Medicine, 35*(3), S261–S271.

Shropshire, C. (2006). Robotics startup AssistWare brought out by Mass Firm. Retrieved April 1, 2013, from http://www.post-gazette.com/stories/business/technology/robotics-startup-assistware-bought-out-by-mass-firm-435171/.

Simons-Morton, B. G., Ouimet, M. C., Zhang, Z., Klauer, S. E., Lee, S. E., Wang, J., et al. (2011). The effect of passengers and risk-taking friends on risky driving and crashes/near crashes among novice teenagers. *Journal of Adolescent Health, 49*(6), 587–593.

Sleep Research Society. Section by Section Analysis of Drowsy Driving Bill: An Act Relative to Drowsy Driving. Retrieved on 2/13/2012 from http://www.sleepresearchsociety.org/PDFs/Government/SecbySecDrowsyDrivingBill.pdf

State of New Jersey 210th Legislature. (2002). *Assembly No. 1347* Retrieved on 2/1/2012 from http://www.njleg.state.nj.us/2002/Bills/A1500/1347_I1.PDF.

Steinberg, L. (2004). Risk taking in adolescence: What changes, and why? [Review]. *Annals of the New York Academy of Sciences,* 1021, 51–58.

Taylor, D. J., Jenni, O. G., Acebo, C., & Carskadon, M. A. (2005). Sleep tendency during extended wakefulness: Insights into adolescent sleep regulation and behavior. *Journal of Sleep Research, 14*(3), 239–244.

Taylor, D. J., & Bramoweth, A. D. (2010). Patterns and consequences of inadequate sleep in college students: Substance use and motor vehicle accidents. *Journal of Adolescent Health, 46*(6), 610–612.

Teran-Santos, J., Jimenez-Gomez, A., Cordero-Guevara, J., & Burgos-Santander, C. G. (1999). The association between sleep apnea and the risk of traffic accidents. *New England Journal of Medicine, 340*(11), 847–851.

Thomas, M., Sing, H., Belenky, G., Holcomb, H., Mayberg, H., Dannals, R., et al. (2000). Neural basis of alertness and cognitive performance impairments during sleepiness. I. Effects of 24 h of sleep deprivation on waking human regional brain activity. *Journal of Sleep Research, 9*(4), 335–352.

Thorleifsdottir, B., Bjornsson, J. K., Benediktsdottir, B., Gislason, T., & Kristbjarnarson, H. (2002). Sleep and sleep habits from childhood to young adulthood over a 10-year period. *Journal of Psychosomatic Research, 53*(1), 529–537.

Vakulin, A., Baulk, S. D., Catcheside, P. G., Anderson, R., van den Heuvel, C. J., Banks, S., & McEvoy, R. D. (2007). Effects of moderate sleep deprivation and low-dose alcohol on driving simulator performance and perception in young men. *Sleep, 30*(10), 1327–1333.

Vakulin, A., Baulk, S. D., Catcheside, P. G., Antic, N. A., van den Heuvel, C. J., Dorrian, J., & McEvoy, R. D. (2011). Driving simulator performance remains impaired in patients with severe OSA after CPAP treatment. *Journal of Clinical Sleep Medicine, 7*(3), 243–250.

Vorona, R. D., Szklo-Coxe, M., Wu, A., Dubik, M., Zhao, Y., & Ware, J. C. (2011). Dissimilar teen crash rates in two neighboring southeastern Virginia cities with different high school start times. *Journal of Clinical Sleep Medicine, 7*(2), 145–151.

Wang, Q., Yang, J. Y., Ren, M. W., & Zheng, Y. J. (2006). Driver fatigue detection: A survey. *Conference Proceedings Sixth World Congress on Intelligent Control and Automation,* 8587–8591. Retrieved from <Go to ISI>://000241773209152

Williams, A. F., & Ferguson, S. A. (2002). Rationale for graduated licensing and the risks it should address. [Research Support, Non-U.S. Gov't]. *Injury Prevention, 8*(Suppl 2), ii9–14; discussion ii14–16.

Williams, A. F. (2003). Teenage drivers: Patterns of risk. *Journal of Safety Research, 34*(1), 5–15.

Yoo, S. S., Gujar, N., Hu, P., Jolesz, F. A., & Walker, M. P. (2007). The human emotional brain without sleep—a prefrontal amygdala disconnect. *Current Biology, 17*(20), R877–R878.

Zador, P. L., Krawchuk, S. A., & Voas, R. B. (2000). Alcohol-related relative risk of driver fatalities and driver involvement in fatal crashes in relation to driver age and gender: An update using 1996 data. *Journal of Studies on Alcohol, 61*(3), 387–395.

Zeitzer, J. M., Dijk, D. J., Kronauer, R. E., Brown, E. N., & Czeisler, C. A. (2000). Sensitivity of the human circadian pacemaker to nocturnal light: melatonin phase resetting and suppression. *Journal of Physiology-London, 526*(3), 695–702.

PART 6

Sleep Difficulties Associated with Developmental and Behavioral Risks

CHAPTER

32 Asthma, Allergies, and Sleep

Daphne Koinis Mitchell *and* Robin Everhart

Abstract

Children with chronic illnesses often experience sleep problems as a result of disease symptoms (e.g., itching, wheezing) or nighttime disease management (e.g., blood glucose monitoring). Poor sleep has negative implications for daytime functioning, including academic performance and quality of life. As asthma and allergic diseases (e.g., allergic rhinitis) are the most common chronic diseases in childhood, associations between sleep and these chronic conditions are of particular concern for researchers and health care providers. Disease-specific factors associated with asthma and allergic disease (e.g., severity, treatment adherence), as well as factors associated with cultural background and the family context (e.g., urban poverty, sleep practices, caregiver functioning) can affect child sleep patterns. Given the consequences of poor sleep on child functioning, clinical recommendations and interventions for children with asthma and allergic disease should focus not only on disease management, but also on family and environmental factors that may impact child sleep.

Key Words: chronic illness, allergic rhinitis, asthma, pathophysiology, adherence, culture, family context, sociocontextual factors

Introduction: Sleep and Chronic Illness in Children

As emphasized throughout this book, sleep is important for all children for promoting optimal physical health, mental health, daytime functioning, learning, and development. Sleep deprivation can negatively influence immune function in healthy children (Ozturk et al., 1999) and it has been shown to delay wound healing in animal models (Gumustekin et al., 2004). Conversely, adequate sleep may assist recovery from illness or injury through secretion of melatonin, which increases the immune response, and growth hormone, which promotes healing (Yarrington & Mehta, 1998). Pediatric populations with acute or chronic medical conditions are at increased risk for sleep disruption. Over 26.6% of children experience a chronic illness in the United States (Van Cleave, Gortmaker, & Perrin, 2010). Children with chronic illnesses are found to have less parent-reported daytime and nighttime sleep than healthy children (Mindell, Spirito, & Carskadon, 1990). Children with chronic disease are vulnerable to sleep disruptions due to factors related to the illness and illness management process, including the variability in symptom pattern that may be more pronounced during nighttime hours and the potential for poor adherence to treatment recommendations (see Meltzer & Walsh, Chapter 13). Such factors (e.g., variability in symptom pattern, poor adherence) can disrupt nighttime sleep patterns and challenge children's abilities to initiate and maintain sleep.

A growing body of research has attempted to further understanding of the impact of chronic illnesses on sleep in children, and several factors that may influence variations in sleep in pediatric populations have been identified. These factors have focused on biological mechanisms (e.g., change in inflammatory mediators at night), illness-related factors (e.g., severity, treatment components), family factors (e.g., caregiver functioning) and, to a lesser extent, environmental factors (e.g., poverty, neighborhood context, cultural factors). Understanding how chronic illnesses can affect sleep patterns and behaviors is a topic of developmental and clinical importance; it provides a context for understanding an important influence that can affect children's sleep behaviors and offers an opportunity to identify avenues for intervention to enhance the quality of sleep in children with specific health needs.

In this chapter, we focus on the most common pediatric health conditions that are chronic in nature, asthma and allergies, and examine the influence of these illnesses on sleep in children. We also focus on asthma because of the alarming racial and ethnic health disparities that exist in the prevalence levels and morbidity of the illness, and sleep quality may be at particular risk in these groups. We begin with a review of the pathophysiology of asthma and the unique way in which asthma can affect nighttime sleep due to the presence of allergic symptoms during the night. Specific focus is on the pathophysiological mechanisms involved with allergic diseases that may be relevant at night for children and adolescents, and how adherence to treatment is critical to improve illness control and, in turn, sleep quality. We then review the current state of the literature on allergic disease and sleep in children. The unique issues related to the family and social context, which may play a role in sleep disruption in chronically ill children, are also highlighted. We end with a discussion of future directions for research and interventions focusing on allergic conditions and sleep in children and adolescents.

How Do Chronic Illnesses Affect Sleep in Children?

Chronic illness may affect sleep in children through various pathways of influence. Some illnesses (e.g., asthma and epilepsy) may have worsening symptoms at night, and others (e.g., diabetes) may require nighttime medication (see review by Boergers & Koinis Mitchell, 2010). Further, pain, hospitalization, and side effects of medications may all interfere with sleep (Valrie, Gil, Redding-Lallinger, & Daeschner, 2007). Unique features of the hospital environment, such as noise, light, and nocturnal disruptions related to nursing care, can interfere with children's sleep routines (Boergers & Koinis Mitchell, 2010). Because of the challenges related to managing chronic illnesses, sleep problems are more common in children with illnesses compared to healthy children.

Asthma and Allergic Disease in Children: Prevalence and Morbidity

Before examining how asthma may influence sleep in children, it is important to review its prevalence in US children and the burden that it may present to children's functioning. Over 12.6% of children in the United States have asthma. Children over the age of 5 years seem to be most affected, and males are at increased risk for asthma prevalence and morbidity compared to female children (14.7% vs. 10.7%; Centers for Disease Control and Prevention, 2010). Asthma burden (e.g., emergency department use) is particularly high in African-American and Latino children compared to non-Latino White children (Lara et al., 2006). Puerto Rican children have the highest rates of asthma morbidity of children from any other ethnic group (Lara et al., 2006). Allergic rhinitis (AR) is a common comorbid condition in children with asthma. For example, approximately 80% of all children with asthma have coexisting AR, and nearly 40% of those with AR have coexisting asthma (Grossman, 1997). AR affects up to 40% of children (Derebery et al., 2008). Roughly one-third of all individuals with AR are less than 17 years of age (Blaiss, 2004). Similarly, other atopic diseases, such as atopic dermatitis (AD), are common and increasing in prevalence in children (Kelsay, 2006).

Morbidity Associated with Allergic Disorders

The burden from allergic disorders such as asthma in the United States has increased over the past two decades, despite advances in asthma treatment. Increases in asthma morbidity and mortality are overrepresented in the pediatric population (Centers for Disease Control, 2002). Uncontrolled asthma can also impose serious limitations on daily life. For example, asthma is the leading cause of school absenteeism due to chronic illness, with approximately 14.7 million school days missed per year due to asthma symptoms in children 5–17 years of age (National Institutes of Health, 2002). Guidelines-based treatment for asthma and AR in children (National Heart, Lung, and Blood Institute, 2007; Bousquet et al., 2008) identified missed sleep due to symptoms as a key indicator of morbidity. Clinical guidelines for AR use the degree of sleep impairment due to symptoms to classify AR severity. Furthermore, the National Center on Sleep Disorders Research has recognized sleep disturbances as an important factor contributing to racial/ethnic and socioeconomic disparities in health outcomes (National Institutes of Health, 2003). Poor sleep quality is an indicator that allergic disease is in poor control given the potential presence of nocturnal symptoms, and has particular relevance for children's daytime functioning and overall quality of life (Blaiss, 2004; Juniper, Buist, Cox, Ferrie, & King, 1999; Koinis Mitchell, Craig, Esteban & Klein, 2012; see reviews Mullol, Maurer, & Bousquet, 2008; Nathan, 2007).

Pathophysiological Characteristics of Allergic Diseases

To provide more context for how asthma may affect sleep in children, it is important to first describe briefly the hallmark characteristics of the disease. Asthma is a complex disease of the airways, characterized by both episodic and chronic features. The guidelines for the diagnosis and management of asthma, developed by the National Heart, Lung, and Blood Institute, define asthma as a chronic inflammatory airway disorder, in which many cells and cellular elements play a role (National Heart, Lung, and Blood Institute, 2007). Asthma involves bronchial hyperresponsiveness (i.e., an exaggerated bronchoconstrictor response to stimuli) and bronchospasm, leading to airflow limitation and intermittent and variable periods of airway obstruction. Chronic inflammation of the airways, even in milder forms of the disease, is also recognized as a core feature. Guidelines-based asthma treatment approaches highlight the need for ongoing management for all forms of the disease to enhance lung function and minimize the burden of nighttime asthma symptoms on sleep, participation in activities, and overall functioning.

Specifically, the pathophysiology of asthma involves multiple overlapping processes, including smooth muscle dysfunction, airway inflammation, airway hyperresponsiveness to various triggers, swelling of the airways, and mucus production (National Institutes of Health, 1997). Smooth muscle contraction causes bronchial constriction. An influx of inflammatory cells (i.e., mast cells, eosinophils, and Type 2 helper T lymphocytes) is associated with airway inflammation. Airway inflammation and bronchoconstriction can result in a range of symptoms, including coughing, wheezing, breathlessness, and chest tightness, particularly at night or early in the morning. If not properly treated, symptoms of asthma and allergic diseases can persist and can impose limitations on physical functioning, including a restriction of activities, missed sleep, and overall quality of life (National Heart, Lung, and Blood Institute, 2007). Other outcomes of illness-related morbidity that can be affected by frequent symptoms include an increase in school absences for children, missed work for adults, and an increase in emergency department visits and hospitalizations. For children and adults, the presence of symptoms can also impair concentration. If untreated and/or severe, asthma, in particular, can result in death (Lara et al., 2006).

Allergic rhinitis (Bousquet, Van Cauwenberge, & Khaltaev, 2001) and atopic dermatitis (Fernandez-Mayoralas, Caballero, & Garcia-Marcos, 2004) have been shown to be risk factors for asthma. Asthma and allergic rhinitis (AR) have the same underlying immunopathology because a range of inflammatory mediators (e.g., histamine, leukotrienes) contribute to inflammation in both the upper and lower airways (Grossman, 1997). Both conditions are affected by similar allergens (e.g., molds) and involve similar treatment procedures: consistent use of medications and trigger control. Despite the similarities between asthma and AR, there are important distinctions. AR results in upper airway compromise because of nasal congestion, rhinorrhea, postnasal drainage, sneezing, and pruritus of the eyes, nose, ears, and throat (Fisher, Ghaffari, Davies, & Craig, 2005). The impact of asthma is more focused on lower airway compromise. AR symptoms may add a unique burden to individuals with asthma and can contribute to increased disruptions in sleep in children (Koinis Mitchell et al., 2012).

Atopic dermatitis appears to result from the complex interplay between defects in skin barrier function, environmental and infectious agents, and immune abnormalities (Watson & Kapur, 2011). Successful management of the disorder involves optimal skin care practices, anti-inflammatory treatment with topical corticosteroids and/or topical calcineurin inhibitors (TCIs), the use of first-generation antihistamines to help manage sleep disturbances, and the treatment of skin infections. Individuals with concomitant atopic conditions such as asthma and AR are at an increased risk for sleep disruption because of both the burden associated with managing multiple diseases and the higher potential for symptoms to occur during sleep if the illnesses are poorly managed (Watson & Kapur, 2011).

Pathophysiological Mechanisms of Allergic Disorders Affecting Sleep

Symptoms related to allergic disease are more frequently experienced during nighttime hours

(Meijer et al., 1995). A dip in cortisol levels at night can increase inflammatory cytokines and other mediators, which can bring on nighttime symptoms. Further, there is an association between inflammation and circadian rhythms; there is an increased inflammation during the night which can influence airway obstruction in asthma, more nasal congestion in allergic rhinitis, and more itching/scratching in atopic dermatitis (Martin & Banks-Schlegel, 1998). Histamine, an inflammatory mediator released during allergic reactions, may contribute to sleep disruption as it is involved in the regulation of the sleep–wake cycle and arousal (Tashiro et al., 2002). Circadian rhythms in nasal mucosa congestion have also been found to peak in adults during early morning hours, adversely affecting sleep quality (Ferguson, 2004).

Sleep posture can also facilitate an increase in mucus production for individuals with asthma and increased nasal congestion for individuals with AR (Craig, Sherkat, & Safaee, 2010). Additional factors in asthma include increased airway resistance at night and increased pollen counts during the nighttime hours. Typical sleep-related problems seen in AR include sleep disordered breathing, sleep apnea, and snoring, all of which are associated with nasal congestion/obstruction (Rappai, Collop, Kemp, & deShazo, 2003; see Craig et al., 2010, and Mullol et al., 2008 for a detailed explanation of mechanisms of sleep impairment involved in AR). For children with atopic dermatitis, disease flare-ups can result in itching and discomfort for the patient and, as a result, sleep can be disrupted (Leung et al., 2007).

Nonadherence to Treatment

Adherence to recommended treatment is an integral component for promoting sleep quality in children who are chronically ill. For children with allergic disorders, effective management requires acceptance of the chronic, episodic nature of the illness, and belief in the efficacy of medications used for treatment (McQuaid et al., 2005). Typical recommendations for asthma include separate medications for symptom control and for management of exacerbations, and identification of environmental triggers and measures to avoid or minimize exposure to them (National Heart, Lung, and Blood Institute, 2007). Quick-relief medications (e.g., short-acting $beta_2$–agonists, and systemic corticosteroids for more severe asthma episodes) are used to provide prompt relief of symptoms associated with bronchoconstriction, a core feature of asthma episodes. Long-term control medications are intended for daily use for extended periods of time to control persistent asthma symptoms. Children and adolescents with persistent asthma symptoms are typically prescribed both quick-relief medication and some form of long-term control medication, and adherence to these medications is crucial for control of symptoms at night (National Heart, Lung, and Blood Institute, 2007).

Child and adolescent patients are instructed that adherence to these treatment recommendations can lead to greater symptom control, decreased need for urgent health care visits, better sleep quality, and enhanced overall quality of life (National Heart, Lung, and Blood Institute, 2007). The more complex a treatment regimen becomes, however, the more challenging it becomes for patients and families to follow it effectively. If individuals with allergic disease do not adhere to daily treatment, whether it be daily use of a topical corticosteroid or daily controller medication use, or if individuals are symptomatic prior to bedtime and avoid using rescue medication, this can also result in increased symptoms during nighttime hours. In general, if nighttime symptoms related to allergic disorders are not well controlled, children can experience sleep loss and secondary daytime fatigue, which may contribute to missed school days, missed work for parents, diminished quality of life, decreased activity participation, and concentration and learning problems (International Conference on Allergic Rhinitis in Childhood, 1999; Juniper, Guyatt, & Dolovich, 1994). When controller medications are used consistently in children with asthma, lower levels of sleep problems have been observed (Garrison, Lozano, & Christakis, 2011).

Studies Examining Sleep and Allergic Disease in Children

Despite wide recognition that night waking due to allergic symptoms is a common problem with potentially significant consequences, sleep disturbance in individuals as a result of nighttime symptoms, particularly in pediatric populations, has been relatively neglected (Strachan, Anderson, Limb, O'Neill, & Wells, 1994).

Asthma

Few studies have examined sleep in children with asthma, despite the high potential for disrupted sleep due to nocturnal symptoms (National Heart, Lung, and Blood Institute, 2007). In one study, data from a night of polysomnography indicated that the primary sleep abnormality associated with asthma symptoms at night is the disruption of sleep due to frequent awakenings (Stores, Ellis, Wiggs, Crawford, & Thomson, 1998). This study also showed that awakenings due to asthma were associated with impairments in children's quality of life.

Fewer studies include representative groups of children, despite the fact that asthma prevalence and morbidity is disproportionately present in children of Puerto Rican and African-American descent (Lara, Akinbami, Flores, & Morgenstern, 2006). One study including non-Hispanic White and African-American children from middle to upper class backgrounds showed associations among the number of asthma-related awakenings (1–7 times per week), more school absences, and poorer school performance (Diette, Markson, Skinner, Nguen, & Algatt-Bergstrom, 2000). Other studies including representative samples of children show that nocturnal symptoms (Strunk, Sternberg, Bacharier, & Szefler, 2002) and parent report of poorer sleep quality are more likely in children with more severe asthma (Fagnano, Bayer, Isensee, Hernandez, & Halterman, 2011). Poor sleep in children with asthma has also been linked with high levels of behavioral problems by caregiver report (e.g., disruptive behaviors; Fagnano et al., 2009), worse asthma control, and poorer quality of life (Dean et al., 2010; Luyster et al., 2011). Finally, asthma symptoms such as wheezing and coughing have been associated with parent report of the child's difficulty falling asleep, disturbed sleep, and daytime sleepiness (Desager, Nelen, Weyler, & De Backer, 2005).

Rhinitis

Several large-scale survey studies have been conducted in the area of rhinitis and sleep. One study estimated that up to 88% of pediatric patients with AR have sleep problems (Juniper et al., 1994). In a recent survey of individuals with AR, 68% of respondents with perennial allergic rhinitis and 48% with seasonal AR reported that their condition interfered with sleep (Blaiss, 2004). In the *Pediatrics Allergies in America Survey*, sleep in individuals with rhinitis was altered with 40% reporting that allergies affected their sleep, 32% reporting having difficulty getting to sleep, and 26% reporting being awakened in the night due to symptoms (Meltzer et al., 2009). As a consequence of poor sleep due to AR symptoms, individuals with rhinitis have been shown to be more likely to have chronic excessive daytime sleepiness or chronic nonrestorative sleep than those who rarely or never have such symptoms (Young, Finn, & Kim, 1997). As in studies with asthma, sleep quality as assessed by subjective measurement is worse in individuals with more severe AR (Bousquet et al., 2006; Colas et al., 2012).

Studies using objective methods to assess sleep, such as actigraphy, are less common. One study demonstrated that adults with perennial allergic rhinitis have more sleep disturbance than healthy control participants (Rimmer, Downie, Bartlett, Gralton, & Salome, 2009). Another prospective study compared questionnaire responses to a sleepiness scale and polysomnography results between children with AR and 25 controls (Stuck et al., 2004). Results indicated an association between daytime sleepiness and quality of life measurements correlating with severity of rhinosinusitis.

It appears that individuals with AR are more prone to poor sleep because of an increase in the number of micro-arousals during sleep that are attributable to disordered breathing, upper airway resistance, and increased nasal discharge (Craig et al., 2010). Some early studies also point to nasal congestion associated with AR as a primary contributor to disturbed sleep and daytime fatigue (e.g., Lavie, Gertner, Zomer, & Podoshin, 1981). A common measure used to assess the impact of AR symptoms on quality of life is The Nocturnal Rhinoconjunctivities Quality of Life Questionnaire (NRQLQ; Juniper, Rohrbaugh, & Meltzer, 2003). Results from studies using this assessment have linked sinus congestion caused by AR with sleep disturbances (Juniper et al., 2003). Other symptoms such as sneezing, rhinorrhea, and nasal pruritus may also contribute to reduced sleep quality and sleep disturbances in AR (Camhi, Morgan, Pernisco, & Quan, 2000). Further, individuals with concomitant asthma and AR appear at greater risk for poor sleep (Janson et al., 1996).

Atopic Dermatitis

Fewer studies have focused on sleep quality and atopic dermatitis. Disturbed sleep in individuals with AD has been corroborated by several observational studies demonstrating that children with AD awaken more often and sleep less during the night, and adults with AD show a similar pattern (Bender & Leung, 2005). One small study examined sleep efficiency and scratching by polysomnography, actigraphy, and self-report in 20 adults with atopic dermatitis (Bender, Ballard, Canono, Murphy, & Leung, 2008). Decreased sleep efficiency was related to disease severity and increased scratching. Associations between poorer sleep by self-report and actigraphy and increased daytime fatigue in adults with AD compared to healthy controls has also been shown (Bender, Leung, & Leung, 2003). Dahl and colleagues (Dahl, Bernhisel-Broadbent, Scanlon-Holdford, Sampson, & Lupo, 1995) found that children with atopic dermatitis reported more nighttime waking, frequent daytime sleepiness, and irritability compared to children without atopic dermatitis. The severity of child dermatitis symptoms was also correlated with more daytime behaviors that were indicative of disturbed sleep (Dahl et al., 1995).

In summary, children with allergic disease are more susceptible to disrupted sleep due to the presence of potential nighttime symptoms and/or poor disease control. Children with more severe disease are at further risk for sleep impairment. Disrupted sleep due to nocturnal symptoms has negative consequences for daytime functioning, particularly quality of life. Compared to studies including individuals with asthma and AD, more research has been conducted in the area of AR and disrupted sleep.

Sleep Disorders

Sleep disordered breathing (SDB), snoring, and obstructive sleep apnea (OSA) are common sleep conditions in individuals with asthma and AR (Craig et al., 2010; Leger et al., 2006; Mullol et al., 2008) based on subjective criteria, although more studies are needed in this area. Moreover, current findings suggest wide racial and ethnic differences in sleep-related disorders, although these specific studies have not examined incidence of asthma or AR in these samples. SDB (snoring, upper airway resistance, obstructive sleep apnea) is twice as likely in young African Americans as in non-Latino Whites (Redline, Tichler, Hans, Tosteson, & Strohl, 1997). Furthermore, parental reports of witnessed apneas, snoring, and excessive daytime sleepiness are significantly more likely in Latino than non-Latino White children (Goodwin et al., 2003).

In studies of asthma, individuals with SDB have an increased risk of having severe asthma (Ross et al., 2012) and AR (Canova et al., 2004). Children with SDB in this study also had more behavioral problems compared with children without SDB. In studies assessing sleep using polysomnography in adults with seasonal allergic rhinitis and healthy adults, differences were found in an increased apnea and hypopnea index, increased snoring time, amount of REM sleep, and sleep latency in individuals with seasonal AR (e.g., Craig, Teets, Lehman, Chinchilli, & Zwillich, 1998; Stuck et al., 2004).

Several other studies have linked AR and allergic sensitization with snoring in children (e.g., Sogut et al., 2005). One study found atopy was the strongest risk factor for habitual snoring; the effect was cumulative, such that a child with comorbid asthma, allergic rhinitis, and atopic dermatitis was seven times more likely to snore (Sogut et al., 2005). Children with asthma and AR are at increased risk for sleep disordered breathing, particularly children with more severe disease. This has implications for children's daytime functioning, although more studies are needed in this area.

Sleep Behaviors and Duration

Limited studies have examined specific sleep behaviors and the quantity of sleep in children with asthma and allergic diseases. In the context of children's sleep practices, rates of napping among children without chronic illnesses have been found to vary by race and ethnicity, with African-American and Latino children often napping more frequently than non-Latino White children (Crosby, LeBourgeois, & Harsh, 2005; Lavigne et al., 1999). Caregivers also reported that African-American children slept less on weekday nights and had shorter nocturnal sleep durations. Less time sleeping at night among African-American children, as well as differences in the cultural acceptance of naps, may explain differences in napping by cultural background (Crosby et al., 2005). Napping also appears to be a more common behavior than expected in children with asthma of minority ethnicity, potentially related to later bedtimes and inadequate nighttime sleep (Kieckhefer, Ward, Tsai, & Lentz, 2008). Further research including ethnic minority children with asthma is needed to examine whether napping behaviors may be more likely in this group to make up for inadequate sleep, or due to more severe disease.

A host of factors associated with allergic disorders (e.g., variability in symptom pattern, potential for nocturnal symptoms, higher severity level, nonadherence to medications) can affect sleep patterns in children. The general consensus among findings indicates that children with allergic disorders are more susceptible to disrupted sleep due to the presence of potential nighttime symptoms that can awaken children and affect sleep quality. There are additional factors related to the family such as the family climate, caregiver functioning, and family cultural background and socioeconomic status that may be affected by the child's allergic disease (and vice versa), and, in turn, influence the child's sleep behaviors, routines, and sleep quality.

The Family Context

The family plays a paramount role in managing the child's allergic disorder (McQuaid, Walders, Kopel, Fritz, & Klinnert, 2005), especially for children who are younger than school age. As children develop, they gain increasing independence managing the illness; however, the family still strongly affects daily decisions about illness management, and consistent findings show that effective family management behaviors are linked with lower levels of illness-related morbidity (e.g., McQuaid et al., 2005). In the context of sleep, aspects of the family environment, such as the family climate, have emerged as contributing factors in sleep disturbances among children with chronic illnesses. For instance, in pediatric asthma, the negative mood of the caregiver, parenting hassles, and disruptions in bedtime routines increase the risk of child awakenings at night (Fiese, Winter, Sliwinski, & Anbar, 2007). Using daily diary data collected via the telephone, Fiese and colleagues (2007) found that the degree to which a parent felt hassled by a daily event (e.g., changing plan because of unexpected child need, children not listening), but not the daily event itself, was associated with the greater likelihood that a child with asthma would awaken at night. A parent who is already sleep deprived from nighttime awakening due to the child's asthma symptoms may have a lower threshold for children's misbehaviors, which may contribute to a caregiver's negative mood. Children may also sense such changes in the parent and may resist bedtime at night or may experience fluctuations in mood as a result of an unhappy parent, which can make it more difficult for the child to fall asleep at night (Fiese et al., 2007).

Caregiver Emotional Distress Related to the Child's Illness and Caregiver Sleep

Results from other studies also highlight the importance of caregiver functioning when considering the sleep of chronically ill children. It is well established that across chronic conditions, the stress of caring for a child with a chronic illness can lead to higher rates of parent emotional distress (Frankel & Wamboldt, 1998). Caregiver mood and stress have been linked to poor sleep quality in caregivers, which may have adverse consequences for a child's daily illness management (Dobbin, Bartlett, Melehan, Grunstein, & Bye, 2005). As compared to a control group of caregivers of children without a chronic illness, caregiver depression and anxiety were found to disrupt caregivers' sleep in those who had children with asthma (Yilmaz et al., 2008). The burden and worry associated with caring for a child with a chronic illness, as well as the task of managing the child's symptoms through the night may contribute to poor sleep in caregivers (Ziaian et al., 2006). Sleep loss in parents has been associated with a parent's ability to adequately manage a child's illness and to make important medical decisions (Scott, Hwang, & Rogers, 2006; Yilmaz et al., 2008), as well as with missed days of work and lost wages for parents (Diette et al., 2000).

As the association between caregiver sleep and caregiver mood is likely cyclical, poor sleep quality in caregivers may intensify poor psychological functioning and increase their sensitivity to depression and anxiety (Meltzer & Mindell, 2006). Studies have found a significant association between sleep and psychological functioning in caregivers of children with asthma (Yuksel et al., 2007). The presence of depressive symptoms in mothers of children with asthma has also been associated with decreased adherence and increased rates of emergency department visits (Bartlett et al., 2004). Consideration of the caregiver's distress level and psychological functioning is important when attempting to address sleep disruption in children with allergic disorders. Caregiver level of distress can likely challenge the effective management of children's disease, which may disrupt the child's and the caregiver's sleep if more symptoms are experienced at night. Furthermore, parent distress leads to fluctuations in family climate, which has the potential to impact child sleep (Fiese et al., 2007; see Meltzer and Walsh, Chapter 13). In addition to caregiver mood, frequent disruptions in the caregiver's sleep are also likely due to the child's asthma and allergy symptoms experienced throughout the night (Ziaian et al., 2006). More nocturnal asthma symptoms have also been related to poorer caregiver quality of life, with caregivers reporting feeling more burdened by their child's asthma (Fagnano, Bayer, Isensee, Hernandez, & Halterman, 2011). The sleep of caregivers with children who have severe illness is an important area of focus, as more support in maintaining adherence to the child's treatment may be warranted.

Caregiver Monitoring at Night

Chronic illnesses that require medical monitoring during the night have also been found to disturb caregiver sleep, including those who have children with asthma (Diette et al., 2000; Horner, 1997). In fact, nighttime monitoring may lead to multiple nighttime visits to check on their child's illness status. This has also been observed in studies including children with diabetes (Monaghan, Hilliard, Cogen, & Streisand, 2009; Sullivan-Bolyai, Deatrick, Gruppuso, Tamborlane, & Grey, 2003) and epilepsy (Williams et al., 2000). Co-sleeping behaviors may be more likely in these circumstances, when caregivers are fearful of their children's breathing problems during the night and, as a result, choose to sleep with the child. This pattern has been observed in caregivers of children with epilepsy; increased rates of co-sleeping following diagnosis have been found, which can affect both parent and child sleep (Becker, Fennell, & Carney, 2003).

In summary, overall family climate, caregiver emotional stress, and caregiver sleep have emerged as areas within the family context that ultimately have implications for child sleep and daily illness management (see Meltzer and Walsh, Chapter 13). In particular, caregiver sleep may be disturbed by nighttime management of symptoms or by monitoring the child's illness during the night. Interventions to improve sleep among children with chronic illnesses should focus on factors related to the family, especially caregiver functioning. Findings related to child sleep in chronic illnesses speak to the need for health care providers to focus on the parent in addition to the child, and make referrals and recommendations for the parent as appropriate.

Family's Cultural Background

Limited studies have considered cultural-related processes related to sleep behaviors among children with chronic illnesses (Boergers & Koinis-Mitchell, 2010). Specific groups of families may experience factors related to ethnic background, such as discrimination, acculturative stress, and health care system challenges (e.g., language barriers) that may affect child health and sleep (Boergers & Koinis-Mitchell, 2010; see Super and Harkness, Chapter 9). Cultural beliefs may impact how the child's illness is managed, which ultimately can have an influence on the quality of a child's sleep. For example, cultural beliefs related to co-sleeping and sleep behaviors (e.g., napping) have emerged as important aspects of sleep that can differ by cultural background. As ethnic minority families are often more likely to live in urban settings, daily stressors such as lack of financial resources, neighborhood safety, child level of stress, and lack of social support may affect the family climate and psychological functioning of parents. Although factors related to the family's sociocontextual background are not often included as cultural factors, they do play an important role in child health and sleep behaviors. Thus, in addition to studies focused on co-sleeping and sleep behaviors, we also include a review of the literature focused on sociocontextual factors and sleep in children with allergic disease.

Co-sleeping (see Burnham, Chapter 12). Most of the literature focused on co-sleeping in ethnically diverse families has found that African American families are more likely to co-sleep than other ethnic groups (Fu, Moon, & Hauck, 2010; Joyner, Oden, Ajao, & Moon, 2010; Shields, Hunsaker, Muldoon, Corey, & Spivack, 2005). Further, bed sharing has been associated with a higher risk of SIDS and risk of accidental suffocation, especially among African American infants (Fu et al., 2010). Reasons for co-sleeping often include parental work schedules, limited space due to financial constraints, and a belief in interdependence over autonomy (Morgan & Johnson, 2001).

There are limited studies specifically focused on co-sleeping among children with chronic illnesses. Co-sleeping in children with health conditions appears to arise in response to a need to keep an eye on the child, such as in children who have developed seizures (Williams et al., 2000). For instance, Williams et al. (2000) found that parents were more likely to co-sleep after an initial diagnosis of epilepsy (22%) versus diabetes (8%). Parents may have been motivated to co-sleep by their own anxiety about their child's condition. Furthermore, 38% of the sample that initiated co-sleeping following diagnosis was African American whereas 19% of the sample that co-slept was non-Latino White.

Co-sleeping in pediatric chronic illness has also emerged as a way to help manage symptoms during the night. In a study of children with atopic dermatitis, 30% of parents reported co-sleeping (Chamlin et al., 2005). Further, 66% of these parents described being bothered by co-sleeping and that doing so helped their child manage symptoms such as itching and scratching. With respect to ethnic differences, Chamlin et al. (2005) found that co-sleeping was more prevalent among Asian-American families of a child with atopic dermatitis versus African-American, Caucasian, or Hispanic families. Although the literature on co-sleeping in families with a child with asthma and allergic disease is sparse, it appears that co-sleeping is mostly utilized to keep a closer watch on the child and to assist with the child's symptoms. It is also likely that cultural values related to co-sleeping or sociocontextual factors related to crowding may lead to higher rates of co-sleeping among ethnic minority families, although more research is needed to determine such associations.

Sociocontextual Factors

Family Socioeconomic Status

In considering factors related to the context within which a child lives, socioeconomic status (SES; see Hale, Parente, and Phillips, Chapter 10) can affect poorer sleep outcomes in children with a chronic illness. For example, in pediatric obesity, neighborhood income and short sleep duration emerged as important predictors of increased odds of child obesity status (Ievers-Landis, Storfer-Isser, Rosen, Johnson, & Redline, 2008). The stress of limited family resources may contribute negatively to the overall family climate and level of stressors, perhaps making sleep routines and maintaining good sleep hygiene as well as illness control difficult among children with chronic illnesses. Limited financial resources have been linked with poorer medication adherence in children with asthma (McQuaid et al., 2009), which can affect the potential for nighttime symptoms.

A higher proportion of poor families tend to live in urban environments where asthma prevalence rates are higher, and there is greater exposure to allergens and low-quality housing, which can make it difficult for families to control asthma symptoms (Koinis-Mitchell et al., 2009; Koinis Mitchell et al., 2007). Such conditions have been found to relate to more psychological distress and more symptoms in children with asthma (Wright et al., 2004). Mechanisms underlying the associations between SES and sleep in children with chronic illnesses are not well understood in the literature and require future research to investigate potential targets for intervention. It is likely that stress levels related to living in an impoverished context may challenge consistent bedtime routines, appropriate sleep hygiene, and effective management behaviors, which are all necessary ingredients to high quality sleep in children with asthma and allergic diseases.

Child Stress Level

Another important factor that can explain poor sleep among children from lower SES families might be related to the increased level of stress the child is experiencing. Stress can affect psychological functioning and in fact, children with chronic illnesses are often at risk for increased levels of depression and anxiety (Lavigne & Faier-Routman, 1992; McQuaid, Kopel, & Nassau, 2001). Ethnic minority children and children from urban settings are also at risk for increased psychological problems, often due to acculturative stress and discrimination as well as limited financial resources (Vera et al., 1991). Behavioral and emotional difficulties have been associated with problems in falling and staying asleep among children with chronic illnesses (Hysing, Sivertsen, Stormark, Elgen, & Lundervold, 2009). Taken together, these findings suggest children with asthma and allergic conditions may be at increased risk for sleep problems and may benefit from behavioral strategies to decrease stress and anxiety, which may in turn decrease psychological as well as illness-related symptoms.

Future Directions for Research

Pathophysiological mechanisms associated with asthma and allergic disease can contribute to disrupted sleep in children. Although research has furthered our understanding on the impact of these conditions on sleep quality, there are many important avenues to pursue in future research. Given the risk for poorer health outcomes in children with comorbid atopic conditions, examining the effects of co-occurring symptoms on sleep quality in children is an important research priority to determine how to reduce the impact of each disease and identify appropriate and specific targets for intervention (e.g., identifying which symptoms to treat first).

Many of the studies reviewed tend to be cross-sectional in nature and involve short time periods of assessment. There is a need for prospective, longitudinal studies examining the co-occurrence of symptoms and sleep patterns in children in order to provide more causal evidence for the effects of allergic disease on sleep. Further, more focus on the consequences of impaired sleep on different areas of functioning relevant to various developmental levels, beyond quality of life, are needed.

Studies including children with asthma and allergic diseases tend to use a range of terminology to describe sleep affected by nighttime symptoms, such as sleep impairment, sleep disturbances, sleep problems, sleep efficiency, sleep quality, and so forth. This is likely influenced by the range of methods used to assess sleep (subjective vs. objective methods) and the specific issues relevant to these illnesses (e.g., sleep disruptions or number of wakings due to symptoms). More clarity is needed with how sleep is defined and measured, as each term used has a specific meaning and may have a different impact on health outcomes.

Most methods for assessing both symptoms and sleep rely on self-report assessments, which are subject to poor recall and bias. These include assessments of daily atopic symptoms, sleep problems, daytime somnolence, fatigue, and quality of life. On the other hand, there are benefits to using these instruments; subjective questionnaires are easy to use, inexpensive and have demonstrated reliability, validity, and reproducibility.

The use of more objective assessments of sleep quality in the form of actigraphy and polysomnography in children with chronic diseases, such as asthma, is less common. Although these methods are expensive and increase burden to participants and on study resources, they do allow for more sophisticated indicators that are relevant to asthma and allergic disease (frequency and duration of night wakings lasting a particular length of time; number of minutes spent asleep). These methods also allow for a more precise assessment of changes in sleep quality across specific sleep periods (sleep onset latency, rest period, sleep period). Further, an accurate diagnosis of asthma and/or AR and classification of disease severity and control are necessary to inform the most appropriate therapeutic interventions determined by guidelines-based approaches and minimize nocturnal symptoms.

Sample sizes in the studies focusing on allergic disease and sleep in children tend to be small, and not representative of specific ethnic groups at high risk for illness-related morbidity. Further study of differences in sleep patterns, timing and duration of sleep, sleep disruptions and sleep disorders in specific ethnic groups is needed. Mechanisms across multiple levels (pathophysiological, cultural/family, individual/psychological, environmental) that may underlie ethnic and racial differences in sleep in children with allergic disease need to be pursued in further depth in order to guide more tailored interventions. In addition, given sleep behaviors are highly variable across the developmental period, studies should focus on whether sleep disruptions or patterns differ across specific age groups in individuals with allergic disease. For example, caregivers may monitor younger children more closely, and bed sharing may be more common in families where children have more persistent disease.

Psychological problems are also more prevalent in children who have atopic conditions such as asthma, yet they have been overlooked in sleep research. Future research is needed to examine whether illness-related symptoms may influence the presence of psychological conditions and, in turn, affect quality of sleep. Medications used to treat conditions such as ADHD (e.g., stimulants) need to also be considered.

Treatments that improve symptoms (of nasal congestion in AR particularly), such as intranasal corticosteroids can enhance children's sleep (Craig et al., 2010) and may improve daytime sleepiness and quality of life (Lunn & Craig, 2011). For children with asthma, fewer sleep problems have been observed in children who are more adherent to daily controller medications (Lunn & Craig, 2011). In contrast, sedating antihistamines can increase daytime sedation and fatigue (Craig et al., 2010). In general, the role of effective management behaviors in promoting high quality sleep practices in children with allergic disease needs to be studied further in research. More attention to the role of medication adherence on sleep quality in children with allergic diseases, who are at increased risk, is clearly needed. For children who have overlapping asthma and AR symptoms, balancing the management of both disorders through effective trigger control and continued medication adherence may be key to preventing impairments in sleep and improving daytime functioning.

Focusing sleep research on other comorbidities of asthma and AR, such as obesity, which seems to be linked with sleep disordered breathing, is an important area for further research (Gozal & Kheirandish-Gozal, 2009). Treating these comorbidities, such as SDB, may improve asthma morbidity and sleep.

Conclusions

In summary, sleep impairment associated with allergic diseases such as asthma, AR, and atopic dermatitis can have a significant impact on children's quality of life and on their concentration and physical activity levels. The sleep disturbance can be caused by symptoms associated with the illness such as wheezing or coughing in asthma, nasal congestion in AR, and itching in AD. Inflammatory cytokines and other mediators can also directly disturb sleep and cause daytime somnolence in children, fatigue, decreased cognitive and psychomotor abilities, and increased difficulty concentrating.

Therapeutic interventions related to guidelines-based treatment for asthma and allergic disorders have demonstrated improvement in symptoms and quality of life. Bolstering adherence to specific treatment recommendations that may be particularly relevant to sleep (medication use and trigger control) is important for future interventions with children, particularly those with more severe disease or comorbid atopic conditions. A range of factors associated with allergic disease and treatment behaviors (e.g., severity, adherence to treatment), as well as a child's and family's cultural background and context (e.g., caregiver functioning, factors related to urban poverty, and family sleep practices) can disrupt sleep and affect sleep patterns and need to be considered when working with children who have allergic disorders. Multilevel interventions that focus on improving adherence to treatment recommendations, enhancing sleep hygiene and behaviors related to sleep quality through behavioral approaches, and attending to family and environmental factors that may affect sleep, are necessary given the multidetermined nature of asthma and allergic disorders and the array of consequences that sleep can have on children's functioning.

Future Research Questions

- The impact of co-occurring symptoms related to asthma and allergic disease on sleep quality in children should be investigated to identify specific targets for interventions to reduce disease impact and improve sleep quality.
- Prospective, longitudinal studies examining the co-occurrence of symptoms and sleep patterns in children are needed to provide more causal evidence for the effects of allergic disease on sleep.
- Studies should also aim to address the consequences of impaired sleep on different areas of child functioning, as well as how these consequences may differ by developmental level.
- As studies including children with asthma and allergic diseases tend to use a range of terminology to describe sleep affected by nighttime symptoms, more clarity is needed as to how sleep is defined and measured across studies.
- Researchers should strive to incorporate objective assessments of sleep quality (e.g., actigraphy) as they allow for more precise assessments of changes in sleep quality across specific sleep periods.
- Studies focused on the mechanisms underlying ethnic and racial differences in sleep in children with allergic disease are needed, as specific ethnic groups are often at high risk for illness-related morbidity.
- Future research is needed to examine whether illness-related symptoms may influence the presence of psychological conditions and, in turn, affect quality of sleep.
- The role of effective management behaviors, including medication adherence, in promoting high quality sleep practices in children with allergic disease needs to be studied further.
- Researchers should consider the impact of comorbid conditions, such as pediatric obesity, on sleep in children with asthma and allergic disease as treating these comorbidities may improve asthma morbidity and sleep.

References

Bartlett, S., Krishnan, J., Riekert, K., Butz, A., Malveaux, F., & Rand, C. (2004). Maternal depressive symptoms and adherence to therapy in inner-city children with asthma. *Pediatrics, 113*(2), 229–237.

Becker, D. A., Fennell, E. B., & Carney, P. R. (2003). Sleep disturbance in children with epilepsy. *Epilepsy & Behavior, 4*, 651–658.

Bender, B. G., Leung, S. B., & Leung, D. Y. (2003). Actigraphy assessment of sleep disturbance in patients with atopic dermatitis: an objective life quality measure. *Journal of Allergy and Clinical Immunology, 111*(3), 598–602.

Bender, B. G., & Leung, D. Y. (2005). Sleep disorders in patients with asthma, atopic dermatitis, and allergic rhinitis. *Journal of Allergy and Clinical Immunology, 116*(6), 1200–1201.

Bender, B. G., Ballard, R., Canono, B., Murphy, J. R., & Leung, D. Y. (2008). Disease severity, scratching, and sleep quality in patients with atopic dermatitis. *Journal of the American Academy of Dermatology, 58*(3), 415–420.

Blaiss, M. (2004). Allergic rhinitis and impairment issues in schoolchildren: A consensus report. *Current Medical Research and Opinions, 20*, 1937–1952.

Bousquet, J., Khaltaev, N., Cruz, A., Denburg, J., Fokkens, W., Togias, A., et al. (2008). Allergic rhinitis and its impact on asthma (ARIA) 2008 update (in collaboration with the World Health Organization, GA2LEN and AllerGen). *Allergy, 63*(Suppl. 86), 8–160.

Bousquet, J., Van Cauwenberge, P., & Khaltaev, N. (2001). Allergic rhinitis and its impact on asthma: Aria workshop report. *Journal of Allergy and Clinical Immunology, 108*(5), S147–S334.

Bousquet, J., Neukirch, F., Bousquet, P. J., Gehano, P., Klossek, J. M., Le Gal, M., et al. (2006). Severity and impairment of allergic rhinitis in patients consulting in primary care. *Journal of Allergy and Clinical Immunology, 117*(1), 158–162.

Boergers, J., & Koinis-Mitchell, D. (2010). Sleep and culture in children with medical conditions. *Journal of Pediatric Psychology, 35*, 915–926.

Camhi, S. L., Morgan, W. J., Pernisco, N., & Quan, S. F. (2000). Factors affecting sleep disturbances in children and adolescents. *Sleep Medicine, 1*(2), 117–123.

Canova, C. R., Downs, S. H., Knoblauch, A., Andersson, M., Tamm, M., & Leuppi, J. D. (2004). Increased prevalence of perennial allergic rhinitis in patients with obstructive sleep apnea. *Respiration, 71*(2), 138–143.

Centers for Disease Control. (2002). Surveillance for asthma—United States, 1980–1999. *Morbidity and Mortality Weekly Report, 51*(SS01), 1–13.

Centers for Disease Control and Prevention. (2010). *Behavioral Risk Factor Surveillance System Survey Questionnaire*. Atlanta, GA: US Department of Health and Human Services.

Chamlin, S. L., Mattson, C. L., Frieden, I. J., Williams, M. L., Mancini, A. J., Cella, D., et al. (2005). The price of pruritus: Sleep disturbance and cosleeping in atopic dermatitis. *Archives of Pediatrics & Adolescent Medicine, 159*, 745–750.

Colas, C., Galera, H., Anibarro, B., Soler, R., Navarro, A., Jauregui, I., et al. (2012). Disease severity impairs sleep quality in allergic rhinitis (The SOMNIAAR study). *Clinical & Experimental Allergy, 42*(7), 1080–1087.

Craig, T. J., Teets, S., Lehman, E. B., Chinchilli, V. M., & Zwillich, C. (1998). Nasal congestion secondary to allergic rhinitis as a cause of sleep disturbance and daytime fatigue and the response to topical nasal corticosteroids. *Journal of Allergy and Clinical Immunology, 101*(5), 633–637.

Craig, T. J., Sherkat, A., & Safaee, S. (2010). Congestion and sleep impairment in allergic rhinitis. *Current Allergy and Asthma Reports, 10*(2), 113–121.

Crosby, B., LeBourgeois, M. K., & Harsh, J. (2005). Racial differences in reported napping and nocturnal sleep in 2- to 8-year-old children. *Pediatrics, 115*, 225–232.

Dahl, R. E., Bernhisel-Broadbent, J., Scanlon-Holdford, S., Sampson, H. A., & Lupo, M. (1995). Sleep disturbances in children with atopic dermatitis. *Archives of Pediatrics & Adolescent Medicine, 149*, 856–860.

Dean, B. B., Calimlim, B. C., Sacco, P., Aguilar, D., Maykut, R., & Tinkelman, D. (2010). Uncontrolled asthma among children: Impairment in social functioning and sleep. *Journal of Asthma, 47*(5), 539–544.

Derebery, J., Meltzer, E., Nathan, R. A., Stang, P. E., Campbell, U. B., Corrao, M., et al. (2008). Rhinitis symptoms and comorbidities in the United States: Burden of rhinitis in America survey. *Otolaryngology – Head and Neck Surgery, 139*(2), 198–205.

Desager, K. N., Nelen, V., Weyler, J. J., & De Backer, W. A. (2005). Sleep disturbance and daytime symptoms in wheezing school-aged children. *Journal of Sleep Research, 14*, 77–82.

Diette, G. B., Markson, L., Skinner, E. A., Nguen, T. T., & Algatt-Bergstrom, P. (2000). Nocturnal asthma in children affects school attendance, school performance and parents' work attendance. *Archives of Pediatric Adolescent Medicine, 154*, 923–928.

Dobbin, C. J., Bartlett, D., Melehan, K., Grunstein, R. R., & Bye, P. T. (2005). The effect of infective exacerbations on sleep and neurobehavioral function in cystic fibrosis. *American Journal of Respiratory and Critical Care Medicine, 172*, 99–104.

Fagnano, M., van Wijngaarden, E., Connolly, H. V., Carno, M. A., Forbes-Jones, E., & Halterman, J. S. (2009). Sleep-disordered breathing and behaviors of inner-city children with asthma. *Pediatrics, 124*(1), 218–225.

Fagnano, M., Bayer, A. L., Isensee, C. A., Hernandez, T., & Halterman, J. S. (2011). Nocturnal asthma symptoms and poor sleep quality among urban school children with asthma. *Academic Pediatrics, 11*(6), 493–499.

Ferguson, B. (2004). Influences of allergic rhinitis on sleep. *Otolaryngology – Head and Neck Surgery, 130*, 617–629.

Fernandez-Mayoralas, M., Caballero, J. M. M., & Garcia-Marcos, A. L. (2004). Association between atopic dermatitis, allergic rhinitis and asthma in schoolchildren ages 13–14 years old. *Anales de Pediatría (Barcelona, Spain), 60*, 236–242.

Fiese, B. H., Winter, M. A., Sliwinski, M., & Anbar, R. D. (2007). Nighttime waking in children with asthma: An exploratory study of daily fluctuations in family climate. *Journal of Family Psychology, 21*, 95–103.

Fisher, L., Ghaffari, G., Davies, M., & Craig, T. (2005). Effects of poor sleep in allergic rhinitis. *Current Opinion in Allergy and Clinical Immunology, 5*, 11–16.

Frankel, K., & Wamboldt, M. Z. (1998). Chronic childhood illness and maternal mental health—Why should we care? *Journal of Asthma, 35*(8), 621–630.

Fu, L. Y., Moon, R. Y., & Hauck, F. R. (2010). Bed sharing among Black infants and sudden infant death syndrome: Interactions with other known risk factors. *Academic Pediatrics, 10*, 376–382.

Garrison, M. M., Lozano, P., & Christakis, D. A. (2011). Controller medication use and sleep problems in pediatric asthma: A longitudinal case-crossover analysis. *Archives of Pediatrics & Adolescent Medicine, 165*(9), 826–830.

Goodwin, J., Barber, S., Kaemingk, K., Rosen, G., Morgan, W., Sherrill, D., et al. (2003). Symptoms related to sleep-disordered breathing in white and Hispanic children. *Chest, 124*, 196–203.

Gozal, D., & Kheirandish-Gozal, L. (2009). Obesity and excessive daytime sleepiness in prepubertal children with obstructive sleep apnea. *Pediatrics, 123*(1), 13–18.

Grossman, J. (1997). One airway, one disease. *Chest, 111*, 11S–16S.

Gumustekin, K., Seven, B., Karabulut, N., Aktas, O., Gursan, N., Aslan, S., et al. (2004). Effects of sleep deprivation, nicotine, and selenium on wound healing in rats. *International Journal Neuroscience, 114*(11), 1433–1442.

Horner, S. D. (1997). Uncertainty in mothers' care for their ill children. *Journal of Advanced Nursing, 26*, 658–663.

Hysing, M., Sivertsen, B., Stormark, K. M., Elgen, I., & Lundervold, A. J. (2009). Sleep in children with chronic illness, and the relation to emotional and behavioral problems—a population-based study. *Journal of Pediatric Psychology, 34*, 665–670.

Ievers-Landis, C., Storfer-Isser, A., Rosen, C., Johnson, N. L., & Redline, S. (2008). Relationship of sleep parameters, child psychological functioning, and parenting stress to obesity status among preadolescent children. *Journal of Developmental and Behavioral Pediatrics, 29*, 243–252.

International Conference on Allergic Rhinitis in Childhood. (1999). Allergic rhinitis in childhood. *Allergy, 54*, S7–S34.

Janson, C., De Backer, W., Gislason, T., Plaschke, P., Bjornsson, E., Hetta, J., et al. (1996). Increased prevalence of sleep disturbances and daytime sleepiness in subjects with bronchial asthma: a population study of young adults in three European countries. *European Respiratory Journal, 9*(10), 2132–2138.

Joyner, B. L., Oden, R. P., Ajao, T. I., & Moon, R. Y. (2010). Where should my baby sleep: A qualitative study of African-American infant sleep location decisions. *Journal of the National Medical Association, 102*, 881–889.

Juniper, E., Guyatt, G., & Dolovich, J. (1994). Assessment of quality of life in adolescents with allergic rhinoconjunctivitis: Development and testing of a questionnaire for clinical trials. *Journal of Allergy and Clinical Immunology, 93*, 413–423.

Juniper, E. F., Buist, A. S., Cox, F. M., Ferrie, P. J., & King, D. R. (1999). Validation of a standardized version of the Asthma Quality of Life Questionnaire. *Chest, 115*(5), 1265–1270.

Juniper, Rohrbaugh, T., & Meltzer, E. O. (2003). A questionnaire to measure quality of life in adults with nocturnal allergic rhinoconjunctivitis. *Journal of Allergy and Clinical Immunology, 111*(3), 484–490.

Kelsay, K. (2006). Management of sleep disturbance associated with atopic dermatitis. *Journal of Allergy and Clinical Immunology, 118*(1), 198–201.

Kieckhefer, G. M., Ward, T. M., Tsai, S. Y., & Lentz, M. J. (2008). Nighttime sleep and daytime nap patterns in school age children with and without asthma. *Journal of Developmental and Behavioral Pediatrics, 29*(5), 338–344.

Koinis Mitchell, D., Craig, T., Esteban, C. A., & Klein, R. B. (2012). Sleep and allergic disease: a summary of the literature and future directions for research. *Journal of Allergy and Clinical Immunology, 130*(6), 1275–1281.

Koinis Mitchell, D., McQuaid, E., Seifer, R., Kopel, S., Esteban, C., Canino, G., et al. (2007). Multiple urban and asthma-related risks and their association with asthma morbidity in children. *Journal of Pediatric Psychology, 32*(5), 582–595.

Koinis-Mitchell, D., McQuaid, E. L., Kopel, S., Esteban, C., Ortega, A., Seifer, R., et al. (2009). Cultural-related, contextual, and asthma-specific risks associated with asthma morbidity in urban children. *Journal of Clinical Psychology in Medical Settings, 17*, 38–48.

Lara, M., Akinbami, L., Flores, G., & Morgenstern, H. (2006). Heterogeneity of childhood asthma among Hispanic children: Puerto Rican children bear a disproportionate burden. *Pediatrics, 117*, 43–53.

Lavie, P., Gertner, R., Zomer, J., & Podoshin, L. (1981). Breathing disorders in sleep associated with "microarousals" in patients with allergic rhinitis. *Acta Otolaryngologica, 92*(5–6), 529–533.

Lavigne, J. V., & Faier-Routman, J. (1992). Psychological adjustment to pediatric physical disorders: A meta-analysis. *Journal of Pediatric Psychology, 17*(2), 133–157.

Lavigne, J. V., Arend, R., Rosenbaum, D., Smith, A., Weissbluth, M., Binns, H. J., et al. (1999). Sleep and behavior problems among preschoolers. *Journal of Developmental and Behavioral Pediatrics, 20*, 164–169.

Leger, D., Annesi-Maesano, I., Carat, F., Rugina, M., Chanal, I., Pribil, C., et al. (2006). Allergic rhinitis and its consequences on quality of sleep: An unexplored area. *Archives of Internal Medicine, 166*(16), 1744–1748.

Leung, A. K., Hon, K. L., & Robson, W. L. (2007). Atopic dermatitis. *Advances in Pediatrics, 54*, 241–273.

Lunn, M., & Craig, T. (2011). Rhinitis and sleep. *Sleep Medicine Reviews, 15*(5), 293–299.

Luyster, F. S., Teodorescu, M., Bleecker, E., Busse, W., Calhoun, W., Castro, M., et al. (2011). Sleep quality and asthma control and quality of life in non-severe and severe asthma. *Sleep & Breathing, 16*(4), 1129–1137.

Martin, R., & Banks-Schlegel, S. (1998). Chronobiology of asthma. *American Journal of Respiratory and Critical Care Medicine, 158*, 1002–1007.

McQuaid, E., Walders, N., Kopel, S., Fritz, G., & Klinnert, M. (2005). Pediatric asthma management in the family context: The family asthma management system scale. *Journal of Pediatric Psychology, 30*, 492–502.

McQuaid, E. L., Kopel, S. J., & Nassau, J. H. (2001). Behavioral adjustment in children with asthma: A meta-analysis. *Journal of Developmental and Behavioral Pediatrics, 22*, 430–439.

McQuaid, E. L., Vasquez, J., Canino, G., Fritz, G. K., Ortega, A. N., Colon, A., et al. (2009). Beliefs and barriers to medication use in parents of Latino children with asthma. *Pediatric Pulmonology, 44*(9), 892–898.

Meijer, G., Postma, D., Wempe, J., Gerristen, J., Knol, K., & van Aadleren, W. (1995). Frequency of nocturnal symptoms in asthmatic children attending a hospital out-patient clinic. *European Respiratory Journal, 8*, 2076–2080.

Meltzer, E. O., & Mindell, J. A. (2006). Impact of a child's chronic illness on maternal sleep and daytime functioning. *Archives of Internal Medicine, 166*, 1749–1755.

Meltzer, E. O., Blaiss, M. S., Derebery, M. J., Mahr, T. A., Gordon, B. R., Sheth, K. K., et al. (2009). Burden of allergic rhinitis: Results from the Pediatric Allergies in America survey. *Journal of Allergy and Clinical Immunology, 124*, S43–70.

Mindell, J. A., Spirito, A., & Carskadon, M. A. (1990). Prevalence of sleep problems in chronically ill children. *Sleep Research, 19*, 337.

Monaghan, M. C., Hilliard, M. E., Cogen, F. R., & Streisand, R. (2009). Nighttime caregiving behaviors among parents of young children with Type 1 diabetes: Associations with illness characteristics and parent functioning. *Families, Systems, & Health: The Journal of Collaborative Family Healthcare, 27*, 28–38.

Morgan, S. K., & Johnson, C. M. (2001). Infant sleep: Resident recommendations and socioeconomic status differences in patient practices. *Family Medicine, 33*, 614–620.

Mullol, J., Maurer, M., & Bousquet, J. (2008). Sleep and allergic rhinitis. *Journal of Investigational Allergology and Clinical Immunology, 18*(6), 415–419.

Nathan, R. A. (2007). The burden of allergic rhinitis. *Allergy & Asthma Proceedings, 28*(1), 3–9.

National Heart, Lung, and Blood Institute. (2007). *Guidelines for the Diagnosis and Management of Asthma.* Bethesda, MD: National Institutes of Health.

National Institutes of Health. (1997). *National Asthma Education and Prevention Program (National Heart, Lung, and Blood Institute) Second Expert Panel on the Management of Asthma. Expert panel report 2: Guidelines for the diagnosis and management of asthma.* Bethesda, MD: National Institutes of Health.

National Institutes of Health. (2002). *National Asthma Education and Prevention Program, Expert Panel, Report. Guidelines for the Diagnosis and Management of Asthma—Update on Selected Topics 2002.* Bethesda, MD: National Institutes of Health.

National Institutes of Health. (2003). *2003 National Sleep Disorders Research Plan.* U.S. Department of Health and Human Services, National Heart, Lung, and Blood Institute, National Center on Sleep Disorders Research, Trans-NIH Sleep Research Coordinating Committee, Bethesda, MD: National Institutes of Health.

Ozturk, L., Pelin, Z., Karadeniz, D., Kaynak, H., Cakar, L., & Gozukirmizi, E. (1999). Effects of 48 hours sleep deprivation on human immune profile. *Sleep Res Online, 2*(4), 107–111.

Rappai, M., Collop, N., Kemp, S., & deShazo, R. (2003). The nose and sleep-disordered breathing: What we know and what we do not know. *Chest, 124*(6), 2309–2323.

Redline, S., Tichler, P., Hans, M., Tosteson, T., & Strohl, K. (1997). Risk factors for sleep-disordered breathing in children. *American Journal of Respiratory and Critical Care Medicine, 155*, 186–192.

Rimmer, J., Downie, S., Bartlett, D. J., Gralton, J., & Salome, C. (2009). Sleep disturbance in persistent allergic rhinitis measured using actigraphy. *Annals of Allergy, Asthma & Immunology, 103*(3), 190–194.

Ross, K. R., Storfer-Isser, A., Hart, M. A., Kibler, A. M., Rueschman, M., Rosen, C. L., et al. (2012). Sleep-disordered breathing is associated with asthma severity in children. *Journal of Pediatrics, 160*(5), 736–742.

Scott, L. D., Hwang, W. T., & Rogers, A. E. (2006). The impact of multiple care giving roles on fatigue, stress, and work performance among hospital staff nurses. *Journal of Nursing Administration, 36*, 86–95.

Shields, L. B., Hunsaker, D. M., Muldoon, S., Corey, T. S., & Spivack, B. S. (2005). Risk factors associated with unexplained infant death: A prospective study of infant care practices in Kentucky. *Pediatrics, 116*, e13–e20.

Sogut, A., Altin, R., Uzun, L., Ugur, M. B., Tomac, N., Acun, C., et al. (2005). Prevalence of obstructive sleep apnea syndrome and associated symptoms in 3–11-year-old Turkish children. *Pediatric Pulmonology, 39*(3), 251–256.

Stores, G., Ellis, A., Wiggs, L., Crawford, C., & Thomson, T. (1998). Sleep and psychological disturbance in nocturnal asthma. *Archives of Disease in Childhood, 78*(5), 413–419.

Strachan, D., Anderson, H., Limb, E., O'Neill, A., & Wells, N. (1994). A national survey of asthma prevalence, severity and treatment in Great Britain. *Archives of Disease in Childhood, 70*, 174–178.

Strunk, R. C., Sternberg, A. L., Bacharier, L. B., & Szefler, S. J. (2002). Nocturnal awakening caused by asthma in children with mild to moderate asthma in the childhood asthma management program. *Journal of Asthma and Clinical Immunology, 110*, 395–403.

Stuck, B., Czaikowski, J., Hagner, A., Lkimek, L., Verse, T., Hormann, K., et al. (2004). Changes in daytime sleepiness, quality of life, and objective sleep patterns in seasonal allergic rhinitis: A controlled clinical trial. *Journal of Allergy and Clinical Immunology, 113*, 663–668.

Sullivan-Bolyai, S., Deatrick, J., Gruppuso, P., Tamborlane, W., & Grey, M. (2003). Constant vigilance: Mothers' work parenting young children with type 1 diabetes. *Journal of Pediatric Nursing, 18*, 21–29.

Tashiro, M., Mochizuki, H., Iwabuchi, K., Sakurada, Y., Itoh, M., Watanabe, T., et al. (2002). Roles of histamine in regulation of arousal and cognition: functional neuroimaging of histamine H1 receptors in human brain. *Life Sciences, 72*(4–5), 409–414.

Valrie, C. R., Gil, K. M., Redding-Lallinger, R., & Daeschner, C. (2007). Brief report: Sleep in children with sickle cell disease: An analysis of daily diaries utilizing multilevel models. *Journal of Pediatric Psychology, 32*(7), 857–861.

Van Cleave, J., Gortmaker, S. L., & Perrin, J. M. (2010). Dynamics of obesity and chronic health conditions among children and youth. *The Journal of the American Medical Association, 303*, 623–630.

Vera, M., Alegria, M., Freeman, D., Robles, R. R., Rios, R., & Rios, C. F. (1991). Depressive symptoms among Puerto Ricans: Island poor compared with residents of the New York City area. *American Journal of Epidemiology, 134*(5), 502–510.

Watson, W., & Kapur, S. (2011). Atopic dermatitis. *Allergy, Asthma & Clinical Immunology, 7*(Suppl 1), S4.

Williams, J., Lange, B., Sharp, G., Griebel, M., Edgar, T., Haley, T., et al. (2000). Altered sleeping arrangements in pediatric patients with epilepsy. *Clinical Pediatrics, 39*, 635–642.

Wright, R. J., Mitchell, H., Visness, C. M., Cohen, S., Stout, J., Evans, R., et al. (2004). Community violence and asthma morbidity: the Inner-City Asthma Study. *American Journal of Public Health, 94*(4), 625–632.

Yarrington, A., & Mehta, P. (1998). Does sleep promote recovery after bone marrow transplantation?—A hypothesis. *Pediatric Transplantation, 2*(1), 51–55.

Yilmaz, O., Sogut, A., Gulle, S., Can, D., Ertan, P., & Yuksel, H. (2008). Sleep quality and depression-anxiety in mothers of children with two chronic respiratory diseases: Asthma and cystic fibrosis. *Journal of Cystic Fibrosis, 7*, 495–500.

Young, T., Finn, L., & Kim, H. (1997). Nasal obstruction as a risk factor for sleep-disordered breathing. The University of Wisconsin Sleep and Respiratory Research Group. *Journal of Allergy and Clinical Immunology, 99*(2), S757–762.

Yuksel, H., Sakar, A., Dinç, G., Yilmaz, O., Gozmen, S., Yorgancioglu, A., et al. (2007). The frequency of wheezing phenotypes and risk factors for persistence in Aegean region of Turkey. *Journal of Asthma 44*, 89–93.

Ziaian, T., Sawyer, M. G., Reynolds, K. E., Carbone, J. A., Clark, J. J., Baghurst, P. A., et al. (2006). Treatment burden and health-related quality of life of children with diabetes, cystic fibrosis and asthma. *Journal of Pediatrics and Child Health 42*, 596–600.

CHAPTER

33 Autism and other Developmental Disabilities

Amanda L. Richdale

Abstract

Parents of children with a developmental disability more commonly report sleep problems than parents of typically developing children. These sleep problems include difficulties getting their child to bed, and that their child takes a long time to fall asleep, wakes frequently, and/or wakes for long periods during the night. These reports are generally supported by objective findings. Sleep-disordered breathing is more common in children with specific developmental disorders such as Down syndrome and Prader-Willi syndrome, where craniofacial features associated with the disorder place them at high risk. Poor sleep in children with a developmental disability is generally associated with more severe daytime behavior difficulties, lower IQ, poorer adaptive behavior, compromised parent sleep, and increased parent stress, placing parents at risk for increased symptoms of anxiety and depression. Such sleep problems are likely to be multifactorial and are best viewed within a biopsychosocial context. Further research on the etiology, impact and intervention for sleep problems in children with a developmental disability is required.

Key Words: autism, sleep disorders, developmental disability, children, sleep

Introduction

This chapter considers sleep issues in children with developmental disorders, including children with an intellectual disability (i.e., IQ < 70 and poor adaptive behavior). The disorders included here are not exhaustive, but serve to illustrate similarities and differences in sleep problems across a range of developmental disorders. A primary focus is sleep in autism spectrum disorders, as they are more common than other developmental disorders and poor sleep is a common comorbid condition (American Psychiatric Association [APA], 2000; Richdale & Schreck, 2009). Effects on families and approaches to intervention for common sleep problems in children with developmental disabilities are also addressed. Readers are directed to Stores (2001) for a description and overview of sleep issues associated with a range of disorders of development, including developmental disabilities not covered here.

Sleep, as has been discussed in other sections of this book, is a developmental phenomenon (see Part 1) which is important for children's physical development, learning, behavioral regulation, and emotional well-being (e.g., Dewald, Meijer, Oort, Kerkhof, & Bögels., 2010; Gregory & Sadeh, 2012; see Part 5). Children's sleep is also influenced by family and environmental factors and, when problematic, can negatively impact families, especially mothers (e.g., Meltzer & Mindell, 2007). As readers already will have noted from other chapters in this book, sleep disturbances are a common occurrence in childhood and adolescence, being most prevalent in infants and young children, decreasing in middle childhood, and increasing in prevalence again with the onset of the physiological and social changes that begin with puberty. At all ages, evidence suggests that sleep problems are more common in children with a developmental disability than in children who are typically developing (Quine, 2001). Physiological features intrinsic to some developmental disorders (e.g., Down syndrome, Prader-Willi syndrome, Smith-Magenis syndrome) carry with them a high risk for specific sleep disorders. Nevertheless, in general the most common sleep problems reported by parents of children with a developmental disability relate to settling and night waking—that is, they are sleep problems and behaviors associated with insomnia, in particular the Behavioral Insomnias of Childhood (International Classification of Sleep Disorders, 2nd Ed. [ICSD-2]; American Academy of Sleep Medicine [AASM], 2005).

Sleep Problems in Developmental Disabilities

Children aged 6 years and over with an IQ < 70 and who have similarly poor adaptive behavior have an intellectual disability (or mental retardation), while a similar presentation in younger children is generally referred to as a *global developmental delay*. These are a heterogeneous group of children, including children who are presumed to have low IQ and adaptive behavior in the absence of any comorbid condition that may explain their delay as well as children with disorders known to be associated with low IQ and poor adaptive behavior, such as Down syndrome or Fragile X syndrome. As most sleep research regarding children with an intellectual disability or developmental disability uses heterogeneous groups of children and adolescents, the term *developmental disability* is used in this chapter to refer to this mixed group regardless of their age or specific developmental disorder.

Reports of high but variable rates of parent-reported sleep disturbance in children with a developmental disability have appeared in the literature for over 30 years. Prevalence figures range from 23.7% (Didden, Korzillius, van Aperlo, van Overloop, & de Vries, 2002), 34% (Clements, Wing, & Dunn, 1986), 57.7% (Richdale, Francis, Gavidia-Payne, & Cotton, 2000), and 77%–86%, with the higher rate in those under 6 years of age (Bartlett, Rooney, & Spedding, 1985). Similarly, Quine (2001) reported that the rate of sleep onset (41%) and night waking (45%) problems was much higher in children with a developmental disability than in children who were typically developing (27% and 13% respectively); restless sleep (53%) and bedwetting (33%) were also common (Quine, 2001). Unlike typically developing children, where sleep problems generally resolve after early childhood, sleep problems can continue for many years in children with a developmental disability (Robinson & Richdale, 2004; Wiggs & Stores, 1996a) and may be lifelong (Bramble, 1996). Keenan, Wild, McArthur, and Espie (2007) reported that parents believe that sleep problems are "chronic" with "severe consequences." The average parent-reported duration of sleep difficulties in children with a developmental disability is up to 8.8 years (Robinson & Richdale, 2004).

In a structured review of 61 papers examining sleep problems in children with a range of disorders of development, excluding autism spectrum disorders, Tietze et al. (2012) concluded that more than two-thirds of children with developmental disabilities presented with sleep problems, exceeding the rates of sleep difficulties reported in typically developing children and children with psychiatric disorders. Children with severe neurodegenerative disorders were almost universally likely to have sleeping difficulties. Insomnia was most common; sleep apnea and severe sleep–wake cycle disturbances were also frequent, with the latter more common in children with severe global brain damage; there did not appear to be any disorder-specific sleep problems. The authors thus concluded that degree of brain damage was more likely to be related to sleep disturbances. The heterogeneity of sleep problem definitions and methods of sleep ascertainment made comparisons difficult, and they noted a clear need for well-validated assessment tools to facilitate both etiological and intervention research.

Impact of Poor Sleep on Daytime Functioning

Poor sleep can have a range of negative consequences for children with a developmental disability (Doran, Harvey, & Horner, 2006), and in particular more severe behavioral difficulties are associated with sleep problems (Clements et al., 1986, Didden et al., 2002, Quine, 1991; Richdale et al., 2000; Wiggs & Stores; 1996a). Poor sleep has also been associated with a range of child factors, including communication, poor adaptive behavior, and poor academic skills (Quine, 1991; Stores, 1992). Quine's 1991 study remains the most comprehensive, examining the interrelationships between sleep, child, and family factors in children with a developmental disability. However, in a sample of 76 children, Robinson (2007) found that while children with a developmental disability and parent-reported sleep problems had poorer adaptive behavior and more behavior problems, these were not significantly worse than those reported for children who did not have a sleep problem.

Impact of Poor Child Sleep on Families

Parents of children with a developmental disability report that their own sleep is disrupted by their child's sleep difficulties (Didden et al., 2002; Robinson & Richdale, 2004) and express concern over the impact that their child's sleep problems may be having on both the child and other family members (Cotton & Richdale, 2006). These parents are also more likely to report fatigue, irritability, and difficulty coping (Didden et al., 2002). Maternal sleep and psychological well-being have been associated with poor sleep and difficult behavior (Chu & Richdale, 2009) in children with a developmental disability, and with parental stress (Gallagher, Phillips, & Carroll, 2010). In mothers of children with a developmental disability, children's sleep quality and behavior problems predicted maternal sleep, while mothers' sleep and children's behavior together predicted maternal stress with mothers' sleep predicting both maternal anxiety and maternal depression (Chu & Richdale, 2009).

Conclusion

Overall, the available evidence leads to the conclusion that for children with a developmental disability, poor sleep is related to a range of adverse consequences for both the children and their families. Nevertheless, in considering mixed disability groups researchers may be confounding a range of child and parent issues related to poor child sleep (Stores, 1992). First, the intrinsic behavioral or medical conditions associated with a specific developmental disorder (e.g., sleep apnea in Down Syndrome) will affect the sleep or behavioral issues reported in any study depending on the composition of the sample under study. Similarly, parents will be under varying degrees of stress associated with support needs, including behaviors associated with their child's developmental disability, social supports, child-related stress, associated medical conditions, education needs and supports, and finances; family income and professional support are of particular importance (Davis & Gavidia-Payne, 2009). For example, families in which a child has autism are more likely to suffer significant economic burden than families of children with other developmental disorders (Cidav, Marcus, & Mandell, 2012). These factors will likely affect parent psychological well-being and sleep.

Thus, it is preferable to investigate sleep within specific developmental disorders. This approach may provide some understanding of the etiology of specific developmental disorders and any commonly associated comorbid conditions, thus assisting in formulating approaches to prevention and intervention. Tietze et al. (2012) also noted the need to consider the impact of physical and psychosocial factors on sleep in children with developmental disorders to better understand poor sleep and develop effective treatments. However, when developmental disorders have a very low prevalence or incidence (rare chromosomal disorders), obtaining larger sample sizes to investigate sleep may be difficult. The following sections will address the sleep issues currently reported for specific developmental disorders and autism spectrum disorder.

Sleep in Specific Developmental Disorders

Down Syndrome

Down syndrome results from the presence of an extra 21st chromosome (trisomy 21) and is the most common noninherited cause of intellectual disability, averaging 1.08 births per 1000 (Irving, Basu, Richmond, Burn, & Wren, 2008); a majority of children with Down syndrome have an intellectual disability. As well as the characteristic facial features, physical characteristics include short stature, poor muscle tone, tendency to excess weight gain, and a protruding tongue. Children are also at risk for a range of medical conditions associated with the disorder, including heart defects, visual and auditory problems, pulmonary hypertension, and lowered immunity (R. Stores, 2001).

In Down syndrome, physical characteristics and poor muscle tone predispose these children to obstructive sleep apnea (OSA). This will generally require medical treatment (see Mclaughlin Crabtree, Rach, and Gamble, Chapter 19). Parents commonly also report behavioral sleep disorders (see R. Stores, 2001, for an early review). While not significantly different from parent-reported rates for comparison groups, rates of sleep problems in children with Down syndrome range from 40% (Cotton & Richdale, 2006) to 65% (Stores & Stores, 2004) and these children were likely to be reported as sleepy during the day (Cotton & Richdale, 2010).

Stores, Stores, and Buckley (1996) surveyed the population of children with Down syndrome (age 4 to 19 years) in one English county, compared with their siblings, with typically developing children, and with a mixed group of children with developmental disabilities. Both disability groups slept less than the siblings and typically developing children. Increased settling, night waking, early morning waking, and co-sleeping problems were found in Down syndrome as compared with siblings and typically developing children, but high levels of these sleep issues also occurred in the children with a developmental disability. Behaviors associated with sleep disordered breathing (SDB) and OSA were more common in Down syndrome. Both disability groups had more settling and sleep maintenance problems, bedwetting, and daytime sleepiness behaviors than the two typically developing groups. Sleep issues were more common in the 4- to 7-year-old children with Down syndrome.

Subsequent research by the same group (Stores, Stores, Fellows, & Buckley, 1998) confirmed that children with Down syndrome may present with sleep problems in three primary areas: *(1)* settling to sleep, *(2)* night waking, and *(3)* SDB and OSA, with sleep difficulties being associated with poorer daytime behavior and increased maternal stress. Further actometry (Stores & Stores, 2004) showed that children with Down syndrome slept less, had poorer sleep efficiency, spent longer awake after sleep onset, and had a higher activity score than typically developing children. In a recent survey of 255 (241 completed all questions) parents of children with Down syndrome (median age 5 years) the high rate of sleeping difficulties was confirmed (Rosen et al., 2011). Over half the parents (59.2%) had discussed their child's sleep with their family doctor; 51.8% of children were reported to have at least some settling difficulties, 69.4% at least some difficulty maintaining sleep, 54% had excessive daytime sleepiness, and 44% of parents had discussed their child's breathing with the family doctor (Rosen et al., 2011).

In children, the removal of tonsils and adenoids is typically undertaken to treat more severe OSA (see McLaughlin Crabtree, Rach, and Gamble, Chapter 19). However, this procedure has been reported as a less effective treatment in Down syndrome than in non–Down syndrome children, with only 3 of 11 Down syndrome children requiring no further treatment for OSA following the operation (Shete, Stocks, Sebelik, & Schoumacher, 2010). Similarly, Rosen and colleagues (2011) reported that of children who had undergone adenotonsillectomy, 47.5% still had apneas and 28.9% still gasped and choked during sleep. Nevertheless, while night waking episodes in Down syndrome may be associated with SDB or OSA, whether or not the child settles easily to sleep at bedtime or is able to return to sleep after waking without disturbing others in the household is a generally likely to be a behavioral issue and may be amenable to behavioral treatment.

In one case (Thackeray & Richdale, 2002), actigraphy showed that sleep in a 5-year-old boy with Down syndrome was highly fragmented and his apnea subscale score on a standardized sleep questionnaire was high. His parents reported that the boy had previously had his adenoids removed to treat sleep apnea. A behavioral intervention improved settling, co-sleeping, and sleep latency, as well as sleep efficiency, but night waking did not improve, actigraphy indicated highly fragmented sleep, and his apnea score on the questionnaire remained high. Thus, both a behavioral and a medical component appeared to contribute to this child's sleep issues, and earlier sleep apnea treatment may not have been successful. This is consistent with Shete et al.'s (2010) report regarding often poor long-term success of adenotonsillectomy to treat OSA in Down syndrome.

Behavior management for sleep issues surrounding settling and night waking can assist parents in the management of their child with Down syndrome. Psychologists and other health professionals need to be aware of the potential contribution of medical issues associated with Down syndrome to any presenting sleep difficulties, including that removal of tonsils and adenoids may not ultimately be successful in addressing sleep apnea. Thus, a medical referral may be needed.

Fragile X Syndrome

Fragile X syndrome is the most common inherited cause of intellectual disability and involves a mutation on the X chromosome where there is a CGG trinucleotide repeat expansion. There are both full and partial mutation forms; the full mutation involves >200 CGG repeats, while the partial mutation involves >50 CGG repeats. This mutation silences the *FMRI* gene resulting in suppression of the production of the FMRP protein, which appears to be the causative factor in the expression of intellectual disability or learning difficulties that occur in Fragile X (Kronk, Dahl, & Noll, 2009). The estimated prevalence of Fragile X full mutation carriers is 1:2500 (Hagerman, 2008). Males are generally more severely affected than females, and there is a high risk for comorbid diagnoses including anxiety and autistic disorder. In a 2001 review, G. Stores noted that there was little research on sleep problems in Fragile X even though sleep difficulties were reported to be common. This situation has not improved.

Two studies give a parent-reported prevalence of current sleep problems of around 30% in children with Fragile X (Kronk, Bishop, Raspa, Bickel, Mandel, & Bailey, 2010; Richdale, 2003). Parents primarily reported that their child had difficulties with sleep onset and night waking. Kronk and colleagues (2009) investigated sleep in 90 children (ages 3–17 years) with Fragile X using a 14-day sleep diary as well as a standardized sleep questionnaire. Clinically relevant sleep difficulties on the questionnaire were exhibited by 47% of their sample and, on the 14-day diary, 50% of children had sleep onset delay and 53% exhibited night waking. Irregular bedtimes (86%) and irregular morning arousal (83%) were very common across the diary period. Furthermore, on the questionnaire, caregivers reported that 79% of children woke once (52%) or more (27%) per night, 41% had sleep onset delay, and 57% were restless sleepers.

Kronk et al. (2010) examined 1295 children and adults with Fragile X full mutation but only gathered further sleep information about those individuals (32%) with a current, parent-reported sleep problem. There was some variability in sleep problems with age; in particular, younger children were more likely to wake at night. Poor sleep was associated with poorer behavioral development and poorer health. Difficulty falling asleep, night waking, and restless sleep were common in both males and females, but males were more likely to wake up to early (68%) and females (21%) were more likely to have difficulty waking in the morning. Richdale examined parent-reported sleep issues in 13 children with Fragile X and found that despite only 4 parents (30%) reporting a sleep problem, 10 (77%) children had evidence of current sleep difficulties. According to parents, 7 (53.8%) children had had a sleep problem in the past, with sleep problems beginning in infancy in 6 cases. Parent-report of a current sleep problem was associated with more severe child behavior problems and increased levels of parent stress.

Using a 14-day sleep diary, Gould, Loesch, Martin, Hagerman, Armstrong, and Huggins (2000) reported that 13 boys with Fragile X exhibited more variable sleep patterns than a comparison group of children. Melatonin levels were also examined in eight of the Fragile X boys and compared with typically developing boys, and melatonin showed an elevated night peak as well as elevation during the day. Normally melatonin levels begin to rise prior to sleep onset, peaking in the early hours of the morning (dark), and production is suppressed by daylight. This finding of elevated melatonin requires replication and its relationship with sleep difficulties in Fragile X remains unclear.

Overall, these findings indicate that poor sleep is quite common in children with Fragile X, with sleep problems being severe enough in at least 30% of cases for parents to report their child's sleep as problematic. Given that Kronk et al. (2010) noted an association between sleep problems and health problems, practitioners should remain alert to the potential need for a medical referral when treating sleep issues in these children.

Chromosome 15 Disorders

PRADER-WILLI SYNDROME

Prader-Willi syndrome results from a failure in the expression of specific paternally derived genes at 15q11–13 with deletion in 70%–75% of cases and maternal uniparental disomy in the majority of remaining cases (Bruni, Verrillo, Novelli, & Ferri, 2010; Õiglane-Shlik et al., 2006). A recent population study found a population prevalence of 1 in 30,606 children and adolescents (Õiglane-Shlik et al., 2006). Children have poor muscle tone, are short with small hands and feet, obese, and have an intellectual disability. Disruption in hypothalamic development and function occurs. Due to the physical features of Prader-Willi syndrome, the hypotonia, and the hypothalamic dysfunction, these infants and children are at risk for sleep apnea (see Chapter 19, this volume), which can be of central origin (Schlüter, Buschatz, Trowitzsch, & Aksu, 1997; Bruni et al., 2010), and excessive daytime sleepiness (Cassidy, McKillop, & Morgan, 1990; Bruni et al., 2010). There are also abnormalities in REM sleep (Bruni et al., 2010; Joo et al., 2009).

Research on sleep in Prader-Willi syndrome is largely confined to an examination of sleep EEG (REM and NREM sleep) and the sleep apnea associated with the disorder (Joo et al., 2009; Bruni et al., 2010; Verrillo et al., 2009). Verrillo et al. (2009) found abnormalities in sleep architecture including sleep microstructure in children with Prader-Willi syndrome. They concluded that sleep microstructure differed from normal, supporting a general hypoarousal state in Prader-Willi syndrome associated with hypothalamic dysfunction. A comparison of children with Prader-Willi syndrome and same-aged obese but otherwise typically developing children showed that children with Prader-Willi syndrome fell asleep more quickly, with an earlier onset of their first REM sleep episode, than the comparison group. Increased total sleep, decreased REM sleep latency, and decreased NREM sleep in the Prader-Willi syndrome children were associated with increased adiponectin levels (the hormone involved in glucose regulation and fat catabolism; Joo et al., 2009).

Report of sleep behaviors and daytime behavior in children and adults with Prader-Willi syndrome (Richdale, Cotton, & Hibbit, 1999) found excessive daytime sleepiness (EDS), more severe snoring, and early morning waking in Prader-Willi syndrome compared with age- and gender-matched controls. Excessive daytime sleepiness distinguished those with Prader-Willi syndrome from the comparison group; EDS began prior to 1 year of age on average and was associated with significant daytime behavior difficulties. An examination of the children and adolescents from Richdale et al. (1999) as compared with other developmental disorders and typically developing children found that 44% of parents reported a sleep problem (Cotton & Richdale, 2006) and that children with Prader-Willi syndrome woke earlier and were more likely to nap than other children (Cotton & Richdale, 2010).

Thus, the primary sleep issues in Prader-Willi syndrome are associated with central sleep apnea and hypothalamic dysfunction, abnormalities in the structure of the sleep EEG, and EDS (Bruni et al., 2010), and the latter may be associated with significant behavior problems. From a nonmedical perspective, psychologists and other health professionals may be able to assist with behavior management but the primary sleep complaints in Prader-Willi syndrome are biological in origin.

ANGELMAN SYNDROME

Angelman syndrome is also a disorder associated with chromosome 15q11–13. There is disruption in the expression of the *UBE3A* gene caused by the deletion of maternally derived genes at 15q11–13 (70% of cases). In a further 15% of cases paternal uniparental disomy, a mutation of the maternal *UBE3A* gene, or an imprinting failure of the maternally derived gene resulting in the expression of the paternally derived gene occurs, while the molecular abnormality has not been determined in 10%–15% of cases (Õiglane-Shlik et al., 2006; Williams, 2010). Children have a severe developmental delay, a disorder of movement or balance, severely impaired speech, and a unique behavioral phenotype that includes excessive laughter and excitability; epilepsy is also common (Williams, 2010). The population prevalence of Angelman syndrome is estimated as 1 in 56,112 children and adolescents (Õiglane-Shlik et al., 2006).

Significant sleep problems are one of the associated conditions reported as present in Angelman syndrome (Williams, 2010). Parents report sleep onset and maintenance difficulties, parasomnias, sleep-related breathing problems, and excessive daytime sleepiness, with overall sleep quality being poor (Bruni et al., 2004; Didden et al., 2004; Walz et al., 2005). Between a fifth and a third of individuals may require sleep medication to fall asleep (Bruni et al., 2004; Didden et al., 2004). Only a weak association between sleep problems and epilepsy has been reported (Didden et al., 2004).

Fifty-four percent of individuals (M = 15.2 years) with Angelman syndrome were reported to have a current severe sleep problem. Night waking (3 or more nights per week) occurred in 37% of children and adults, and about half remained awake for an hour or more; 93% of the sample had incontinence at night. Parents (40%) rated night waking as the most problematic of their child's sleeping difficulties. Sleep problems were present on average for 9.7 years, and parents reported that their own sleep was significantly affected (Didden et al., 2004). Similarly, Bruni et al. (2004) reported that compared with typically developing children, children with Angelman syndrome (2.3–14.8 years) woke frequently (62.2%). Difficulty with going to bed (59.5%), sleep transition behaviors, restlessness (67.6%) and unusual movements (48.6%), enuresis (35%), bruxism (21.6%), snoring (32.4%), shortened night sleep (70.3% slept < 8 hours), and daytime sleepiness (24%) were among other common issues reported. Restlessness and movement, along with EDS, were suggested to be specifically associated with Angelman syndrome. Walz et al. (2005) reported a similar range of sleep issues, with the exception of waking screaming; sleep problems were present in 50% of their sample of 300 children, adolescents, and young adults with Angelman syndrome.

The most recent survey of 16 children and adolescents with Angelman syndrome (Goldman et al., 2012) collected both PSG and actigraphy data, as well as using a standardized sleep questionnaire to confirm sleep problems. Both objective measures of sleep indicated problems with sleep onset (sleep latency >30 minutes), night waking of an hour or more, poor sleep efficiency, and high sleep fragmentation index. Average scores on all subscales on the sleep questionnaire exceeded normative values, as did the total score. Poor child sleep was associated with insomnia and daytime sleepiness in parents, and increased parent stress.

Despite the presence of significant sleep problems, only a minority of parents (33%) of children with Angelman's syndrome are offered treatment for their child's sleep difficulties (Didden et al., 2004).

Medication was the most common treatment and few had received psychological (behavioral) intervention, which was rated as most effective. However, no intervention was highly endorsed by these parents. Thus, there appears to be scope to address at least some aspects of poor sleep in Angelman syndrome (e.g., settling) using behavioral approaches.

Williams Syndrome

Williams syndrome occurs as a result of a deletion of about 25 to 30 genes on chromosome 7q11.23 (Annaz, Hill, Ashworth, & Holley, 2011; Mason et al., 2011). Characteristic facial features and medical abnormalities, including cardiovascular abnormalities, are generally present (Annaz et al., 2011; Gombos, Bódizs, & Kovács, 2011). Children with Williams syndrome are likely to have a mild to moderate intellectual disability with significant visual-spatial abnormalities, relative strengths in expressive language, anxiety, and comorbid ADHD; children with Williams syndrome are generally highly sociable (Goldman, Malow, Newman, Roof, & Dykens, 2009; Gombos et al., 2011). Incidence estimates vary from 1:20,000 live births (Annaz et al., 2011) to 1:7500 live births (Mason et al., 2011).

While sleep problems are not reported in descriptions of abnormalities and behaviors associated with Williams syndrome, given the high rate of sleep difficulties found in children with developmental disabilities, sleep patterns and sleep problems have become a focus of interest in recent years (Annaz et al., 2011; Goldman et al., 2009; Gombos et al., 2011; Mason et al., 2011). Goldman and colleagues (2009) examined sleep in 23 adolescents and adults (17–35 years) with Williams syndrome. Problems with sleep were acknowledged by 36.4% of participants and while they averaged 7.6 hours sleep, sleep efficiency was poor. Daytime sleepiness was reported by 77.3% of the cohort, 34.8% had EDS, and 90.5% had nocturia.

In 2011, two papers were published examining sleep patterns in children with Williams syndrome (Annaz et al., 2011; Mason et al., 2011). Annaz et al. looked at parent-reported sleep problems on a standard sleep questionnaire in 64, 6–12-year-old children with Williams syndrome as compared with 93 similar-age typically developing children. Children with Williams syndrome had a significantly higher total sleep score and significantly higher subscale scores for bedtime resistance, sleep onset delay, sleep anxiety, night waking, and daytime sleepiness than the typically developing children; daytime tiredness was reported for 61% of the Williams syndrome children. While a high rate of medical issues was reported, in general these were not significantly associated with poor sleep. The presence of asthma and allergies was perhaps not surprisingly associated with sleep onset delay, and cardiac problems affected sleep duration. Parents also reported high rates of snoring and enuresis. Total night sleep was highly variable for the Williams syndrome group, and 55% of parents felt that their child got insufficient sleep.

In the second child study (Mason et al., 2011), overnight PSG and parent sleep questionnaires were used to examine sleep in 35 children (M = 9.34 years) with Williams syndrome as compared with 35 gender- and ethnicity-matched typically developing children (M = 9.52 years); symptoms of ADHD were also examined. According to parents, children with Williams syndrome had more difficulty falling asleep, and had restless sleep with leg movements and prolonged night waking. Behavioral symptoms associated with ADHD were also significantly more common in the Williams syndrome group. PSG confirmed parent reports of night waking, with poorer sleep efficiency, higher respiratory-related arousal index, and more slow wave sleep occurring in children with Williams syndrome. Parental reports of restless legs and restless sleep were variously associated with periodic limb movement measurements during PSG for the Williams syndrome children, but the presence or absence of ADHD did not differentiate the sleep of the Williams syndrome children. Decreased total sleep and REM sleep, increased slow wave sleep, lower sleep efficiency, and increased leg movements as compared with a control group were also reported by Gombos et al. (2011) in a smaller group of 9 young people with Williams syndrome aged 14–28 years.

Thus, the available evidence suggests a pattern of sleep problems in Williams syndrome that likely continue into adulthood. These include settling issues, restless sleep with periodic limb movements, and prolonged night waking with consequent decreased total sleep, sleep efficiency, and increased daytime sleepiness. While limited, data also suggest that the sleep EEG may differ from age-matched typically developing young people. The role of associated medical conditions in exacerbating or causing sleep difficulties is uncertain, but cardiac problems have been implicated. It is likely that behavioral interventions will be helpful in addressing some of these sleep issues, but the potential for comorbid medical conditions or ADHD to affect sleep should not be ignored.

Smith-Magenis Syndrome

Smith-Magenis syndrome involves chromosome 17 with interstitial deletion at 17p11.2, resulting in distinctive craniofacial features, short stature, hypertonia and failure to thrive in infancy, language delay, significant behavioral problems, intellectual disability, and significant sleep disturbances which begin early in life; other medical problems may also occur (De Leersnyder, 2006; Smith, Dykens, & Greenberg, 1998). Sleep problems in Smith-Magenis syndrome are almost universal and have been attributed to an inverted melatonin rhythm, which has been found in almost all cases (Boudreau et al., 2009; De Leersnyder, 2006). Additionally, total sleep problems have been reported as the most significant predictor of maladaptive behaviors on the CBCL in 35 children and adolescents (M = 9 years) with Smith-Magenis syndrome (Dykens & Smith, 1998).

Early bedtime, night waking, early morning waking, and daytime sleepiness were reported in 39 children, adolescents, and young adults (M = 10.5 years) with Smith-Magenis syndrome (Smith et al., 1998). Most commonly, parents reported bedtime rituals, enuresis, night waking, napping and daytime sleepiness, and snoring; taking sleep medication was common. Morning waking could occur as early as 2:00 am with the average wake time being 5:30 am. Similar sleep problems have been reported by other researchers (G. Stores, 2001); thus, sleep is phase-advanced in these children.

Subsequent research showed that children with Smith-Magenis syndrome have a phase-shifted melatonin rhythm. The normal pattern of a melatonin peak at night after sleep onset and low levels during the day is inverted, and this is associated with the sleep and daytime behavior problems (De Leersnyder, 2006). De Leersnyder and colleagues (2003) showed that a single bedtime dose of controlled-release melatonin in conjunction with a morning dose of a β-adrenergic antagonist to block daytime melatonin production resulted in relatively normal melatonin rhythms. The treatment phase delayed sleep onset by about 30 minutes and wake time by an hour, reduced night waking and increased total night sleep, improving sleep in 8 of 10 children ages 4 to 18 years. Daytime behavior also reportedly improved with this treatment.

Thus, the usual behavioral approaches to assist sleep in children may not have a significant impact in children with Smith-Magenis syndrome; these children will primarily need a pharmacological intervention. However, not all individuals with Smith-Magenis syndrome and poor sleep may show an inversion of the normal melatonin rhythm associated with their sleeping difficulties (Boudreau et al., 2009).

Rett Syndrome

Rett syndrome is currently classified as a pervasive developmental disorder (APA, 2000), but does not appear in the draft revisions of the fifth edition of the *Diagnostic and Statistical Manual of Mental Disorders* (APA, http://www.dsm5.org/proposedrevision/Pages/NeurodevelopmentalDisorders.aspx). Rett syndrome predominantly occurs in females with an estimated prevalence of 1.09 per 10,000 females (Young et al., 2007). The disorder is progressive, with a loss of skills. Stereotypic movements, slowing of head growth, gait abnormalities, and autistic behaviors commonly occur (Glaze 2004; Young et al., 2007). Thus, Rett syndrome needs to be considered in young, more severely delayed girls who may be suspected of having autism. Rett syndrome involves mutations in the *MECP2* gene, with at least 200 identified mutations to date, and the specific mutation found affects the severity of the clinical picture (Young et al., 2007).

Sleep problems have been identified as associated with Rett syndrome for over 20 years (Glaze, Frost, Zoghbi, & Percy, 1987), though there is surprisingly little research. Piazza, Fisher, Kiesewetter, Bowman and Moser (1990) conducted an examination of sleep in 20 females (1–32 years, median age 8 years) with Rett syndrome, training parents to undertake momentary time sampling of behaviors during the day and at night. Parents also recorded when they were woken up or disturbed by their child during the night. Late sleep onset (11:00 pm), night waking and early morning waking (4:00 am) were observed, as was more frequent daytime napping. Additionally, the expected decrease in total sleep with age did not occur due to a tendency for increased daytime naps with age. The girls slept less at night than expected for their age. Delayed sleep onset was the most prominent feature and was shown by 85% of girls.

Using a questionnaire format, Young et al. (2007) examined sleep at three time points over a 4-year period in 237 cases of girls with Rett syndrome, with 131 completed questionnaires returned at all time points. Sleep was examined across four age groups: 0–7, 8–12, 13–17, and 18+ years. Sleep problems were frequent in all age groups, at all time points (range 71.7% to 95.2%), with 90.4%, 82.4%, and 83.1% of girls having sleep problems at each time examined. Laughing at night (58.9%), night screaming (35.6%), teeth grinding (55%), night seizures (26.2%), and frequent daytime naps (77%) were most commonly reported across the sample. Night laughing decreased and daytime naps increased with age.

Sleep EEG studies have been conducted, mostly in the 1990s. For example, Marcus et al. (1994) examined overnight PSG including both respiratory patterns (hyperventilation and breath-holding have been reported in Rett syndrome) and sleep architecture in 30 girls (ages 1–32 years) and 30 matched controls (ages 1–17 years). Overall they found no difference in sleep architecture or sleep efficiency between the two groups, though a small number of Rett syndrome participants exhibited decreased REM or slow wave sleep or abnormalities associated with Stage 2 K-complexes and sleep spindles (see Lushington, Pamula, Martin, and Kennedy, Chapters 5 and 6, this volume). Normal respiratory patterns were found in NREM sleep and near-normal patterns in REM sleep, but Rett syndrome girls showed abnormal breathing patterns when awake. The authors postulated that hyperventilation was from an "organic defect" (p. 223) rather than being a behavioral manifestation. Glaze et al. (1987) noted similar normal breathing patterns at night but abnormal breathing during wakefulness, but also found a reduction in REM sleep.

Thus, girls with Rett syndrome have distinctive features to their sleep problems, laughing and screaming during night waking, as well as daytime sleepiness and difficulties with sleep onset and sleep problems, and these problems occur across age ranges. Treatment studies in this population are few and have largely been confined to the use of melatonin (McArthur & Budden, 1998; Miyamoto, Oki, Takahashi, & Okuno, 1999). It is likely that behavioral approaches would assist with bedtime and settling issues.

Autism Spectrum Disorders

The term *autism spectrum disorder* refers to three pervasive developmental disorders—autistic disorder (autism), Asperger's disorder, and pervasive developmental disorder-not otherwise specified (PPDNOS)—that involve delayed and/or deviant development in three areas of development: communication, social interaction and repetitive, stereotyped or ritual behaviors (APA, 2000). The global median reported prevalence of autism spectrum disorder is 0.62% (Elsabbagh et al., 2012). Children with Asperger's disorder typically do not have an intellectual disability, whereas around 70% of children with autistic disorder and many children with PDDNOS have a comorbid intellectual disability (APA, 2000). Poor sleep is among a number of comorbid conditions reported to occur in autism or autism spectrum disorder (APA, 2000, Richdale & Schreck, 2009). Regardless of age or intellectual ability, sleep problems are common with half or more of these children having a parent-reported sleep problem at some time (Miano & Ferri, 2010; Richdale & Schreck, 2009); for example, 86.2% of 167 children with an autism spectrum disorder were reported to have a sleep problem in one recent study (Liu, Hubbard, Fabes, & Adam, 2006). The most common problems meet ICSD-2 (AASM, 2005) criteria for behavioral insomnia of childhood (Richdale & Schreck, 2009; Souders et al., 2009).

Insomnia, including difficulties with sleep onset, sleep maintenance, and co-sleeping are most commonly found (Allik, Larsson, & Smedje, 2006a, 2006b; Liu et al., 2006; Malow et al., 2006; Souders et al., 2009; Wiggs & Stores, 2004). Sleep onset difficulties differentiated children with autism from children with Down syndrome, Prader-Willi syndrome, developmental disability, and typically developing children (Cotton & Richdale, 2006). At bedtime children with autism spectrum disorder are less likely to be sleepy, are likely to be noncompliant, may follow problematic bedtime routines, and may have reduced night sleep (Malow et al., 2006; Patzold, Richdale, & Tonge, 1998, Paavonen et al., 2008). Other sleep problems include extended periods of night waking, often accompanied by behaviors that disturb the rest of the family (e.g., laughing, screaming, playing; Richdale, 1999); irregular sleep/wake patterns with variability in sleep onset and waking (Inamura, 1984); early morning waking (Richdale & Prior, 1995); and reduced sleep efficiency (Allik, Larsson, & Smedje, 2006b; Malow et al., 2006; Wiggs & Stores, 2004) compared with typically developing peers. Using both actigraphy and a sleep questionnaire to compare sleep in autism spectrum disorder and typically developing children aged 4 to 10 years, Souders et al. (2009) concluded that in autism spectrum disorder sleep problems were likely to be associated with the disorder; that is, these children had insomnia due to pervasive developmental disorder.

Settling and Sleep Onset

Settling and sleep onset issues, including increased sleep latency, occur more frequently in children and adolescents with autism spectrum disorder than they do in typically developing children (Cotton & Richdale, 2006; Malow et al., 2006) or children with Prader-Willi syndrome, Down syndrome, or intellectual disability (Cotton & Richdale, 2006). Nevertheless, similar rates of sleep problems in young children with autism and young children with a developmental disability have been reported (Goodlin-Jones et al., 2009). Difficult and challenging bedtime behaviors, nonfunctional or challenging bedtime routines or rituals (Liu et al., 2006; Marquenie et al., 2011), sleep habits, or comfort objects, and long sleep latency (>30 minutes)—that is, difficulty settling in bed and readily falling asleep—are most frequently reported by parents (Liu et al., 2006; Patzold et al., 1998). For example, a parent wrote in a sleep diary: "He won't sleep at night until conditions are right for him—this usually means his older brother must have walked past his room to go to bed." Children with high-functioning autism spectrum disorder (i.e., the children do not have an intellectual disability) also self-report difficulty falling asleep with longer sleep latency than typically developing children and adolescents (Paavonen et al., 2008).

Night Waking

While night waking is commonly reported by parents of children with autism spectrum disorder (Malow, Marzec, et al., 2006; Krakowiak, Goodlin-Jones, Picciotto, Croen, & Hansen, 2008, 2012; Schreck & Mulick, 2000), the frequency of night waking appears similar to that reported by parents of children with other developmental disabilities (Richdale & Schreck, 2009). On waking, some children with autism spectrum disorder also engage in a range of disturbing night waking behaviors with waking periods that last an hour or more. Behaviors that parents report include screaming, talking, singing and laughing, crying, getting up and roaming the house, playing (Patzold et al., 1998), or co-sleeping with parents (Cotton & Richdale, 2006; Liu et al., 2006). These behaviors appear to represent a subgroup of night wakers and when they occur, obviously are very disturbing. Reasons for their occurrence remain unknown, but these behaviors may be associated with night terrors, other parasomnias, or epilepsy in some children, as such phenomena occur in association with these disorders in pediatric populations (Sheldon & Glaze, 2005). Night waking also occurs in conjunction with enuresis or toileting, and the child may then find it difficult to return to sleep, further disturbing the household.

Other Sleep Disturbances

Besides the more common settling and night waking difficulties, parents of children with autism spectrum disorder also report a number of other sleep difficulties. Recent research using sleep questionnaires containing subscales measuring behaviors associated with parasomnias suggest that these sleep phenomena may be relatively common in children with autism spectrum disorder (Goldman et al., 2011; Liu et al., 2006; Polimeni, Richdale, & Francis, 2005; Schreck & Mulick, 2000). Parent concerns about a range of behaviors including symptoms of psychopathology, sensory issues, self-injurious behavior, and attention were related to elevated parasomnia scores in children and adolescents with autism spectrum disorder (Goldman et al., 2011). Parasomnias may also relate to parent reports that some of these children wake screaming, possibly suggesting a susceptibility to night terrors.

Total Sleep

On average, children with autism spectrum disorder show a reduction in total night sleep compared with compared with typically developing children or age- and IQ-matched controls, and this difference is often significant (Inamura, 1984; Paavonen et al., 2008; Patzold, Richdale, & Tonge, 1998; Richdale & Prior, 1995). However, not all studies report significantly reduced night sleep time in comparison to other children (Malow, et al. 2006; Schreck & Mulick, 2000; Souders et al., 2009). Total 24-hour sleep may also be significantly reduced in children with autism (Cotton & Richdale, 2010; Inamura, 1984; Krakowiak et al., 2008, 2012). Thus, there is likely to be a subgroup of children with autism spectrum disorder that get insufficient sleep.

Naps

According to sleep diary studies, nap frequency may be lower in young children with autism, though reports can be contradictory and are likely related to age variation in the samples, the use of mixed disability groups for comparison, sample size, and the time period over which data are collected. Children with autism aged 4 years or younger slept less in a 24-hour period than typically developing children, despite napping (Inamura, 1984), and young children with autism spectrum disorder (< 6 years) napped less frequently and for a shorter period than children with mixed disabilities or typically developing children (Schwichtenberg et al., 2011). However, when children with autism (mean age 7.2 years) were compared to similar-age children with specific disabilities or who were typically developing, nap frequency only differed from children with Prader-Willi syndrome, while total 24-hour sleep was significantly less than for typically developing children (Cotton & Richdale, 2010). Therefore, young children with autism spectrum disorder may take shorter naps or fewer naps, thus sleeping less over a 24-hour period than other children. This is important in terms of determining the origin of sleep problems and whether the child is getting sufficient sleep, as it is the total sleep each 24 hours that determines whether the child's sleep is sufficient.

ETIOLOGY OF SETTLING AND NIGHT WAKING PROBLEMS IN AUTISM SPECTRUM DISORDER

It is likely that sleep problems in autism spectrum disorder are multifactorial and will include biological, behavioral, and/or environmental contributions. Thus, causal factors may vary from child to child. The communication, social, and ritualistic behaviors that form the basis of a diagnosis of autism spectrum disorder may also predispose these children to sleeping difficulties (Richdale & Schreck, 2009). As illustrated in a recent examination of 1784 children and adolescents with autism spectrum disorder, poor sleep was significantly associated with a range of parent-reported difficult behaviors, symptoms associated with autism spectrum disorder, and psychopathology (Goldman et al., 2011).

Daytime Behavior

The high incidence of comorbid behavioral problems in autism spectrum disorder—comorbid intellectual disability, poor communication, and poor adaptive behavior—are likely to differentiate cases with autism spectrum disorder from typically developing cases and to result in sleep problems in autism spectrum disorder that continue long after they have resolved in most typically developing children. Significant behavioral difficulties are associated with poor sleep in children with autism (Goldman et al., 2011; Patzold et al., 1998); moreover, daytime behavioral difficulties have been reported as associated with parent-report of both current and past sleeping problems (Patzold et al., 1998). Parents of 1784 children with autism spectrum disorder aged 2 to 18 years who reported behavioral concerns and, in particular self-injury, aggression, mood swings and compulsive behaviors in their child, were more likely to report that their child was a poor sleeper (Goldman et al., 2011).

Psychopathology

Anxiety and depression are associated with sleeping difficulties in typically developing children (Gregory & Sadeh, 2012; see also Chapter 35), and sleeping problems are common in children with attention deficit hyperactivity disorder (ADHD; Owens, 2005; see also Corkum and Coulombe, Chapter 34). Thus, comorbid anxiety, depression, or ADHD symptoms may precipitate or maintain sleep difficulties, particularly symptoms of insomnia. High levels of anxiety and depression are common in autism spectrum disorder (DeVincent, Gadow, Delosh, & Geller, 2007; Liu et al., 2006; Mayes & Calhoun, 2009; Mayes, Calhoun, Murray, Ahuja, & Smith, 2011; van Steensel, Bögels, & Perrin, 2011). Parents reported that in 117 low-functioning and 233 high-functioning children with autism aged 6–16 years, anxiety (67% and 79% respectively) and depression (42% and 54% respectively) symptoms were highly prevalent compared with typically developing children or children with brain injury or intellectual disability; anxiety symptoms were more frequent than in children with depression (Mayes et al., 2011a). Similarly, while an ADHD co-diagnosis cannot be given (APA, 2000), around 50% of children with autism spectrum disorder nevertheless meet DSM-IV-TR criteria (APA, 2000) for ADHD (Gadow, DeVincent, & Pomeroy, 2006; Leyfer et al., 2006).

Several studies have reported that ADHD symptoms and sleep problems are associated in children with autism spectrum disorder, in particular symptoms of hyperactivity or ADHD (DeVincent et al., 2007; Liu et al., 2006; Mayes & Calhoun, 2009). Children with autism spectrum disorder aged 8–12 years and insomnia had more teacher-reported hyperactive behaviors than did those without insomnia (Allik, Larsson, & Smedje, 2006a). Parent-reported symptoms of anxiety, depression, or emotional problems are reported as associated with sleep problems or insomnia in children and adolescents with autism spectrum disorder (Allik et al., 2006a; Mayes & Calhoun, 2009; Wiggs & Stores, 2004), while self-reported sleep fears and negative attitudes toward sleeping have been found in children aged 5–17 years with Asperger's disorder (Paavonen et al., 2008). Successful treatment of sleep problems has also been reported to improve both internalizing and externalizing behavior in children and adolescents with Asperger's disorder (Paavonen, Nieminen-von Wendt, Vanhala, Aronen, & von Wendt, 2003). However, Mayes, Calhoun, Murray, and Zahid (2011b) reported that increased autism severity, older age, and higher verbal IQ were the best predictors of anxiety or depression in autism spectrum disorder, but not sleep.

Cognition and Adaptive Behavior

Using questionnaires (Krakowiak et al., 2008, 2012), sleep diaries (Patzold et al., 1998; Richdale & Prior, 1995) and actigraphy (Wiggs & Stores, 2004), research has consistently found that sleep problems in autism spectrum disorder are common regardless of the child's age or IQ. Most recently, Mayes and Calhoun (2009b) reported that IQ did not differentiate poor and good sleepers with autism spectrum disorder.

However, in examining specific areas of problematic sleep, Taylor, Schreck, and Mulick (2012) found that children with autism spectrum disorder and poorer cognitive skills were more likely to have reduced nocturnal sleep. Risk for sleep problems in autism spectrum disorder was higher in toddlers with autism or PDDNOS as compared with atypically developing children (Kozlowski, Matson, Belva, & Rieske, 2012), and toddlers with autism were the most likely to have sleep difficulties. While sleep problems were associated with lower DQs, those with an autism spectrum disorder diagnosis (autism or PDDNOS) still had more sleep problems than atypical children after developmental quotient was accounted for. What has not been systematically investigated is whether the etiology or type of sleep problem with which children present differs with IQ.

The impact of adaptive behavior on sleep has been less consistently examined, but Krakowiak et al. (2008, 2012) found no association between adaptive behavior and sleep in autism spectrum disorder. Conversely, in 335 children with autism spectrum disorder with IQ in both the intellectual disability and normal range, children with better adaptive behavior had more sleep over 24 hours; children who slept more per night with less disturbed sleep had better communication skills (Taylor et al., 2012).

Thus, while it seems clear that at all cognitive levels children with autism spectrum disorder are at an increased risk for sleep problems compared with typically developing children, the relationships between sleep, cognitive skills, and adaptive behavior within the autism spectrum disorder population are unclear and require further examination.

Symptoms of Autism Spectrum Disorder

Increased autism severity symptoms are associated with poor sleep (Mayes & Calhoun, 2009a) including reduced night sleep, parasomnias, and sleep disordered breathing (Hoffman et al., 2005; Schreck, Mulick, & Smith, 2004). Autism severity as measured by the Gilliam Autism rating scale was reported as associated with reduced night sleep (Hoffman et al., 2005; Schreck et al., 2004). Poor sleep has also been associated with communication abnormalities (Elia et al., 2000; Schreck et al., 2004), social-relatedness, or socialization (Hoffman et al., 2008; Malow, Marzic et al., 2006; Malow, McGrew, Harvey, Henderson, & Stone, 2006, Schreck et al., 2004), and repetitive behaviors and rituals (Gabriels, Cuccaro, Hill, Ivers, & Goldson, 2005; Hoffman et al., 2008; Liu et al., 2006; Schreck et al., 2004). However, Gabriels et al. (2005) found that once IQ was controlled for, the association between sleep and repetitive behaviors was removed.

About a third of children with autism show regression or loss of previously acquired skills, usually during latter half of their second year. This has been associated with more severe sleep problems than in the non-regressed autism group. Both autism groups had more sleep problems than typically developing children (Giannotti, Cortesi, Cerquiglini, Vagnoni, & Valente, 2011).

Age

While research has primarily examined preschool and primary school-aged children with autism spectrum disorder, sleep problems are common regardless of age (Richdale & Schreck, 2009; Goldman, Richdale, Clemens, & Malow, 2012), while the type of sleep difficulty may change with age (Goldman et al., 2012) and may persist into adulthood (Tani et al., 2003). The 2012 Goldman study examined parent-reported sleep problems using a sleep questionnaire, with data available from 1859 children and adolescents available for analysis. Issues including bedtime resistance, sleep anxiety, parasomnias, and night waking were more common in younger children, while symptoms of sleep reduction including shortened night sleep, long sleep latency, and daytime sleepiness were more common in those ≥ 11 years.

Families

Mothers of children with autism report higher levels of stress and depression compared to mothers of other children (Ingersoll et al., 2011). Stress has been shown to independently predict depression in these mothers, and reduced parenting efficacy may result (Hastings, 2002). Parents report high levels of stress when their child with autism has sleep difficulties (Doo & Wing, 2006). Research by Marquenie, Rodger, Mangohig, and Cronin (2011) has shown that settling and challenging bedtime routines can be difficult and stressful for mothers if they are not performed exactly. Parents of children with autism spectrum disorder also report poor sleep quality and quantity (Lopez-Wagner et al., 2008; Meltzer, 2008). Mothers' poor sleep and increased stress are, in turn, are associated with poor sleep and behavior problems in children with autism (Doo & Wing, 2006; Hoffman et al., 2008). The impact on parents of their child's sleep problem therefore needs consideration when nonpharmacological sleep interventions are proposed. Parents may be too exhausted to implement any strategies.

Biological Mechanisms Underlying Sleep

Over a period of about 40 or more years, a number of studies have examined the sleep EEG in children, adolescents, and adults with autism spectrum disorder. Findings vary; sample sizes are generally small and often heterogeneous with regard to age and intellectual functioning, which may confound findings and makes conclusions difficult to draw. Researchers have found reduced REM latency, reduced REM eye movement, decreased sleep spindles in stage 2 sleep, alterations in the amount of stage 1 sleep (mainly increased), decreased slow wave sleep, and alterations to sleep microstructure (Richdale & Schreck, 2009). Giannotti et al. (2011) reported that young children with autism had reduced REM latency, less slow wave sleep, more stage 2 sleep, less time in REM sleep and altered sleep microstructure compared with age- and gender-matched typically developing children, with the differences generally more pronounced in children with autistic regression. Thus, current evidence suggests altered sleep EEG in children with autism but how this is related to problematic sleep remains to be determined.

Several authors have also speculated that the neurotransmitter serotonin may be implicated in the poor sleep patterns found in autism spectrum disorder. Hypersecretion of serotonin is one of the most replicable neurotransmitter findings, and researchers have speculated about the role of serotonin or other neurotransmitters that may be implicated in autism spectrum disorder (e.g., GABA) in the development and maintenance of sleep difficulties (Johnson, Giannotti, & Cortesi, 2009). Serotonin is also a precursor to melatonin, a neurohormone that is involved in signaling sleep onset and synchronizing circadian rhythms to their normal 24-hour cycle. It has been hypothesized that alterations in melatonin synthesis, a phase-advanced melatonin rhythm, or reduced night melatonin secretion may be related to insomnia in autism spectrum disorder (Bourgeron, 2007; Johnson et al., 2010; Richdale & Schreck, 2009; Souders et al., 2009). It also has been hypothesized that circadian timing is altered in autism spectrum disorder. Circadian timing involves the Clock Genes *Per1* and *NPAS2* (Bourgeron, 2007; Richdale & Schreck, 2009; Souders et al., 2009), variants of which have been associated with autism (Nicholas et al., 2007).

Medical Factors

As well as the factors described above, children with autism spectrum disorder may present with sleep problems associated with comorbid medical conditions. Like all children, children with autism spectrum disorder may have asthma, allergy, SDB, or OSA, and these and other medical conditions may disturb their sleep (see Koinis-Mitchell and Everhart, Chapter 32). The resolution of acute medical conditions or the control of chronic conditions may not lead to a resolution of sleep difficulties, as new routines, habits, and expectations will have been set during the illness. Given the communication and social difficulties that are present in autism spectrum disorder it is likely that changing these sleep associations will require the support of a health professional, particularly when symptoms of autism spectrum disorder are severe. Treatment of OSA may lead to significant behavioral improvement (Malow et al., 2006).

About 20%–40% of children with autism spectrum disorder have epilepsy (seizure disorder; Giannotti et al., 2008), and this may be associated with sleeping difficulties. Additionally, sleep deprivation can provoke seizures (Malow, 2004). However, the role of epilepsy in the precipitation or maintenance of sleep problems in autism spectrum disorder has received little attention. Both sleep problem severity and epilepsy have been associated with regression in autism (Giannotti et al., 2008). Recently, Tsai et al. (2012) reported that sleep problems were more common in children with autism spectrum disorder than in children with epilepsy. Malow (2004) provides a review of the potential role of epilepsy in the sleep problems found in autism spectrum disorder.

Treating Sleep Problems in Children with a Developmental Disability

Although sleep problems in children with a developmental disability are common, there is a lack of evidence-based treatments targeting insomnia or other sleep difficulties in these children. In particular, clinical trials examining pharmacological treatments are required (Mindell, Emslie et al., 2006;). Behavioral interventions are the primary treatment for common causes of pediatric insomnia in typically developing children and have best empirical support (Mindell, Kuhn, Lewin, Meltzer, & Sadeh, 2006). Tikotzky and Sadeh (2010) concluded that cognitive-behavioral treatments had *strong empirical support* (p. 690) for treating childhood insomnia and improving parent well-being. However, despite the limitations of current evidence, medications are often prescribed for common pediatric sleep problems, especially for children with a developmental disability (Mindell, Emslie et al., 2006).

Research on behavioral interventions for sleep problems in children with a developmental disability is still "in its infancy" (Richdale & Wiggs, 2005). The best support is for behavioral interventions for insomnia based on extinction procedures, with little research on interventions for other sleep disorders including parasomnias. In a review of behavioral treatments for sleep problems in children with autism spectrum disorder, Vriend, Corkum, Moon, and Smith (2011) similarly concluded that: "despite the high prevalence of sleep problems in children with autism, evidence for effective treatment is sparse (p. 10). And further that: The high prevalence of sleep problems in children with autism, and the negative consequences of inadequate sleep, make appropriate intervention an urgent priority for many families" (p. 10). Melatonin is the only pharmacological intervention for which some evidence of efficacy is reported for children with a developmental disability (e.g., Rossignol & Frye, 2011; Sajith & Clarke, 2007).

In the absence of evidence-based guidelines for treating insomnia, parents of children with a developmental disability often try, or are recommended, a range of interventions (pharmacological, behavioral, or complementary and alternative treatments) to alleviate their child's sleep problems. Many of these treatments have little or no empirical support, and parents do not always rate their effectiveness highly (Keenan et al., 2007; Kronk et al., 2010; Robinson & Richdale, 2004; Williams, Sears, & Allard, 2006; Wiggs & Stores, 1996b). Williams et al. (2006) reported that 204 parents of children with an autism spectrum disorder used a variety of nonpharmacological approaches to assist their child's sleep. Common treatments used included a range of sleep hygiene practices, bedtime stories, taking a toy to bed, music, adjusting light levels, and co-sleeping with parents. Regular bedtime, co-sleeping with parents, wrapping the child in a blanket, and noise masking were rated as the most effective. There is little or no objective research on the use of most of these approaches to treat sleep in autism spectrum disorders or other developmental disorders.

Parent beliefs about child sleep problems influence how parents cope with these problems and how they respond to them emotionally (McDougall, Kerr, & Espie, 2005). Parents may believe that sleep problems are part of the disability or medical condition (Didden et al., 2004; Keenan et al., 2007; Robinson & Richdale, 2004); may be offered poor treatment advice or support (Robinson & Richdale, 2004; Wiggs & Stores, 1996b); may not know how they might obtain treatment, may think the child gets sufficient sleep, or may believe they can "fix" the problem themselves (Robinson & Richdale, 2004); or the treatment may be unacceptable (Wiggs & Stores, 1996a). As a result, many children go untreated (Robinson & Richdale, 2004; Wiggs & Stores, 1996b). Perceived control over the child's sleep behavior has also been found to influence whether or not they report that their child has a sleep problem (Wiggs & Stores, 1998; Robinson, 2007). Additionally, parent knowledge about normal sleep development, children's sleep problems, and good sleep hygiene is reported to be poor, and parent education is needed (Jan et al., 2008; Owens & Jones, 2011; Schreck & Richdale, 2011). Thus, parent education should be a component of any sleep intervention.

Of further concern is that pediatric sleep is not a prominent topic in health professionals' training (Meltzer, Phillips, & Mindell, 2009; Owens, 2001). While health professionals may rely on parents reporting their child's sleep problems, parents often fail to discuss this with a health professional (Blunden et al., 2004) and health professionals may not enquire about sleep in older children (Owens, 2001). Thus, there may be a failure by both parents and health professionals to: *(1)* recognize when significant sleep problems are present; *(2)* the contribution that poor sleep, including sleep apnea, can make to presenting daytime behavioral problems; and *(3)* a tendency to think that little can be done to assist children with a developmental disability and their families. It is therefore important to question parents of children with a developmental disability regarding their child's sleep. Given that parents have poor knowledge of childhood sleep, a simple question such as 'Does your child have any sleep problems?" (p. 4, Owens, 2001) is unlikely to suffice. More detailed questioning about the child's sleep habits and patterns is required if children are to receive appropriate treatment (Schreck & Richdale, 2011).

BEHAVIORAL TREATMENTS

Before any choice can be made about an appropriate sleep treatment, a thorough assessment of the presenting issues and a diagnosis of the sleep problem is required (see Part 3). As noted under specific developmental disabilities, settling and night waking (insomnia) are common sleep complaints and are likely to have a behavioral origin or component. Behavioral interventions, including standard extinction, are acceptable to parents of children with a developmental disability (Bramble, 1996; Keenan et al., 2007; Wiggs & Stores, 1996b), autism, or Fragile X (Weiskop et al., 2005), and have been shown to be successful in treating behavioral insomnia in children with developmental disabilities (Richdale & Wiggs, 2005) or autism (Vriend et al., 2011). Compared with medication, behavioral treatments for children's sleep are generally, but not always, rated more highly by parents of children with a developmental disability (Keenan et al., 2007; Robinson & Richdale, 2004; Wiggs & Stores, 1996b).

Children may learn to fall asleep under specific conditions and if these are not present at bedtime, or if the child wakes at night, then the child is likely to disturb his/her family (see Polimeni, Richdale, & Francis, 2007). Like typically developing children, children with a developmental disability may: *(1)* be attached to comfort objects (e.g., falling asleep with a bottle); *(2)* have learned to fall asleep with a parent present; *(3)* not have well-established routines around sleep, or have dysfunctional routines (e.g., requiring specific pajamas; only accepting a bedtime drink from a specific person); or *(4)* Only be able to sleep if their regular bedtime routine is followed exactly. If the child wakes during the night and, for example, a parent is not present then the child may not be able to self-soothe and return to sleep. Therefore, many children with a developmental disability and sleep problems will meet ICSD-2 criteria (AASM, 2005) for behavioral insomnias of childhood. Like typically developing children, children with a developmental disability may also be anxious or fearful at night (e.g., Wiggs & Stores, 2004) or exhibit nightmares, night terrors, or other parasomnias (e.g., Liu et al., 2006).

Reed et al. (2009) used a 3-session manualized parent education program, which taught parents of children with autism spectrum disorder and insomnia symptoms about sleep and sleep problems as well as a range of behavioral techniques, followed by individual consultation in Session 3 about their child. The intervention produced improvements in sleep in 20 children with autism spectrum disorder, and there was some evidence for improvement in behavior (Reed et al., 2009). A random controlled trial (RCT) of a behavior intervention for 66 children with a developmental disability and sleep problems compared a booklet teaching about children's sleep, behavior management, and behavioral approaches to sleep treatment (media intervention) with a face-to-face session with the therapist directly teaching these principles. Results showed that the media intervention was as effective as the therapist session (Montgomery et al., 2004), with about 67% of children showing improvement in their sleep. A 90-minute group session plus information booklet (media) on children's sleep for mothers of children with Down syndrome that included opportunity for the discussion of individual problems showed that as measured by a composite sleep problems score, children's sleep improved at a 6-month follow-up compared with children whose mothers did not receive training. Information that the mothers found useful included consistency, learning about sleep structure, behavioral reinforcement, bedtime routines, and persistence of their efforts to address the sleep issues (Stores & Stores, 2004).

Thus, these group and media programs demonstrate the potential usefulness of teaching parents about children's sleep, behavior management, and the application of behavior intervention principles to improve insomnia. However, most sleep intervention research in children with a developmental disability uses single case study designs; there are few RCTs. Richdale and Wiggs (2005) provide a comprehensive review of behavioral interventions for children with a developmental disability and sleep problems up to 2005.

Sleep Hygiene

As for other children, the first important consideration for any sleep intervention for children with a developmental disability is the implementation of good sleep hygiene (appropriate sleep habits). Good sleep hygiene—in particular appropriate bedtime, a comfortable bedroom and bed, and a regular bedtime routine—is an important part of any intervention and in some cases may be sufficient to resolve less severe sleep difficulties. A sleep intervention may fail if children's daytime and pre-sleep habits that can impact night sleep are not changed (Jan et al., 2008). However, published behavioral intervention case studies suggest that sleep hygiene alone may not be sufficient for improving sleep in children with a developmental disability. For example, Weiskop, Richdale, and Matthews (2005) and Thackeray and Richdale (2002) provided data on bedtime routines prior to the introduction of extinction and found that with the exception of one child with Fragile X, sleep hygiene alone was not successful in alleviating sleep problems in children with autism, Fragile X, Down syndrome, or intellectual disability. Nevertheless, sleep hygiene principles should be incorporated in any sleep intervention (Jan et al., 2008).

Parent Education

Given that parents have poor knowledge of normal sleep development and children's sleep problems (Owens et al., 2011; Schreck & Richdale, 2011), parent education is an important component of any sleep intervention. Many sleep interventions that have reported successful treatment outcomes have therapist/parent manuals and incorporate parent education about pediatric sleep into their intervention programs (Cortesi et al., 2012; Montgomery et al., 2004; Moon, Corkum, & Smith, 2011; Reed et al., 2009; Stores & Stores, 2004; Thackeray & Richdale, 2002; Weiskop et al., 2005).

Behaviorally Based Procedures

Extinction and graduated extinction (ignoring problematic behaviors; see Part 7) have been shown to be successful in treating settling and night waking in children with a range of developmental disabilities, primarily using single case designs, and thus may be considered as probably efficacious treatments (Richdale & Wiggs, 2005). In children with autism, Vriend et al. (2011) rated both extinction and faded bedtime with response cost as possibly efficacious treatments.

Behavioral interventions, based on a functional assessment of the presenting problems, that use extinction or graduated extinction techniques and incorporate a bedtime routine have been shown to successfully address settling and night waking problems in children with a range of developmental disabilities (e.g., Bramble, 1997; Didden, Curfs, Sikkema, & de Moor, 1998; Didden, de Moor, & Curfs, 2004; Durand, Gernott-Dott, & Mapstone, 1996; Thackeray & Richdale, 2002; Weiskop et al., 2005) as well as in an RCT (Montgomery et al., 2004). Bedtime disturbances, sleep latency, night waking, and co-sleeping variously improved, and changes were usually maintained at follow-ups varying from 2 to 12 months.

There is also a range of other behavioral interventions that have been shown to be efficacious for treating insomnia in children with a developmental disability. These include faded bedtime with and without response cost (Piazza, Fisher, & Sherer, 1997, Moon et al., 2011), sleep restriction (Christodulu & Durand, 2004), stimulus fading (Howlin, 1984), and desensitization for bedtime fears (Didden et al., 1998).

In a variation on extinction, Moore (2004) used a social story about bedtime in conjunction with implementing the bedtime routine and graduated extinction and reported it was successful for a child with autism. Reed et al. (2009) incorporated use of the bedtime pass into their parent training program for children with autism and sleep problems. The bedtime pass has been found effective in addressing sleep onset issues in young typically developing children by providing children with a pass that can be exchanged for one pre-sleep disturbance (Moore, Friman, Fruzzetti, & MacAleese, 2007).

Two recent papers have reported improved sleep latency in children with autism spectrum disorder when using a behavioral treatment (Cortesi, Giannotti, Sebastiani, Panunzi, & Valente, 2012; Moon et al., 2011). Moon et al. found that sleep latency was improved in three children with autism using a faded bedtime with response cost, and gains were maintained 12 weeks later. In such procedures children are put to bed when they would be expected to be very tired (later than typical sleep onset time) and if not asleep within 20 minutes are removed from bed for 20 minutes (response cost). When a bedtime is established where the child falls asleep within 20 minutes over a two consecutive nights, the child's bedtime is moved 20 minutes earlier. This procedure is repeated until the child reaches the desired bedtime and is able to fall asleep within 20 minutes.

A 4-week behavior intervention based on Montgomery et al. (2004) and Weiskop et al. (2005) formed part of a large RCT trial (160 children with autistic disorder aged 4–10 years) comparing a behavior intervention and melatonin alone and in combination (Cortesi et al., 2012) to treat insomnia in children with autistic disorder. The behavior intervention was successful in improving sleep latency in particular, while melatonin in conjunction with a behavioral intervention was superior to either treatment alone in treating symptoms of insomnia.

Despite these reports of effective treatments for insomnia in children with a developmental disability the literature remains limited, with few intervention papers published concerning sleep treatments for parasomnias and circadian rhythm sleep disorders in this population. Richdale and Wiggs (2005) provide a review of these interventions.

MEDICATION

Medication is appealing because it is ostensibly a faster and simpler alternative to a behavioral treatment and may result in an immediate, positive impact on sleep. However, sleep medications lack appropriate management guidelines for pediatric use and require research into safety and efficacy (Mindell, Emslie, et al., 2006). Thus, there is no strong evidence base to support the long-term use of sleep medications for the treatment of insomnia in children (Mindell, Emslie et al., 2006) or children with a developmental disability (Holloway & Aman, 2011). Additionally, parents of children with a developmental disability may not like their child being prescribed medications (Keenan et al., 2007).

Parents in Williams et al.'s (2006) survey also reported on medication use for sleep problems in children with autism spectrum disorder: Medication was used less frequently than other treatments. While Benadryl (diphenhydramine) was the most commonly used (35% of cases), it was not rated as effective as Catapres (clonidine), Noctec (chloral hydrate) and Atarax (hydroxyzine), which were most frequently reported as effective. Melatonin and Desyrel (trazodone) were least effective. Parents in Keenan et al.'s (2007) study rated behavioral intervention and melatonin as equally acceptable, but were likely to endorse the use of melatonin for more severe sleep problems. Other than melatonin there is little sound evidence to support the use of medications to treat sleep problems in the developmental disabilities, which is consistent with pharmacological treatment for pediatric sleep problems in general (Mindell, Emslie et al., 2006).

Melatonin

Most research attention has been given to melatonin for treating sleep in children with a developmental disability (see Guénolé et al. 2011; Jan & Freeman, 2004; Phillips & Appleton, 2004; Rossignol & Frye, 2011; Sajith & Clarke, 2007 for reviews), and it has better empirical support than other medications for treating sleep in children with a developmental disability (Holloway & Aman, 2011).

Randomized, crossover, double-blind placebo-controlled trials have shown that melatonin can be useful for treating insomnia (e.g., Cortesi et al., 2012; Malow et al., 2012; Wasdell et al., 2008; Wirojanan et al., 2009). Fifty children with a developmental disability and chronic and severe sleep problems, including sleep latency >30 minutes and/or significant night-waking, and who had not responded to a sleep hygiene intervention, completed a randomized, placebo-controlled, double-blind crossover trial of 5mg of controlled-release melatonin to treat their insomnia. There were significant improvements in both total night sleep and sleep latency in response to treatment (Wasdell et al., 2008). In Wirojanan and colleague's (2009) study 12 children with autism and/or Fragile-X also completed a randomized, placebo-controlled, double-blind crossover trail using 3mg melatonin and again, improvements were seen in sleep latency and total night sleep for these children. Using a placebo-controlled RCT across 160 children with autistic disorder, Cortesi et al. (2012) showed that a dose 3 mg of controlled release melatonin treatment at 21:00 hours each night was superior to a behavior intervention but not a combined behavior/melatonin treatment for insomnia. Similarly, Malow et al. (2012) showed that either 1 mg or 3 mg of melatonin was useful for treating sleep latency difficulties in 21 children with autism spectrum disorder, with three children responding to 6 mg.

Thus, there is some support for using melatonin to treat insomnia in children with a developmental disability. Nevertheless, in relation to its use in autism spectrum disorder, Guénolé et al. (2011) concluded that the small number of melatonin studies to date, limitations associated with study research design, lack of large scale multisite RCTs, and the lack of long-term safety data mean that melatonin presently cannot be considered as an evidence-based treatment for insomnia. These issues likely apply to the use of melatonin to treat sleep insomnia in other developmental disabilities. Additionally, melatonin has both soporific and circadian altering properties and its mode of action in children with a developmental disability and sleep problems has not been determined.

Conclusions

Sleep problems in children with a developmental disability may be complex, with medical, psychological, behavioral, and/or environmental components potentially needing to be considered. Factors associated with specific developmental disorders may predispose children to some sleep problems, in particular SDB and OSA. Even when a medical condition that affects sleep is present, other factors including anxiety or bedtime fears, parental attention, poor sleep routines, or the sleeping environment can contribute to the presentation of poor sleep patterns. These psychological, behavioral, and environmental factors, if resolved, may improve the child's sleep or at least the child may no longer disturb other family members, thus resulting in improved sleep for them.

There is a growing body of evidence supporting the usefulness of behavioral interventions that include sleep hygiene and parent education components to successfully treat insomnia in children with a developmental disability, particularly settling and sleep onset issues. However, intervention research on treatment of parasomnias is sparse. Melatonin is the only pharmacological intervention that has some support as useful for insomnia treatment in these children, and it may be more effective in combination with a behavioral treatment (Cortesi et al., 2012). As has been stressed in other sections of this book it is most important that a thorough assessment and diagnosis of the presenting sleep issues, as well as family preferences and stressors, forms the basis of intervention choices. Currently, best support is found for the use of behavioral techniques based on extinction principles or melatonin to treat insomnia in young children with a developmental disability. Intervention is an area badly in need of research.

Few intervention studies have examined improvement in children's daytime behavior in response to sleep intervention, and any effects of intervention on children's behavior remain unclear. Positive impacts on mothers and children have been reported (e.g., Reed et al., 2009), but others have found no consistent change in children's daytime behavior (e.g., Thackeray & Richdale, 2002; Wiggs & Stores, 1999). The impact of a child sleep intervention on parents' sleep, parenting efficacy, or parents' mental health in response to improvements in sleep for children with a developmental disability, requires further exploration.

Future Directions

Definitions of sleep problems, standardization of measures:

Studies use a range of definitions to define sleep problems and their severity; ICSD-2 (AASM, 2005) criteria are rarely used to examine the presence of specific sleep disorders. Definitions of sleep problems are often based on questionnaires, which have been developed based on sleep in typically developing children and may fail to meet adequate criteria for questionnaire development. Readers are referred to Spruyt and Gozal for advice on sleep questionnaire development (2011a) and a critical review of published pediatric sleep questionnaires (2011b). Standardization of definitions and approaches to measurement would facilitate comparison of research findings across studies and developmental disorders and aid in the development of prevention and intervention strategies.

Randomized controlled trials (RCTs):

A focus on prevention and intervention research for sleep problems in children with developmental disability is needed. RCTs that examine the efficacy of pharmacological and behavioral interventions to treat sleep problems/disorders in children with a developmental disability are required; effectiveness studies are also needed. Case study designs can also provide good evidence about the efficacy of behavioral interventions. Targeted pediatric sleep research funding is needed that places a high priority on sleep problems in children with a developmental disability.

Etiology may inform practice/intervention:

A clearer understanding of the etiology of the sleep problems/disorders found in children with specific developmental disorders is required. Whether or not there are disorder-specific etiological factors would inform assessment protocols and the development of more effective prevention and intervention strategies.

Families and children:

Families of children with a developmental disability are often under more stress than other families, and poor child sleep is associated with increased vulnerability to fatigue, anxiety, and mood disorders in mothers. More needs to be understood about the impact of these children's poor sleep on family functioning and individual family members. In addition, as children's development is already compromised by their disability, we need to understand more about the impact of poor sleep on their daytime functioning.

Education:

Education needs to occur in two areas. First, health professionals require information about the assessment and treatment of sleep problems in children with a developmental disability. Second, parents need information about normal pediatric sleep development and common sleep problems, as well as knowledge of basic sleep hygiene principles and how to apply them with their child. Such education may assist in preventing common and often less severe settling and night waking problems.

References

Allik, H., Larsson, J. O., & Smedje, A. (2006a). Insomnia in school-age children with Asperger syndrome or high-functioning autism. *BMC Psychiatry, 6*, 6–18.

Allik, H., Larsson, J. O., & Smedje, A. (2006b). Sleep patterns of school-age children with Asperger syndrome or high-functioning autism. *Journal of Autism and Developmental Disorders, 36*, 585–595.

American Academy of Sleep Medicine (2005). *International Classification of Sleep Disorders* (2nd ed.). Westchester, IL: Author.

American Psychiatric Association (2000). *Diagnostic and Statistical Manual of Mental Disorders.* (Text Rev., 4th ed.). Washington, DC: Author.

Annaz, D., Hill, C. M., Ashworth, A., & Holley, S. (2011). Characterisation of sleep problems in children with Williams syndrome. *Research in Developmental Disabilities, 32*, 164–169

Bartlett, L. B., Rooney, V., & Spedding, S. (1985). Nocturnal difficulties in a population of mentally handicapped children. *British Journal of Mental Subnormality, 31*, 54–59

Blunden, S., Lushington, K., Lorenzen, B., Ooi, T., Fung, F., & Kennedy, D. (2004). Are sleep problems under-recognised in general practice? *Archives of Disability in Childhood, 89*, 708–712.

Boudreau, E. A., Johnson, K. P., Jackman, A. R., Blancato, J., Huizing, M., Bendavid, C., Jones, M. P., et al. (2009). Review of disrupted sleep patterns in Smith–Magenis syndrome and normal melatonin secretion in a patient with an atypical interstitial 17p11.2 deletion. *American Journal of Medical Genetics, Part A, 149A*, 1382–1391.

Bourgeron T. (2007). The possible interplay of synaptic and clock genes in autism spectrum disorders. *Cold Spring Harbor Symposium Quarterly Biology, LXXII*, 1–10.

Bramble D. (1996). Consumer opinion concerning the treatment of a common sleep problem. *Child: Care, Health and Development, 22*, 355–366.

Bramble, D. (1997). Rapid-acting treatment for a common sleep problem. *Developmental Medicine & Child Neurology, 39*, 543–547.

Bruni, O., Ferri, R., D'Agostino, G., Miano, S., Roccella, M., & Elia, M. (2004). Sleep disturbances in Angelman syndrome: A questionnaire study. *Brain & Development, 26*, 233–240.

Bruni, O., Verrillo, E., Novelli, L., & Ferri, R. (2010). Prader-Willi syndrome: Sorting out the relationships between obesity, hypersomnia, and sleep apnea. *Current Opinion in Pulmonary Medicine, 16*, 568–573

Cassidy, S. B., McKillop, J. A., & Morgan, W. J. (1990). Sleep disorders in Prader-Willi syndrome. *Dysmorphology and Clinical Genetics, 4*, 13–17.

Christodulu, K. V., & Durand, M. V. (2004). Reducing bedtime disturbance and night waking using positive bedtime routines and sleep restriction. *Focus on Autism and Other Developmental Disabilities, 19*, 130–139.

Chu, J., & Richdale, A. L. (2009). Sleep quality and psychological wellbeing in mothers of children with developmental disabilities. *Research in Developmental Disabilities, 30*, 1512–1522.

Cidav, Z., Marcus, S. C. & Mandell, D. S. (2012). Implications of childhood autism for parental employment and earnings. *Pediatrics, 129*, 617–623

Clements, J., Wing, L., & Dunn G. (1986). Sleep problems in handicapped children: A preliminary study. *Journal of Child Psychology & Psychiatry, 27*, 399–407.

Cortesi, F., Giannotti, F., Sebastiani, T., Panunzi, S., & Valente, D. (2012). Controlled-release melatonin, singly and combined with cognitive behavioural therapy, for persistent insomnia in children with autism spectrum disorders: A randomized placebo-controlled trial. *Journal of Sleep Research. 21*(6), 700–709.

Cotton, S., & Richdale, A. (2006). Brief report: Parental descriptions of sleep problems in children with autism, Down syndrome, and Prader-Willi syndrome. *Research in Developmental Disabilities, 27*, 151–161.

Cotton S. M., & Richdale A. L. (2010). Sleep patterns and behaviour in typically developing children and children with autism, Down syndrome, Prader-Willi syndrome and intellectual disability. *Research in Autism Spectrum Disorders, 4*, 490–500.

Davis, K., & Gavidia-Payne, S. (2009). The impact of child, family, and professional support characteristics on the quality of life in families of young children with disabilities. *Journal of Intellectual and Developmental Disability, 34*, 153–162.

De Leersnyder H., Bresson, J. L., de Blois, M-C., Souberbielle, J-C., Mogenet, A., Delhotal-Landes, B., et al. (2003). β1-adrenergic antagonists and melatonin reset the clock and restore sleep in a circadian disorder, Smith-Magenis syndrome. *Journal of Medical Genetics, 40*, 74–78.

De Leersnyder, H. (2006). Inverted rhythm of melatonin secretion in Smith–Magenis syndrome: From symptoms to treatment. *TRENDS in Endocrinology and Metabolism, 17*, 291–298.

DeVincent, C. J., Gadow, K. D., Delosh, D., & Geller, L. (2007). Sleep disturbance and its relation to DSM-IV psychiatric symptoms in preschool-age children with pervasive developmental disorder and community controls. *Journal of Child Neurology, 22*, 161–171.

Dewald, J. F., Meijer, A. M., Oort, F. J., Kerkhof, G. A., & Bögels, S. M. (2010). The influence of sleep quality, sleep duration and sleepiness on school performance in children and adolescents: A meta-analytic review. *Sleep Medicine Reviews, 14*, 179–189.

Didden, R., Curfs, L. M. G., Sikkema, S. P. E., & de Moor, J. M. H. (1998). Functional assessment and treatment of sleep problems with developmentally disabled children: Six case studies. *Journal of Behavior Therapy and Experimental Psychiatry, 29*, 85–97.

Didden R., Korzillius H., van Aperlo B., van Overloop C., & de Vries, M. (2002). Sleep problems and daytime problem behaviours in children with intellectual disability. *Journal of Intellectual & Developmental Disability, 46*, 537–547.

Didden, R, de Moor, J. M. H., & Curfs, L. M. G. (2004a). Behavioural treatment of sleep problems in three children with developmental disabilities. *The British Journal of Developmental Disabilities, 50*, 13–19.

Didden, R., Korzillius H., Smits, M. G., & Curfs, L. M. G. (2004b). Sleep problems in individuals with Angelman sydrome. *American Journal on Mental Retardation, 109,* 275–284.

Doo S., & Wing Y. K. (2006). Sleep problems of children with pervasive developmental disorders: Correlation with parental stress. *Developmental Medicine & Child Neurology, 48,* 650–655.

Doran, S. M., Harvey, M. T., & Horner, R. H. (2006). Sleep and developmental disabilities: Assessment, treatment and outcome measures. *Mental Retardation, 44,* 13–27.

Durand, V. M., Gernott-Dott, P., & Mapstone, E. (1996). Treatment of sleep disorders in children with developmental disabilities. *Journal of the Association for Persons with Severe Handicaps, 21,* 114–122.

Dykens, E. M., & Smith, A. C. M. (1998). Distinctiveness and correlates of maladaptive behaviour in children and adolescents with Smith-Magenis syndrome. *Journal of Intellectual Disability Research, 42,* 481–489.

Elia, M., Ferri, R., Musumeci, S. A., Del Gracco, S., Bottitta, M., Scuderi, C. et al. (2000). Sleep in subjects with autistic disorder: A neurophysiological and psychological study. *Brain & Development, 22,* 88–92.

Elsabbagh, M., Divan, G., Koh, Y-J., Kim, Y. S., Kauchali, S., Marcín, C., et al. (2012). Global presence of autism and other pervasive developmental disorders. *Autism Research, 5*(3), 160–179.

Gabriels R. L., Cuccaro M. L., Hill, D. E., Ivers B. J., & Goldson, E. (2005). Repetitive behaviors in autism: Relationships with associated clinical features. *Research in Developmental Disabilities, 26,* 169–181.

Gadow, K. D., DeVincent, C. J., & Pomeroy, J. (2006). ADHD symptoms subtypes in children with pervasive developmental disorder. *Journal of Autism and Developmental Disabilities, 36,* 271–283.

Gallagher, S., Phillips, A. C., & Carroll, D. (2010). Parental stress is associated with poor sleep quality in parents caring for children with developmental disabilities. *Journal of Pediatric Psychology, 35,* 728–737, 2010.

Giannotti, F., Cortesi, F., Cerquiglini, A., Miraglia, D., Vagnoni, C., Sebastiani, T., et al. (2008). An investigation of sleep characteristics, EEG abnormalities and epilepsy in developmentally regressed and non-regressed children with autism. *Journal of Autism and Developmental Disorders, 38,* 1888–1897

Giannotti, F., Cortesi, F., Cerquiglini, A., Vagnoni, C. & Valente, D. (2011). Sleep in children with autism with and without autistic regression. *Journal of Sleep Research, 20,* 338–347.

Glaze, D. G., Frost Jr., J. D., Zoghbi, H. Y., & Percy, A. K. (1987). Rett's syndrome: Characterization of respiratory patterns and sleep. *Annals of Neurology, 21,* 377–382.

Glaze, D. G. (2004). Rett syndrome: Of girls and mice—lessons for regression in autism. *Mental Retardation and Developmental Disabilities Research Reviews, 10,* 154–158

Goldman, S. E., Malow, B. A., Newman, K. D., E. Roof, E., & Dykens, E. M. (2009). Sleep patterns and daytime sleepiness in adolescents and young adults with Williams syndrome. *Journal of Intellectual Disability Research, 53,* 182–188.

Goldman, S. E., McGrew, S., Johnson, K. P., Richdale, A. L., Clemons, T., & Malow, B. A. (2011). Sleep is associated with problem behaviors in children and adolescents with autism spectrum disorders. *Research in Autism Spectrum Disorders, 5,* 1223–1229.

Goldman, S. E., Richdale, A. L., Clemens, T., & Malow, B. A. (2012). Parental sleep concerns in autism spectrum disorders: Variations from childhood to adolescence, *Journal of Autism and Developmental Disorders, 42,* 531–538

Goldman, S. E., Bichell, T. J., Surdyka, K., & Malow, B. A. (2012). Sleep in children and adolescents with Angelman syndrome: Association with parent sleep and stress.. *Journal of Intellectual Disability Research, 56*(6), 600–608.

Gombos, F., Bódizs, R., & Kovács, I. (2011). Atypical sleep architecture and altered EEG spectra in Williams syndrome. *Journal of Intellectual Disability Research, 55,* 255–262.

Goodlin-Jones, B., Schwichtenberg, A. J., Iosif, A-M., Tang, T., Liu, J., & Anders, T. F. (2009). Six-month persistence of sleep problems in young children with autism, developmental delay, and typical development. *Journal of the American Academy of Child & Adolescent Psychiatry, 48,* 847–854.

Gould, E. L., Loesch D. Z., Martin M. J., Hagerman R. J., Armstrong S. M., & Huggins, R. M. (2000). Melatonin profiles and sleep characteristics in boys with Fragile X syndrome: A preliminary study. *American Journal of Medical Genetics, 95,* 307–315.

Gregory, A. M., & Sadeh, A. (2012). Sleep, emotional and behavioral difficulties in children and adolescents. *Sleep Medicine Reviews, 16,* 129–136.

Guénolé F., Godbout, R., Nicolas, A. Franco, P. Claustrat, B., & Baleyte, J. M. (2011). Melatonin for disordered sleep in individuals with autism spectrum disorders: Systematic review and discussion. *Sleep Medicine Reviews, 15,* 379–387.

Hagerman, R. (2008). The Fragile X prevalence paradox. *Journal of Medical Genetics, 45,* 498–499.

Hastings, R. P. (2002). Behavior problems in children with autism, parental self-efficacy and mental health. *American Journal on Mental Retardation, 107,* 222–232

Hoffman, C. D., Sweeny, D. P., Gilliam, J. E., Apodaca, D. D., Lopez-Wagner, M. C., & Castillo, M. M. (2005). Sleep problems and symptomology in children with autism. *Focus on Autism and Other Developmental Disabilities, 20,* 194–200.

Hoffman C. D., Sweeney, D. P., Lopez-Wagner, M. C., Hodge, D., Nam, C. Y., & Botts, B. H. (2008). Children with autism: Sleep problems and mothers' stress. *Focus Autism and Other Developmental Disabilities, 23,* 155–165.

Holloway, J. A., & Aman, M. G. (2011). Pharmacological treatment of sleep disturbance in developmental disabilities: A review of the literature. *Research in Developmental Disabilities, 32,* 939–962.

Howlin, P. (1984). A brief report on the elimination of long term sleeping problems in a 6-year-old autistic boy. *Behavioural Psychotherapy, 12,* 257–260.

Inamura, K. (1984). Sleep-wake patterns in autistic children. *Japan Journal of Child & Adolescent Psychiatry, 25,* 205–217 (In Japanese).

Ingersoll B., Myer, K., & Becker, M. W. (2011). Increased rates of depressed mood in mothers of children with autism spectrum disorder associated with the presence of the broader autism phenotype. *Autism Research, 4,* 143–148.

Irving, C., Basu, A., Richmond, S., Burn, J., & Wren, C. (2008). Twenty-year trends in prevalence and survival of Down syndrome. *European Journal of Human Genetics, 16,* 1336–1340

Jan, J. E., & Freeman, R. D. (2004). Melatonin therapy for circadian rhythm sleep disorders in children with multiple disabilities: What have we learned in the last decade? *Developmental Medicine & Child Neurology, 46,* 776–782.

Jan J. E. Owens, J. A., Weiss, M. D., Johnson, K. P., Wasdell, M. B., Freeman, R. D., & Ipsiroglu, O. S. (2008). Sleep hygiene for children with neurodevelopmental disabilities. *Pediatrics, 122*, 1343–1350.

Johnson, K. P., Giannotti, F., & Cortesi, F. (2009). Sleep patterns in autism spectrum disorders. *Child and Adolescent Psychiatric Clinics of North America, 18*, 917–928.

Joo, E. Y., Hong, S. B., Sohn, Y. B., Kwak, M. J., Kim, S. J., Choi, Y. O., et al. (2009). Plasma adiponectin level and sleep structures in children with Prader–Willi syndrome. *Journal of Sleep Research, 19*, 248–254.

Keenan R. A., Wild, M. R., McArthur, I., & Espie, C. A. (2007). Children with developmental disabilities and sleep problems: parental beliefs and treatment acceptability. *Journal of Applied Research in Intellectual Disabilities, 20*, 455–465.

Kozlowski A., Matson, J. L., Belva, B., Rieske, R. (2012). Feeding and sleep difficulties in toddlers with autism spectrum disorders. *Research in Autism Spectrum Disorders, 6*, 385–390.

Krakowiak, P., Goodlin- Jones, B., Picciotto, I. Z., Croen, L. A., & Hansen, R. L. (2008). Sleep problems in children with autism spectrum disorders, developmental delays, and typical development: A population-based study. *Journal of Sleep Research, 17*, 197–206.

Krakowiak, P., Goodlin-Jones, B., Picciotto, I. Z., Croen, L. A., & Hansen, R. L. (2012). Corrigendum: Sleep problems in children with autism spectrum disorders, developmental delays, and typical development: a population-based study. *Journal of Sleep Research, 21*, 231.

Kronk, R., Dahl, R., & Noll, R. (2009). Caregiver reports of sleep problems on a convenience sample of children with Fragile X syndrome. *American Journal on Intellectual and Developmental Disabilities, 114*, 383–392.

Kronk, R., Bishop, E. E., Raspa M., Bickel, J. O., Mandel, D. A., & Bailey, D. B. (2010). Prevalence, nature, and correlates of sleep problems among children with Fragile X syndrome based on a large scale parent survey. *Sleep, 33*, 679–687.

Leyfer, T. O., Folstein, S. E., Bacalman, S., Davis, N. O., Dinh, E., Morgan, J., et al. (2006). Comorbid psychiatric disorders in children with autism: Interview development and rates of disorders. *Journal of Autism and Developmental Disorders, 36*, 849–861.

Liu, X., Hubbard, J. A., Fabes, R. A., & Adam, J. B. (2006). Sleep disturbances and correlates of children with autism spectrum disorders. *Child Psychiatry and Human Development, 37*, 179–191.

Lopez-Wagner, M. C., Hoffman, C. D., Sweeney, D. P., Hodge, D., & Gilliam, J. E. (2008). Sleep problems of parents of typically developing children and parents of children with autism. *Journal of Genetic Psychology, 169*, 245–259.

Malow, B., Adkins, K. W., McGrew, S. G., Wang, L., Goldman, S. E., Fawkes, D., & Burnette, C. (2012). Melatonin for sleep in children with autism: A controlled trial examining dose, tolerability, and outcomes. *Journal of Autism and Developmental Disorders, 42*(8), 1729–1737.

Malow, B. A. (2004). Sleep disorders, epilepsy, and autism. *Mental Retardation and Developmental Disabilities Research Reviews, 10*, 122–125

Malow, B. A., Marzec, M. L., McGrew, S. G., Wang, L., Henderson, L. M., & Stone, W. L. (2006). Characterizing sleep in children with autism spectrum disorders: A multidimensional approach. *Sleep, 29*, 1563–1571.

Malow B. A., McGrew, S. G., Harvey, M., Henderson, L. M., & Stone, W. E. (2006). Impact of treating sleep apnea in a child with autism spectrum disorder. *Pediatric Neurology, 34*, 325–328.

Marcus, C. L., Carroll, J. L., McColley, S. A., Loughlin, G. M., Curtis, S., Pyzik, P., & Naidu, S. (1994). Polysomnographc characteristics of patients with Rett syndrome. *The Journal of Pediatrics, 125*, 218–224.

Marquenie, K., Rodger, S. Mangohig, K., & Cronin, A. (2011). Dinnertime and bedtime routines and rituals in families with a young child with an autism spectrum disorder. *Australian Occupational Therapy Journal, 58*, 145–154.

Mason, T. B. A., Arens, R., Sharman, J., Bintliff-Janisak, B., Schultz, B., Walters, A. S., et al. (2011). Sleep in children with Williams syndrome. *Sleep Medicine, 12*, 892–897.

Mayes, S. D., & Calhoun, S. L. (2009). Variables related to sleep problems in children with autism. *Research in Autism Spectrum Disorders, 3*, 931–941.

Mayes, S. D., Calhoun, S. L., Murray, M. J., Ahuja, M., & Smith, L. A. (2011a). Anxiety, depression, and irritability in children with autism relative to other neuropsychiatric disorders and typical development. *Research in Autism Spectrum Disorders, 5*, 474–485.

Mayes, S. D., Calhoun, S. L., Murray, M. J., & Zahid, J. (2011b). Variables associated with anxiety and depression in children with autism. *Journal of Developmental and Physical Disabilities, 23*, 325–337

McArthur, A. J., & Budden, S. S. (1998). Sleep dysfunction in Rett syndrome: A trial of exogenous melatonin treatment. *Developmental Medicine & Child Neurology, 40*, 186–192.

McDougall, A., Kerr, A. M., & Espie, C. A. (2005). Sleep disturbance in children with Rett syndrome: A qualitative investigation of the parental experience. *Journal of Applied Research in Intellectual Disabilities, 18*, 201–215.

Meltzer, L. J., & Mindell, J. A. (2007). Relationship between child sleep disturbances and maternal sleep, mood, and parenting stress: A pilot study. *Journal of Family Psychology, 21*, 67–73.

Meltzer, L. J. (2008). Brief report: Sleep in parents of children with autism spectrum disorders. *Journal of Pediatric Psychology, 33*, 380–386.

Meltzer, L. J., Phillips, C., & Mindell, J. A. (2009). Clinical psychology training in sleep and sleep disorders. *Journal of Clinical Psycholology, 65*, 305–318.

Miano, S. & Ferri, S. (2010). Epidemiology and management of insomnia in children with autistic spectrum disorders. *Pediatric Drugs, 12*, 75–84.

Mindell J. A., Emslie G. Blumer, J., Myron Genel, M., Daniel Glaze, D., Ivanenko, A., et al. (2006). Pharmacologic management of insomnia in children and adolescents: Consensus statement. *Pediatrics, 117*, 1223–1232.

Mindell, J. A., Kuhn, B., Lewin, D. S., Meltzer, L. J., & Sadeh, A. (2006). Behavioral treatment of bedtime problems and night wakings in infants and young children. *Sleep, 29*, 1264–1276.

Miyamoto, A., Oki, J., Takahashi, S., & Okuno, A. (1999). Serum melatonin kinetics and long-term melatonin treatment for sleep disorders in Rett syndrome. *Brain and Development, 21*, 59–62

Montgomery, P., Stores, G., & Wiggs, L. (2004). The relative efficacy of two brief treatments for sleep problems in young learning disabled (mentally retarded) children: A randomised controlled trial. *Archives of Diseases of Childhood, 89*, 125–130

Moon, E. C., Corkum, P., & Smith, I. M. (2011). Case study: A case-series evaluation of a behavioral sleep intervention for three children with autism and primary insomnia. *Journal of Pediatric Psychology, 36*, 47–54.

Moore, B. A., Friman, P. C., Fruzzetti, A. E., & MacAleese, K., (2007). Brief report: Evaluating the bedtime pass program for child resistance to bedtime—a randomized, controlled trial. *Journal of Pediatric Psychology, 32*, 283–287.

Moore, P. S. (2004). The use of social stories in a psychology service for children with learning disabilities: A case study of a sleep problem. *British Journal of Learning Disabilities, 32*, 133–138.

Nicholas, B. Rudrasingham, V., Nash, S., Kirov, G., Owen, M. J., & Wimpory, D. C. (2007). Association of per1 and Npas2 with autistic disorder: Support for the clock genes/social timing hypothesis. *Molecular Psychiatry, 12*, 581–592.

Õiglane-Shlik, E., Talvik, T., Zordania, R., Põder, H., Kahre, T., Raukas, E. et al. (2006). Prevalence of Angelman syndrome and Prader–Willi syndrome in Estonian children: Sister syndromes not equally represented. *American Journal of Medical Genetics Part A 140A*, 1936–1943.

Owens, J. (2005). The ADHD sleep conundrum: A review. *Journal of Developmental and Behavioral Pediatrics, 26*, 312–323.

Owens, J. A. (2001). The practice of pediatric sleep medicine: Results of a community survey. *Pediatrics, 108*(3), E51. Accessed April 6, 2013 from http://www.pediatrics.org/cgi/content/full/108/3/e51.

Owens, J. A., Jones, C., & Nash, R. (2011). Caregivers' knowledge, behavior, and attitudes regarding healthy sleep in young children. *Journal of Clinical Sleep Medicine, 7*(4), 345–350.

Owens, J. A., & Jones, C. (2011). Parental knowledge of healthy sleep in young children: Results of a primary care clinic survey. *Journal of Developmental and Behavioral Pediatrics, 32*, 447–453.

Paavonen, J. E., Nieminen-von Wendt, T., Vanhala, R., Aronen, E. T., & von Wendt, L. (2003). Effectiveness of melatonin in the treatment of sleep disturbances in children with Asperger disorder. *Journal of Child and Adolescent Psychopharmacology, 13*, 83–95.

Paavonen, J. E., Vehkalahti, K., Vanhala, R., von Wendt, L., Nieminen-von Wendt, T., & Aronen, E. T. (2008). Sleep in children with Asperger syndrome. *Journal of Autism and Developmental Disorders, 38*, 41–51.

Patzold, L., Richdale, A., & Tonge, B. (1998). An investigation into the sleep characteristics of children with autism and Asperger's disorder. *Journal of Paediatrics and Child Health, 34*, 528–533.

Phillips, L., & Appleton, R. E. (2004). Systematic review of melatonin treatment in children with neurodevelopmental disabilities and sleep impairment. *Developmental Medicine & Child Neurology, 46*, 771–775.

Piazza, C. C., Fisher, W., Kiesewetter, K., Bowman, L., & Moser, H. (1990). Aberrant sleep patterns in children with the Rett syndrome. *Brain & Development, 12*, 488–493.

Piazza, C. C., Fisher, W. W., & Sherer, M. (1997). Treatment of multiple sleep problems in children with developmental disabilities: Faded bedtime with response cost versus bedtime scheduling. *Developmental Medicine & Child Neurology, 39*, 414–418.

Polimeni, M. A., Richdale, A. L., & Francis, A. J. P. (2005). A survey of sleep problems in autism, Asperger's disorder and typically developing children. *Journal of Intellectual Disability Research, 49*, 260–268

Polimeni, M. A., Richdale, A. L., & Francis, A. J. P. (2007). The impact of children's sleep problems on the family and behavioural processes related to their development and maintenance. *E-Journal of Applied Psychology, 3*, 76–85.

Quine, L. (1991). Sleep problems in children with mental handicap. *Journal of Mental Deficiency Research, 35*, 269–290.

Quine, L. (2001). Sleep problems in primary school children: Comparison between mainstream and special school children. *Child: Care, Health and Behavior, 27*, 201–221.

Reed, H. E., McGrew, S. G., Artibee, A., Surdkya, K., Goldman, S. E., Frank, K., Wang, L. & Malow, B. A. (2009). Parent-based sleep education workshops in autism. *Journal of Child Neurology, 24*, 936–945.

Richdale A., Francis, A., Gavidia-Payne, S., & Cotton, S. (2000). Stress, behaviour, and sleep problems in children with an intellectual disability. *Journal of Intellectual & Developmental Disability, 25*, 147–161.

Richdale, A. (2003). A descriptive analysis of sleep behaviour in children with Fragile X. *Journal of Intellectual & Developmental Disability, 28*, 135–144.

Richdale, A., & Wiggs, L. (2005). Behavioral approaches to the treatment of sleep problems in children with developmental disorders. What is the state of the art? *International Journal of Behavioral & Consulting Therapy, 1*, 165–189.

Richdale, A. L., & Prior, M. R. (1995). The sleep/wake rhythm in children with autism. *European Child and Adolescent Psychiatry, 4*, 175–186.

Richdale, A. L. (1999). Annotation: Sleep problems and autism: Comparison with other disabilities, causes, and intervention. *Developmental Medicine and Child Neurology, 41*, 60–66.

Richdale, A. L., Cotton, S., & Hibbit, K. (1999). Sleep and behaviour difficulties in the Prader-Willi syndrome. A questionnaire study. *Journal of Intellectual Disability Research, 43*, 380–392.

Richdale, A. L., & Schreck, K. A. (2009). Sleep problems in autism spectrum disorders: Prevalence, nature, and possible biopsychosocial etiologies. *Sleep Medicine Reviews, 13*, 403–411.

Robinson, A. M., & Richdale, A. L. (2004). Sleep problems in children with an intellectual disability: Parental views of treatment, satisfaction and effectiveness. *Child: Care, Health and Development, 30*, 139–150

Robinson, A. M. (2007). *Children with an intellectual disability and sleep problems: The role of child and parent factors and treatment efficacy using the Signposts program.* Doctoral dissertation, RMIT University, Melbourne, Australia.

Rosen, D., Lombardo, A., Skotko, B., & Davidson, E. J. (2011). Parental perceptions of sleep disturbances and sleep-disordered breathing in children with Down syndrome. *Clinical Pediatrics, 50*, 121–125.

Rossignol, D. A., & Frye, R. E. (2011). Melatonin in autism spectrum disorders: A systematic review and meta-analysis. *Developmental Medicine & Child Neurology, 53*, 783–792.

Sajith, S. G., & Clarke, D. (2007). Melatonin and sleep disorders associated with intellectual disability: A clinical review. *Journal of Intellectual Disability Research, 51*, 2–13.

Schlüter, B., Buschatz, D., Trowitzsch, E., & Aksu, F. (1997). Respiratory control in children with Prader-Willi syndrome. *European Journal of Pediatrics, 156*, 65–68.

Schreck, K. A., & Mulick, J. (2000). Parental report of sleep problems in children with autism. *Journal of Autism and Developmental Disorders, 30*, 127–135.

Schreck, K. A., Mulick, J., & Smith, A. (2004). Sleep problems as possible predictors of intensified symptoms of autism. *Research in Developmental Disabilities, 25*, 57–66.

Schreck, K. A., & Richdale, A. L. (2011). Knowledge of childhood sleep: A possible variable in under or misdiagnosis of childhood sleep problems. *Journal of Sleep Research, 20,* 598–597.

Schwichtenberg, A. J., Iosif, A. M., Goodlin-Jones, B., Tang, K., & Anders, T. (2011). Daytime sleep patterns in preschool children with autism, developmental delay, and typical development. *American Journal on Intellectual and Developmental Disabilities, 116,* 142–152.

Sheldon, S. H., & Glaze, D. G. (2005). Sleep in neurologic disorders. In S. H. Sheldon, R. Ferber, & M. H. Kryger (Eds.), *Principles and Practice of Pediatric Sleep Medicine* (pp. 269–292). Philadelphia, PA: Elsevier Saunders.

Shete, M. M., Stocks, R. M. S., Sebelik, M. E., & Schoumacher, R. A. (2010). Effects of adeno-tonsillectomy on polysomnography patterns in Down syndrome children with obstructive sleep apnea: A comparative study with children without Down syndrome. *International Journal of Pediatric Otorhinolaryngology, 74,* 241–244.

Smith, A. C. M., Dykens, E., & Greenberg, F. (1998). Sleep disturbance in Smith-Magenis syndrome (del 17 p11.2). *American Journal of Medical Genetics (Neuropsychiatric Genetics), 81,* 186–191.

Souders, M. C., Mason, T. B. A., Valladares, O., Bucan, M., Levy, S. E., Mandell, D. S., et al. (2009). Sleep behaviors and sleep quality in children with autism spectrum disorder. *Sleep, 32,* 1566–1578.

Spruyt, K., & Gozal, D. (2011a). Development of pediatric sleep questionnaires as diagnostic or epidemiological tools: A brief review of Dos and Don'ts. *Sleep Medicine Reviews, 15,* 7–17.

Spruyt, K., & Gozal, D. (2011b). Pediatric sleep questionnaires as diagnostic or epidemiological tools: A review of currently available instruments. *Sleep Medicine Reviews, 15,* 19–32.

Stores, G. (1992). Annotation: Sleep studies in children with a mental handicap. *Journal of Child Psychology and Psychiatry, 33,* 1303–1317.

Stores, G. (2001). Aspects of sleep in other neurodevelopmental disorders. In G. Stores & L. Wiggs (Eds.), *Sleep Disturbances in Children and Adolescents with Disorders of Development: Its Significance and Management* (pp. 87–94). London, UK: McKeith Press.

Stores, R., Stores, G., & Buckley, S. (1996). The pattern of sleep problems in children with Down syndrome and other intellectual disabilities. *Journal of Applied Research in Intellectual Disabilities, 9,* 145–158.

Stores, R., Stores, G., Fellows, B., & Buckley, S. (1998). A factor analysis of sleep problems and their psychological associations in Down syndrome. *Journal of Applied Research in Intellectual Disabilities, 11,* 345–354.

Stores, R. (2001). Sleep and Down syndrome. In G. Stores & L. Wiggs (Eds.), *Sleep Disturbances in Children and Adolescents with Disorders of Development: Its Significance and Management* (pp. 53–59). London, UK: McKeith Press.

Stores, R., & Stores, G. (2004). Evaluation of brief group-administered instruction for parents to prevent or minimize sleep problems in young children with Down syndrome. *Journal of Applied Research in Intellectual Disabilities, 17,* 61–70.

Tani, P., Lindberg, N., Nieman-von Wendt, T., von Wendt, L., Alanko, L., Appelberg, B., & Porkka-Heiskanen, T. (2003). Insomnia is a frequent finding in adults with Asperger syndrome. *BMC Psychiatry, 3,*12..

Taylor, M. A., Schreck, K. A., & Mulick, J. A. (2012). Sleep disruption as a correlate to cognitive and adaptive behavior problems in autism spectrum disorders. *Research in Developmental Disabilities, 33,* 1408–1417.

Thackeray E., & Richdale, A. (2002). The behavioural treatment of sleep difficulties in children with an intellectual disability. *Behavior Interventions, 17,* 211–231

Tietze, A-L., Blankenburg, M., Hechler, T., Michel, E., Koh, M., Schlüter, B., & Zernikow, B. (2012). Sleep disturbances in children with multiple disabilities. *Sleep Medicine Reviews, 16*(2), 117–127.

Tikotzky L., & Sadeh, A. (2010). The role of cognitive-behavioral therapy in behavioral childhood insomnia. *Sleep Medicine, 11,* 686–691.

Tsai, F-J., Chiang, H-L., Lee, C-M., Gau, S. S-F., Lee, W-T., Fan, P-C., et al. (2012). Sleep problems in children with autism, attention-deficit hyperactivity disorder, and epilepsy. *Research in Autism Spectrum Disorders, 6,* 413–421.

van Steensel, F. J. A., Bögels, S. M., & Perrin, S. (2011). Anxiety disorders in children and adolescents with autistic spectrum disorders: A meta-analysis. *Clinical Child & Family Psychology Reviews, 14,* 302–317.

Verrillo, E., Bruni, O., Franco, P., Ferri, R., Gerard Thiriez, G., Pavone, M., et al. (2009). Analysis of NREM sleep in children with Prader–Willi syndrome and the effect of growth hormone treatment. *Sleep Medicine, 10,* 646–650.

Vriend, J. L., Corkum, P. V., Moon, E. C., & Smith, I. M. (2011). Behavioral interventions for sleep problems in children with autism spectrum disorders: current findings and future directions. *Journal of Pediatric Psychology, 36*(9), 1017–1029.

Walz, N., Beebe, D., & Byars, K. (2005). Sleep in individuals with Angelman syndrome: Parent perceptions of patterns and problems. *American Journal on Mental Retardation, 110,* 243–252.

Wasdell, M. B., Jan, J. E., Bomben, M. M., Freeman, R. D., Rietveld, W. J., Tai, J., et al. (2008). A randomized, placebo-controlled trial of controlled release melatonin treatment in delayed sleep phase syndrome and impaired sleep maintenance in children with neurodevelopmental disabilities. *Journal of Pineal Research, 44,* 57–64.

Weiskop S., Richdale, A., & Matthews, J. (2005). Treatment to reduce sleep problems in children with autism or Fragile X syndrome. *Developmental Medicine & Child Neurology, 47,* 94–104

Wiggs, L., & Stores, G. (1996a). Severe sleep disturbance and challenging daytime behaviour in children with severe learning disabilities. *Journal of Intellectual Disability Research, 40,* 518–528.

Wiggs, L., & Stores, G. (1996b). Sleep problems in children with severe intellectual disabilities: What help is being provided? *Journal of Applied Research in Intellectual Disabilities, 9,* 159–164.

Wiggs, L., & Stores, G. (1998). Factors affecting parental reports of the sleep patterns of children with severe learning disabilities. *British Journal of Health Psychology, 3,* 345–359.

Wiggs, L., & Stores, G. (1999). Behavioural treatment for sleep problems in children with severe learning disabilities and challenging daytime behaviour: Effect on daytime behaviour. *Journal of Child Psychology and Psychiatry, 40,* 627–635.

Wiggs, L., & Stores, G. (2004). Sleep patterns and sleep disorders in children with autistic spectrum disorders: Insights using parent report and actigraphy. *Developmental Medicine & Child Neurology, 46,* 372–380.

Williams, C. A. (2010). The behavioral phenotype of the Angelman syndrome. *American Journal of Medical Genetics Part C (Seminars in Medical Genetics), 154C,* 432–437.

Williams G., Sears, L., & Allard, A. M. (2006). Parent perceptions of efficacy for strategies used to facilitate sleep in

children with autism. *Journal of Developmental and Physical Disabilities, 18*, 25–33.
Wirojanan, J., Jacquemont, S., Diaz, R., Bacalman, S., Anders, T. F., Hagerman, R. J., & Goodlin-Jones, B. L. (2009). The efficacy of melatonin for sleep problems in children with autism, Fragile X syndrome, or autism and Fragile X syndrome. *Journal of Clinical Sleep Medicine, 5*, 145–150.
Young, D., Nagarajan, L., de Klerk, N., Jacoby, P., Ellaway, C., & Leonard, H. (2007). Sleep problems in Rett syndrome. *Brain & Development, 29*, 609–616.

CHAPTER

34

Sleep in the Context of ADHD: A Review of Reviews to Determine Implications for Research and Clinical Practice

Penny Corkum *and* J. Aimée Coulombe

Abstract

The relationship between sleep and ADHD is not well understood. To identify research and practice priorities, meta-analytic, systematic, and narrative reviews were examined. Consistent findings across meta-analyses and systematic reviews (Level 1) included a discrepancy between parent-reported sleep problems and those identified on objective measures, increased motor movements during sleep, the absence of an ADHD-specific sleep architecture profile, and the need to consider confounding variables (e.g., age, comorbidity). Findings with some consistency across reviews (Level 2) included negative effects of medication on sleep, increased daytime sleepiness, and higher, but nonpathological, increases in sleep apnea indices in children with ADHD. Narrative reviews give comparable emphasis to Level 1 and 2 findings, underplaying confounding or moderating variables. Given the results of our review, we believe that it is important to conceptualize ADHD as a chronic and pervasive disorder that affects children not only during the day but also during the night. That is, ADHD is a 24-hour disorder.

Key Words: ADHD, sleep, children, assessment, intervention

Introduction

Few topics in the pediatric sleep literature have received the level of interest as the questions of whether and how sleep and attention-deficit/hyperactivity disorder (ADHD) are related and the implications of this for clinical practice. Despite this focus and effort, an understanding of the relationship of sleep to ADHD remains elusive. The purpose of the present chapter is to review the existing literature on sleep in children with ADHD and provide an integrated method of assessing and addressing sleep problems in this population. First, we provide an overview of ADHD and its treatment. We then explore the research specific to sleep in children with ADHD. Given the large number of studies and reviews conducted in this area, we decided to conduct a *review of reviews*, comparing results presented in meta-analyses, qualitative systematic reviews, and narrative reviews. Our final section presents a discussion of clinical implications and recommendations for future directions. These recommendations include a call for future research to include large-scale studies that adequately address confounding variables, and increased involvement of psychologists and other behavioral specialists in the provision of sleep-related care for children with ADHD.

Attention-Deficit/Hyperactivity Disorder

ADHD is a common and complex neurobiological disorder occurring in approximately 5% of school-age children (Schachar, 2009). Males are diagnosed more frequently than females, with sex ratios ranging between 4:1 and 9:1, although these rates may be somewhat controversial given that there is some evidence that girls are underdiagnosed (Reid et al., 2000).

Diagnostic Criteria

According to DSM-IV TR (American Psychiatric Association [APA], 2000) criteria, a diagnosis of ADHD can be made when an individual *often* experiences six or more symptoms of inattention (ADHD-predominantly inattentive subtype; e.g., difficulty organizing tasks, easily distracted), six or more symptoms of hyperactivity/impulsivity (ADHD-predominantly hyperactive/impulsive subtype; e.g., fidgets), or six or more symptoms in both domains (ADHD-combined subtype). Symptoms must have persisted for at least 6 months, be maladaptive, and be inconsistent with developmental level. Although these symptoms are frequently the focus of research—where group membership is often based on questionnaire data that assesses symptoms only—their presence is only the first of five criteria that must be met for diagnosis. Evidence of symptoms *causing impairment* must have appeared before the age of 7 years (criterion B), impairment must be present in two or more settings (e.g., school and home; criterion C), and evidence of clinically significant impairment in social, academic, or occupational functioning—as a result of ADHD symptoms—must be clear (criterion D). ADHD-related impairments in children include difficulties interacting with parents, teachers, and peers; poor emotion regulation (Wehmeier, Schacht, & Barkley, 2010); difficulties in daily living and adaptive skills (Anastopoulos et al., 2011); and poor academic achievement (Daley & Birchwood, 2010). Sleep is also an area that might be impaired by ADHD and, as will be discussed, inadequate sleep may also contribute to many of the impairments just listed. Finally, to meet criterion E, ADHD symptoms should not occur exclusively during the course of a pervasive developmental disorder or psychotic disorder, or be better accounted for by another disorder. As effects of inadequate sleep may mimic symptoms and impairments often associated with ADHD, sleep disorders should always be included in the list of potential differential diagnoses (Corkum, Davidson, & Macpherson, 2011).

Heterogeneity, Comorbidity, and ADHD

A notable clinical and research challenge in the field of ADHD, relevant to understanding the association between sleep and ADHD, is the heterogeneity of its presentation. This is reflected in its current diagnostic criteria, which include the three recognized subtypes described above. Thus, it is important to consider that associations between sleep and ADHD may not be consistent across subtypes. This is an area requiring further research. Differences and fluctuations in the expression of ADHD symptoms across contexts, developmental periods, and between sexes also add to the complexity of understanding this disorder (see Barkley, 2003) and its association(s) with sleep. High rates of psychological comorbidity present a further challenge. Most children with ADHD have at least one comorbid psychological disorder (for review see Taurines, Schmitt, Renner, Conner, Warnke, & Romanos, 2010). In addition to sleep problems, the most common comorbidities associated with ADHD in children and adolescents are oppositional defiant disorder (ODD), conduct disorder (CD), anxiety and mood disorders, and learning disorders (see Gau, Shang, Soong, Wu, Lin, & Chiu, 2010; Schachar, 2009). Many of these disorders have themselves been associated with poor sleep (e.g., Alfano & Gamble, 2009). Associations between sleep and internalizing problems (e.g., anxiety, depression) are fairly well established (e.g., Lofthouse, Gilchrist, & Splaingard, 2009); however, relationships between sleep and externalizing problems (e.g., ODD, CD) have received much less research attention and require further investigation (Lindberg, Tani, Sailas, Virkkala, Urrila, & Virkkunen, 2008). As such, the potential influence of both comorbid internalizing and externalizing problems on sleep and ADHD should always be considered.

Etiology and Risk

The etiology of ADHD is complex, with multiple hypotheses proposed at the neurochemical, genetic, and cognitive levels (e.g., Schachar, 2009). Although the disorder is highly heritable, environmental factors also contribute to the development and manifestation of ADHD (e.g., parental psychopathology and distress, low parental involvement, family conflict; see Deault, 2010; Schachar, 2009). From a theoretical perspective, the cognitive-energetic model provides a relatively comprehensive explanation of ADHD (Sergeant, Geurts, Huijbregts, Scheres, & Oosterlaan, 2003), integrating deficits in top-down control (i.e., executive functions), specific cognitive processes, and state or energetic factors (i.e., effort, arousal, activation). This theory may be of particular relevance to researchers whose interests in sleep and ADHD include the effects of sleep deprivation on executive functions and cognitive, affective, and behavioral regulation (e.g., Corkum, Panton, Ironside, Macpherson, & Williams, 2008). The hypoarousal (Weinberg & Brumback, 1990) theory is also relevant to a discussion of sleep and ADHD.

This theory suggests that children with ADHD are hypoaroused, and hyperactive behaviors are manifestations of stimulus-seeking attempts to regulate arousal and stay alert. It is often presented as a rationale underlying the effectiveness of stimulant medication. Studies examining daytime sleepiness in children with ADHD draw upon this theory (e.g., Cortese, Faraone, Konofal, & Lecendreux, 2009).

Treatment of ADHD

Empirically supported treatments for ADHD include stimulant medications (Kaplan & Newcorn, 2011) and behavioral interventions (e.g., parent training, school-based interventions, peer interventions; Chronis, Jones, & Raggi, 2006). An important consideration in the use of medication is their perceived and documented side effects (Katragadda & Schubiner, 2007), particularly in regard to sleep (Corkum, Moldofsky, Hogg-Johnson, Humphries, & Tannock, 1999). Side effects include reductions in total sleep time and increased sleep onset latency (Corkum et al., 2008) and may be influenced by the timing of medication administration (Ironside, Davidson, & Corkum, 2010). Parent training, which teaches parents how to alter negative interactional patterns and child behavior by altering their parenting strategies, has demonstrated success in treating not only ADHD (Chronis et al., 2006; Eiraldi, Mautone, & Power, 2012), but also many of its comorbid psychopathologies (e.g., conduct problems and behavior problems; Dretzke et al., 2009). Parents are taught behavior modification techniques such as making changes to the environment to encourage positive child behavior (e.g., structure and routines), planned ignoring, and using rewards. Very similar behavioral techniques are employed in evidence-based sleep interventions (Vriend & Corkum, 2011). Once they have developed a working knowledge of sleep and its measurement, psychologists and clinicians who are comfortable with the behavioral treatment of ADHD should not have difficulty applying these concepts to improve their patients' sleep.

Review of the Literature on ADHD and Sleep

We conducted a review of the literature focusing on sleep problems in children with ADHD (but did not include the literature examining sleep disorders resulting in ADHD-like symptoms). Moreover, we did not provide a general overview of sleep, as this can be found in Section 1 of this book. Rather than reviewing individual research studies examining sleep in children with ADHD, we decided to conduct a *review of reviews*. This approach was taken because systematic reviews provide the highest level of evidence to direct clinical practice (Canadian Psychological Association, 2012). After an extensive literature search, we found eight systematic reviews (i.e., three quantitative and five qualitative). We then extracted relevant information from the systematic reviews. A narrative overview of these findings is provided below. (The systematic reviews are indicated by double asterisks in the reference list.)

In addition to reviewing the eight systematic reviews, we also thought it would be important to evaluate the existing narrative reviews, given that these types of reviews are often read by clinicians and as such may have a greater impact on clinical practice (Loke & Derry, 2003). After an extensive literature search we found 16 narrative reviews published in peer-reviewed journals. (The 16 narrative reviews are identified with a single asterisk in the reference list.) Each of the narrative reviews was first read by the authors of this chapter to ensure appropriateness of including the narrative review in the review of reviews. Next each narrative review was read by two university students in Dr. Corkum's research lab, who rated the article in terms of the main messages presented about the relationship between ADHD and sleep and the potential confounding variables. The students who reviewed the narrative reviews included both undergraduate and graduate students. The main findings are described below.

Systematic Reviews

Systematic reviews provide a summary of the research literature using an objective and transparent approach for research synthesis and can be divided into two broad categories: quantitative (i.e., meta-analyses) and qualitative. We located three quantitative and five qualitative reviews of ADHD and sleep. It is important to note that the authors of these reviews did not indicate if they had followed the reporting standards set forth by PRISMA (Preferred Reporting Items for Systematic Reviews and Meta-Analyses), or its predecessor QUOROM (Quality of Reporting of Meta-analyses), which outline the necessary components and content required for a systematic review. Therefore, the quality of these meta-analyses cannot be readily assessed. Across these eight systematic reviews, there were a total of 78 studies reviewed. No single study was included in all eight reviews. In fact, more than half of the studies (44 studies, 56%) were included in only one review, 18 (23%) in two reviews, 7 (9%) in three reviews, 4 (5%) in four reviews, 3 (4%) in five reviews and 2 (3%) in six reviews. This sets the stage for inconsistent findings across reviews.

QUANTITATIVE SYSTEMATIC REVIEWS (META-ANALYSES)

Meta-analyses use statistical approaches to combine data across a number of studies in order to determine which findings are consistent. Typically, the literature is thoroughly reviewed to find relevant research studies and then the methodological rigor of each study is evaluated. Only those studies considered to be high quality research are included in the analyses. Meta-analyses provide the highest level of research evidence (CPA, 2012). Three meta-analyses were found in our literature search (Cortese et al., 2009; Cortese, Konofal, Yateman, Mouren, & Lecendreux, 2006; Sadeh, Pergamin, & Bar-Haim, 2006).

An overview of the three meta-analyses can be found in Table 34.1. The first meta-analysis, conducted by Cortese and colleagues in 2006, consisted of a meta-analysis of objective measures and a qualitative analysis of subjective measures. The meta-analysis consisted of eight studies that used a range of objective measures, including PSG, actigraphy, and videosomnography. The analyses were collapsed across these different types of sleep assessment. As can be seen in Table 34.1, children with ADHD, relative to the control group, did not evidence any differences in their sleep architecture. However, children with ADHD did have more daytime sleepiness and higher mean values on a measure of sleep apnea. As well, more movements during sleep were noted, although this variable was not included in the actual meta-analyses. While these are interesting results, it is important to note that these findings were based on a small number of studies; for example, two studies addressing daytime sleepiness and three studies addressing sleep apnea. Moreover, the mean values for the sleep apnea variable were all in the nonpathological range and so while the mean apnea score for the ADHD groups were elevated relative to the normal controls, these were not indicative of clinical levels of sleep apnea.

Also published in 2006 was another meta-analysis of objective measures (Sadeh, Pergamin, & Bar-Haim, 2006). In this meta-analysis, Sadeh and colleagues included only PSG studies, but from a wider time frame relative to the meta-analysis by Cortese and colleagues et al. (2006). The selection criteria was also different in that Cortese and colleagues et al. (2006) controlled for some potential confounds by excluding studies from their analyses, whereas Sadeh and colleagues included all high quality studies but examined the moderating effects as part of their analyses. In total, Sadeh and colleagues included 12 samples of children with ADHD and normal controls. The only significant difference found between the ADHD and control groups was that the ADHD groups had higher rates of periodic limb movements. There were no differences in any other sleep variable, including sleep architecture.

Importantly, the analyses conducted by Sadeh et al. underscore the role of a number of important moderating variables (e.g., sex, age, comorbidities, sleep lab adjustment). For example, these authors found that although there was no overall difference between ADHD and normal control groups on sleep duration, there was in fact a difference if broken down by age (e.g., groups with younger children with ADHD had longer sleep durations and groups with older children with ADHD had shorter sleep durations compared to controls), sex (e.g., ADHD groups with just males had a greater effects than ADHD groups with both males and females), comorbidity (e.g., sleep onset latency was longer in groups of children with ADHD without comorbidities), and sleep lab adaptation night (e.g., when there was an adaptation night, the ADHD groups had longer sleep duration than control groups, but this was not the case when there was no adaptation night).

In 2009, Cortese and colleagues published an updated meta-analysis of findings from objective measures as well as conducted a meta-analysis of subjective measures. In regard to objective measures, 13 studies were analyzed, which included the eight studies from their 2006 paper (Cortese et al., 2006) along with four additional studies. Unlike their previous meta-analysis, Cortese et al., (2009) reported the analyses separately for PSG and actigraphy. The results of the meta-analysis of the PSG studies were similar to those in Cortese et al., (2006), in that the sleep apnea index and daytime sleepiness measure were both higher for ADHD groups than control groups. This is not surprising, as these results are based on the same studies as in the previous meta-analysis. Also similar to their previous results, it is reported that children with ADHD have more movements in sleep. Again, this was based on a qualitative review, as this variable was not included in their meta-analysis. The main differences in findings between the two meta-analyses conducted by Cortese and colleagues is that in

Table 34.1 Overview of key design criteria and findings of objective measures from the three meta-analyses

	Cortese, Faraone, Konofal, & Lecendreux, 2009	Sadeh, Pergamin, & Bar-Haim, 2006	Cortese, Konofal, Yateman, Mouren, & Lecendreux, 2006
Search criteria	Searched PubMed (1987–Nov 2008) using keywords. As well, searched references from obtained articles and references from known systematic reviews and meta-analyses for relevant studies. Also searched abstracts from relevant conference proceedings and contacted experts in the field to find relevant articles. Used, after confirming, articles utilized for their 2006 meta-analyses.	Searched PsycInfo, PubMed, and ISI Web of Science (Jan 1980–Oct 2005) using keywords and authors' names. As well, searched all references of the obtained articles and references of relevant review papers for relevant studies.	Searched PubMed (Jan 1987–Oct 2005) using keywords. References from relevant papers were reviewed to find any additional studies.
Selection criteria	Participants 18 yrs or under; DSM diagnosis of ADHD based on standardized criteria (DSM-III-R or later); inclusion of a control group; at least one subjective and one objective measure of sleep; study provided data conducive to a meta-analysis; only included studies that excluded comorbid psychiatric disorders that would have impact on sleep (e.g., anxiety, depression); excluded studies where participants were treated with medication; excluded studies that looked at specific populations (e.g., obese children).	Compared sleep parameters between an ADHD/ADD group and normal control group; ADHD group could not be first selected due to sleep problem; PSG recordings of relevant variables; study provided data needed to conduct meta-analysis.	Needed to have completed rigorous clinical interviews according to DSM-III-R or DSM-IV criteria; study had to exclude or control for psychiatric comorbidity and medication; no case reports or descriptive reports; studies that examined sleep in medicated participants were not included.
Final sample	16 samples from 16 journal articles – PSG (9 studies) – 271 ADHD, 200 NC – Actigraphy (4 studies) – 160 ADHD, 228 NC – Subjective (6 studies) – 404 ADHD, 372 NC 722 children with ADHD, 638 NC children Note: Meta-analysis of both objective and subjective measures was conducted by authors. Only the meta-analysis for objective measures is reported in this table.	12 samples from 11 journal articles 333 children with ADHD, 231 NC children Note: Meta-analysis of PSG studies only.	13 studies, both objective (8) and subjective (5), retained 280 children with ADHD, 228 NC children – 6 PSG (2 also had MLST, 1 also had video analyses) – 218 ADHD, 139 NC – 2 actigraphy – 62 ADHD, 89 NC Note: Subjective measures were not included in meta-analysis, but rather a qualitative review was conducted of these studies.

(*continued*)

Table 34.1 (Continued)

	Cortese, Faraone, Konofal, & Lecendreux, 2009		Sadeh, Pergamin, & Bar-Haim, 2006	Cortese, Konofal, Yateman, Mouren, & Lecendreux, 2006
RESULTS ON OBJECTIVE MEASURES				
	PSG/Video	**Actigraphy**	**PSG only**	**Mix of PSG, actigraphy, & video**
Sleep onset latency	ADHD=NC (n=7)	ADHD>NC (n=4)	NS (n=10)	ADHD=NC (n=6)
Total Sleep time (TST)	N/A	"True Sleep" ADHD<NC (n=3)	ADHD=NC (n=10)	N/A
Sleep efficiency	ADHD<NC (n=7)	ADHD=NC (n=3)	ADHD=NC (n=11)	ADHD=NC (n=6)
Night Wakings	N/A	ADHD=NC (n=3)		
PLM	N/A	N/A	ADHD>NC (n=7)	ADHD>NC (n=?)
Sleep Apnea (AHI)	ADHD>NC (n=3)	N/A	ADHD=NC (n=5)	ADHD>NC (n=3)
Arousals	N/A	N/A	ADHD=NC (n=6)	N/A
MSLT	ADHD<NC (n=2)	N/A	N/A	ADHD>NC (n=2)
# stage shifts in TST	ADHD=NC (n=3)	N/A	N/A	ADHD=NC (n=3)

# stage shifts/hr	ADHD>NC (n=2)	N/A	N/A	N/A
% stage 1	ADHD=NC (n=7)	N/A	ADHD=NC (n=8)	ADHD=NC (n=4)
% stage 2	ADHD=NC (n=7)	N/A	ADHD=NC (n=8)	ADHD=NC (n=4)
% SWS	ADHD=NC (n=7)	N/A	ADHD=NC (n=11)	ADHD=NC (n=4)
REM latency	ADHD=NC (n=6)	N/A	ADHD=NC (n=10)	ADHD=NC (n=4)
% REM	ADHD=NC (n=7)	N/A	ADHD=NC (n=11)	ADHD=NC (n=4)
MAIN FINDINGS				
	Children with ADHD have more sleep problems than controls based on most of the subjective measures and some objective measures. Hypothesized that sleep in children with ADHD was more fragmented, potentially as a result of abnormal movements.		Children with ADHD are more likely to have PLMS. No other variable was significantly different between ADHD and controls. Moderator analyses indicated the important role of confounding factors (e.g., age, sex, comorbidity).	Children with ADHD have more sleepiness during the day, more movements at night and increased AHI, but no differences in macro-architecture or continuity of sleep.

Notes: In the "Results on objective measures" section of the table: N/A=not assessed, ADHD>ND = ADHD displays more/longer of (sleep variable) than normal controls; ADHD<ND = ADHD displays less/shorter of (sleep variable) than normal controls; (n=X) = number of studies that examined the specific sleep variable.

the 2009 review they found that the ADHD group had poorer sleep efficiency (although this change from a nonsignificant to significant finding happened as the result of one additional study being added) and more stage shifts per hour (which was not examined in the earlier meta-analysis). Similar to Cortese et al., 2006, there were no differences in sleep architecture between the groups.

Interestingly, for some variables the findings from the meta-analysis of actigraphy variables were in contrast to the findings from PSG. Based on actigraphy, children with ADHD had longer sleep onset latency and shorter sleep duration but no difference in sleep efficiency and night wakings. This is in contrast to the PSG results, which found that children with ADHD had lower sleep efficiency and no difference in sleep onset latency. The reason for these contradicting findings is unknown; however, it may be that there were too few studies included in the meta-analyses (only 3–4 actigraphy studies depending on the variable assessed), or it may be that the validity of actigraphy relative to PSG is not as strong in children with ADHD as it has been shown to be in typically developing children.

Cortese and colleagues et al. (2009) conducted a separate meta-analysis of subjective measures, which included six studies. Based on this analysis, the ADHD groups were reported to have many more sleep problems compared to the normal control groups (i.e., more bedtime resistance, night wakings, and difficulties with morning awakenings, as well as longer sleep onset latency, increased daytime sleepiness, and higher rates of sleep apnea).

The only consistent findings across the three meta-analyses were that in comparison to normal controls, children with ADHD: *(1)* have higher rates on a wide range of parent-reported sleep problems, *(2)* evidence increased nocturnal movements, and *(3)* do not present with differences in sleep architecture. Although there were other significant findings in the two meta-analyses by Cortese (e.g., ADHD groups having lower sleep efficiency, higher mean sleep apnea index scores, and increased daytime sleepiness), these were not found in the meta-analysis by Sadeh and as such are not consistent across the meta-analytic reviews. It is also important to underscore that the authors of the three meta-analytic reviews all caution the reader that their results are tentative given the small number of samples included in the analyses and the high level of variability.

QUALITATIVE SYSTEMATIC REVIEWS

Qualitative systematic reviews apply similar review standards as meta-analytic reviews, but use qualitative methods (e.g., comparing and contrasting) rather than statistical approaches to determine which results are consistent across studies. An overview of the five qualitative reviews can be found in Table 34.2. In 1998, the first systematic review was conducted by Corkum and colleagues. This review included 16 peer-reviewed studies published after 1970 and used a box-score approach to examine findings across studies. The only consistent finding across studies was an increase in nocturnal movements in children with ADHD. Also, medication was found to negatively impact sleep. The review also highlighted the differences in findings between subjective and objective measures, with parents reporting many more sleep problems than what was confirmed based on objective measures. Moreover, this review underscored the important role of some potential confounding variables, such as ADHD diagnostic procedures and ADHD subtype, comorbidity, and treatment with stimulant medication.

Since this initial review, three other qualitative systematic reviews have been published, one in 2004 (Cohen-Zion & Ancoli-Israel), one in 2005 (Bullock & Schall), and most recently in 2011 (Jan, Yang, & Huang). These three reviews echo the conclusions reached by Corkum et al. (1998) and underscore the significant differences in rates of sleep problems based on parent-report compared to objective measures of sleep, as well as the findings of increased motor movements during sleep in children with ADHD. However, some differences in findings between these qualitative reviews are also evident. Cohen-Zion and Ancoli-Israel (2004) concluded that there was also evidence for reduced REM sleep and daytime sleepiness in children with ADHD. Bullock and Schall (2005) also report decreased REM as well as increased sleep latency. These authors, in contrast to Corkum et al. (1998), report that treatment with medication for ADHD (i.e., stimulant medications) does not affect objective measures of sleep. The most recent systematic review by Jan et al. (2011) concludes that although sleep problems and ADHD symptoms are often comorbid, there is little objective evidence for a unique pattern of sleep problems in medication-naïve children with ADHD.

The only other systematic review was one conducted by Cortese et al. in 2005, but this review was focused exclusively on restless leg syndrome. Samples ($n = 8$) from seven studies (one of which consisted of adult ADHD participants) were reviewed. The

Table 34.2 Overview of five qualitative systematic reviews

	Corkum et al., 1998	Cohen-Zion & Ancoli-Israel, 2004	Bullock & Schall, 2005	Jan et al., 2011	Cortese et al., 2005
Search criteria	Searched Medline using key words, cross-checked references of articles found	Searched Medline and PsycInfo, used keywords, cross-checked references in articles found	Searched National Library of Medicine and the Cochrane Library, used keywords	Searched PubMed; used keywords; cross-checked references in articles found, including existing review articles	Searched PubMed, used keywords, cross-checked references in articles found. Review focused on **RLS & ADHD only.**
Selection criteria	English; 1970 onward; peer-reviewed journals	English; Published between 1980 (DSM-III) and March 2004; participants ages 3–19; English; Articles were excluded if they were single case reports, descriptive reports with no statistical analyses of data, or open-label clinical trials. Studies excluded if comorbidity (except LD, ODD, CD). Studies excluded that did not follow a preset data collection protocol or in which sleep may have been artificially affected by external stimuli (e.g. auditory stimuli); Treatment studies were limited to those using stimulant medications.	English; published between 1999–June 2004; employed objective measures of sleep, alone or in combination with objective measures	Published between 1994–May 2011; case reports and descriptive reports without data analysis were excluded from the review	Up to Feb 2005, child and adult; studies excluded if no measure of RLS
Final sample	16 studies	47 studies – naturalistic studies with no planned intervention (n=34) and stimulant intervention studies (n=13); total of 1138 children with ADHD and 1133 controls were included. Note: 9 of these studies were counted twice, therefore, n=38.	10 articles which used objective measures (6 PSG, 2 actigraphy, 1 both, 1 video-recording and PSG; (16 studies met criteria but 6 of these included only subjective reports of sleep)	33 studies included in tables in the paper	8 samples in 7 studies; 1 adult study, remaining 7 studies included child participants

(*continued*)

Table 34.2 (Continued)

	Corkum et al., 1998	Cohen-Zion & Ancoli-Israel, 2004	Bullock & Schall, 2005	Jan et al., 2011	Cortese et al., 2005
MAIN FINDINGS					
	Although many parents-reported sleep problems, these were not verified on objective measures. The only consistent findings were that children with ADHD move more in their sleep and their sleep duration was not different than TD children. Stimulant medication led to some changes.	High rates of parental reports of sleep disturbances; majority not confirmed by objective data. Unmedicated children with ADHD demonstrated increased nighttime activity, decreased REM sleep, and increased daytime sleepiness in comparison to TD controls.	Parents report high levels of sleep difficulties that were not verified by PSG or actigraphy. It was concluded that while children with ADHD do show increased sleep latency and noctural activity, along with decreased REM sleep, initial evidence suggests that stimulant medication for ADHD does not have a significant impact on objective sleep characteristics.	Sleep problems and ADHD-related symptoms frequently co-occur; not much objective support for unique relationship of sleep and "pure unmedicated" ADHD.	Found an association between RLS and ADHD, with up to 44% of subjects with ADHD exhibiting RLS or RLS symptoms, and up to 26% of subjects with RLS exhibiting ADHD or ADHD symptoms.

Notes: (n=X) = number of studies that examined the specific sleep variable.

authors concluded that there was a link between RLS and ADHD, with up to 44% of participants with ADHD presenting with RLS or symptoms.

CONCLUSIONS FROM SYSTEMATIC REVIEWS

Our *review of reviews* was able to capture the consistent findings across eight systematic reviews, including three meta-analyses and five qualitative reviews. We grouped the findings into two levels: Level 1, where there is consistent evidence across all meta-analyses and qualitative systematic reviews; and Level 2, for which there is some evidence in at least one of the meta-analyses and in one or more of the qualitative systematic reviews.

Level 1: Findings that are consistent across systematic reviews

1. Parents of children with ADHD report many more sleep problems than what is verified based on objective measures.
2. Children with ADHD have abnormal levels of motor movements during the night.
3. There is no specific sleep architecture profile that is consistently found in children with ADHD.
4. There are many confounding variables that moderate the results of studies (e.g., sex, age, diagnostic procedures, ADHD subtype, comorbidity, treatment with medication, sleep lab adaptation differences).

Level 2: Findings with some consistency across reviews

1. Medication may result in some sleep problems, but the severity and chronicity of these problems is unknown.
2. Daytime sleepiness in children with ADHD compared to controls has been found, but there have only been two studies addressing this.
3. Sleep apnea index is higher in ADHD groups, but the elevation is not clinical. Moreover, the meta-analyses were inconsistent in their findings with this variable and only included a few well-designed studies addressing this variable.

Narrative Reviews

Narrative reviews are generally not as rigorous as systematic reviews, but rather provide a general summary of the relevant literature based on the author's perspective. There is usually no attempt to locate all relevant literature or to evaluate primary research studies for quality, but rather pivotal papers known to the authors are included in the review. Despite the fact that narrative reviews are not as scientifically rigorous as systematic reviews, these are often read by clinicians and as such may influence practice. We were interested in determining whether the information contained in the 16 narrative reviews that we found in peer-reviewed journals was consistent with the findings of the systematic reviews, as described above. (The 16 narrative reviews are identified with a single asterisk in the reference list.) Each of the 16 narrative review articles was read by two students familiar with the field of ADHD and sleep, but not experts in this field. After reading each article, these individuals completed a survey about the narrative review. The survey included two primary questions—the first focused on the main messages put forth in the paper in terms of the relationship between ADHD and sleep, and the second question focused on the emphasis the authors placed on the role of potential moderators of this relationship.

In terms of main messages of these reviews (see Table 34.3), students rated ten statements about sleep in children with ADHD using a four-point Likert scale. A low score indicated that the students believed that the authors of the reviews presented the variable as having strong research evidence, whereas a high score indicated that the authors presented the variable as having limited evidence (i.e., based on speculation). As can be seen by examining Table 34.3, no variable was rated as being presented as a confirmed fact, which is appropriate given the current state of the literature. The variable that was rated as being the most factual (i.e., parents of children with ADHD report that their children have many sleep problems compared to parents of typically developing children) was appropriate given that this statement would be considered a Level 1 finding based on the systematic reviews. However, the variable rated second as the most factual was daytime sleepiness in children with ADHD, which is considered a Level 2 finding. Importantly, the variable considered to have the least evidence (i.e., children with ADHD have different sleep architecture) was consistent with a Level 1 finding from the systematic reviews. Based on the students' ratings, it would seem that both Level 1 and Level 2 findings are being given equal weighting in terms of significance across the narrative reviews. As such, there were some variables that were under-endorsed (i.e., the relationship between ADHD and PLM/restless legs/nocturnal movements; the discrepancy between subjective and objective measures in terms of identifying sleep problems in children with ADHD) and some variables that were over-endorsed

Table 34.3 *Student Ratings of Narrative Reviews in terms of their Impressions of the Evidence for Ten Potential Findings related to ADHD and Sleep*

Question	Mean Rating	Ranking
1. For a significant number of children, ADHD might be caused by sleep apnea	2.83	8
2. For a significant number of children, ADHD might be caused by periodic limb movement disorder and/or restless leg syndrome	2.54	6
3. For a significant number of children, ADHD might be caused by another intrinsic sleep disorder (e.g., narcolepsy)	2.84	9
4. Children with ADHD have different sleep architecture (i.e., REM/NREM) than typically developing children	3.11	10
5. The parents of children with ADHD report that their children have lots of sleep problems (e.g., bedtime resistance, sleep onset, night wakings, trouble waking in the morning, poor sleep efficiency) in comparison to typically developing children	1.58	1
6. Objective measures of sleep (such as actigraphy and polysomnography) demonstrate that children with ADHD have lots of sleep problems (e.g., bedtime resistance, sleep onset, night wakings, trouble waking in the morning, poor sleep efficiency) in comparison to typically developing children	2.54	7
7. Daytime sleepiness is a problem for children with ADHD	1.84	2
8. Children with ADHD move more during the night	2.03	3
9. Medication for ADHD often causes sleep problems	2.31	4
10. Sleep duration is different in children with ADHD	2.47	5

Note. Mean Rating based on the following rating scale: 1. This finding was clear and presented as a fact. Based on the author(s) statements, it would appear that the evidence for this finding must be very good; 2. This finding was presented as a fact, with some potential limitations in interpretation. It would appear that the evidence for this finding must be good; 3. This finding was presented as a potential finding that required more research. It appeared that there was some evidence, but not enough to draw any conclusions; 4. This finding was presented as a speculation. It would appear that there is limited research to draw any conclusions. Rank: Each statement was given a ranking, with the statement that was thought to have the most evidence ranked as "1" and each following rank was given to the next closest number down to a rank of 10 which indicated the least evidence for the statement.

(e.g., objective measures demonstrating sleep problems in children with ADHD).

Students also rated 12 potential confounding variables as to the importance they believed that the author inferred to each variable in understanding and evaluating the literature on sleep in ADHD (see Table 34.4). It is important to note that our student reviewers indicated that some of the potential confounding variables were rarely discussed in the reviews (i.e., where the research participants were recruited from [e.g., sleep clinic, ADHD clinic], child's age, sex, and ADHD subtype). Unfortunately, many of the variables rarely discussed in the narratives are the variables known to have a significant impact based on the meta-analyses by Sadeh and colleagues et al (2006). Based on the students' mean ratings, the majority of variables identified in previous research as potential confounds were presented by the authors as important to consider when interpreting the results of research in this field. The two highest rated variables were the diagnostic procedures used to identify children for the ADHD group and the comorbidities associated with ADHD, both which have been underscored as important in the systematic reviews.

CONCLUSIONS FROM NARRATIVE REVIEWS

Narrative reviews in this field appear to be giving significance to both Level 1 and 2 findings. This is concerning, as these reviews may be underemphasizing Level 1 findings that have been consistently found through systematic reviews and overemphasizing Level 2 findings that have not been consistently found. Moreover, some of the key confounding variables are often not noted in the narrative reviews. It is important to underscore that the students' ratings

Table 34.4 *Student Ratings of Narrative Reviews in terms of their Impressions of the Relevance of Twelve Potential Confounding Variables*

Variable	Number of Studies Noting Variable	Mean Rating
1. Recruitment sources for participants	3	2.13
2. Diagnostic procedures used to determine ADHD	12	1.94
3. Comorbidities related to ADHD	14	1.68
4. Using polysomnography to measure sleep	15	1.99
5. Using actigraphy to measure sleep	14	2.33
6. Using questionnaires completed by parents to measure children's sleep	15	2.39
7. Using questionnaires completed by the child to measure his/her sleep	10	2.41
8. Using sleep diaries as a way of measuring sleep	10	2.38
9. Whether the child was on medication or not	13	2.04
10. Child age	6	2.97
11. Child sex	4	3.00
12. Possible differences associated with ADHD sub-type	7	2.22

Note. Ratings based on the following scale: 1. This variable was mentioned as **one of the most important** variables to consider when evaluating the research on sleep in ADHD; 2. This variable was mentioned as an **important** variable to consider when evaluating the research on sleep in ADHD; 3. This variable was **mentioned but no importance was given** in terms of relevance to understanding sleep in children with ADHD; 4. This variable was **mentioned but presented as not relevant** in terms of understanding sleep in children with ADHD

were across narrative reviews, and therefore some reviews may be presenting information very accurately while others may not be as accurate.

Conclusions from the Review of Reviews

There is no doubt that parents report frequent and pervasive sleep problems in their children with ADHD. Despite this high rate of parent-reported sleep problems, verification of these sleep problems on objective measures of sleep has not been consistently documented. In fact, the only consistent finding across all systematic reviews is that children with ADHD not only move more during the day but also move more during the night. This highlights the importance of viewing ADHD as a chronic and pervasive disorder that affects children not only during the day but also during the night. The significance of this increase in nocturnal movements has not been determined. It may be that these nocturnal movements disrupt sleep, which in turn reduces overall sleep quality. This could result in increased daytime impairment, thus exacerbating existing ADHD core and associated symptoms.

Given that there is no convincing evidence for a unique and specific sleep profile for children with ADHD, it is important to conceptualize sleep problems/disorders as one would conceptualize any other potential differential or comorbid disorder. Therefore, the full range of sleep problems and sleep disorders should be included in the differential diagnosis related to ADHD and should be considered as potential comorbid disorders. Clinicians can use the results of the ADHD and sleep literature to guide their assessment and treatment practices.

Clinical Implications

We believe that, with some increased knowledge of sleep and sleep measurement, psychologists and other behavioral clinicians who work with children with ADHD should have no difficulty addressing many of the sleep-related service needs of their patients (see Chapter 19, this volume). In fact, where sleep problems are behavioral in nature it may be preferable for a single clinician (or clinical team) to provide services addressing children's daytime and nighttime difficulties (vs. referral to a separate clinician or clinical team)[1]. This should increase efficiencies at multiple levels of service delivery, as there is likely substantial overlap between the factors associated with the maintenance and treatment of sleep problems and those associated with the maintenance and treatment of ADHD at the individual and family level (e.g., temperament, parenting, influence of comorbidity). In this section, we focus on the development of diagnostic and clinical formulations and treatment plans that integrate ADHD and sleep.

Screening, Assessment, and Diagnostic and Clinical Formulation

The diagnostic approach should begin with screening for the primary disorder(s) of interest (i.e., ADHD) and other problems that present with it or contribute to a differential diagnosis (i.e., sleep problems, internalizing and externalizing problems), followed by in-depth assessment as indicated by the results of the screener.

SCREENING

All children with ADHD or suspected of having ADHD should be screened for sleep problems (see Spruyt, Chapter 18). An example of a popular screening measure is described in Owens and Dalzell (2005). Clinicians who suspect that a child might have an organic sleep problem (e.g., snoring/apnea, restless legs/periodic limb movements) should arrange for further investigation. Where available, referral should be made to a pediatric sleep clinic with access to PSG technology. Similarly, clinicians who believe that sleep problems may be related to an underlying medical condition (e.g., asthma, epilepsy, pain) should also make a referral to a health professional who can assess and treat the underlying condition. Psychologists and other behavioral clinicians who suspect that a child might have a behavioral insomnia,[2] however, will have many of the core competencies to permit further assessment (e.g., skill at integrating multiple sources of information, interviewing). The competencies that they may not possess as part of traditional clinical training are most likely knowledge-based (i.e., knowledge of sleep processes) rather than skill-based and as such can be easily acquired.

ASSESSMENT

If screening provides evidence of behavioral sleep problems, further evaluation can be conducted using questionnaires, sleep diaries, and video recordings. Assessment should include information about sleep history, sleep problems, sleep quality, sleep beliefs and knowledge, and sleep hygiene and routines. Video recordings can assist with the evaluation of behaviors that occur outside of parents' awareness or exist within the context of parent–child interactions and can be useful in the identification of environmental factors contributing to children's sleep problems (e.g., pets, noise, light, media). Clinical interviews can provide further clarification about the information contained in subjective measures and behaviors observed in the videos (e.g., underlying cognitions, motivations, history, patterns). Sleep diaries, which can be used to document how often and when target behaviors occur, are particularly useful for treatment planning and tracking treatment progress. For a thoughtful discussion and review of pediatric sleep questionnaires (see Spruyt, Chapter 18), clinicians may refer to Lewandowski, Toliver-Sokol, and Palermo (2011). For a measure of parents' sleep-related knowledge, clinicians may wish to read Owens and Jones (2011). Measures of parents' beliefs about sleep (Bessey, Coulombe, Smith, & Corkum, 2013) and about sleep strategies (e.g., Coulombe & Reid, 2012) have also recently been developed.

DIAGNOSTIC AND CLINICAL FORMULATIONS

At the end of the information-gathering process, the clinician should have enough data for a diagnostic formulation related to sleep and ADHD. There are many formulations possible, including but not limited to the following: (a) ADHD, no sleep problems; (b) sleep problems, no ADHD; (c) ADHD and sleep problems; (d) ADHD, sleep problems, and comorbid psychopathology. For the remainder of this chapter we will assume that either scenario C or D is true. The clinician should also be able to describe a typical day and night for the child and his or her family, as well as a typical week. This description will serve as the foundation for an integrated clinical formulation. The primary objective of the clinical formulation is to better understand the nature of the sleep difficulty experienced within the context of the child (e.g., temperament, psychological comorbidity), his or her ADHD, and the family environment over the full 24-hour period. This would include consideration of how sleep problems and symptoms of ADHD may overlap and interact, including the role that sleep problems may play in further impairing the functioning of children with ADHD. Experimental restriction of sleep in children and adolescents without ADHD has been found to result in poorer performance on tasks related to attention, learning, memory, executive function, and emotion regulation (e.g., Fallone, Acebo, Seifer, & Carskadon,

2005; Gruber, Wiebe, Montecalvo, Brunetti, Amsel, & Carrier, 2011; Kopasz, Loessl, Hornyak, Riemann, Nissen, Piosczyk, & Voderholzer, 2010; Vriend, Davidson, Corkum, Rusak, McLaughlin, & Chambers, 2012).[3] Given the impact of inadequate sleep on healthy children, it is likely that inadequate sleep may increase the impairment experienced by children with ADHD.

The role of ADHD medication in the development or exacerbation of sleep problems should also be considered, as should any overlap between sleep problems, ADHD, and symptoms of comorbid psychopathology. A child with ADHD who experiences difficulty falling asleep at night due to worries associated with comorbid anxiety, for example, may require a different treatment approach than a child with ADHD who has difficulty falling asleep at night due to restlessness, or a child with ADHD whose refusal to go to bed is consistent with oppositional behavior. Further, because parental reports of sleep problems in children with ADHD are often higher than sleep problems measured using objective measures, efforts should be made to identify factors that could contribute to parents' increased perceptions of their child's sleep as problematic (e.g., parenting stress, fatigue). Clinicians who are familiar with the child and family may have already built a significant portion of their clinical formulation through the process of completing an existing ADHD assessment. One way of integrating sleep problems into an existing clinical formulation may be to ask, "What might this child's symptoms look like at bedtime, through the night, and in the morning?"

Treatment

Medication is generally not recommended as a first line of intervention for behavioral sleep problems in children (for discussion of pharmacotherapy, see Mindell et al., 2006). Behavioral interventions are highly effective in treating behavioral sleep problems in typically developing children (Meltzer, 2010; Vriend & Corkum, 2011)[4] and may be effective in treating behavioral sleep problems in children with ADHD (Mullane & Corkum, 2006). Some modifications, however, are advisable.

At the core of behavioral sleep interventions is the principle that healthy sleep is a behavior that must be learned. This is achieved in several steps, each of which is consistent with the behavioral techniques used in psychosocial interventions for ADHD and its psychological comorbidities. There are a number of excellent resources describing these techniques in more detail (e.g., Meltzer, 2010; Vriend & Corkum, 2011; Weiss, 2006). To illustrate how they can be integrated into ADHD treatment, we will group the strategies according to the following levels: (a) psychoeducation, (b) providing an environment that fosters success, (c) using behavioral contingencies, and (d) teaching coping skills. Additional information about modifying evidence-based sleep interventions for children with ADHD can be found in Corkum et al. (2011).

PSYCHOEDUCATION

It is likely that parents' sleep-related knowledge influences their sleep-related beliefs, strategies, and, as a result, children's sleep (Coulombe, Corkum, Reid, & Bessey, 2012; Owens & Jones, 2011; see Chapter 39, this volume). Providing parents with psychoeducation about sleep is an important component of behavioral sleep interventions (Vriend & Corkum, 2011). Psychoeducation is also routinely provided to parents as a component of effective interventions for ADHD in children (Young & Amarasinghe, 2010). Psychoeducation provided to parents of children with ADHD and sleep problems should be integrative and include a discussion of potential relationships between sleep and ADHD, potential effects of ADHD medication on sleep, and the role that treating sleep problems may play in improving children's overall functioning. Parents should be informed about what to expect during treatment, including discussion of the additional effort required when making changes to children's sleep, the typical response burst that can be expected prior to extinction of maladaptive sleep behaviors, and how symptoms of ADHD and comorbid psychopathologies may be exacerbated during the initial treatment period. Psychologists and other behavioral clinicians with cognitive and affective training (e.g., motivational interviewing, behavior change) will also be able to help parents identify any beliefs or concerns that may interfere with treatment. For example, parents of children with ADHD have been found to hold stronger beliefs that their children's sleep problems are less modifiable, more intrinsically driven, and less responsive to treatment than parents of typically developing children (Bessey et al., 2013); these beliefs may make parents less likely to see a role for behavioral sleep interventions in their child's treatment plan. Research does suggest, however, that behavioral sleep interventions can work for children with ADHD (Mullane & Corkum, 2006; Sciberras, Fulton, Efron, Oberklaid & Hiscock, 2012).

PROVIDING AN ENVIRONMENT THAT FOSTERS SUCCESS

Evidence-based psychosocial interventions for ADHD often require changes to the home and school environment that facilitate the child's ability to regulate his or her behavior (e.g., Eiraldi et al., 2012). Examples include designating separate areas within the child's home for play and for work; routines; and the consistent use of techniques such as leaving time for transitions, giving short and direct instructions when making requests, and using "when-then" statements. Sleep hygiene, a core component of evidence-based sleep interventions, can be easily integrated with daytime modifications to the environment. The "ABCs of SLEEPING"[5] can be used to remember key sleep hygiene principles: (1) ***A***ge appropriate ***B***edtimes and wake-times with ***C***onsistency, (2) ***S***chedule (including meal times) and routines, (3) ***L***ocation (dark, quiet room; comfortable bed; consistent location), (4) ***E***xercise (regular exercise, nothing too exciting close to bed) and diet (no caffeine, no big meals before bed), (5) no ***E***lectronics in the bedroom or before bed, (6) ***P***ositivity and relaxation (positive time together during the day, positive and relaxing routines at bedtime), (7) ***I***ndependence when falling asleep (after a relaxing routine and pleasant goodnight), (8) ***N***eeds of child met during the day (e.g., affection, attention, activity), and (9) all together equals ***G***reat sleep!

Parents should be encouraged to use the same principles to help children learn bedtime and morning routines that they use to help them learn and adhere to daytime routines (e.g., visual reminders). Further, routines should follow a logical, goal-oriented sequence that minimizes distractions and opportunities to get "off track"; this can be particularly important for children with ADHD, who can be particularly vulnerable to distraction. For example, a bedtime routine should move closer to the child's bedroom with each step. A notable challenge for some families, particularly those with comorbid externalizing problems, may be maintaining a positive and relaxing tone to bedtime routines; this is critical, however, to helping a child settle to sleep. Similarly, children should not be sent to bed or to their bedroom as a punishment; nor should children who become frustrated with academic challenges be expected to complete homework in their bedrooms or immediately before bed.

Children who continue to have difficulty settling to sleep at night, after sleep hygiene and consistent routines have been applied, may benefit from bedtime fading (Meltzer, 2010). In this strategy, a child's bedtime is moved closer to the time that he or she typically falls asleep, reducing prolonged time in bed before sleep onset and providing less opportunity for bedtime struggles. A consistent wake time is maintained to ensure, in part, that the child is sufficiently tired at night to fall asleep quickly; napping is discouraged unless age-appropriate. Once the child is falling asleep with less difficulty, the bedtime is moved earlier by 15 minutes every 2 to 3 nights, until the child is settling easily at the target bedtime. There are several factors to consider. First, this technique is partially dependent on temporary sleep deprivation. Given the effects of sleep deprivation on children's functioning, parents of children with ADHD should be prepared to expect some additional daytime challenges during the course of the protocol. Parents should also be careful to ensure that children do not engage in sleep-interfering behaviors prior to the later bedtime (e.g., watching television or playing video games, engaging in rough or exciting play), thereby circumventing treatment mechanisms. Further, clinicians will need to work closely with parents to ensure that the later bedtime is not reinforcing for the child. This said, it should be noted that bedtime fading was included as a key component in one of the only published intervention studies of sleep problems in children with ADHD (Mullane & Corkum, 2006). A clinically significant decrease in insomnia severity was reported in this study.

USING BEHAVIORAL CONTINGENCIES

Behavioral contingencies (i.e., planned ignoring, rewards) are at the core of behavioral interventions for sleep (see Meltzer, 2010) and for ADHD (see Young & Amarasinghe, 2010; see Blampied, Chapter 15). When applied at night, and in response to sleep-interfering behaviors (e.g., calling out, leaving the bedroom), planned ignoring is known as *limit setting* or *extinction* (see Meltzer, 2010). After the bedtime routine has been completed, parents should say goodnight to their child and minimize further interactions. Permissible interactions include simple and non-reinforcing reminders of what is expected (e.g., walking a child back to his or her room, reminding him or her that it is time to sleep). Parents should avoid arguments or explanations. Children with ADHD who leave the room frequently or who make multiple requests may benefit from a concrete reminder about what is appropriate (e.g., a "bedtime pass" that allows one glass of water or trip to the bathroom; Moore, Friman, Fruzzetti, & MacAleese, 2007). Careful attention to sleep hygiene, such as taking electronic devices out of the bedroom, may minimize the opportunities for children to engage in inappropriate behaviors at night. Rewards for appropriate sleep-facilitating behaviors (e.g., staying in bed, not calling out, lying in bed with eyes closed) should also be used. A detailed discussion of the development of reward systems is beyond the scope of this chapter; however, Meltzer (2010) provides an excellent overview of the use of rewards in the treatment of behavioral sleep problems. Psychologists and other behavioral clinicians working with children with ADHD should be well-versed in the successful use of rewards in this population and, with professional guidance, parents who are already using rewards as part of a behavioral program during the day should have little difficulty applying similar principles to encourage sleep-promoting behaviors at night. A recent meta-analysis of nonpharmacological interventions for children with ADHD (Hodgson, Hutchinson, & Denson, 2012) found behavior modification techniques to be effective across a range of functional domains; unfortunately, sleep and sleep behaviors were not examined as outcomes in this study.

TEACHING COPING SKILLS

Although pediatric sleep interventions do not usually include the use of coping skills (e.g., relaxation, cognitive restructuring, emotional regulation), these skills are often components of other psychosocial interventions for children (e.g., Simpson, Suarez, & Connolly, 2012) as well as behavioral interventions for insomnia in adults (Taylor & Roane, 2010). They have also been successfully included in interventions for children with ADHD (e.g., Waxmonsky et al., 2012; Webster-Stratton, Reid, & Beauchaine, 2011). Clinicians who are working with children with ADHD, particularly those with comorbid psychopathology, may wish to help their patients apply these strategies to their sleep problems. For example, school-age children with anxiety may benefit from opportunities to discuss and address daytime worries as well as maladaptive cognitions about sleep before they begin their bedtime routine. Many children will dislike some of the sleep hygiene principles (e.g., removal of electronic devices from the bedroom) and changes to bedtime routines (e.g., independent settling) required to ensure healthy sleep; the use of coping skills may assist parents and children with these changes.

Conclusion

The exact nature of the relationship between ADHD and sleep has continued to elude us, even after more than a decade of fairly intensive investigation into this area. At this point in time, there is no convincing evidence for a unique and specific sleep profile for children with ADHD. However, parents of children with ADHD report significant sleep problems in their children and objective measures provide consistent evidence of increased movement during the night. It is likely that the behaviors and processes underlying the daytime challenges experienced by children with ADHD present comparable challenges at night. As such, we believe that it is important to conceptualize ADHD as a chronic and pervasive disorder that affects children not only during the day but also during the night (i.e., ADHD is a 24-hour disorder). Therefore, sleep problems/disorders should be conceptualized similarly to other potential differential or comorbid disorders. The full range of sleep problems and sleep disorders should be included in the differential diagnosis related to ADHD as well as be considered as potential comorbid disorders. Sleep problems/disorders should be integrated into the treatment plan for ADHD. Psychologists and other behavior specialists are in a perfect position to treat sleep problems in children with ADHD, given their expertise in the area of behavioral interventions. Opportunities to enhance knowledge of sleep and sleep problems would allow more psychologists to treat ADHD as a disorder that results in impairments not only during the daytime but also at nighttime.

Future Directions

Additional research needs to be conducted in order to better understand the relationship between ADHD and sleep; however, it is important that future research moves the field ahead rather than continuing to conduct studies that have similar limitations in terms of methodology. To this end, we recommend that upcoming research include the following:

- Large-scale studies powered and designed to statistically address potentially confounding and moderating variables (e.g., can test the role of each confounding variable in this relationship, such as sex differences, subtypes of ADHD, and comorbidities).
- Studies that have strong methodology and controls for confounding variables (e.g., samples with narrower age ranges, more closely age- and sex-matched samples, rigorous diagnostic procedures for ADHD, gold standard sleep assessment procedures such as inclusion of an adaptation night when using PSG).

• Studies that examine why different results are found with different sleep measures (i.e., PSG, actigraphy, sleep diaries, parent questionnaires).

• Experimental studies that manipulate sleep to determine the impact on children with ADHD. This would include treatment intervention studies that target sleep and evaluate the outcome in regard to sleep and daytime functioning.

Clinically, it is important that psychologists and other behavioral specialists learn more about sleep problems and sleep disorders and include sleep in their assessment and treatment plans for children with ADHD. To this end, we recommend the following practices:

• All children being assessed for ADHD should also be screened for sleep problems/disorders.

• ADHD be conceptualized as a 24-hour disorder and that sleep as well as daytime behaviors be taken into consideration when conducting an assessment and developing and implementing treatment plans.

• Training programs for psychologists and other behavioral specialists include curriculum and practicum experiences in order to build knowledge and skills in the area of sleep. This training will allow the practitioner to address sleep problems across a range of mental health and physical health problems.

• Intervention research should focus on the impact of psychological comorbidity on treatment of sleep problems in children with ADHD, as well as determine what order treatments should be delivered in; for example, should sleep problems be addressed first?

• There is a paucity of research regarding sleep in children with behavioral problems (i.e., Conduct Disorder, Oppositional Defiant Disorder). Further research is needed, and these studies should be designed to avoid the problems that have been identified in the ADHD and sleep literature, as noted above.

Notes

1. Given the limited access to behavioral sleep specialists and clinics, the most realistic scenario is not a choice between (a) "treat both ADHD and sleep in this clinic" or (b) "treat ADHD in this clinic and have sleep treated by a behavioral sleep specialist," but rather a choice between (a) and not having a child's sleep addressed at all.
2. In some cases, parasomnias (e.g., nightmares, night terrors, sleepwalking) might also be addressed without immediate referral to specialty clinics. These problems are beyond the scope of this chapter but may be ameliorated with basic/foundational interventions (e.g., sleep hygiene) and the reduction of anxiety and stress. Video recording and diaries are very helpful in their assessment.
3. Notably, experimental sleep restriction in children has not been consistently observed to result in symptoms of hyperactivity/impulsivity (Fallone et al., 2005; Poirer, Gendron, & Corkum, 2012).
4. The most common sleep problems experienced by children are behavioral in nature. Given that this type of sleep problem can be addressed effectively in non–sleep specialty settings, we will restrict our discussion of treatment to these problems.
5. The "ABCs of SLEEPING" mnemonic was created by Ms. Melissa Gendron, MSc. Project Coordinator, Corkum LABS, Dalhousie University.

References

Alfano, C.A., & Gamble, A.L. (2009). The role of sleep in childhood psychiatric disorders. *Child Youth Care Forum, 38*, 327–340.

American Psychiatric Association. (2000). *Diagnostic and Statistical Manual of Mental Disorders.* (4th ed., Text Revision). Washington, DC: Author.

Anastopoulos, A. D., Smith, T. F., Garrett, M. E., Morrissey-Kane, E., Schatz, N. K., Sommer, J. L., et al. (2011). Self-regulation of emotion, functional impairment, and comorbidity among children with AD/HD. *Journal of Attention Disorders, 15*(7), 583–592.

Archbold, K. (2006). Sleep disorders and attention-deficit hyperactivity disorder in children: A missing differential diagnosis. *Journal of the American Psychiatric Nurses Association, 12*(4), 216–224.

Ball, J. D., & Koloian, B. (1995). Sleep patterns among ADHD children. *Clinical Psychology Review, 15*(7), 681–691.

Barkley, R.A. (2003). Issues in the diagnosis of attention-deficit/hyperactivity disorder in children. *Brain & Development, 25*, 77–83.

Bessey, M., Coulombe, A., Smith, I. & Corkum, P. (2013). Assessing parental sleep attitudes and beliefs in typically developing children and children with ADHD and ASD. *Children's Health Care. 42*(2), 116–133.

Bullock, G. L., & Schall, U. (2005). Dyssomnia in children diagnosed with attention deficit hyperactivity disorder: A critical review. *Australian and New Zealand Journal of Psychiatry, 39*(5), 373–377.

Canadian Psychological Association, Task Force on Evidence-Based Practice. (2012). *Report of the CPA Task Force on the Definition of Evidence-Based Practice of Psychological Treatment.* Retrieved April 3, 2012, from: http://www.cpa.ca/docs/file/Science/CPA_Definition_of_Evidence-Based_Practice_of_Psychological_Treatments.pdf.

Chronis, A. M., Jones, H. A., & Raggi, V. L. (2006). Evidence-based psychosocial treatments for children and adolescents with attention-deficit/hyperactivity disorder. *Clinical Psychology Review, 26*(4), 486–502.

Cohen-Zion, M. & Ancoli-Israel, S. (2004). Sleep in children with attention-deficit hyperactivity disorder (ADHD): A review of naturalistic and stimulant intervention studies. *Sleep Medicine Reviews, 8*(5), 379–402.

Corkum, P., Tannock, R. & Moldofsky, H. (1998). Sleep disturbances in children with attention-deficit/hyperactivity disorder. *Journal of the American Academy of Child & Adolescent Psychiatry, 37*(6), 637–646.

Corkum, P., Moldofsky, H., Hogg-Johnson, S., Humphries, T., & Tannock, R. (1999). Sleep problems in children with attention-deficit/hyperactivity disorder: Impact of subtype, comorbidity, and stimulant medication. *Journal of the American Academy of Child and Adolescent Psychiatry, 38*(10), 1285–1293.

Corkum, P., Panton, R., Ironside, S., Macpherson, M., & Williams, T. (2008). Acute impact of immediate release methylphenidate administered three times a day on sleep in children with attention-deficit/hyperactivity disorder. *Journal of Pediatric Psychology, 33*(4), 368–379.

Corkum, P., Davidson, F., & Macpherson, M. (2011). A framework for the assessment and treatment of sleep problems in children with attention-deficit/hyperactivity disorder. *Pediatric Clinics of North America, 58*(3), 667–683.

Cortese, S., Konofal, E., Lecendreux, M., Arnulf, I., Mouren, M., Darra, F., & Dalla Bernardina, B. (2005). Restless legs syndrome and attention-deficit/hyperactivity disorder: A review of the literature. *Sleep: Journal of Sleep and Sleep Disorders Research, 28*(8), 1007–1013.

Cortese, S., Konofal, E., Yateman, N., Mouren, M., & Lecendreux, M. (2006). Sleep and alertness in children with attention-deficit/hyperactivity disorder: A systematic review of the literature. *Sleep: Journal of Sleep and Sleep Disorders Research, 29*(4), 504–511.

Cortese, S., Faraone, S. V., Konofal, E., & Lecendreux, M. (2009). Sleep in children with attention-deficit/hyperactivity disorder: Meta-analysis of subjective and objective studies. *Journal of the American Academy of Child & Adolescent Psychiatry, 48*(9), 894–908.

Coulombe, J. A., Corkum, P., Reid, G. J., & Bessey, M. (June, 2012). *A theoretical model of parental cognitions and children's sleep.* Poster presented at SLEEP 2012, the 26th Annual Meeting of the Associated Professional Sleep Societies (APSS), Boston, MA.

Coulombe, J. A. & Reid, G. J. (2012). Agreement with night-waking strategies among community mothers of preschool-aged children. *Journal of Pediatric Psychology, 37*(3), 319–328.

Daley, D., & Birchwood, J. (2010). ADHD and academic performance: Why does ADHD impact on academic performance and what can be done to support ADHD children in the classroom? *Child: Care, Health and Development, 36*(4), 455–464.

Deault, L. C. (2010). A systematic review of parenting in relation to the development of comorbidities and functional impairments in children with attention-deficit/hyperactivity disorder (ADHD). *Child Psychiatry and Human Development, 41*(2), 168–192.

Dretzke, J., Davenport, C., Frew, E., Barlow, J., Stewart-Brown, S., Bayliss, S., et al. (2009). The clinical effectiveness of different parenting programmes for children with conduct problems: A systematic review of randomised controlled trials. *Child and Adolescent Psychiatry and Mental Health, 3*(1), 7.

Eiraldi, R. B., Mautone, J. A., & Power, T. J. (2012). Strategies for implementing evidence-based psychosocial interventions for children with attention-deficit/hyperactivity disorder. *Child and Adolescent Psychiatric Clinics of North America, 21*(1), 145–159, x.

Fallone, G., Acebo, C., Seifer, R., & Carskadon, M. A. (2005). Experimental restriction of sleep opportunity in children: Effects on teacher ratings. *Sleep, 28*(12), 1561–1567.

Gau, S. S., Ni, H. C., Shang, C. Y., Soong, W. T., Wu, Y. Y., Lin, L. Y., & Chiu, Y. N. (2010). Psychiatric comorbidity among children and adolescents with and without persistent attention-deficit hyperactivity disorder. *The Australian and New Zealand Journal of Psychiatry, 44*(2), 135–143.

Gruber, R. (2009). Sleep characteristics of children and adolescents with attention deficit-hyperactivity disorder. *Child and Adolescent Psychiatric Clinics of North America, 18*(4), 863–876.

Gruber, R., Wiebe, S., Montecalvo, L., Brunetti, B., Amsel, R., & Carrier, J. (2011). Impact of sleep restriction on neurobehavioral functioning of children with attention deficit hyperactivity disorder. *Sleep, 34*(3), 315–323.

Hoban, T. F. (2004). Assessment and treatment of disturbed sleep in attention deficit hyperactivity disorder. *Expert Review of Neurotherapeutics, 4*(2), 307–316.

Hoban, T. F. (2008). Sleep disturbances and attention deficit hyperactivity disorder. *Sleep Medicine Clinics, 3*(3), 469–478.

Hodgson, K., Hutchinson, A. D., & Denson, L. (2012). Nonpharmacological treatments for ADHD: A meta-analytic review. *Journal of Attention Disorders*, epub ahead of print. doi:10.1177/1087054712444732

Ironside, S., Davidson, F. & Corkum, P. (2010). Circadian motor activity affected by stimulant medication in children with ADHD. *Journal of Sleep Research, 9*, 546–551.

Jan, Y. W., Yang, C. M., & Huang, Y. S. (2011). Comorbidity and confounding factors in attention-deficit/hyperactivity disorder and sleep disorders in children. *Psychology Research and Behavior Management, 4*(1), 139–150.

Kaplan, G., & Newcorn, J. H. (2011). Pharmacotherapy for child and adolescent attention-deficit hyperactivity disorder. *Pediatric Clinics of North America, 58*(1), 99–120.

Katragadda, S., & Schubiner, H. (2007). ADHD in children, adolescents, and adults. *Primary Care: Clinics in Office Practice, 34*(2), 317–341.

Konofal, E., Lecendreux, M., & Cortese, S. (2010). Sleep and ADHD. *Sleep Medicine, 11*(7), 652–658.

Kopasz, M., Loessl, B., Hornyak, M., Riemann, D., Nissen, C., Piosczyk, H., & Voderholzer, U. (2010). Sleep and memory in healthy children and adolescents—a critical review. *Sleep Medicine Reviews, 14*(3), 167–177.

Lewandowski, A. S., Toliver-Sokol, M., & Palermo, T. M. (2011). Evidence-based review of subjective pediatric sleep measures. *Journal of Pediatric Psychology, 36*(7), 780–793.

Lindberg, N., Tani, P., Sailas, E., Virkkala, J., Urrila, A., & Virkkunen, M. (2008). Sleep in conduct-disordered adolescents- a polysomnographic and spectral power analysis. *Psychiatry Research, 159*, 339–345.

Lofthouse, N., Gilchrist, R., & Splaingard, M. (2009). Mood-related sleep problems in children and adolescents. *Child and Adolescent Psychiatric Clinics of North America, 18*(4), 893–916.

Loke, Y. K., & Derry, S. (2003). Does anybody read "evidence-based" articles? *BMC Medical Research Methodology, 3*, 14–19.

Meltzer, L. J. (2010). Clinical management of behavioral insomnia of childhood: Treatment of bedtime problems and night wakings in young children. *Behavioral Sleep Medicine, 8*(3), 172–189.

Mindell, J. A., Emslie, G., Blumer, J., Genel, M., Glaze, D., Ivanenko, A., et al. (2006). Pharmacologic management of insomnia in children and adolescents: Consensus statement. *Pediatrics, 117*(6), e1223–1232.

Moore, B. A., Friman, P. C., Fruzzetti, A. E., & MacAleese, K. (2007). Brief report: Evaluating the bedtime pass program for child resistance to bedtime—a randomized, controlled trial. *Journal of Pediatric Psychology, 32*(3), 283–287.

Mullane, J.C. & Corkum, P. (2006). Case Series: Evaluation of a behavioral sleep intervention for three children with attention deficit hyperactivity disorder and dyssomnia. *Journal of Attention Disorders, 10(2),* 217–227.

Owens, J. A. (2005). The ADHD and sleep conundrum: A Review. *Journal of Developmental and Behavioral Pediatrics, 26*(4), 312–322.

Owens, J. A., & Dalzell, V. (2005). Use of the "BEARS" sleep screening tool in a pediatric residents' continuity clinic: A pilot study. *Sleep Medicine, 6,* 63–69.

Owens, J. A. (2008). Sleep disorders and attention-deficit/hyperactivity disorder. *Current Psychiatry Reports, 10*(5), 439–444.

Owens, J. A. (2009). A clinical overview of sleep and attention-deficit/hyperactivity disorder in children and adolescents. *Journal of the Canadian Academy of Child and Adolescent Psychiatry, 18*(2), 92–102.

Owens, J.A. & Jones, C. (2011). Parental knowledge of healthy sleep in young children: Results of a primary care clinic survey. *Journal of Developmental and Behavioral Pediatrics, 32,* 447–453.

Poirer, A., Gendron, M., & Corkum, P. (June, 2012). *The Impact of Sleep Restriction on Daytime Movement in Typically Developing Children.* Poster Presentation at Canadian Psychological Association Convention 2012, Halifax, NS.

Reid, R., Riccio, C. A., Kessler, R. H., DuPaul, G. J., Power, T. J., Anastopoulos, A. D., et al. (2000). Gender and ethnic differences in ADHD as assessed by behavior ratings. *Journal of Emotional & Behavioral Disorders, 8*(1), 38.

Sadeh, A., Pergamin, L., & Bar-Haim, Y. (2006). Sleep in children with attention-deficit hyperactivity disorder: A meta-analysis of polysomnographic studies. *Sleep Medicine Reviews, 10*(6), 381–398.

Schachar, R. (2009). Attention deficit hyperactivity disorder in children, adolescents, and adults. *Continuum Lifelong Learning Neurology, 15*(6), 78–97.

Sciberras, E., Fulton, M., Efron, D., Oberklaid, F., & Hiscock, H. (2012). Managing sleep problems in school aged children with ADHD: A pilot randomised controlled trial. *Sleep Medicine, 12,* 932–935.

Sergeant, J. A., Geurts, H., Huijbregts, S., Scheres, A., & Oosterlaan, J. (2003). The top and the bottom of ADHD: A neuropsychological perspective. *Neuroscience and Biobehavioral Reviews, 27*(7), 583–592.

Simpson, D., Suarez, L., & Connolly, S. (2012). Treatment and outcomes for anxiety disorders among children and adolescents: A review of coping strategies and parental behaviors. *Current Psychiatry Reports, 14*(2), 87–95.

Spruyt, K., & Gozal, D. (2011). Sleep disturbances in children with attention-deficit/hyperactivity disorder. *Expert Review of Neurotherapeutics, 11*(4), 565–577.

Taurines, R., Schmitt, J., Renner, T., Conner, A. C., Warnke, A., & Romanos, M. (2010). Developmental comorbidity in attention-deficit/hyperactivity disorder. *Attention Deficit and Hyperactivity Disorders, 2*(4), 267–289.

Taylor, D. J., & Roane, B. M. (2010). Treatment of insomnia in adults and children: A practice-friendly review of research. *Journal of Clinical Psychology, 66*(11), 1137–1147.

Tsai, M. H., & Huang, Y. S. (2010). Attention-deficit/hyperactivity disorder and sleep disorders in children. *The Medical Clinics of North America, 94*(3), 615–632.

Van der Heijden, K. B., Smits, M. G., & Gunning, W. B. (2005). Sleep-related disorders in ADHD: A review. *Clinical Pediatrics, 44*(3), 201–210.

Vriend, J. & Corkum, P. (2011). Clinical management of behavioral insomnia of childhood. *Psychology Research and Behavior Management, 4,* 69–79.

Vriend, J. L., Davidson, F. D., Corkum, P. V., Rusak, B., McLaughlin, E. N., & Chambers, C. T. (2012). Sleep quantity and quality in relation to daytime functioning in children. *Children's Health Care, 41*(3), 204–222.

Walters, A. S., Silvestri, R., Zucconi, M., Chandrashekariah, R. & Konofal, E. (2008). Review of the possible relationship and hypothetical links between attention deficit hyperactivity disorder (ADHD) and the simple sleep related movement disorders, parasomnias, hypersomnias, and circadian rhythm disorders. *Journal of Clinical Sleep Medicine, 4*(6), 591–600.

Waxmonsky, J. G., Wymbs, F. A., Pariseau, M. E., Belin, P. J., Waschbusch, D. A., Babocsai, L., et al. (2012). A novel group therapy for children with ADHD and severe mood dysregulation. *Journal of Attention Disorders,* epub ahead of print. doi:10.1177/1087054711433423

Webster-Stratton, C., Reid, M. J., & Beauchaine, T. (2011). Combining parent and child training for young children with ADHD. *Journal of Clinical Child & Adolescent Psychology, 40*(2), 191–203.

Wehmeier, P. M., Schacht, A., & Barkley, R. A. (2010). Social and emotional impairment in children and adolescents with ADHD and the impact on quality of life. *Journal of Adolescent Health, 46*(3), 209–217.

Weinberg, W. A., & Brumback, R. A. (1990). Primary disorder of vigilance: A novel explanation of inattentiveness, daydreaming, boredom, restlessness, and sleepiness. *The Journal of Pediatrics, 116*(5), 720–725.

Weiss, M. D., & Salpekar, J. (2010). Sleep problems in the child with attention-deficit hyperactivity disorder: Defining aetiology and appropriate treatments. *CNS Drugs, 24*(10), 811–828.

Weiss, S. K. (2006). *Better Sleep for your Baby & Child: A Parent's Step-by-Step Guide to Healthy Sleep Habits.* Toronto: Robert Rose Inc.

Yoon, S. Y. R., Jain, U., & Shapiro, C. (2012). Sleep in attention-deficit/hyperactivity disorder in children and adults: Past, present, and future. *Sleep Medicine Reviews, 16*(4), 371–388.

Young, S. & Amarasinghe, J. M. (2010). Practitioner review: Non-pharmacological treatments for ADHD: A lifespan approach. *The Journal of Child Psychology and Psychiatry, 51*(2), 116–133.

CHAPTER

35 Mood Disorders

Allison G. Harvey, Candice A. Alfano, *and* Greg Clarke

Abstract

Mood disorders are prevalent and concerning, particularly among children and adolescents. Sleep disturbances, particularly insomnia and hypersomnia (but also delayed sleep phase and sleep need), often co-occur with the mood disorders. Evidence has accrued suggesting that sleep disturbances are important pathways contributing to the mood disorders. The risk of depression is increased by preexisting insomnia, sleep problems interfere with depression treatment success, and in depressed adults treating the depression and insomnia is markedly better relative to treating depression alone. An evidence base is growing for the use of psychosocial treatments for sleep disturbance in youth. We describe the protocol we have developed for treating insomnia in depressed youth. Potential advantages for delivering psychosocial treatments for sleep disturbance, over medication treatments, are reviewed. We also discuss the importance of working with parents, the slight tip toward eveningness with the onset and progression through puberty, and the role of technology (cell phones, video games, etc.) in contributing to sleep disturbance.

Key Words: depression, bipolar disorder, insomnia, hypersomnia, adolescence, children

Mood disorders in youth are alarmingly common. The goal of this chapter is to review the growing literature indicating the importance of disturbed sleep in the mood disorders. This is important because sleep disturbances are among the most prominent correlates of mood episodes and inadequate recovery. Moreover, the evidence is increasingly compelling that sleep disturbances may be important pathways contributing to mood problems.

Mood Disorders Among Youth: A Critical Public Health Problem

Mood disorders are severe, impairing, and potentially life threatening conditions. The two most studied mood disorders will be our focus; namely, depression and bipolar disorder. *Major depressive disorder* (MDD) is characterized by one or more episodes of depressed mood or loss of interest for at least 2 weeks, along with symptoms like weight loss or gain, agitation or retardation, fatigue or loss of energy, difficulty concentrating, and feelings of worthlessness. Bipolar (BP) disorder is characterized by episodes of mood shifts. *Bipolar I disorder* is characterized by one or more manic or mixed episodes, and usually episodes of depression, too. A manic episode lasts for at least 1 week and can include the following symptoms: inflated self-esteem, talkativeness, distractibility, and excessive involvement in pleasurable activities with high potential for negative consequences. A mixed episode is diagnosed when the criteria for both mania and depression are met. *Bipolar II disorder* is characterized by one or more episodes of depression as well as one hypomanic episode which is a period of 4 days in which the symptoms of mania are experienced (American Psychiatric Association, 2000). Note that early-onset bipolar disorder is often characterized by very rapid cycling (Geller et al., 1998), with coexisting irritability and elation (Geller et al., 2003), as well as significant mood lability and aggression (Faedda, Baldessarini, Glovinsky, & Austin, 2004b; Geller, Zimmerman, et al., 2002). In fact, many child and adolescent BP cases appear to be marked less by "classic" cycles of mania and depression and more by rather chronic displays of irritable, explosive, and "mixed" mood states (Biederman, Faraone, Wozniak, Mick, Kwon, & Megan, 2004).

In this chapter, we focus on mood disorders during adolescence because the age of onset for these disorders is often during this developmental phase. Indeed, it is well established that adolescence is a high-risk time for the onset of mental health difficulties, with at least 50% of all adult disorders having their onset during the adolescent years (Belfer, 2008). Mood disorders among youth have become a significant public health priority because early onset of unipolar and bipolar depression is associated with poorer prognosis (Klein et al., 1999). Also, several complex biological, psychological, and social interactions render this a particularly important phase for mechanistic and clinical research relating to associations between sleep and the mood disorders.

Unipolar depression is one of the most common disorders in adolescence; 20% of adolescents will have had a depressive episode by age 18 (Lewinsohn, Hops, Roberts, Seeley, & Andrews, 1993) with as many as 75% of these experiencing a second episode within 5 years (Kovacs, Fienberg, Crouse-Novak, Paulaukas, & Finkelstein, 1984a, 1984b). Depression is associated with substantial impairment in all domains and an alarming 30-fold increased risk of completed suicide (Birmaher et al., 1996; Brent, 1993; Brent et al., 1988). It is important to also note that preadolescent children can and do experience depression as well, although rates are much lower. Prevalence of unipolar depression in school-age children ranges from .03% to 3.0% (Costello, Foley, & Adrian, 2006). Depression not otherwise specified (NOS) appears to be diagnosed more commonly than MDD or dysthymia in preteens (Costello, et al., 2006), suggesting that symptom profiles may be more varied in this age group. Depression rates in adolescent and adult females are approximately two times that of males, whereas boys and girls are equally likely to be diagnosed with depression during the preteen years (Angold & Rutter, 1992; Twenge & Nolen-Hoeksema, 2002).

Prevalence rates of early onset bipolar disorder are similar to adults and stand at 1%–2% (Lewinsohn, Klein, & Seeley, 1995). However, only 11% of bipolar adolescents meet full criteria for bipolar I, with the remainder meeting diagnostic criteria on the bipolar spectrum (bipolar II disorder, cyclothymia or bipolar disorder NOS). Even with the inclusion of those who did not meet full criteria for bipolar I disorder, youth with bipolar spectrum disorders have twice the rate of suicide attempts and significantly worse levels of overall functioning compared to adolescents with major depressive disorder. Diagnosis of bipolar spectrum disorders in young children remains controversial. However, youth meeting criteria for bipolar disorder NOS appear to be similar to those with bipolar 1 disorder on many factors, including age of onset, duration of illness, rates of comorbid diagnoses, suicidal ideation, prior major depressive episodes, family history, and the types of manic symptoms that were present during the most serious lifetime episode (Axelson et al., 2006).

Sleep Disturbance is a Prominent Feature of Mood Disorders

Sleep disturbances are among the most prominent correlates of mood episodes and inadequate recovery (Ehlers, Kupfer, Frank, & Monk, 1993; Harvey, 2008b; Kupfer, 1995; Wehr, Sack, & Rosenthal, 1987). There are various types of sleep disturbances that co-occur with the mood disorders. *Insomnia* and *hypersomnia* are listed in the *Diagnostic and Statistical Manual of Mental Disorders* (DSM-IV-TR) as symptoms of major depressive disorder, and *reduced need for sleep* is listed as a symptom for a manic episode (American Psychiatric Association, 2000). It may seem impossible for insomnia and hypersomnia to co-occur, but it's clear that they often do (Liu et al., 2007). Although not listed in the DSM-IV-TR, other sleep difficulties that commonly co-occur with the mood disorders include *night-to-night variability in sleep* and *delayed sleep phase.* Moreover, given the phasic nature of the mood disorders—there are depressed episodes, manic episodes, hypomanic episodes, and mixed episodes as well as inter-episode periods—the nature of the sleep disturbance may be different across these phases.

It's very clear that sleep disturbances are frequently comorbid with depression (Brunello et al., 2000; Dahl & Harvey, 2007), and there is evidence that these conditions have bidirectional, mutually maintaining influences (Harvey, 2008a, 2008b; Wehr et al., 1987). In a recent study of 553 youth with major depression, 72.7% also reported a sleep disturbance, mostly insomnia; these youth (age range 7.3 to 14.9 years) were also more severely depressed. More specifically, 73% reported sleep problems including insomnia (54%), hypersomia (9%) and both insomnia and hypersomnia (10%; Liu, et al., 2007). Estimates of hypersomnia in the mood disorders vary widely across ages and studies, ranging from as low as 8.9% in childhood (Williamson et al., 2000) to as high as 75.8% in young adulthood (Parker, Malhi, Hadzi-Oavlovic, & Parker, 2006).

Objective sleep data do not always correlate with subjective reports of sleep (Harvey & Tang, 2012). In a comprehensive review of studies that included polysomnography (PSG), only 15 out of 27 reported the presence of significant PSG differences in depressed compared to healthy adolescents (Ivanenko, McLaughlin Crabtreec, & Gozald, 2005). Even fewer studies reported PSG abnormalities among depressed children. These findings stand in contrast to the well-established trait-like sleep abnormalities found in adults with MDD, including an increased percentage of rapid eye movement (REM) sleep, shortened latency to REM, increased REM density, and reduced slow wave sleep (Reynolds & Kupfer, 1987). Although not the focus of this chapter, developmental differences in objective sleep patterns likely relate to a number of potentially synergistic factors including, most prominently, perceptual issues as well as neurodevelopment and sleep–wake processes (Harvey & Tang, 2012; Pillai, Kalmbach, & Ciesla, 2011). Overall, it is clear that associations between objective sleep abnormalities and depression become stronger as children mature into adolescents and adults.

Sleep disturbance is also a prominent feature of bipolar disorder in youth, with rates estimated between 40% and 60% (Harvey, Mullin, & Hinshaw, 2006). A decreased need for sleep is common with a weighted average of 72% across studies (Kowatch, Youngstrom, Danielyan, & Findling, 2005). Among preadolescent children with bipolar spectrum disorders, sleep difficulties most frequently occurred during depressive periods (82%) but were also common in relation to mania symptoms (58%; Lofthouse, Fristad, Splaingard, & Kelleher, 2007). Objective estimates of sleep (i.e., PSG, actigraphy) have been included in only a few studies. Findings indicate that compared to healthy controls, youth with bipolar disorder exhibit lower sleep efficiency, longer slow wave sleep, and reduced REM sleep (Mehl et al., 2006).

A number of methodological issues arise from research on sleep and mood disorders in teens (Harvey, et al., 2006). First, there is a need for psychometrically validated self-report and/or observational methods of assessing sleep disturbance in youth, as discussed earlier in this handbook. In addition, there is a need for more studies to include objective estimates of sleep such as PSG and actigraphy. Other limitations include the absence of comparison groups to tease out specificity of findings, as well as limited assessments of comorbidity. Given high comorbidity rates in youth, it will be important for future studies to track comorbidity so as to determine interactions with sleep disturbance. Finally, the strategies for dealing with medication confounds vary across studies, with several studies not reporting these details. The impact of medications on sleep is an important methodological issue (Harvey, Talbot, & Gershon, 2009).

Is Sleep Disturbance a Mechanism in the Mood Disorders?

As already highlighted, sleep disturbance is highly comorbid with the major mood disorders. An important shift in perspective has taken hold over the past decade. The accumulated evidence has refuted the idea that the sleep symptoms are merely an epiphenomenon of mood disorders, but instead supports the view that sleep is an important yet understudied mechanism in the complex and multifactorial causation of the symptoms and functional disability associated with the mood disorders (for review see Harvey, 2001b; Harvey, et al., 2009; McCrae & Lichstein, 2001; NIH, 2005; Smith, Huang, & Manber, 2005). Although the research reviewed below has tended to emphasize the importance of insomnia as a mechanism contributing to mood disorders, there's increasing interest in the possibility that hypersomnia, delayed sleep phase and reduced sleep need may also be mechanisms (Kaplan & Harvey, 2009).

Several lines of evidence have emerged in support of the hypothesis that sleep disturbances may contribute mechanistically to mood disorders. Several aspects of the relationship between sleep disturbances and child/adolescent mood disorders are briefly reviewed below.

Insomnia Contributes to Risk of Depression Onset/Severity

Evidence has steadily accrued indicating that insomnia is an independent risk factor for first and recurrent episodes of depression (Ford & Kamerow, 1989; Harvey, 2001a; Perlis et al., 2006; Riemann, Berger, & Voderholzer, 2001; Taylor, Lichenstein, & Durrence, 2003). For example, community residing youth (N = 4500) who reported frequent trouble sleeping were more likely than normal-sleeping controls to report anxiety or depression (odds ratio = 22.7; Johnson, Breslau, Roehrs, & Roth 1999). A similar study of 1014 teens found that chronologically primary insomnia significantly predicted future depression (hazard rate = 3.8) but that primary depression did not predict subsequent insomnia (Johnson, Roth, & Breslau, 2006). Insomnia symptoms also predicted subsequent depression in another large adolescent community panel (Roberts, Roberts, & Chen, 2002); elevated insomnia at Wave 1 predicted greater depression severity at Wave 2 even when controlling for Wave 2 insomnia. There also is substantial evidence that sleep problems emerging during early childhood are independently predictive for the later onset of depression (Gregory et al., 2005; Ong, Wickramaratne, Tang, & Weissman, 2006).

Sleep Disturbance as an Early Marker for Bipolar Disorder

There is evidence that sleep disturbance may be an early marker for bipolar spectrum disorders in youth. Compared to children of control parents, children of parents with bipolar disorder exhibited shorter sleep latency measured via actigraphy but lower Pittsburgh Sleep Quality Index score, as well as a trend toward less variable sleep and greater sleep duration via actigraphy (2006). This discrepancy between subjectively perceived sleep and objectively estimated sleep is an ongoing puzzle in the field (Harvey & Tang, 2012). On the one hand, it may be that objective estimates of sleep, like actigraphy, are not capturing the subjective sleep complaint. Or perhaps these findings reflect a tendency toward hypersomnia or a mechanism related to sleep pressure. In a study of early onset bipolar disorder (n = 82), sleep disturbance was reported by about half of the parents as one of the earliest symptoms observed (Faedda, Baldessarini, Glovinsky, & Austin, 2004a). In another study, sleep disturbances (and anxiety disorders) were identified as an antecedent to the onset of bipolar disorder in a subset of high-risk youth (Duffy, Alda, Crawford, Milin, & Grof, 2007). Further evidence is provided by findings reported in a study (Shaw, Egeland, Endicott, Allen, & Hostetter, 2005) of 100 at-risk children with a parent with bipolar I and a control group of 112 children with well parents. Decreased sleep was one of the distinguishing features of the high-risk group.

Specific Types of Sleep Disturbance May Be a Distinguishing Feature of Bipolar Disorder

Several studies raise the possibility that sleep disturbances may help to distinguish manifestations of bipolar illness from the early development of other psychopathology. First, compared to children with ADHD and healthy controls, children diagnosed with bipolar disorder have significantly higher rates of sleep difficulties (Geller, Zimerman, et al., 2002). Second, a decreased need for sleep is more common among children with bipolar profile symptoms than in children with comparable levels of psychopathology excluding bipolar disorder symptoms (Holtmann et al., 2007). Finally, youth with unipolar depression who had undergone PSG assessment as adolescents (1990) were followed up for 7 years (into their early 20s). Clinical interviews were administered to determine disease course (Rao et al., 2002). Five of the 26 patients who were diagnosed with unipolar depression at the first assessment had switched to bipolar disorder by the time of the follow-up. Based on these new categorizations, the original PSG data were reanalyzed. The results indicated that depressed participants who followed a unipolar course showed reduced REM latency, higher REM density, and increased overall REM sleep, whereas those who moved to a bipolar course demonstrated increased stage 1 sleep and decreased stage 4 sleep. These findings raise the possibility that sleep abnormalities, in adults, may distinguish bipolar from unipolar trajectories.

Sleep Disturbance Contributes to Relapse

There are several lines of evidence, mostly based on adults, suggesting that sleep disturbance contributes to relapse. First, a systematic review of 73 reports of prodromal symptoms in bipolar disorder and unipolar depression (Jackson, Cavanagh, & Scott, 2003) finds that the majority of patients (over 80%) reported sleep disturbance as one of the most common of early symptoms. In a follow-up study of children and adolescents successfully treated for MDD, longer sleep onset latency and lower sleep efficiency at post-treatment predicted recurrence of depression within 1 year (Emslie et al., 2001). Second, a handful of experimental studies and case reports have found induced sleep deprivation to be associated with the onset of hypomania or mania in a proportion of patients (Colombo, Benedetti, Barbini, Campori, & Smeraldi, 1999; Wehr, et al., 1987). There is an urgent need for research programs to test the presumed generalizability of these findings to youth with a mood disorder.

Sleep is Critical for Affect Regulation

There is robust evidence in adults that sleep deprivation undermines emotion responding and regulation the following day (Pilcher & Huffcutt, 1996; Yoo, Gujar, Hu, Jolesz, & Walker, 2007), with similar findings in fewer studies with youth (McGlinchey et al., 2011; Talbot, McGlinchey, Kaplan, Dahl, & Harvey, 2010). A study by Zohar et al. (2005) suggests that the context in which the emotion is experienced is important for determining the direction of the effect of sleep disturbance on affective functioning. Studies experimentally restricting sleep in healthy youth have reported decrements in affective functioning as a function of sleep loss (Leotta, Carskadon, Acebo, Seifer, & Quinn, 1997; McGlinchey et al., 2011; Talbot et al., 2010). Conversely, better quality sleep may buffer against affective risk. For example, a prospective study of children at high risk for MDD found that a greater percentage of slow wave sleep during childhood was protective against the development of depression during adolescence and young adulthood (Silk et al., 2007). The reciprocal relationships between sleep, early brain development, and affective regulation may in part explain these findings.

Sleep is Important for Cognitive Functioning

Deficits in neuropsychological performance have been demonstrated in youth with a mood disorder (Dickstein et al., 2004; Doyle et al., 2005). The extent to which sleep disturbance partially accounts for these findings should be examined. It seems plausible that sleep disturbance may contribute, given that adverse and severe effects of sleep deprivation on cognitive functioning have been clearly demonstrated (Van Dongen, Maislin, Mullington, & Dinges, 2003; Walker & Stickgold, 2006). In addition to the acute effects of sleep loss, cognitive impairments may persist over time. In one prospective study, parent-reported sleep problems during childhood significantly predicted neuropsychological functioning in early adolescence (Gregory, Caspi, Moffitt, & Poulton, 2009). Adverse effects in this domain are likely to be particularly critical for youth diagnosed with a mood disorder, whose educational achievements (so reliant on cognitive function) will have far reaching and long-term consequences.

Sleep and Obesity

Mood disorders are associated with a wide range of medical problems in adults, with the most common being cardiovascular disease, diabetes mellitus, and thyroid disease (Krishnan, 2005; Patten et al., 2008; Whooley et al., 2008). The physical health of youth with mood disorders has been less studied, although there is evidence of weight problems and obesity and indications that obesity is associated with worse outcomes (Jolin, Weller, & Weller, 2007). Detecting an association between mood disorder and medical problems is difficult in youth because most disorders of interest have a later life onset; in adolescence they may only present as elevated prodromal states. Further, it is unclear whether the observed association is attributable to depression itself, or the treatment (particularly antidepressants) or other epiphenomena. For example, many of the medications used to treat mood disorders are associated with weight gain (Elmslie, Silverstone, Mann, Williams, & Romans, 2000; Zimmermann, Kraus, Himmerich, Schuld, & Pollmacher, 2003). It also seems likely that depressive symptoms may be associated with physical inactivity, which is also a contributor to obesity (Whooley, et al., 2008). Another possible explanation, given that sleep deprivation increases appetite, weight gain, and insulin tolerance (Spiegel, Tasali, Penev, & Van Cauter, 2004), is that sleep disturbance may be an additional contributor. Indeed, in a recent meta-analysis involving 30 studies (12 in children) and 634,511 participants, an association between short sleep and obesity was observed across the age range. Specifically, there was a 60%–80% increase in the odds of being a short sleeper among children who were obese (Cappuccio et al., 2008). Further, experimentally induced short-term sleep deprivation in normal weight college-age volunteers is associated with disturbed appetite hormones (grehlin, leptin) in a direction associated with obesity (Spiegel, Tasali, Penev, & Van Cauter, 2004).

Sleep Deprivation is Associated with Substance Use

Several studies indicate that the presence of a mood disorder in adolescence is associated with elevated risk for alcohol abuse, drug abuse, and cigarette smoking. This finding cannot be attributed to comorbid conduct disorder (Wilens et al., 2004), attention deficit and hyperactivity disorder, or multiple anxiety disorders (Wilens et al., 2008). Again, the contributors to these high rates of comorbidity with substance use problems are going to be complex and multifactorial. One possibility is that the sleep disturbance characteristic of the mood disorders may be one contributor. Indeed, among a Finnish sample of adolescents, irregular sleep schedules and daytime sleepiness accounted for 26% of the variance in substance use in 15-year-old boys and 12% in 15-year-old girls (Tynjala, Kannas, & Levalahti, 1997). Another large study of 4500 adolescents ages 12 to 17 year found that those who had trouble sleeping reported greater use of alcohol (odds ratio of 2.6), marijuana (odds ratio of 2.4), and cigarettes (odds ratio of 2.2; Johnson, Breslau, Roehrs, & Roth, 1999). It is possible that the effects of drugs and alcohol may be sought out for the sedation and/or emotional regulatory effects or for rewarding and/or stimulating effects.

Sleep Deprivation Contributes to Suicidality

Youth with mood disorders have high rates of suicide attempts (Bellivier, Golmard, Henry, & Leboyer, 2001; Tsai, Lee, & Chen, 1999). Sleep disturbance may be relevant. Teens with more insomnia and nightmares reported more suicidal ideation (Choquet & Menke, 1989), and insomnia and hypersomnia were independently associated with suicidal ideation (Choquet, Kovess, & Poutignat, 1993). Poor sleep has also been associated with suicide attempts. Eighty-one percent of teens presenting to an emergency room following a suicide attempt reported difficulty falling asleep or early morning waking immediately preceding the attempt. Nightmares were associated with increased risk for suicide attempts and those who slept less than 8 hours were three times more likely to attempt suicide (Liu & Buysse, 2006). Poor sleep has also been associated with suicide completion. Insomnia also predicts adolescent hospitalization for suicide attempt (Gasquet & Choquet, 1994).

Using a psychological autopsy protocol in which parents, siblings, and friends were interviewed between 4 and 6 months after the suicide, Goldstein et al. (2008) compared adolescent suicide completers (n = 140) to an age/sex matched control group (n = 131). Suicide completers had higher rates of overall sleep disturbance, insomnia, and hypersomnia within the past week.

Taken together, these lines of evidence indicate that sleep disturbance may contribute in several direct and indirect ways to core problems and symptoms of mood disorders among youth. Accordingly, treatments targeting sleep may represent unique opportunities for intervention that may improve sleep, health, and cognitive functioning, and reduce risk for suicide and improve mood.

Current Options and Practices for Treatment of Sleep Disturbance

The adult cognitive-behavior therapy for insomnia (CBT-I) treatment literature is relatively well established, with numerous clinical trials conducted over the past few decades. The evidence base for CBT for adults with insomnia has been summarized in multiple meta-analyses (Morin, Culbert, & Schwartz, 1994; Murtagh & Greenwood, 1995; Smith et al., 2002) and two practice parameters papers commissioned by the American Academy of Sleep Medicine (Morin et al., 2006; Morin et al., 1999). The clear conclusion is that CBT for insomnia produces reliable and durable changes in sleep.

The research literature on the treatment of sleep disturbance using psychological interventions in children and adolescents is small but promising, as are the data on the behavioral and/or emotional improvements after the treatment of sleep problems. Bootzin and colleagues developed a 6-session (90 minutes per session) group treatment for sleep disturbance in adolescents with substance-related problems (ages 12 to 19). The intervention was based on CBT-I for adults but was developmentally adapted to enhance the motivation, commitment, and compliance of the youth. In an uncontrolled pilot study participants who completed four or more sessions showed improved sleep (Bootzin & Stevens, 2005), and improving sleep led to a reduction in substance abuse problems at the 12-month follow-up. In a separate report, improvements in sleep were associated with significant decreases in aggressive thoughts and actions (Haynes et al., 2006). Another small (n = 18) uncontrolled pilot (Schlarb, Liddle, & Hautzinger, 2010) of a 6-session insomnia behavioral therapy (BT-I) found improvement in numerous sleep parameters. While both of these trials have been limited by the lack of a randomized control condition, the generally positive results are encouraging. These data show the feasibility of improving sleep through a short-term psychological intervention in adolescents and provide promising preliminary results suggesting that improved sleep in youth can contribute to improvements in behavioral and emotional functioning. Gradisar et al. (2011) evaluated 6 sessions of CBT-I plus morning bright light therapy to advance sleep onset (CBT-I plus BLT) versus waitlist for adolescents diagnosed with delayed sleep phase disorder (DSPD). CBT-I plus BLT was associated with reduced sleep latency, earlier sleep onset and rise times, total sleep time (school nights), wake after sleep onset, sleepiness, and fatigue. At 6-month follow-up, these improvements were sustained. Also, Cain et al. (2011) attempted to address common problems of low motivation for treatment, poor treatment adherence, and attrition among adolescent patients by using the school classroom as an alternative arena for sleep intervention. A total of 104 youth from intervention or control classrooms were included in the sample. Students receiving the motivation-based sleep intervention attended four 50-minute sleep education classes once per week for one month. At post-treatment, students in intervention classes reported significantly increased knowledge about sleep relative to the control group. Despite self-reported increases in motivation to improve their sleep, sleep patterns and daytime functioning were not significantly different between the groups at post-treatment. Although promising, these findings might be interpreted to suggest that even in the face of adequate motivation, adolescents require parental and/or clinician assistance in regulating and maintaining healthy sleep schedules.

The use of medications to promote sleep onset is perhaps the most contentious issue in treating sleep problems in children and adolescents with difficulty going to sleep (Owens, Rosen, & Mindell, 2003). Adult sleep pharmacology has seen numerous advances, including new-generation agents with a much better specificity for sleep, duration of action, and relatively low risk and side effects. However, much of this research has yet to be conducted in youth beyond a few small trials of melatonin supplementation for childhood insomnia (Smits, Nagtegaal, van der Heijden, Coenen, & Kerkhof, 2001; Smits et al., 2003; Weiss, Wasdell, Bomben, Rea, & Freeman, 2006). One might argue that some of these medications represent better treatment options for insomnia in children and adolescents. However, until there are empirical data and controlled trials using these medications in youth (including dosing, side effects, and efficacy) it seems unwise to advocate any specific medication at this time. Indeed, it's possible that pharmacologically induced sleep may not provide the health benefits that humans have specifically evolved to obtain from sleep. For example, Seibt et al. (2008) investigated the impact of zolpidem (Ambien) on the development of the visual system in kittens 28–41 days old. As expected, zolpidem *increased* NREM sleep by 27% and *increased* total sleep over the 8-hour period. However, rather alarmingly, zolpidem *reduced* cortical plasticity by 50%. The authors concluded that *hypnotics that produce more "physiological" sleep based on EEG may actually impair critical sleep-dependent brain processes during development.* This finding should stimulate new research into the safety of certain pharmacologic agents, particularly regarding impacts on the developing bodies and brains of children and adolescents. There may also be implications for adults who continue to need sleep for growth, repair, learning, plasticity, and optimal emotional functioning.

Other advantages of developing psychological interventions such as CBT-I to improve sleep in adolescents with mood disorder, as compared to pharmacological interventions, include: *(1)* the absence of adverse side effects; *(2)* the fact that youth with a mood disorder are often already taking one or more psychotropic medications, so adding an additional medication to target sleep has the potential to lead to drug interactions and complicated medication regimens; *(3)* evidence that depressed youth and their parents favor psychotherapy over pharmacotherapy (Jaycox, Asarnow, Sherbourne, & et al., 2006); and *(4)* lacking evidence of efficacy and feasibility for sleep medications in youth. For these reasons our discussion below will focus on psychosocial treatments.

Current Options and Practices for Treatment of Sleep Disturbance in Adults with a Mood Disorder

There are already encouraging findings on treating sleep among adults with major depressive disorder. Manber, Edinger, Gress, et al. (2008) recruited patients who were currently depressed. All patients received the antidepressant medication escitalopram. Half also received CBT-I, while the other half received placebo psychotherapy for sleep. CBT-I is a multicomponent treatment typically comprising various components including stimulus control, sleep restriction, sleep hygiene education, relaxation, and cognitive therapy (Morin et al., 2006). The addition of CBT-I to the antidepressant treatment resulted in greater remission from insomnia (50% vs. 7.7% in the control condition) *and* a substantially higher rate of remission of depression (61.5% vs. 33.3%). These are startling outcomes that add to the already large evidence base indicating the efficacy and effectiveness of CBT-I (Morin et al., 2006) and the value of joint treatment of sleep disturbance and depression where they coexist.

To the best of our knowledge there are no clinical trials of interventions for sleep disturbance in adults or youth with bipolar disorder. However, several of the psychological adjunctive interventions for bipolar disorder include one or more components targeting sleep. Interpersonal and social rhythm therapy includes instruction in behavioral techniques designed to regularize routines and reduce social rhythm disruption (Frank, Swartz, & Kupfer, 2000). Cognitive-behavior therapy provides education about the importance of a regular social routine and sleep–wake cycle via the monitoring of mood and sleep as well as the use of activity scheduling. It also involves identifying prodromes or trigger situations, which typically include sleep disturbance, and developing effective coping strategies for such prodromes (e.g., Lam et al., 2003; Patelis-Siotis et al., 2001). Family interventions (Miklowitz & Goldstein, 1997), group psychoeducation, and individual psychoeducation (Miklowitz & Johnson, 2006) also encourage sleep/wake stabilization. Although these approaches have been shown to reduce relapse in adults and youth (Craighead, Miklowitz, Frank, & Vajk, 2002; Frank et al., 2005; Lam, Hayward, Watkins, Wright, & Sham, 2005; Miklowitz et al., 2000), at present there are no data on sleep-specific outcomes. Also, these approaches have yet to draw from advances in knowledge on the psychological treatment of sleep disturbance in adults with insomnia (Morin et al., 2006).

Toward a Psychological Intervention for Sleep Disturbance in Adolescents with Mood Disorders

Given the prevalence of sleep disturbance among youth with mood disorders, the associated adverse consequences, and the lack of empirically tested treatments, a high priority for future research is to develop an intervention for the sleep disturbance experienced by youth with mood disorders. An intervention for sleep may be particularly acceptable to youth as the payoffs of improving sleep are immediate, and sleep is often perceived by patients to be an aspect of health that is free of the strong stigma associated with mental health. In fact, delivering such an intervention to youth with a current or past mood disorder may help protect this high-risk group against the potential negative vicious cycles of escalating sleep disturbance and emotion dysregulation leading to school failure, unemployment, and withdrawal of social supports, along with reducing the other hypothesized adverse outcomes we described earlier.

Given all of the above plus the evidence that insomnia interferes with depression treatment, and that residual insomnia is a major component of incompletely remitted depression, we have hypothesized that treating youth insomnia simultaneously with depression treatment may improve both sleep and mood outcomes (Clarke & Harvey, 2012). Elsewhere we have described our careful process of developmentally adapting insomnia treatments for teens with depression (Clarke & Harvey, 2012). We have also been working on developing sleep treatment for bipolar disorder (Harvey, 2008b) and hypersomnia (Kaplan & Harvey, 2009).

In the section that follows we review three developmental considerations. We then summarize the general treatment themes covered within the treatment approaches, including some of the special considerations for adaptations for youth with bipolar disorder. Several formal evaluations of these treatments are in progress, the results of which are eagerly awaited.

Developmental Considerations

1. Parents. The extent to which parents are involved in bedtimes and choice of evening activities and bedtimes varies across development. Sleep disturbance is often amplified during adolescence vis-à-vis increasing levels of independence from parental and adult influences on sleep-relevant decisions. Clinical decision making about the extent of involvement in the intervention should be made on the basis of the youth's age and level of maturity, although an emphasis must be placed on the young person taking responsibility and initiative and inviting the parent or caregiver for support and/or structure when needed.

2. Eveningness. Eveningness is an important contributor to, and maybe even cause of vicious cycles of escalating vulnerability and increased risk for mood problems and disorders among youth (Caci, Bouchez, & Bayle, 2009; Chelminski, Ferraro, Petros, & Plaud, 1999; Gaspar-Barba et al., 2009; Gau et al., 2007; Kitamura et al., 2010). A biological shift in the circadian system at puberty in the direction of a delayed sleep phase (later onset of sleep) (Carskadon, Acebo, & Jenni, 2004; Lee, Hummer, Jechura, & Mahoney, 2004) is compounded by social changes such as less parental control, increased access to stimulating social activities (music, Internet, text messaging etc.), the importance of peers and socialization, and increased use of alcohol and substances that contribute to sleep disruption. Together, the social influences are synergistic with biological tendencies toward phase delay and can spiral quickly into a pattern of extremely delayed bedtimes. Yet, school/work usually requires a fixed early wake-up time (Hansen, Janssen, Schiff, Zee, & Dubocovich, 2005). These biopsychosocial and behavioral forces converge to constrain time available for sleep, resulting in very high rates of youth obtaining insufficient sleep (Carskadon, 2002; Carskadon, Mindell, & Drake, 2006; Hansen et al., 2005). This tendency toward eveningness necessitates components of an intervention for sleep to incorporate timed light exposure and use of powerful nonphotic cues such as regularizing meal times and exercise.

3. Technology. The National Sleep Foundation (NSF) Poll focused on technology this year. In the 13–19-year-old age group, 54% watched television, 72% used their cell phones, 60% their laptops, 64% their music player, and 23% played video games every night or almost every night within the hour before going to sleep. These behaviors have multiple potential adverse impacts in sleep. The artificial light exposure suppresses release of the sleepiness-promoting hormone melatonin, enhances alertness, and shifts circadian rhythms to a later hour. Technology is also highly arousing and engaging and facilitates the much-loved contact with peers. These influences are so potent that it is very difficult for many teens to switch media devices off at night, delaying bedtimes still further (National Sleep Foundation, 2011). Moreover, cell phones are, too often, a source of sleep disturbance during the night. About 1 in 10 of 13–19-year-olds in the NSF poll reported being awakened after they go to bed every night or almost every night by a phone call, text message, or email. Clearly, these are *modifiable* sources of sleep disturbance.

Treatment Components

As will become evident, the sections below are derived from various sources of empirical evidence. However, it must be emphasized that we are still awaiting the evaluation of the full multicomponent approach, and there is a need to determine which of the components are responsible for any positive outcome that is reported.

1. Functional Analysis and Case Formulation. This involves a detailed clinical interview in which the clinician probes the frequency, intensity, and duration of the sleep disturbance as well as its antecedents, behaviors, and consequences (see Blampied, Chapter 15). For homework we ask youth to complete a daily sleep diary, supplementing standard sleep diary questions with additional probes to enable the collection of information on the psychological and contextual variables that might be contributing. If available, actigraphy can be a useful adjunct. It may be helpful to enlist a parent's help in sleep diary completion, particularly for early adolescents and younger children.

2. Motivational Interviewing. This involves a straightforward review with the young person to explore how he or she sees the pros and cons of working toward managing the sleep disturbance (Miller & Rollnick, 2002). By using motivational interviewing techniques, the patient's motivation can be clarified and enhanced. Many sleep-incompatible/interfering behaviors are rewarding, such as text messaging with friends into the nighttime hours or freely surfing the Internet once parents have gone to bed. Moreover, parental influence over bedtime and bedroom activities wanes during adolescence. Hence, following other treatments for youth with sleep disturbance, it is likely to be necessary to begin treatment with a motivational component designed to assist the young person to find his or her internal motivation for enhancing sleep.

The search for motivating influences is inevitably influenced by the factors relevant to and meaningful for the individual adolescent (as opposed to the clinician or parent). Given the intense focus on physical appearance, peer perceptions, and romantic relationships that characterizes adolescence, results from a recent experimental study provide one example of a possible innovative avenue for increasing motivation to improve sleep. Axelsson et al. (2010) asked participants to rate the perceived health and attractiveness of participants photographed after a normal night's sleep and after a night of sleep deprivation. Sleep-deprived participants were consistently perceived as less attractive and less healthy, with effects mediated in large part by apparent tiredness. Although adequate sleep is associated with a host of benefits, socially relevant benefits such as these may serve to facilitate motivational enhancements in youth.

3. Sleep and Circadian Education. This module aims to target specific factors and behaviors that interfere with good sleep (Stepanski & Wyatt, 2003). Erratic sleep/wake schedules, including large discrepancies between wake time on school days (typically 6:00–7:00 am) versus weekends and holidays (typically 11:00 am–2:00 pm) constitute a weekly experience of severe "jetlag" and contribute to high rates of insufficient sleep in adolescents in general, and may represent a particularly important target for youth with a mood disorder. This module has three core aims: to correct unhelpful sleep habits (e.g., surfing the Internet until late) while developing new healthy sleep habits (e.g., on waking up be active and, if possible during the day, have bright light exposure such as walking outdoors), and to maintain these new healthier habits. After an initial education session, we follow two steps to correct habits: behavioral contracting, and monitoring healthy sleep behaviors and sleep-interfering behaviors on a daily basis. The maintenance of healthy habits will be achieved by regular check-ins on progress throughout the remaining sessions and by including the targets of change in the relapse prevention plan.

There are two additional core parts to this module for youth with a mood disorder. These are added in recognition of two sets of empirical findings on sleep in the mood disorders. First, based on the finding that sleep disturbance is the most common prodrome of mania and the sixth most common prodrome of depression (Jackson, et al., 2003), we include a discussion of sleep disturbance as an early warning of an episode and aim to develop effective coping strategies for such prodromes (drawing on Lam & Wong, 2005). This needs to be individualized for each patient, as some youth with bipolar disorder appear to be characterized by less "classic" cycles of mania and depression and more by chronic displays of irritable, explosive and "mixed" mood states (Biederman, Faraone, Wozniak, Mick, Kwon, & Aleardi, 2004). Second, on the basis that bipolar disorder is a disorder of emotion regulation (Hyman, 2000), along with the evidence suggesting that sleep has a key mood regulatory function (Cartwright, Luten, Young, Mercer, & Bears, 1998; Perlis & Nielsen, 1993), we draw a link between sleep disturbance and daytime mood dysfunction. In the patients treated thus far, these two aspects have been addressed by education and appear to serve to increase the internal motivation for working to enhance sleep.

For those with hypersomnia it can also be helpful to educate the young person about two additional domains (Kaplan & Harvey, 2009). The first involves education about the operation of the circadian system, the environmental influences acting on it (e.g., light), the tendency if left unchecked to move toward a delayed phase, and the difficulty of achieving fast shifts in circadian patterns. The second involves education about sleep inertia. This includes the fact that that among adults as well as youth, most mornings there is a period between 5 and 20 minutes when we feel dazed and sleepy, and that this is a normal transitional state between a state of sleep and a state of wakefulness. Acknowledging that these feelings are not pleasant and that the feelings are not necessarily indicative of having had a poor night of sleep can be helpful.

4. Regularizing the Sleep–Wake Schedule. Delayed sleep phase is common in teenagers, particularly those with bipolar disorder. Indeed, a significant delay in the circadian sleep–wake cycle has been hypothesized to be a core deficit of pediatric bipolar disorder (Staton, 2008). It often begins with a tendency to stay up late at night, sleeping in late, and/or taking a late afternoon nap. This process often starts on weekends, holidays, or summer vacations. Problems become apparent when school schedules result in morning wake-up battles and difficulties in getting to school. Often, these adolescents cope by taking afternoon naps and getting catch-up sleep on the weekends. Although some of these behaviors occur in many adolescents, in extreme cases the circadian system can become set to such a late time that even highly motivated adolescents can have difficulty shifting their sleep back to an earlier time.

An adapted version of Bootzin's stimulus control intervention (Bootzin, 1972), which was a core component of the sleep intervention administered to youth with substance-related difficulties (Bootzin & Stevens, 2005), is an important component for regularizing the sleep–wake cycle. The aim of this intervention is strengthening the association between the bed and sleeping by limiting sleep-incompatible behaviors within the bedroom environment, while developing a consistent sleep–wake schedule (Bootzin, 1972). The traditional components of the intervention involve the therapist providing a detailed rationale for and assisting the patient to achieve the following: (a) use the bed only for sleep (i.e., no TV watching or talking on cell phones); (b) go to bed only when sleepy, (c) get out of bed and go to another room when unable to fall asleep or return to sleep within approximately 15–20 minutes, and return to bed only when sleepy again; and (d) arise in the morning at the same time each day (no later than plus-2 hours on weekends; Bootzin & Stevens, 2005). The goal is to gradually move toward a regular schedule 7 days a week. In the bipolar and unipolar depression youth we have treated thus far, we have retained (a) and (d) but considered, on a case-by-case basis, omitting

(b) and (c). Point (b) is sometimes omitted because patients with bipolar disorder often need to get into bed, even though not yet sleepy, in order to begin the process of down-regulating sufficiently to fall off to sleep. Point (c) was omitted to avoid sleep deprivation during the early phase of treatment; getting out of bed risks getting caught up in rewarding and arousing activities that reduce the potential for sleep. The latter is key for patients with bipolar disorder where hypomania and mania is often related to elevated achievement motivation, ambitious goal setting, and excessive goal pursuit (Johnson, 2005). To achieve (a) and (d) we use the standard CBT manualized methods (Morin & Espie, 2003) that include providing a rationale, setting goals for bedtime and wake time, a daily sleep diary to monitor progress toward goals, and a review of the diary on a weekly basis. For difficulty falling asleep we sometimes replace the traditional stimulus control instruction (e.g., get up out of bed) with training in imagery (Harvey & Payne, 2002), savoring (McMakin, Siegle, & Shirk, 2011), and relaxation/mindfulness (Bootzin & Stevens, 2005; Morin & Espie, 2003) with the goal of reducing arousal and promoting sleep onset.

5. Hypersomnia. In our experience, excessive daytime sleepiness is common among youth, especially youth with a mood disorder. In addition, during phases of depression patients commonly suffer from periods of hypersomnia (Kupfer et al., 1972). Hypersomnia has adverse consequences for school attendance and performance, relationships, mood, and sense of self-worth. There is very little existing literature on the mechanisms that contribute to hypersomnia in mood disorder, nor the methods to treat it (Kaplan & Harvey, 2009). In our clinical experience, treating hypersomnia is likely to begin with goal setting, which involves reducing nightly sleep as well as setting goals for life. The latter is based on our clinical experience that "having nothing to get up for" can be a key contributor to hypersomnia in patients with mood disorders. Often the combination of the mood disorder and the sleep disorder has led to school disengagement/drop-out, unemployment, and/or disrupted social networks. After setting the "sleep" and "life" goals for the treatment, the young person is asked to identify one small step toward these goals for the coming week. After a detailed discussion of how to achieve those goals, possible obstacles are identified. We engage in problem solving to limit the impact of these obstacles on reaching the goal, and a method is developed for monitoring the extent to which the goal is achieved (see Kaplan & Harvey, 2009, for further details).

6. Wind-down, Wake-up, and Regularity. Often youth need assistance to devise a "wind-down" period of 30–60 minutes prior to sleep in which to engage in relaxing, sleep-enhancing activities. A central issue influencing bedtime is the use of electronic media (Internet, cell phones, MP3 players) for entertainment and social interaction at night. A crucial aspect of achieving earlier sleep onset requires a behavioral contract by each individual wherein they voluntarily *choose* a time for turning off all access to these devices; e.g., in the hour just prior to bedtime. Equally important is the "wake-up protocol" (e.g., not hitting snooze on the alarm, making the bed so the incentive to get back in is reduced, get in the shower, take a quick brisk walk, get sunlight). Finally, we emphasize the importance of minimal fluctuation in the sleep–wake schedule across weekday and weekend nights.

7. Behavioral Experiments. Educational approaches are often very helpful, but there is evidence that arranging situations that allow clients to experience the issues being discussed can bring about more profound change (Bennett-Levy et al., 2004). To give one example, hypersomnia patients typically believe that the only way they can feel less tired is to try to sleep more. *Telling* them that being active can generate energy is less effective than setting up an experience that allows them to *experience* the energy-generating effects of activity. Here is a brief description of a behavioral experiment we recently conducted with a hypersomnia patient to provide them with *experience*. Over two days the patient tested his belief that the only way to get energy is to keep sleeping or go back to sleep. On the first day he spent one 3-hour block *conserving* energy (e.g., sleeping in each morning, going back to bed, when out of bed attempting only mundane tasks) and then a 3-hour block *using* energy (e.g., taking a 10-minute walk, arranging to see a friend). The following day he did this in the reverse order. Contrary to his beliefs, his mood and energy were *improved* by "using" energy. As a result of this experiment, "using" energy became synonymous with "generating" energy and this became one strategy for managing daytime tiredness. There are many behavioral experiments already developed for treating sleep (Ree & Harvey, 2004), with much room for further innovation.

8. Unhelpful Beliefs about Sleep. Holding dysfunctional beliefs about sleep is an important maintainer of insomnia in adults (Edinger, Wohlgemuth,

Radtke, Marsh, & Quillian, 2001). In our clinical work with youth it has become clear that altering beliefs about the sleep–wake cycle is important for reducing sleep disturbance. Typical unhelpful beliefs about sleep held by youth include: "there is no point going to bed earlier because I won't be able to fall asleep," "sleep is a waste of time," "sleep is boring," and "getting more sleep doesn't help me." Hence, we suggest that including a module to target such beliefs will be important. The intervention for dysfunctional beliefs typically involves a 4-step process: (a) identification of dysfunctional beliefs; (b) use of guided discovery and Socratic questioning to challenge the beliefs; (c) individualized experiments to test the validity and utility of dysfunctional beliefs and to collect data on new beliefs; and (d) the identification and dropping of safety behaviors that prevent disconfirmation of dysfunctional beliefs. The foundation of this module is manualized (Harvey, 2005a; Ree & Harvey, 2004). Adaptations for adolescents include several vignettes of youth describing their sleep problems and the unrealistic beliefs that maintain them; youth are asked to identify the beliefs and generate realistic alternative thoughts.

9. Bedtime Worry, Rumination, and Vigilance. Youth with a mood disorder often attribute difficulty getting to sleep to excessive negative (worry/rumination) and positive cognitive activity (Harvey, Schmidt, Scarna, Semler, & Goodwin, 2005). As anxiety (Espie, 2002) and cognitive activity (Harvey, 2005b) are antithetical to sleep onset, it will be important to include a module to help the young person manage bedtime worry, rumination, and anxiety. This intervention includes Beckian cognitive therapy to teach methods to assist the patient to evaluate worry and rumination, diary writing or scheduling a "worry period" to encourage the processing of worries several hours prior to bedtime, creating a "to do" list prior to getting into bed to reduce worry about future plans/events, training to disengage from pre-sleep worry, use of savoring to redirect attention to pleasant (distracting) imagery, and/or demonstrating the adverse consequences of thought suppression while in bed, and scheduling a pre-sleep "wind-down" period prior to bedtime to promote disengagement from daytime concerns. The foundation of this module is already manualized (Harvey, 2005a; Morin & Espie, 2003).

10. Relapse Prevention. The goal is to consolidate and maximize maintenance of gains and to set the young person and his or her parent(s) on a trajectory for continued improvement. It is guided by an individualized summary of learning and achievements. Areas needing further intervention are addressed by setting specific goals and creating a specific plan for achieving each goal. The overarching aim of this relapse prevention module is to ensure progress continues into the future.

Finally, it is often necessary to highlight that different behavioral strategies may be needed for the current sleep problem versus other sleep problems that have been experienced in the past and will possibly be experienced again in the future (e.g., hypersomnia, reduced sleep need, delayed phase). Hence, we seek to adapt each sleep principle for current sleep problems as well as other sleep problems that may emerge. By the end of treatment we aim to have a well developed decision tree and menu of options for managing sleep problems. This is particularly pertinent for mood disorders.

Summary and Conclusion

Sleep disturbance in youth with a mood disorder is critically important, yet surprisingly understudied. We have reviewed evidence on the prevalence and nature of sleep disturbance in youth with depressive and bipolar disorders. Evidence pointing to the importance of sleep includes that sleep disturbance *(1)* appears to be an early marker; *(2)* is a distinguishing feature; *(3)* contributes to relapse, affect dysregulation, and deficits in cognitive functioning; and *(4)* may also contribute to weight problems, comorbid substance use problems, and suicide. The implications for intervention are explained and a multicomponent sleep intervention is outlined. At a simple pragmatic level, one can make a compelling argument for the advantages of implementing cognitive and behavioral interventions to improve sleep and regularize sleep/wake schedules in ways that are likely to have a positive impact on mental and physical health (and affect regulation) in youth with a mood disorder. At a scientific level, there is an equally compelling case regarding the potential advances for mechanistic understanding of the interactions between sleep and affect regulation in the mood disorders. Clearly, there is an urgent need for research to delineate the specific genetic, neurobiological, and psychosocial contributors to sleep disturbance in youth.

Future Directions

- While an initial multicomponent treatment approach is presented, future research is needed to evaluate efficacy and effectiveness.
- Treatment "experiments" to determine which components within the multicomponent package

are effective is one pathway toward developing a more efficient approach.

• Treatment adaptations for younger children and for the various sleep problems will be needed.

• Given that mood disorders and sleep problems appear to be bidirectionally and mutually maintaining, it is important to determine whether the treatment approach should be sequential (i.e., treat the depression then insomnia or insomnia then depression) versus interwoven (i.e., 25 minutes of each therapy session for targeting the insomnia, 25 minutes of each therapy session targeting the depression).

• The impact of treating or preventing sleep problems in the mood disorders on mood, cognition, and health should be determined.

References

American Psychiatric Association. (2000). *Diagnostic and Statistical Manual of Mental Disorders (4th Edition, Text revision)*. Washington, DC: American Psychiatric Association.

Angold, A., & Rutter, M. (1992). The effects of age and pubertal status on depression in a large clinical sample. *Development and Psychopathology, 4*, 5–28.

Axelson, D., Birmaher, B., Strober, M., Gill, M. K., Valeri, S., Chiappetta, L., et al. (2006). Phenomenology of children and adolescents with bipolar spectrum disorders. *Archives of General Psychiatry, 63*, 1139–1148.

Axelsson, J., Sundelin, T., Ingre, M., Van Someren, E. J., Olsson, A., & Lekander, M. (2010). Beauty sleep: Experimental study on the perceived health and attractiveness of sleep deprived people. *British Medical Journal, 341*, c6614.

Belfer, M. L. (2008). Child and adolescent mental disorders: The magnitude of the problem across the globe. *Journal of Child Psychology and Psychiatry, 49*, 226–236.

Bellivier, F., Golmard, J.-L., Henry, C., & Leboyer, M. (2001). Admixture analysis of age at onset in bipolar I affective disorder. *Archives of General Psychiatry, 58*, 510–512.

Bennett-Levy J. B. G., Fennell, M., Hackmann, A., Mueller, M., & Westbrook, D. (2004). *The Oxford Handbook of Behavioural Experiments*. Oxford: Oxford University Press.

Biederman, J., Faraone, S. V., Wozniak, J., Mick, E., Kwon, A., & Megan, A. (2004). Further evidence of unique development phenotypic correlates of pediatric bipolar disorder: Findings from a large sample of clinically referred preadolescent children assessed over the last 7 years. *Journal of Affective Disorders, 82*(Suppl1), S45–S58.

Birmaher, B., Ryan, N. D., Williamson, D. E., Brent, D. A., Kaufman, J., Dahl, R. E., et al. (1996). Childhood and adolescent depression: A review of the past 10 years. Part I. *Journal of the American Academy of Child and Adolescent Psychiatry, 35*, 1427–1439.

Bootzin, R. R. (1972). Stimulus control treatment for insomnia. *Proceedings of the American Psychological Association, 7*, 395–396.

Bootzin, R. R., & Stevens, S. J. (2005). Adolescents, substance abuse, and the treatment of insomnia and daytime sleepiness. *Clinical Psychology Review, 25*, 629–644.

Brent, D. A., Perper, J. A., Goldstein, C. E., Kolko, D. J., Allan, M. J., Allman, C. J., et al. (1988). Risk factors for adolescent suicide. A comparison of adolescent suicide victims with suicidal inpatients. *Archives of General Psychiatry, 45*, 581–588.

Brent, D. A. (1993). Depression and suicide in children and adolescents. *Pediatric Review, 14*, 380–388.

Brunello, N., Armitage, R., Feinberg, I., Holsboer-Traschler, E., Leger, D., Linkowiski, P., et al. (2000). Depression and sleep disorders: Clinical relevance, economic burden and pharmacological treatment. *Neuropsychobiology, 42*, 107–119.

Caci, H., Bouchez, J., & Bayle, F. J. (2009). Inattentive symptoms of ADHD are related to evening orientation. *Journal of Attention Disorders, 13*, 36–41.

Cain, N., Gradisar, M., & Moseley, L. (2011). A motivational school-based intervention for adolescent sleep problems. *Sleep Medicine, 12*, 246–251.

Cappuccio, F. P., Taggart, F. M., Kandala, N. B., Currie, A., Peile, E., Stranges, S., et al. (2008). Meta-analysis of short sleep duration and obesity in children and adults. *Sleep, 31*, 619–626.

Carskadon, M. A. (2002). *Adolescent Sleep Patterns Biological, Social, and Psychological Influences*. Cambridge: Cambridge University Press.

Carskadon, M. A., Acebo, C., & Jenni, O. G. (2004). Regulation of adolescent sleep: Implications for behavior. In R. E. Dahl & L. P. Spear (Eds.), *Adolescent Brain Development Vulnerabilities and Opportunities* (Vol. 1021, pp. 276–291). New York: Annals of the New York Academy of Sciences.

Carskadon, M. A., Mindell, J. A., & Drake, C. (2006). *Sleep in America Poll*. The National Sleep Foundation.

Cartwright, R., Luten, A., Young, M., Mercer, P., & Bears, M. (1998). Role of REM sleep and dream affect in overnight mood regulation: A study of normal volunteers. *Psychiatry Research, 81*, 1–8.

Chelminski, I., Ferraro, F. R., Petros, T. V., & Plaud, J. J. (1999). An analysis of the "eveningness–morningness" dimension in "depressive" college students. *Journal of Affective Disorders, 52*, 19–29.

Choquet, M., & Menke, H. (1989). Suicidal thoughts during early adolescence: Prevalence, associated troubles, and help-seeking behavior, 81, 170–177. *Acta Psychiatrica Scandinavia (Suppl), 81*, 170–177.

Choquet, M., Kovess, V., & Poutignat, N. (1993). Suicidal thoughts among adolescents: An intercultural approach. *Adolescence, 28*, 649–659.

Clarke, G., & Harvey, A. G. (2012). The complex role of sleep in adolescent depression. *Child and Adolescent Psychiatric Clinics of North America, 21*(2): 385–400.

Colombo, C., Benedetti, F., Barbini, B., Campori, E., & Smeraldi, E. (1999). Rate of switch from depression into mania after therapeutic sleep deprivation in bipolar depression. *Psychiatry Research, 86*, 267–270.

Costello, J., Foley, D., & Adrian, A. (2006). 10-year research update: The epidemiology of child and adolescent psychiatric disorders: II. Developmental epidemiology. *Journal of the American Academy of Child and Adolescent Psychiatry, 45*, 8–25.

Craighead, W. E., Miklowitz, D. J., Frank, E., & Vajk, F. C. (2002). Psychosocial treatments for bipolar disorder. In P. E. Nathan & J. M. Gorman (Eds.), *A Guide to Treatments that Work* (2nd ed., pp. 263–275). London: Oxford University Press.

Dahl , R. E., Puig-Antich, J., Ryan, N. D., Nelson, B., Dachille, S., Cunningham, S. L., et al. (1990). EEG sleep in adolescents with major depression: The role of suicidality and inpatient status. *Journal of Affective Disorders, 19*, 63–75.

Dahl, R. E., & Harvey, A. G. (2007). Sleep in children and adolescents with psychiatric or emotional disorders. *Sleep Medicine Clinics, 2,* 501–511.
Dickstein, D. P., Treland, J. E., Snow, J., McClure, E. B., Mehta, M. S., Towbin, K. E., et al. (2004). Neuropsychological performance in pediatric bipolar disorder. *Biological Psychiatry, 55*(1), 32–39.
Doyle, A. E., Wilens, T. E., Kwon, A., Seidman, L. J., Faraone, S. V., Fried, R., et al. (2005). Neuropsychological functioning in youth with bipolar disorder. *Biologial Psychiatry, 58,* 540–548.
Duffy, A., Alda, M., Crawford, L., Milin, R., & Grof, P. (2007). The early manifestations of bipolar disorder: A longitudinal prospective study of the offspring of bipolar parents. *Bipolar Disorders, 9,* 828–838.
Edinger, J. D., Wohlgemuth, W. K., Radtke, R. A., Marsh, G. R., & Quillian, R. E. (2001). Does cognitive-behavioral insomnia therapy alter dysfunctional beliefs about sleep? *Sleep, 24,* 591–599.
Ehlers, C. L., Kupfer, D. J., Frank, E., & Monk, T. H. (1993). Biological rhythms and depression: The role of zeitgebers and zeitstorers. *Depression, 1,* 285–293.
Elmslie, J. L., Silverstone, J. T., Mann, J. I., Williams, S. M., & Romans, S. E. (2000). Prevalence of overweight and obesity in bipolar patients. *Journal of Clinical Psychiatry, 61,* 179–184.
Emslie, G. J., Armitage, R., Weinberg, W. A., Rush, A. J., Mayes, T. L., & Hoffmann, R. F. (2001). Sleep polysomnography as a predictor of recurrence in children and adolescents with major depressive disorder. *International Journal of Neuropsychopharmacology, 4*(2), 159–168.
Espie, C. A. (2002). Insomnia: Conceptual issues in the development, persistence, and treatment of sleep disorder in adults. *Annual Review of Psychology, 53,* 215–243.
Faedda, G. L., Baldessarini, R. J., Glovinsky, I. P., & Austin, N. B. (2004a). Pediatric bipolar disorder: phenomenology and course of illness. *Bipolar Disorders, 6,* 305–313.
Faedda, G. L., Baldessarini, R. J., Glovinsky, I. P., & Austin, N. B. (2004b). Pediatric bipolar disorder: Phenomenology and course of illness. *Bipolar Disorders, 6,* 305–313.
Ford, D. E., & Kamerow, D. B. (1989). Epidemiologic study of sleep disturbances and psychiatric disorders. An opportunity for prevention? *Journal of the American Medical Association, 262,* 1479–1484.
Frank, E., Swartz, H. A., & Kupfer, D. J. (2000). Interpersonal and social rhythm therapy: Managing the chaos of bipolar disorder. *Biological Psychiatry, 48,* 593–604.
Frank, E., Kupfer, D. J., Thase, M. E., Mallinger, A., Swartz, H., Fagioli, A., et al. (2005). Two year outcomes for interpersonal and social rhythm therapy in individuals with bipolar I disorder. *Archives of General Psychiatry, 62,* 996–1004.
Gaspar-Barba, E., Calati, R., Cruz-Fuentes, C. S., Ontiveros-Uribe, M. P., Natale, V., De Ronchi, D., et al. (2009). Depressive symptomatology is influenced by chronotypes. *Journal of Affective Disorders, 119,* 100–106.
Gasquet, I., & Choquet, M. (1994). Hospitalization in a pediatric ward of adolescent suicide attempters admitted to general hospitals. *Journal of Adolescent Health, 15,* 416–422.
Gau, S. S., Shang, C. Y., Merikangas, K. R., Chiu, Y. N., Soong, W. T., & Cheng, A. T. (2007). Association between morningness-eveningness and behavioral/emotional problems among adolescents. *Journal of Biological Rhythms, 22,* 268–274.
Geller, B., Williams, M., Zimmerman, B., Frazier, J., Beringer, L., & Warner, K. L. (1998). Prepubertal and early adolescent bipolarity differentiate from ADHD by manic symptoms, grandiose delusions, ultra-rapid or ultradian cycling. *Journal of Affective Disorders, 51,* 81–91.
Geller, B., Zimerman, B., Williams, M., Delbello, M. P., Bolhofner, K., Craney, J. L., et al. (2002). DSM-IV mania symptoms in a prepubertal and early adolescent bipolar disorder phenotype compared to attention-deficit hyperactive and normal controls. *Journal of Child and Adolescent Psychopharmacology, 12,* 11–25.
Geller, B., Zimmerman, B., Williams, M., DelBello, M. P., Frazier, J., & Beringer, L. (2002). Phenomenology of prepubertal and early adolescent bipolar disorder: Examples of elated mood, grandiose behaviors, decreased need for sleep, racing thoughts and hypersexuality. *Journal of Child and Adolescent Psychopharmacology, 12,* 3–9.
Geller, B., Craney, J. L., Bolhofner, K., DelBello, M. P., Axelson, D., Luby, J., et al. (2003). Phenomenology and longitudinal course of children with a prepubertal and early adolescent bipolar disorder phenotype. In B. Geller & M. P. DelBello (Eds.), *Bipolar Disorder in Childhood and Early Adolescence* (pp. 25–50). New York: Guilford.
Goldstein, T. R., Bridge, J. A., & Brent, D. A. (2008). Sleep disturbance preceding completed suicide in adolescents. *Journal of Consulting and Clinical Psychology, 76,* 84–91.
Gradisar, M., Dohnt, H., Gardner, G., Paine, S., Starkey, K., Menne, A., et al. (2011). A randomized controlled trial of cognitive-behavior therapy plus bright light therapy for adolescent delayed sleep phase disorder. *Sleep, 34*(12), 1671–1680.
Gregory, A. M., Caspi, A., Eley, T. C., Moffitt, T. E., Oconnor, T. G., & Poulton, R. (2005). Prospective longitudinal associations between persistent sleep problems in childhood and anxiety and depression disorders in adulthood. *Journal of Abnormal Child Psychology, 33*(2), 157–163.
Gregory, A. M., Caspi, A., Moffitt, T. E., & Poulton, R. (2009). Sleep problems in childhood predict neuropsychological functioning in adolescence. *Pediatrics, 123,* 1171.
Hansen, M., Janssen, I., Schiff, A., Zee, P. C., & Dubocovich, M. L. (2005). The impact of school daily schedule on adolescent sleep. *Pediatrics, 115,* 1555–1561.
Harvey, A. G. (2001a). Insomnia: Symptom or diagnosis? *Clinical Psychology Review, 21,* 1037–1059.
Harvey, A. G., & Payne, S. (2002). The management of unwanted pre-sleep thoughts in insomnia: Distraction with imagery versus general distraction. *Behaviour Research and Therapy, 40,* 267–277.
Harvey, A. G., Schmidt, D. A., Scarna, A., Semler, C. N., & Goodwin, G. M. (2005). Sleep-related functioning in euthymic patients with bipolar disorder, patients with insomnia, and subjects without sleep problems. *American Journal of Psychiatry, 162,* 50–57.
Harvey, A. G. (2005a). A cognitive theory of and therapy for chronic insomnia. *Journal of Cognitive Psychotherapy, An International Quarterly, 19,* 41–60.
Harvey, A. G. (2005b). Unwanted intrusive thoughts in insomnia. In D. A. Clark (Ed.), *Intrusive Thoughts in Clinical Disorders: Theory, Research, and Treatment* (pp. 86–118). New York: Guilford Press.
Harvey, A. G., Mullin, B. C., & Hinshaw, S. P. (2006). Sleep and circadian rhythms in children and adolescents with bipolar disorder. *Development and Psychopathology, 18,* 1147–1168.
Harvey, A. G. (2008a). Insomnia, psychiatric disorders, and the transdiagnostic perspective. *Current Directions in Psychological Science, 17,* 299–303.

Harvey, A. G. (2008b). Sleep and circadian rhythms in bipolar disorder: Seeking synchrony, harmony, and regulation. *American Journal of Psychiatry, 165,* 820–829.

Harvey, A. G., Talbot, L. S., & Gershon, A. (2009). Sleep disturbance in bipolar disorder across the lifespan. *Clinical Psychology: Science and Practice, 16,* 256–277.

Harvey, A. G., & Tang, N. K. Y. (2012). (Mis)perception of sleep in insomnia: A puzzle and a resolution. *Psychological Bulletin, 138,* 77–101.

Haynes, P. L., Bootzin, R. R., Smith, L., Cousins, J., Cameron, M., & Stevens, S. (2006). Sleep and aggression in substance-abusing adolescents: Results from an integrative behavioral sleep-treatment pilot program. *Sleep, 29,* 512–520.

Holtmann, M., Bolte, S., Goth, K., Dopfner, M., Pluck, J., Huss, M., et al. (2007). Prevalence of the Child Behavior Checklist-pediatric bipolar disorder phenotype in a German general population sample. *Bipolar Disorders, 9,* 895–900.

Hyman, S. E. (2000). Goals for research on bipolar disorder: The view from NIMH. *Biological Psychiatry, 48,* 436–441.

Ivanenko, A., McLaughlin Crabtreec, V., & Gozald, D. (2005). Sleep and depression in children and adolescents. *Sleep Medicine Reviews, 9*(2), 115–129.

Jackson, A., Cavanagh, J., & Scott, J. (2003). A systematic review of manic and depressive prodromes. *Journal of Affective Disorders, 74,* 209–217.

Jaycox, L. H., Asarnow, J. R., Sherbourne, C. D., Rea, M. M., LaBorde, A. P., & Wells, K. B. (2006). Adolescent primary care patients' preferences for depression treatment. *Administrative Policy and Mental Health, 33*(2), 198–207.

Johnson, E. O., Breslau, N., Roehrs, T., & Roth, T. (1999). Insomnia in adolescence: Epidemiology and associate problems. *Sleep, 22*(S1), S22.

Johnson, E. O., Roth, T., & Breslau, N. (2006). The association of insomnia with anxiety disorders and depression: exploration of the direction of risk. *Journal of Psychiatric Research, 40*(8), 700–708.

Johnson, S. L. (2005). Mania and dysregulation in goal pursuit: A review. *Clinical Psychology Review, 25,* 241–262.

Jolin, E. M., Weller, E. B., & Weller, R. A. (2007). The public health aspects of bipolar disorder in children and adolescents. *Current Psychiatry Reports, 9,* 106–113.

Jones , S. H., Tai, S., Evershed, K., Knowles, R., & Bentall, R. (2006). Early detection of bipolar disorder: A pilot familial high-risk study of parents with bipolar disorder and their adolescent children. *Bipolar Disorders, 8,* 362–372.

Kaplan, K. A., & Harvey, A. G. (2009). Hypersomnia across mood disorders: A review and synthesis. *Sleep Medicine Reviews, 13*(4), 275–285.

Kitamura, S., Hida, A., Watanabe, M., Enomoto, M., Aritake-Okada, S., Moriguchi, Y., et al. (2010). Evening preference is related to the incidence of depressive states independent of sleep-wake conditions. *Chronobiology International, 27,* 1797–1812.

Klein, N. K., Schatzberg, A. F., McCullough, J. P., Dowling, F., Goodman, D., Howland, R. H., et al. (1999). Age of onset in chronic major depression: Relation to demographic and clinical variables, family history, and treatment response. *Journal of Affective Disorders, 55,* 149–157.

Kovacs, M., Fienberg, T. L., Crouse-Novak, M. A., Paulaukas, S. T., & Finkelstein, R. (1984a). Depressive disorders in childhood. I. A longitudinal prospective study of characteristics and recovery. *Archives of General Psychiatry, 41,* 229–237.

Kovacs, M., Fienberg, T. L., Crouse-Novak, M. A., Paulaukas, S. T., & Finkelstein, R. (1984b). Depressive disorders in childhood. II. A longitudinal study of the risk for a subsequent major depression. *Archives of General Psychiatry, 41,* 643–649.

Kowatch, R. A., Youngstrom, E. A., Danielyan, A., & Findling, R. L. (2005). Review and meta-analysis of the phenomenology and clinical characteristics of mania in children and adolescents. *Bipolar Disorders, 7*(6), 483–496.

Krishnan, K. R. R. (2005). Psychiatric and medical comorbidity of bipolar disorder. *Psychosomatic Medicine, 67,* 1–8.

Kupfer, D. J., Himmelhoch, J. M., Swartzburgh, M., Anderson, C., Byck, R., & Detre, T. P. (1972). Hypersomnia in manic-depressive disease: A preliminary report. *Diseases of the Nervous System,* 720–724.

Kupfer, D. J. (1995). Sleep research in depressive illness: Clinical implications—a tasting menu. *Biological Psychiatry, 38*(6), 391–403.

Lam, D., & Wong, G. (2005). Prodromes, coping strategies and psychological interventions in bipolar disorders. *Clinical Psychology Review. Special Issue: The Psychology of Bipolar Disorder, 25,* 1028–1042.

Lam, D. H., Watkins, E. R., Hayward, P., Bright, J., Wright, K., Kerr, N., et al. (2003). A randomized controlled study of cognitive therapy for relapse prevention for bipolar affective disorder: Outcome of the first year. *Archives of General Psychiatry, 60,* 145–152.

Lam, D. H., Hayward, P., Watkins, E. R., Wright, K., & Sham, P. (2005). Relapse prevention in patients with bipolar disorder: Cognitive therapy outcome after 2 years. *American Journal of Psychiatry, 162,* 324–329.

Lee, T. M., Hummer, D. L., Jechura, T. J., & Mahoney, M. M. (2004). Pubertal development of sex differences in circadian function: An animal model. *Annals of the New York Academy of Science, 1021,* 262–275.

Leotta, C., Carskadon, M. A., Acebo, C., Seifer, R., & Quinn, B. (1997). Effects of acute sleep restriction on affective response in adolescents: Preliminary results. *Sleep Research, 26,* 201.

Lewinsohn, P. M., Hops, H., Roberts, R. E., Seeley, J. R., & Andrews, J. A. (1993). Adolescent psychopathology: I. Prevalence and incidence of depression and other DSM-III-R disorders in high school students. *Journal of Abnormal Psychology, 102,* 133–144.

Lewinsohn, P. M., Klein, D. N., & Seeley, J. R. (1995). Bipolar disorders in a community sample of older adolescents: Prevalence, phenomenology, comorbidity, and course. *Journal of the American Academy of Child and Adolescent Psychiatry, 34,* 454–463.

Liu, X., & Buysse, D. J. (2006). Sleep and youth suicidal behavior: A neglected field. *Current Opinion in Psychiatry, 19,* 288–293.

Liu, X., Buysse, D., Gentzler, A. L., Kiss, E., Mayer, L., Kapomai, K., et al. (2007). Insomnia and hypersomnia associated with depressive phenomenology and comorbidity in childhood depression. *Sleep, 30,* 83–90.

Lofthouse, N., Fristad, M., Splaingard, M., & Kelleher, K. (2007). Parent and child reports of sleep problems associated with early-onset bipolar spectrum disorders. *Journal of Family Psychology, 21,* 114–123.

Manber, R., Edinger, J. D., Gress, J. L., San Pedro-Salcedo, M. G., Kuo, T. F., & Kalista, T. (2008). Cognitive behavioral therapy for insomnia enhances depression outcome in patients with comorbid major depressive disorder and insomnia. *Sleep, 31,* 489–495.

McCrae, C. S., & Lichstein, K. L. (2001). Secondary insomnia: Diagnostic challenges and intervention opportunities. *Sleep Medicine Reviews, 5,* 47–61.

McGlinchey, E. L., Talbot, L. S., Chang, K. H., Kaplan, K. A., Dahl, R. E., & Harvey, A. G. (2011). The effect of sleep deprivation on vocal expression of emotion in adolescents and adults. *Sleep, 34*, 1233–1241.

McMakin, D. L., Siegle, G. J., & Shirk, S. R. (2011). Positive affect stimulation and sustainment (PASS) module for depressed mood: A preliminary investigation of treatment-related effects. *Cognitive Therapy and Research, 35*, 217–226.

Mehl, R. C., O'Brien, L. M., Jones, J. H., Dreisbach, J. K., Mervis, C. B., & Gozal, D. (2006). Correlates of sleep and pediatric bipolar disorder. *Sleep, 29*, 193–197.

Miklowitz, D. J., & Goldstein, M. J. (1997). *Bipolar Disorder: A family-focused treatment approach.* New York, NY: Guilford Press.

Miklowitz, D. J., Simoneau, T. L., George, E. L., Richards, J. A., Kalbag, A., Sachs-Ericsson, N., et al. (2000). Family-focused treatment of bipolar disorder: 1-year effects of a psychoeducational program in conjunction with pharmacotherapy. *Biological Psychiatry, 48*, 582–592.

Miklowitz, D. J., & Johnson, S. L. (2006). The psychopathology and treatment of bipolar disorder. *Annual Review of Clinical Psychology, 2*, 199–235.

Miller, W. R., Rollnick, S. (2002). *Motivational Interviewing: Preparing People for Change.* New York: Guilford Press.

Morin, C. M., Culbert, J. P., & Schwartz, S. M. (1994). Nonpharmacological Interventions for insomnia: A meta-analysis of treatment efficacy. *American Journal of Psychiatry, 151*, 1172–1180.

Morin, C. M., Hauri, P. J., Espie, C. A., Spielman, A. J., Buysse, D. J., & Bootzin, R. R. (1999). Nonpharmacologic treatment of chronic insomnia. An American Academy of Sleep Medicine review. *Sleep, 22*, 1134–1156.

Morin, C. M., & Espie, C. A. (2003). *Insomnia: A Clinical Guide to Assessment and Treatment.* New York: Kluwer Academic/Plenum Publishers.

Morin, C. M., Bootzin, R. R., Buysse, D. J., Edinger, J., D., Espie, C. A., & Lichstein, K. L. (2006). Psychological and behavioral treatment of insomnia: An update of recent evidence (1998–2004). *Sleep, 29*, 1396–1406.

Murtagh, D. R., & Greenwood, K. M. (1995). Identifying effective psychological treatments for insomnia: A meta-analysis. *Journal of Consulting and Clinical Psychology, 63*, 79–89.

National Sleep Foundation. (2011). 2011 *Sleep in America Poll: Communications Technology and Sleep.* from The Foundation

NIH. (2005). National Institutes of Health State of the Science Conference Statement: Manifestations and management of chronic insomnia in adults. June 13–15, 2005. *Sleep, 28*, 1049–1057.

Ong, S. H., Wickramaratne, P., Tang, M., & Weissman, M. M. (2006). Early childhood sleep and eating problems as predictors of adolescent and adult mood and anxiety disorders. *Journal of Affective Disorders, 96*(1–2), 1–8.

Owens, J. A., Rosen, C. L., & Mindell, J. A. (2003). Medication use in the treatment of pediatric insomnia: Results of a survey of community-based pediatricians. *Pediatrics, 111*(5 Pt 1), 628–635.

Parker, G., Malhi, G. S., Hadzi-Oavlovic, D., & Parker, K. (2006). Sleeping in? The impact of age and depressive sub-type on hypersomnia. *Journal of Affective Disorders, 90*, 73–76.

Patelis-Siotis, I., Young, L. T., Robb, J. C., Marriott, M., Bieling, P. J., Cox, L. C., et al. (2001). Group cognitive behavioral therapy for bipolar disorder: A feasibility and effectiveness study. *Journal of Affective Disorders, 65*, 145–153.

Patten, S. B., Williams, J. V. A., Lavorato, D., Modgill, G., Jette, N., & Eliasziw, M. (2008). Major depression as a risk factor for chronic disease incidence: longitudinal analyses in a general population cohort. *General Hospital Psychiatry, 30*, 407–413.

Perlis, M. L., & Nielsen, T. A. (1993). Mood regulation, dreaming and nightmares: Evaluation of a desensitization function for REM sleep. *Dreaming, 3*, 243–257.

Perlis, M. L., Smith, L. J., Lyness, J. M., Matteson, S. R., Pigeon, W. R., Jungquist, C., et al. (2006). Insomnia as a risk factor for onset of depression in the elderly. *Behavioral Sleep Medicine, 4*, 104–113.

Pilcher, J. J., & Huffcutt, A. I. (1996). Effects of sleep deprivation on performance: A meta-analysis. *Sleep, 19*, 318–326.

Pillai, V., Kalmbach, D. A., & Ciesla, J. A. (2011). A meta-analysis of electroencephalographic sleep in depression: Evidence for genetic biomarkers. *Biological Psychiatry, 70*, 912–919.

Rao, U., Dahl, R. E., Ryan, N. D., Birmaher, B., Williamson, D. E., Rao, R., et al. (2002). Heterogeneity in EEG sleep findings in adolescent depression: Unipolar versus bipolar clinical course. *Journal of Affective Disorders, 70*, 273–280.

Ree, M., & Harvey, A. G. (2004). Insomnia. In J. Bennett-Levy, G. Butler, M. Fennell, A. Hackman, M. Mueller, & D. Westbrook (Eds.), *Oxford Guide to Behavioural Experiments in Cognitive Therapy* (pp. 287–305). Oxford: Oxford University Press.

Reynolds, C. F., & Kupfer, D. J. (1987). Sleep research in affective illness: State of the art circa 1987. *Sleep, 10*(3), 199–215.

Riemann, D., Berger, M., & Voderholzer, U. (2001). Sleep and depression—results from psychobiological studies: An overview. *Biological Psychology, 57*, 67–103.

Roberts, R. E., Roberts, C. R., & Chen, I. G. (2002). Impact of insomnia on future functioning of adolescents. *Journal of Psychosomatic Research, 53*, 561–569.

Schlarb, A., Liddle, C., & Hautzinger, M. (2010). JuSt—a multimodal program for treatment of insomnia in adolescents: a pilot study. *Nature and Science of Sleep, 3*, 13–20.

Seibt, J., Aton, S. J., Jha, S. K., Coleman, T., Dumoulin, M. C., & Frank, M. G. (2008). The non-benzodiazepine hypnotic zolpidem impairs sleep-dependent cortical plasticity. *Sleep, 31*, 1381–1391.

Shaw, J. A., Egeland, J. A., Endicott, J., Allen, C. R., & Hostetter, A. M. (2005). A 10-year prospective study of prodromal patterns for bipolar disorder among Amish youth. *Journal of the American Academy of Child & Adolescent Psychiatry, 44*(11), 1104–1111.

Silk, J., Vanderbilt-Adriance, E., Shaw, D., Forbes, E., Whalen, D., Ryan, N., et al. (2007). Resilience among children and adolescents at risk for depression: Mediation and moderation across social and neurobiological contexts. *Development and Psychopathology, 19*, 841–865.

Smith, M. T., Perlis, M. L., Park, A., Smith, M. S., Pennington, J., Giles, D. E., et al. (2002). Comparative meta-analysis of pharmacotherapy and behavior therapy for persistent insomnia. *American Journal of Psychiatry, 159*, 5–11.

Smith, M. T., Huang, M. I., & Manber, R. (2005). Cognitive behavior therapy for chronic insomnia occurring within the context of medical and psychiatric disorders. *Clinical Psychology Reviews, 25*, 559–592.

Smits, M. G., Nagtegaal, E. E., van der Heijden, J., Coenen, A. M., & Kerkhof, G. A. (2001). Melatonin for chronic sleep onset insomnia in children: A randomized placebo-controlled trial. *Journal of Child Neurology, 16*, 86–92.

Smits, M. G., van Stel, H., van der Heijden, K. B., Meijer, A. M., Coenen, A. M., & Kerkhof, G. A. (2003). Melatonin improves health status and sleep in children with idiopathic sleep onset insomnia. *Journal of the American Academy Child and Adolescent Psychiatry, 42*, 1286–1293.

Spiegel, K., Tasali, E., Penev, P., & Van Cauter, E. (2004). Brief communication: Sleep curtailment in healthy young men is associated with decreased leptin levels, elevated ghrelin levels, and increased hunger and appetite. *Annals of Internal Medicine, 141*, 846–850.

Staton, D. (2008). The impairment of pediatric bipolar sleep: hypotheses regarding a core defect and phenotype-specific sleep disturbances. *Journal of Affective Disorders, 108*(3), 199–206.

Stepanski, E. J., & Wyatt, J. K. (2003). Use of sleep hygiene in the treatment of insomnia. *Sleep Medicine Reviews, 7*, 215–225.

Talbot, L. S., McGlinchey, E. L., Kaplan, K. A., Dahl, R. E., & Harvey, A. G. (2010). Sleep deprivation in adolescents and adults: Changes in affect. *Emotion, 10*(6), 831–841.

Taylor, D. J., Lichenstein, K. L., & Durrence, H. H. (2003). Insomnia as a health risk factor. *Behavioral Sleep Medicine, 1*, 227–247.

Tsai, S.-Y., Lee, J.-C., & Chen, C.-C. (1999). Characteristics and psychosocial problems of patients with bipolar disorder at high risk for suicide attempt. *Journal of Affective Disorders, 52*, 145–152.

Twenge, J. M., & Nolen-Hoeksema, S. (2002). Age, gender, race, socioeconomic status, and birth cohort difference on the children's depression inventory: A meta-analysis. *Journal of Abnormal Psychology, 111*, 578–588.

Tynjala, J., Kannas, L., & Levalahti, E. (1997). Perceived tiredness among adolescents and its association with sleep habits and use of psychoactive substances. *Journal of Sleep Research, 6*, 189–198.

Van Dongen, H. P., Maislin, G., Mullington, J. M., & Dinges, D. F. (2003). The cumulative cost of additional wakefulness: Dose-response effects on neurobehavioral functions and sleep physiology from chronic sleep restriction and total sleep deprivation. *Sleep, 26*, 117–126.

Walker, M. P., & Stickgold, R. (2006). Sleep, memory, and plasticity. *Annual Reviews in Psychology, 57*, 139–166.

Wehr , T. A., Goodwin, F. K., Wirz-Justice, A., Breitmaier, J., & Craig, C. (1982). 48-hour sleep-wake cycles in manic-depressive illness: Naturalistic observations and sleep deprivation experiments. *Archives of General Psychiatry, 39*, 559–565.

Wehr, T. A., Sack, D. A., & Rosenthal, N. E. (1987). Sleep reduction as a final common pathway in the genesis of mania. *American Journal of Psychiatry, 144*, 201–204.

Weiss, M. D., Wasdell, M. B., Bomben, M. M., Rea, K. J., & Freeman, M. D. (2006). Sleep hygiene and melatonin treatment for children and adolescents with ADHD and initial insomnia. *Journal of the American Academy Child and Adolescent Psychiatry, 45*, 512–518.

Whooley, M. A., de Jonge, P., Vittinghoff, E., Otte, C., Moos, R., Carney, R. M., et al. (2008). Depressive symptoms, health behaviors, and risk of cardiovascular events in patients with coronary heart disease. *Journal of the American Medical Association, 300*, 2379–2388.

Wilens, T. E., Biederman, J., Kwon, A., Ditterline, J., Forkner, P., Moore, H., et al. (2004). Risk of substance use disorders in adolescents with bipolar disorder. *Journal of the American Academy of Child and Adolescent Psychiatry, 43*, 1380–1386.

Wilens, T. E., Biederman, J., Adamson, J. J., Henin, A., Sgambati, S., Gignac, M., et al. (2008). Further evidence of an association between adolescent bipolar disorder with smoking and substance use disorders: A controlled study. *Drug and Alcohol Dependence, 95*, 188–198.

Williamson, D. E., Birmaher, B., Brent, D. A., Balach, L., Dahl, R. E., & Ryan, N. D. (2000). Atypical symptoms of depression in a sample of depressed child and adolescent outpatients. *Journal of the American Academy of Child & Adolescent Psychiatry, 39*(10), 1253–1259.

Yoo, S., Gujar, N., Hu, P., Jolesz, F., & Walker, M. (2007). The human emotional brain without sleep: A prefrontal-amygdala disconnect? *Current Biology, 17*, R877–878.

Zimmermann, U., Kraus, T., Himmerich, H., Schuld, A., & Pollmacher, T. (2003). Epidemiology, implications and mechanisms underlying drug-induced weight gain in psychiatric patients. *Journal of Psychiatric Research, 37*, 193–220.

Zohar, D., Tzischinsky, O., Epsten, R., & Lavie, P. (2005). The effects of sleep loss on medical residents' emotional reactions to work events: A cognitive-energy model. *Sleep, 28*, 47–54.

CHAPTER

36 Substance Use: Caffeine, Alcohol, and Other Drugs

Richard R. Bootzin, Jennifer C. Cousins, Monica R. Kelly, *and* Sally Stevens

Abstract

Sleep plays a central role in physical, emotional, and cognitive development. The increasing exposure to and use of substances has major effects on sleep and thus on development. In this chapter, we review the current status of illicit substance use and abuse in adolescents, the effects of prenatal and postnatal exposure and use of substances on the sleep of infants, children, and adolescents, the effect of disturbed sleep on subsequent substance use, and the effect of substance use and disturbed sleep on mental health. Expanded attention is given to substances that are widely available to adolescents including caffeine, nicotine, alcohol, and marijuana. The chapter concludes with a description of a successful demonstration project in which sleep disturbances in adolescents with a substance abuse history were treated.

Key Words: substance use, substance abuse, prenatal exposure, sleep disturbance, insomnia, cognitive behavioral therapy, caffeine, nicotine, alcohol, marijuana

There has been an expanding adult literature on the effects of substance use and abuse on sleep and circadian rhythms (e.g., see reviews by Hasler, Smith, Cousins, & Bootzin, 2012; Roehrs & Roth, 2011). In this chapter we will review the literature for infants, children, and adolescents of both the effects of substance use on sleep and the effect of disturbed sleep on subsequent substance use (see Bootzin & Stevens, 2005, for an earlier review). We will give expanded attention to caffeine, nicotine, alcohol, and marijuana, as these are substances commonly available to adolescents.

Illicit Substance Use and Abuse in Adolescents

Before discussing the bidirectional effects of substance use on sleep and vice versa, it will be helpful to examine the extent to which substance abuse is a current problem among adolescents. Recent data from the 2011 *Monitoring the Future* study (Johnston, O'Malley, Bachman, & Schulenberg, 2012), a large longitudinal study that included 46,700 students in 8th, 10th, and 12th grades in 400 schools nationwide, indicates that while alcohol use among adolescents generally decreased in recent years, marijuana use has increased. During the prior 3 years marijuana use increased for all three grades surveyed, resulting in a total of 6.6% of adolescent marijuana users reporting daily use—the highest percent since 1981 (Johnston, et al., 2012). Use of illegal drugs other than marijuana had gradually declined since 2001, but there have been only slight or no declines since 2009 (Johnston, et al., 2012).

In 2011, 15.2% of high school seniors used prescription drugs for nonmedical purposes in the past year. Data indicate that the most commonly abused prescription drugs by adolescents were Vicodin, a brand name pharmaceutical pain reliever, and Adderall, a brand name pharmaceutical psychostimulant typically used to treat attention-deficit/hyperactivity disorder (ADHD; National Institute on Drug Abuse, 2012). Illicit use of psychostimulants is of particular concern given the recent increase in abuse by both high school and college students (Clegg-Kraynok, McBean, & Montgomery-Downs, 2011; National Institute of Mental Health, 2011). Use of psychostimulants has numerous negative side effects, including effects on sleep. Research indicates that college students who use psychostimulants more frequently engage in additional risk behaviors, such as the use of other illicit substances (McCabe, Knight, Teter, & Wechsler, 2005) and report worse subjective sleep quality and more sleep disturbance (Clegg-Kraynok, McBean, & Montgomery-Downs, 2011).

Data from adolescents entering substance abuse treatment programs indicate that youth are predominately marijuana and alcohol users, although a substantial percentage of youth entering inpatient treatment centers are being treated for harder drugs (Dennis, Muck, Dawud-Noursi, & McDermeit, 2003). This trend has continued for the past decade. Treatment entry data continues to show that marijuana is the primary substance for which adolescents enter treatment. In 2005, on any given day 68% of adolescents age 12 to 17 admitted to treatment presented with marijuana as the primary substance of abuse (Substance Abuse and Mental Health Services Administration, 2007), and in 2009 this percent increased slightly to 70% for 12- to 14-year-olds and 72% for those 15 to 17 years of age. However, adolescents entering inpatient treatment continue to report higher rates of harder drug use, including both heroin and nonmedical use of prescription opioids, along with higher rates of substance abuse disorders and dependency (Fishman, Winstanley, Curren, Garrett & Subramaniam, 2010; Stevens, 2004).

The younger the person is at drug use onset, the more likely he or she is to develop a substance use disorder and to have the disorder continue into adulthood (Dennis, et al., 2003). In fact, the risk of addiction goes up to about one in six among those who start using as adolescents, and upwards of 25%–50% for daily users (National Institute on Drug Abuse, 2011).

With regard to sex differences in adolescent substance use, data from *Monitoring the Future* (Johnston et al., 2012) indicates that among 12th-grade students, males are more likely to use most illicit drugs and with higher frequency levels. In 2010, daily marijuana use was 8.8% for males compared to 3.6% for females. Recent research indicates differences in reasons, motivation, use, and consequences of use between male and female substance users (Walitzer & Dearing, 2006; Stevens, 2006; Stevens, Andrade & Ruiz, 2009) and there is some evidence of a faster transition from marijuana initiation to regular use in females when compared to males (Schepis et al., 2011).

Substance abuse treatment outcomes for adolescents have generally demonstrated reductions in use following treatment exposure (Dennis et al., 2003; Hser et al., 2001). Recent outcome data supports earlier findings. Those who remain in treatment show greater positive outcomes (Austin & Wagner, 2010; Stevens, Schwebel & Ruiz, 2007; White & McLellan, 2008). In addition, for those who have completed substance abuse treatment, engagement in continuing care is important. As noted by Ruiz, Korchmaros, Greene, and Hedges (2011) and Scott and Dennis (2009), each continuing care session counts; the greater the engagement in continuing care the less likelihood of relapse to substance use.

The outcomes from treatment of substance abuse in adolescents are important to consider when developing treatments for sleep disturbances in those with a substance abuse history. The next two sections will focus on issues of risk and resilience by examining the reciprocal effects of substances on sleep and of disturbed sleep on the development of substance abuse.

Effects of Substances on the Sleep of Children and Adolescents

In this section we will discuss the effects that different substances have on sleep and sleepiness with a focus on caffeine, nicotine, alcohol, and marijuana.

Caffeine

We are in an era of new and seemingly endless and exciting energy-boosting drink options that are targeted directly to youth populations. Consequently, it should be no surprise that children and adolescents are the fastest growing population of caffeine users with an estimated 75% of adolescents using caffeine daily (National Sleep Foundation, 2006). According to self-report evaluations, energy drinks are consumed by 30% to 50% of adolescents and young adults in the United States (Seifert, Schaechter, Hershorin, & Lipshultz, 2011). Caffeine is the most readily available and commonly consumed psychoactive substance throughout the world. It is considered a stimulant, as it has arousal effects on the central and peripheral nervous system (Roehrs & Roth, 2008). Caffeine is an antagonist for adenosine receptors, and the blockade of these receptors is related to caffeine's stimulating effects. Thus, adenosine promotes sleep and when caffeine blocks adenosine, sleep disruptions can occur (Roehrs & Roth, 2008).

In adults, caffeine can have effects that last 6 to 8 hours after consumption; however, this rate is not fully known in children or even adolescents. Many children and adolescents consume caffeine in the afternoon and evenings (Temple, 2009), which is likely to impact their quality of sleep. The primary effect of caffeine is to increase arousal (Temple, 2009), and many people who consume caffeine use it as a means to increase energy and arousal and to combat daytime sleepiness (Temple, 2009; Ludden & Wolfson, 2010). Moderate doses of caffeine (200–300 mg), which is approximately two to three cups of coffee, may produce improved concentration and cognitive performance, increased arousal and energy, as well as good feelings in children and adults (Bernstein et al., 1994; Smit & Rogers; 2000). However, high doses (>400 mg) can produce feelings of anxiety, nausea, and jitteriness (Garrett & Griffiths, 1997). As a reference, a typical soft drink in the United States contains approximately 45 mg of caffeine (Orbeta, Overpeck, Ramcharran, Kogan & Ledsky, 2006)—substantially less than even one cup of coffee. On average in the United States, the caffeine intake is around 60 to 70 mg/day but can extend up to 800 mg/day; most of this is from soft drinks, but the use of energy drinks continues to grow (Seifert, et al., 2011).

Warzak, Evans, Floress, Gross, and Stoolman (2011) found that in a small Canadian sample of children ages 5–12, the younger children ages 5–7 consumed approximately 52 mg of caffeine per day and the older children ages 8–12 consumed approximately 109 mg of caffeine per day. The Canadian guidelines of daily caffeine use are ages 4–6 = 45 mg/day, ages 7–9 = 62 mg/day, and ages 10–12 = 85 mg/day. Although the differences between the average use by age and the Canadian guidelines are relatively small, many children were consuming caffeine at higher than the average levels, and even small differences are likely to add up to significant effects over the long run. There are only a handful of countries that provide caffeine consumption guidelines, and the specificity of the guidelines also varies. The European Union, for example, requires a "high caffeine content" label on energy drinks.

In the United States, if caffeine is considered "food" as it is in soft drinks, the FDA deems it safe and limits the amount of caffeine in soft drinks to 0.02% or 71 mg/12 fluid oz. (Food and Drug Administration, 2013). However, energy drinks have not been monitored as well. Many energy drinks exceed the 0.02% limit and can range from 50 mg to 505 mg of caffeine. Some manufacturers of energy drinks can skirt the limit by using the 1994 Dietary Supplement Health and Education Act, which states that substances that derive from natural sources or herbs, such as guarana, are dietary supplements not psychoactive substances. Currently, the US FDA does not require warning labels or guidelines of proper caffeine use and has not regulated the amount of caffeine in energy drinks (Reissig, Strain, & Griffiths, 2009).

Bernstein, Carroll, Thuras, Cosgrove, and Roth (2002) examined the likelihood of caffeine dependence based on criteria from the DSM-IV in a US adolescent population. They found that adolescents between the ages of 13–17 were consuming 3.2 caffeinated beverages daily (244.4 mg/day). Over 22% of the adolescents met three of the four criteria for substance dependence based on the DSM-IV criteria. Furthermore, those adolescents reporting higher levels of caffeine use were more likely to also use other substances such as marijuana and nicotine. A 1-year follow-up study from the same research group focused on those adolescents who used caffeine indicated that out of 21 adolescents, 23.8% met criteria for caffeine dependence according to the DSM-IV. In addition, similar to adults, adolescents reported withdrawal symptoms that included tiredness, sluggishness, and headaches (Oberstar, Bernstein, & Thuras, 2002). Giannotti, Cortesi, Sebastiani, and Ottaviano (2002) examined circadian preferences in a large sample of Italian high school students. They found that those who described themselves as having evening rather than morning preferences in activities reported more caffeine use, naps, daytime sleepiness, attention problems, and emotional disruptions. Partially, this may be due to those with evening preferences consuming more caffeine later in the day. Further evidence has shown that evening types may display more risk-taking behaviors such as the use of and higher amounts of illegal substances, nicotine, and caffeine compared to morning-types (Negriff, Dorn, Pabst & Susman, 2011; Preckel et al., 2013).

The amount of caffeine consumed on a daily or regular basis appears to have an impact on sleep outcomes. Heavy caffeine use during a particular day was associated with more reports of sleep disturbance that night in an early adolescent population (Pollak & Bright, 2003). High school students who reported high caffeine use from multiple sources (i.e., soda and/or coffee) were more likely to use caffeine earlier in the day, get up early on school days, and report more daytime sleepiness (Ludden & Wolfson, 2010). Orbeta and others (2006) found in a sample of over 4000 adolescents in the United States that a high caffeine intake, greater than one caffeinated beverage daily, was associated with a two-fold increase in difficulty sleeping and more morning tiredness compared to adolescents with very low caffeine use, one or fewer caffeinated beverages a week. A large national Icelandic poll (n = 7377) of 9th- and 10th-graders found that increased caffeine consumption, as measured by types of beverages consumed per day, was associated with greater reports of daytime sleepiness assessed with the Epworth Sleepiness Scale and worse academic achievement scores (James, Kristjansson & Sigfusdottir, 2011).

Furthermore, an inverse relationship was found for caffeine consumption and reported hours of sleep at night. According to the National Sleep Foundation (2006), adolescents who consumed two or more caffeinated beverages per day were more likely to report more sleep disturbance, less sleep time during the week, and more sleepiness than those adolescents who drank less than one caffeinated beverage per day.

COGNITIVE PERFORMANCE

Caffeine is commonly used to boost attention, has been shown to increase cognitive performance in adults in a dose-dependent manner (Smit & Rogers, 2000), and reduce cognitive deficits and spontaneous sleep episodes during extended periods of wakefulness (Wyatt, Cajochen, Ritz-De Cecco, Czeisler, & Dijk, 2004). Less is known, however, about the cognitive effects of caffeine on children and adolescents. Heatherley, Hancock, and Rogers (2006) examined outcomes on a number search cognitive task before and after the administration of 50 mg of caffeine. The sample of 9-11-year-olds was divided into groups based on high and low caffeine use. After one night of abstaining from caffeine, children who were considered habitual or high-dose users performed worse on the task than the low or non–caffeine users prior to caffeine intake. After caffeine intake, the high-dose users had improved performance, but not better than the low-dose or non–caffeine users. In this case, caffeine may have improved performance in the high-caffeine users that was at suboptimal levels due to overnight withdrawal effects.

COMBINED EFFECTS OF CAFFEINE AND TECHNOLOGY

The use of technology in youth populations has increased dramatically (see Gradisar and Short, Chapter 11). For many adolescents there is a constant presence of communication with friends via cell phones, Internet, and social media. These technologies have an impact on sleep and on behaviors that negatively influence sleep. In a sample of United States school children (6–10 years of age), children who consumed caffeinated beverages had an average of 15 minutes less total sleep time during the night. Those children who consumed caffeine and had a TV, computer, and telephone in their bedroom had 45 minutes less total sleep time than children with no technology in their rooms (Calamaro, Yang, Ratcliffe & Chasens, 2012). In a study of adolescents, caffeine consumption combined with technology-related activities, such as watching TV, texting, being on the Internet, and so forth, was associated with a marked increase in reports of falling asleep during school, increased reports of difficulty falling asleep on school nights, and feeling tired as they drove, which is a risk for vehicular accidents (Calamaro, Mason & Ratcliffe, 2009).

CAFFEINE AND MENTAL HEALTH DISORDERS

Mental health disorders such as anxiety and depression often are associated with sleep difficulties in adults and, consequently, disturbed sleep is listed as one of the diagnostic criteria for some mental health disorders (American Psychiatric Association, DSM-IV-TR, 1997). In youth, sleep problems have been found to increase anxiety and depressive symptoms and contribute to further sleep problems (Cousins et al., 2011; Luebbe & Bell, 2009). Children and adolescents with depression may be drawn to caffeine for its uplifting effects (Bernstein, Carroll, Thuras, Cosgrove, & Roth, 2002), but when caffeine is added to the mix it can cause even worse sleep patterns. Whalen and colleagues (2008) examined the effect of caffeine consumption in youth between the ages of 7 and 17, with and without major depressive disorder, on subjective reports of nighttime sleep. The youth with major depressive disorder reported more caffeine use, more feelings of anxiety associated with caffeine use, and more sleep problems compared to healthy controls. Adolescents aged 13–17 with frequent migraines and/or chronic headaches had more sleep problems and depressive symptoms and reported more caffeine use (Pakalnis, Splaingard, Splaingard, Kring, & Colvin, 2009). In addition, increased daily caffeine consumption was positively correlated with reports of morning headache as assessed from the Pediatric Sleep Questionnaire, but not sleep disordered breathing as assessed from the Child Sleep Habits Questionnaire (Pakalnis, et al. 2009).

A particularly vulnerable population for the effects of caffeine may be youth with attention-deficit/hyperactivity disorder (ADHD; see Corkum and Coulombe, Chapter 34,). There are numerous reports that youth with ADHD often report sleep disturbance; however, the data are mixed (Mayes et al., 2009; Owens, 2005). The type and extent of sleep problem may be associated with the subtype of ADHD and the presence of comorbidities rather than just having an ADHD diagnosis (Mayes, et al., 2009). Since the most common method to treat ADHD is with the use of a stimulant, most often methylphenidate and atomoxetine, the effect of caffeine on sleep in this population may compensate for lower levels of arousal and may even enhance cognitive performance compared to youth without ADHD (Walker, Abraham, & Tercyak, 2010). Mayes and colleagues (2009) found that the medicated children from kindergarten to 5th grade with a diagnosis of ADHD had higher total sleep problems at night compared to children who were not being medicated; however, those children who were being medicated tended to have more severe ADHD symptoms, which may be a contributing factor to the sleep disruptions. Barry, Clarke, McCarthy, and colleagues (2012) examined the effect of a single oral dose of caffeine (.9 to 3.2 mg/kg based on weight) on arousal as measured by skin conductance level (SCL) in a controlled double-blind study in children (ages 8–13) with and without a diagnosis for ADHD. The youth with ADHD had a lower SCL across the conditions compared to controls, suggestive of hypoarousal. It was also noted that the increase in arousal induced by caffeine for youth with ADHD was positively related to their Connor's hyperactivity/impulsivity score. A review of recent literature of ADHD and cognitive performance by Leon (2000) found that children with ADHD often show improvements from caffeine on measures of impulsivity, hyperactivity, aggression, cognitive functioning, and adult reports of behavior when compared to no treatment. However, commonly prescribed stimulant medications produced more improvement than caffeine only (Leon, 2000).

The data for the effects of caffeine on sleep disordered breathing is unclear. It has been reported that children with ADHD have a higher apnea/hypopnea index (Huang et al., 2004); however, a nonsignificant relationship has been found for sleep disordered breathing and ADHD symptoms (Melendres, Lutz, Rubin, & Marcus, 2004). In a community sample of over 500 children between the ages of 5 and 8, parent reports of caffeine intake was not associated with excessive daytime sleepiness, a common symptom of sleep disordered breathing. Objective measures of sleep derived from polysomnography were also not associated with excessive daytime sleepiness (Calhoun et al., 2011).

Caffeine can be quite detrimental to sleep in children and adolescents. The studies reviewed have reported negative associations between increased caffeine use and fewer reported hours of sleep at night, reduced sleep quality, increased self-reported sleep problems, difficulty falling asleep, difficulty waking, and more daytime sleepiness. Despite these general findings, there are still research problems to be addressed. For example, there are few studies employing objective measures of sleep or administering or more accurately measuring the amount of caffeine being consumed.

There have been many laboratory studies that examined caffeine and sleep in adult populations. Caffeine in moderate amounts results in increased sleep latency, reduced sleep efficiency, and reduced slow wave sleep as assessed by polysomnography (Roehrs & Roth, 2008). In studies with children and adolescents, however, there are relatively few studies that use objective assessments of sleep such as actigraphy or polysomnography. Research on the effects of caffeine on sleep and performance is particularly important given the abundance of food and beverage products that contain caffeine and are being marketed specifically to youth populations.

Nicotine

Nicotine, like caffeine, is a stimulant and individuals who smoke experience a dose-related increase in wakefulness during sleep (Roehrs & Roth, 2011). In a 4-year longitudinal, population-based study of 7960 adolescents, 28% of the 4866 adolescents who did not report sleep problems at time 1 reported sleep problems 4 years later (Patten, Choi, Gillin, & Pierce, 2000). Cigarette smoking status at time 1 showed a dose-response relationship with the development and maintenance of self-reported sleep disturbances, as did being female and having depressive symptoms. The social context in which smoking occurs is also important. In a study of 6553 Hong Kong adolescents aged 13 to 18, the smoking status of parents and having a best friend who smoked were independently associated with the adolescent's smoking behaviors including current smoking, history of ever smoking, and the intention to smoke (Mak, Ho, & Day, 2012).

Smokers attempting to withdraw from nicotine experience increased sleep disturbance over those who continue to smoke or who use nicotine patches overnight (Roehrs & Roth, 2011). Because sleep involves withdrawing from smoking each night, sleep disruptions appear to be due to both the stimulant effect of nicotine and withdrawal-caused disturbances. Adolescent self-reported nicotine withdrawal symptoms are consistent with adult self-reported nicotine withdrawal symptoms. However, adolescent boys report higher levels of sleep-related problems during attempts to quit and adolescent girls report more irritability and hunger (Pergadia et al., 2010).

In a study of 219 asthmatic children 6 to 12 years of age, second-hand smoke exposure was related to parent-reported sleep problems of their children. These problems include increased sleep onset latency (especially in girls), parasomnias, sleep disordered breathing, daytime sleepiness, and general sleep disturbance, as well as sleep anxiety in boys (Yolton, Xu, Khoury, et al., 2010). In a study of 29,397 Chinese adolescents, current and infrequent smokers had a higher odds ratio of snoring and difficulty breathing compared to nonsmokers (Mak et al., 2010). Current smokers also experienced an increase in sleep maintenance problems.

The effect of both prenatal and postnatal nicotine exposure on sleep has been studied in infants. Evidence is accumulating that there is a negative impact on the sleep of infants whose mothers smoke. Neonates born to heavy-smoking mothers had a birth weight that was 21% less than those born to nonsmoking mothers (Stéphan-Blanchard, Telliez, Léké, et al., 2008). Prenatal exposure resulted in reduced total sleep time and quiet sleep, as well as increased active sleep and sleep fragmentation in newborns.

Long-lasting effects into childhood of prenatal exposure to nicotine, cocaine, and other drugs on sleep have also been found. Prenatal nicotine and cocaine exposure predicts later maternal-reported sleep problems in children 18 months to 9 years of age (Stone, High, Miller-Loncar, LaGasse, & Lester 2009); children 1 month to 12 years of age experience a dose-response effect specifically from prenatal nicotine exposure on later development of maternal reported sleep problems. This effect was observed even when controlling for postnatal nicotine exposure (Stone et al., 2010).

In a study of postnatal nicotine exposure, infants were studied polysomnographically, at 2–4 weeks, 2–3 months, and 5–6 months of age (Richardson, Walker, & Horne, 2009). Infant exposure to maternal smoking was associated with decreased cortical arousal and increased subcortical activation. A similar pattern of arousal processes is seen in infants who die from sudden infant death syndrome (SIDS). The authors hypothesize that this pattern may be related to impairment in the brainstem-cortex arousal process.

In a study of the effect of smoking during breastfeeding, infant sleep was assessed by actigraphy 3.5 hours after breast feeding. Results were obtained when mothers were asked to smoke as usual compared to when they were asked to refrain from smoking prior to breast feeding. Infants consuming breast milk containing nicotine experienced a reduction in quiet, active, and total sleep time (Mennella, Yourshaw, & Morgan, 2007).

Alcohol

Alcohol is a central nervous system depressant. Alcohol, like other depressants, suppresses rapid eye movement (REM) sleep. Acute effects involve sedation at the beginning of the night followed by sleep fragmentation later in the night. Tolerance develops and the individual may increase alcohol intake leading to an increase in sleep fragmentation. Withdrawal from heavy drinking produces a REM rebound effect that is accompanied by restless sleep and nightmares (Bootzin, Manber, Loewy, Kuo, & Franzen, 2001).

In a study of 4187 boys and girls 15 years of age, use of nicotine and alcohol was associated with delayed and erratic sleep schedules as well as perceived tiredness (Tynjälä, Kannas, & Levälahti, 1997). Similarly, Johnson and Breslau (2001) found that use of alcohol, cigarettes, and other substances (i.e., marijuana, cocaine, inhalants) was related to self-reported sleep disturbance in adolescents between 12 and 17 years of age. When internalizing and externalizing symptoms were statistically controlled, this relationship was maintained for polydrug use and regular alcohol use, defined as having used alcohol more than 12 days per month.

In addition to the effects on sleep of the use of alcohol in children and adolescents, the effects on sleep of prenatal and postnatal alcohol exposure has been studied in infants. Infants of mothers classified as heavy drinkers throughout pregnancy demonstrated reduced total sleep time versus infants of mothers who reduced or abstained from alcohol by the 3rd trimester. Additionally, infants of mothers who drank heavily experienced more fragmented, restless sleep than infants of mothers who abstained from alcohol (Rosett, Louis, Sander, et al., 1979). In other studies of the prenatal effects of alcohol, infants exposed to alcohol prenatally experience alterations in sleep-state cycling compared to infants of mothers who abstained from alcohol during pregnancy (Stoffer, Scher, Richardson, Day, & Coble, 1988), and infants exposed to alcohol prenatally demonstrate EEG hypersynchrony in all stages of sleep (D'Angiulli, Grunau, Maggi, & Herdman, 2006).

In mothers who used alcohol or marijuana daily versus mothers who abstained from these substances during pregnancy, prenatal alcohol exposure during the 1st and 2nd trimester was related to increased arousals and increased transitional sleep (Scher, Richardson, Coble, Day, & Stoffer, 1988). Prenatal marijuana exposure, regardless of trimester, was related to increased nocturnal body movements and reduced quiet sleep.

There are long-term effects of the prenatal exposure to alcohol and marijuana. Children at 8 years of age who were prenatally exposed to alcohol are at greater odds of short sleep and reduced sleep efficiency than children who were not exposed to alcohol prenatally (Pesonen, Räikkönen, Matthews, et al., 2009).

Marijuana

Although marijuana often has a reputation for being sedating, physiological arousal during sleep has been observed in both children exposed in utero and adolescent marijuana users. At 3 years of age, children prenatally exposed at least weekly to marijuana demonstrated increased arousals, wake after sleep onset, and reduced sleep efficiency compared to children who either were not exposed or were exposed less than once per week to marijuana (Dahl, Scher, Williamson, Robles, & Day, 1995). Studies of objective changes in sleep have found that marijuana use in adolescents is associated with a reduction in slow wave sleep and an increase in periodic limb movements during sleep, a sleep disorder that produces frequent arousals during sleep (Jacobus, Bava, Cohen-Zion, Mahmood, & Tapert (2009).

Sleep disturbances are also observed during withdrawal from marijuana, as seen in substance abuse treatment programs. In a marijuana treatment study for adolescents, the four withdrawal symptoms endorsed by more than 30% of the adolescents as being of moderate or greater severity were craving for marijuana, irritability, sleep difficulty, and depressed mood (Vandrey, Budney, Kamon, & Stanger, 2005). In addition, severity of sleep difficulty was highly related to the severity of other withdrawal symptoms. Withdrawal symptoms, including sleep disturbance, may result in an increased likelihood of relapse if effective sleep interventions are not provided.

The Effects of Sleep on Substance Use

Sleep problems can become part of a vicious cycle in which substance abuse leads to sleep disturbance, and daytime sleepiness leads to further substance use to counter these effects. In a long-term longitudinal study of sons of alcoholic men, Wong, Brower, Fitzgerald, and Zucker (2004) found that sleep and overtiredness problems as rated by mothers when the boys were 3 to 5 years old predicted the early onset of cigarette, alcohol, and other drug use, as well as the development of attention problems and anxiety or depression at 12 to 14 years of age. As part of a follow-up to this study, daughters were recruited to participate when they were between the ages of 6 and 11. A majority of the eligible daughters joined the study. Analysis of the full sample, 292 boys and 94 girls, found that those with trouble sleeping in childhood were twice as likely to have the same sleep problems in adolescence (Wong, Brower, Nigg, & Zucker, 2010). Importantly, overtiredness in childhood predicted poor response inhibition in adolescence as well as increased alcohol use and alcohol-related problems in young adulthood.

Similarly, in a 1-year longitudinal study of 11- to 17-year-old adolescents sampled from managed care rosters, Roberts, Roberts, and Chen (2002) found that sleep disturbances were significantly associated with a wide range of health, interpersonal, and psychological variables one year later. Moreover, once sleep problems developed they tended to be maintained. These results indicate that the treatment of sleep disorders may be of benefit as prevention before problems develop and as treatment if problems do develop. Since many adolescents who abuse substances are also anxious and depressed, targeting sleep disturbance for treatment has the potential benefit of increasing treatment success for both substance abuse and emotional regulation.

Parental involvement with their children has been found to be a protective factor reducing substance use, particularly among younger adolescents (Ellickson, Tucker, Klein, & Saner, 2004; Tang & Orwin, 2009). In an analysis from our research with adolescents (Cousins, Bootzin, Stevens, Ruiz, &

Haynes, 2007), we found that lower levels of parental involvement were associated with higher levels of psychological distress in adolescents. Higher distress was associated with lower sleep efficiency and more time in bed.

Distress and sleep, like substance abuse and sleep, has bidirectional causal pathways. As described earlier, adolescents who were depressed were more likely to develop subsequent sleep problems than controls (Patten, et al., 2000) and, as described in this section, sleep problems in adolescents have been found to increase the risk for anxiety disorders, depression, and substance abuse.

Substance Abusing Adolescents and Mental Health

As seen in the previous section, disturbed sleep leads to a broad range of subsequent problems including increased risk for substance abuse, anxiety, depression, and other mental health problems. In contrast, improved sleep could lead to resilience in the face of stress and reduced risk for developing mental health symptoms. Consequently, sleep disturbance could be a critical target for the treatment of adolescents who have a substance abuse history.

Many adolescents enrolled in substance abuse treatment report that they have mental health symptoms (Oshri, Tubman, & Jaccard, 2011; Stevens, Estrada, Murphy, McKnight, & Tims, 2004). Those enrolled in treatment represent a heterogeneous population and vary not only with regard to substance use patterns but also in psychiatric symptoms and maltreatment experiences (Tubman, Oshri, Taylor, & Morris, 2011). Dennis and colleagues (2012) report that 50% of substance using youth enrolled in juvenile drug courts present with 5 to 12 major clinical problems based on self-report count of alcohol use disorder, cannabis use disorder, other drug use disorder, depression, anxiety, trauma, suicide, ADHD, conduct disorder, and violence/illegal activity.

The prevalence of psychiatric disorders among adolescents in substance abuse treatment programs not only varies by type of treatment, but also by age and sex. In childhood, rates of depression are equivalent in boys and girls, but by adolescence, girls show dramatic increases in anxiety and mood disorders while boys are more likely than girls to exhibit externalizing symptoms such as anger and conduct problems (as reported in Cauffman, Lexcen, Goldweber, Shulman, & Grisso, 2007). Females with substance abuse disorders are twice as likely to be diagnosed with depression (Grella, Hser, Joshi, & Rounds-Bryant, 2001), while younger substance using adolescents have higher rates of comorbid psychiatric disorder and are at higher risk for "injury to self" (Unger, Kipke, Simon, Montgomery, & Johnson, 1997).

Mental health issues among adolescent substance users enrolled in treatment are often linked with past experiences of traumatic stress (Cavaiola & Schiff, 2000; Titus, Flores, Perez, & Stevens, 2012). Stevens and Murphy (2000) found that adolescents presenting for substance abuse treatment who reported traumatic stress also reported problems associated with their sleep (i.e., daytime sleepiness, not able to fall asleep, nightmares). In fact, 76% of males and 88% of females reported sometimes using alcohol or drugs to help them sleep.

As seen throughout this chapter, disturbed sleep, substance use, and mental health symptoms are often intertwined. The successful treatment of sleep disturbances in adolescents who abuse substances may also have beneficial effects on mental health symptoms and emotion regulation.

Treating the Sleep Disturbances of Adolescents with a Substance Abuse History

To evaluate whether treating the sleep and daytime sleepiness problems of adolescents who have had a history of substance abuse could result, first, in improved sleep, and second, in lowered risk for substance abuse relapse, our research laboratory embarked on an evaluation of a multicomponent cognitive-behavioral treatment program for insomnia and daytime sleepiness in adolescents (Bootzin & Stevens, 2005).

Participants were 55 adolescents, both male and female, average age of 16.09 years, of whom 23 (42%) attended four or more sessions and were classified as completing the sleep treatment. Participants all had completed outpatient substance abuse treatment programs within the previous 12 months but continued to have sleep or sleepiness problems. The sleep treatment was a 6-session multicomponent small group cognitive-behavioral therapy for insomnia with two to six adolescents in each group. The sessions were 90 minutes long and were held weekly, with a 2-week break between the fifth and sixth sessions to help shift the focus to the maintenance of gains made during the treatment period. Treatment components were selected to have maximal impact on the sleep problems of adolescents. The components included stimulus control therapy (Bootzin & Epstein, 2011), the use of bright light to change sleep/wake circadian rhythms (Lack &

Bootzin, 2003), sleep education, cognitive therapy (Morin, 1993), and mindfulness-based stress reduction (MBSR) including mindfulness meditation (Kabat-Zinn et al., 1992).

To measure the adolescents' sleep–wake circadian rhythms, dim-light melatonin onset (DLMO) was assessed before and after treatment (Hasler, Bootzin, Cousins, Fridel, & Wenk, 2008). The median DLMO was 9:45 pm with many earlier than 9:00 pm, suggesting that there may be different etiologies for the sleep problems in those who had early and late DLMOs (see Chapters 17 and 23, this volume). Those with early DLMOs may regularly stay up, due to social activities, past their optimal biological time to fall asleep. In contrast, those adolescents with late DLMOs may be exhibiting the more typical sleep phase delay and have trouble falling asleep because they are not yet at their biological time to fall asleep. The phase-delayed adolescents are also likely to have to awaken before they are biologically ready to do so because of school schedules. Having a late DLMO appears to be a signal of vulnerability because those with late DLMOs had more severe substance abuse problems than those with early DLMOs (Hasler et al., 2008).

Among those who completed at least four of the six sessions, there was significant improvement in sleep on total sleep time, time to fall asleep, minutes of wake time after sleep onset, and the adolescents' ratings of sleep quality (Britton et al., 2010).

Although the multicomponent sleep therapy was not designed to be a substance abuse treatment, it is possible that there would be positive effects on drug use and recidivism. The participants were interviewed before and after the multi-component sleep treatment, and at three and 12 months following treatment. There was a sex difference on the two major measures of substance use, i.e., the number of days in the preceding month that the adolescent used substances and on a measure of problems caused by substance use (Britton, et al., 2010). Female completers showed decreases on both measures from pretreatment through the 3-month follow-up, but returned to baseline at the 12-month follow-up. The male completers, although showing considerable improvement in sleep, did not improve on the substance use measures. Rather, they increased substance use and substance problem scores throughout the study. Noncompleters, whether female or male, similarly had increased substance use and substance problem scores at the end of the sleep treatment period and at the follow-up interviews.

Two additional analyses were done to evaluate changes in emotional and mental health functioning. Because conduct disorder problems are sometimes associated with substance abuse, the first analysis was on the relationship between increased total sleep duration as a result of treatment and the adolescents' reports of aggressive thoughts and behaviors. Those who reported decreased aggressive thoughts and behavior at the end of treatment had improved their total sleep by more than an hour to an average of more than 8.5 hours of sleep a night at the post-treatment assessment. In contrast, those who reported that they still had aggressive thoughts or engaged in aggression toward others at the end of treatment did not improve their total sleep significantly from baseline (Haynes et al., 2006). These findings suggest that adolescents may require at least 8 hours of nightly sleep to effectively regulate aggressive ideation and behavior.

The second analysis of mental health functioning examined anxiety symptoms as a result of the multicomponent sleep treatment. Both the amount of initial baseline total sleep and the amount of improvement in time to fall asleep during the treatment period were associated with improvement in symptoms such as fear of sleeping and having nightmares (Stevens, Haynes, Ruiz, & Bootzin, 2007). Improvement in falling asleep is a goal of the stimulus control component of the treatment. In this instance, improvement in falling asleep had a powerful effect in reducing emotional distress in those who had already been getting more total sleep at baseline. Thus, more total sleep provided the opportunity, either directly or in combination with falling asleep faster, for improvement of both aggression and emotional distress.

An important component of our multicomponent treatment was the incorporation of mindfulness meditation practice. An analysis of the mindfulness component of the treatment (Britton et al., 2010) found that the frequency of mindfulness meditation practice was related to increased sleep duration during treatment and improvement in self-efficacy about substance use. Increased sleep duration was associated with improvements in psychological distress, relapse resistance, and reductions in substance use–related problems.

In this exploratory study there were a number of positive, encouraging findings, including substantial improvement of the sleep of both female and male treatment completers, improvement on substance abuse measures through the 3-month follow up assessment for females, and reductions in thoughts of aggression, aggressive actions, and emotional distress in both female and male treatment completers. For this study, adolescents had been recruited after they had completed outpatient treatment for substance abuse but were still reporting sleep disturbances. More powerful effects on substance use may occur if the sleep and substance abuse treatments are integrated and occur together. This project was but a first step. It is critical to continue to develop sleep treatments for children and adolescents with comorbid problems such as substance abuse.

Conclusion

As seen throughout this chapter, there are bidirectional causal pathways between substance use and sleep in infants, children, and adolescents. Substance use, whether it is caffeine, nicotine, alcohol, marijuana, or other drugs, produces disturbed sleep and places limits on resilience. Strikingly, even prenatal exposure to caffeine, nicotine, alcohol, and marijuana produce sleep disturbances in infants. Caffeine, which is legally available to children, has been shown to have some benefits for cognitive functioning, but these are outweighed by the disadvantages associated with shortened and disturbed sleep. Poor sleep, at every developmental stage, increases the risk for substance abuse, health disorders, emotional and mental health problems, and cognitive and academic difficulties.

Substance use and abuse has reached crisis proportions during adolescence. Preventing and treating sleep problems in childhood is an important gateway to strengthen resilience and reduce risk across areas of functioning. In that regard, the results from the multicomponent treatment for sleep and sleepiness of adolescents with a history of substance abuse was particularly encouraging. Sleep was improved even in a sample of adolescents with a history of substance abuse, and there was improvement in emotion regulation and distress. Improvement in substance abuse and recidivism was better for females than males and is similar to what has been reported in substance abuse treatment programs. Integrating the sleep treatment with substance abuse treatment is a future direction that needs to be evaluated.

There is still much to be done to advance knowledge about sleep and substance use in children and adolescents. This is a critical area for investigation, as improved sleep at early developmental stages promises to provide a pathway for beneficial gains.

Future Directions

- Can stimulant use by children and adolescents be reduced to the point that sleep is not disturbed?
- Can programs for mothers and families be developed that will reduce prenatal and postnatal exposure to caffeine, nicotine, alcohol, marijuana, and other drugs?
- Can prevention programs be developed that involve child and adolescent peers in improving sleep and decreasing use of psychoactive substances?
- Is an integrated treatment for sleep and substance abuse in adolescents more efficacious than sequential treatments?

References

American Psychiatric Association. (1997). *Diagnostic and Statistical Manual of Mental Disorders*, 4th Ed., Text Revision. Washington, DC: Author.

Austin, A., & Wagner, E. F. (2010). Treatment attrition among racial and ethnic minority youth. *Journal of Social Work Practice in the Addictions, 10*, 63–80.

Barry, R. J., Clarke, A. R., McCarthy, R., Selikowitz, M., MacDonald, B., & Dupuy, F. E. (2012). Caffeine effects on resting-state electrodermal levels in AD/HD suggest an anomalous arousal mechanism. *Biological Psychology, 89*, 606–608.

Bernstein, G. A., Carroll, M. E., Crosby, R. D., Perwien, A. R., Go, F. S., & Benowitz, N. L. (1994). Caffeine effects on learning, performance, and anxiety in normal school age children. *Journal of American Academy of Child and Adolescent Psychiatry 33*, 407–415.

Bernstein, G. A., Carroll, M. E., Thuras, P. D., Cosgrove, K. P., & Roth, M. E., (2002). Caffeine dependence in teenagers. *Drug and Alcohol. Dependence, 66*, 1–6.

Bootzin, R. R., Manber, R., Loewy, D. H., Kuo, T. F., & Franzen, P. L. (2001). Sleep disorders. In H. E. Adams & P. B. Sutker (Eds.), *Comprehensive Handbook of Psychopathology*, 3rd ed. (pp. 671–711). New York: Plenum Press.

Bootzin, R. R. & Stevens, S. J. (2005). Adolescents, substance abuse, and the treatment of insomnia and daytime sleepiness. *Clinical Psychology Review, 25*, 629–644.

Bootzin, R. R., & Epstein, D. R. (2011). Understanding and treating insomnia. *Annual Review of Clinical Psychology, 7*, 435–458.

Britton, W. B., Bootzin, R. R., Cousins, J. C., Hasler, B. P., Peck, T., & Shapiro, S. L. (2010). The contribution of mindfulness practice to a multicomponent behavioral sleep intervention following substance abuse treatment in adolescents: A treatment-development study. *Substance Abuse, 31*, 86–97.

Calamaro, C. J., Mason, T. B. A., & Ratcliffe, S. J. (2009). Adolescents living the 24/7 lifestyle: Effects of caffeine and technology on sleep duration and daytime functioning. *Pediatrics, 123*, 1005–1010.

Calamaro, C. J., Yang, K., Ratcliffe, S. & Chasens, E. R. (2012). Wired at a young age: The effect of caffeine and technology on sleep duration and body mass index in school-aged children. *Journal of Pediatric Health Care, 26*, 276–282.

Calhoun, S. L., Vgontzas, A. N., Fernandez-Mendoza, J., Mayes, S. D., Tsaoussoglou, M., Basta, M. & Bixler, E. O. (2011). Prevalence and risk factors of excessive daytime sleepiness in a community sample of young children: The role of obesity, asthma, anxiety/depression, and sleep. *Sleep, 34,* 503–507.

Cauffman, E., Lexcen, F.J., Goldweber, A., Shulman, E. P., & Grisso, T. (2007). Gender differences in mental health symptoms among delinquent and community youth. *Youth Violence and Juvenile Justice, 5,* 287–306.

Cavaiola, A. A. & Schiff, M. M. (2000). Psychological distress in abused, chemically dependent adolescents. *Journal of Child & Adolescent Substance Abuse, 10,* 81–92.

Clegg-Kraynok, M. M., McBean, A. L., & Montgomery-Downs, H. E. (2011). Sleep quality and characteristics of college students who use prescription psychostimulants nonmedically. *Sleep Medicine, 12,* 598–602.

Cousins, J. C., Bootzin, R. R., Stevens, S. J., Ruiz, B. S, & Haynes, P. L. (2007). Parental involvement, psychological distress, and sleep: A preliminary examination in sleep-disturbed adolescents with a history of substance abuse. *Journal of Family Psychology, 21,* 104–113.

Cousins, J. C., Whalen, D., Dahl, R., Forbes, E., Olino, T., Ryan, N. & Silk, J. (2011). The daily bi-directional association between daytime mood and nighttime sleep in youth with anxiety and depression. *Journal of Pediatric Psychology, 36,* 969–979.

Dahl, R. E., Scher, M. S., Williamson, D. E., Robles, N., & Day, N. (1995). A longitudinal study of prenatal marijuana use: Effects on sleep and arousal at age 3 years. *Archives of Pediatrics and Adolescent Medicine, 149,* 145–150.

D'Angiulli, A., Grunau, P., Maggi, S., & Herdman, A. (2006). Electroencephalographic correlates of prenatal exposure to alcohol in infants and children: A review of findings and implications for neurocognitive development. *Alcohol, 40,* 127–133.

Dennis, M. L., Muck, R. D., Dawud-Noursi, S., & McDermeit, M. (2003). The need for developing and evaluating adolescent treatment models. In S. J., Stevens & A. R. Morral (Eds.), *Adolescent Substance Abuse Treatment in the United States: Exemplary models from a national evaluation study* (pp. 3–34). Binghampton, NY: The Haworth Press.

Dennis, M. L., Moritz, M. A., Meckley, R., Jones, N., Richardson, S., Crary, C., et al. (2012). *Evaluating the Impact of Adding the Reclaiming Futures Approach to Juvenile Treatment Drug Courts.* Normal, IL: Chestnut Health Systems.

Ellickson, P. L., Tucker, J. S., Klein, D. J., & Saner, H. (2004). Antecedents and outcomes of marijuana use initiation during adolescence. *Preventive Medicine, 39,* 976–984.

Fishman, M. J., Winstanley, E. L., Curren, E., Garrett, S., & Subramaniam, G. (2010). Treatment of opioid dependence in adolescent and young adults with extended release naltrexone: Preliminary case-series and feasibility. *Addiction, 105,* 1669–1676.

Food and Drug Administration (2013). Substances Generally Recognized as Safe. Code of Federal Regulations. Title 21, volume 3, 21CFR182.1180. Accessed April 22, 2013, from http://www.accessdata.fda.gov/scripts/cdrh/cfdocs/cfcfr/CFRSearch.cfm?fr=182.1180

Garrett, B. E., & Griffiths, R. R. (1997). The role of dopamine in the behavioral effects of caffeine in animals and humans. *Pharmacological Biochemical Behavior, 57,* 533–541.

Giannotti, F., Cortesi, F., Sebastiani, T., & Ottaviano, S. (2002). Circadian preference, sleep and daytime behavior in adolescence. *Journal of Sleep Research, 11,* 191–199.

Grella, C. E., Hser, Y. I., Joshi, V., & Rounds-Bryant, J. (2001). Drug treatment outcomes for adolescents with comorbid mental and substance use disorders. *Journal of Nervous and Mental Distress, 189,* 384–392.

Hasler, B. P., Bootzin, R. R., Cousins, J. C., Fridel, K., & Wenk, G. L. (2008). Circadian phase in sleep-disturbed adolescents with a history of substance abuse: A pilot study. *Behavioral Sleep Medicine, 6,* 55–73.

Hasler, B. P., Smith, L. J., Cousins, J. C., & Bootzin, R. R. (2012). Circadian rhythms, sleep, and substance abuse. *Sleep Medicine Reviews, 16,* 67–81.

Haynes, P. L., Bootzin, R. R., Smith, L., Cousins, J. Cameron, M., & Stevens, S. (2006). Sleep and aggression in substance abusing adolescents: Results from an integrative, behavioral sleep treatment pilot program. *Sleep, 29,* 512–520.

Heatherley, S. V., Hancock, K. M. F., & Rogers, P. J. (2006). Psychostimulant and other effects of caffeine in 9- to 11-year-old children. *Journal of Child Psychology and Psychiatry, 47,*135–142.

Hser, Y. I., Grella, C. E., Hubbard, R. L., Hsieh, S. C., Fletcher, B. W., Brown, B. S., & Anglin, M. D. (2001). An evaluation of drug treatment for adolescents in four US cities. *Archives of General Psychiatry, 58,* 689–695.

Huang, Y-S., Chen, N-H., Li, H-Y., Wu, Y-Y., Chao, C-C., & Guilleminault, C. (2004). Sleep disorders in Taiwanese children with attention deficit/hyperactivity disorder. *Journal of Sleep Research, 13,* 269–277.

Jacobus, J., Bava, S., Cohen-Zion, M., Mahmood, O., & Tapert, S. F. (2009). Functional consequences of marijuana use in adolescents. *Pharmacology Biochemistry and Behavior, 92,* 559–565.

James, J. E., Kristjansson, A. L., & Sigfusdottir, I. D. (2011). Adolescent substance use, sleep, and academic achievement: Evidence of harm due to caffeine. *Journal of Adolescence, 34,* 665–673.

Johnson, E. O., & Breslau, N. (2001). Sleep problems and substance use in adolescence. *Drug and Alcohol Dependency, 64,* 1–7.

Johnston, L. D., O'Malley, P. M., Bachman, J. G., & Schulenberg, J. E. (2012). *Monitoring the Future — National Results on Adolescent Drug Use: Overview of key findings, 2011.* Ann Arbor: Institute for Social Research, The University of Michigan.

Kabat-Zinn, J., Massion, A. O., Kristeller, J., Peterson, L. G., Fletcher, K. E., Pbert, L., Lenerking, W. R., & Santorelli, S. F. (1992). Effectiveness of a meditation based stress reduction program in the treatment of anxiety disorders. *American Journal of Psychiatry, 149,* 936–943.

Lack, L., & Bootzin, R. R. (2003). Phase disorders: Diagnostic issues, behavioral treatment, future directions. In M. Perlis & K. Lichstein (Eds.), *Handbook of Sleep Disorders: Principles and Practice of Behavioral Sleep Medicine* (pp. 305–343). New York: John Wiley & Sons.

Leon, M. R. (2000). Effects of caffeine on cognitive, psychomotor, and affective performance of children with attention-deficit/hyperactivity disorder. *Journal of Attention Disorders, 4,* 27–47.

Ludden, A. B., & Wolfson, A. R. (2010). Understanding adolescent caffeine use: Connecting use patterns with expectancies, reasons, and sleep. *Health Education & Behavior, 37,* 330–342.

Luebbe, A. M., & Bell, D. J. (2009). Moutain Dew or mountain don't?: A pilot investigation of caffeine use parameters and relations to depression and anxiety symptoms in 5th- and 10th- grade students. *Journal of School Health, 79*, 380–387.

Mak, K.-K., Ho, S.-Y., Thomas, G. N., Lo, W.-S., Cheuk, D. K.-L., Lai, Y.-K., & Lam, T.-H. (2010). Smoking and sleep disorders in Chinese adolescents. *Sleep Medicine, 11*, 268–273.

Mak, K.-K., Ho, S.-Y., & Day, J. R. (2012). Smoking of parents and best friend—independent and combined effects on adolescent smoking and intention to initiate and quit smoking. *Nicotine and Tobacco Research, 14*, published online: doi: 10.1093/ntr/nts008.

Mayes, S. D., Calhoun, S. L., Bixler, E. O., Vgontzas, A. N., Mahr, F., Hillwig-Garcia, J., et al. (2009). ADHD subtypes and comorbid anxiety, depression, and oppositional-defiant disorder: Differences in sleep problems. *Journal of Pediatric Psychology, 34*, 328–337.

McCabe, S. E., Knight, J. R., Teter, C. J., & Wechsler, H. (2005). Non-medical use of prescription stimulants among US college students: Prevalence and correlates from a national survey. *Addiction, 99*, 99–106.

Melendres, M. C., Lutz, J. M., Rubin, E. D., & Marcus, C. L. (2004). Daytime sleepiness and hyperactivity in children with suspected sleep disordered breathing. *Pediatrics, 114*, 768–775.

Mennella, J. A., Yourshaw, L. M., & Morgan, L. K. (2007). Breastfeeding and smoking: Short-term effects on infant feeding and sleep. *Pediatrics, 120*, 497–502.

Morin, C. M. (1993). *Insomnia: Psychological Assessment and Management*. New York: Guilford Press.

National Institute of Mental Health (2011). *Prescribed Stimulant Use for ADHD Continues to Rise Steadily.* Accessed August 16, 2012 from http://www.nih.gov/news/health/sep2011/nimh-28.htm

National Institute on Drug Abuse (2011). Topics in Brief. Accessed June 5, 2012, from http://www.drugabuse.gov/publicationa/topic-in-brief/marijuana.

National Institute on Drug Abuse (2012). Drug Facts: High School and Youth Trends. Accessed August 8, 2012, from http://www.drugabuse.gov/publications/drugfacts/high-school-youth-trends.

National Sleep Foundation. (2006). 2006 Sleep in America poll: Summary of findings. Washington, DC: National Sleep Foundation.

Negriff, S., Dorn, L. D., Pabst, S. R., & Susman, E. J. (2011). Morningness/eveningness, pubertal timing and substance use in adolescent girls. *Psychiatry Research, 185*, 408–413.

Oberstar, J. V., Bernstein, G. A., & Thuras, P. D. (2002). Caffeine use and dependence in adolescents: One-year follow-up. *Journal of Child and Adolescent Psychopharmacology, 12*, 127–135.

Orbeta, R. L., Overpeck, M. D., Ramcharran, D., Kogan, M. D., & Ledsky, R. (2006). High caffeine intake in adolescents: Associations with difficulty sleeping and feeling tired in the morning. *Journal of Adolescent Health, 38*, 451–453.

Oshri, A., Tubman, J. G., & Jaccard, J. (2011). Psychiatric symptoms typology in a sample of youth receiving substance abuse treatment services: Associations with self-reported child maltreatment and sexual risk behavior. *Aids and Behavior, 15*, 1844–1856.

Owens, J. A. (2005). The ADHD and sleep conundrum: A review. *Developmental and Behavioral Pediatrics, 26*, 312–322.

Pakalnis, A., Splaingard, M., Splaingard, D., Kring, D., & Colvin, A. (2009). Serotonin effects on sleep and emotional disorders in adolescent migraine. *Headache, 49*, 1486–1492.

Patten, C. A., Choi, W. S., Gillin, J. C., & Pierce, J. P. (2000). Depressive symptoms and cigarette smoking predict development and persistence of sleep problems in US adolescents. *Pediatrics, 106*, E23.

Pergadia, M. L., Agrawal, A., Heath, A. C., Martin, N. G., Bucholz, K. K., & Madden, P. A. F. (2010). Nicotine withdrawal symptoms in adolescent and adult twins. *Twin Research and Human Genetics, 13*, 359–369.

Pesonen, A.-K., Räikkönen, K., Matthews, K., Heinonen, K., Paavonen, J. E., Lahti, J., Komsi, N., et al. (2009). Prenatal origins of poor sleep in children. *Sleep, 32*, 1086–1092.

Pollak, C. P., & Bright, D. (2003). Caffeine consumption and weekly sleep patterns in US seventh-, eighth-, and ninth-graders. *Pediatrics, 111*, 42–46.

Preckel, F., Lipnevich, A. A., Boehme, K., Brandner, L., Georgi, K., K¨onen, T., Mursin, K. & Roberts, R. D. (2013). Morningness-eveningness and educational outcomes: The lark has an advantage over the owl at high school. *British Journal of Educational Psychology, 83*(Pt 1), 114–134.

Reissig, C. J., Strain, E. C., & Griffiths, R. R. (2009). Caffeinated energy drinks—A growing problem. *Drug and Alcohol Dependence, 99*, 1–10.

Richardson, H. L., Walker, A. M., & Horne, R. S. C. (2009). Maternal smoking impairs arousal patterns in sleeping infants. *Sleep, 32*, 515–521.

Roberts, E. R., Roberts, C. R., & Chen, I. G. (2002). Impact of insomnia on future functioning of adolescents. *Journal of Psychosomatic Research, 53*, 561–569.

Roehrs, T., & Roth, T. (2008). Caffeine: Sleep and daytime sleepiness. *Sleep Medicine Reviews, 12*, 153–162.

Roehrs, T., & Roth, T. (2011). Medication and substance abuse. In. M. H. Kryger, T. Roth, & W. C. Dement (Eds.), *Principles and Practice of Sleep Medicine*, 5th Ed. (pp. 1512–1523). St. Louis, MO: Elsevier-Saunders.

Rosett, H. L., Louis, P.S., Sander, W., Lee, A., Cook, P., Weiner, L., & Gould, J. (1979). Effects of maternal drinking on neonate state regulation. *Developmental Medicine and Developmental Medicine & Child Neurology, 21*, 464–473.

Ruiz, B. S., Korchmaros, J. D., Greene, A. & Hedges, K. (2011). Evidence-based substance abuse treatment for adolescents: Engagement and outcomes. *Practice: Social Work in Action, 23*, 215–233.

Schepis, T. S., Desai, R. A., Cavallo, D. A., Smith, A. E., McFetridge, A., Liss, T. B., Potenza, M. N., & Krishnan-Sarin, S. (2011). Gender differences in adolescent marijuana use and associated psychosocial characteristics. *Journal of Addictive Medicine, 5*, 65–73.

Scher, M. S., Richardson, G. A., Coble, P. A., Day, N. L., & Stoffer, D. S. (1988). The effects of prenatal alcohol and marijuana exposure: Disturbances in neonatal sleep cycling and arousal. *Pediatric Research, 24*, 101–105.

Scott, C. & Dennis, M. L. (2009). Results from two randomized clinical trials evaluating the impact of quarterly recovery management checkups with adult chronic substance users. *Addiction, 104*, 959–971.

Seifert, S. M., Schaechter, J. L., Hershorin, E. R. & Lipshultz, S. E. (2011). Health effects of energy drinks on children, adolescents, and young adults. *Pediatrics, 127*, 511–528.

Smit, H. J., & Rogers, P. J. (2000). Effects of low doses of caffeine on cognitive performance, mood and thirst in low and higher caffeine consumers. *Psychopharmacology, 152*, 167–173.

Stéphan-Blanchard, E., Telliez, F., Léké, A., Djeddi, D., Bach, V., Libert, J.-P., & Chardon, K. (2008). The Influence of in utero exposure to smoking on sleep patterns in preterm neonates. *Sleep, 31,* 1683–1689.

Stevens, S., Estrada, B., Murphy, B. S., McKnight, K. M., & Tims, F. (2004). Gender differences in substance use, mental health, and criminal justice involvement of adolescents at treatment entry and at 3, 6, 12, and 30 month follow-up. *Journal of Psychoactive Drugs, 36,* 13–25.

Stevens, S. (2006). *Women and substance abuse: A gendered perspective.* Fifth Annual Women's Mental Health Symposium, Tucson, AZ. January 7, 2006.

Stevens, S., Schwebel, R., & Ruiz, B. (2007). Seven challenges: An effective treatment for adolescents with co-occuring substance abuse and mental health problems. *Journal of Social Work in the Addictions, 7,* 29–49.

Stevens, S., Andrade, R. A. C., & Ruiz, B. S. (2009). Women and substance abuse: Gender, age and cultural considerations. *Journal of Ethnicity in Substance Abuse, 8,* 341–358.

Stevens, S. J., & Murphy, B. S. (2000). *Ethnic and gender differences in drug use and sleep disorders among adolescent drug users.* Presented at the Center for Substance Abuse Treatment Adolescent Treatment Models Grantee Meeting, Washington, DC, September 25–27, 2000.

Stevens, S. J. (2004). *Adolescent treatment models: Program models and client descriptions.* Workshop presented at the Substance Abuse and Mental Health Service Administration and Robert Wood Johnson Foundation Annual Grantee Meeting, Baltimore, MD., February 25, 2004.

Stevens, S. J., Haynes, P. L., Ruiz, B. S., & Bootzin, R. R. (2007). Effects of a behavioral sleep medicine intervention on trauma symptoms in adolescents recently treated for substance abuse. *Substance Abuse, 28,* 21–31.

Stoffer, D. S., Scher, M. S., Richardson, G. A., Day, N. L., & Coble, P. A. (1988). A Walsh-Fourier analysis of the effects of moderate maternal alcohol consumption on neonatal sleep-state cycling. *Journal of the American Statistical Association, 83,* 954–963.

Stone, K. C., High, P. C., Miller-Loncar, C. L., Lagasse, L. L., & Lester, B. M. (2009). Longitudinal study of maternal report of sleep problems in children with prenatal exposure to cocaine and other drugs. *Behavioral Sleep Medicine, 7*(4), 196–207.

Stone, K. C., LaGasse, L. L., Lester, B. M., Shankaran, S., Bada, H. S., Bauer, C. R., & Hammond, J. A. (2010). Sleep problems in children with prenatal substance exposure. *Archives of Pediatric Adolescent Medicine, 164,* 452–456.

Substance Abuse and Mental Health Services Administration, Office of Applied Statistics (2007). *The OAS report: A day in the life of American adolescents: Substance use and facts.* Rockville, MD: Author.

Tang, Z., & Orwin, R. G. (2009). Marijuana initiation among American youth and its risks as dynamic processes: Prospective findings from a national longitudinal study. *Substance Use and Misuse, 44,* 195–211.

Temple, J. L. (2009). Caffeine use in children: What we know, what we have left to learn and why should we worry. *Neuroscience and Biobehavioral Reviews, 33,* 793–806.

Titus, J., Flores, L., Perez, G., & Stevens, S. (2012). *Trauma-informed care for diverse adolescents with co-occurring trauma and substance abuse: Interventions and outcomes.* Joint Meeting on Adolescent Treatment Effectiveness, Washington D.C., April 10–12, 2012.

Tubman, J. G., Oshri, A., Taylor, H. L., & Morris, S. L. (2011). Maltreatment clusters among youth in outpatient substance abuse treatment: Co-occurring patterns of psychiatric symptoms and sexual risk behaviors. *Archive of Sex Behaviors, 40,* 301–309.

Tynjälä, J., Kannas, L., & Levälahti, E. (1997). Perceived tiredness among adolescents and its association with sleep habits and use of psychoactive substances. *Journal of Sleep Research, 6,* 189–198.

Unger, J. B., Kipke, M. D., Simon, T. R., Montgomery, S. B., & Johnson, C. J. (1997). Homeless youth and young adults in Los Angeles: Prevalence of mental health problems and the relationship between mental health and substance abuse disorders. *American Journal of Community Psychology, 25,* 371–394.

Vandrey, R., Budney, A. J., Kamon, J. L., & Stanger, C. (2005). Cannabis withdrawal in adolescent treatment seekers. *Drug and Alcohol Dependence, 78,* 205–210.

Walitzer, K. S., & Dearing, R. L. (2006). Gender differences in alcohol and substance use relapse. *Clinical Psychology Review, 26,* 128–148.

Walker, L. R., Abraham, A. A., & Tercyak, K. P. (2010). Adolescent caffeine use, ADHD, and cigarette smoking. *Children's Health Care, 39,* 73–90.

Warzak, W. J., Evans, S., Floress, M. T., Gross, A. C., & Stoolman, S. (2011). Caffeine consumption in young children. *Journal of Pediatrics, 158,* 508–509.

Whalen, D., Silk, J., Semel, M., Forbes, E., Ryan, N., Axelson, D., Birmaher, B., & Dahl, R. E. (2008). Caffeine consumption, sleep, and affect in the natural environments of depressed youth and healthy controls. *Journal of Pediatric Psychology, 33,* 358–367.

White, W. L., & McLellan, A. T. (2008). Addiction as a chronic disorder. *Counselor Magazine,* June, 24–33.

Wong, M. M., Brower, K. J., Fitzgerald, H. E., & Zucker, R. A. (2004). Sleep problems in early childhood and early onset of alcohol and other drug use in adolescence. *Alcoholism: Clinical and Experimental Research, 28,* 578–587.

Wong, M. M., Brower, K. J., Nigg, J. T., Zucker, R. A. (2010). Childhood sleep problems, response inhibition, and alcohol and drug outcomes in adolescence and young adulthood. *Alcoholism: Clinical and Experimental Research,34,* 1–12.

Wyatt, J. K., Cajochen, C., Ritz-De Cecco, A., Czeisler, C. A., Dijk, D-J. (2004). Low-dose repeated caffeine administration for circadian-phase-dependent performance degradation during extended wakefulness. *Sleep, 27,* 374–381.

Yolton, K., Xu, Y., Khoury, J., Succop, P., Lanphear, B., Beebe, D. W., & Owens, J. (2010). Associations between secondhand smoke exposure and sleep patterns in children. *Pediatrics, 125,* e261–e268.

PART 7

Prevention and Intervention

CHAPTER

37 The Impact of Behavioral Interventions for Sleep Problems on Secondary Outcomes in Young Children and Their Families

Melisa Moore *and* Jodi A. Mindell

Abstract

Childhood sleep problems are common, occurring in up to one-third of young children. Although behavioral treatments are effective at decreasing night wakings and bedtime problems, parents and clinicians may have concerns about the impact of these interventions on the child and on the parent–child relationship. Empirical evidence of the impact of behavioral interventions on other domains of the child and family is less well documented. Thus, an investigation of child sleep interventions reporting outcomes beyond child sleep was conducted. Significant improvements in child domains including mood and daytime behavior were found post-intervention. Parental factors, including sleep, well-being, marital satisfaction, mood, and mental health were also found to be improved following treatment of young children's sleep disturbances. Additionally, improvements in the parent–child relationships, bonding, and attachment were found. No systematic negative effects were described for parents or children. This review indicates that improving child sleep via behavioral interventions has implications that go far beyond sleep.

Key Words: sleep, bedtime problems, night waking, child sleep, behavioral intervention, treatment

Introduction

It is estimated that sleep problems occur in about 30% of children (Liu, Liu, Owens, & Kaplan, 2005; Mindell & Owens, 2009), with bedtime difficulties and frequent night wakings, two of the most common issues, occurring in 20%–30% of children under the age of 3 (Mindell, Kuhn, Lewin, Meltzer, & Sadeh, 2006; Sadeh, Mindell, Luedtke, & Wiegand, 2009). A myriad of studies have provided solid evidence that sleep problems affect emotional, cognitive, behavioral, and academic functioning (Fallone, Acebo, Seifer, & Carskadon, 2005; Sadeh, Gruber, & Raviv, 2002, 2003) and also relate to critical public health concerns such as pediatric obesity (Hart, Cairns, & Jelalian, 2011). In addition, sleep problems in children and adolescents can affect both parent sleep and parent daytime functioning (Meltzer & Mindell, 2007).

Sleep problems in young children tend not to go away on their own. Kataria, Swanson, and Trevathan (1987) found that 84% of 1–2-year-olds with a sleep problem had the same problem at age 3, indicating the importance of intervention. There is a vast literature that has shown behavioral interventions to be efficacious. Mindell and colleagues' (2006) review of 52 treatment studies for bedtime problems and frequent night wakings found that 94% of studies were efficacious, with over 80% of children treated demonstrating clinically significant improvement. These improvements were maintained for 3 to 6 months.

Despite this evidence, there are many who are resistant to behavioral interventions because of beliefs about iatrogenic effects. Anecdotally, they cite concerns about the impact on attachment, security, and mental health (Blunden, Thompson, &

Dawson, 2011; Narvaez, 2011). Many parents worry about the effects of interventions that involve infant crying (Tse & Hall, 2008), and thus the popularity of parenting books promising approaches that improve children's sleep without crying. Semantics also likely play a role in these beliefs, given that behavioral sleep interventions are often referred to in terms that have negative connotations. For example, extinction is often referred to as the "cry it out" method, implying that babies are being left to cry on their own for long stretches (see Blampied, Chapter 15). Others refer to "sleep training," which at times leads to parents equating these behavioral approaches to "animal training."

Thus, while it is known that behavioral interventions decrease bedtime problems and night wakings, as well as increase sleep duration, empirical evidence of the impact of behavioral interventions on other domains of the child and family is less well documented. For this chapter, Medline and Psych info searches for pediatric behavioral sleep intervention studies were conducted and the bibliographies of each study were further culled. Studies were excluded if the intervention was not clearly behavioral or if no outcomes were reported beyond child sleep outcomes, and the 35 studies that remained are discussed in this review. Secondary outcomes were grouped according to the effect on the child, parent(s), parent–child relationship, and interventions conducted in special populations will be discussed. Furthermore, a section is devoted to studies that have specifically looked at potential negative effects of behavioral sleep interventions.

Child

As previously cited, research has clearly demonstrated that behavioral interventions are effective in treating behaviorally based sleep issues in young children (Mindell et al., 2006). Some studies, however, have also looked at the impact in other domains, including any negative sequelae of treatment. All studies reported here found significant improvements in sleep. Although the specifics of these improvements are not presented, positive sleep outcomes should be assumed for all studies unless otherwise stated.

Mood

Only one study has assessed child mood in relation to behavioral interventions for sleep disturbances. Skuladottir and Thome (2003) found improvement in sleep outcomes in 33 infants (ages 6–23 months) who participated in an inpatient behavioral treatment program. The researchers reported significant improvement in mood in 15 of the 19 infants who were described as irritable prior to the start of treatment. These infants were described as being "happier, more playful, more calm, more cheerful, and more easy to please" at 2-month follow-up. There was no control group in this study, and all results are based on pre- and post-testing; however, the existing evidence suggests improved mood following a behavioral sleep intervention.

Daytime Behavior

Improvements in daytime behavior concurrent with improvements in sleep have been evaluated in a number of studies. Seymour, Bayfield, Brock, and During (1983) found that based on parental report, 73% of a sample of 208 children (ages 0–6 years) were found to have positive changes in their child's daytime behavior once their child's sleep improved, including being "happier," "easier to handle," and "less aggressive." Only one parent (2%) reported a negative outcome ("more grizzly"). Sanders et al. (1984) also found positive outcomes in daytime behavior in the four children they treated, with significant improvements reported in both home and community settings. France (1992) found improvements in agreeableness, likeability, and emotionality/tension, based on the Child Behavior Characteristics Scale, in a group of 35 infants (6–24 months) compared to no changes seen in controls. These improvements were seen during the treatment phase and up to 18 months post-treatment.

Richman, Douglas, Hunt, Lansdown, and Levere (1985) conducted a study of 35 children (ages 1–5 years) with severe sleep disorders treated with behavioral strategies (e.g., positive reinforcement of appropriate behaviors, implementation of a bedtime routine). They found that although there were too few children with concomitant behavioral problems to statistically assess outcomes, of the nine children with behavioral problems three also showed marked improvement in behavior with sleep improvement, three continued to have behavioral difficulties but no longer sleep problems, and three had no improvement in sleep or general behavioral problems.

Eckerberg (2004) utilized visual analogue scales to assess five behavioral dimensions (alert-tired; good-poor appetite; happy-depressed; secure-anxious; accommodating-obstinate) at baseline, 2 weeks after intervention implementation, and at 1-month and 3-month follow-ups. They found in the 95 families studied that parents rated their children (ages 4 to 45 months) as significantly more alert, happy, secure, and accommodating at 2 weeks post-intervention, with continued improvements in alertness and security at 3-month follow-up. In a small sample study of the use of positive routines for bedtime noncompliance in low-income families whose children attended Head Start, improvements were noted in daytime behavior based on parent-report using the Eyberg Child Behavior Inventory at post-treatment and 2-month follow-up (Ortiz & Bodkin, 2008). No significant changes at either time point, however, were seen in teacher report on the Sutter-Eyberg Behavior Inventory-Revised.

A number of studies have utilized the Child Behavior Checklist (CBCL) to assess general behavioral outcomes. In one study (Burke, Kuhn, & Peterson, 2004), a storybook that modeled appropriate bedtime behavior with tangible rewards was used to successfully treat four children (ages 2 to 7 years) with disruptive bedtime behaviors. In addition to the significant improvements in bedtime behaviors and night wakings, parents reported significant improvements in daytime behavior in three of the four children. At baseline, all four children scored in the clinical range for total problems on the CBCL. At post-treatment, scores were in the normal range for two of the four children, improved in one child, and unchanged for one child. Another study (Reid, Walter, & O'Leary, 1999) included CBCL to assess side effects of treatment of sleep disturbances on daytime behaviors in 43 children (ages 16–48 months) utilizing standard or graduated ignoring treatment. No changes in internalizing or externalizing behaviors were found for either intervention between baseline and post-treatment. A study of 28 toddlers with serious sleep problems who were treated with the institution of a bedtime routine and a checking method also utilized the CBCL to assess behavioral outcomes (Minde, Faucon, & Falkner, 1994). At baseline these children had significantly higher scores on the CBCL and Child Behavior Checklist compared to 30 matched controls, with scores significantly improving at 3-month and 6-month follow-up. Finally, Hiscock et al. (2008) assessed longer-term outcomes of a behavioral intervention conducted at 8–10 months of age. At 2 years of age, no differences in internalizing or externalizing behaviors based on the CBCL were found between the intervention group and control group. At 6 years of age, there continued to be no differences between groups on the Strength and Difficulties Questionnaire (emotional problems and conduct problems subscale), nor on psychosocial functioning based on the Pediatric Quality of Life Inventory. Thus, successful behavioral treatment of sleep disturbances in all these studies was found to have a positive effect on both sleep and general behavior.

Although unusual in the United States, other countries such as Australia provide residential facilities that help parents in the early years with infant and child problems such as sleep and feeding. One study assessed infant behavior following behavioral treatment in a residential center (Fisher, Feekery, & Rowe, 2004). One hundred ninety mothers of infants up to age 12 months reported that infant crying and fussing behavior in 24 hours decreased from 151 minutes at baseline to 72.5 minutes 1 month post-discharge.

Thus, improvements in daytime behavior have been found in a number of studies, using a variety of methods and measures concomitant with behavioral treatment of sleep disturbances. Of all child outcomes investigated, daytime behavior is well studied and the most robust.

Temperament

Temperament is another child outcome of interest, as behavioral interventions should not negatively affect a child's disposition. Pinilla and Birch (1993) investigated the efficacy of behavioral entrainment (including a focal feed, increasing intervals between feeds, and maximizing day/night environmental cues) in 26 newborns randomly assigned to intervention or control over the first 8 weeks of life. By 3 weeks of age, significant differences were seen in longer sleep episodes of the intervention group. By 8 weeks, 100% of the treatment infants were sleeping through the night compared to just 23% of controls. Assessment of infant temperament (Bates' Infant Characteristics Questionnaire) by mothers and fathers was conducted at 1 week and 8 weeks of age. No differences were found across time and across groups; however, the infants in the intervention group were rated as more predictable at both week 1 and week 8. Hiscock et al. (2007) also assessed temperament in their study of the efficacy of behavioral interventions for infants recruited at 7 months of age (n = 174 intervention; n = 154 matched controls). At 10 months and 12 months there were no significant differences in temperament ratings using a 5-point Global Infant Temperament Scale between intervention and control infants. The findings that behavioral sleep interventions resulted in either no change in temperament or an increase in predictability make sense given that temperament is considered a relatively stable trait.

Health Outcomes

There has been very limited research on health outcomes following treatment of behaviorally based sleep disturbances. One particular area of focus, given the recent epidemic of childhood obesity, is the link between obesity and sleep. A recent pilot study (Paul et al., 2011) found that a behavioral intervention targeting feeding as well as sleep resulted in lower weight-for-length percentiles at 1 year of age. Given that obesity has become an epidemic in the United States, with more than 20% of children between the ages of 2 and 5 being overweight, it is recommended that measures of obesity such as BMI (body mass index) be included as outcomes of behavioral sleep interventions in children. With regard to illness, Skuladottir and Thome (2003) found fewer recurring illnesses in 33 infants (ages 6–23 months) who participated in an inpatient behavioral treatment program. Those infants whose sleep improved more were reported to have fewer illnesses, such as ear infections, asthma, and reflux, 2 months post-treatment. Because there was no control group, it is difficult to assess the impact of intervention on health outcomes in this study. It can be argued that sleep problems persisted as a result of these health issues, rather than improved sleep leading to fewer illnesses. Although there is little evidence in this area, given the potential impact on areas of public health concern such as obesity, health and illness variables should be considered in future research.

Parent–Child Relationship

A primary concern for parents and practitioners is whether interventions will negatively impact parent–child relationships. This issue has received attention in academic journals (Blunden et al., 2011) and even more so in blogs and magazines aimed at the public (Narvaez, 2011), with claims that behavioral interventions cause long-term damage. Several studies have looked specifically at security/attachment, maternal bonding, parenting style, maternal confidence/competence/efficacy, perception of behavioral control, and parent cognitions.

A number of studies have examined the issues of security and attachment as outcomes of behavioral sleep interventions, primarily during infancy. For example, France and colleagues (France, 1992; France, Blampied, & Wilkinson, 1991) looked at the impact of behavioral treatment on security as a primary aim. Utilizing the Flint Infant Security Scale (excluding sleep items), she found a significant improvement in security scores at day 3 of treatment, with further improvements at the end of treatment (week 6). No changes in security were noted in untreated and normal sleep controls. Eckerberg (2004) also utilized the revised Flint Infant Security Scale in assessing security at baseline, during intervention, and at follow-up. Compared to a nonreferred community comparison group, the 95 infants referred for treatment in their study had significantly lower scores at baseline. After the intervention, at 1-month follow-up, these differences were eliminated, with significant improvements in dependent trust and self-trust, as well as total security. Interestingly, the lower the security score at baseline the greater the increase after intervention. Additionally, as mentioned above, parents reported significant improvements on a visual analogue scale for "secure-anxious" by 2 weeks post-intervention.

Parent–child interactions have also been evaluated. Minde et al. (1994) assessed play and feeding interactions of toddlers with their mothers using the Parent-Child Early Relational Assessment Scale. Following treatment for sleep disturbances utilizing a graduated extinction approach with 28 toddlers (and 30 matched controls), improvements were seen in child characteristics including "infant organization, attentional, and social skills" and "infant dysregulation, irritability, and negative behavior." Similar results were found for mother–child interactions, with significant improvements seen for "dyadic mutuality and reciprocity" and "dyadic tension." Additionally, the sleep-disturbed toddlers scored lower at baseline on these indices indicating poorer initial child behavior and dyadic interactions, with treatment of sleep issues ameliorating these interactional difficulties. Furthermore, those children who were most problematic at baseline in terms of their sleep and daytime behaviors showed the largest improvements in their interactions 6 weeks post-treatment.

Following a 5-day inpatient intervention (Matthey & Speyer, 2008), items from the Being a Mother and Bonding Scale (BaMB) were assessed including "I have felt close to my baby," "My baby seemed to like me," and "I have regretted having this baby." Scores on these three items improved significantly at 5 weeks post-discharge, and this change remained stable at 4 months post-discharge. Hiscock et al. (2008) also asked mothers 17 months post-recruitment whether behavioral interventions had affected their relationship with their child.

Of those mothers who responded, 84% indicated that behavioral interventions had a positive effect on their relationship with their child. Additionally, there was no difference in parenting style (harsh discipline or nurturing) between the intervention and control groups at this long-term follow-up time point. These same children were followed up at age 6 to assess for any long-term negative implications (Price, Wake, Ukoumunne, & Hiscock, 2010). Again, there were no differences on the Child-Parent Relationship Scale between the intervention and control group, suggesting no negative outcomes regarding attachment.

In terms of parenting style, one small study (Reid et al., 1999) found that mothers of infants in a standard extinction group reported less verbose parenting (a positive effect), and mothers in a graduated extinction group reported improved interactions with their children. Both of these effects were found post-treatment within subjects, as well as compared to waitlist controls.

Another study investigated parental cognitions around sleep (Hall et al., 2006). They used the Maternal Cognitions about Infant Sleep Scale (MCISQ) within a pre–post design of a group intervention. At 6-week follow-up they found significant improvements in parental cognitions regarding limit setting around infant sleep, feeding at night, anger about infant sleep, and doubts about handling infant sleep. At 16 weeks, however, the parents unexpectedly had a significant increase in anger around their infant's sleep. The authors' potential explanation is that parents initially experienced an improvement, which they thought would be a "magic bullet" for their child's sleep and behavior. At 16 weeks new problems may have emerged, such as teething, which interfered with the child's sleep.

Maternal competence has also been assessed. Wolfson, Lacks, and Futterman (1992) found that an intervention consisting of two prenatal and two postnatal sessions resulted in higher parental efficacy scores for the intervention group as compared with controls. From the prenatal period to the follow-up period, both the control and intervention groups significantly increased their sense of competence. Mindell et al.'s (2011a) study of an Internet-based intervention also found a significant increase in maternal confidence from baseline to week 2 and from week 2 to week 3. At 1-year follow-up, maternal confidence was still significantly improved as compared to baseline, though in the Internet-plus-routine group this improvement was not as large as it was at week 3 (Mindell et al., 2011b).

Finally, parental behavioral control has been evaluated in one study. Pritchard and Appleton's (1988) study of a health visitor intervention for infants and toddlers with bedtime problems and frequent night wakings found that at week 3, mothers felt their level of behavioral control significantly increased compared to baseline. This was also true at 3-month follow-up (although slightly decreased from week 3).

As reviewed here, the data refute the frequent claims and suppositions that behavioral interventions harm security, attachment, and parent–child interactions. Rather, young children and their families with sleep disturbances score lower on these factors compared to good sleepers and treatment actually improves security, attachment, and parent–child interactions. Denying or avoiding treatment may actually result in *more* problems instead of causing them. That is, not treating sleep problems may result in continued problems with parent–child relationships, whereas treatment results in rectifying not only sleep but also improving family relationships.

Parent

As with the child outcomes previously discussed, all studies reported here found significant improvements in *child* sleep, although results are not presented. When the child's sleep improves via a behavioral intervention, studies demonstrate that aspects of *parent* sleep improve as well. The forthcoming sections review the impact of sleep-related behavioral interventions on parent sleep and health, parent well-being, and parent mood and mental health.

Parent Sleep and Health

A child's sleep problem clearly impacts domains of parent sleep and health including duration, frequency of night wakings, sleepiness, fatigue, and general health. Thome and Skuladottir (2005) looked at both mothers' and fathers' responses to an inpatient intervention for infants ages 6–23 months who were hospitalized for sleep problems in Australia. Pediatric nurses, who met with the families 2–4 hours per night for 4 nights, carried out the behaviorally based intervention. The parents left the hospital each night while the infants stayed. They found decreased fatigue and stress related to fatigue compared to baseline in both mothers and fathers 2 months following this inpatient intervention.

The majority of other studies in this area have assessed outpatient interventions. One study of

39 families pre- and post-intervention included group education, phone calls, and completion of sleep charts, and found significant improvements in parent self-reported sleep quality (Pittsburgh Sleep Quality Index, PSQI) and a reduction in fatigue via the Multidimensional Assessment of Fatigue Scale (MAF), but not on the Epworth Sleepiness Scale (Hall et al., 2006). A Swedish study of 95 children (ages 4–45 months) divided the intervention into two steps: bedtime behavior (step 1) and night wakings (step two). Both mothers and fathers reported being less tired as early as 2 weeks after the first step (Eckerberg, 2004). Mindell and Durand (1993) found significant improvements in maternal and paternal sleep following an intervention with six children including implementing a bedtime routine and graduated extinction. First, participants received treatment for bedtime problems and then night wakings were addressed. Five families received one session and one family received two sessions. All of the mothers reported night wakings (average of 1.38 per night), and these were significantly decreased following treatment and sustained at 1-month follow up. No significant change was found in mothers' sleep onset latency or total duration of nighttime sleep. Fathers' number of night wakings was also significantly reduced, but there was little improvement in duration of night wakings, sleep onset latency, or nighttime sleep duration.

Randomized trials include Hiscock et al.'s (2007) infant sleep intervention including extinction and found that fewer mothers in the intervention group reported poor sleep quality and insufficient sleep at both 10 and 12 months compared to the control group. An unexpected finding was that with regard to physical health on the SF-12, the groups were the same at 10 months but intervention mothers had poorer health at 12 months. A behaviorally based Internet intervention designed to improve infant and toddler sleep (Mindell et al., 2011a) in a nonclinical population randomly assigned 264 participants to an Internet intervention alone, Internet intervention plus a prescribed bedtime routine, or a control group. The investigators found significant improvements for both intervention groups in maternal sleep, including sleep onset latency, duration, sleep efficiency, and total sleep quality as measured by the PSQI. No changes in bedtime or wake time were found. Mothers in the control group were also found to have fewer night wakings and improved global sleep quality at week 3 compared to baseline, though the effect sizes were smaller for the control group (ES = 0.27) as compared with the intervention groups (ES = 0.51). One-year follow-up of this same cohort found improvements as compared to baseline, but these improvements were not as high as at week 3 (Mindell et al., 2011b).

Only one study utilized actigraphy for estimating maternal sleep outcomes. Stremler et al. (2006) investigated a 45-minute behavioral/educational intervention delivered by a nurse in a hospital postpartum unit to 15 first-time mothers. In addition to the meeting, participants were provided with a booklet reviewing this information and with weekly phone contact to reinforce the information and problem-solve. At 6 weeks postpartum, the mothers in the intervention group averaged 57 minutes more nighttime sleep than controls (433 vs. 376 minutes) via actigraphy. Additionally, significantly fewer rated their sleep as problematic on the General Sleep Disturbance Scale as compared with controls. Many other variables were studied, including nocturnal awakenings, longest nocturnal sleep period, daytime sleep, fatigue, and bed sharing, and none of these yielded significant differences.

The studies reviewed here demonstrate that improvements in children's sleep via behavioral interventions relate to improvements in parent sleep including longer sleep duration, fewer night wakings and sleep problems, and better overall sleep quality, although potentially not to parents' general health.

Parental Well-Being

Indicators of parental well-being, including distress, stress, and marital satisfaction, are common parental outcome measures in studies of child behavioral sleep interventions and generally improve concurrent with improvements in children's sleep. Both total stress and "role restriction" (e.g., not having time for oneself, feelings of restraint) were reduced in a Swedish study following improvements in the sleep of 4–45-month-olds (Eckerberg, 2004). Similarly, a study (Reid et al., 1999) of 16–48-month-olds with sleep problems randomly assigned to standard extinction (n = 16), graduated extinction (n = 17), or an age- and sex-matched control group (n = 16), found that for both intervention groups, parenting-related distress was significantly reduced post-intervention as compared to waitlist controls. Thome and Skuladottir (2005), in their previously described inpatient intervention, found that 83% of parents in the study reported reduced distress (as measured by a composite construct including parenting stress, symptoms of depression and anxiety, and fatigue and stress regarding fatigue) at 2-month follow-up. Specifically, they found a reduction in parenting stress for both mothers and fathers on the Parenting Stress Index (PSI).

Wolfson and colleagues (1992) also assessed parental stress as a secondary outcome to behavioral intervention. They randomly assigned first-time parents to a 4-session training group (2 sessions prenatally, 2 booster sessions when the infants were "settling age") or a control group. Mothers' and fathers' stress and marital satisfaction were measured via the Hassles and Uplifts Scale. While both groups reported increased hassles from the prenatal time point to post-birth, only the control group demonstrated a statistically significant increase. No significant increases were found in uplifts.

Parental emotional state and marital satisfaction have also been assessed. A study of 31 children (ages 9 months to 3.5 years) referred for bedtime problems and/or frequent wakings utilized an individualized behaviorally based program (Pritchard & Appleton, 1988). Health visitors visited the families every 2–3 days for 3 weeks in one group, and in the second group families were seen only at week 3. There were no differences between the groups on any of the outcome measures, and they were combined for the analyses. Maternal emotional state as measured by the General Health Questionnaire was significantly improved from baseline to the end of the 3-week intervention. At 3 months, mothers' emotional state was also significantly improved from baseline, though slightly poorer compared to 3 weeks post-intervention.

With regard to the parental relationship, a South African study of 20 families (Leeson, Barbour, Romaniuk, & Warr, 1994) found that 68% of parents reported that their relationship was "better" or "much better" 1 month after a residential behavioral sleep intervention for their 8–12-month-old infants; 32% reported it was the same, and none reported it was worse. A study of 36 toddlers and preschoolers (Adams & Rickert, 1989) who were assigned to a positive routines intervention, a graduated extinction intervention, or a control group found that parents in the positive routines group reported a significant positive change in marital satisfaction on the Dyadic Adjustment Scale (DAS). They attributed this improvement to less family stress and more time spent together. Finally, Durand and Mindell's (1990) single case design of a behavioral sleep intervention with a 14-month-old found increased maternal and paternal marital satisfaction on the DAS, and this improvement was concurrent with improvements in the child's sleep. The investigators expanded this approach to six children with similar findings (Mindell & Durand, 1993). Though the parents did not report significant marital distress at baseline, significant increases in marital satisfaction were found.

In sum, the studies reviewed found increases in parental sleep and well-being, decreases in stress, and increased marital satisfaction. Thus, interventions for pediatric sleep issues result not only in improved sleep for the child but also subsequent improvements in parental well-being, including not only sleep but other general measures of well-being.

Parent Mood and Mental Health

While not studied as often as parental well-being or distress, parent mental health (specifically symptoms of anxiety and depression) has also been shown to improve with improvements in child sleep, especially for mothers who have more symptoms at baseline. A study (Hiscock & Wake, 2002) investigating the impact of a 3-session infant sleep intervention including graduated extinction found improvements in depression via the Edinburgh Postnatal Depression Scale (EPDS) for all mothers at 2-month and 4-month follow-up, with greater improvement in the intervention group. When looking more specifically at baseline scores, the mothers who met criteria for depression (EPDS $\geq$ 10) experienced significantly greater improvements than those who were less depressed. In fact, controlling for other professional services and other factors typically associated with depression, the only factor that predicted an *increase* in depressive symptoms was the persistence of the infant's sleep problem.

A similar intervention (Hiscock et al., 2007) again found significant improvements in EPDS scores for mothers in the intervention group compared to controls, but this improvement was most significant in those with baseline scores $\geq$ 10. Mothers in the intervention group also had higher mental health scores at both 10 and 12 months on the SF-12 (indicating better mental health) post-intervention when compared with controls. This research group has conducted the only studies investigating the long-term effects of infant behavioral sleep interventions. At 2 years of age (Hiscock et al., 2008) the odds of reporting depressive symptoms was 59% lower for mothers in the intervention group as compared to controls. When the children were age 6 years, there were no differences between the intervention group and controls (Price et al., 2010) with regard to maternal depression. This latter finding was interpreted by the researchers as implying no long-term negative effects of behavioral interventions that occurred during infancy. The Swedish study previously mentioned also found both mothers and fathers to be significantly happier, more hopeful, and less depressed 2 weeks after the intervention (Eckerberg, 2004). Of note, prior to the intervention mothers reported feeling more depressed, tired, and discouraged than fathers, and after the intervention there was no difference between mothers and fathers. These improvements were stable at 3-month follow up. Similarly, France and colleagues (1991) studied mothers of 35 children (ages 7–27 months) using extinction (n = 13), extinction plus a placebo (n = 12), or extinction plus medication (n = 10) for infant night wakings. One week post-intervention, the mothers in the intervention groups were significantly less anxious. Interestingly, fathers were not significantly anxious at baseline and there were no significant differences in anxiety post-intervention.

At least one single case study (Durand & Mindell, 1990) of a 14-month-old found improvements in both maternal and paternal depressive symptoms on the Beck Depression Inventory (BDI) that occurred following decreases in the child's night wakings. Similarly, the same investigators in a multiple baseline study of six children found significant improvements in both maternal and paternal depressive symptoms on the BDI, even though the parents had not been clinically depressed (Mindell & Durand, 1993).

Even a behavioral sleep intervention as simple as instituting a bedtime routine has been found to improve maternal mood. In one study of both infants and toddlers, mothers were randomly assigned to an intervention group (3-step bedtime routine for 2 weeks) or a control group (Mindell, Telofski, Wiegand, & Kurtz, 2009). Following 1 week of baseline data collection, mothers of intervention infants (n = 134) were told to give their baby a bath, a massage, and quiet activities (lullaby, cuddle, sing) with lights out within 30 minutes of the end of the bath. The infants were then put to bed as usual. Intervention toddlers (n = 133) received the same intervention with the exception of the massage, which was replaced by putting on of lotion. Improvements in maternal mood (Profile of Moods Scale) were found for both the infant and toddler intervention groups from baseline to both week 2 and week 3, while no changes were noted in the mothers in the control groups. Significant improvements for mothers of infants were found on all subscales: tension, depression, anger, fatigue, vigor, and confusion. Mothers of toddlers significantly improved on tension, anger, fatigue, and confusion.

Matthey and Speyer (2008) studied 116 mothers in Australia who were recruited following admission for a 5-day inpatient stay for infant sleep problems. In addition to education about infant sleep and parenting support, nursing staff encouraged "progressive waiting," a strategy similar to controlled crying or graduated extinction but with a quicker response time. Following the intervention, mothers had significantly improved with regard to symptoms of anxiety and depression as measured by the Edinburgh Postnatal Depression Scale and the Hospital Anxiety and Depression Scale (HADS) anxiety subscale. Of the 55% who had clinically significant scores on either the EPDS or the HADS anxiety subscale at baseline, more than half had recovered at 5 weeks post-discharge and this improvement was stable at 4 months.

Other studies conducted in other countries utilizing a residential model have also noted significant improvements in parental outcomes. A South African study involving a residential 4-night intervention (Leeson et al., 1994) followed 23 infants (ages 8–12 months) and their families and found a decrease in depressive symptoms (via the CES-D) at 1-month follow-up as compared to baseline for both mothers and fathers. Another study utilizing the CES-D found decreases in depressive symptoms for mothers, but not for fathers, following a group sleep intervention for 6–12-month-old infants, with follow-up phone calls (Hall et al, 2006). Thome and Skuladottir's (2005) inpatient intervention at an Icelandic hospital found parents' depressive symptoms (as measured by the Edinburgh Postnatal Depression Scale) and symptoms of anxiety (measured by the State Trait Anxiety Inventory) were at clinically elevated levels prior to the intervention. In their pre–post design previously described, parents demonstrated significant improvement 2 months post-intervention, with the participants returning to nonclinical levels on both measures.

Contrary to the previously reviewed studies, one study (Stremler et al., 2006) did not find any change in maternal depression (via the Edinburgh Postnatal Depression Scale) or anxiety (via the State Trait Anxiety Inventory) following a sleep intervention as compared to controls. Thirty mothers and their newborn infants from a postpartum unit were randomized to either an intervention (n = 15) or control group (n = 15). The sleep intervention involved an individual meeting where sleep was discussed in addition to provision of an 11-page booklet about infant sleep. Families were called each week for 5 weeks post-discharge to discuss sleep difficulties. The control group was given individual information about maternal sleep hygiene and basic information about infant sleep, and a 1-page handout reviewing this information. They were also called at weeks 3 and 5 post discharge. Though the infants in the intervention group had improved sleep at 6 weeks, there was no difference between groups on maternal depression or anxiety. This result may be due to the fact that the intervention was conducted during the newborn period, prior to the entrainment of the infants' circadian rhythm.

The data from multiple studies show that not only do behavioral sleep interventions improve secondary outcomes in children, but they also lead to positive outcomes in parents. As might be expected, improvements in children's sleep relate to improvements in parent sleep (duration, quality, and night wakings). In addition, better child sleep relates to improved parental well-being, decreased stress, increased marital satisfaction, and better mood and mental health. It is likely that the positive effects of improving children's sleep lead not only to better parent health and functioning but also to better parenting.

Special Populations

While sleep disturbances are common in typically developing children, children with conditions such as autism spectrum disorders (ASDs) and attention-deficit/hyperactivity disorder (ADHD) are at increased risk for problems with sleep. Thus, investigating child and parent outcomes of interventions to improve sleep in children with ASDs and ADHD is critical.

Autism

Though behavioral interventions may be less well-studied, more difficult to implement, and offered less frequently than medications, parents of children with ASDs prefer behavioral interventions to sleep medications (Stores & Wiggs, 1998; Wiggs & Stores, 1999). One study evaluated the efficacy of faded bedtime with response cost, combined with positive reinforcement, in three children with ASD (Moon, Corkum, & Smith, 2011). Sleep onset latency improved in all cases during treatment and 12 weeks later. Daytime behavior as measured by the CBCL improved, with scores moving from borderline clinical range to average range in two of the three children. Another study (Reed et al., 2009) of 20 children with ASDs (ages 3–10 years), whose parents attended a 3-part workshop on treatment of sleep issues, found significant improvements in hyperactivity and self-stimulatory behavior subscales as measured by the Parental Concerns Questionnaire (13 total subscales), in addition to significant improvements in sleep. On the Repetitive Behavior Scale, the restricted behavior scale total score improved with treatment, without significant improvement in the total score or the other 5 subscale scores.

Regarding parent outcomes of behavioral sleep interventions for children with ASDs, Reed et al. (2009) conducted an intervention (three 2-hour intervention sessions focusing on education) with parents of 20 children with autism (ages 3–10 years). No improvements in parenting stress, parental distress, or parent–child interactions were found despite improvements in the children's sleep and daytime behavior.

Although not limited to children with autism, Wiggs and Stores (2001) conducted a randomized controlled trial of a behavioral sleep intervention in 15 children with severe intellectual disabilities compared with 15 controls. This intervention was based on a functional analysis of the sleep problem and was tailored to the family using a variety of behavioral techniques (e.g., extinction, positive reinforcement, and stimulus control). Compared with controls, mothers had significantly reduced stress (Malaise Inventory), increased satisfaction with their own sleep (on a Likert scale asking about sleep satisfaction), and increased ability to cope with their child's sleep (Internality/Externality Control Scale). Fathers demonstrated increased satisfaction with their own sleep, though they reported feeling less control over their child's sleep (visual analog scale asking about perceived control of the child's sleep problem) following the intervention. Maternal sleepiness (Epworth Sleepiness Scale) and maternal perception of control over their child's sleep improved in both the intervention and control groups.

ADHD

Even fewer studies have been conducted on behavioral interventions for sleep problems in children with ADHD, with minimal assessment of other outcomes beyond sleep. There has been one recent randomized control trial of behavioral intervention for 27 children (ages 5–14 years) that found minimal change in ADHD symptom scores from baseline to 5-month post-treatment following either a brief or extended treatment of sleep issues (Sciberras, Fulton, Efron, Oberklaid, & Hiscock, 2011).

Parent outcomes have only been studied in one small pilot study of children (ages 5–14) with ADHD. A brief behavioral sleep intervention (1 session, n = 13) was compared to an extended session (2–3 sessions, n = 14). While both interventions improved the child's sleep, only the extended intervention resulted in improvements in parent anxiety at 5 months and better work attendance at 2 months post-intervention (Sciberras et al., 2011).

Negative Effects

There have been very few studies that have specifically investigated the negative side effects of behavioral sleep interventions. No studies in this review had a priori hypotheses that negative effects of behavioral sleep interventions would be found; however, all studies presented here assessed for potential negative secondary outcomes using the measures described. Sanders, Bor, and Dadds (1984) treated four children (ages 2–5 years) for bedtime difficulties, utilizing a planned bedtime cue, planned ignoring, time out, and rewards for not waking during the night. Based on the Child Behavior Problem Checklist, three of four children had a reduction in problem behaviors in the home and community setting, with one child having a slight increase in the number of problem behaviors in the community but not at home. France (1992; 1991) specifically looked at negative effects of behavioral interventions in 35 infants (ages 6–24 months) treated with extinction compared with 13 untreated and 15 normal sleep controls. Negative impact was assessed in terms of security (Flint Security Scale) and behavior (Child Behavior Characteristics Scale). Improved security scores were found for the treatment group, with no similar change in the two control groups. For behavior, there were no changes in the two control groups but a significant improvement for the intervention group both at the end of treatment and at follow-up (up to 18 months). Thus, this study did not find any negative effects, but rather that infants were more secure, less emotional/tense, and more likeable after treatment. Eckerberg (2004) similarly aimed to investigate potential negative effects of sleep training, given the claim of harmful effects. However, in their study of 95 families they also found positive effects on daytime behavior and family well-being as early as 2 weeks after implementation of the intervention, again refuting claims that behavioral treatments are detrimental to children.

With regard to negative effects of behavioral sleep interventions on parents, no systematic conclusions can be drawn, as the negative findings are inconsistent across studies. The only study to specifically investigate negative parent outcomes of a behavioral intervention found that parents did not become more anxious from implementing the intervention (France et al., 1991), even when using standard extinction. Hiscock et al. (2007) found that with regard to physical health on the SF-12, the intervention mothers had slightly poorer health at 12 months as compared to controls. This finding was thought to be unrelated to the intervention. Hall et al. (2006) found at 16 weeks post-intervention that parents unexpectedly had a significant increase in cognitions relating to anger around their infants' sleep, although earlier follow-up time points found an improvement. As previously mentioned, the authors suggest the parents may have thought the improvement in their child's sleep was a "magic bullet" and that further disruptions in the child's sleep due to such issues as teething, illness, and family stress were unexpected. Finally, Wiggs and Stores (2001) found that fathers of children with severe intellectual disabilities reported feeling less control over their child's sleep (visual analog scale asking about perceived control of the child's sleep problem) following the intervention.

Conclusion

While it is clear that behavioral interventions are effective at increasing sleep duration, decreasing night wakings, and decreasing bedtime problems in young children, such interventions also positively impact multiple other domains of child and parent functioning. Overall, looking at the literature in its entirety (e.g., 35 studies that measured secondary outcomes), almost every study found significant improvements rather than negative effects. Furthermore, in certain domains (e.g., depression, infant security) the research to date indicates that those with more symptoms or more problematic relationships prior to the intervention improve the most across all domains. In other domains (marital satisfaction), it may be that even those who do not report significant dissatisfaction at baseline experience improvements post-intervention. In sum, while parents and practitioners may be concerned about the implications of behavioral approaches to childhood sleep problems, few if any negative effects were uncovered in this systematic review. In terms of child and child–parent relationship factors, there were no negative outcomes described immediately post-intervention or at long-term follow-up. The only parental negative effects (increased cognitions about anger related to infant sleep, longer-term maternal health, and decreased paternal control) described across the plethora of studies conducted were inconsistent and, in fact, none of the negative effects were replicated in any other study. Given the solid foundation of evidence, it is clear that improving child sleep via behavioral interventions has widespread positive effects on the child and the family. Furthermore, as previously stated, not intervening may actually result in more negative outcomes for children and their relationships with their parents.

Future Directions

Studies, as noted above, have primarily assessed longer-term outcomes in children, whether weeks or months or later. No studies to date, though, have assessed immediate outcomes. That is, does sleep training on a given night result in negative outcomes the next day or next several days. However, although studies specifically designed to measure negative outcomes, such as the one just described, may seem to be a logical next step, given the existing evidence it would be difficult to generate a priori hypotheses that sleep interventions have any negative effects. A different future direction is to conduct a meta-analysis across all intervention studies, as is currently being conducted by the authors, which will provide objective evidence to the strength of these behavioral interventions as well as the lack of harm to children and families. Furthermore, the results of such analysis may show that not only are these interventions not harmful, but that they actually lead to overall improvements across multiple child and family domains. In addition, as is evidenced by the few studies conducted with children with special needs, more studies of behavioral interventions for sleep issues in children with autism, ADHD, obesity, and other chronic conditions are needed.

References

Adams, L. A., & Rickert, V. I. (1989). Reducing bedtime tantrums: Comparison between positive routines and graduated extinction. *Pediatrics, 84*(5), 756–761.

Blunden, S. L., Thompson, K. R., & Dawson, D. (2011). Behavioural sleep treatments and night time crying in infants: challenging the status quo. *Sleep Medicine Reviews, 15*(5), 327–334.

Burke, R. V., Kuhn, B. R., & Peterson, J. L. (2004). Brief report: A "storybook" ending to children's bedtime problems—the use of a rewarding social story to reduce bedtime resistance and frequent night waking. *Journal of Pediatric Psychology, 29*(5), 389–396.

Durand, V. M., & Mindell, J. A. (1990). Behavioral treatment of multiple childhood sleep disorders. Effects on child and family. *Behavior Modification, 14*(1), 37–49.

Eckerberg, B. (2004). Treatment of sleep problems in families with young children: Effects of treatment on family well-being. *Acta Paediatrica, 93*(1), 126–134.

Fallone, G., Acebo, C., Seifer, R., & Carskadon, M. A. (2005). Experimental restriction of sleep opportunity in children: Effects on teacher ratings. *Sleep, 28*(12), 1279–1285.

Fisher, J., Feekery, C., & Rowe, H. (2004). Treatment of maternal mood disorder and infant behaviour disturbance in an Australian private mothercraft unit: a follow-up study. *Archives of Women's Mental Health, 7*(1), 89–93.

France, K. G., Blampied, N. M., & Wilkinson, P. (1991). Treatment of infant sleep disturbance by trimeprazine in combination with extinction. *Journal of Developmental and Behavioral Pediatrics, 12*(5), 308–314.

France, K. G. (1992). Behavior characteristics and security in sleep-disturbed infants treated with extinction. *Journal of Pediatric Psychology, 17*(4), 467–475.

Hall, W. A., Clauson, M., Carty, E. M., Janssen, P. A., & Saunders, R. A. (2006). Effects on parents of an intervention to resolve infant behavioral sleep problems. *Pediatric Nursing, 32*(3), 243–250.

Hart, C. N., Cairns, A., & Jelalian, E. (2011). Sleep and obesity in children and adolescents. *Pediatric Clinics of North America, 58*(3), 715–733.

Hiscock, H., & Wake, M. (2002). Randomised controlled trial of behavioural infant sleep intervention to improve infant sleep and maternal mood. *British Medical Journal, 324*(7345), 1062–1065.

Hiscock, H., Bayer, J., Gold, L., Hampton, A., Ukoumunne, O. C., & Wake, M. (2007). Improving infant sleep and maternal mental health: A cluster randomised trial. *Archives of Disease in Childhood, 92*(11), 952–958.

Hiscock, H., Bayer, J. K., Hampton, A., Ukoumunne, O. C., & Wake, M. (2008). Long-term mother and child mental health effects of a population-based infant sleep intervention: cluster-randomized, controlled trial. *Pediatrics, 122*(3), e621–627.

Kataria, S., Swanson, M. S., & Trevathan, G. E. (1987). Persistence of sleep disturbances in preschool children. *Behavioral Pediatrics, 110*, 642–646.

Leeson, R., Barbour, J., Romaniuk, D., & Warr, R. (1994). Management of inflant sleep problems in a residential unit. *Child: Care, Health and Development, 20*, 89–100.

Liu, X., Liu, L., Owens, J. A., & Kaplan, D. L. (2005). Sleep patterns and sleep problems among schoolchildren in the United States and China. *Pediatrics, 115*(1), 241–249.

Matthey, S., & Speyer, J. (2008). Changes in unsettled infant sleep and maternal mood following admission to a parentcraft residential unit. *Early Human Development, 84*(9), 623–629.

Meltzer, L. J., & Mindell, J. A. (2007). Relationship between child sleep disturbances and maternal sleep, mood, and parenting stress: A pilot study. *Journal of Family Psychology, 21*(1), 67–73.

Minde, K., Faucon, A., & Falkner, S. (1994). Sleep problems in toddlers: Effects of treatment on their daytime behavior. *Journal of the American Academy of Child and Adolescent Psychiatry, 33*(8), 1114–1121.

Mindell, J. A., & Durand, V. M. (1993). Treatment of childhood sleep disorders: Generalization across disorders and

effects on family members. *Journal of Pediatric Psychology, 18*(6), 731–750.
Mindell, J. A., Kuhn, B., Lewin, D. S., Meltzer, L. J., & Sadeh, A. (2006). Behavioral treatment of bedtime problems and night wakings in infants and young children. *Sleep, 29*(10), 1263–1276.
Mindell, J. A., & Owens, J. A. (2009). *A Clinical Guide to Pediatric Sleep: Diagnosis and Management of Sleep Problems* (2nd ed.). Philadelphia: Lippincott Williams & Wilkins.
Mindell, J. A., Telofski, L. S., Wiegand, B., & Kurtz, E. (2009). A nightly bedtime routine: Impact on sleep problems in young children and maternal mood. *Sleep, 32*, 599–606.
Mindell, J. A., Du Mond, C. E., Sadeh, A., Telofski, L. S., Kulkarni, N., & Gunn, E. (2011a). Efficacy of an internet-based intervention for infant and toddler sleep disturbances. *Sleep, 34*(4), 451–458.
Mindell, J. A., Du Mond, C. E., Sadeh, A., Telofski, L. S., Kulkarni, N., & Gunn, E. (2011b). Long-term efficacy of an internet-based intervention for infant and toddler sleep disturbances: One year follow-up. *Journal of Clinical Sleep Medicine, 7*(5), 507–511.
Moon, E. C., Corkum, P., & Smith, I. M. (2011). Case study: A case-series evaluation of a behavioral sleep intervention for three children with autism and primary insomnia. *Journal of Pediatric Psychology, 36*(1), 47–54.
Narvaez, D. (December 11, 2011). Dangers of "crying it out": Damaging children and their relationships for the longterm. *Psychology Today.* http://www.psychologytoday.com/blog/moral-landscapes/201112/dangers-crying-it-out
Ortiz, C., & Bodkin, L. M. (2008). *One-session group parent training in positive routines for bedtime non-compliance in Head Start children.* Paper presented at the Pediatric Sleep Medicine conference, Amelia Island, FL.
Paul, I. M., Savage, J. S., Anzman, S. L., Beiler, J. S., Marini, M. E., Stokes, J. L., et al. (2011). Preventing obesity during infancy: A pilot study. *Obesity, 19*(2), 353–361.
Pinilla, T., & Birch, L. L. (1993). Help me make it through the night: Behavioral entrainment of breast-fed infants' sleep patterns. *Pediatrics, 91*(2), 436–444.
Price, A., Wake, M., Ukoumunne, O. C., & Hiscock, H. (2010). Impact of "controlled crying" on child and parent mental health to 6 years: Randomised clinical trial. *Journal of Paediatrics and Child Health, 46*, 1–16.
Pritchard, A. & Appleton, P. (1988). Management of sleep problems in pre-school children: Effects of a behavioural programme on sleep routines, maternal depression and perceived control. *Early Child Development and Care, 34*, 227–240.
Reed, H. E., McGrew, S. G., Artibee, K., Surdkya, K., Goldman, S. E., Frank, K., et al. (2009). Parent-based sleep education workshops in autism. *Journal of Child Neurology, 24*(8), 936–945.
Reid, M. J., Walter, A. L., & O'Leary, S. G. (1999). Treatment of young children's bedtime refusal and nighttime wakings: A comparison of "standard" and graduated ignoring procedures. *Journal of Abnormal Child Psychology, 27*(1), 5–16.
Richman, N., Douglas, J., Hunt, H., Lansdown, R., & Levere, R. (1985). Behavioural methods in the treatment of sleep disorders—a pilot study. *Journal of Child Psychology and Psychiatry, and Allied Disciplines, 26*(4), 581–590.
Sadeh, A., Gruber, R., & Raviv, A. (2002). Sleep, neurobehavioral functioning, and behavior problems in school-age children. *Child Development, 73*(2), 405–417.
Sadeh, A., Gruber, R., & Raviv, A. (2003). The effects of sleep restriction and extension on school-age children: What a difference an hour makes. *Child Development, 74*(2), 444–455.
Sadeh, A., Mindell, J. A., Luedtke, K., & Wiegand, B. (2009). Sleep and sleep ecology in the first 3 years: A web-based study. *Journal of Sleep Research, 18*(1), 60–73.
Sanders, M. R., Bor, B., & Dadds, M. (1984). Modifying bedtime disruptions in children using stimulus control and contingency management techniques. *Behavioural Psychotherapy, 12*, 130–141.
Sciberras, E., Fulton, M., Efron, D., Oberklaid, F., & Hiscock, H. (2011). Managing sleep problems in school aged children with ADHD: A pilot randomised controlled trial. *Sleep Medicine, 12*(9), 932–935.
Seymour, F. W., Bayfield, G., Brock, P., & During, M. (1983). Management of night-waking in young children. *Australian Journal of Family Therapy, 4*, 217–223.
Skuladottir, A., & Thome, M. (2003). Changes in infant sleep problems after a family-centered intervention. *Pediatric Nursing, 29*(5), 375–378.
Stores, G., & Wiggs, L. (1998). Clinical services for sleep disorders. *Archives of Disease in Childhood, 79*(6), 495–497.
Stremler, R., Hodnett, E., Lee, K., MacMillan, S., Mill, C., Ongcangco, L., et al. (2006). A behavioral-educational intervention to promote maternal and infant sleep: A pilot randomized, controlled trial. *Sleep, 29*(12), 1609–1615.
Thome, M., & Skuladottir, A. (2005). Evaluating a family-centred intervention for infant sleep problems. *Journal of Advanced Nursing, 50*(1), 5–11.
Tse, L., & Hall, W. (2008). A qualitative study of parents' perceptions of a behavioural sleep intervention. *Child: Care, Health, and Development, 34*, 167–172.
Wiggs, L., & Stores, G. (1999). Behavioural treatment for sleep problems in children with severe learning disabilities and challenging daytime behaviour: Effect on daytime behavior. *Journal of Child Psychology and Psychiatry, 40*(4), 627–635.
Wiggs, L., & Stores, G. (2001). Behavioural treatment for sleep problems in children with severe intellectual disabilities and daytime challenging behaviour: Effect on mothers and fathers. *British Journal of Health Psychology, 6*(Pt 3), 257–269.
Wolfson, A., Lacks, P., & Futterman, A. (1992). Effects of parent training on infant sleeping patterns, parents' stress, and perceived parental competence. *Journal of Consulting and Clinical Psychology, 60*(1), 41–48.

CHAPTER

38 Systematic Strategies: Case of School Start Times

Rhoda Au, Erica R. Appleman, *and* Karina Stavitsky

Abstract

Insufficient sleep in adolescents is widely regarded as a public health concern that can negatively affect students' academic achievement, as well as impact physical and emotional wellbeing. While a number of social and biological dynamics contribute to sleep deprivation in this population, research is increasingly pointing to early school start times as a significant modifiable factor. The consensus across researchers is that delaying school start times is an effective intervention in successfully attenuating sleep deprivation and may foster positive benefits for physical and mental health, student safety, and academic performance. Despite compelling results, the issue remains emotionally and politically contentious, with both pragmatic considerations and passionately held beliefs acting as barriers to change. Future research is needed to dispel myths and provide sufficient objective data to elucidate the benefits of later start times for both students and communities.

Key Words: school start times, sleep deprivation, sleep patterns, adolescents, education

Introduction

While the developmental process during childhood and adolescence is defined by biological change, daily life is more fixed, structured in large part by the ubiquitous school schedule. Although schools within the United States and throughout the world differ in many ways, the vast majority of schools follow a highly choreographed schedule of activities determined by a specific start time. A number of financial and logistical factors are involved in determining school start times, with many districts having their high schools start the earliest. Empirical data often plays an underrepresented role in school start-time decisions, even though research has indicated that adolescents biologically need approximately 9.25 hours of sleep a night, which is consistently not being met (Wolfson & Carskadon, 1998; National Sleep Foundation, 2006). Studies have further indicated that early school start times may exacerbate the challenge of adolescents obtaining the needed amount of sleep on school nights (Wolfson & Carskadon, 1998).

Within the United States there is, however, a rising trend of school leaders and the lay community recognizing that school start times are contributing to the documented sleep deprivation of adolescents across the country and, as a result, schools have begun to consider implementing changes to their schedule (Kirby, Maggi, & D'Angiulli, 2011). Calls to change school start times often ignite a firestorm of emotions both within the school system and the community it serves, which has brought to light serious barriers to enacting change. Despite the inexplicable turmoil that frequently ensues, a growing number of schools have successfully implemented later middle school and high school start times, and the evidence supportive of these changes is consistently growing (Kirby, Maggi & D'Angiulli, 2011).

Yet, even with the growing amount of research touting the benefits of later start times, public opinion remains divided on the plausibility and need for change. Thus, as researchers continue to build the case for later school start times for adolescents, the question is not if schools should change their start times but whether proponents of this change can overcome the numerous competing fiscal, logistical, and psychological factors.

Adolescent Sleep Patterns and Sleep Deprivation

The biological evidence is clear that an individual's sleep needs change significantly from infancy through childhood and from adolescence to adulthood (Wolfson & Carskadon, 1998). It was once believed that children required fewer hours of sleep as they progressed through puberty, and that by their late teens they needed equal amounts of sleep as adults (Carskadon, Harvey, Duke, Anders, Litt, & Dement, 1980). In 1980, Carskadon and colleagues conducted the first study to refute this commonly held belief. As discussed at length in Carksadon's chapter in this volume (Carskadon and Tarokh, Chapter 8), they conducted a 6-year longitudinal study that demonstrated adolescents' biological need for 9.2 hours of sleep across the entire pubertal stage, substantially more time than the 8 hours recommended for adults (Carskadon et al., 1980). Additional research has confirmed these findings in both the United States (Mercer, Merritt, & Cowell, 1998) and across 11 European countries (Tynjala, Kannas, & Valimaa, 1993).

Since the seminal Carskadon study, subsequent investigations have consistently demonstrated that adolescents are not getting enough sleep on school days (Carskadon, 1990; Eaton, McKnight-Eily, Lowry, Perry, Presley-Cantrell, & Croft, 2010; Hansen, Janssen, Schiff, Zee, & Dubocovich, 2005). Total reported sleep time of children reliably decreases with age, with high school students reporting significantly shorter total sleep times than younger children. Sleep times are found to dwindle from 10 hours in middle childhood to less than 7.5–8 hours by age 16 (Allen, 1992; Carskadon, 1982, 1990; Wolfson & Carskadon, 1998); National Sleep Foundation, 2006; Au, 2010). In their large-scale survey of 1602 adolescents, the 2006 *Sleep in America* poll reported that respondents were getting an average of 7.6 hours of sleep per night, well short of the 9 recommended hours of sleep each night (National Sleep Foundation, 2006). Similarly, the average total sleep time for over 3000 high school students surveyed in Rhode Island was only 7 hours, 20 minutes (Wolfson & Carskadon, 1998). Further, the problems of sleep deprivation appear to extend to the college years, with reports from students of excessive daytime sleepiness (Wolfson, 2010).

One factor that accounts for the diminishing amount of sleep is that as students go through the adolescent years, they report increasingly later bedtimes. Within the Rhode Island sample, 45% of 10th–12th-graders reported going to bed after midnight on school nights; this number increased to 90% for weekend nights (Wolfson & Carskadon, 1998). The gap between weekday and weekend total sleep time widens with increasing age, with a 30–60 minute differential in 10–14 year olds to over 2 extra weekend hours in 18 year olds (Bearpark & Michie, 1987; Petta, Carskadon & Dement, 1984; Strauch & Meier, 1988). The students surveyed in the Rhode Island study reported weekend bedtimes that were 2 hours later than weeknight bedtimes, with weekend wake-up times up to 3.5 hours later than weekdays (Wolfson & Carskadon, 1998). This research provides evidence that adolescents are attempting to recuperate from weeknight sleep deprivation through increased weekend sleep, which is counter to the recommendation that sleep/wake cycles should remain consistent throughout the week to maximize the restorative benefits of sleep (Dahl & Carskadon, 1995; Dahl & Lewin, 2002).

Other social and environmental factors have been implicated in the increasingly late bedtimes for adolescents. These include decreased parental regulation such as enforced bedtimes, increased scholastic and extracurricular demands, part-time employment, use of caffeine, alcohol, and other drugs, increased participation in later night social engagement and activities, and most recently use of technology that further exacerbates the problem of late-night social interactions (Carskadon, Wolfson, Tzischinsky, & Acebo, 1995; Wolfson, 2002; Calamaro, Mason, & Ratcliffe, 2009).

Consistent sleep deprivation on school nights leads to the development of significant sleep debt during the week, measured as lengthening of weekend sleep durations, as students try to make up for insufficient sleep during the weekdays. Research indicates that extra sleep on the weekend cannot solely make up for reduced sleep during the week (Petta, Carskadon, & Dement, 1984). But advocating for earlier bedtimes to combat sleep deprivation is not a feasible solution given the biological evidence that many teenagers are simply unable to fall asleep before 11:00 pm or later (delayed sleep phase) due to developmental shifts in their melatonin levels, the hormone that regulates sleep/wake cycles. Thus, the compendium of scientific results supports Carskadon's recommendation that middle school and high school start times should occur after 8:00 am (Carskadon, Acebo, Richardson, Tate, & Seifer, 1997; Wolfson, Spaulding, Dandrow, & Baroni, 2007).

Researchers in other countries have also found evidence of sleep deprivation and its effects in their respective adolescent populations. A survey of students in a Japanese international school utilized the Epworth Sleepiness Scale and found that 25% of students reported excessive daytime sleepiness (Ng, Ng, & Chan, 2009). Further, sleep deprivation was negatively associated with performance in mathematics. Specific sleepiness variables, such as sleepiness upon rising and sleepiness during third and fourth lessons, were associated with poorer English and Math grades.

A survey including over 3000 Canadian high school students also utilized the Epworth Sleepiness Scale and found that scores indicating greater sleepiness were associated with students reporting falling grades, being late for school, being extremely sleepy in school, and participating in fewer extracurricular activities (Gibson et al., 2006). A group of Korean students in grades 5 through 12 were administered the School Sleep Habits Survey, a modified version of Wolfson and Carskadon's (1998) instrument, and results showed similar patterns to American adolescent sleep habits, including increasing bedtimes with age and profound sleep deprivation on school nights (Yang, Kim, Patel, & Lee, 2005). Early school start time was one of the most commonly cited reasons for sleep deprivation for students in 10th, 11th, and 12th grades.

These international studies agree largely with those of the United States, and indicate that the problem of sleep deprivation is epidemic across the world. The implications are generations of students not being permitted to achieve their full academic, physical, and mental health potential.

Early High School Start Times: Decades of Precedence

Little research exists to explain why high schools historically start earliest, followed by middle schools or junior high schools, and why elementary schools traditionally start the latest (Wolfson & Carskadon, 2005). High school start times across the United States have been informally and formally surveyed on several occasions in recent years. One pilot study compared data from 1975–1996 for 59 early-starting (before 8:00 am) and late-starting (8:00 am and later) high schools. Early-starting schools maintained their early status over the 20-year time period (Carskadon & Acebo, 1997). A sampling of 1996–1997 school year schedules posted on the Internet from 40 high schools throughout the United States found that 48% had start times of 7:30 am or earlier, with only 12% starting between 8:15 am–8:55 am (Wolfson, 2002). Another assessment of 50 high schools from around the country for the 2001–2002 school year found 35% of schools posted start times before 7:30 am and 16% between 8:15 am–8:55 am (Acebo & Wolfson, 2005).

In 2005, Wolfson and Carskadon conducted a comprehensive analysis of factors that contributed significantly to the determination of high school start times and whether these times changed across the decades (Wolfson & Carskadon, 2005). Over 4000 public high schools representing 10% of public high schools in the United States were randomly selected from the National Center for Education Statistics' online database and asked to complete a brief survey regarding the pattern of school schedules and student demographics. Additionally, schools were asked about whether or not they had considered changing the school start times and perceived barriers to making the change. The final data set yielded information from 345 schools, for academic years 1986–1987 through 2001–2002. Results indicated that school start and end times remained stable across this 15-year time span. Factors associated with earlier start times were higher socioeconomic status, urban environment, and larger student populations with busing systems that operate multiple routes at different times each day (Wolfson & Carskadon, 2005).

Research on Delayed High School Start Times

Since the 1990s, researchers have examined the effects of school start times on measures of sleepiness and academic performance. Dexter and colleagues (2003) compared high school students in early-starting (7:50 am) versus late-starting (8:35 am) schools and reported reduced total sleep time and increased daytime sleepiness based on the Epworth Sleepiness Scale. Allen and colleagues have demonstrated that students from early-starting compared to late-starting schools reported shorter sleep times and a longer sleep phase delay (Allen, 1991). A follow-up study indicated that students at an earlier-starting school (7:40 am) slept less on weeknights and woke up later on weekends than students at a later-starting school (8:30 am; Allen, 1992). Later weekend bedtimes were associated with poorer grades in all students, with a higher percentage of students with "average grades" reporting bedtimes after 2:30 am compared to students that reported receiving the highest grades. Another investigation examining early (7:20 am) versus late (9:30 am) starting schools found that students at both schools reported similar bedtimes, but students at the earlier-starting schools had shorter total sleep times and more irregular sleep schedules, which were also related to poorer grades (Kowalski & Allen, 1995). A large sample of Rhode Island students who reported that they were failing or struggling academically (receiving Cs, Ds, and Fs) also reported later bedtimes, increased sleepiness, and more irregular sleep schedules than students who reported receiving higher grades (e.g., As and Bs; Wolfson & Carskadon, 2003).

The first longitudinal study to examine the effect of school start times on sleep patterns in adolescents did an initial evaluation of 9th-grade students in a junior high with a start time of 8:25 am and repeated the examination when they were in 10th grade at a high school with a start time of 7:20 am (Carskadon, Wolfson, Acebo, Tzischinsky, & Seifer, 1998). The study protocol included both actigraphy and sleep diaries completed at home, as well as 22-hour evaluations in the sleep laboratory with saliva sampling, sleep monitoring, and the multiple sleep latency test (MSLT). Results found that while these students reported similar bed times in the 9th and 10th grades, they woke up earlier in 10th grade to accommodate the earlier school start time and thus experienced shorter sleep durations. These students were also found to have significantly greater daytime sleepiness as evidenced by results of the MSLT in 10th grade compared to when they were in the 9th grade. For some students, sleepiness levels reached pathological levels similar to those suffering from narcolepsy.

The groundbreaking prospective study examining effects of delaying school start times on school performance was conducted in the mid-1990s in Minneapolis-St. Paul, Minnesota. Initial data were gathered from a suburban school district in Edina, Minnesota, that delayed start times at their high school by 65 minutes (from 7:25 am to 8:30 am). In comparison to the year before the change was implemented, they found improved performance in attendance, mood, and academics. This initial study was expanded into the full-scale School Start Time Study, with the goal of documenting the effects of a start-time delay from 7:15 am to 8:40 am during the 1996–1997 school year in seven public high schools within an urban district. The district enlisted the Center for Applied Research and Educational Improvement (CAREI) in the College of Education and Human Development at the University of Minnesota to oversee the data collection and analysis effort. The strength of the methodology was in its comprehensiveness, which included data from over 18,000 students spanning 2 years prior to and up to 3 years after the delay in school start times. Measures included both self-report outcomes (e.g., the norm-referenced School Sleep Habits Survey), as well as objective indices provided by the district, such as grades and enrollment and attendance records. Importantly, it focused on the effects of school start time changes on the community as a whole, analyzing results from focus groups with students, teachers, and other community members.

Self-reported sleep variables were assessed through two administrations of the School Sleep Habits Survey after the time change in year 1 (December 1997) and year 4 (January 2001). Additionally, a random sample of high school students from an anonymous but demographically similar district with a school start time of 7:30 am was also surveyed at both time points for comparison purposes. Importantly, wake-up and bedtimes did not statistically differ from 1997 to 2001. Students in the urban Minneapolis high schools were documented to sleep an average of 1 hour more per night than students from the district with a start time at 7:30 am in 1997, and this difference remained significant in year 4 after the change. This translates into students in the Minneapolis high schools getting 5 extra hours of sleep per week compared to students at the schools with an earlier start time. This finding countered the concerns of parents at the outset of the study that later start times would lead to later bedtimes in students; survey data obtained the year following the change, as well as 4 years later, refuted this belief.

Other significant differences in survey responses were found for students with earlier versus later school start times. Students at the Minneapolis high schools reported less overall daytime sleepiness, more frequent alertness in class, and fewer feelings of sleepiness while in class, during tests, and while completing homework. Additionally, students at later-starting schools noted fewer depressive feelings on a questionnaire querying their overall emotional state compared to students at schools with earlier start times (CAREI, 1998).

Further analyses uncovered positive relationships between later start times and student enrollment, attendance, and academic performance. The percentage of high school students who remained continuously enrolled in the same school or same district increased significantly in the years following the time change. While students may elect to change schools for a variety of reasons, the policy within this district mandated that students with excessive tardiness to class be dropped from those classes, prompting students to switch schools to avoid documentation of dropped classes on transcripts. The later school start time was postulated to contribute to decreased tardiness and subsequently fewer students needing to switch schools to cover up dropped classes.

Results concerning enrollment in a high–risk population were also encouraging. Although 9th–11th-graders who were continuously enrolled in the same school for 2 or more years demonstrated high and relatively unchanged attendance rates before and after the change, a different pattern emerged for students with discontinuous enrollment. Students who moved between multiple high schools throughout their 4 years had increased attendance after the change in school start times, with the most significant gains seen in the 11th-graders. A gain in attendance rates for students in 12th grade, however, was not seen after the change in school start times. Since many students in 12th grade are above the age of mandatory school attendance, the greater variability in attendance for this age may mask the more modest gains attributable to school start times.

Grades were a highly anticipated source of objective data; however, results only indicated a trend toward improved academic performance after the time change. The study revealed a number of challenges to utilizing grades as an outcome measure, including difficulty of comparing courses, schedules, and grading periods across various schools; student transience between schools; data entry errors on the part of school personnel; and missing data within the recording system.

Focus groups were also conducted with students, and a number of other groups were also surveyed and interviewed, including teachers, coaches, administrators, principals, counselors, parents, and other members of the community. For comparison purposes, similar surveys and focus groups were conducted with the suburban Edina schools that initially delayed their school start times. These interviews elucidated both negative and positive consequences of the change. Students from the urban high schools cited that they could not imagine returning to the earlier start times and anecdotally reported less sleepiness and morning stress. Reports of negative consequences from the urban schools largely focused on the impact to athletics, in which students occasionally were required to leave school early in order to travel to competitions in neighboring areas.

The survey of teachers was particularly comprehensive. Before the change, in 1996, 578 high school teachers in 17 suburban school districts responded to a survey in which 64% classified between 8:00 and 8:30 am as the optimal start time, despite the fact that most were teaching in high schools that started between 7:15 and 7:35 am. In a survey administered to the urban Minneapolis high school teachers after the start change, 57% reported more alert students during the first two periods of the day and 51% believed fewer students were sleeping at their desks. Teachers were, however, evenly divided on opinion as to whether students were positive toward the change and if it positively affected their teaching. In contrast to urban teachers, those surveyed from the suburban schools in Edina were nearly unanimous in the positive effects it had on their schools. Coaches' responses were more variable, with some vocal about their dislike for the change and its effect on practice and travel, but a majority was supportive and believed students were more alert at the end of the day after the change. Despite the fact that some programming was shortened and students returned home later than before the change, participation in extracurricular activities remained consistent across the 4 years after the change.

A sample of eight high school principals in the urban schools were interviewed and cited increased calmness in their schools, with 5 of the 8 reporting fewer disciplinary referrals. Seventeen school counselors and three nurses in the urban schools were also interviewed and agreed with this assessment, reporting fewer students expressing problems with peer or parent relationships. Reactions from parents in the urban schools were mixed during focus groups, while suburban parents who completed written surveys were overwhelmingly positive, with 93% reporting being "pleased" with the later start time for high school students. Both sets of parents did indicate that their children were "easier to live with" after the change and that the morning household routine was positively impacted as well.

Since this set of studies in urban and suburban Minnesota, only a limited number of other published results exist that document the effects of changes in school start times, and no other studies examine changes on such a widespread scale. However, a handful of more recent studies have reported similar findings within the past decade.

Students at Wilton High School in Wilton, Connecticut, were surveyed in 2001 and 2002 and again in 2004 after a school start time change from 7:35 am to 8:15 am (O'Malley & O'Malley, 2008). Average total sleep times increased by 34 minutes after the change. Although student bedtimes did not change, additional sleep was gained from students being able to extend their morning sleep time. These results suggested again that parental fears of students delaying bedtimes due to later start times were unfounded. While there was an overall reduction in self-reported daytime sleepiness in students, one-third of students still frequently reported occasional "problem sleepiness" even after the change, pointing to the magnitude of the sleep deprivation problem in adolescent students.

In 2010, Owens and colleagues examined the impact of a 30-minute start delay on sleep durations of students attending a Rhode Island private boarding high school. Students were surveyed utilizing the Sleep Habits Survey (Wolfson & Carskadon, 1998) both before and after a school start-time change from 8:00 to 8:30 am. Total average school night sleep times increased 45 minutes, from 7 hours 7 minutes to 7 hours 52 minutes. In addition to students sleeping later in the morning (6:54 am vs. 7:25 am), they also reported significantly earlier bedtimes (11:39 pm vs. 11:21 pm). This finding contrasts with reports from the Minnesota sample, which found consistent bedtimes before and after the change. Researchers postulated that results may have been impacted by seasonal variations in bedtimes and cited anecdotal reports from students that a heightened awareness of potential benefits from increased sleep may have been a motivating factor in changing sleep habits. Importantly, the percentage of students reporting 8 or more hours of sleep increased, from 16.4% to 54.7%, while the percentage reporting less than 7 hours of sleep decreased by 79.4%.

Additional self-reported survey results demonstrated that students felt less daytime sleepiness, feelings of fatigue, and depressed mood. The number of students requiring some type of assistance to wake significantly decreased. Feelings of fatigue or lack of motivation were also reported by fewer students after the change. The Student Health Center documented that between the before and after surveys, fewer students came to the health center with fatigue-related complaints; but medical and psychological complaints did not differ between the two survey time points.

Although the New England boarding school plans were for a temporary change in school start time, there was an overwhelming consensus among teachers, parents, and students to make the delay in start time permanent. While this particular school population is not typical of large urban school districts, results corroborated previous reports demonstrating that sleep deprivation problems are widespread and the start time solution can be beneficial. While this study sample may not generalize to those of public schools, the relative control this school had over students' sleep and wake schedules provided useful insights.

Recent research suggests that the age range in which sleep deprivation occurs among adolescents is widening to include middle school–age students. A study of students from one early-starting (7:15 am) and one late-starting (8:37 am) middle school within the same public northeastern district found that students at the late-starting school obtained 50 more minutes of sleep each night (Wolfson, Spaulding, Dandrow, & Baroni, 2007). Students at the late-starting school reported wake times over 1 hour later than those at the early-starting school, and also reported less sleepiness and tardiness than students at the early-starting school.

The issue of school start times and its role in adolescent sleep deprivation is not limited to research within the United States. A case control study in Israel examined the effects of a temporary delay in school start times for middle school students on measures of attention (Lufi, Tzischinsky & Hadar, 2011). Students in an experimental group had school start times delayed by one hour for one week and then reverted to their original schedule for a second week, while the control group remained at the original schedule for both weeks of the study. Students were assessed using measures of sustained attention at the end of each week. All students were instructed to maintain the same bedtimes they were accustomed to before the change. Students wore actigraphs and kept sleep diaries throughout the two weeks of the study. Results demonstrated that students in the experimental group slept an average of 55 minutes longer each night during the week of delayed school start time. Those students who slept longer demonstrated better performance on measures of attention, impulsivity, and performance rate on the sustained attention tasks.

The previously described studies provide consistent evidence that delaying school start times can lead to increased total sleep time for adolescents, and counters the myth that later start times lead to later bedtimes. Changing school start times can also have a constructive influence on students' academic and emotional well-being, and does relatively quickly garner support from administrators, parents, teachers, and students.

While there is much consensus on the benefits of delayed high school start times from a limited number of research studies, analyses are based on self-reported surveys, which carry inherent response bias. The volatile nature of this issue also makes systematic longitudinal studies difficult to conduct. Lack of parental and school cooperation, scalability, and costs have been barriers to studies seeking to use more objective assessments such as academic performance or cognitive performance on neuropsychological tests.

Additional Benefits of Later High School Start Times

Sleep deprivation in adolescents contributes to a range of negative outcomes that include poorer cognitive functioning, disruptive sleep patterns, and physical and mental health issues (Anderson, Petros, Beckwith, Mitchell, & Fritz, 1991; Dahl, 1996; Carskadon, 1994; Wolfson & Carskadon, 1996; Poirel & Larouche, 1987; Maas, 1995; Wolfson & Carskadon, 1998; O'Brien & Mindell, 2005; Pack, Pack, Rodgman, Cucchiara, Dinges, & Schwab, 1995). Most recently, studies have examined the link between school start times and sleep deprivation and its impact on risky behaviors in adolescents, such as drowsy driving and juvenile delinquency. A study in Virginia found that schools with later start times reported lower teen car crash rates than schools with earlier start times (Vorona, Szklo-Coxe, Wu, Dubik, Zhao, & Ware, 2011). Researchers in Kentucky found that average teen crash rates decreased 16.5% in the two years following a 1-hour delay in high school start times when compared to the 2 years prior to the change, while rates for the rest of the state increased during the same period (Danner & Phillips, 2008). Another study reported a positive correlation between sleep deprivation in adolescents and the volume of violent and property crime (Clinkinbeard, Simi, Evans, & Anderson, 2011). Sleeping just one hour less (7 hours) than the recommended reference group (8–10 hours of sleep) contributed to increased likelihood of property delinquency, and the effect increased for each hour of sleep missed. The hours immediately following school release times have been found to have the highest rates of juvenile delinquency (National Archive of Criminal Justice Data, 2008). Thus, later release times may lead to some reduction in community crime.

Recent educational policy research has examined data surrounding school start times and academic achievement in an attempt to construct a cost-benefit ratio for later start times. In the Hamilton Report, (Jacob & Rockoff, 2011) economists calculated a 9:1 benefit to cost ratio for later start times. They utilized studies conducted by Carrell and colleagues (2011) and Edwards (2011) to show that delaying start times by one hour could increase test scores by an average of 0.175 standard deviations. Carrell and colleagues utilized first-year students in the Air Force academy who have varying regimented schedules and standardized assessment examinations and found that students beginning classes before 8:00 am performed worse in all of their courses. A 1-hour delay corresponded to a 0.5 standard deviation increase in performance. Edwards (2011) examined data for a number of schools with varying start times in Wake County, North Carolina, and found that variation in start times at schools over time corresponded to a 2-point percentile gain in math and 1-point percentile gain in reading performance, with increased benefits seen for disadvantaged students. The report calculated the potential increase in academic achievement to correspond to an 8% rise in future earnings per student, or $17,500 annually in today's value. Transportation costs for changing school start times were estimated based on recent research to range from $0 to $1950 per student over their entire school career, putting the benefit to cost ratio at a minimum of 9:1.

Barriers to Changing School Start Times

Despite research evidence on the significant benefits of delaying middle and high school start times, there are also documented challenges associated with implementing a change, particularly in a large public school district. The School Start Time Study in Minnesota identified a diverse group of individuals that would be affected by school schedules, including teachers, administrators, custodial staff, transportation and food service employees, community members involved in before- and after-school childcare, and local business owners that employ students (Center for Applied Research and Educational Improvement [CAREI], 1998). School start times evolved, in part, to accommodate these various scheduling needs, which in turn affected the schedule of the surrounding community. Thus, the prospect of changing start times is not something that can be undertaken without an extensive, time-consuming effort involving various stakeholders.

The School Start Time Study conducted interviews with a broad range of affected individuals who voiced concerns ranging from the impact on local traffic patterns to the use of shared community facilities for athletics and extracurricular activities. In addition to interviewing those in the suburban Edina district and urban Minneapolis high schools that delayed their start times, a total of 17 suburban districts were included in an analysis to determine potential barriers to change. Many schools share the use of facilities with community groups, such as adult continuing education, services for seniors, and independent organizations for athletics and the arts. Schools usually take priority for use of these facilities in the hours immediately following school dismissal times. Later school start times consequently delay the start times of community activities that share these spaces, which can limit the amount of programming that can be offered.

Costs also are a significant barrier for change that affects the district as a whole, with student busing costs being one of the most commonly cited expenses (Kirby, Maggi, & D'Angiulli, 2011). Multi-tiered busing schedules used to lower transportation costs can be difficult to alter; however, the School Start Time Study found that delaying start times did not increase transportation costs in either the suburban district in Edina or the urban district in Minneapolis (Wahlstrom, 2002). The 2005 survey published by the National Sleep Foundation found that switching bus schedules between elementary and high schools can eliminate an increase in transportation cost, and one district reported saving money by eliminating the busing for high school students in favor of utilizing public transportation, a potential option for urban schools but not likely for suburban schools. Transportation options and costs vary significantly across the country and require analysis by each individual district considering a change in school start times. Other financial considerations include school schedule shifts that can misalign hours specified in teacher contracts, leading to increased costs to accommodate new schedules (CAREI, 1998).

For older students, the scheduling of before-school and after-school extracurricular activities is one of their most salient concerns (CAREI, 1998). Any change in school start times would necessitate corresponding changes to these activities. This is also a particular issue for athletic directors who are faced with the challenge of coordinating inter-school collaboration and competition with other districts. Results from the School Start Time Study in Minnesota indicated that later start times did not alter student participation in after-school activities; however, there were reports of students leaving school early to allow travel time to events when competing against schools with earlier dismissal times.

The School Start Time Study also examined concerns of local business owners that employ students after school. Students with later start times worked fewer hours at paid jobs compared to students from earlier starting schools; however, future research is necessary to eliminate other factors that may have contributed to this difference.

Parental biases that persist despite contrary scientific evidence offer another significant barrier to enacting change within a district. One of the most salient parental biases is the belief that later start times will simply lead to later bedtimes for older students, eliminating any increase in total sleep time (Au, 2009). Although research has not supported this contention (Wolfson, 2002; Wolfson, Spaulding, Dandrow, & Baroni, 2007; O'Malley & O'Malley, 2008; Owens, Belon, & Moss, 2010), the belief persists among parents in communities considering making a change.

The decision to delay high school start times while minimizing costs to the school system often involves changing to earlier start times for younger students, generating another set of concerns and additional barriers from parents of these students. While this solution may keep costs minimal for the school, it can lead to higher before- and after-school childcare costs. Teachers who are parents to young children may find their new work schedule askew from existing childcare options. Other working parents may confront similar childcare scheduling mismatches, particularly for those that have relied on high school students for after-school babysitting.

Low-light conditions due to early start times or late dismissal times prompt parental concerns over safety (CAREI, 1998). Some states and districts have implemented structured bus pick-ups and drop-offs around "civil twilight," which is defined as when the geometric center of the sun is 6 degrees below the horizon (Fairfax County School Board Transportation Task Force Final Report, 2008). Practically, this time period is the limit of illumination at which objects can be sufficiently distinguished in clear weather conditions and varies day to day throughout the school year (Fairfax County School Board Transportation Task Force Final Report, 2008). Reports from the Minnesota sample indicated that transportation directors did not voice any problems regarding safety in low-light conditions (CAREI, 1998). A Fairfax County Virginia Task force that was investigating a possible change in school start times found that the majority of participants wanted civil twilight to be considered, but not utilized as a barrier when establishing busing schedules (Fairfax County School Board Transportation Task Force Final Report, 2008).

In addition to safety, parents of elementary-age children facing the possibility of earlier start times express a number of other fears. One of their central arguments is that this switch simply transfers the problem of sleep deprivation from the older students to the younger ones. Consequently, younger students' ability to learn will be diminished because they will be too sleepy to be alert and attentive throughout the school day (Au, 2009). When called upon, sleep researchers and experts, in an effort to dispel these parental reservations, offer the observation that there is no biological rationale that prevents younger children from falling asleep earlier. They posit that parents can establish consistent bedtime routines to ensure that their children obtain enough sleep each night. The science, however, falls short in allaying parental anxieties because, to date, there are no published studies of the impact of early school start times on elementary-age students.

The research community's recommendation of earlier bedtimes for younger students to offset earlier school start times creates another potential issue for parents, particularly for those who work outside of the home. These parents cite that the altered routine will disrupt family time and decrease the already limited number of hours they can spend with their children (Au, 2009). Additionally, if parents rely on older siblings to watch their younger children during the initial after-school hours, they may be faced with new childcare needs during the gap between elementary and high school release times (Au, 2009). Schools may want to consider how to alleviate these particular concerns by offering convenient options for before- and after-school childcare.

Wolfson and Carskadon (2005) and others have corroborated the initial findings of the Minnesota School Start Time Study addressing barriers to change, particularly the issues related to scheduling and financial concerns affecting the school as a whole and the impact on high school students' after-school schedules (Wahlstrom, 2002). Additional research has documented the relationship of school start times and school bus safety, transportation costs, and energy efficiency (Humphres & Vincent, 1981; Mawdsley, 1996; Miller, 1988; Transportation Research Board, 1989).

Taken together, the studies suggest that schools make policy decisions based on historical precedent, perceived and demonstrated efficacy, and cost-effectiveness. Of less import to the decision-making processes is consideration of health and science research (Wolfson & Carskadon, 2005). Having to accommodate many stakeholders including parents, teachers, administrators, childcare providers, coaches, instructors, employers, bus drivers, other school employees, community organizations, community facilities used and shared with the schools—not to mention the students themselves—it is not surprising that policy makers often overlook research, particularly when its findings are at odds with majority opinion. To enact any type of change requires compromise and acceptance of potential consequences (including disadvantages to some, which may or may not be temporary) as well as willingness to wait for longer-term benefits to become evident.

These barriers to change create a politically contentious environment that present obstacles to researchers as well as administrators (Wolfson, 2002). Implementing scientifically appropriate study designs that will generate results generalizable to the larger population depends on identifying heterogeneous study samples, using validated instruments, and administering these tests on a time-sensitive schedule longitudinally. While school districts around the country share the common problem of too-early start times, each district and its community feels that its situation is contending with its own unique barriers and thus cannot be subjected to the rigorous conditions of a research-based evaluation. Researchers must balance the demands of proper research methodology to produce reliable and valid results with the realities of trying to do so in an emotionally charged environment. As research in this area continues to evolve, future projects will need to share both the strengths and limitations of their findings, and likely pool their results to generate a comprehensive database comprising districts from varying geographical regions and students from different socioeconomic backgrounds. Also necessary is the inclusion of other mitigating factors, such as parental demographics and schools' academic standing.

Wolfson (2002) further counsels that researchers need to be open to developing collaborations with educators focused on interdisciplinary communication, mutual respect, and support from others in the fields of sleep research and medicine. While researchers may find daunting the task of designing a scientific protocol that aligns with the goals of the district while trying to maintain the integrity and validity of the data collection process, achieving this balance will likely require compromises on the part of both the district and the research group. However, Wolfson contends working toward accomplishing these goals should both strengthen the field and lead to more informed decision making regarding educational reforms. The experiences of researchers in the School Start Time Study demonstrated that successful implementation of a change involves coordinated communication between all parties involved and a focus on hard data rather than theories and assumptions about what is possible within a school district (Wahlstrom, 1999).

Conclusion

The research described in this chapter has documented consistent and significant positive effects on academic performance and on social and psychological behaviors when middle school and high school start time delays have been implemented. Anecdotal and subjective reports from opinion surveys and focus groups have echoed these encouraging results with generally affirmative sentiments. While some dissenting voices remain in each group, negative opinions largely center on discomfort with the idea of a change in general, or on specific concerns with disruptions in the before-/after-school schedules, particularly related to athletics. Even those that maintain opinions in opposition to changes in start times are frequently willing to admit to positive effects on student behavior (CAREI, 1998).

Apart from the demonstrated increased sleep durations that occur when high school start times are delayed, the pragmatic factors create challenges that the beneficial findings cannot overcome. For many school administrators, the emotional toll that is exacted from trying to overcome the many real and perceived barriers is too high a cost, regardless of the potential benefit. Administrators also have to assess other proposed district-wide policy changes and make decisions as to which are of greatest priority. How these battles for change are fought also sets a precedent of conduct for addressing other education policy issues. Effective administrators seek to institute policy change with minimal conflict between themselves, teachers, students, and families. The educational system is designed on a foundation of routine, with school start times acting as the bedrock. Wahlstrom (2002), in describing her experiences with the School Start Time Study, noted that it could be particularly unsettling to change something as fundamentally accepted as local school start times. Natural resistance leads otherwise rational, well-meaning people to succumb to myths rather than facts. For example, despite consistent contrary evidence, parents and administrators still frequently cite that a reason for not delaying high school start times is because students will stay awake later if they are allowed to sleep in later. Another common assumption is that changing start times will be costly because it often involves altering busing schedules; however, research in a number of districts has shown that busing transportation can be modified to accommodate the changes without increasing costs.

Despite the noteworthy work to date, there are still significant gaps in the research literature related to school start times and its impact on sleep in school-age children. There are few longitudinal studies in general and fewer that have data on the effects of a change in school start times beyond the initial year or so. Further, most of the studies center around schools in the Midwest and Northeast. The paucity of studies lends to the problem of not enough representative samples of different types of school districts and of demographically diverse student populations. The lack of representative data exacerbates the disconnection between what sleep researchers are finding and what information school policy decisions are based on.

As more communities examine the issue of school start times, the lack of data on younger children is creating an almost insurmountable barrier for differentiating real versus perceived impact. Since many school districts operate on a multiple bell schedule in which elementary, middle, and high school start times are staggered, a frequent solution to delaying high school start times is to swap the start times between high schools and elementary schools. This allows districts to leave busing schedules intact and avoid any significant increase in costs, removing a key financial barrier to change. Research on prepubescent children indicate that earlier rise times are not problematic for younger students, but additional research looking at the impact of school start times on younger-age students would reinforce the biological data. The availability of objective evidence across the school-age spectrum would be of benefit to school administrators, school committee members, teachers, and parents, in addressing the needs of their entire school population. Currently, lack of data on the impact of school start times on younger children is resulting in far fewer schools willing to consider or able to enact change.

Researchers, policy makers, educators, and health providers each have an important role in moving forward the debate of school start times for younger and older students. For researchers, continued advancement in the understanding of the benefits and consequences of delayed start times for high school students will enhance the objective data already available today. But there should be a call for studies focused on the impact of school start times on younger children as well. While the biological changes that motivate the argument for delayed start times for adolescents do not uniformly apply for these younger students (Werner, LeBourgeois, Geiger, & Jenni, 2009), the public policy consequences of not doing this research can be equally compelling. Policy makers need to be vigilant in the separation of real from perceived consequences. Careful scrutiny and dissemination of research findings may help attenuate the emotional volatility of the debate and allow for objective cost-benefit assessment to determine the true value of a change in school start times to the community.

Educators and health providers provide the best line of communication to students and their parents. Students of all ages need to obtain adequate amounts of sleep to maintain both physical and mental health. Getting both students and parents to understand how school start times may be impacting their ability to get proper amounts of sleep is just one step. Teaching students proper day and bedtime practices (e.g., sleep hygiene) that promote sufficient hours as well as quality of sleep and encouraging parents to help their child, even during the teenage years, establish and maintain good sleep hygiene practices can lead to lifelong positive benefits even in the absence of a change in school start times.

Future Directions

- Studies investigating the impact of early school start times in younger students are needed to provide objective data that documents the full school-age spectrum.
- More research examining the longer-range longitudinal effects of delaying start times is warranted, using methods that include valid measures of sleep habits, emotional and physical well-being, risky behaviors, attendance and enrollment, and indices of academic achievement collected more years before and after a change is implemented.
- To increase the generalizability of data, investigations need to cast a larger net to better capture a wider range of demographics, particularly in geography, school size, socioeconomic status, and other related variables.
- As communities consider whether to change their school start times, it is important to have available scientific data that addresses the range of perceived as well as biological, psychosocial, and academic concerns.
- Proper and comprehensive education of all stakeholders is an important initial step. Researchers must find effective methods for disseminating study outcomes, and educators and health providers should promote the importance of developing healthy sleep habits in students of all ages.

References

Acebo, C., & Wolfson, A. R. (2005). Inadequate sleep in children and adolescents. In C. A. Kushida (Ed.), *Sleep Deprivation* (pp. 151–175). New York: Marcel Dekker.

Allen, R. (1992). Social factors associated with the amount of school week sleep lag for seniors in an early starting suburban high school. *Sleep Research, 21*, 114.

Allen, R. P. (1991). School-week sleep lag: Sleep problems with earlier starting of senior high schools. *Sleep Research, 20*, 198.

Anderson, M. J., Petros, T. V., Beckwith, B. E., Mitchell, W. W., & Fritz, S. (1991). Individual differences in the effect of time of day on long-term memory access. *American Journal of Psychology, 104*(2), 241–255.

Au, R. (2009). *Changing School Start Times: Report for Duxbury Public Schools.* Unpublished manuscript.

Au, R. (2010). *The reality of changing school start times.* Presentation at National Sleep Foundation Conference., Washington D.C.

Bearpark, H. M., & Michie, P. T. (1987). Prevalence of sleep/wake disturbances in Sydney adolescents. *Sleep Research, 16*, 304.

Calamaro, C. J., Mason, T. B. A., & Ratcliffe, S. J. (2009). Adolescents living the 24/7 lifestyle: Effects of caffeine and technology on sleep duration and daytime functioning. *Pediatrics, 123*(6), e1005–e1010.

Carrell, S. E., Maghakian, T., & West, J. E. (2011). A's from ZZZZ's? The causal effect of school start time on the academic achievement of adolescents. *American Economic Journal, 3*(3), 62–71.

Carskadon, M. A., Harvey, K., Duke, P., Anders, T. F., Litt, I. F., & Dement, W. C. (1980). Pubertal changes in day-time sleepiness. *Sleep, 19*, 453–460.

Carskadon, M. A. (1982). In the second decade. In C. Guilleminault (Ed.) *Sleeping and Waking Disorders: Indications and Techniques* (pp. 99–125). Menlo Park, CA: Addison-Wesley.

Carskadon, M. A. (1990). Patterns of sleep and sleepiness in adolescents. *Pediatrician, 17,* 5–12.

Carskadon, M. A. (1994). Measuring daytime sleepiness. In M. H. Kryger, T. Roth, & W. C. Dement (Eds.), *Principles and Practice of Sleep Medicine* (2nd ed., pp. 961–962). Philadelphia: W.B. Saunders.

Carskadon, M. A., Wolfson, A. R., Tzischinsky, O., & Acebo, C. (1995). Early school schedules modify adolescent sleepiness. *Sleep Research, 24,* 92.

Carskadon, M. A., & Acebo, C. (1997). Historical view of high school start time: Preliminary results. *Sleep, 26,* 184.

Carskadon, M. A., Acebo, C., Richardson, G. S., Tate, B. A. & Seifer, R. (1997). An approach to studying circadian rhythms of adolescent humans. *Journal of Biological Rhythms, 12*(3), 278–289.

Carskadon, M. A., Wolfson, A. R., Acebo, C., Tzischinsky, O. & Seifer, R. (1998). Adolescent sleep patterns, circadian timing, and sleepiness at a transition to early school days. *Sleep, 21*(8), 871–881.

Center for Applied Research and Educational Improvement (CAREI) College of Education and Human Development University of Minnesota School Start Time Study Full Report. (1998). http://conservancy.umn.edu/bitstream/4221/1/CAREI%20SST-1998VI.pdf

Clinkinbeard, S. S., Simi, P., Evans, M. K., & Anderson, A. L. (2011). Sleep and delinquency: Does the amount of sleep matter? *Journal of Youth and Adolescents, 40*(7), 916–930.

Dahl, R. E., & Carskadon, M. A. (1995). Sleep and its disorders in adolescence. In R. Ferber & M. H. Kryger (Eds.), *Principles and Practices of Sleep Medicine in the Child* (pp. 19–27). Philadelphia: Saunders.

Dahl, R. E. (1996). The impact of inadequate sleep on children's daytime cognitive functioning. *Seminars in Pediatric Neurology, 3*(1), 44–50.

Dahl, R. E., & Lewin, D. S. (2002). Pathways to adolescent health: Sleep regulation and behavior. *Journal of Adolescent Health, 31,* 175–184.

Danner, F., & Phillips, B. (2008). Adolescent sleep, school start times, and teen motor vehicle crashes. *Journal of Clinical Sleep Medicine, 4*(6), 533–535.

Dexter, D., Bijwadia, J., Schilling, D., & Applebaugh, G. (2003). Sleep, sleepiness and school start times: A preliminary study. *Wisconsin Medical Journal, 102,* 44–46.

Eaton, D. K., McKnight-Eily, L. R., Lowry, R., Perry, G. S., Presley-Cantrell, L., & Croft, J. B. (2010). Prevalence of insufficient, borderline, and optimal hours of sleep among high school students—United States, 2007. *Journal of Adolescent Health, 46,* 399–401.

Edwards, F. (2011). *Early to rise: The effect of daily start times on academic performance.* Working paper, University of Illinois at Urbana-Champaign.

Fairfax County School Board Transportation Task Force Final Report, 2008. http://www.fcps.edu/fts/taskforce07/documents/finalreport/majorityfinalreport.pdf

Gibson, E. S., Powles, A. C., Thabane, L., O'Brien, S., Molnar, D. S., Trajanovic, N., et al. (2006). "Sleepiness" is serious in adolescence: Two surveys of 3235 Canadian students. *BMC Public Health, 6,* 116.

Hansen, M., Janssen, I., Schiff, A., Zee, P. C., & Dubocovich, M. L. (2005). The impact of school daily schedule on adolescent sleep. *Pediatrics, 115,* 1555–1161.

Humphres, K. W., & Vincent, R. (1981). Five tips for cutting transportation costs. *American School Board Journal, 168*(11), 25.

Jacob, B. A., & Rockoff, J. E. (2011) Organizing schools to improve student achievement: start times, grade configurations, and teacher assignments. Supra pp. 5–11. http://www.brookings.edu/~/media/research/files/papers/2011/9/organization%20jacob%20rockoff/092011_organize_jacob_rockoff_paper.pdf

Kirby, M., Maggi, S. & D'Angiulli, A. (2011). School start times and the sleep-wake cycle of adolescents: A review and critical evaluation of available evidence. *Educational Researcher, 40*(2), 56–61.

Kowalski, N. A., & Allen, R. P. (1995). School sleep lag is less but persists with very late starting high school. *Sleep Research, 24.*

Lufi, D., Tzischinsky, O. & Hadar, S. (2011). Delaying school starting time by one hour: Some effects on attention levels in adolescents. *Journal of Clinical Sleep Medicine, 7*(2), 137–143.

Maas, J. B. (1995). *Power Sleep.* New York: Villard-Random House.

Mawdsley, R. D. (1996). *Pupil Transportation and the Law.* (Monograph Series No. 55). (2nd ed.) Topeka, KS: National Organization on Legal Problems of Education.

Mercer, P. W., Merritt, S. L., & Cowell, J. M. (1998). Differences in reported sleep need among adolescents. *Journal of Adolescent Health, 2,* 453–460.

Miller, A.R. (1988). *Pupil Transportation Management.* Thousand Oaks, CA: Ramsburg and Roth.

National Archive of Criminal Justice Data, 2008. http://www.icpsr.umich.edu/icpsrweb/content/NACJD/guides/ucr.html

National Sleep Foundation. (2006). *Sleep in America Poll. Teens and Sleep.* National Sleep Foundation website. Available at http://www.sleepfoundation.org/article/sleep-america-polls/2006-teens-and-sleep/html.

Ng, E. P., Ng, D. K., & Chan, C. H. (2009). Sleep duration, sleep/wake symptoms, and academic performance in Hong Kong Secondary School Children. *Sleep and Breathing, 13*(4), 357–367.

O'Brien, E. M., & Mindell, J. A. (2005). Sleep and risk-taking behaviors in adolescents. *Behavioral Sleep Medicine, 3*(3), 113–133.

O'Malley, E. B., & O'Malley, M. B. (2008). School start time and its impact on learning and behavior. In A. Ivanenko (Ed.), *Sleep and Psychiatric Disorders in Children and Adolescents* (pp. 28–72). New York, London: Information Heathcare Publisher.

Owens, J. A., Belon, K. & Moss, P. (2010). Impact of delaying school start time on adolescent sleep, mood, and behavior. *Archives of Pediatrics and Adolescent Medicine, 164*(7), 608–614.

Pack, A. I., Pack, A. M., Rodgman, D., Cucchiara, A., Dinges, D. F., & Schwab, C. W. (1995). Characteristics of crashes attributed to the driver having fallen asleep. *Accident Analysis and Prevention, 27,* 769–775.

Petta, D., Carskadon, M., & Dement, W. C. (1984). Sleep habits in children aged 7–13 years. *Sleep Research, 13,* 86.

Poirel, C., & Larouche, B. (1987). Human circadian patterns of memory processes: chronopsychology of rates of forgetting, a rhythmometric study. *Psychological Reports, 61*, 3–12.

Strauch, I., & Meier, B. (1988). Sleep need in adolescents: A longitudinal approach. *Sleep, 11*(4), 378–386.

Transportation Research Board. (1989). *Improving School Bus Safety: Special report.* Washington, DC: National Research Council.

Tynjala, J., Kannas, L., & Valimaa, R. (1993). How young Europeans sleep. *Health Education Research, 8*, 69–80.

Vorona, R. D., Szklo-Coxe, M., Wu, A., Dubik, M., Zhao, Y., & Ware, J. C. (2011). Dissimilar teen crash rates in two neighboring southeastern Virginia cities with different high school start times. *Journal of Clinical Sleep Medicine, 7*(2), 145–151.

Wahlstrom, K. (1999). The prickly politics of school starting times. *Phi Delta Kappan, 80*(5), 344–347.

Wahlstrom, K. (2002). Changing times: findings from the first longitudinal study of later high school start times. *NASSP Bulletin, 86*(633), 3–21.

Werner, H., LeBourgeois, M., Geiger, A., & Jenni, O. G. (2009). Assessment of chronotype in four-to eleven-year-old children: Reliability and validity of the children's chronotype questionnaire (CCTQ). *Chronobiology International, 26*(5), 992–1014.

Wolfson A. (2002). Bridging the gap between research and practice: What will adolescents' sleep/wake patterns look like in the 21st century. In M. A. Carskadon (Ed.), *Adolescent Sleep Patterns: Biological, Social and Psychological Influences* (pp. 198–219). New York: Cambridge University Press.

Wolfson, A. R., & Carskadon, M. A. (1996). Early school start times affect sleep and daytime functioning in adolescents. *Sleep Research, 25*, 117.

Wolfson, A. R. & Carskadon, M. A. (1998). Sleep schedules and daytime functioning in adolescents. *Society for Research in Child Development, 69*(4), 875–887.

Wolfson, A. R., & Carskadon, M. A. (2003). Understanding adolescents' sleep patterns and school performance: a critical appraisal. *Sleep Medicine Review, 7*(6), 491–506.

Wolfson, A. R., & Carskadon, M. A. (2005). A survey of factors influencing high school start times. *NASSP Bulletin, 89*, 47–66.

Wolfson, A. R., Spaulding, N. L., Dandrow, C., & Baroni, E. M. (2007). Middle school start times: The importance of a good night's sleep for young adolescents. *Behavioral Sleep Medicine, 5*, 194–209.

Wolfson, A. R. (2010). Adolescents and emerging adults' sleep patterns: New developments. *Journal of Adolescent Health, 46*(2), 97–99.

Yang, C-K., Kim, J. K., Patel, S. R., & Lee, J-H. (2005). Age-related changes in sleep-wake patterns among Korean teenagers. *Pediatrics, 115*(1), 250–256.

CHAPTER

39 Preventative Intervention: Curricula and Programs

Reut Gruber, Evelyn Constantin, Jamie Cassoff, *and* Sonia Michaelsen

Abstract

A substantial body of evidence indicates that an appropriate quantity and quality of sleep is necessary for healthy physical development as well as optimization of cognitive growth, academic success, and emotional well-being. These are key features of successful development. Inadequate or poor sleep impairs health, emotional regulation, and cognitive development. The many negative impacts of sleep deprivation and disturbance emphasize the need to provide health care professionals with the education and tools required to assist parents and their children to achieve the sleep required for healthy development. In the present review, therefore, we include sections for each of the traditional pediatric age groups: early postpartum and infancy, toddlers and preschoolers, school-age children, and adolescents. For each age period, we first briefly describe normal sleep behavior (which is more extensively reviewed in the first section of this book) and identify primary sleep issues of particular importance during different developmental periods that should be the focus of educational interventions. We then review and evaluate evidence-based pediatric sleep intervention curricula and programs that target such sleep issues. Next we suggest sleep promotion strategies that may be effective within particular areas of need. Finally, we discuss potential future directions for relevant health care professionals, including pediatricians and psychologists.

Key Words: sleep promotion, preventative interventions, prevention, sleep deprivation, sleep education, sleep hygiene, pediatric health care, sleep programs, sleep curricula

Introduction

A substantial body of evidence indicates that an appropriate level of sleep is necessary for healthy physical development, optimization of cognitive growth, academic success, and emotional well-being, which are key elements of successful development. Sufficient sleep ensures that metabolism is normal and physiological functioning is appropriate, whereas sleep deprivation has been empirically linked to an increased risk for the development of obesity and, in adulthood, diabetes, hypertension, metabolic syndrome, and cardiovascular problems (Dinges & Chugh, 1997; Hasler, Buysse, Klaghofer, Gamma, Ajdacic, et al., 2004; Magee, Huang, Iverson, & Caputi, 2010; Shigeta, Shigeta, Nakazawa, Nakamura, & Yoshikawa, 2001). In addition, poor sleep has been shown to impair *learning, memory, and* general cognitive ability as reflected by IQ test scores and other measures, especially in the context of activities essential for academic success (Alhola & Polo-Kantola, 2007; BaHammam, Al-Faris, Shaikh, & Saeed, 2006; Horne, 1988; Linde & Bergströme, 1992; Meijer, 2008; Meijer, Habekothé, & Van Den Wittenboer, 2000; Nilsson, Söderström, Karlsson, Lekander, Åkerstedt, et al., 2005; Shin, Kim, Lee, Ahn, & Joo, 2003). Inadequate sleep creates a low threshold for expression of negative affect (irritability and frustration) and is associated with difficulty in modulation of impulse and emotion. Earlier research showed that short sleep duration and sleep disruption are associated with emotional dysregulation (Gruber, Cassoff, Frenette, Wiebe, & Carrier, 2012a; Walker & Van Der Helm, 2009) and development of psychiatric disorders (Lin, Tung, Hsieh, & Lin, 2011) in children. Collectively, therefore, the multiple negative impacts of sleep deprivation emphasize the need to provide health care professionals with education and tools that assist parents and their children to achieve the extent and quality of sleep required for healthy physical and emotional development, and that optimize the cognitive potential of the child.

An understanding of what constitutes a normal sleep pattern during development and the identification of factors affecting child sleep, are prerequisites if healthy sleep is to be achieved and maintained. The goals of the present review are, therefore, *(1)* to use a developmental perspective to review and evaluate current evidence-based pediatric sleep intervention curricula and programs that target such sleep issues; *(2)* to suggest potential sleep promotion strategies that may be effective when no evidence-based program is yet available within a particular area of need; and *(3)* to discuss potential future directions for research and for relevant health care professionals, including pediatricians and psychologists.

Review And Evaluate Current Evidence-Based Pediatric Sleep Intervention Curricula And Programs That Target Sleep Concerns

In the following section we will briefly describe normal sleep behavior at various ages (which are covered in detail in the chapters of the first section of this book) to highlight sleep issues that are relevant during particular developmental periods. Next, we will review and evaluate current evidence-based pediatric sleep intervention curricula and programs that target such sleep issues. Key features sought were first, identifiable interventional components and second, methodological issues (study design, use of a control group, randomization, and reporter blinding). Studies employing randomization, with control groups, and wherein informants reporting on outcome measures were blinded, were rated as the strongest. An intervention that did not feature any of the above qualities was considered to yield only marginal or weak evidence. In terms of the significance of primary and secondary outcomes, we distinguished between measurement of sleep knowledge and sleep behavior. Measurement of both factors was considered the strongest, whereas measurement of changes in sleep knowledge in the absence of measurement of sleep behavior was considered to be weaker. We further distinguished between objective (e.g., actigraphy) and subjective (e.g., parental reporting) measurement of sleep behavior. Inclusion of both measures was considered to be a feature of the strongest design; use of objective measures only was considered to be quite strong, whereas inclusion of subjective measures only was viewed as less strong. Reports were considered weaker if no blinding occurred and stronger if the reporter of the outcome measure was blinded to the intervention. We also considered the reported levels of effectiveness in terms of changes in outcome measures and durability of any effects noted.

Evidence-Based Pediatric Intervention Curricula Targeting Early Postpartum and Infancy

Normative Pattern of Sleep

In humans, the most rapid shift in terms of sleep consolidation occurs during the first year of life (Davis, Parker, & Montgomery, 2004). The sleep loss tolerance of newborns is rather low; infants cannot endure long periods of wakefulness. A major developmental milestone achieved by most infants by age 6 to 9 months is the ability to "sleep through the night" (i.e., to sleep for at least 8 hours a night). In addition to intrinsic changes in the circadian and homeostatic timing systems, behaviorally guided changes in the timing of light exposure, changes in family habits, and changes in environmental cues associated with sleep and wakefulness may interact directly with the phase-resetting mechanism of the circadian timing system. Such changes affect sleep timing and consolidation and, hence, the ability of a child to fall asleep at a desired time and to sleep through the night.

Primary Sleep Issues to be Targeted in a Sleep Intervention/Prevention Program

The development of the infant's circadian system and the process of sleep consolidation, which leads to a gradual reduction in sleep need and an increase in wake periods, highlight this period. Therefore, prevention strategies during this developmental stage are aimed at helping parents make behavioral choices that support the infant's ability to develop a sleep pattern that is consistent with the consolidation of longer sleep during the night. As further described below, there is evidence to support the idea that sleep intervention programs and sleep promotion strategies are effective in improving sleep in infants and their families.

Evidence-Based Sleep Intervention/Prevention Programs

Several studies have been conducted aimed at assessing the impact of behavioral and/or educational interventions designed to improve both maternal and infant sleep in the early postpartum period—these studies have highlighted the positive impact of early prevention (Mindell, Du Mond, Sadeh, Telofski, Kulkarni, & Gunn, 2011b; Mindell, Telofski, Wiegand, & Kurtz, 2009; Pinilla & Birch, 1993; St James-Roberts & Gillham, 2001; Stremler, Hodnett, & Lee, 2006; Symon, Marley, Martin, & Norman, 2005; Wolfson, Lacks, & Futterman, 1992).

In particular, four well-designed randomized controlled trials have demonstrated effectiveness of sleep behavior and education intervention programs for parents of newborns (Pinilla & Birch, 1993; St James-Roberts & Gillham, 2001; Symon et al., 2005; Wolfson et al., 1992). There is robust evidence that these intervention programs lead to improvements in sleep outcome measures, particularly more consistent sleep patterns and longer sleep duration (Pinilla & Birch, 1993; St James-Roberts & Gillham, 2001; Symon et al., 2005; Wolfson et al., 1992). One study also showed a positive impact on parents, with the parents who received the education intervention reporting improved self-efficacy and decreased stress (Wolfson et al., 1992). All of the studies offered parents personalized sessions (individual or in groups) with individuals trained in sleep education, and several of the studies provided parents with written documentation on sleep. The outcome measures for all of the studies were subjective reporting from parents using parent diaries/logs and/or questionnaires. Although the subjective parent reporting provides rich data, there are inherent weaknesses to subjective measures. Further studies are needed and would be strengthened by using both subjective and objective measures for determining sleep quality and quantity.

Evidence-Based Pediatric Intervention Curricula Targeting Toddlers and Preschool-aged children

Normative Pattern of Sleep

Following rapid development during the first year, a gradual decline in daytime napping is evident and sleep becomes consolidated into a single nighttime period (Weissbluth, 1995; Wolfson, 1996). In addition, although a longer period of consolidated sleep is achieved, night awakening is common (Acebo, Sadeh, Seifer, Tzischinksy, Hafer, & Carskadon, 2005). Whereas night awakening is "normative" (Davis, Parker, & Montgomery, 2004), the ability of the child to return to sleep without parental intervention determines whether a sleep disorder might develop. Several defining characteristics of this developmental period impact sleep behavior, as well as the manner in which parents respond to their child's nighttime behavior. First, rapid cognitive development may lead to development of normative nighttime fears (Moore, Meltzer, & Mindell, 2008), and the development of normative emotional attachments can create separation anxiety at bedtime (Blum & Carey, 1996). Such emerging themes may lead to development of dependency on a caregiver and, thus, problematic nighttime behavior may ensue; either sleep onset association insomnia or "reactive" co-sleeping may develop (Miller & Commons, 2010). Whether such behaviors become "problematic" or they are addressed in a manner allowing for the development of healthy sleep behavior depends greatly on parental expectations and responses. The normative developmental issues that can affect sleep behavior must be considered when planning a preventative sleep intervention (see Burnham, Chapter 12).

Primary Sleep Issues to be Targeted in a Sleep Intervention/Prevention Program

Developmental milestones particular to toddlers and preschoolers that may impact sleep and sleep behavior include rapid cognitive development leading to nighttime fears (Moore et al., 2007) and separation anxiety (Chorney, Detweiler, Morris, & Kuhn, 2008) at bedtime and, ultimately, to difficulties in sleep onset and more frequent night waking. With the developmental onset of independent locomotion (Jenni & Carskadon, 2005), children have the tendency to seek consolation for these nighttime fears (Moore et al., 2007) and anxieties through co-sleeping with their parents or guardians (Chorney et al., 2008). Alteration of napping schedules also comes into play in this age group, with gradual weaning of the daytime nap. Most children no longer have scheduled naps by age 3 to 5 years (Blum & Carey, 1996).

There are some important signs that require particular attention, where parents and clinicians must be vigilant to assess for symptoms of underlying sleep disorders that may hinder toddlers and preschoolers from quality sleep. Symptoms of snoring, difficulty breathing at night, mouth breathing, and observed obstructive pauses during sleep, as well as daytime hyperactivity or daytime fatigue, can be related to obstructive sleep apnea (American Thoracic Society, 1999). The American Academy of Pediatrics (AAP) recommends that primary care physicians routinely inquire about snoring and sleep symptoms for all children 1 year of age or older and, furthermore, that primary care physicians should send referrals to a sleep specialist for diagnostic tests (see McLaughlin Crabtree, Rach, and Gamble, Chapter 19) for children who have symptoms or signs suggestive of obstructive sleep apnea (Farber, 2002).

Environmental factors and family dynamics, such as those previously discussed, are also important in this particular age group of toddlers and preschool-aged children and should be emphasized in preventative interventions strategies.

Impact on Maternal and Infant Sleep

Two research groups studied the impact on maternal health (Hiscock, Bayer, Hampton, Ukoumunne, & Wake, 2008; Stremler et al., 2006). Using a cluster-randomized trial design, Hiscock and colleagues (2008) examined the impact of a brief behavior modification program to improve sleep in 8–10-month-old infants on symptoms of maternal depression. They demonstrated that at a 2-year follow-up, only 15% of mothers of infants who received the sleep intervention reported symptoms of clinical depression compared to 26% of mothers who did not receive the sleep intervention.

In addition, Stremler and colleagues assessed the impact of a behavior and educational intervention on both maternal and infant sleep (2006). The intervention, called TIPS (Tips for Infant and Parent Sleep), included a 45-minute behavioral and educational session with a trained research nurse, as well as an 11-page booklet highlighting the sleep issues discussed. Stremler and colleagues' randomized controlled trial demonstrated that such an intervention implemented to primiparous mothers during the early postpartum period (first 6 weeks) improved both maternal and infant sleep with longer sleep duration and fewer night awakenings.

Although these are essential studies highlighting the importance of maternal sleep on maternal health and maternal and infant sleep behavior, further studies need to be done focusing on fathers and other family members.

Evidence-Based Sleep Intervention/ Prevention Programs

Similar to the sleep intervention/prevention programs for infants, the education programs implemented for toddlers and preschool-aged children have demonstrated improvements in sleep patterns and behaviors (Martin, Barajas, Brooks-Gunn, & Hale, 2011a; Mindell, Du Mond, Sadeh, Telofski, Kulkarni, & Gunn, 2011a; Mindell et al., 2011b; Mindell et al., 2009). The parenting programs for this age group have focused on establishment of a regular bedtime and nightly bedtime routines; for example, the three-step program by Mindell and colleagues: (1) bath; (2) massage; (3) quiet activities (Mindell et al., 2009); and the Early Head Start Program by Martin and colleagues (Martin, Barajas, Brooks-Gunn, & Hale, 2011b). With the widespread availability and accessibility of the Internet, Internet-based behavioral interventions have been recently implemented and have shown significant improvements in quality of sleep (i.e., less night waking, improved sleep continuity, more rapid sleep onset; Mindell et al., 2011a). Although these studies were well designed and demonstrate solid results for these innovative programs, there are only a few published studies. Future studies are needed to further evaluate sleep education programs for this age group. Two studies are currently underway. Corkum and colleagues' Canadian Pediatric Sleep Team has recently developed another web-based intervention, the Better Nights/Better Days program, (Corkum, Coulombe, Chambers, Godbout, Gruber, et al., 2012). The program targets children with behavioral insomnia ages 1 to 10 years and will be delivered over the Internet, with added telephone support. Corkum and colleagues will examine whether parents make good use of this program, whether it is effective in improving sleep among children, and whether improved sleep results in better daytime functioning for children and for the sleep and functioning of parents. Reid and colleagues have completed a study evaluating a parenting intervention for parents of children 2 to 5 years old (Reid, 2011). Their trial intervention, called the *Parenting Matters Treatment Program*, included self-help treatment booklets—one on sleep issues, the other on discipline problems—and two telephone coaching calls at the second and fifth week of the program. To our knowledge, the results of this study have not yet been published.

Of the six interventional studies that have been conducted with toddlers and preschool children, all examined sleep behavior and none explored sleep knowledge. Only one study used an objective measure to document changes in sleep behavior; two studies employed randomization and two studies had control groups. All studies reported positive outcomes. Future research should feature randomization, comparison of outcomes to those of a control group, the use of objective measures of sleep, and blinding of evaluators yielding subjective outcome measures. This is challenging, as the parents are both the reporters and those who perform the intervention. Potential ways to overcome this problem include the use of video photography to document both the intervention and the outcome. The video would be viewed and scored by an observer blinded to the intervention and who had no personal connection with the parents or the child. Of the four studies conducted in the interval from just after birth to infancy, all had a strong research design; control groups were used and randomization was performed. No study used objective measures to evaluate sleep outcomes.

Evidence-Based Pediatric Sleep Intervention Curricula Targeting School-Age Children

Normative Patterns of Sleep

The school-age years are a period of transition of neural systems that govern the capacity for self-regulation (Grolnick & Farkas, 2002). Because these changes occur just before development of a biological tendency toward phase delay, this period affords a unique window of opportunity to help children to learn, refine, and consolidate good sleeping habits. Such work may prevent the establishment of unhealthy habits that can spiral into a pattern of extremely delayed bedtimes and the associated sleep deprivation that is seen in many adolescents (Dahl, 2004). Sleep education should seek to provide children and their caregivers (i.e., parents, school officials [see Buckhalt, Chapter 21], and health care professionals) with the knowledge and tools needed to help children prioritize sleep as "child" life becomes characterized by an increasing level of autonomy, participation in an increasing number of extracurricular activities, the beginnings of a social life, and the increasing demands of schoolwork.

Primary Sleep Issues to be Targeted in a Sleep Intervention/Prevention Program

In consideration of the developmental milestones of school-age children, including the development of circadian sleep phase preference and the growing "competition" between a variety of activities for the child's time, such as social life and extracurricular activities, it is crucial to develop sleep promotion strategies that empower children to make sleep a priority in their life (Carskadon, Vieira, & Acebo, 1993; Kataria, 2004). Additionally, it is important to involve influential individuals such as parents and teachers in these sleep promotion initiatives, as they play a strong role in behaviors related to sleep for children at this age (Meltzer & Mindell, 2007). Finally, *because sleep* is the result of bidirectional interactions among various characteristics of the child, their family, school, community, and societal levels, it is recommended that proposed interventions target multiple contexts, among which both schools and families are important (Gruber, Wiebe, Wells, Cassoff, & Monson, 2010).

Sleep promotion strategies for school-age children feature the imparting of sleep knowledge via interactive experiential learning activities. Methods of delivery include interactive discussion using a variety of teaching tools, such as PowerPoint presentations (Blunden, 2007b) or animated cartoon narratives with characters demonstrating the importance of sleep (Gruber, Sommerville, Brouillette, & Monson, 2009). Programs targeting school-age children have engaged the children only (Blunden, 2007b), or children and some or all of their parents, teachers, and school administrators (Gruber et al., 2009). Although few evidence-based interventions have been conducted in health care settings, the results of school-based interventions are promising.

Strong empirical evidence supports the notion that healthy sleep improves academic performance (Gruber et al., 2010), mood regulation (Dahl & Lewin, 2002), and the general health and well-being (Cappuccio, Taggart, Kandala, & Currie, 2008; Smaldone, Honig, & Byrne, 2007) of school-age children. However, to the best of our knowledge, evidence-based sleep promotion programs targeting individual children or their parents are lacking. School-based sleep promotion programs (Blunden, 2007b; Gruber et al., 2009) that target classrooms of students show promise; such programs seem to prevent sleep deprivation by delivery of education on healthy sleep to school-age children. Although health care professionals cannot implement such programs acting alone, it might be beneficial if they collaborated with school personnel to facilitate program implementation.

Evidence-Based Sleep Prevention/ Intervention Programs

To date, only two known sleep promotion programs have been created for school-age children and both have been evaluated in pilot studies (Blunden, 2007b; Gruber, Sommerville, Bergmame, Enros, Kestler, et al., 2012b). Both programs targeted elementary school students in the school setting, and one study featured a control group. The sleep education program delivered by Blunden and colleagues (2007b) successfully improved sleep knowledge. The sleep promotion program of Gruber and colleagues (2012b) effectively improved sleep behavior, as measured by parental reporting and actigraphy, and positively affected daytime functioning and mood. Current research focuses on primary developmental considerations for this age group, including the need to establish healthy sleep habits and a sleep knowledge base during the primary school years to potentially minimize sleep problems in adolescence. Future work should seek to replicate existing promising findings and to expand on such preliminary evidence by using appropriate sample sizes and by employing both objective and subjective measures of sleep behavior and knowledge. Given that school-age children become increasingly busier as they develop, and assume more responsibility, it may be useful if future work addresses such developmental issues by offering school-age children rationales for making sleep a priority in life, and strategies to assist toward this end.

Evidence-Based Pediatric Sleep Intervention Curricula Targeting Adolescents

Normative Sleep Patterns

Puberty is a critical maturational phase characterized by delayed sleep phase, where adolescents show an endogenous preference for much later bedtimes than children and adults (see Carskadon and Tarokh, Chapter 8). This phase delay may result in insufficient sleep time during the school week and a need for "catch-up sleep" on weekends. Similarities among adolescent sleep patterns across various cultures suggest that maturational changes in biological sleep processes underlie the sleep phase delay associated with adolescence (Carskadon, 2002). However, such changes are augmented by psychosocial influences. These include variation in family configuration, adolescent need for increased autonomy and independence, elevated academic demands, influence of peer culture, social expectations, employment opportunities, time spent on extracurricular activities, and use of electronic devices (Andrade, Benedito-Silva, Domenice, Arnhold, & Menna-Barreto, 1993; Carskadon, 2005; Carskadon & Acebo, 2002; Dahl & Lewin, 2002; Edgar, Dement, & Fuller, 1993; Saarenpää-Heikkilä, Rintahaka, Laippala, & Koivikko, 1995).

Primary Sleep Issues to be Targeted in a Sleep Intervention/Prevention Program

Adolescence is a developmental period during which individuals become increasingly independent. Adolescents, and not their parents, determine when they go to sleep (Wolfson & Carskadon, 1998). Because of this decrease in parental influence, it is important to create sleep promotion strategies that help adolescents internalize the importance of sleep, permitting the making of decisions that are conducive to healthy sleep hygiene. It is not enough to provide adolescents with sleep education alone (Blunden, 2012); it is important to include other cognitive-behavioral and/or motivational strategies enhancing the desire to prioritize sleep over other activities including social gatherings, participation in online chat rooms, playing of computer games, watching television, doing homework, engaging in extracurricular activities, and enjoyment of social media, all of which often occur at late at night. This concern is supported by other research on health promotion; the results suggest that enhancement of knowledge on the negative effects of alcohol use is not enough to make adolescents sufficiently motivated to make healthy behavioral changes (Tobler, 2000).

Strategies used to promote sleep have been explored in studies with early-stage adolescents (Johnson, Harkins, Marco, Ludden, & Wolfson, 2012) and/or those who were older (Moseley & Gradisar, 2009). Using a social learning, self-efficacy approach, the *Young Adolescent Sleep-Smart Pacesetter Program* for early-stage adolescents (Johnson et al., 2012) included the delivery of a sleep curriculum to 7th–8th-grade students, the completion of sleep diaries by adolescents, and the distribution of sleep newsletters for parents to review and reinforce their child's sleep education. The work with older adolescents (Moseley & Gradisar, 2009) featured sleep education delivered via collaborative and experiential learning and/or conventional teacher instruction with the aid of cognitive-behavioral techniques. Specific strategies included reducing the anxiety associated with good sleep behavior (Meltzer & Mindell, 2004); the imparting of stimulus control tools such as removal of stimulating technological devices from the bedroom (thus ensuring that use of the bedroom was associated solely with sleep (Meltzer & Mindell, 2008); and delivery of strategies allowing adolescents to overcome barriers associated with getting to sleep at an early hour despite the demands of competing activities (Noland, Price, Dake, & Telljohann, 2009). Recently, motivational interviewing, a nonconfrontational therapy that attempts to facilitate the intrinsic motivational capacity within each individual to allow that individual to personally decide to change behavior, has been integrated in school-based sleep promotion programs. This approach seeks to translate sleep knowledge acquisition into actual sleep behavior improvements (Cain, Gradisar, & Moseley, 2011). Although the preventative strategies discussed above can be implemented in both health care and school settings, most have been delivered in school settings. This may be because health care professionals have less contact with adolescents than do teachers, and the former professionals are thus not in a position to impart preventative health care strategies to adolescents (Elster, 1993; Gans, Alexander, Chu, & Elster, 1995; Klein, McNulty, & Flatau, 1998).

Evidence-Based Sleep Intervention/ Prevention Programs

Of the eight sleep promotion programs that have been created for adolescents, three programs only assessed sleep knowledge (Bakotić, Radošević-Vidaček, & Košćec, 2009; Blunden, 2007a; Cortesi, Giannotti, Sebastiani, Bruni, & Ottaviano, 2004); two evaluated sleep behavior only (De Sousa, Araujo, & De Azevedo, 2007; Wolfson et al., 2012); and three programs assessed both sleep knowledge and behavior (Brown, W. C., & Soper, 2006; Cain et al., 2011; Moseley & Gradisar, 2009). Although most studies featured control groups, all such groups were "classes as usual" (i.e., no alternative educational program was offered). One intervention (Brown et al., 2006) featured an attention control group consisting of a presentation about the scientific method conducted by the same interventionist from the experimental condition. When sleep knowledge was assessed, it appeared that the level of knowledge improved during and after the sleep promotion program. The impact of programs in terms of improving sleep behavior have been less consistent; some studies failed to document any significant improvement in such behavior despite the fact that sleep knowledge was enhanced (Cain et al., 2011). A few programs have attempted to enhance personal motivation toward improvement of adolescent sleep habits (Cain et al., 2011). Future work should prioritize motivation as a key element of such programs (Blunden, Chapman, & Rigney, 2011); motivation is uniquely an adolescent challenge. Specifically, given that many activities more inherently enjoyable than sleep (e.g., socializing with friends, computer use, participation in extracurricular sports) are available to adolescents, it is essential that adolescents are intrinsically motivated to change sleep habits; sleep must be accorded priority over competing activities. In addition, future adolescent sleep promotion programs should consider employing an objective measure of sleep behavior (e.g., actigraphy or polysomnography), in addition to self-report, to validate and enrich the quality of research findings. To the best of our knowledge, objective assessments of sleep have yet to be conducted within the context of sleep interventional programs targeting adolescents. Finally, future work should seek to fill gaps evident in current programs; both sleep knowledge and behavior should be recognized as important outcome measures. Also, the experimental design should always be meaningful, in that control and experimental groups treated identically (except for delivery of the sleep program) must be employed.

General Summary

Overall, across all age groups from postpartum to adolescence, 20 interventional studies have been conducted. Most studies documented positive changes in either sleep knowledge or sleep behavior, suggesting that promotion of sleep knowledge, education on healthy sleep, and prevention of sleep problems are indeed feasible. Whereas interventional studies in the early postpartum period used research designs yielding high-quality evidence (control groups were included and participants were randomly allocated to control and interventional groups), studies with children of other age groups have been less rigorous. With a few exceptions, most studies did not use objective measures to evaluate changes in sleep behavior and no study blinded reporters of subjective sleep data. Again with a few exceptions, the studies did not include outcome measures of daytime functioning of children or their families. Future studies would benefit from the use of a research design that allows interventional effectiveness to be determined and that yields high-quality evidence. Control groups should be included; randomization of participants to control and interventional groups is required; reporters should be blinded; objective methods should be employed; and daytime measures that improved sleep should affect (mood, attention, and behavior) should be evaluated.

Sleep Hygiene Strategies

The following section will review developmentally appropriate sleep hygiene strategies. Health care professionals have suggested sleep hygiene strategies that can be used by parents to help their child develop healthy sleep habits. In addition, resources for information about sleep that healthcare professionals can use to reinforce and supplement the proposed sleep hygiene strategies are described below.

Sleep Hygiene Recommendations to Parents of Newborns and Infants

1. Place your baby in the crib when they are sleepy, not when they are already asleep (Blum & Carey, 1996), and encourage your baby to fall asleep on his/her own (Meltzer & Mindell, 2008).
2. Ensure that your baby's room is quiet and dark (Blum & Carey, 1996).
3. Ensure that the room is at a comfortable temperature and place your baby on his/her back with his/her face and head free from blankets and other items (part of the "Back to Sleep Campaign" and other recommendations to help in prevention of sudden infant death syndrome; Pollack & Frohna, 2002).
4. Be aware of your child's sleep patterns in order to identify signs of sleepiness. It is important to note your child may manifest fatigue not just by yawning and slowing down, but by being hyperactive and less able to control their emotions, which may be misleading when trying to identify their fatigue levels (Muñiz, 2012).
5. Create a consistent and enjoyable bedtime routine for your baby (Blum & Carey, 1996).
6. Develop a consistent daily bedtime and wake time schedule for your baby (Blum & Carey, 1996).

Sleep Hygiene Recommendations to Parents of Toddlers

1. Continue developing a regular sleep–wake schedule for your toddler that is consistent on both weekdays and weekends (Meltzer & Mindell, 2008).
2. Continue developing a regular and relaxing bedtime routine for your child (Blum & Carey, 1996).
3. Your toddler's sleep environment should be consistent every night and throughout the night (i.e., he/she should not be moving from a crib to a bed or from one bed to another throughout the night; Mindell, 2005).
4. Encourage your toddler's use of a security transitional object throughout the night to help with the transition from crib to bed (Blum & Carey, 1996).
5. If your toddler stalls at bedtime, be sure to set clear limits (Mindell, 2005).

Sleep Hygiene Recommendations to Parents of Preschoolers

1. Follow through with a consistent sleep schedule (Blum & Carey, 1996).
2. Follow through with a consistent bedtime routine every night (Blum & Carey, 1996).
3. Your child should have a sleep-friendly environment every night, which should be cool, quiet, dark, and without electronic devices such as computers and televisions (Blum & Carey, 1996).
4. Observe your child's sleep and watch for difficulty breathing, unusual nighttime awakenings, chronic sleeping difficulties, and behavioral and attention problems throughout the day and night (Muñiz, 2012).

Sleep Hygiene Recommendations to School-Age Children and Adolescents

1. A fixed bedtime and wake time is important. The body adapts to falling asleep at a certain time, but only if the sleep schedule is relatively consistent, with no more than 1 hour of bedtime difference between school nights and weekends or holidays (Meltzer & Mindell, 2008).
2. Recommend a consistent, calm, bedtime routine that includes relaxing activities over the span of about 20 to 30 minutes in the room where the child sleeps (Morgenthaler, Owens, Alessi, Boehlecke, Brown, et al., 2006).
3. The ideal sleeping environment is quiet, dark, and cool in the evening, and well lit in the morning. It is important that the sleeping environment should be associated with positive experiences and emotions and, therefore, parents should not use the bedroom or going to bed early as punishments (Meltzer & Mindell, 2008).
4. Heavy meals within the 2 hours before bedtime should be avoided, but a small snack close to bedtime is acceptable so that the child does not go to bed hungry (Kataria, 2004).
5. Caffeine should be avoided in the late afternoon and evening. Examples of caffeinated beverages and foods include coffee, tea, energy drinks, sodas, hot chocolate, and solid chocolate (Meltzer & Mindell, 2008).
6. Television, computers, and cell phones should not be present in the bedroom. Furthermore, Internet use should be kept to a

minimum in the evening (Cain & Gradisar, 2010; Meltzer & Mindell, 2008).

7. Napping during the day may create difficulty in nighttime sleeping (Meltzer & Mindell, 2008).

8. Regular exercise in the afternoon can help deepen sleep, but intense exercise (e.g., soccer practice) within 2 hours before bedtime can prevent the ability to fall asleep (Bowden, Lorenc, Robinson, Quintanilha, Cruz, Corso, et al., 2010).

9. Each child should attempt to maximize bright light exposure in the morning and limit it in the evening, as this will help align their internal circadian rhythm with the external environment thus rendering them more alert during the day and fatigued at night (El-Sheikh, 2011).

10. Be aware of signs of chronic difficulty sleeping, excessive and loud snoring, breathing problems, unusual nighttime awakenings, and recurrent daytime sleepiness (Kataria, 2004).

Sleep promotion strategies appropriate for adolescents are similar to those suitable for school-age children (see list above), but include a few additional components specific to the adolescent lifestyle.

1. Given the high prevalence of sleep deprivation in adolescence and the natural tendency toward delayed rising and bedtime, it is important to advise adolescents on the importance of healthy sleep habits over the weekend. Although waking up late on the weekends is reasonable, it should be limited to no more than 90 minutes past the usual wake time in order to prevent sleep onset difficulties and erratic sleep/wake schedules (Wolfson & Carskadon, 1998)

2. Adolescents should avoid stimulating activities and the use of stimulants (e.g., caffeine, difficult homework, text messaging, online chatting, computer games) in the hour before bedtime (Cain & Gradisar, 2010; see Gradisar and Short, Chapter 11).

3. It is important for adolescents and their parents/guardians to understand the increased risk for and dangers associated with drowsy driving in adolescence (see Hershner, Chapter 31). The combination between an increased prevalence of sleep deprivation, an increased sleep need, and an age at which a driver's license can be obtained renders adolescents prone to being drowsy while driving during the morning, afternoon, and/or evening (Curry, Hafetz, Kallan, Winston, & Durbin, 2011).

Resources Regarding Pediatric Sleep for Psychologists, Educators, and Health Care Professionals

Many resources (e.g., online information, pamphlets, sleep education curricula, books, articles, conference proceedings, health recommendations) regarding pediatric sleep are currently available and continue to be developed for psychologists, educators, and health care professionals by organizations in the United States, Canada, and Europe. For example, the American Academy of Pediatrics (AAP; www.aap.org), the American Academy of Sleep Medicine (AASM; www.aasmnet.org/), and the National Sleep Foundation (NSF; http://www.sleepfoundation.org/) are in the United States. Canadian initiatives include the Canadian Sleep Society (CSS; www.canadiansleepsociety.ca/) and Canadian Pediatric Society (CPS; http://www.cps.ca/). The European Sleep Research Society (ESRS; www.esrs.eu) has developed materials as well.

Future Directions

The goals of this section are, first, to discuss potential future directions that could be taken to improve the effectiveness of sleep promotion programs; second, to identify methodological concerns and barriers that should be considered in future studies; third, to discuss potential strategies facilitating dissemination of such programs and enhancing collaboration among health care professionals, to promote healthy sleep and the benefits thereof and to combat pediatric sleep problems.

Potential Future Directions Aimed at Improving the Effectiveness of Sleep Promotion Programs

- **Acquiring Empirical Evidence to Support Widely Used Sleep Hygiene Recommendations that are not Evidence-Based**

"Sleep hygiene" is a set of key practical strategies frequently recommended to parents and to subjects of all ages to optimize sleep and to prevent sleep deprivation (Hauri, 1969; Hauri, 1992). Although these strategies seem sensible and are considered to be effective in improving sleep and preventing sleep deprivation and associated problems, substantial empirical evidence supporting these recommendations, or allowing adjustment of recommendations to suit the changing developmental needs of children of different ages, is lacking. Future research is needed to support existing sleep hygiene recommendations, to provide a scientific rationale for such suggestions, to better describe how the recommendations should be implemented, and to introduce a developmental perspective. This research may potentially identify ways in which the recommendations could be optimized and adjusted to suit children of different ages.

• Individualizing Standard Recommendations to Accommodate the Varied Needs Of Parents

Parenting and attachment styles, parental cognition and beliefs, parents' personalities, and family situations vary considerably (Sigel, McGillicuddy-De Lisi, & Goodnow, 1992). These factors may influence how parents follow routine recommendations regarding nighttime behavior. This is particularly true when parents respond to children who cry during the night; when handling children's protests (again, frequently articulated by crying behavior); and when a clinician recommends that parents create and follow consistent routines. It is therefore important that future research identify family and parental factors that might affect the implementation of preventative interventional strategies and then develop strategies tailored to accommodate individual differences in parental styles and family backgrounds.

• Individualizing Standardized Recommendations to Accommodate Adolescent Needs and the Ability of Adolescents to Implement Preventative Strategies

Given the high prevalence of sleep deprivation during adolescence and the natural tendency of adolescents to delay both bed and rise times, it is important to help adolescents develop healthy sleep habits. A key barrier impeding preventative sleep interventions in adolescence is the development of increased autonomy (associated with less parental supervision and reduced parental involvement in the setting of bedtime) combined with a reluctance to prioritize sleep over social activities and schoolwork. Given this combination of factors, a key challenge in developing effective sleep promotion programs for adolescents, and an important future research direction, is the identification of strategies that motivate adolescents to prioritize sleep and healthy sleep behavior on the one hand, but support the natural development of autonomy and independence on the other. Furthermore, it is necessary that the environment reinforce healthy sleeping habits among adolescents. This would involve making schools more "sleep friendly" by having later start times (Owens, Belon, & Moss, 2010; Wolfson, Spaulding, Dandrow, & Baroni, 2007) as well as earlier extracurricular activities and school-sponsored social events (e.g., school dances).

Methodological Concerns and Barriers

1. Measuring the Impact of Sleep Promotion Programs on the Health and Success of Children and Parents.

Whereas several prevention programs developed to improve sleep in infants and newborns have used empirical approaches to document changes in sleep behavior, and a few have measured maternal mood, research into the beneficial impact of such programs on the daytime functioning of children and their parents is lacking. Studies exploring parental productivity at work; family relationships; parental mood and attention levels; and child daytime behavior, mood, and performance, are needed to measure and document the impact of sleep promotion programs on the health and success of children and their families.

2. Distinction between Changing Sleep Knowledge and Changing Sleep Behavior

Sleep promotion programs that seek to change the sleep behavior of parents, and programs constructed to help school-aged children and adolescents, frequently include a sleep education component. Although this is important, it is critical to draw a distinction between increasing knowledge on the one hand, and instilling actual change in behavior on the other. Whereas knowledge acquisition provides an important basis for behavioral change, mere learning is not sufficient to ensure behavioral change and can indeed be frequently noted in the absence of such change. It is therefore important to clearly distinguish between sleep knowledge and sleep behavior, and to measure and carefully document the effectiveness of sleep promotion programs in changing actual sleep behavior or sleep priorities.

3. Facilitating Dissemination of Sleep Promotion Programs to Parents, Psychologists, Nurses, Pediatricians, and Educators

Despite the extent and strength of evidence demonstrating the critical importance of sleep, and the adverse impacts of sleep deprivation, such knowledge is not widely available to children or their families. The existence of problems that may potentially be remedied upon application of healthy sleep education, and the difficulties currently experienced in addressing such problems, constitute a "translation gap." Given the critical nature of the domains adversely affected by sleep restriction, the delivery of sleep education within the community and in the consulting rooms of primary care pediatricians, psychologists, nurses, and school personnel offers unique opportunities to close the gap in sleep education. This would significantly improve youth health and well-being and reduce the preventable burden of disease caused by sleep deprivation. Key information and resources to be disseminated include general information on the importance of sleep, best-practice papers for health care providers, and evidence-based educational tools. Professional collaboration, involving the exchange of information among health care professionals who have ongoing natural contact with parents, and whom parents consult if problems develop in their children, would increase the availability and use of preventative sleep interventions, thus improving the health and well-being of youth and their families.

Conclusion

In the present chapter we emphasize the importance of sufficient and high-quality sleep in terms of the health and success of youth. We identify specific developmental milestones in the development of sleep, describe a variety of sleep promotional programs and strategies that can be used to facilitate healthy sleep, and also consider the specific sleep needs and developmental characteristics of children of different ages. An emphasis is placed on the importance of transferring relevant knowledge of the impact of sleep on health and academic performance, along with useful tools, to parents, health care providers, and educators. It is important for doctors, nurses, and psychologists to engage with their clients in a way that is developmentally appropriate. For example, it is important to deliver information regarding best sleep practices in a way that would be engaging to children (e.g., with cartoon animations; Gruber et al., 2009) to motivate improved sleep in a way that is age-appropriate. Furthermore, given the cultural differences of families with which health care professionals will interact, it is encouraged for health care professionals to act in a collaborative manner in order to identify the most appropriate and effective way to target each child and his or her family in an individualized manner. We expect that a rise in the use of preventative sleep intervention approaches will yield several important benefits. First, youth sleep would fundamentally improve with positive effects on the health of both children and parents, including enhanced daytime functioning. Also, such work would advance the development of partnerships among health care providers, educators, and the families such professionals serve. Future work should focus on the building of skills enabling health care providers, parents, and youth to facilitate and maintain child and adolescent sleep behavioral changes. In addition, the acquisition of empirical evidence supporting recommended sleep hygiene strategies, and the tailoring of individual programs to the unique needs and characteristics of particular families, would enhance the effectiveness of the work.

References

Acebo, C., Sadeh, A., Seifer, R., Tzischinksy, O., Hafer, A., & Carskadon, M. A. (2005). Sleep/wake patterns derived from activity monitoring and material report for health 1- to 5-year-old children. *Sleep, 28*(12), 1568.

Alhola, P., & Polo-Kantola, P. (2007). Sleep deprivation: Impact on cognitive performance. *Neuropsychiatric Disease and Treatment, 3*(5), 553.

American Thoracic Society. (1999). Cardiorespiratory sleep studies in children. Establishment of normative data and polysomnographic predictors of morbidity. *American Journal of Respiratory and Critical Care Medicine, 160*, 1381–1387.

Andrade, M. M. M., Benedito-Silva, A. A., Domenice, S., Arnhold, I. J. P., & Menna-Barreto, L. (1993). Sleep characteristics of adolescents: A longitudinal study. *Journal of Adolescent Health, 14*(5), 401–406.

BaHammam, A., Al-Faris, E., Shaikh, S., & Saeed, A. B. (2006). Sleep problems/habits and school performance in elementary school children. *Sleep and Hypnosis, 8*(1), 12.

Bakotić, M., Radošević-Vidaček, B., & Košćec, A. (2009). Educating adolescents about healthy sleep: Experimental study of effectiveness of educational leaflet. *Croatian Medical Journal, 50*(2), 174–181.

Blum, N. J., & Carey, W. B. (1996). Sleep problems among infants and young children. *Pediatrics in Review, 17*(3), 87–92.

Blunden, S. (2007a). The implementation of a sleep education program in adolescents. *Sleep Biological Rhythms, 5*, A31.

Blunden, S. (2007b). The implementation of a sleep education program in primary school children. *Sleep Biological Rhythms, 5*, A32.

Blunden, S. L., Chapman, J., & Rigney, G. A. (2011). Are sleep education programs successful? The case for improved and consistent research efforts. *Sleep Medicine Reviews, 16*(4), 355–370.

Blunden, S. L. (2012). Behavioural sleep disorders across the developmental age span: An overview of causes, consequences and treatment modalities. *Psychology, 3*(3), 249–256.

Bowden, A., Lorenc, A., Robinson, N., Quintanilha, S. M., Cruz, C. P. T., Corso, G., et al. (2010). Clinical roundup: How do you treat insomnia in your practice?—Part 2. *Alternative and Complementary Therapies, 16*(5), 299–305.

Brown, F. C., W.C., B., & Soper, B. (2006). Development and evaluation of the Sleep Treatment and Education Program for Students (STEPS). *Journal of American College Health 54*(4), 231–237.

Cain, N., & Gradisar, M. (2010). Electronic media use and sleep in school-aged children and adolescents: A review. *Sleep Medicine, 11*(8), 735–742.

Cain, N., Gradisar, M., & Moseley, L. (2011). A motivational school-based intervention for adolescent sleep problems. *Sleep Medicine 12*, 246–251.

Cappuccio, F. P., Taggart, F. M., Kandala, N. B., & Currie, A. (2008). Meta-analysis of short sleep duration and obesity in children and adults. *Sleep, 31*(5), 619–629.

Carskadon, M. A., Vieira, C., & Acebo, C. (1993). Association between puberty and delayed phase preference. *Sleep, 16*(3), 258–262.

Carskadon, M. A. (2002). *Adolescent Sleep Patterns: Biological, Social, and Psychological Influences.* Cambridge: Cambridge University Press.

Carskadon, M. A., & Acebo, C. (2002). Regulation of sleepiness in adolescents: Update, insights, and speculation. *Sleep, 25*(6), 606–616.

Carskadon, M. A. (2005). Sleep and circadian rhythms in children and adolescents: Relevance for athletic performance of young people. *Clinics in Sports Medicine, 24*(2), 319–328.

Chorney, D. B., Detweiler, M. F., Morris, T. L., & Kuhn, B. R. (2008). The interplay of sleep disturbance, anxiety, and depression in children. *Journal of Pediatric Psychology, 33*(4), 339–348.

Corkum, P., Coulombe, A., Chambers, C., Godbout, R., Gruber, R., Hall, W., & Witmans, M. (2012). *Innovations in Sleep Research: Development of a Canadian, web-based project for the treatment of behavioral insomnias in 1- to 10-year old children.* Paper presented at the SLEEP 2012, 26th Annual Meeting of the Associated Professional Sleep Societies Boston, MA.

Cortesi, F., Giannotti, F., Sebastiani, T., Bruni, O., & Ottaviano, S. (2004). Knowledge of sleep in Italian high school students: Pilot-test of a school-based sleep educational program. *Journal of Adolescent Health, 34*(4), 344–351.

Curry, A. E., Hafetz, J., Kallan, M. J., Winston, F. K., & Durbin, D. R. (2011). Prevalence of teen driver errors leading to serious motor vehicle crashes. *Accident Analysis & Prevention, 43*(4), 1285–1290.

Dahl, R. E., & Lewin, D. S. (2002). Pathways to adolescent health sleep regulation and behavior. *Journal of Adolescent Health 31*(6), 175–184.

Dahl, R. E. (2004). Adolescent brain development: A period of vulnerabilities and opportunities. *Annals of the New York Academy of Sciences,* 1021(1), 1–22.

Davis, K. F., Parker, K. P., & Montgomery, G. L. (2004). Sleep in infants and young children: Part One: Normal sleep. *Journal of Pediatric Health Care, 18*(2), 65–71.

De Sousa, I., Araujo, J., & De Azevedo, C. (2007). The effect of a sleep hygiene education program on the sleep-wake cycle of Brazilian adolescent students. *Sleep and Biological Rhythms, 5*(4), 251–258.

Dinges, D., & Chugh, D. (1997). Physiologic correlates of sleep deprivation. In J. Kinney & H. Tucker (Eds.), *Physiology, Stress, and Malnutrition: Functional Correlates, Nutritional Intervention* (p. 668). New York: Lippincott-Raven Philadelphia.

Edgar, D. M., Dement, W. C., & Fuller, C. A. (1993). Effect of SCN lesions on sleep in squirrel monkeys: Evidence for opponent processes in sleep-wake regulation. *The Journal of Neuroscience, 13*(3), 1065–1079.

El-Sheikh, M. (2011). *Sleep and Development: Familial and Socio-Cultural Considerations.* New York: Oxford University Press.

Elster, A. B. (1993). Confronting the crisis in adolescent health: Visions for change. *Journal of Adolescent Health, 14*(7), 505–508.

Farber, J. M. (2002). Clinical practice guideline: Diagnosis and management of childhood obstructive sleep apnea syndrome. *Pediatrics, 110*(6), 1255–1257.

Gans, J. E., Alexander, B., Chu, R. C., & Elster, A. B. (1995). The cost of comprehensive preventive medical services for adolescents. *Archives of Pediatrics and Adolescent Medicine, 149*(11), 1226.

Grolnick, W. S., & Farkas, M. (2002). Parenting and the development of children's self-regulation. *Handbook of Parenting, 5*, 89–110.

Gruber, R., Sommerville, G., Brouillette, D., & Monson, E. (2009). *Sleep for Success Overview.* McGill University, Montreal

Gruber, R., Wiebe, S. T., Wells, S., Cassoff, J., & Monson, E. (2010). Sleep and academic success: Mechanisms, empirical evidence, and interventional strategies. *Adolescent Medicine: State of the Art Reviews, 21*(3), 522–541.

Gruber, R., Cassoff, J., Frenette, S., Wiebe, S., & Carrier, J. (2012a). Impact of Sleep Extension and Restriction on Children's Emotional Lability and Impulsivity *Pediatrics, IN PRESS.*

Gruber, R., Sommerville, G., Bergmame, L., Enros, P., Kestler, M., Gillies-Poitras, E., et al. (2012b). *The impact of a school-based program on the sleep and daytime functioning of school-aged children.* Paper presented at the Sleep 2012, 26th Annual Meeting of the Associated Professional Sleep Societies Boston, MA.

Hasler, G., Buysse, D. J., Klaghofer, R., Gamma, A., Ajdacic, V., Eich, D., et al. (2004). The association between short sleep duration and obesity in young adults: A 13-year prospective study. *Sleep, 27*(4), 661.

Hauri, P. (1969). The influence of evening activity on the onset of sleep. *Psychophysiology, 5*(4), 426–430.

Hauri, P. J. (1992). Sleep hygiene, relaxation therapy, and cognitive interventions. In Hauri, P.J. (Ed.), *Case Studies in Insomnia* (pp. 65–84). New York: Plenum Publishing Corporation.

Hiscock, H., Bayer, J. K., Hampton, A., Ukoumunne, O. C., & Wake, M. (2008). Long-term mother and child mental health effects of a population-based infant sleep intervention: Cluster-randomized, controlled trial. *Pediatrics, 122*(3), 621–627.

Horne, J. (1988). Sleep loss and "divergent" thinking ability. *Sleep, 11*(6), 528–536.

Johnson, M., Harkins, E., Marco, C., Ludden, A., & Wolfson, A. (2012). Effects of the Sleep-Smart Program on early adolescents' sleep patterns and hygiene, emotional health, and academic performance. Presented at the annual meeting of the Associated Professional Sleep Societies. Boston, Massachusetts.

Kataria, S. (2004). A clinical guide to pediatric sleep: Diagnosis and management of sleep problems. *Journal of Developmental & Behavioral Pediatrics, 25*(2), 132–133.

Klein, J. D., McNulty, M., & Flatau, C. N. (1998). Adolescents' access to care: Teenagers' self-reported use of services and perceived access to confidential care. *Archives of Pediatrics and Adolescent Medicine, 152*(7), 676.

Lin, J. D., Tung, H. J., Hsieh, Y. H., & Lin, F. G. (2011). Interactive effects of delayed bedtime and family-associated factors on depression in elementary school children. *Research in Developmental Disabilities, 32*(6), 2036–2044.

Linde, L., & Bergströme, M. (1992). The effect of one night without sleep on problem-solving and immediate recall. *Psychological Research, 54*(2), 127–136.

Magee, C. A., Huang, X. F., Iverson, D. C., & Caputi, P. (2010). Examining the pathways linking chronic sleep restriction to obesity. *Journal of Obesity*, 2010.

Martin, A., Barajas, R. G., Brooks-Gunn, J., & Hale, L. (2011a). Parenting services may be an opportunity for improving bedtime routines among at-risk preschoolers. *Behavioral Sleep Medicine*, *9*(4), 237–242.

Martin, A., Barajas, R. G., Brooks-Gunn, J., & Hale, L. (2011b). Parenting services may be an opportunity for improving bedtime routines among at-risk preschoolers. *Behavioral Sleep Medicine*, *9*(4), 237–242.

Meijer, A., Habekothé, H., & Van Den Wittenboer, G. (2000). Time in bed, quality of sleep and school functioning of children. *Journal of Sleep Research*, *9*(2), 145.

Meijer, A. (2008). Chronic sleep reduction, functioning at school and school achievement in preadolescents. *Journal of Sleep Research*, *17*(4), 395–405.

Meltzer, L. J., & Mindell, J. A. (2004). Nonpharmacologic treatments for pediatric sleeplessness. *Pediatric Clinics of North America*, *51*(1), 135–152.

Meltzer, L. J., & Mindell, J. A. (2007). Relationship between child sleep disturbances and maternal sleep, mood, and parenting stress: A pilot study. *Journal of Family Psychology*, *21*(1), 67–73.

Meltzer, L. J., & Mindell, J. A. (2008). Behavioral sleep disorders in children and adolescents. *Sleep Medicine Clinics*, *3*(2), 269–279.

Miller, P. M., & Commons, M. L. (2010). The Benefits of Attachment Parenting for Infants and Children: A Behavioral Developmental View. *Behavioral Developmental Bulletin*, 1–14.

Mindell, J. A. (2005). *Sleeping Through the Night: How infants, toddlers, and their parents can get a good night's sleep*. New York: HarperCollins Publishers.

Mindell, J. A., Telofski, L. S., Wiegand, B., & Kurtz, E. S. (2009). A nightly bedtime routine: Impact on sleep in young children and maternal mood. *Sleep*, *32*(5), 599–606.

Mindell, J. A., Du Mond, C., Sadeh, A., Telofski, L., Kulkarni, N., & Gunn, E. (2011a). Long-term efficacy of an internet-based intervention for infant and toddler sleep disturbances: One year follow-up. *Journal of Clinical Sleep Medicine*, *7*(5), 507–511.

Mindell, J. A., Du Mond, C. E., Sadeh, A., Telofski, L. S., Kulkarni, N., & Gunn, E. (2011b). Efficacy of an internet-based intervention for infant and toddler sleep disturbances. *Sleep*, *34*(4), 451–458.

Moore, M., Meltzer, L. J., & Mindell, J. A. (2008). Bedtime problems and night wakings in children. *Primary Care: Clinics in Office Practice*, *35*(3), 569–581.

Morgenthaler, T., Owens, J., Alessi, C., Boehlecke, B., Brown, T., Coleman, J., et al. (2006). Practice parameters for behavioral treatment of bedtime problems and night wakings in infants and young children. *Sleep*, *29*(10), 1277–1281.

Moseley, L., & Gradisar, M. (2009). Evaluation of a school-based intervention for adolescent sleep problems. *Sleep*, *32*(3), 334–341.

Muñiz, E. I. (2012). A clinical guide to pediatric sleep: diagnosis and management of sleep problems. *Journal of Developmental & Behavioral Pediatrics*, *33*(1), 95.

Nilsson, J. P., Söderström, M., Karlsson, A. U., Lekander, M., Åkerstedt, T., Lindroth, N. E., & Axelsson, J. (2005). Less effective executive functioning after one night's sleep deprivation. *Journal of Sleep Research*, *14*(1), 1–6.

Noland, H., Price, J. H., Dake, J., & Telljohann, S. K. (2009). Adolescents' sleep behaviors and perceptions of sleep. *Journal of School Health*, *79*(5), 224–230.

Owens, J. A., Belon, K., & Moss, P. (2010). Impact of delaying school start time on adolescent sleep, mood, and behavior. *Archives of Pediatrics and Adolescent Medicine*, *164*(7), 608–614.

Pinilla, T., & Birch, L. L. (1993). Help me make it through the night: Behavioral entrainment of breastfed infants' sleep patterns. *Pediatrics*, *91*(2), 436–444.

Pollack, H. A., & Frohna, J. G. (2002). Infant sleep placement after the Back to Sleep campaign. *Pediatrics*, *109*(4), 608–614.

Reid, G. J. (2011). Parenting matters: Helping parents with young children. Retrieved from http://clinicaltrials.gov/ct2/show/NCT00133055. Last accessed May 22, 2013.

Saarenpää-Heikkilä, O. A., Rintahaka, P. J., Laippala, P. J., & Koivikko, M. J. (1995). Sleep habits and disorders in Finnish schoolchildren. *Journal of Sleep Research*, *4*(3), 173–182.

Shigeta, H., Shigeta, M., Nakazawa, A., Nakamura, N., & Yoshikawa, T. (2001). Lifestyle, obesity, and insulin resistance. *Diabetes Care*, *24*(3), 608–608.

Shin, C., Kim, J., Lee, S., Ahn, Y., & Joo, S. (2003). Sleep habits, excessive daytime sleepiness and school performance in high school students. *Psychiatry and Clinical Neurosciences*, *57*(4), 451–453.

Sigel, I. E., McGillicuddy-De Lisi, A. V., & Goodnow, J. J. (1992). *Parental Belief Systems: The Psychological Consequences for Children*. New Jersey: Lawrence Erlbaum.

Smaldone, A., Honig, J. C., & Byrne, M. W. (2007). Sleepless in America: Inadequate sleep and relationships to health and well-being of our nation's children. *Pediatrics*, *119*(Supplement 1), S29–S37.

St James-Roberts, I., & Gillham, P. (2001). Use of a behavioural programme in the first 3 months to prevent infant crying and sleeping problems. *Journal of Paediatrics and Child Health*, *37*(3), 289–297.

Stremler, R., Hodnett, E., & Lee, K. (2006). A behavioral-educational inter-vention to promote maternal and infant sleep: A pilot randomized, controlled trial. *Sleep*, *29*(12), 1609–1615.

Symon, B. G., Marley, J. E., Martin, A. J., & Norman, E. R. (2005). Effect of a consultation teaching behaviour modification on sleep performance in infants: A randomised controlled trial. *The Medical Journal of Australia*, *182*(5), 215–218.

Tobler, N. (2000). Lesson learned. *Journal of Primary Prevention*, *20*, 261–274.

Walker, M. P., & Van Der Helm, E. (2009). Overnight therapy? The role of sleep in emotional brain processing. *Psychological Bulletin*, *135*(5), 731.

Weissbluth, M. (1995). Naps in children: 6 months–7 years. *Sleep*, *18*(2), 82–87.

Wolfson, A., Lacks, P., & Futterman, A. (1992). Effects of parent training on infant sleeping patterns, parents' stress, and perceived parental competence. *Journal of Consulting and Clinical Psychology*, *60*(1), 41–48.

Wolfson, A., Johnson, M., Harkins, E., & Marco, C. (2012). Effects of the Sleep-Smart Pacesetter Program on young teens' sleep hygiene, emotional well-being, and sleep-health competence. Presented at the annual meeting of the Associated Professional Sleep Societies. Boston, Massachusetts.

Wolfson, A. R. (1996). Sleeping patterns of children and adolescents: Developmental trends, disruptions, and adaptations. *Child and Adolescent Psychiatric Clinics of North America, 5*(3), 549–568.

Wolfson, A. R., & Carskadon, M. A. (1998). Sleep schedules and daytime functioning in adolescents. *Child Development, 69*(4), 875–887.

Wolfson, A. R., Spaulding, N. L., Dandrow, C., & Baroni, E. M. (2007). Middle school start times: The importance of a good night's sleep for young adolescents. *Behavioral Sleep Medicine, 5*(3), 194–209.

CHAPTER

40 Late Adolescence and Emerging Adulthood: A New Lens for Sleep Professionals

Pamela V. Thacher

Abstract

Researchers have increasingly identified the ages of 17–23 as a separate developmental stage, referred to as "emerging adulthood," distinct from our understanding of what it is to be in adolescence or to have reached adulthood. This chapter extends and deepens what is known about treating adults and middle adolescent patient populations to clarify the practice parameters in treating the late adolescent/emerging adult (LA/EA). With a focus on sleep disorders that will appear in this population, the chapter also highlights important developmental elements such as the LA/EA's consideration of risk and reward, approaches to decision making, and goal-directed behaviors. Both practical and contextual aspects of clinical practice are outlined for the clinician with respect to the unique demands of this clientele.

Key Words: adolescence, late adolescence, emerging adulthood, sleep disorders, young adult, risk, reward, decision making

"…I would there were no age between ten and three-and-twenty, or that youth would sleep out the rest; for there is nothing in the between but getting wenches with child, wronging the ancientry, stealing, fighting…"

W. Shakespeare, "The Winter's Tale," 3.3.58–61.

Developmental approaches to sleep and mental health have recognized the passage out of high school and into a new and more independent setting as a unique and important transitional stage, not well characterized by either of the terms "young adult" or "adolescent." Arnett has offered the term *emerging adulthood* to better describe this very dynamic stage of life (Arnett, 2000). Arnett conceptualizes emerging adulthood as distinct from late adolescence ("the second decade of life," Arnett, 2000, p. 476) and from young adulthood because individuals in this life phase (between 17 and 25) largely do *not* self-identify as "adults" (Arnett, 2001). As Arnett first noted, many variables that characterize adulthood are still in flux during emerging adulthood as contrasted to young adulthood. In emerging adulthood, stability in occupational path and financial independence have not been achieved; marital status is typically "single" during this time—although meaningful romantic relationships are more common (Giordano, Manning, & Longmore, 2010)—and those who have had a child are exceptions to the rule at this age (Arnett, 2000, p. 477). In most ways, including other less tangible aspects (e.g., non-role-oriented identifications), individuals in this group feel less than fully adult and yet not children, either.

They cherish independence, yet also engage in many behaviors that betray lingering immaturity.

Parental control over behavior in the late adolescent/emerging adult (LA/EA) group is incomplete at best, and thus parents cannot compel their children to cooperate with the family's health care provider. Thus clients in this group may need to be encouraged to move closer to accepting the responsibilities of adulthood and to participate in the treatment suggestions. Providers working with this age group need to understand not only the psychiatric and behavioral problems that LA/EAs bring to their practice, but must also comprehend the developmental aspects that are salient as this group moves fully into adulthood.

This chapter will consider three broad areas to help providers anticipate and manage the challenges and the rewards of working with this age group who evidence problems with sleep. Because some readers will be primarily sleep clinicians interested in expanding practice parameters to include the LA/EA clientele, and others will be clinicians who treat adolescents and wish to develop expertise in addressing sleep problems, the information of interest may vary. Thus the chapter is organized so that first I present a general overview of sleep requirements and consequences of inadequate sleep. In this section, psychologists and other clinicians who do not have primary expertise in sleep can gain the necessary "basics," so that the remainder of the chapter is more coherent. The second section of the chapter directly addresses diagnostic and treatment issues that arise *in this age group;* that is, the late teen and emerging adult. Lastly, and potentially of interest to all readers, I offer a brief review of the context of the brain and mind in this age group, sometimes loosely referred to as the "neuroscience" of development and psychopathology.

Overview of the Sleep/Wake Cycle in the Late Adolescent/Emerging Adult

Sleep Requirements of the Late Adolescent and Emerging Adult

Although sleep requirements can be generally described for children, adolescents, and adults as "between 6 and 9 hours per night," in fact, sleep requirements vary significantly and systematically by both age and developmental stage: children in early and middle adolescence (ages 7–11 and 12–16 years old, respectively) need about 9 hours of sleep at night (Carskadon, Harvey, Duke, Anders, & Dement, 1980); the late adolescent/emerging adult (LA/EA; about ages 17–23), on the other hand, apparently resembles adults more closely in the range of their sleep need, and need closer to 8 hours (Wehr, 1991). More research on the specific parameters of sleep in this population is needed, however, as this group has only recently emerged as a distinct developmental stage. In fact, considerable research has focused on college students who fit into the LA/EA demographic, as their ages range from 17–23 years old, and thus we do have useful data regarding the middle range of this demographic. Studies on college and university students consistently report that total sleep time is between 6.7 and 7.7 hours of sleep per night (Pilcher & Ott, 1998; Pilcher, Ginter, & Sadowsky, 1997), suggesting that the majority are not getting enough sleep. Few studies have examined sleep in the emerging adult who has entered the working world (or who is both working full-time and attending college). For the purposes of this discussion, the emerging adult who is working will be considered as needing the same amount of sleep as a college student in this age group.

Chronotype and Circadian factors

Circadian systems affect virtually all of the body's functions (see Auger and Crowley, Chapters 17 and 23). The system that has the most immediate relevance to circadian influence is the sleep/wake cycle. One of the easiest markers of the circadian system's ebb and flow is found in the times that a person chooses for bedtime and for rise time). Individual differences influence bedtime/rise times, such that some of us consider ourselves "night owls" and some "morning larks"; these preferences are operationalized in scores obtained from questionnaires and other measures and are usually referred to as "morningness" and "eveningness" (Roenneberg, Wirz-Justice, & Merrow, 2003).

In addition to individual differences that persist throughout adulthood, developmental influences are also prominent, particularly in the first three decades. Throughout early and middle childhood, "morning preference" dominates. For the LA/EA population, circadian preference steadily delays due to changes in both biological and social systems (Carskadon Vieira, & Acebo, 1993; Carskadon, Acebo, Richardson, Tate, & Seifer, 1997). The gradual development of earlier circadian preference (an "advance" in the circadian clock) may provide a rough estimate of the true onset of adulthood, at least with respect to the sleep/wake cycle as it interacts with the adulthood phenotype in the circadian system (Roenneberg, Kuehnle, Pramstaller, Ricken, Havel et al., 2004). *Chronotype* refers to metabolic or hormonal markers (e.g., melatonin) of this biological system; circadian *preference* is the behavioral feature of this system, in which individuals arrange their schedules (if possible) to coincide with preferred hours of wake and sleep. The provider should consider circadian preference whenever possible when treating the LA/EA.

Circadian preference moderates many aspects of sleep schedule choices, particularly among students who can choose their own schedules. Those with a morning circadian preference have earlier bedtimes, earlier rise times, and complain of fewer sleep-related problems (Giannotti, Cortesi, & Ottaviano, 1997, Giannotti, Cortesi, Sebastiani, & Ottaviano 2002; Onyper, Thacher, Gilbert, & Gradess, 2012; Wolfson & Carskadon, 2003). "Larks," as those with morning circadian preference are sometimes called, have better scores on formal tests of cognitive ability and have higher GPAs (Gray & Watson, 2002; Trockel, Barnes, & Eggett, 2000). The provider may want to inquire, therefore, about the direction and strength of the client's circadian preference (e.g., "Owl" or "Lark"), especially if the client shows a strong preference for one extreme chronotype or the other.

Providers should also directly inform students with strong tendencies towards "owlish" preference—staying up late and rising later—of the impact that this behavior may have on their academic performance. Although it is unlikely that these students will be able to change their circadian preference simply by being informed, they should know that actions which may exacerbate this preference (frequent or extreme delays of bedtime on weekends; excessive oversleeping on the weekends) are likely worsen daytime function, which for the majority of this age group coincides with times they are in class. Providers working with this age group should engage their clients in a focused conversation about findings that suggest earlier rise times are associated with higher GPA (Gray & Watson, 2002; Onyper et al., 2012; Trockel et al., 2000; Wolfson & Carskadon, 1998). In this way, although they may not be able to "choose" to be "larks," individuals may take measures to keep sleep schedules similar to those that larks might choose. This choice is more likely to occur if the client is aware of the repercussions of delayed schedule on weekends than if he or she remains ignorant of these connections.

Sleep Schedules in the LA/EA

School schedules—high school start times or college class times—largely determine the parameters of the sleep cycle. Providers who treat LAs/EAs will likely encounter clients whose mental health issues may be in part exacerbated by inflexible schedules. For high school students (late adolescents), the single most important factor that determines RT is their *school start time*; the length of their sleep cycle follows this variable closely (Carskadon, Wolfson, Tzichinsky, & Acebo, 1995; Owens, Belon, & Moss, 2010; Szymczak, Jasinska, Pawlak, & Swierzykowska,1993; Wahlstrom, 2002; Wolfson, Spaulding, Dandrow & Baroni, 2007; also see Au, Appleman, and Stavitsky, Chapter 38). When students have more freedom to set bedtimes (vacations, weekends), most keep later bedtimes and also stay asleep for a longer duration (Wolfson & Carskadon, 1998). This is true for both high school students (Owens et al., 2010; Szymczak et al., 1993; Wahlstrom, 2002) and college students (Onyper et al., 2012).

In this age group, then, sleep schedules follow from academic schedules. Later class times result in delayed bedtimes and rise times but also longer sleep and reduced daytime sleepiness. Specifically, for every one hour of delay in class start time, college students gained, on average, 22 minutes of sleep on weekday nights (Onyper et al., 2012), consistent with findings from studies that utilized high school students. Later start time for academics (school start times or college class start times) increases the total sleep time, improves daytime energy and motivation for academics, and improves school attendance for both late adolescents and for emerging adults (Carskadon, Wolfson, Acebo, Tzischinsky, & Seifer 1998; Onyper et al., 2012; Owens et al., 2010; Wahlstrom, 2002; Wolfson et al., 2007).

Later circadian preferences generally accompany increased difficulty in early rise times. Nonetheless, in most communities school start times are set earlier as students move from middle school to high school (e.g., Wahlstrom, 2002). As a result, students report that they get less sleep than they need beginning at about age 13 (Wolfson & Carskadon, 1998).

Rise times are set by school or work, and bedtimes are driven later by biological and social influences. The treating professional must keep these contextual aspects—biological and social—in awareness as they devise treatment plans. Despite the client's possible reluctance to change their weekend pattern (e.g., sleeping in late), the LA/EA who habitually delays his or her bedtime, and sleeps later on weekends, is likely to experience problems, some quite serious, during the week. These include increased sleepiness, poorer motivation to engage in classwork and other academic or work-related tasks, irritability, anxiety and depression, more truancy and tardiness, increased drop-out rates, and problems in regulating mood (Dahl & Lewin, 2002; Manber, Bootzin, Acebo, & Carskadon, 1996; Onyper et al., 2012; Talbot, McGlinchey, Kaplan, Dahl, & Harvey, 2010); Wolfson & Carskadon, 1998). Although little research has examined work absences in this age group, it may be the case that emerging adults who have obtained a job are more likely to either lose that job or miss work if they, too, delay sleep on weekends. Because of these consistent links between poor or inadequate sleep and mood dysregulation, providers should ask clients who complain of these daytime sequelae about their sleep, even if clients do not identify sleep deprivation as a concern. The provider cannot afford to ignore the disparity between weekend and weekday patterns for the teen or emerging adult client who complains of daytime sequelae that typically accompany this pattern.

LA/EA and School Schedules: Total Sleep Time and Sleepiness

For both high school students and college students, later school or class start times improve functioning across many of the same domains. Daytime sleepiness lessens, total sleep time increases, and depressed mood, irritability, and stress concerns all decrease. For college students, however, a later class start time may not be critical. Findings from one study found that class schedules were only weakly associated with semester GPA when the influence of other variables was controlled: Onyper et al. (2012) found in a path analysis that for every hour that classes started later, GPA *declined* slightly. Earlier class start times thus were associated with improved academic performance, although this relationship was small, about two-tenths of a point (the difference between, for example, a 78% for a course, which might equate to a grade of a C+, and an 80%, which might equate to a B-. Note however that for many students, this kind of difference—the difference between a "B" and a "C"—is meaningful across many domains. For example, GPA cut-offs are invoked for such diverse resources as financial aid, scholarships, and special programs (e.g., applications to study abroad). Thus, although the absolute difference in grade may be slight, it may be important to individual students.

This difference may only be important, then, when student grades are at the border of one grade and another. The overall message might be that students should not necessarily choose later classes in hopes of increasing their GPA, as is somewhat more likely to occur with a younger student (e.g., a high school student). Onyper et al.'s findings (2012) indicated that fatigue and alcohol use, rather than absolute length of sleep, contributed the most to low GPA. For some clients, fatigue should be addressed directly rather than focusing the client on when a college class is offered. In other words, students should be encouraged to consider attending earlier classes, eschewing drinking to the greatest extent possible, and addressing issues of fatigue through regular, adequate sleep schedules, rather than simply trying to sleep longer in the mornings (Onyper et al., 2012) Many studies have identified the dramatic and negative effects of sleepiness and fatigue on academic performance (Link & Ancoli-Israel, 1995; Rodrigues, Viegas, Abreu e Silva, & Tavares, 2002; Singleton & Wolfson, 2009).

Moving beyond simple GPA, other studies have demonstrated that shorter sleep—rather than sleepiness—has important implications for well-being. Shorter sleep and lower quality sleep are both strongly tied to subjective reports of decreased health (Pilcher et al., 1997; Pilcher & Ott, 1998) as well as poorer immunological response in both experimental (Spiegel, Sheridan, & Van Cauter, 2002) and naturalistic studies (Prather, Hall, Fury, Ross, Muldoon et al.2012). More recently, reports of the role that total sleep time plays in cellular and metabolic health have begun to appear in the literature (Buboltz, Loveland, Jenkins, Brown, Soper et al., 2006; Spiegel, Leproult, & Van Cauter, 1999). Poor quality sleep also results in problems in mental health and mood regulation (Dahl & Lewin, 2002; Talbot et al., 2010). For some clients the academic issue may be more important than issues of health, specifically. For others, whose complaints focus more on adequate sleep, the fatigue, depressed mood, or frequent illnesses may be more pressing. The client and provider together might have a conversation that weighs the various issues when designing a treatment plan.

Certainly, then, inconsistencies between effects of decreased total sleep time (TST) and increased sleepiness introduce some uncertainty into this literature. It may be the case that sample characteristics and/or specific definitions of the variables and their measurement might account for the findings that suggest TST and sleepiness have different, and not entirely consistent, effects on well-being and academic performance. These subtly different variables should be examined further to ascertain more about how they operate to affect the client whose daily functioning is the focus of intervention or medication.

Affective, Cognitive, and Academic issues Related to Sleep Loss and Sleepiness

Some students deny feeling sleepy after short TST, or deny any particular cognitive or emotional strain from losing sleep. Results from studies that examine sleep loss under controlled conditions and with careful attention to valid dependent measures, however, commonly detect serious problems: worsening reaction time, poorer mood regulation, and increased attention/memory deficits among others (Durmer & Dinges, 2005; Nilsson, Derstro, Andreas, Karlsson, Akerstedt et al.,2005; Pilcher & Huffcutt, 1996). Deficits in cognition build both acutely (after a single night of total sleep deprivation) and over time (chronic sleep deprivation). No evidence for accommodation to sleep loss is seen in experimental protocols (Van Dongen, Maislin, Mullington, & Dinges, 2003).

These cognitive deficits mount in most (although not all) experimental participants in spite of confidence in their continued abilities. The provider should keep in mind that the client may deny possible problems from sleep deprivation, even going so far as to claim that they have become accustomed to less sleep in spite of evidence to the contrary (e.g., irritability, poor memory, mood dysregulation, etc.; Orzech, Salafsky, & Hamilton, 2011). Although the combination of inadequate sleep and increasing academic, social, and emotional demands on the LA/EA may be difficult to negotiate, most LAs/EAs do not develop major psychopathology (Merikangas, He, Burstein, Swanson, Avenevoli, et al., 2010). However, some types of psychopathology develop at this stage, with unipolar and bipolar depression, anxiety, impulse control disorders, eating disorders, and substance abuse being the most common (Kessler, Berglund, Demler, Jin, Merikangas, et al., 2005; Swanson, Crow, le Grange, Swendsen, & Merikangas, 2011). The electronic media in which many LAs/EAs immerse themselves, furthermore, create permanent records of the choices, outcomes, and disasters that occur. Thus, although there is room for hope and positive expectations, the provider needs to quickly determine the best path and the interventions most likely to succeed.

For later adolescents, peer influence is strong and interacts with parental influence, especially in families where parents both monitor their adolescents' activities and value time spent with them (Laible, Carlo, & Roesch, 2004; Wood, Read, Mitchell, & Brand, 2004). Peers influence the LA/EA's choices regarding activities in a number of domains. Decisions about when and how much to sleep, when and how many substances to ingest, in fact whether and when to engage in virtually all activities that are not mandatory (e.g., school attendance) will likely bear the stamp of the peer group's influence. High school and college settings may inadvertently increase the salience of the peer group, as the ratio of student to adult tends to be skewed heavily toward the student. Students have fewer opportunities to experience the guidance or influence of adults when ratios are so one-sided. Furthermore, research regarding parental influence on college students' choices is nearly nonexistent, despite the common lament in the popular media about the involvement of parents in college student's lives (Hofer, 2010).

In working with this age group, therefore, interventions and recommendations should take into account the client's strong ties to a variety of social networks including friends, fellow team members, and workplace friends or acquaintances. Providers may want to include a brief inventory of the sleep schedules of the client's closest friends, romantic partners, or teammates, in order to anticipate and respond to potential peer influences on bedtime (and, less commonly, on rise time). For example, as providers are likely well aware, bedtime may be quite delayed in order to both send and receive electronic communications from a close friend or from larger groups of peers. If the clinician can engage the client in a serious discussion about texting, and arrange for the client to choose a "cut-off" time, late-night texting can be anticipated and managed if not eliminated. Even moderate reductions in this behavior may improve sleep and should not be overlooked as a point of intervention

Cognitive Functioning and Academic Achievement

Students who sleep less, who have more irregular sleep, and who have the latest bedtimes typically have lower grade point average (GPA; Kelly, Kelly, & Clanton, 2001; Trockel et al., 2000; Wolfson & Carskadon, 1998, 2003) but the effect sizes can be small. In addition, insufficient sleep leads to detriments in sustained attention (Kamdar, Kaplan, Kezirian, & Dement, 2004), critical thinking (Pilcher & Walters, 1997), problem solving (Campos-Morales, Valencia-Flores, Castano-Meneses, & Castaneda-Figueira et al., 2005; Wagner, Gais, Halder, Verleger, & Born, 2004), and overall cognitive ability (Buboltz et al., 2006).

Students with an evening circadian preference find it particularly challenging to perform well in morning schedules (Fernandez-Mendoza, Ilioudi, Montex, Olavarrieta-Bernardino, Aguirre-Berrocal, et al., 2010; Guthrie, Ash, & Bendapudi, 1995). Unmet sleep needs have the potential to affect a wide range of behaviors critical to success in academic settings in ways that include but certainly also go beyond GPA.

Role of Substance Use and Alcohol

Similar to younger students, college students complain that their sleep is too short, is of poor quality, and is quite irregular (Carney, Edinger, Meyer, Lindman, & Istre, 2006; Manber et al., 1996). Providers may find that increased substance abuse parallels these complaints. Students in college report using more substances than students in high school (White, Lavouvie, & Papadaratsakis, 2005, White, McMorris, Catalano, Fleming, Haggerty et al., 2006), including alcohol (see Bootzin, Cousins, Kelly, & Stevens, Chapter 36), stimulants generally, caffeinated beverages and substances specifically, tobacco, and also more illegal substances including marijuana and sedative/depressant substances. Emerging adults both use and abuse more prescription medication, particularly pain medications, than younger or older groups (SAMHSA, 2006). Prescriptions target problems with pain and also sleep, attention deficits, mood, and anxiety most commonly (SAMHSA, 2006). One in five admit to using prescription medications that were intended for others or that were for different purposes than originally prescribed (e.g., methylphenidate prescribed for ADHD being used to help study; Clegg-Kraynok, McBean, & Montgomery-Downs, 2011; Wu, Pilowsky, & Patkar, 2008). Many substances disrupt both the quantity and quality of sleep (Galambos, Dalton & Maggs, 2009; Jacobus, Bava, Cohen-Zion, Mahmood, & Tapert, 2009; Morin & Wooten, 1996). Sedatives, which may also decrease the quality of sleep, are habit forming and may create dependency and addiction.

Alcohol use in particular has a dramatic effect on both sleep and academics: alcohol use commonly leads to poor sleep and poorer academic achievement (e.g., Onyper et al., 2012; Singleton & Wolfson, 2009). Thus, one of the most important questions a provider can ask of a student who is complaining of problems in college or in a first job must be with respect to substance use, particularly alcohol, as this is by far the most common drug for this age group to abuse (White et al., 2006). Alcohol worsens sleep and depression (Galambos et al., 2009; Jacobus et al., 2009), and depression is certainly among the most common reasons that a student is referred for professional help to a sleep center. Furthermore, alcohol is associated with both delayed sleep schedules and lowered GPA (Onyper et al., 2012; Wolaver, 2002) although some studies report mixed results for these variables and their relationships to academic performance (e.g., Paschall & Freisthler, 2003). In many studies, the number of drinks consumed on a typical weekend night is the strongest predictor of academic performance—Onyper et al. (2012) found that an increase of 1 standard deviation in alcohol use (approximately 4 drinks) was associated with a .28 SD decline in semester GPA (approximately .13 points).

If students in college drink heavily during the weekends, further compensatory actions during the week may become necessary. For students who drink to the point of inebriation on the weekends, sleep/wake and study/recreate schedules become irregular and ineffective for continued academic achievement (Taylor, Wright, & Lack, 2008). One compensatory strategy for some students might be "pulling an all-nighter" to make up for lost study time over the weekend. In one study examining this practice, about 60% reported engaging in this form of sleep deprivation at least once during the previous semester. Use of "all-nighters" predicted lower GPA, a more "evening" circadian preference, and a later BT. Students who endorsed this practice also reported they were "sure" that they could "recover" from a night of total sleep deprivation in "about a day" (Thacher, 2008), although other research suggests this is unlikely (Van Dongen et al., 2003). The use of all-nighters, in fact, may disadvantage the student's ability to function for several days and may worsen attention, memory, and motivation in important ways. Effects in these domains may comprise the mechanism of lower GPA for students who engage in this behavior, and further research in this practice is needed. (Thacher, 2008; Onyper et al., 2012). All-nighters may serve as a marker for other poor sleep habits that together increase risk for poor sleep. If the provider asks about sleep habits and the client cites numerous all-nighters, this may be an entrée into a longer conversation about how the client's weekly study patterns are being affected by an irregular and unpredictable sleep/wake cycle.

Other compensatory actions for lost sleep may include taking naps, or delaying rise time and advancing bedtime (that is, going to bed earlier) to extend sleep. If other tasks are pressing and tests or other assignments are looming, students may miss class in order to complete an assignment or study for an exam, or may miss class unintentionally because of falling into an unscheduled nap or sleeping past an alarm (Thacher, 2008). All of these events suggest that a student is not in control of his or her schedule. Likewise, frequent and binge types of drinking worsen sleep and increase sleepiness and fatigue on the days following a drinking episode, secondary to alcohol's depressive effects (Roehrs & Roth, 2001). One way that students may compensate for subsequent alcoholic "hangovers" could be the choice to sleep in later on weekdays (hence possibly missing class) or to miss study time during the evening hours or weekend days and instead make up the lost sleep in extended nights or naps (Wolaver, 2002).

Interventions Regarding Sleep Schedules in the LA/EA

How have providers addressed these problems? In one prospective longitudinal study, the authors asked students to "regularize" their sleep–wake schedule in addition to other, more general, suggestions to improve sleep hygiene (e.g., decrease use of caffeine) for 4 weeks. Compliance was good and participants reported significant improvements in both sleep quality and quantity (Manber et al., 1996). In a similar study that utilized e-mail communications to students with sleep complaints, fewer depressive symptoms and better quality sleep were both reported, and at extremely low cost (Trockel, Manber, Chang, Thurston, & Tailor, 2011). Thus it seems clear that the LA/EA is capable of seeking out and executing suggestions to improve their sleep quality and quantity.

Treatment Issues for Sleep and Sleep-Related Disorders in the Late Adolescent/Emerging Adult

Most clients in this age group bring into treatment a number of issues unique to adolescence and emerging adulthood. Providers who work with this client population on a regular basis will find the issues familiar, but for the sleep specialist who is new to the LA/EA population these considerations could prove helpful as they begin to work with them. For providers who are familiar with the population but who are new to sleep treatments, I provide a brief overview of the most common elements of disordered sleep that might be encountered. These deserve careful consideration from the treating provider.

Health Insurance Portability and Accountability Act (HIPAA), Confidentiality and Record-Keeping Considerations

One arena in which critical differences arise when comparing treatment of children and adolescents versus emerging adults is that of record-keeping and confidentiality. For clinicians who are accustomed to seeing clients exclusively from a pediatric or family population it is axiomatic that records and appointment details are, of necessity, open to the parent/guardian and access to the child's records is granted as a matter of course. In adult practice, by contrast, only the client himself or herself has access to the records without written consent, and this practice is also a matter of course. Practitioners who work with a late adolescent population from high school, college, or early adulthood, however, may need to become either more or less flexible with record access as the legal constraints and requirements differ and become more complex. The adolescent client may have one set of expectations, while his or her parents or guardians may have different expectations regarding access. For example, in the case of a client who is 17 years old—legally a minor—parents may expect to have continued access to all records on demand. However, depending on the country, state, and the practice, some minor children (especially during the late teen years) may have certain rights with respect to keeping details of their treatment private and confidential. A minor client, therefore, may raise issues about privacy that do not arise with either pediatric or adult populations, necessitating careful navigation on the part of the treating professional about how to handle these different expectations and preferences. In each case of a minor or a client who recently reached the age of majority (e.g., a child who has turned 18), the provider must familiarize himself or herself with the relevant laws regarding access to records. The Health Insurance Portability and Accountability Act of 1996 (HIPAA; http://www.hhs.gov/ocr/privacy/hipaa/administrative) provides guidelines for practitioners to follow with respect to privacy of records. These vary by state and change as new legislation is adopted. In cases where state law is more restrictive than federal law, state laws will prevail (English & Ford, 2004). Providers must understand and apply appropriate practice guidelines if in private practice, or must familiarize themselves with their sites' application of relevant laws regarding access, confidentiality, and exceptions. In addition to the provider's needing absolute clarity regarding these legal guidelines, both parents/guardians and the LA/EA should be made explicitly aware of who has access to the records, under what conditions access to records will occur, how the issues of confidentiality regarding therapy and records about therapy will be handled, and possible exceptions to these decisions and guidelines.

In most cases, any client over the age of 18 will be presumed to be an adult and although parents may be paying for treatment (or the treatment may be covered under a parent's or guardian's health insurance plan), the records remain protected under both state and federal law. Written consent from the LA/EA is required before records can be shared with parents/guardians. This should also be made explicit, as parents or guardians may be accustomed to a pattern of access to records which they experienced before children reached majority age. Although they are designated adults in some settings (e.g., in the provider's office or at college), in other settings, such as in their parents' home and in an insurance company's records, the client is designated as a "dependent." With care to delineate the relationship up front and before disclosure has begun, however, providers can avoid or lessen problems that might arise as a result. Although most parents will not be surprised to learn that guidelines and restrictions change when children reach 18, clear explanations and statements, documented in writing if possible, will help to avoid possible misunderstandings, misplaced expectations, or complications more generally.

General Diagnostic and Treatment Factors in LA/EA: Contexts of Treating for Sleep Disorders

Although providers may focus practice parameters on sleep disorders generally, many LA/EA clients who present for treatment may have other complaints in addition to sleep dysfunction. Prevalence data for disorders in adolescent and adult populations reveal similar patterns: mood disorders, anxiety disorders, and substance abuse problems represent the diagnoses with the highest rates for both adolescents (13–18 year olds in this study; Merikangas et al., 2010) and for adults (DHHS, 2006). Providers should keep in mind that adolescents are likely to have experienced fewer years of symptoms, although some adolescents exhibit symptoms, especially for anxiety and depressive disorders, in the pubertal and even prepubertal stage (e.g., from age 6–13; Merikangas et al., 2010). In some cases the provider may be seeing the client soon after the first symptoms appeared. During this stage of life, the LA/EA considers issues of selfhood, contemplates future goals for occupation, and engages in a balancing act as he or she considers demands from family of origin and his/her own desire for more autonomy. An important consideration during this developmental time includes emerging sexual identity and the consideration of possibly "coming out" as a gay or lesbian individual, and the LA/AE may be actively considering how to go about this process. Lastly, a new feature of identity at this time in life is frequently how to create and sustain a lasting, intimate relationship, as opposed to exploration of sexuality per se (Giordano et al., 2010). All of these avenues to increased independence carry the risk for missteps, false starts, painful mistakes, and the chance of rich and rewarding experiences.

Some LA/EA clients are eager to begin the experience of counseling. Providers will be able to intervene directly and effectively. Others, however, may not arrive at the first appointment with as much motivation. For these clients, conversations about eating disorders, suicidal thoughts, etc., can be difficult. The client may be reluctant to broach or sustain a conversation around these topics. With these clients, a more indirect or general approach will be called for. One possible starting point lies with the sleep/wake cycle, and the provider may want to begin there, using sleep as a kind of gentle starting point to reach into areas that otherwise might feel too contested, fraught or otherwise "tender."

Sleep may be uniquely situated for this kind of indirect therapeutic approach. Sleep-related problems in adolescents with anxiety complaints, for example, may be as high as 90% (Chase & Pincus, 2011); sleep related problems for depression are a close second at about 80% (Taylor, Lichstein, Durrence, Riedel, & Bush, 2005), and both of these (anxiety and depression) often are comorbid with substance abuse. Given the increased stigma attached to major mental illness, and to substance abuse/addiction (Hinshaw & Stier, 2008), the provider may find an easier path to begin a therapeutic alliance and treatment suggestions that center on sleep-related symptoms as a starting point. Furthermore, treating sleep can have a cascading effect on other problems. For example, treatment of insomnia and daytime sleepiness has been shown to reduce substance use problems even after 12-month follow-up (Bootzin & Stevens, 2005). In a study that examined rates of anxiety after sleep deprivation, both self-reports of anxiety and ratings of the likelihood of catastrophic events occurring increased

(Talbot et al., 2010), suggesting that restoring sleep to clients who are anxious may be an effective way to address that disorder as well.

In any case, since many older adolescents and emerging adults are getting insufficient sleep or have erratic sleep/wake patterns, providers and counselors can use sleep factors to begin a conversation about well-being without immediately having to ask about behaviors that touch on more stigmatized or defended symptoms, such as purging, obsessive-compulsive rituals, and so forth. Other topics to introduce as entrees to a broader discussion of psychiatric functioning could include usual bedtimes, wake times, and incidents of middle-of-the-night awakenings. These discussions can open conversations about jobs, sports, homework/project and work time, and evening pre-bedtime rituals, including any problems that regularly arise during these activities. The provider can suggest to the LA/EA that the techniques for addressing anxious aspects of the sleep/wake cycle can or could be used to address anxiety in other situations as well, such as at a job or at school.

Another disorder that can be treated under the umbrella of sleep is depression. Many LAs/EAs who are at risk of developing a mood disorder will experience their first episode of depression and/or mania during adolescence and early adulthood (Dahl, Ryan, Matty, Birmaher, Al-Shabbout et al., 1996; Benca, Obermeyer, Thisted, & Gillin,1992). Because stigma is always a consideration when a client describes psychiatric symptoms (Sirey, Bruce, Alexopoulos, Perlick Raue et al., 2001) it may feel less shameful for some clients if the clinician initially asks about sleep rather than, for example, depression or binge eating. oadly, the provider has a variety of topics with which to start off discussion, but for most clients the following variables should be inquired about as part of a thorough intake session.

Brief Summary of Intake Foci for Treatment of the LA/EA with Primary Sleep Complaints

Sleep Schedule

- Bedtime [BT] and Rise time[RT]
  - Ask about BT and RT for both weekdays and weekends (e.g., when school/work constrains BT/RT and when little or nothing constrains BT/RT)
  - Calculate the difference between weekdays and weekends;
- Differences of about two or more hours indicate that the client may be experiencing difficulties secondary to the shift back and forth between weekday and weekend patterns, sometimes referred to as "social jet lag"

Other Sleep-Related Symptoms/Foci

– Snoring (other family members are more reliable reporters of this than the client) (see McLaughlin Crabtree, Rach, and Gamble, Chapter 19)

– Nightmares (see Ivanenko and Larson, Chapter 24)

– Hypnogogic/hypnopompic hallucinations with or without sleep paralysis

– Obsessive/compulsive bedtime rituals

Past trauma may continue to influence sleep, creating sleep phobia, nightmares, etc.

Asking about trauma may help alleviate symptoms, through respect and acknowledgement ofpast traumatic events (Felitti & Anda, 2009). The provider is not obligated to make the trauma history the focus of the treatment (unless abuse is ongoing), but research suggests that acknowledgement that such a history may be affecting one's health can provide significant relief to clients, without in-depth discussion or treatment focus.

Sleep Complaints as a "24 hour" Phenomena

It can be helpful to conceptualize sleep disorders, and the symptoms that are described by clients, as covering the full 24 hours of a day. With this approach the client can more easily grasp the impact that sleep disorders can have on their lives. In any case, the provider needs to ask about both day and night features.

Daytime Sleep Problems

As with adults, the teen and emerging adult should be asked to describe any problems in these arenas:

– Tardiness to class or school on a regular basis due to sleeping too late to leave the house and arrive on time

– Falling asleep during the day

– Mood instability that is interfering with daytime functioning. This can take the form of irritability, feeling very sad, feeling very "raw" or reactive.

– Strong afternoon "dip" in alertness, interfering with ability to function

– Frequent napping during the week (especially if unintended)

• Excessive reliance on caffeine or other stimulant to "get through the day," especially if used in the later afternoon/evening.

The LA/EA may not believe that caffeine is interfering with sleep because they fall asleep and stay asleep during the night. They may, therefore, resist suggestions to decrease the amount of caffeine they are ingesting, or suggestions to cease using caffeine after some point in the early afternoon. Thus the provider should be ready to ask "do you think caffeine use is interfering with your sleep?" in order to highlight the findings in sleep research that although sleep may be initiated without noticeable problems, or that it may not be noticeably interrupted during the night (see Bootzin, Cousins, Kelly and Stevens, Chapter 36), nevertheless problems in the depth and quality of sleep are common and may be marked. The provider should ask about caffeine products and substances with care, as this may be underestimated by many late adolescents and emerging adults. When caffeine intake is higher than about 400 mg per day (about 4 caffeinated sodas), it is important for the clinician to discuss how caffeine use maybe interfering with sleep and to work with the client on slowly weaning him/her from caffeinated products. Although many clients may believe that since they can fall asleep with relative ease they must not be affected by caffeine, caffeine's effects on sleep depth and on sleep architecture can be described. Once the client understands the cycle of fatigue → caffeine use → poor sleep quality → increased fatigue (Roehrs & Roth, 2008), he or she may be more willing to cut back or eliminate caffeine use.

Nighttime Sleep Problems

- Early morning awakenings
- Extreme lethargy upon rising; inability to function adequately after WT+30 minutes
- Use of multiple alarms to waken/sleeping past two or more alarms
- Getting in bed earlier than one otherwise might in order to "leave enough time to sleep"
    - This behavior contributes to excessive sleep onset latency periods. Early BT is often chosen for an evening following a bad night. Thus, once in a while this behavior may be rewarded with rapid onset of sleep.
- Shortened SOL (<5–10 minutes) paired with later fragmentation during the night—often followed by one or more periods of extended wake periods after sleep onset (WASO), frequently accompanied by worry and apprehension about total sleep time (TST), etc., when awake, including clock watching; catastrophizing; changing plans for the next day ("I won't be able to go out with friends [for example] now that I'm getting so little sleep, I'll just be too tired, so I'd better cancel that activity"). See Harvey, 2002 for an excellent summary of cognitive contributions to insomnia.
- "Bad dreams" and nightmares
- Nighttime eating
- Sleepwalking
- Panic attacks that arise or waken the client from sleep

Daytime sequelae of all sleep issues mentioned may be immediately tied together by the LA/EA as he or she describes the difficulties in the 24-hour sleep cycle. It may also be the case, however, that these connections are opaque to the teen and the client may even strongly resist that daytime problems are in any way related to sleep.

Daytime sequelae include moodiness, irritability, general feelings of malaise or tiredness, problems with attention, memory difficulties, difficulties with impulsivity, problems with inhibiting responses that are pre-potent (shouting/fighting, aggressive behavior generally), and difficulty in arriving to class or other appointment on time, especially if scheduled for the morning (afternoon tardiness may be much less of a problem or nonexistent, so that the client can arrive on time to sports/team activities, work-related activities, etc.).

Substance Use

- Caffeine intake: type, (including soda, caffeine-concentrated beverages such as *Rock Star*, *Monster*, etc; "energy drinks"); amount; timing
- Nicotine: type (including cigarettes/cigars, chewing tobacco); amount; timing
- Alcohol: Frequency and amount, including asking about binge drinking; including combinations of alcohol and caffeine
- Marijuana
- Sedatives: inquire regarding benzodiazepines sedatives (e.g., diazepam [Valium®], etc., and non-benzodiazepine sedativesme.g., Eszopiclone [Lunesta®], etc.)
- Herbal substances
- Melatonin; amount, timing

It is not necessary to decide whether or not the presenting problem is primarily due to sleep problems or to depression. The fortunate fact is that treating sleep—making it longer if it is too short and making it better quality if it is unsatisfying—can yield changes in mood, decreased anxiety (especially as nighttime/BT approaches) and less daytime tiredness. Increasing the teen's sense of control, or at the very least their understanding of how these symptoms are interrelated, can help decrease subjective stress levels, which may also help the overall picture and increase the client's ability to function during the day and night.

For each of the above scenarios, the teen/emerging adult may be having multiple problems during the day that are consequences of lost sleep, part of a symptom profile that may not be primarily a sleep disorder. Although the diagnosis itself may need to be pinned down for a variety of reasons, the relative unambiguously positive goal of improving sleep quality and sleep quantity can give the provider a straightforward path to a therapeutic alliance and progress toward improved function. For an excellent summary of behavioral treatments of sleep and related disorders, several texts can be of use to the professional working with sleep patients. Each of these texts provides the reader with case studies, clinical examples, specific protocols, and treatment procedures that can be followed in lieu of formal training (or as guides during formal training. Texts include:

1. *Behavioral Treatments for Sleep Disorders: A Comprehensive Primer of Behavioral Sleep Medicine Interventions.* (2011). M. Perlis, M. Aloia, & B. Kuhn, eds. San Diego, CA: Elsevier.

2. *Cognitive Behavioral Treatment of Insomnia: A Session-by-Session Guide.* (2008). 2nd edition. M L. Perlis, C. Jungquist, M. T. Smith, & D. Posner, eds. New York: Springer.

3. Anxiety and Sleep. (2008) A. G. Harvey, I. S. Hairston, J. Gruber & A. Gershon. In *Oxford Handbook of Anxiety and Related Disorders.* M. M. Antony & M. B. Stein, eds. New York: Oxford University Press.

Social and Behavioral Neuroscience: Context of Working with Late Adolescents and Emerging Adults

When clients arrive at a sleep clinic, mental health clinic, or general health clinic they typically have one or two "presenting complaints" that provide a crisp focus for the provider. Because most providers have only three to four sessions to convince a client that the time and money spent on therapy are worthwhile (McCay & Bannon, 2004), providers need to very quickly gather information and explore whether other problems may serve as more meaningful targets for any interventions. Context is also important: consideration of the LA/EA's cognitive and emotional development, how they see their problems, and how they weigh their choices going forward can make an enormous difference to the success of the therapy.

Health choices, including choices about how to manage sleep and the sleep/wake cycle, are the focus of much of the literature with respect to decision making because poor decision making can have long-term consequences—and even may result in death. In many instances, the decision-making process fails to consider poor outcome as a real possibility. Fortunately, the decision-making process that adolescents use with respect to risky behaviors is often "outgrown"—abandoned without any specific intervention to help this to occur. Driving without seatbelts, choices about drinking (binge drinking, driving drunk, etc.), failing to use protection during sexual activity, and so on, all become less common as the LA/EA grows in age and experience into a full adult role.

Age as a Proxy for Adulthood

In examining how issues of the law and various legal aspects of roles that society regulates, it may be helpful to realize that many considerations of "adulthood" take capabilities—both cognitive and emotional—into account. For example, the ages and restrictions for marriage, alcohol purchase, voting, and driving are presented. These represent just a few of the roles and obligations that society legislates carefully with consideration of age to be the dominant defining variable.

In considering this age group, providers can choose between two general approaches. The first might be described as a "wait and support" stance, given that the LA/EA client may "outgrow" or simply leave behind the behavior. In this approach, the provider may monitor the LA/EA's decisions, but in general act more as a supportive trusted adult, encouraging judicious limit setting and monitoring by parents or other adults. When adults can mentor or supervise adolescents through their transition to adulthood, the hope is that adults will help the client to avoid catastrophic results. If this path is chosen for therapy, providers should encourage parents especially, but all adults generally, to "weigh in" where possible in frequent, supportive, and constructive ways on the kinds of decisions that the LA/EA is making. This can be difficult (perhaps more so with some teens than others), to say the least. The input of adults into the decision-making process may help the late adolescent understand and emulate a more adult decision-making approach.

If the client is unwilling to discuss decisions with a parent or coach, the provider can serve as a model for the client, using the session to engage in appropriate and supportive conversations that explore the possibility of a catastrophic outcome of a poor choice. On the other hand, if the client is reluctant to engage in a discussion of decision making with the provider, the provider can encourage the client to broach the subject with another trusted adult.

A second approach lies in helping the adolescent to understand and directly emulate the pathways and processes that adults use to identify problem behaviors and set goals for the future. The provider can strategically and transparently help the LA/EA to use these same component processes to help them achieve adult goals such as increased independence, better employment, more success at such tasks as academic achievement or athletic performance, and so on. To help in this process, the provider should understand both adolescent and adult decision-making rubrics. One important difference between adolescent and adult approaches is how these two groups consider cost-benefit and risk, especially with respect to sleep-related decisions.

Providers working with the LA/EA to improve sleep may find that their approach to scheduling decisions regarding bedtime and rise time may fall prey to a clear cost-benefit approach. Most of the time, of course, we don't consciously "weigh" costs versus benefits. The decision is made beneath the level of consciousness, ingrained in habits. In any case, when the provider raises the topic of sleep schedule for a consideration of how choices and consequences may be linked, the LA/EA will need the provider's guidance to slow the decision making down so that different choices might be considered.

Changes that might be discussed include changing usual bedtime or rise time, or thinking more carefully about naps, delayed schedules on the weekends, and use of substances. The provider should be prepared for the LA/EA to weigh the "risk" of continuing to go about their daily activities in a chronically sleep-deprived state against the "rewards" of doing so.

For some clients, the willingness to make changes will be slow or even nonexistent. As with any client population, the provider needs to be willing to point out that the *client* must make these changes, and if the client is simply not willing to make changes the therapy is essentially over.

Example: Sleepy Driving

One example of a health-related behavior that can be very risky is that of driving in a sleep-deprived state. (see Hershner, Chapter 31) Professional drivers (for example, long-haul truck drivers) describe the intense fear they experience after falling asleep while driving and narrowly avoiding a catastrophic accident. The truck driver will not need to be convinced by a provider of the risk of sleep deprivation and the connection of choices regarding sleep schedules to the risk of falling asleep at the wheel. By contrast, for the LA/EA the risks of driving sleepy may feel so trivial that a conversation about them may not register as real risk at all. Thus, such a conversation may very well be required in order to motivate the LA/EA client toward changing this behavior.

In this example, the LA/EA may require a summary of statistics of fall-asleep accidents, the increased cost of car insurance that results, time away from school or work, and possible injury or death. It is unlikely that one conversation will change the client's mind, but with repeated conversations and when other considerations are added—the chance of improved grades, of better mood, of decreased feelings of stress, better ability to get to class or work on-time—the likelihood of changed behavior increases.

Sleep Schedule Decisions

In a less dramatic—but perhaps more common—example, the LA/EA may consider an earlier BT as he or she begins to understand the costs of inadequate sleep. However, the LA/EA is likely to be more conversant with the benefits of a late bedtime, which might include increased connection with peers, decreased likelihood of having the conversation turn to gossip about himself or herself, increased knowledge about the events and opinions that are important to the client and his or her friends, and the release of tension from trying to fall asleep. Although any or all of these may be trivial or minimal on a given night, from time to time the value of one of these factors will spike, providing an unpredictable—and thus highly reinforcing—pattern of reward for having stayed up later in order to stay "in the loop." The costs—increased tiredness, decreased motivation, low energy, or emotional dysregulation—may be important only under specific circumstances, such as anticipation of taking an important test or participating in an athletic contest.

Without conveying, at least in part, the poor outcomes that become likely—including risk of death or injury that might accompany the choices that are made with respect to sleep—the provider will find that motivating change will be difficult at best. At the same time, once that risk is communicated it is likely that the teen will then use the same approach to this risk as is used to weigh the risk of death or injury when driving fast or driving under the influence. In these situations, the teen doesn't just ask him or herself about the cost/benefit. They also ask: what are the chances? Several studies show evidence that teens actually overestimate risk rates as compared to accurate real-world statistics about risk (Reyna & Farley, 2006; Reyna, Estrada, Demarinis, Myers, Stanisz,et al., 2011). The challenge for the provider is to encourage the client to eschew the riskier schedule and commit to a more regular and generous sleep schedule in order to enable the sleepiness to dissipate over time. This can be difficult for this age client to endorse and execute, partly because of the nature of many of their decision-making processes.

Assessment of Risk

Much has been written of the teen's relationship to risk (for an excellent review on the extensive literature, see Reyna & Farley, 2006). Early research focused on attempts to educate, and for many decades adolescent researchers remained convinced that education could improve decision making in adolescents and alter the adolescent's apparent disregard for safety. It seemed as if teens simply did not grasp the risks involved in, for example, excessive speed or dangerous driving, frequent or excessive drug use and experimentation, risky sexual-emotional relationships, or seeking out intense novelty. Current research indicates that statements such as "They think they're invincible!" or "They think they'll live forever!" fail to capture the adolescent perspective and comprehension of risk. In fact, as Steinberg (2008) has observed, "Adolescents' greater involvement in risk-taking does not stem from ignorance, irrationality, delusions or invulnerability, or faulty calculations." (p. 80) Adolescents' greater involvement in risk-taking is the logical outcome of an affective system that seeks out and values reward far more than it fears punishment (Steinberg, 2004). The cost-benefit calculus is over-weighted to the benefit of risk: not "What happens if I fail—crash, die, lose?" but rather, "What happens if I succeed—connect, discover, achieve?"

In assessing risk, then, LA/EA are also assessing reward: here they weigh the benefit/good of a successful engagement with, for example, excessive speed in the vehicle they drive: "If I drive as fast as possible and I get into an accident, I could suffer pain, legal consequences, loss of the car... but if I *don't* have an accident, I gain peer approval, self-esteem, confidence in driving; I gain a better reputation in the school at large, which may increase my choice of friends, romantic partners; either way, my sense of boredom is removed... " and so forth. Both positive reinforcement (gain of reputation, for example) and negative reinforcement (relief of boredom) are engaged as they weigh possible benefits. The risk of failure seems real, but at any rate avoiding it is not the main goal: *the primary goal at this age is the gain of the good, not, as is the case for adults, the avoidance of the bad.*

Late adolescents and emerging adults see the risk clearly, but may decide to "play the odds." The "play the odds" approach is much rarer in adult populations. Adults base decisions more commonly on a process called *gist-based decision making.* This is the type of decision making process that the LA/EA should be guided toward by a strategic and empathic provider.

Gist-Based Decision Making

The ability to make decisions based on "gist" understanding increases with age. Making decisions based on gist means to use the underlying meaning or risky outcome of the behavior under consideration without deliberating about tradeoffs; adults say "no" to the entire process of deliberating about engaging in risky behaviors, whereas the LA/EA is likely to weigh cost/benefit and make decisions based on the risk for having a bad outcome in a particular instance, rather than on a general principle (Reyna & Farley, 2006; Reyna et al., 2011).

The ability to avoid risk, especially to avoid engaging in what is assessed as a *small* risk for a *potentially catastrophic* outcome increases with age.

By contrast to analytic decision making, in which we see that the "odds" of a bad outcome are quite small, gist-based decision making uses experience to construct *impressions* of the memory, on the whole. Examples include "I go to bed at midnight" or "I could get into an accident when I drive sleepy," both of which describe the "gist" of a decision or an outcome. In contrast, analytic thinking uses specific instances. Examples include the experience as a sample of one possible choice: "Last night, I went to bed at midnight" and "I did not get into an accident the last time I drove when I was very sleepy." Adolescent decision making is different than that of adults on a number of features: specifically, it leads to more risk taking, especially as experiences wherein the "cost" was not incurred mount in frequency, as is likely to happen (until it doesn't).

Encouraging a More Adult Perspective on Behavior in the LA/EA: A Specific Role for the Treating Professional

The adult world presents goals for the adolescent: jobs, independence, freedom of choice in a myriad of domains (what to wear, what to do as a job, peer groups with whom the adolescent chooses to associate). These appealing goals are leveraged for influence by parents, teachers, and employers to support the adolescent in his or her attempts to move into adult roles. In other words, parents offer (for one example) the use of a car if the college student can drive themselves back and forth to school, obviating the time spent by the parent on such a task. In this way the parent uses the LA/EA's desire for a more adult role—having access to a car—in order to encourage increasing responsibility.

When working with the LA/EA on issues of bedtime or rise time, the provider may also leverage the emerging adult's desire for a more fully adult persona. Although the client may not want to admit that sleep habits need to be changed to address problems in mood or fatigue, the provider would do well to address the issue as one of adult choices to attain adult goals.

In general, then, the context in which older adolescents and emerging adults function can be a powerful stimulus, either to move the teen toward, or hold the teen back from, a more mature and considered action. Roles that might enhance the adult values and adult ways of making decisions will only move the adolescent toward a more adult way of behaving when the adolescent can closely witness, observe, and utilize the processes used by an adult—whether that adult is a provider, teacher, coach, employer, college professor, or even a parent.

Future Directions

A primary consideration for comprehensive progress in understanding the sleep and wake issues in this population is that of navigating the transition to adulthood. To help clients in this age group to successfully navigate the transition into adulthood with healthy sleep patterns, clinicians need to know more about the challenges of getting adequate sleep in this age group, as well as more about the benefits of doing so. Not known is whether patterns developed in college or at one's first job persist into adulthood for any length of time or whether these habits and problems fall by the wayside. Are adult patterns natural extensions of sleep patterns in late adolescence, or are adults as distinct from LA/EA clients as pediatric clients are from adults? What are the health implications of a transition to adulthood in which sleep is subordinated to all other activities? Do these individuals take longer to reach adult goals? Does their health suffer? Answers to these questions would inform both practice and policy, potentially, for schools and colleges.

Another area in which future research might focus is the success of current efforts to educate and persuade this age group to have respect and care for their sleep. Educational outreach could help at the high school level as well as education at the college level if it is effective and if it is targeted to individuals who are open to such communications. Research that addresses how and when education and preventive educational approaches influence sleep habits, currently rare, would help to point educators, parents, and practitioners in the right direction (see Gruber, Constantin, Cassoff, and Michaelsen, Chapter 39).

In formal research protocols, one improvement that could be made with relatively little cost would be to assign participants in this age group—17–23—a separate participant category distinct from both "adolescence" and from "adulthood." If results for research studies and experimental protocols included a category for "emerging adult," results might then be broken out for this developmental stage. With more precision about this population's habits, preferences, and challenges, progress in developing a deeper understanding of this age group would come faster.

Conclusion

In this chapter I have considered treatment of sleep problems in the late adolescents and the emerging adults so that providers may find areas of interest whether their primary area of expertise is in the field of sleep disorders or in working with late adolescents/emerging adults. For both sets of readers, certainly, it is clear that sleep is a complex behavior with far-reaching consequences for young and developing adults. Clients in this developmental stage often experience therapeutic change as life altering, certainly, as the late adolescent is just beginning to experience adult life with all of its complications and rewards, and improvements to their health may set the stage for good habits and good health for decades to come.

The sleep professional who is new to working with this age group and the therapist who is new to the field of sleep disorders will both find that the challenges and rewards of clients in this developmental stage provide a practice that is both complex and rich—in spite of their admitted tendency to want to "wrong the ancientry" as they learn to right their sleep.

References

Arnett, J. J. (2000). Emerging adulthood: A theory of development from the late teens through the twenties. *American Psychologist, 55*(5), 469–480.

Arnett, J. J. (2001). Conceptions of the transition to adulthood: Perspectives from adolescence through midlife. *Journal of Adult Development, 8(2),* 133–143.

Benca, R. M., Obermeyer, W. H., Thisted, R. A., & Gillin, J. C. (1992). Sleep and psychiatric disorders. A meta-analysis. *Archives of General Psychiatry, 49,* 651–668; discussion 669–670.

Bootzin, R. R., & Stevens, S. J. (2005). Adolescents, substance abuse, and the treatment of insomnia and daytime sleepiness. *Clinical Psychology Review, 25,* 629–644.

Buboltz, W. C., Loveland, J., Jenkins, S. M., Brown, F., Soper, B., & Hodges, J. (2006). College student sleep: Relationship to health and academic performance. In M. V. Landow (Ed.), *College Students: Mental Health and Coping Strategies* (pp. 1–39). Hauppauge, NY: Nova Science Publishers.

Campos-Morales, R. M., Valencia-Flores, M., Castano-Meneses, A., Castaneda-Figueiras, S., & Martinez-Guerrero, J. (2005). Sleepiness, performance, and mood state in a group of Mexican undergraduate students. *Biological Rhythm Research, 36(1–2),* 9–13.

Carney, C. E., Edinger, J. D., Meyer, B., Lindman, L., & Istre, T. (2006). Daily activities and sleep quality in college students. *Chronobiology International, 23(3),* 623–663.

Carskadon, M. A., Harvey, K., Duke, P., Anders, T. F., & Dement, W. C. (1980). Pubertal changes in daytime sleepiness. *Sleep, 2,* 453–460.

Carskadon, M. A., Vieira, C., & Acebo, C. (1993). Association between puberty and delayed phase preference. *Sleep, 16,* 258–262.

Carskadon, M. A., Wolfson, A., Tzichinsky, O., & Acebo, C. (1995). Early school schedules modify adolescent sleepiness. *Sleep Research, 24,* 92.

Carskadon M. A., Acebo, C., Richardson, G. S., Tate, B. A. & Seifer, R. (1997). Long nights protocol: Access to circadian parameters in adolescents. *Journal of Biological Rhythms, 12,* 278–289.

Carskadon, M..A., Wolfson, A. R., Acebo, C., Tzischinsky, O., & Seifer, R. (1998). Adolescent sleep patterns, circadian timing, and sleepiness at a transition to early school days. *Sleep, 21*(8), 871–881.

Chase, R. M., & Pincus, D. B. (2011). Sleep-related problems in children and adolescents with anxiety disorders. *Behavioral Sleep Medicine, 9,* 224–236.

Clegg-Kraynok, M. M., McBean, A. L., & Montgomery-Downs, H. E. (2011). Sleep quality and characteristics of college students who use prescription psychostimulants nonmedically. *Sleep Medicine, 12,* 598–602.

Dahl, R. E., Ryan, N. D., Matty, M. K., Birmaher, B., Al-Shabbout, M., Williamson, D. E. & Kupfer D. J. (1996). Sleep onset abnormalities in depressed adolescents. *Biological Psychiatry 39 (6),* 400–410.

Dahl, R. E., & Lewin, D. S. (2002). Pathways to adolescent health: Sleep regulation and behavior. *Journal of Adolescent Health, 31,* 175–184.

Department of Health & Human Services (DHHS). (2012, July 29). Updated last 2006. Re: Does the HIPAA Privacy Rule allow parents the right to see their children's medical records? [online information websource for DHHS]. Retrieved from http://www.hhs.gov/hipaafaq/personal/227.html

Durmer, J. S. & Dinges, D. F. (2005). Neurocognitive consequences of sleep deprivation. *Seminars in Neurology, 25(1),* 117–129, 2005.

English, A., & Ford, C. A. (2004). The HIPAA privacy rule and adolescents: Legal questions and clinical challenges. *Perspectives on Sexual and Reproductive Health, 36(2),* 80–86.

Felitti, V. J., & Anda, R. F. (2009). The relationship of Adverse Childhood Experience to adult medical disease, psychiatric disorders, and sexual behavior: Implications for health care. In R. R. Lanius and E. Vermetten (Eds.), *The hidden epidemic: The impact of early life trauma on health and disease* (pp. 1–18). Boston, MA: Cambridge University Press.

Fernandez-Mendoza, J., Ilioudi, C., Montes, M. I., Olavarrieta-Bernardino, S., Aguirre-Berrocal, A., de la Cruz-Troca, J. J., & Vela-Bueno, A. (2010). Circadian preference, nighttime sleep and daytime functioning in young adulthood. *Sleep and Biological Rhythms, 8,* 52–62.

Galambos, N. L., Dalton, A. L., & Maggs, J. L. (2009). Losing sleep over it: Daily variation in sleep quantity and quality in Canadian students' first semester of university. *Journal of Research on Adolescence, 19,* 741–761.

Giannotti, F., Cortesi, F., & Ottaviano, S. (1997). Sleep pattern, daytime functioning and school performance in adolescence: Preliminary data on an Italian representative sample. *Sleep Research 35,* 196.

Giannotti, F., Cortesi, F., Sebastiani, T., & Ottaviano, S. (2002). Circadian pattern, sleep and daytime behavior in adolescence. *Journal of Sleep Research 11,* 191–199.

Giordano, P. C., Manning, W. D., & Longmore, M. A. (2010). Affairs of the heart: Qualities of adolescent romantic relationships and sexual behavior. *Journal of Research on Adolescence, 20*(4), 983–1013.

Gray, E. K., & Watson, D. (2002). General and specific traits of personality and their relation to sleep and academic performance. *Journal of Personality, 70,* 177–206.

Guthrie, J. P., Ash, R. A., & Bendapudi, V. (1995). Additional validity evidence for a measure of morningness. *Journal of Applied Psychology, 80,*186–190.

Hall, P., Schwartz-Bloom, R. D., & McConnell, E. S. (2008). The current state of teenage drug abuse: Trend toward prescription drugs. *Supplement to the Journal of School Nursing,* retrieved from http://www.nasn.org/Portals/0/resources/pd_toolkit_nurses_supplement.pdf on July 10, 2012.

Harvey, A. G. (2002). A cognitive model of insomnia. *Behavior Research and Therapy, 40,* 869–893.

Hinshaw, S. P., & Stier, A. (2008.) Stigma as related to mental disorders. *Annual Review of Clinical Psychology, 4,* 367–393.

Hofer, B. (2010). *Keeping in Touch (Just Enough).* Retrieved from http://www.parent.wisc.edu/badger-parent/201010/pdf/ParentNews.pdf on September 7,

Jacobus, J., Bava, S., Cohen-Zion, M., Mahmood, O., & Tapert, S. F. (2009). Functional consequences of marijuana use in adolescents. *Pharmacology, Biochemistry and Behavior, 2*(4), 559–565.

Kamdar, B. B., Kaplan, K. A., Kezirian, E. J., & Dement, W. C. (2004). The impact of extended sleep on daytime alertness, vigilance, and mood. *Sleep Medicine, 5*, 441–448.

Kelly, W. E., Kelly, K. E., & Clanton, R. C. (2001). The relationship between sleep length and grade-point average among college students. *College Student Journal, 35*(1), 84–86.

Kessler, R. C., Berglund, P., Demler, O., Jin, R., Merikangas, K. R., Walters, E. E. (2005). Lifetime prevalence and age-of-onset distributions of DSM-IV disorders in the National Comorbidity Survey Replication. *Archives of General Psychiatry 62*(6), 593–602.

Laible, D. J., Carlo, G., & Roesch, S. C. (2004). Pathways to self-esteem in late adolescence: The role of parent and peer attachment, empathy, and social behaviors. *Journal of Adolescence, 27*(6), 703–716.

Link, S., & Ancoli-Israel, S. (1995). Sleep and the teenager. *Sleep Research, 24a*,184.

Manber, R., Bootzin, R. R., Acebo, C., & Carskadon, M. A. (1996). The effects of regularizing sleep-wake schedules on daytime sleepiness. *Sleep, 19*, 432–441.

McKay, M. M., & Bannon, W. M. (2004). Engaging families in child mental health services. *Child and Adolescent Psychiatric Clinics of North America Special Issue: Evidence-Based Practice, Pt. 1: Research Update, 13*, 905–921.

Merikangas, K. R., He, P., Burstein, M., Swanson, S. A., Avenevoli, S., Cui L., et al. (2010). Lifetime prevalence of mental disorders in US adolescents: Results from the National Comorbidity Survey Replication—Adolescent Supplement (NCS-A). *Journal of the American Academy of Child & Adolescent Psychiatry, 49*(10), 980–989.

Morin, C. M., & Wooten, V. (1996). Psychological and pharmacological approaches to treating insomnia: Critical issues in assessing their separate and combined effects. *Clinical Psychology Review, 16*, 521–542.

Nilsson J. P., Derstro, M. O., Andreas, U., Karlsson, M. L., Akerstedt, T., Lindroth, E. N., & Axelsson, J. (2005). Less effective executive functioning after one night's sleep deprivation. *Journal of Sleep Research, 14*, 1–6.

Onyper, S. V., Thacher, P. V., Gilbert, J. W., & Gradess, S. G. (2012). Class start times, sleep and academic performance in college: A path analysis. *Chronobiology International 29(3)*, 318–335.

Orzech, K. M., Salafsky, D. B., & Hamilton, L. A. (2011). The state of sleep among college students at a large public university. *Journal of American College Health, 59 (7)*, 612–619.

Owens, J. A., Belon, K., & Moss, P. (2010). Impact of delaying school start time on adolescent sleep, mood, and behavior. *Pediatric Adolescent Medicine, 167*(7), 608–614.

Paschall, M. J., & Freisthler, B. (2003). Does heavy drinking affect academic performance in college? Findings from a prospective study of high achievers. *Journal of Studies on Alcohol, 64*, 515–519.

Pilcher, J. J., Ginter, D. R., & Sadowsky, B. (1997). Sleep quality versus sleep quantity: Relationships between sleep and measures of health, well-being, and sleepiness in college students. *Journal of Psychosomatic Research, 42*(6), 583–596.

Pilcher, J. J., & Huffcutt, A. I.. (1996). Effects of sleep deprivation on performance: A meta-analysis. *Sleep,19*(4), 318–326.

Pilcher, J. J., & Walters, A. S. (1997). How sleep deprivation affects psychological variables related to college students' cognitive performance. *Journal of American College Health, 46*, 121–126.

Pilcher, J. J., & Ott, E. S. (1998). The relationships between sleep and measures of health and well-being in college students: A repeated-measures approach. *Behavioral Medicine, 23*, 170–178.

Prather, A. A., Hall, M., Fury, J. M., Ross, D. C., Muldoon, M. F., Cohen, S., & Marsland, A. L. (2012). Sleep and antibody response to Hepatitis B vaccination. *Sleep, 35(8)*, 1063–1069.

Reyna, V. F., & Farley, F. (2006). Risk and rationality in adolescent decision-making: Implications for theory, practice and public policy. *Psychological Science in the Public Interest 7*(1), 1–44.

Reyna, V. F., Estrada, S. M., Demarinis, J. A., Myers, R. M., Stanisz, J. M., & Mills, B. A. (2011). Neurobiological and memory models of risky decision-making in adolescents versus young adults. *Journal of Experimental Psychology: Learning, Memory and Cognition 37*(5), 1125–1142.

Rodrigues, R. N., Viegas, C. A., Abreu e Silva, A. A., & Tavares, P. (2002). Daytime sleepiness and academic performance in medical students. *Arquivos de Neuro-Psiquiatria. 60*, 6–11.

Roehrs, T., & Roth, T. (2001). Sleep, sleepiness, sleep disorders and alcohol use and abuse. *Sleep Medicine Reviews, 5*(4), 287–297.

Roehrs, T. & Roth, T. (2008). Caffeine: Sleep and daytime sleepiness. *Sleep Medicine Reviews, 12*(2), 153–162.

Roenneberg, T., Wirz-Justice, A., & Merrow, M. (2003). Life between clocks: Daily temporal patterns of human chronotype. *Journal of Biological Rhythms, 8*, 80–90.

Roenneberg, T., Kuehnle, T., Pramstaller, P., Ricken, J., Havel, M., Guth, A., & Merrow, M. (2004). A marker for the end of adolescence. *Current Biology, 14*, R1038–R1039.

SAMHSA. (Substance Abuse and Mental Health Services Administration). (2006). *National Survey on Drug Use and Health: National Results.* Retrieved from: http://oas.samhsa.gov/nsduh/2k6nsduh/2k6results.cfm on June 10, 2012.

Singleton, R. A., & Wolfson, A. R. (2009). Alcohol consumption, sleep, and academic performance among college students. *Journal of Studies on Alcohol and Drugs, 70*, 355–363.

Sirey, J. A., Bruce, M. L., Alexopoulos, G. S., Perlick, D. A., Raue, P., Friedman, S. J., & Meyers, B. S. (2001). Perceived stigma as a predictor of treatment discontinuation in young and older outpatients with depression. *American Journal of Psychiatry, 158*, 479–481.

Spiegel, K., Leproult, R., & Van Cauter, E. (1999). Impact of sleep debt on metabolic and endocrine function. *The Lancet, 354*,1435–1439.

Spiegel, K., Sheridan, J. F., & Van Cauter, E. (2002). Effect of sleep deprivation on response to immunization. *Journal of the American Medical Association, 288*, 1471–1472.

Steinberg, L. (2004). Risk taking in adolescence: What changes, and why? *Annals of the New York Academy of Sciences, 1021*, 51–58.

Steinberg, L. (2008). A social neuroscience perspective on adolescent risk-taking. *Developmental Reviews 28(1)*, 78–106.

Swanson, S. A., Crow, S. J., le Grange, D., Swendsen, J., & Merikangas, K. (2011). Prevalence and correlates of eating disorders in adolescents. *Archives of General Psychiatry, 68(7)*, 714–723.

Szymczak, J. T., Jasinska, M., Pawlak, E., & Swierzykowska, M. (1993). Annual and weekly changes in the sleep-wake rhythm of school children. *Sleep 16*(5),433–435.

Talbot, L. S., McGlinchey, E. L., Kaplan, K. A., Dahl, R. E., & Harvey, A. G. (2010). Sleep deprivation in adolescents and adults: Changes in affect. *Emotion 10*(6), 831–841.

Taylor, A., Wright, H. R., & Lack, L. C. (2008). Sleeping-in on the weekend delays circadian phase and increases sleepiness the following week. *Sleep and Biological Rhythms, 6(3),* 172–179.

Taylor, D. J., Lichstein, K. L., Durrence, H. H., Riedel, B. W., & Bush, A. J. (2005). Epidemiology of insomnia, depression and anxiety. *Sleep, 28,* 1457–1464.

Thacher, P. V. (2008). University students and the "all-nighter": Correlates and patterns of students' engagement in a single night of total sleep deprivation. *Behavioral Sleep Medicine, 6*(1), 16–31.

Trockel, M. T., Barnes, M. D., & Egget, D. L. (2000). Health-related variables and academic performance among first-year college students: Implications for sleep and other behaviors. *Journal of American College Health, 49*(3), 125–131.

Trockel, M. T., Manber, R., Chang, V., Thurston, A., & Tailor, C. B. (2011). An e-mail delivered CBT for sleep-health program for college students: Effects on sleep quality and depression symptoms. *Journal of Clinical Sleep Medicine, 7*(3), 276–281.

Van Dongen, H. P. A., Maislin, G., Mullington, J. M., & Dinges, D. F.. (2003). The cumulative cost of additional wakefulness: Dose-response effects on neurobehavioral functions and sleep physiology from chronic sleep restriction and total sleep deprivation. *Sleep, 2,* 117–126.

Wagner, U., Gais, S., Halder, H., Verleger, R., & Born, J. (2004). Sleep inspires insight. *Nature, 427,* 352–355.

Wahlstrom, K. L. (2002). Changing times: Findings from the first longitudinal study of later high school start times. *NASSP Bulletin, 86,* 3–21.

Wehr, T. A. (1991). Sleep-loss as a possible mediator of diverse causes of mania. *British Journal of Psychiatry, 159,* 576–578.

White, H. R., Lavouvie, E. W., & Papadaratsakis, V. (2005). Changes in substance use during the transition to adulthood: A comparison of college students and their non-college age peers. *Journal of Drug Issues, Spring,* 281–304.

White, H. R., McMorris, B. J., Catalano, R. F., Fleming, C. B., Haggerty, K. P., & Abbott, R. D. (2006). Increases in alcohol and marijuana use during the transition out of high school into emerging adulthood: The effects of leaving home, going to college, and high school protective factors. *Journal of Studies on Alcohol, 67,* 810–822.

Wolaver, A.M. (2002). Effects of heavy drinking in college on study effort, grade point average, and major choice. *Contemporary Economic Policy, 20,* 415–428.

Wolfson, A. R., & Carskadon, M. A. (1998). Sleep schedules and daytime functioning in adolescents. *Child Development, 69*(4), 875–887.

Wolfson, A. R., & Carskadon, M. A. (2003). Understanding adolescents' sleep patterns and school performance: A critical appraisal. *Sleep Medicine Reviews, 7,* 491–506.

Wolfson, A. R., Spaulding, A. L., Dandrow, C., & Baroni, E. M. (2007). Middle school start times: The importance of a good night's sleep for young adolescents. *Behavioral Sleep Medicine, 5(3),* 194–209.

Wood, M. D., Read, J. P., Mitchell, R. E., & Brand, N. H. (2004). Do parents still matter? Parent and peer influences on alcohol involvement among recent high school graduates. *Psychology of Addictive Behaviors, 18(1),* 19–30.

Wu, L. T., Pilowsky, D. J., & Patkar, A. A. (2008). Non-prescribed use of pain relievers among adolescents in the United States. *Drug and Alcohol Dependence, 94*(1–3), 1–11.

CHAPTER

41 Behavioral Sleep Medicine: Training, Credentialing, and the Role in Sleep Laboratories

S. Justin Thomas, Kristin T. Avis, *and* Kenneth L. Lichstein

Abstract

Behavioral sleep medicine (BSM) is defined by the Society of Behavioral Sleep Medicine (SBSM) as "the field of clinical practice and scientific inquiry that encompasses the study of behavioral, psychological, and physiological factors underlying normal and disordered sleep across the lifespan; and, the development and application of evidence-based behavioral and psychological approaches to the prevention and treatment of sleep disorders and co-existing conditions." BSM plays an integral role in the assessment and treatment of a variety of sleep disorders and patient populations. Thus, training of BSM practitioners has become an increasingly important focus for the field of BSM. Formal training is best accomplished through accredited BSM training programs. In lieu of participating in an accredited BSM training program, two tracks have been established to allow qualified individuals to take the BSM credentialing examination. BSM practitioners have an important role in comprehensive sleep disorders centers, particularly in pediatric populations, and play a critical role in the diagnosis and treatment of sleep disorders. This chapter will provide an overview of BSM, information on BSM training and credentialing, and the role of BSM in sleep laboratories.

Key Words: behavioral sleep medicine, training, credentialing

Introduction

The Society of Behavioral Sleep Medicine (SBSM) defines behavioral sleep medicine (BSM) as "the field of clinical practice and scientific inquiry that encompasses the study of behavioral, psychological, and physiological factors underlying normal and disordered sleep across the lifespan; and, the development and application of evidence-based behavioral and psychological approaches to the prevention and treatment of sleep disorders and co-existing conditions" (Society of Behavioral Sleep Medicine, 2011). BSM plays an integral role in the broader field of sleep medicine by providing a psychological approach to health care, research, and education. Specifically, BSM applies cognitive, behavioral, and developmental approaches to both normal and disordered sleep. Cognitive approaches focus on maladaptive thoughts that often exist in the presence of sleep disorders and may impede the ability to achieve or maintain sleep (e.g., individuals with insomnia who fear that they will *never* sleep well). Behavioral approaches address behaviors that either facilitate or exacerbate sleep disorders (e.g., individuals who linger in bed to make up for a poor night of sleep). Behavioral approaches to sleep disorders may be most helpful in child and adolescent populations, where behavioral perspectives are critical in diagnosis and treatment. Lastly, developmental approaches to both normal and disordered sleep are important across the life span and are critically important in working with children and adolescents.

Overview of Behavioral Sleep Medicine

What Is Behavioral Sleep Medicine?

BSM, as it is known today, was born from early behavioral interventions. Many treatments currently used by BSM clinicians, including stimulus control, sleep compression and restriction, and relaxation training, were initially described and researched within the past 80 years. These treatments may be used individually; however, they are more frequently combined into a treatment package based on an individual's symptoms and treatment preferences (Chesson et al., 1999; Lacks & Morin, 1992; Morin, Bastien, & Savard, 2003; Smith, Smith, Nowakowski, & Perlis, 2003).

Bootzin (1972) introduced stimulus control. Since that time, stimulus control has become the most thoroughly researched of all BSM treatments and is a powerful tool for clinicians treating individuals with difficulties initiating and/or maintaining sleep (Chesson et al., 1999; Lacks, Bertelson, Gans, & Kunkel, 1983; Lacks, Bertelson, Sugerman, & Kunkel, 1983; Lacks & Morin, 1992; Morin, Bastien, & Savard, 2003; Morin, Kowatch, & O'Shanick, 1989; Reidel et al., 1998; Smith, Smith, Nowakowski, & Perlis, 2003). Stimulus control is based on learning theories and limits the amount of time individuals spend awake in the bed/bedroom, thus reducing any association between the bed/bedroom and sleep difficulties. A specific treatment protocol is provided by Bootzin and Perlis (2011).

Sleep restriction therapy (SRT) was introduced by Spielman, Saskin, and Thorpy (1987) and is effective in treating both sleep-onset and sleep-maintenance insomnia (Friedman, Bliwise, Yesavage, & Salom, 1991; Morin, Bastien, & Savard, 2003; Smith, Smith, Nowakowski, & Perlis, 2003; Spielman, Saskin, & Thorpy, 1987). Sleep compression therapy (SCT) is akin to SRT and differs mainly in the method of reducing time in bed (Lichstein, Riedel, Wilson, Lester, & Aguillard, 2001). Both SCT and SRT reduce time in bed closer to an individual's self-reported total sleep time. Treatment protocols for SCT and SRT may be found in Lichstein, Thomas, and McCurry (2011) and in Spielman, Yang, and Glovinsky (2011), respectively.

Jacobson (1929) invented progressive muscle relaxation to address physical arousal as a result of stress. Relaxation techniques are effective in improving sleep in a variety of populations (Lacks, Bertelson, Gans, & Kunkel, 1983; Lacks & Morin, 1992; Lichstein, 2000; Lichstein & Johnson, 1993; Lichstein, Riedel, Wilson, Lester, & Aguillard, 2001). There is no standardized relaxation technique, and many forms of relaxation therapy likely exist. A relaxation treatment protocol may be found in Lichstein, Taylor, McCrae, and Thomas (2011).

Although much of the early research on treatments for sleep disorders focused on insomnia in adult populations, BSM addresses a variety of sleep disorders (e.g., parasomnias and circadian rhythm disorders) and patient populations (both pediatric and adults). In fact, many of the earliest behavioral treatments were developed for pediatric sleep disorders (Mowrer, 1938; Watson, 1928). Kuhn and Elliott (2003) provide a thorough review of the efficacy of behavioral treatments for pediatric sleep disorders.

BSM is a result of early cognitive and behavioral research into both normal and disordered sleep, which is acknowledged by the SBSM definition of BSM. Additionally, according to Stepanski and Perlis (2003), BSM involves "the identification of the psychological (e.g., cognitive and/or behavioral) factors that contribute to the development and/or maintenance of sleep disorders and developing and providing empirically validated cognitive, behavioral, and/or other non-pharmacologic interventions." These two definitions highlight the importance of research into both normal and disordered sleep, evidence-based clinical practice, a developmental approach to sleep research and clinical practice, and the role of psychological principles in sleep medicine.

The development of BSM as a formal field of sleep medicine in the United States essentially began with the creation of a presidential committee, by then American Academy of Sleep Medicine president Daniel Buysse, in 2000. This presidential committee was tasked with the promotion of BSM through accreditation of practitioners, development of BSM training and education, and investigation of reimbursement for BSM services. The formation of this presidential committee ultimately resulted in the creation of the SBSM in 2010. The SBSM currently comprises a number of members who have made significant contributions to the understanding of normal and disordered sleep through research. In 2011, the SBSM announced the adoption of *Behavioral Sleep Medicine*, which reports on a wide range of behavioral sleep research, as its official journal (McCrae, Perlis, Smith, & Taylor, 2011). Grants for BSM research are available from a variety of sources including the National Institutes of Health, the American Sleep Medicine Foundation, and the Sleep Research Society. Overall, research is an important aspect of BSM, as this emphasis on research guides evidence-based clinical practice. BSM has established validated treatments for a number of sleep disorders. Thus, any evidence-based approach to sleep disorders will likely include a number of BSM approaches. For example, image rehearsal therapy (IRT) is a validated approach of using imagery to treat nightmares. Additionally, stimulus control is a validated application of learning theories to treat insomnia (Chesson et al., 1999; Kuhn & Elliott, 2003; Lichstein & Nau, 2003; Morgenthaler et al., 2006).

BSM also relies on a developmental approach to normal and disordered sleep. Thus, BSM focuses on a variety of developmental aspects such as normal sleep development, deviations from normal sleep patterns, changes in sleep across the life span, and the role that one's environment plays in sleep (for additional information, see Gradisar and Short, Chapter 11). Developmental approaches are particularly important in the diagnosis and treatment of pediatric sleep disorders, as much of normal and disordered pediatric sleep must be considered from a developmental perspective (Mindell & Owens, 2010; Sadeh, 2005). For example, a strictly cognitive-based approach to treatment of a sleep disorder would not be helpful in most pediatric populations, as children of young ages have not developed the cognitive skills necessary to carry out the intervention. Ecological systems theory, which considers environmental impacts on development, is also utilized in pediatric sleep disorders diagnosis and treatment (Bronfenbrenner, 1974). It is extremely difficult to separate the child from environmental influences. Therefore, when instituting behavioral changes one should take into account the impact that the child's environment (e.g., immediate family members) may have on treatment. It is often necessary to engage the caregivers in treatment to assist with treatment implementation and to address any environmental factors that affect the child's sleep. Additionally, cultural factors and institutional policies may both play an important role in assessing and treating sleep disorders in pediatric populations. For example, a number of factors such as school enrollment sizes, socioeconomic status, and geographic setting have been found to influence school start times (Wolfson & Carskadon, 2005). In turn, school start times may affect sleep duration and daytime functioning in young children and adolescents (Carskadon, Wolfson, Acebo, Tzischinsky, & Seifer, 1998; Wolfson & Carskadon, 1998). Furthermore, the practice of BSM is not restricted to pediatric populations, as BSM developmental approaches are also important in diagnosing and treating sleep disorders across the life span. For example, BSM plays an important role in the diagnosis and treatment of late-life insomnia (Lichstein & Morin, 2000).

Lastly, psychological principles (both cognitive and behavioral) are important factors governing both normal and disordered sleep. Cognitive and behavioral factors have been associated with the development and maintenance of sleep disorders, and cognitive-behavioral treatments (CBTs) have been shown to be highly effective in a variety of sleep disorders (Edinger & Means, 2005; Kuhn & Elliott, 2003; Morgenthaler et al., 2006; Morin, Culbert, & Schwartz, 1994; Murtagh & Greenwood, 1995; Sadeh, 2005). However, BSM treatments are not restricted to CBT. Psychological principles that play a role in the treatment of both pediatric and adult sleep disorders include learning theories, behavioral extinction, systematic desensitization, imagery, and mindfulness-based treatments. These principles are the basis of a number of empirically validated treatments including IRT, stimulus control, and relaxation techniques (Chesson et al., 1999; Kuhn & Elliott, 2003, Morgenthaler et al., 2006).

Who Practices BSM?

As of the summer of 2012, close to 170 individuals from a variety of health care disciplines have been credentialed through the American Board of Sleep Medicine (ABSM) to practice BSM. A majority of these individuals are psychologists and include practitioners from the United States, Canada, Australia, Taiwan, and Korea (American Board of Sleep Medicine, 2012). For additional information on credentialed BSM practitioners, see the ABSM website (http://www.absm.org/). Additionally, a census project was started in 1997 to identify practitioners of behavioral treatment for insomnia (S. D. Nau, personal communication, January 6, 2012). The individuals identified during the census have been invited to join the *Behavioral Treatment for Insomnia Roster*. The Roster is a referral communications tool for people who see adult, adolescent, or pediatric clients. Posting a request for referral help to the Behavioral Sleep Medicine listserv (http://www.behavsleepmed.com) or contacting Dr. Nau (nau@bellsouth.net) for referral help are the current ways to access the contents of the Roster. Greater dissemination of the Roster to practitioners is planned. The Behavioral Treatment for Insomnia Roster currently lists 160 practitioners, of which 101 practitioners report offering behavioral insomnia treatment for adolescents and/or children. The pediatric practitioners on the Roster are located in 28 US states, Canada, and Australia. Fifty-seven are certified in behavioral sleep medicine (by the

American Board of Sleep Medicine) and 44 are not certified. The Roster is growing.

Sleep disorders are highly prevalent in the general population and in a number of health care settings (Ford & Kamerow, 1989). Therefore, credentialed BSM clinicians may provide a valuable service by assisting in the diagnosis and treatment of a variety of sleep disorders (e.g., insomnia, circadian rhythm disorders, and nightmares). In general, clinicians would likely be interested in BSM training to broaden their scope of practice and improve their efficacy in treating common sleep disorders (Mindell, Moline, Zendell, Brown, & Fry, 1994). For example, primary care clinicians may be interested in incorporating BSM therapies in conjunction with or in place of pharmacotherapy for individuals with sleep disorders. Additionally, a credentialed BSM clinician within a sleep disorders center may allow individuals to receive BSM treatments without requiring additional referrals. Lastly, pediatric sleep laboratories may benefit the most from a credentialed BSM clinician due to the growing prevalence of sleep disorders and the efficacy of behavioral interventions in pediatric populations (Kuhn & Elliott, 2003; Morgenthaler et al., 2006). For more information, see McLaughlin Crabtree, Rach, and Gamble, Chapter 19.

BSM Training

The demand for BSM treatments has far exceeded the supply, prompting a call to increase the number of credentialed BSM practitioners (Taylor, Perlis, McCrae, & Smith, 2010). To answer this call the SBSM, in cooperation with the American Board of Sleep Medicine (ABSM), has created training guidelines and a credentialing examination. At this time there is no consensus on who should be eligible for BSM training and credentialing (Taylor, Perlis, McCrae, & Smith, 2010). Currently, the eligibility requirements for the BSM examination are as follows: possession of a doctoral degree in psychology, nursing, social work, or equivalent health-science field, a valid license to provide mental-health related services, experience as defined in the next section on training, and a supervisor's signed acknowledgement that these criteria have been met (American Board of Sleep Medicine, 2012).

There are currently two routes to fulfill BSM training criteria prior to taking the ABSM certification examination: *(1)* a standard track, requiring the completion of an accredited BSM training program and *(2)* an alternative track, which allows for clinical experience to replace the completion of an accredited BSM training program (American Board of Sleep Medicine, 2012). It should be noted that BSM training and credentialing described in this chapter generally refer to training and practice in the United States. The majority of work toward establishing BSM as a formal field has been accomplished in the United States; however, other countries and regions are also involved in these processes. For example, a Latin America Behavioral Sleep Medicine association has been established. Additionally, an online BSM program has been created at the University of Glasgow. This online program, as developed by Colin Espie, has three levels of training: a certification (a minimum of 400 hours of didactic training), a diploma (1800 didactic hours), and a master's degree in BSM (1800 didactic hours and a research portfolio) (A. Ginda, personal communication, May 24, 2012). Further information may be found at the University of Glasgow Sleep Centre's website (http://www.gla.ac.uk/researchinstitutes/neurosciencepsychology/glasgowsleepcentre/).

The SBSM is responsible for accrediting BSM training programs in the United States and there are currently nine accredited BSM training programs (Table 41.1). The ultimate goal of accrediting BSM training programs is to provide exemplary training while fulfilling the requirements to sit for the BSM certification examination. In general, accredited BSM training programs provide a minimum of 1000 hours of supervised clinical BSM training or 500 hours of BSM training and 500 hours in general behavioral medicine. However, many accredited programs provide more than the minimum required clinical training. For example, the University of Alabama's accredited BSM training program provides approximately 1250 clinical training hours, 700 research hours, and 200 didactic hours for a total of 2150 training hours in sleep research and clinical practice. These training hours are specifically accomplished through the following: participation in a 20-hour per week BSM clinical practicum at an AASM accredited sleep disorders center, supervised by a BSM certified clinical psychologist and a board-certified neurologist and ABSM diplomate; BSM-focused research under the direction of a BSM certified clinical psychologist; and didactic training ranging from sleep physiology and development to sleep diagnosis and treatment. Assessment in this BSM training program is multimodal, incorporating both written and oral examinations on case work and reading assignments. It is important to note that the current accredited BSM

Table 40.1 Accredited Behavioral Sleep Medicine Programs

Program	Address	Contact Information
University of Alabama	Department of Psychology Box 870348 University of Alabama Tuscaloosa, AL 35487–0348	Kenneth Lichstein, Ph.D. (205) 348–4962 lichstein@ua.edu
Stanford University School of Medicine	Stanford Sleep Disorders Clinic 401 Quarry Road, Suite 3301 Stanford, CA 94305–5547	Rachel Manber, PhD (650) 724–2377 rmanber@stanford.edu
Rush University Medical School	Sleep Disorders Center Rush University Medical Center 1653 West Congress Parkway Chicago, IL 60612–3833	Jason Ong, PhD (312) 942–5440 jason_ong@rush. edu
Johns Hopkins University	Behavioral Sleep Medicine Postdoctoral Fellowship 600 N. Wolfe Street/Meyer 1–108 Baltimore, MD 21287–7613	Michael T. Smith, PhD (410) 614–3396 msmith62@jhmi.edu
University of Rochester	Sleep and Neurophysiology Research Laboratory University of Rochester 300 Crittenden Blvd Rochester, NY 14642	Wilfred Pigeon, PhD (585) 275–3374 wilfred_pigeon@urmc.rochester.edu
University of Michigan	University of Michigan Sleep Disorders Center 1500 East Medical Center Dr. Med Inn C728 Ann Arbor, MI 48109–5845	J. Todd Arnedt, PhD Deirdre A. Conroy, PhD (734) 764–1234 tarnedt@med.umich.edu
Hospital of the University of Pennsylvania Children's Hospital of Philadelphia	Penn Sleep Centers 3624 Market Street Philadelphia, PA 19104	Jodi Mindell, PhD Philip Gehrman, PhD (215) 746–3578 gehrman@mail.med.upenn.edu
University of North Texas	Department of Psychology PO Box 311280 Denton, TX 76203–1280	Daniel J. Taylor, PhD (940) 565–4682 djtaylor@unt.edu
Willford Hall Medical Center	San Antonio Military Medical Center Dept. of Behavioral Medicine 59 MHS/SGOWMP 2200 Bergquist Dr. Ste 1 Lackland AFB, TX 78236	Lt. Col. Ann S. Hryshko-Mullen, PhD Phone: (210) 292–5968 ann.hryshko-mullen@lackland. af.mil

Note: Programs in grey indicate pediatric BSM training

training programs differ in clinical experience with varying clinical populations. It is recommended that clinicians contact each BSM training site for an idea of typical clinical populations. There is a paucity of accredited BSM training programs at this time. Therefore, an alternative training track has been established to allow for individuals with less formal supervised BSM training to sit for the BSM certification examination.

The alternative track, which allows for current clinicians to obtain BSM certification, requires a licensed clinician to complete a minimum of two years of clinical practice with 25% of his/her practice consisting of behavioral medicine (e.g., pain management, smoking cessation, stress management, etc.). Under this alternative track, two clinical waivers have been established. In the first, the clinician must complete three months (480 hours) of supervised BSM experience. In the second, clinical activity in BSM is required for at least two years following completion of all internship and postdoctoral experience/training required for licensure, with the cumulative of six months (960 hours) clinical experience in BSM. The activity in behavioral sleep medicine must be comprehensive and sustained throughout the most recent 2-year period—specifically, the equivalent of a half day per week. Both waivers require 32 hours of AASM or SBSM sponsored continuing education units in BSM (8 hours in an overview of sleep, 8 hours in normal sleep and assessment, 8 hours in adult treatment, and 8 hours in child treatment). Detailed information regarding accredited training programs is available on the SBSM website (http://www.behavioralsleep.org).

Both the standard and alternative tracks meet eligibility criteria for taking the BSM certification examination. Although the standard track may be the preferable method for gaining initial supervised experience in BSM, the alternative track allows for established clinicians to gain BSM experience and sit for the BSM certification examination without having to complete an accredited BSM training program. For the latter, the SBSM offers many additional training opportunities, including the annual SBSM meeting, to learn about BSM and maintain knowledge.

Credentialing Through Exam

The ABSM is an independent, nonprofit organization that oversees the credentialing process of sleep clinicians and technologists in the United States. This organization administers three credentialing examinations, one of which is the BSM certification examination (American Board of Sleep Medicine, 2012). The only other formal BSM credentialing process occurs through the University of Glasgow online program that, as discussed previously, provides three levels of training.

The ABSM BSM certification examination is open to applicants who possess a postdoctoral degree or equivalent in a health-related field, a currently valid doctoral license granted by a state, provincial, or federal authority in the United States or Canada to provide mental-heath related clinical services, and experience that fulfills either the Standard Track or Alternate Track requirements. The BSM examination covers clinical aspects (including advanced diagnostic assessments and therapeutic techniques), as well as establishing and maintaining standards, conducting clinical research, assimilating new knowledge and skills into the BSM domain, and supervising BSM certification candidates. The BSM certification examination demonstrates minimum knowledge in BSM; however, the credentialing examination does not convey expertise in the field of BSM. Rather, it is encouraged that taking and passing the BSM credentialing examination is one of many steps to becoming adept at BSM.

Role of BSM in Sleep Laboratories

BSM has an integral role in the assessment and treatment of sleep disorders, as BSM is the optimal treatment, either as monotherapy or in combination with other therapies, for disorders such as insomnia and circadian rhythm disorders (Chesson et al., 1999). Beyond treatments for a variety of sleep disorders, BSM techniques are effective in enhancing other forms of treatments and addressing treatment adherence (e.g., continuous positive airway pressure; Haynes, 2005). The ability to assist in the diagnosis of sleep disorders, act as a first-line treatment, and enhance other forms of treatments makes BSM an integral part of a comprehensive sleep center. In fact, it has been suggested that sleep centers incorporate a BSM clinician to achieve the status of "Academic Program of Distinction" (Taylor, Perlis, McCrae, & Smith, 2010).

BSM is valuable in comprehensive pediatric sleep laboratories in which treatments are designed after consideration of the child, family, environment, and developmental level of the child. Different successful models exist across the country depending on the structure of the sleep center and whether or not the clinic is multidisciplinary in nature or its own behavioral sleep clinic. For example, one model consists of employing a BSM provider to participate in the sleep center in the assessment and diagnosis of pediatric sleep disorders, and then the BSM provider also conducts individual treatment sessions. Typical BSM pediatric services, just to name a few, include CBT for insomnia, behavioral treatments for pediatric insomnias, parasomnias, adherence to positive airway pressure (PAP) therapy in children with sleep-related breathing disorders, and desensitization to the sleep study equipment or PAP therapy. In addition, BSM providers offer a positive training opportunity for the Accreditation Council for Graduate Medical Education accredited fellowship programs in which training in behavioral sleep medicine practices should be provided to future sleep specialists.

Conclusion

The application of psychological principles to both normal and disordered sleep practice, research, and education is a key component of BSM. BSM has proven to be an integral part of any intervention plan addressing a variety of sleep disorders (e.g., insomnia, parasomnias, and circadian rhythm disorders), such that BSM has demonstrated its salience in mainstream sleep medicine.

BSM has grown as a subspecialty in the past decade, primarily with the formation of a society, formal accredited training opportunities, and a credentialing exam. Despite the obvious importance to sleep medicine practice, research, and education, a number of hurdles exist in the application of BSM to the broader field of sleep medicine. Training qualified BSM practitioners remains an obstacle in providing more clinicians. Until this is achieved, there will continue to be a disparity between the limited supply of BSM clinicians and the demand for BSM. Furthermore, despite the obvious efficacy and need for BSM treatments in the sleep disorders center, billing for BSM treatments needs further development.

Future Directions

- Address the disparity in supply and demand for BSM by training qualified BSM practitioners.
- Support growth of current BSM practitioners through education.
- Address billing issues for BSM.
- Increase emphasis on research in areas related to BSM.
- Increase emphasis on dissemination of treatments in a variety of domains.

References

American Board of Sleep Medicine. (2012). *Behavioral Sleep Medicine Specialists.* Retrieved May 2012 from http://www.absm.org/BSMSpecialists.aspx.

Bootzin, R. R. (1972). Stimulus control treatment for insomnia. *Proceedings, 80th Annual Convention, American Psychological Association*, 395–396.

Bootzin, R. R., & Perlis, M. L. (2011). Stimulus control therapy. In M. Perlis, M. Aloia, & B. Kuhn (Eds.), *Behavioral Treatments for Sleep Disorders: A Comprehensive Primer of Behavioral Sleep Medicine Treatment Protocols* (pp. 21–30). Burlington, MA: Elsevier, Inc.

Bronfenbrenner, U. (1974). Developmental research, public policy, and the ecology of childhood. *Child Development, 45*, 1–5.

Carskadon, M. A., & Wolfson, A. R., Acebo, C., Tzischinsky, O., & Seifer, R. (1998). Adolescent sleep patterns, circadian timing, and sleepiness at a transition to early school days. *Sleep, 21*, 871–881.

Chesson, A. L., Anderson, W. M., Littner, M., Davila, D., Hartse, K, Johnson, S., et al. (1999). Practice parameters for the nonpharmacologic treatment of chronic insomnia. *Sleep, 22*, 1128–1133.

Edinger, J. D., & Means, M. K. (2005). Cognitive-behavioral therapy for primary insomnia. *Clinical Psychology Review, 25*, 539–558.

Ford, D. E., & Kamerow, D. B. (1989). Epidemiologic study of sleep disturbances and psychiatric disorders: An opportunity for prevention? *Journal of the American Medical Association, 262*, 1479–1484.

Friedman, L., Bliwise, D.,Yesavage, J. A., & Salom, S. R. (1991). A preliminary study comparing sleep restriction and relaxation treatments for insomnia in older adults. *Journal of Gerontology, 46*, 1–8.

Haynes, P. L. (2005). The role of behavioral sleep medicine in the assessment and treatment of sleep disordered breathing. *Clinical Psychology Review, 25*, 673–705.

Jacobson, E. (1929). *Progressive Relaxation.* Chicago: University of Chicago Press.

Kuhn, B. R., & Elliott, A. J. (2003). Efficacy of behavioral interventions for pediatric sleep disturbance. In K. L. Lichstein & M. L. Perlis (Eds.), *Treating Sleep Disorders: Principles and Practice of Behavioral Sleep Medicine* (pp. 415–451). Hoboken, NJ: John Wiley & Sons, Inc.

Lacks, P., Bertelson, A. D., Gans, L., & Kunkel, J. (1983). The effectiveness of three behavioral treatments for different degrees of sleep onset insomnia. *Behavior Therapy, 14*, 593–605.

Lacks, P., Bertelson, A. D., Sugerman, J. L., & Kunkel, J. (1983). The treatment of sleep maintenance insomnia with stimulus control techniques. *Behaviour Research & Therapy, 21*, 291–295.

Lacks, P., & Morin, C. M. (1992). Recent advances in the assessment and treatment of insomnia. *Journal of Consulting and Clinical Psychology, 60*, 586–594.

Lichstein, K. L., & Johnson, R. (1993). Relaxation for insomnia and hypnotic medication use in older women. *Psychology and Aging, 8*, 103–111.

Lichstein, K. L. (2000). Relaxation. In K. L. Lichstein & C. M. Morin (Eds.), *Treatment of Late-Life Insomnia* (pp. 185–206). Thousand Oaks, CA: Sage Publication, Inc.

Lichstein, K. L., & Morin, C. M. (Eds.) (2000). *Treatment of Late-Life Insomnia.* Thousand Oaks, CA: Sage Publication, Inc.

Lichstein, K. L., Riedel, B. W., Wilson, N. M., Lester, K. W., & Aguillard, R. N. (2001). Relaxation and sleep compression for late-life insomnia: A placebo-controlled trial. *Journal of Consulting and Clinical Psychology, 69*, 227–239.

Lichstein, K. L., & Nau, S. D. (2003). Behavioral-cognitive science: The foundation of behavioral sleep medicine. In K. L. Lichstein & M. L. Perlis, *Treating Sleep Disorders: Principles and Practice of Behavioral Sleep Medicine* (pp. 3–26). Hoboken, NJ: John Wiley & Sons, Inc.

Lichstein, K. L., Taylor, D. J., McCrae, C. S., & Thomas, S. J. (2011). Relaxation for insomnia. In M. Perlis, M. Aloia, & B. Kuhn (Eds.), *Behavioral Treatments for Sleep Disorders: A Comprehensive Primer of Behavioral Sleep Medicine Treatment Protocols* (pp. 45–54). Burlington, MA: Elsevier, Inc.

Lichstein, K. L., Thomas, S. J., & McCurry, S. M. (2011). Sleep compression. In M. Perlis, M. Aloia, & B. Kuhn (Eds.), *Behavioral Treatments for Sleep Disorders: A Comprehensive Primer of Behavioral Sleep Medicine Treatment Protocols* (pp. 55–60). Burlington, MA: Elsevier, Inc.

McCrae, C. S., Perlis, M. L., Smith, M. T., & Taylor, D. J. (2011). Editorial: Society of behavioral sleep medicine announces the adoption of Behavioral Sleep Medicine as the society's official journal. *Behavioral Sleep Medicine, 9*, 1–3.

Mindell, J. A., Moline, M. L., Zendell, S. M., Brown, L. W., & Fry, J. M. (1994). Pediatricians and sleep disorders: Training and practice. *Pediatrics, 94*, 194–200.

Mindell, J. A., & Owens, J. A. (2010). *A Clinical Guide to Pediatric Sleep: Diagnosis and Management of Sleep Problems* (2nd ed.). Philadelphia, PA: Lippincott Williams & Wilkins.

Morgenthaler, T. I., Owens, J., Alessi, C., Boehlecke, B., Brown, T., Coleman, J., et al. (2006). Practice parameters for behavioral treatment of bedtime problems and night wakings in infants and young children. *Sleep, 29*, 1277–1281.

Morin, C. M., Kowatch, R. A., & O'Shanick, G. O. (1989). Behavioral management of sleep disturbances secondary to chronic pain. *Journal of Behavior Therapy and Experimental Psychiatry, 20*, 295–302.

Morin, C. M., Culbert, J. P., & Schwartz, S. M. (1994). Nonpharmacological interventions for insomnia: A meta-analysis of treatment efficacy. *American Journal of Psychiatry, 151*, 1172–1180.

Morin, C. M., Bastien, C., & Savard, J. (2003). Current status of cognitive-behavior therapy for insomnia: Evidence for treatment effectiveness and feasibility. In K. L. Lichstein & M. L. Perlis (Eds.), *Treating Sleep Disorders: Principles and Practice of Behavioral Sleep Medicine* (pp. 3–26). Hoboken, NJ: John Wiley & Sons, Inc.

Mowrer, O. H. (1938). Apparatus for the study and treatment of enuresis. *American Journal of Psychology, 51*, 163–166.

Murtagh, D. R. R., & Greenwood, K. M. (1995). Identifying effective psychological treatments for insomnia: A meta-analysis. *Journal of Consulting and Clinical Psychology, 60*, 79–89.

Reidel, B., Lichstein, K. L., Peterson, B. A., Epperson, M. T., Means, M. K., & Aguillard, R. N. (1998). A comparison of the efficacy of stimulus control for medicated and nonmedicated insomniacs. *Behavior Modification, 22*, 3–28.

Sadeh, A. (2005). Cognitive-behavioral treatment for childhood sleep disorders. *Clinical Psychology Review, 25*, 612–628.

Smith, M. T., Smith, L. J., Nowakowski, S., & Perlis, M. L. (2003). Primary insomnia: Diagnostic issues, treatment, and future directions. In K. L. Lichstein & M. L. Perlis (Eds.), *Treating Sleep Disorders: Principles and Practice of Behavioral Sleep Medicine* (pp. 214–261). Hoboken, NJ: John Wiley & Sons, Inc.

Society of Behavioral Sleep Medicine (2011). *Society of Behavioral Sleep Medicine*. Retrieved May 2012 from http://www.behavioralsleep.org.

Spielman, A. J., Saskin, P., & Thorpy, M. J. (1987). Treatment of chronic insomnia by restriction of time in bed. *Sleep, 10*, 45–56.

Spielman, A. J., Yang, C. M., & Glovinsky, P. B. (2011). Sleep restriction therapy. In M. Perlis, M. Aloia, & B. Kuhn (Eds.), *Behavioral Treatments for Sleep Disorders: A Comprehensive Primer of Behavioral Sleep Medicine Treatment Protocols* (pp. 9–20). Burlington, MA: Elsevier, Inc.

Stepanski, E. J., & Perlis, M. L. (2003). A historical perspective and commentary on practice issues. In K. L. Lichstein & M. L. Perlis (Eds.), *Treating Sleep Disorders: Principles and Practice of Behavioral Sleep Medicine* (pp. 3–26). Hoboken, NJ: John Wiley & Sons, Inc.

Taylor, D. J., Perlis, M. L., McCrae, C. S., & Smith, M. T. (2010). The future of behavioral sleep medicine: A report on consensus votes at the Ponte Vedra behavioral sleep medicine consensus conference, March 27–29, 2009. *Behavioral Sleep Medicine, 8*, 63–70.

Watson, J. B. (1928). *Psychological Care of Infant and Child.* New York: Norton.

Wolfson, A. R., & Carskadon, M. A. (1998). Sleep schedules and daytime functioning in adolescents. *Child Development, 69*, 875–887.

Wolfson, A. R., & Carskadon, M. A. (2005). A survey of factors influencing high school start times. *NASSP Bulletin, 89*, 47–66.

CHAPTER

42 Overview

Hawley E. Montgomery-Downs

Abstract

The overarching purpose of The Oxford Handbook is to both inform readers about the current state of our science in infant, child, and adolescent sleep and behavior, and to inspire additional, innovative contributions. These contributions will come from current members, and ideally also from behavioral scientists in related disciplines who are interested in dedicating energy to this remarkable field. The goal in this concluding chapter is to share a compilation of the chapter authors' collective view on the most urgent future directions in infant, child and adolescent sleep. Represented here are eight cross-cutting goals that were identified by 25% or more of the chapter authors as imperative to advancing the field: increase research using longitudinal and/or experimental designs; more in-depth focus on individual differences; more systems and family-oriented research; more thorough validation of instrumentation and equipment; innovative behavioral interventions; more integration of environmental contributions; and greater sleep education.

Key Words: education, environmental contribution, experimental design, future directions, individual differences, intervention, longitudinal design, systems, validation

It has been a privilege to work on this volume with Amy Wolfson and all of our contributing authors, whose passionate dedication to our field is evident through the care and thoughtful approach in their chapters. By design, each chapter stands alone as a comprehensive state-of-the-science review of each author's area of expertise within infant, child, and adolescent sleep and behavior. To compliment the depth within each chapter, we have worked to ensure that extensive cross-referencing gives our readers the opportunity to follow themes across chapters. Thus, it is our hope that a significant and lasting contribution of this volume will be a pathway through converging topical areas that will facilitate insight into the field.

I have valued the opportunity that reviewing our authors' collective work has given me to update and refine my understanding of several areas distinct from my own laboratory's primary research focus. An additional and unexpected benefit has been that through Oxford's formalized *Future Directions* section for each chapter we were able to capture each author's perspective on where our science needs to go from here. Independently, our authors' Future Directions follow closely from the work they presented in their chapter. Cumulatively they show a pattern that sets an agenda for the field. This where-now and where-to synergy played perfectly into our aim of using this volume not only as a platform to describe the state of the field, but additionally to inspire novel, innovative contributions. Our specific hope is that both long-time contributors and behavioral scientists relatively new to child and adolescent sleep will both find through these chapters that there are tremendous questions remaining, and that their contributions are critical to answering them.

My goal in this concluding chapter is to share with you the results of my compilation and analyses of our authors' collective view on the most urgent future directions in child and adolescent sleep. Here I have represented each of eight cross-cutting Future Direction themes that were identified by 25% or more of our authors.

Longitudinal Studies

The need for longitudinal studies, identified by more than half of our authors, was the most frequently cited priority area. Of note, these authors point not simply to normative, descriptive work (which is certainly needed), but also to the importance of establishing sleep duration needs across the child and adolescent age span, how these needs change over time, developmental trajectories in both macro and micro structure of sleep, and the long-term behavioral and biomedical consequences of early sleep disorders. In other words, knowing how much infants, children, and adolescents sleep is not enough; we need to know what sleep duration, consolidation, and timing are optimal and how these change across development.

Two ends of the age spectrum are worth highlighting. The earliest period of development, prenatal, is generally underrepresented in sleep science and thus excluded almost entirely from this volume. However, new technologies such as high-resolution ultrasound are increasingly used to identify human prenatal physiologic state and development. Importantly, fetal observation can inform us about both the current status of the maternal-fetal system and predict infant outcomes (Salisbury, Fallone & Lester, 2005; Salisbury, Ponder, Padbury & Lester, 2009). In addition, exciting behavioral neuroscience approaches are increasingly applied by investigators using animal models to examine sleep behaviors, as well as waking behaviors that are facilitated by sleep, even during prenatal development (Tiriac, Uitermarkt, Fanning, Sokoloff, & Blumberg, 2012).

The latter end of our age span—adolescence—is equally important. At the intersection between "child" and "adult," work on adolescents and emerging adults continues to emphasize the uniqueness of this developmental period. Specifically, chapters by Mary Carskadon, Shelly Hershner, and Pamela Thatcher and their colleagues highlight the changes that occur during this period to the circadian system of adolescents,, the high-stakes risks to which this exposes them, and the challenges in their treatment, respectively. Amy Wolfson (2007) has long been an advocate for policy changes to benefit adolescents (and, as a consequence, the rest of us) and made a point of encouraging authors to address how sleep issues pertain to adolescents within the chapters as often as possible.

Individual Differences

Closely related to longitudinal work is the need, identified by about a quarter of our authors, for increased empirical evaluation of individual differences within infant, child, and adolescent sleep. This differential psychology approach can yield rich insight into how—and sometimes why—different people have different trajectories or responses. Traditionally seen as error variance, unique responses can instead inspire novel insight into human behavior. It is important to study individual differences from the perspective of normal development, but it is also important when examining risk factors for disorders, protective factors that promote resilience, and factors that may be used to predict responsivity or resistance to behavioral and other treatments. This approach has been infrequently applied to pediatric and adolescent sleep; its ability to reveal interesting truths is exemplified by St James-Roberts and Plewis (1996) in their study describing changes in and relations between infant sleep, feeding, and crying behaviors during the first 40 weeks after birth.

Family Systems, General Systems, and Biopsychosocial Approaches

Nearly half of our authors note that more work reflecting a dynamic systems approach is needed. One example of this is the increasing use of multimodal assessment strategies. Mothers have one perspective on their child's sleep, but the profile becomes much more revealing when both parents report independently, in conjunction with the school or daycare teacher and, for older children and adolescents, their self-report (for example, see Beebe, Ris, Kramer, Long, & Amin, 2010). Another example is that little work has currently been done to address the sleep of postpartum fathers or the impact of sleep disturbance on their contributions to the workplace or family; their potential role for mitigating the impact of sleep disturbance on postpartum mothers is almost entirely unexplored. More work is clearly needed to balance a culturally sensitive and practical approach to co-sleeping when considering infant sleep interventions—both of which are often-controversial issues in our field (see Chapter 37 on interventions by Melisa Moore and Jodi Mindell and Chapter 12 on co-sleeping by Melissa Burnham). A truly biopsychosocial approach that uses a systems approach to include simultaneous assessment of biological, behavioral, and environmental influences on pathology is as important now as when it was originally conceptualized nearly 40 years ago (Engel, 1977). This doesn't make such work any less challenging.

Valid, Standardized Subjective and Objective Assessment Measures

Over one-third of the authors emphasized the urgency of demand for improvement of both objective and subjective assessments we use for screening, assessing, estimating, and measuring sleep behaviors. Since polysomnography became established as the gold standard for identification of sleep states, the field has seen a surge of technologies and approaches to measuring and collecting parent and self-report of child and adolescent sleep. The chapters by Karen Spruyt on survey validation (Chapter 18) and by Rosemary Horne and Sarah Biggs on actigraphy (Chapter 16) indicate how far we have come—and how far we still have to go.

I want to particularly emphasize that the quality of our science depends on the quality of these measurement techniques, so it is in the interest of all sleep researchers that we insist on tools with the strongest validity for use with our infant, child, and adolescent populations—both normative and disordered. This is particularly true for methods such as actigraphy that are now in wide use and, due to decreasing costs, likely to become even more frequently used. However, pediatric and adolescent sensitivity *and especially specificity* are generally very low with these devices, and we currently have no professional standards (Meltzer, Montgomery-Downs, Insana, & Walsh, 2012). This issue is compounded when parent report and child self-report measures are then validated against actigraphy. Researchers and clinicians should insist on the highest standards for their recording equipment and refuse to accept or support anything inferior.

Intervention Efficacy and Novel Therapies

One-third of our authors also highlighted that interventions—and specifically behavioral interventions—should undergo rigorous evaluation for efficacy among pediatric and adolescent populations. In addition, they point out that novel, innovative therapies are needed. As described by Charles Super and Sara Harkness in their chapter on Culture and Children's Sleep, and by Melissa Burnham in her chapter on Co-Sleeping and Self-Soothing during Infancy, it is essential that interventions be developed from a perspective of genuine sensitivity to the family's situation, resources, and history—both developmentally and culturally.

Environmental Contributions

A quarter of our authors noted the need to account for the environment in our science. This point is quite important to me professionally because my training background and way of thinking are in developmental psychobiology; within this field, the need to consider nonobvious influences on the developing system is critical (Miller, 1997). That the context in which sleep takes place influences the sleeper should no longer be nonobvious—but our authors point out that there are much deeper potentials for investigation within "environment." Profoundly important is the broader environment; a marked weakness in our field currently is our lack of understanding of the influences of poverty and social class on sleep duration, quality, and timing. On another level of environment, several authors specifically mentioned epigenetics, the study of how history and environment influence our genome, an impact that can be transmitted across generations (Meaney, 2010; Roth, 2012). A Medline search for the concurrence of the terms "epigenetic*" and "sleep" (on November 28, 2012) revealed that 55 such papers have been published to date, none of which are on young humans or animal models. Investigators with the resources to incorporate developmental sleep into their epigenetic research programs, developmental sleep researchers who can address epigenetics, or (best yet) collaborations between the two, will be well-positioned for discovery and innovation.

Experimental Design

More than one quarter of the chapters discussed the need for more studies that use experimental designs or randomized control trials to establish the mechanisms of action—particularly underlying treatment effects. I suspect that more authors would likely have identified this as prominent gap in our science were it not so challenging to implement this type of study in child and adolescent populations. Obvious ethical concerns aside, the logistics of experimental manipulation and accounting for a multitude of influences (see section on systems approach above) can seem insurmountable. Collaboration and formation of multisite studies is one way to overcome this, which has been done successfully over the past decade by top investigators studying the efficacy of adenotonsillectomy, the current front-line treatment for childhood obstructive sleep apnea (Redline, Amin, Beebe, Chervin,

Garetz, Giordani, et al., 2011). To my knowledge, at this time no such large-scale collaboration on evaluating behavioral therapy of any kind in pediatric and adolescent sleep has been initiated.

Education

Finally, 20% of our authors indicated a greater need for education about infant, child, and adolescent sleep. They specify that the target audiences include parents, children and adolescents, health care providers, and school personnel. To these I will add that legislators also need us to teach them more about sleep and its importance among their youngest constituents. There have been several successful approaches to prevention and education; these are well-described in Chapter 21, Role of Schools in Identification, Treatment, and Prevention of Children's Sleep Problems by Joseph Buckhalt, and in the chapter Preventative Intervention: Curricula and Programs by Reut Gruber and colleagues.

Sleep is well-loved by the media. As sleep scientists we are well poised to take advantage of the public's general fascination with (and, if our generally anti-sleep culture and rampant mythology about sleep is any index, a perseverating ignorance about) our field. Sleep science is fun, sleep facts are cool, and sleep is linked to danger in the form of disorders that cause morbidity and mortality as well as increased risk behaviors. Sleep is also something that *every person* does. In short, our field includes all of the prerequisites to "arouse and fulfill"—the not-so-secret method for effective science communication (Olson, 2009). It is incumbent upon sleep scientists to ensure that the message of the good work we are doing is represented—and represented accurately—to those who need to hear it: the public, health care providers, parents, schools, policy makers. I suggest we find a poster child for pediatric sleep; someone as effective at "getting the message out" about infant, child, and adolescent sleep as Arianna Huffington has been for women's sleep (Huffington, 2011). Such a voice is desperately needed to counter the anti-sleep culture that is endemic in—as a popular example—advertisement campaigns aimed at selling caffeine-laden drinks to adolescents.

Addressing these priority areas is necessary toward advancing our basic behavioral science, as well as translating that science into improved interventions to advance sleep health care. Of note, these priority areas reflect each of the four areas of translational research depicted in the 2003 United States National Institutes of Health roadmap, designed to set the research agenda for the future (Zerhouni, 2003) and that has been incorporated as a way of thinking among researchers around the world (Woolf, 2008). These priorities identified by our chapter authors also reflect current national health care agendas around the world. As an example, three of the four target Sleep Health priorities outlined in the United States objectives for Healthy People 2020 are directly relevant to pediatric and adolescent sleep: *evaluation for obstructive sleep apnea* (including pediatric patients); *vehicular crashes due to drowsy driving* (particularly relevant to adolescents); and *sufficient sleep among 9th through 12th graders* (Healthy People 2020).

As my co-editor, Amy Wolfson, aptly described at the beginning of this handbook, we hope that psychologists and other behavioral scientists who are drawn to this volume will continue to work in sleep and become greater contributors to this fascinating field. There are many ways to get involved with sleep research. Collaborating is great; although I also like to tell, or even warn, colleagues that I don't collaborate... I infiltrate. Sleep researchers are a remarkably friendly group of researchers and clinicians, perhaps owing in some part to the relative newness of our field. There are national and regional sleep societies too numerous to list here—and every year new groups are formed. Attending a nearby conference or joining a professional society is an excellent way to start. There is also an ever-growing list of high-quality peer reviewed journals with editorial boards that are remarkably receptive to receiving submissions from those outside the mainstream sleep field who have incorporated sleep into their research programs. Those looking for information about adult sleep are also referred to our "sister book": *The Oxford Handbook of Sleep and Sleep Disorders*. Our volume was developed to complement the success of Morin and Espie (Eds.) volume, and the interested reader will find there a compendium of the state-of-the-science of adulthood and aging (2012).

In closing, a brief message to trainees in our field. The Sleep Research Society (based in the United States) invests the majority of its revenue in a "Trainee Day" pre-meeting preceding the annual meeting of the Associated Professional Sleep Societies; in 2012 they hosted the 17th annual pre-meeting for undergraduate, graduate, postdoctoral, and medical trainees. While working on this chapter it surprised me to realize that I began attending this conference prior to the first Trainee Day. Two of the most important lessons

I learned were at these training days, both from then-editors-in-chief of the top-tier journal in our field, *SLEEP*, the official journal of the Associated Professional Sleep Societies. The messages were: (1) do *not* do "me too" research that reiterates the work of others and (2) *do* publish your work in journals other than those focused on an exclusively sleep-science readership. In other words, do exciting, risky research and then tell everyone about it—not just your friends.

Currently, pediatric sleep is a field in which important discoveries are rapidly reshaping how we think about sleep development and disorders, their antecedents and consequences. There is tremendous opportunity in the field now, and we have an urgent need for others to lend their time, energy, and expertise toward answering key developmental questions in the field. Above all, it was with the goal of energizing our field by introducing it to others that we began thinking about this volume. It is our hope that this collection of chapters by some of the world's experts will serve as a vehicle for this purpose.

References

Beebe, D. W., Ris, M. D., Kramer, M. E., Long, E., & Amin, R. (2010). The association between sleep disordered breathing, academic grades, and cognitive and behavioral functioning among overweight subjects during middle to late childhood. *Sleep, 33*, 1447–1456.

Engel, G. L. (1977). The need for a new medical model: A challenge for biomedicine. *Science, 196*, 129–136.

Healthy People 2020. Retrieved April 4, 2013, from http://www.healthypeople.gov/2020/

Huffington, A. (2011). *Arianna Huffington: Sleep Your Way to the Top*. The Daily Muse. Retrieved April 4, 2013, from: http://www.thedailymuse.com/career/arianna-huffington-sleep/)

Meaney, M. J. (2010). Epigenetics and the biological definition of gene x environment interactions. *Child Development, 81*, 41–79.

Meltzer, L. J., Montgomery-Downs, H. E., Insana, S. P., & Walsh, C.M. (2012). Use of actigraphy for assessment in pediatric sleep research. *Sleep Medicine Reviews, 16*, 463–475.

Miller, D. B. (1997). The effects of nonobvious forms of experience on the development of instinctive behavior. In C. Dent-Read & P. Zukow-Goldring (Eds.), *Evolving Explanations of Development. Ecological Approaches to Organism—Environment Systems* (pp. 457–507). Washington, DC: American Psychological Association.

Morin, C. M., & Espie, C. A. (Eds.). (2012). *The Oxford Handbook of Sleep and Sleep Disorders (Oxford Library of Psychology)*. New York, NY: Oxford University Press.

Olson, R. (2009). *Don't be Such a Scientist; Talking Substance in an Age of Style*. Washington, DC: Island Press.

Redline, S., Amin, R., Beebe, D., Chervin, R. D., Garetz, S. L., Giordani, B., et al. (2011). The Childhood Adenotonsillectomy Trial (CHAT): rationale, design, and challenges of a randomized controlled trial evaluating a standard surgical procedure in a pediatric population. *Sleep, 34*, 1509–1517.

Roth, T. L. (2012). Epigenetics of neurobiology and behavior during development and adulthood. *Developmental Psychobiology, 54*, 590–597.

Salisbury, A. L., Fallone, M. D., & Lester, B. (2005). Neurobehavioral assessment from fetus to infant: the NICU Network Neurobehavioral Scale and the Fetal Neurobehavior Coding Scale. *Mental Retardation and Developmental Disabilabilities Research Reviews, 11*, 14–20.

Salisbury, A. L., Ponder, K. L., Padbury, J. F., & Lester, B. M. (2009). Fetal effects of psychoactive drugs. *Clinics in Perinatology, 36*, 595–619.

St. James-Roberts, I., & Plewis, I. (1996). Individual differences, daily fluctuations, and developmental changes in amounts of infant waking, fussing, crying, feeding, and sleeping. *Child Development, 67*, 2527–2540.

Tiriac, A., Uitermarkt, B. D., Fanning, A. S., Sokoloff, G., & Blumberg, M. S. (2012). Rapid whisker movements in sleeping newborn rats. *Current Biology, 22*, 2075–2080.

Wolfson, A. R. (2007). Adolescent sleep update: Narrowing the gap between research and practice. *Sleep Review: The Journal for Sleep Specialists, 8*, 28–32.

Woolf, S. H. (2008). The meaning of translational research and why it matters. *Journal of the American Medical Association, 299*, 211–213.

Zerhouni, E. (2003). The NIH Roadmap. *Science, 302*, 63–72.

INDEX

B

C

D

N

Q

R

T

U

V

W

Y

Z